The Acupuncturist's Guide
to Conventional Medicine

of related interest

The Fundamentals of Acupuncture
Nigel Ching
Foreword by Charles Buck
ISBN 978 1 84819 313 0
eISBN 978 0 85701 266 1

Acupuncture and Chinese Medicine
Roots of Modern Practice
Charles Buck
ISBN 978 1 84819 159 4
eISBN 978 0 85701 133 6

Intuitive Acupuncture
John Hamwee
ISBN 978 1 84819 273 7
eISBN 978 0 85701 220 3

The Acupuncture Points Functions Colouring Book
Rainy Hutchinson
Forewords by Richard Blackwell, and Angela Hicks and John Hicks
ISBN 978 1 84819 266 9
eISBN 978 0 85701 214 2

The Acupuncturist's Guide to Conventional Medicine

Second Edition

Clare Stephenson

Foreword by Angela Hicks
and John Hicks

SINGING
DRAGON

LONDON AND PHILADELPHIA

This second edition first published in 2017
by Singing Dragon
an imprint of Jessica Kingsley Publishers
73 Collier Street
London N1 9BE, UK
and
400 Market Street, Suite 400
Philadelphia, PA 19106, USA

www.singingdragon.com

First edition published in 2011 by Churchill Livingstone, Elsevier, London, UK and in 2015
by Singing Dragon, an imprint of Jessica Kingsley Publishers, London, UK

Library of Congress Cataloging in Publication Data
Title: The acupuncturist's guide to conventional medicine / Clare Stephenson.
Other titles: Complementary therapist's guide to conventional medicine.
Description: Second edition. | London ; Philadelphia : Jessica Kingsley
 Publishers, 2017. | Preceded by Complementary therapist's guide to
 conventional medicine / Clare Stephenson. 2011. | Includes bibliographical
 references and index.
Identifiers: LCCN 2016056980 | ISBN 9781848193024 (alk. paper)
Subjects: | MESH: Medicine | Acupuncture Therapy | Medicine, Chinese
 Traditional--methods
Classification: LCC R129 | NLM WB 100 | DDC 610.1/4--dc23 LC record available at
https://lccn.loc.gov/2016056980

British Library Cataloguing in Publication Data
A CIP catalogue record for this book is available from the British Library

ISBN 978 1 84819 302 4
eISBN 978 0 85701 255 5

Printed and bound by CPI Group (UK) Ltd, Croydon, CR0 4YY

Contents

Disclaimer

Knowledge and best practice in this field are constantly changing. As new research and experience broaden our understanding, changes in research methods, professional practices, or medical treatment may become necessary.

Practitioners and researchers must always rely on their own experience and knowledge in evaluating and using any information, methods, compounds, or experiments described herein. In using such information or methods they should be mindful of their own safety and the safety of others, including parties for whom they have a professional responsibility.

With respect to any drugs or pharmaceutical products identified, readers are advised to check the most current information provided (i) on procedures featured or (ii) by the manufacturer of each product to be administered, to verify the recommended dose or formula, the method and duration of administration, and contraindications. It is the responsibility of practitioners, relying on their own experience and knowledge of their patients, to make diagnoses, to determine dosages and the best treatment for each individual patient, and to take all appropriate safety precautions.

To the fullest extent of the law, neither the Publisher nor the authors, contributors, or editors, assume any liability for any injury and/or damage to persons or property as a matter of products liability, negligence or otherwise, or from any use or operation of any methods, products, instructions, or ideas contained in the material herein.

Online material

The online material supporting this text can be downloaded at https://library.singingdragon.com/redeem using the code STEPHENSONACU.

It includes:

- Full-color illustrations from the book.

- Self-assessment questions and answers. These self-assessment questions are designed to support home study of the text. The student is advised to write down answers to each question as they progress through the study of a section. The written answers can then be compared with the model answers, which are also to be found online.

- End of section self-assessment tests. These are designed to help the student review their learning after completion of each of the sections that make up each chapter.

Foreword

The College of Integrated Chinese Medicine brings together two styles of Chinese medicine. We had not thought, however, of bringing together Chinese and Western medicine. Until, that is, Clare Stephenson joined the teaching staff. She saw the potential for something different.

As both a Western doctor and a practitioner of Chinese medicine, Clare immediately recognized the huge areas of similarity, as well as differences, between these two systems of medicine. She graduated from the College, and subsequently became the program leader for conventional medicine. This started her on the path of writing what was later to become this textbook.

From the moment we saw the first texts for the study course, it became clear that she was writing something very special, unique even. The students agreed. Their evaluations sang the praises of the course. Staff who had not done the course clamored for the text. They had recognized its potential for deepening their learning and as a reference tool.

It soon became obvious to us that this should and would become a textbook at some stage. It took over five years for Clare to fully complete what was then an in-depth study course for our students. We are now delighted that, from its first conception as a course at the College, through its extensive development, it was born as a book in 2011 and now, in 2017, is in its second edition.

Before this book the only in-depth texts available were those written for Western medicine practitioners such as doctors, nurses and physiotherapists. Clare's innovative vision for Chinese medicine practitioners was to enable them to learn Western medicine but from their own perspective.

Chinese medicine and Western medicine are two substantial yet very different medical models. Chinese medicine practitioners can often search for connections and relationships between the two models but find more differences than similarities. This book bridges that gap and brings the two closer. This enables practitioners of both medical models to understand how the other thinks.

In this textbook Clare takes complementary practitioners through the basics of Western physiology and pathology, and compares and contrasts it with the underlying theory of Chinese medicine. It helps Chinese medicine practitioners to understand the workings of the mind of a conventional doctor: how they question patients, what tests they might carry out, how the results might be interpreted, as well as possible Western treatments and their effects.

Throughout the text each subject is discussed not only from the Western but also from the Chinese medical perspective. For instance, Clare examines holistic versus reductionist theories, she summarizes the underlying philosophy of both medical models and also explains medications both in Western terms and in terms of their Chinese energetic effects. On top of this, and perhaps most striking, is how she thoughtfully considers each Western disease and compares it to a possible Chinese medicine diagnosis.

For a holistic practitioner, comparing diseases from these two perspectives might be seen as slightly risky. We might worry that it could encourage practitioners to treat only what in Chinese medicine terms is called the *Biao*, or outward manifestation, rather than the *Ben*, or root cause of the problem. Clare's rich understanding prevents this from happening. Whilst remembering that this is primarily a conventional medicine textbook, she comments on Chinese medicine differentiations of disease, without being too prescriptive. This gives practitioners useful insights but doesn't narrow their holistic point of view.

Each part of this clear text is complemented by online learning-points, self-tests and case histories as well as numerous additional comments and comparisons between Western and complementary medicine.

This book will be of use not only to students of Chinese medicine but also to practitioners of all complementary therapies as an in-depth step-by-step study course with timed and specified sections of study. Equally it is extremely useful to qualified practitioners as a reference book. Although this book was not written for Western practitioners, those who read it with an open mind might also find it arouses their interest. The discussion about the Chinese medicine approach might resonate with their experience of patients.

This book is immensely dense and at the same time exceedingly readable. It will be hard for another textbook to match it in its breadth and depth. We have no doubt that it will soon be a standard text for Chinese and other complementary medicine students as well as a standard reference for practitioners. It has so much embedded in the text that the reader might find, as we did, valuable gems popping out at every visit. It has left us more interested in, as well as much more informed about, Western medicine, whilst remaining proud of our own Chinese medicine.

Angela Hicks and John Hicks
Principals, College of Integrated Chinese Medicine, Reading,
Berkshire, UK, September 2010. Updated in 2017.

Acknowledgements

This book is primarily dedicated to all students and practitioners who, through the practice of acupuncture, are committed to enriching the lives of others. Their focus on restoring health through enabling patients to find a place of more balanced living is a profound contribution to human well-being, but is not necessarily recognized as such in this current age of speed and technology.

The creation of this book was inspired by my contact with successive generations of students of acupuncture at the College of Integrated Chinese Medicine in Reading, UK. Over the years of teaching these students, this textbook evolved in response to their expressed need both to understand conventional medicine and also to make sense of how it sat alongside their studies of Chinese medicine. Moreover, this book was very much shaped by the feedback these students gave to the emerging text, and for this I am very thankful.

I also have great gratitude to Angela and John Hicks and Peter Mole, the founders of the College of Integrated Chinese Medicine, who continue to teach and inspire students. From the outset they supported my enthusiasm to develop teaching materials about conventional medicine for their students. They then very generously encouraged me to submit these materials, written for the College, as material to be considered for publication. Without their support this book could not have been published.

In the writing of the first edition of the book I had great help from my colleagues at the time, Di Eckersley and Pam Batten. I am very grateful for their wisdom and encouragement.

I am also indebted to John Wheeler who read through the whole of the First Edition and deftly pruned my long sentences.

Thanks also have to go to Claire Wilson, Jane Evans and all the team at Singing Dragon who have taken on the unenviable task of the production and distribution of this book. It has been a pleasure to work with you all.

In the research for the Second Edition I have turned time and time again to a small number of source texts. I have always been impressed by the breadth and depth of the writings of Giovanni Maciocia and Bob Flaws in particular. I have enormous respect for the dedication of these two masters of Chinese medicine who have enabled so many in the West to have access to the wisdom of both the ancient and current day healers from China.

In terms of sources of up-to-date information on conventional medical practice, I have relied heavily on the internet-based resource, Patient (http://patient.info). This website is regularly updated, thoroughly researched and very accessible. I am also very grateful to the small team of doctors who write the hundreds of articles to be found on this website.

I was first trained in conventional medicine, and this training will always form the foundation of my practice in acupuncture and also in teaching. I have had an ever-deepening education in medicine, spread as it is over many years from medical student to experienced doctor. The opportunity to learn from others never ceases in medicine. Many teachers and doctors I worked alongside with over the years have been sources of inspiration; they include, to name but a few, Alan Weeds, Chris Bunch, Bent Juel-Jensen, Basil Shepstone, Crispin Fisher, Geoff Summerfield, Judith Shakespeare, Angie Anderson and Sally Hope.

Finally I have to express my great admiration for my most recent medical colleagues Matthew Easdale, Robin Carr and Chloe Borton, who are still working extremely long and relentless hours in UK general practice. The commitment and dedication of conventional doctors in the UK National Health Service (NHS) has to be worked alongside to be believed.

I trust that this book will be a source of support for acupuncturists in practice. It is also my hope that it will help to enable constructive dialogue between healers from the conventional and Chinese medical traditions.

Introduction

This textbook has been developed to enable students and practitioners of complementary health disciplines, and acupuncturists in particular, to understand more about the Western medical model of healthcare. It is intended to enable a recognition of how the Western medical approach to interpreting and managing disease can be stood alongside, and to some degree translated, into the terms of a more holistic model, namely, that of Chinese medicine. The ultimate aim is that interactions with patients in the clinic will be enriched by helping both acupuncturist and patient make sense of how the patient's experiences of Western medicine might relate to the treatments they are being offered in the acupuncture clinic. This will have the added benefit of enabling patients to make safe and positive healthcare choices based on this understanding.

My understanding of conventional medicine comes from having trained as a medical doctor and having practiced for a number of years in British hospital medicine and general practice. However, my perspective on healthcare has been fundamentally shaped by stepping aside from conventional practice, and spending over 13 years in the practice of traditional acupuncture. My interest in Chinese medicine was sparked by a brief initial training in clinical acupuncture in Nanjing, China. I followed this by studying the practice of acupuncture at the College of Integrated Chinese Medicine in Reading, UK. I then spent ten years both practicing acupuncture in Oxford and also teaching conventional medicine to students at the College where I had just trained.

As I began to reflect on these two contrasting practices of medicine, and brought these reflections into my clinical practice, I learned how my consultations with patients were positively influenced by the drawing together of information from more than one medical philosophical framework. I found that my increasing fluency in these contrasting languages of medicine, and also the ability to "translate" between them, enabled my patients to benefit from the insights and wisdom inherent in the best aspects of both conventional and "alternative" medical disciplines. I found that also helped them to make more informed choices about what treatments might be best for them.

I now no longer regularly practice conventional medicine. I found the ever-increasing pressures placed on conventional clinicians who work in modern healthcare systems to deliver guideline-based medical treatments (irrespective of the individual needs and preferences of the patients) incompatible with my desire to understand and manage the patient holistically.

This decision was not taken easily. First, I recognize that modern conventional medicine offers so much that is crucial to the well-being of countless individuals. This includes: the management of day-to-day mundane health queries in general practice; the safe management of pregnancy and childbirth and children's developmental problems; so many health promotion programs in the developing and developed worlds; the provision of a robust and safe setting and framework for meeting the needs of the many people who will need nursing care; and also access to high quality emergency care. The very young, the vulnerable, those with serious chronic disease and those at the end of their lives are more than likely to rely on conventional healthcare when they need support. My experience is that the people who work in conventional medicine, the doctors, nurses, paramedics, healthcare assistants, and even administrative staff and cleaners, are more often than not healers in their own right. In a public healthcare system they are often paid low wages, and even then tend to work longer hours than for which they are paid. In the setting of conventional healthcare provision, it is so often the kind words and gentle touch that is remembered by patients in spite of the pressure and speed and underfunding of the system within which the care is offered. I will always have the utmost respect for the dedication and care of so many wonderful colleagues in conventional medicine in the UK.

Second, and regrettably, alternative medical approaches in the West are very often only accessible to those who can afford them. Certain population groups (arguably those most in need of gentle approaches to healing) will never come close to being able to benefit from them. In my practice as a GP I would routinely come into contact with people of all ages and from all walks of life. As an acupuncturist in the UK, however, I do not expect ever to have the privilege of being able to care for such a diverse client group.

I live in hope, though, and I trust that by enabling the patients with whom I do have clinical contact to live a more natural life in tune with their environment, respectful of their own bodies and attentive to the needs of the people around them, this will indeed have an indirect beneficial effect on many more individuals than I could hope to meet as a practitioner. As a holistic practitioner I hope that my patients will be able to manage their own health and, in the most part, have no need for conventional medicine. Of course, in the event of serious disease or at the time of the important transitions of childbirth and death, it is of great comfort to know that conventional medicine is the safety net in place for when people really need to rely on its care and powerful interventions.

With this brief personal history as background, I shall now go on to clarify the rationale and structure of this textbook.

As I have explained, the overarching aim of the book is that acupuncturists might develop an understanding of conventional medicine that will first enable them to make links between conventional and more holistic medical concepts, and as a result this will enrich their consultations with their patients. Further aims are to encourage a clear understanding of why doctors work in the way they do, and to instill greater confidence in the management of "red flag" conditions, those situations when a patient is likely to benefit from, or even urgently need, access to conventional medical treatment.

Many institutions involved in training complementary healthcare practitioners in the conventional medical sciences currently rely on source texts designed for doctors and nurses in training. These texts are, of course, appropriate for detailing the knowledge base of conventional medical practice, but were not intended to answer questions about how medical facts and approaches may relate to a complementary health discipline. For this reason, many students find the conventional medical aspects of their training dry and irrelevant, and the material difficult to retain.

What this text offers in addition to the material found in standard medical texts is a presentation of medical information in the same systematic way, but with continual reference to how this information might relate to the practice of holistic medicine, and Chinese medicine in particular. Whilst the comparisons are largely confined to the language and concepts of Chinese medicine, they illustrate a process of "translation" that it is easily possible to undertake in any of the complementary medical disciplines.

After the introductory chapters in Stages 1 and 2 of the text, all the chapters that follow have a similar structure. In each chapter the following topics relating to a physiological subsystem of the body are explored:

- The physiology of that system.
- The pathology relevant to the system (i.e. what happens when disease causes imbalance).

- The conventional medicine approach to treatment of the diseases that have been described.
- Comparisons with the language of Chinese medicine wherever possible. These "translations" relate to physiology, pathology and the effects of medical treatments. To distinguish these paragraphs from the main part of the text, this information is presented in characteristic text boxes.

The attempt to translate from one medical language to another in this text is based on the premise that there is one reliable constant irrespective of the world view of the health practitioner. This reliable constant is the patient's experience of disease (the symptoms), and how the patient demonstrates a response to the disease process in their body (the signs). All medical approaches respond to these features of illness. Moreover, although conventional and complementary medical approaches may seem to have different languages, they all respond to a patient's symptoms and signs in predictable ways. For this reason, in theory, it is possible to translate from one medical language to another, even when the underlying theoretical framework of the two medical approaches appears to be startlingly different. The patient's symptoms and signs become the point at which a medical description from one discipline, "inflammation," for example, can be mapped onto a medical description from another such as "Wind Heat." This is not to say that inflammation is the same as Wind Heat; it most definitely is not. Instead it means that when a doctor diagnoses inflammation – because of localized redness, pain and swelling – then the Chinese energetic syndrome of Wind Heat is likely to be diagnosed in the same patient by a Chinese medicine practitioner, simply because this is the diagnosis to which these symptoms point. Some principles that underlie this process of translation can be found in the "Note to the Reader" which follows this Introduction.

This text is for the main part, however, a conventional medical textbook. It presents information about clinical medicine that is both up to date and relevant to clinical practice in any developed country and in the UK in particular. The most significant area in which the text may differ from texts written for a readership from other developed countries is in that of drug nomenclature. The names used in this text are based on the International Nonproprietary Name (INN) system recommended by the World Health Organization (WHO 2016)[1] and as used in the *British National Formulary of Medications* (British Medical Association and Royal Pharmaceutical Society 2016).[2]

The book has been designed for two modes of use. First, it will stand alone as a medical textbook, which can be referred to in the course of clinical practice by therapists in a wide range of complementary disciplines. The language in which it is written has been chosen to be accessible to complementary therapists. Ideally it will act as a guide for a practitioner with little or no scientific background in the navigation of what might be written about a patient's medical diagnosis in standard medical texts or online medical resources. Initially designed as a study course for students of acupuncture in the UK, the text has been studied in detail by hundreds of students who have provided valuable feedback and confirmed the readability of the information it presents.

Second, the text has been written in such a way that it can be followed systematically as part of a course in clinical medicine for students of acupuncture. To this end, online study aids such as a list of learning intentions for each chapter, "in-text questions" and end of chapter assessment tests have been designed to relate to the material in each chapter, and these can be found in the online study materials linked to this text.

The online material can be downloaded at https://library.singingdragon.com/redeem using the code STEPHENSONACU.

It includes:

- Full-color illustrations from the book.

- Self-assessment questions and answers. These self-assessment questions are designed to support home study of the text. The student is advised to write down answers to each question as they progress through the study of a chapter. The written answers can then be compared with the model answers, which are also to be found online.

- End of chapter self-assessment tests. These are designed to help the student review their learning after completion of each chapter.

This book is structured in six stages, each of which consists of three to four chapters ordered into topic sections. There are four appendices.

Stages 1 and 2 relate to topics that form the foundation of the study of clinical medicine, and include basic principles of physiology, pathology and pharmacology. These stages also introduce the theoretical basis used throughout the text for the translation of conventional medical language into Chinese medicine language, as described earlier. Stages 3–6 focus on the description of all the important medical conditions and their treatment as they relate to conventionally recognized body systems or patient groups. The conclusions in Chapter 6.3 focus on topics relevant to the practical management of clinical

patients with Western medical diagnoses. This includes guidance on the referral of patients with "red flag" conditions (Section 6.3a), managing the withdrawal from conventional medication (Section 6.3b), and some ethico-legal aspects of treating a patient who is also under the care of a medical practitioner (Section 6.3d).

In terms of using the book as a study course, the online self-assessment tests for each section have been designed to help the student ensure that the specified learning intentions have been met. If teaching institutions choose to adopt this text as a study course, then a pace of one stage per semester (i.e. six semesters in total) provides continual challenge without becoming too overwhelming. Ideally, if the course is taught in this way, home study can be supported by two to four teaching sessions per stage of the course, and by setting the students an end-of-stage written assignment as a form of summative assessment of their learning.

This book is packed with information intended to enrich the clinical encounter with a patient in need of healing. It is always good, however, to retain a degree of perspective when dealing with such information; there may be a danger that the weight of the information distracts the practitioner to the detriment of the potential of the healing encounter. For this reason, this Introduction concludes with the words of a wise healer. These encourage the practitioner engaged in developing a mastery of information to allow those theories to work quietly from only the background of their consciousness during the profound time when the patient has entered the clinic room.

> Practical medicine is, and always has been an art, and the same is true of practical analysis. True art is creation, and creation is beyond all theories. That is why I say to any beginner: learn your theories as well as you can, but put them aside when you touch the miracle of the living soul. No theories but your own creative individuality alone must decide. (Jung *et al.* 1928)[3]

Notes

1   WHO (World Health Organization) (2016) *International Nonproprietary Names*. Available at www.who.int/medicines/services/inn/en, accessed on 3 May 2016.
2   British Medical Association and Royal Pharmaceutical Society (2016) *British National Formulary 71*. London: BMJ Group and Pharmaceutical Press.
3   Jung, C.G. *et al.* (1928) *Contributions to Analytical Psychology*. New York: Harcourt, Brace & Company.

Note to the Reader: Understanding Western Medical Terminology in Chinese Medical Terms

As explained in the Introduction, the primary focus of this book is to introduce practitioners of Chinese medicine to the basic principles, pathological interpretations and clinical approaches of Western medicine. In addition, throughout the text "translations" are offered for expressing some of the signs and symptoms of Western medicine into the descriptive language of Chinese medicine.

Before any translation can be attempted, however, some clarity is required about the use of language and terminology in Chinese medicine. It is unfortunate that Chinese medical terms for organs and substances – which have unique energetic meanings – have been conventionally ascribed Western medical names. Terms such as Heart, Small Intestine, Liver, Blood and Phlegm all have particular meanings in Chinese medicine that bear little relationship to their biological namesakes. Throughout this text Chinese medical terms are ascribed a capital letter to differentiate them from biological terms. Appendix I clarifies in more systematic detail how the Chinese organs and biological organs of the same name are very different entities. The reader is thus counseled to be alert when studying Chinese medicine in the English language not to conflate the Chinese and biological organs and substances, and always to recognize each as constructs as defined within the terms of their originating medical philosophy.

To return to the topic of translation of disease descriptions, all physicians observe and describe symptoms and signs in their patients, whatever their theoretical background. According to this background, they may place different degrees of emphasis on different symptoms and signs. The pulse qualities that are described and considered significant in Chinese medicine, for example, are very different from those considered clinically significant in Western medicine. Nevertheless, physicians from each discipline are unlikely to disagree that a patient has nausea, fever, a rash and swollen joints, if indeed these are the symptoms and signs present in that particular case.

The links suggested between Western and Chinese medicine in this text are forged on the basis that Western and Chinese practitioners share this common ground, that they both recognize the consistency and value of symptoms and signs as indicators of disease. In this text, when a translation is attempted from Western medical terminology to that of Chinese medicine, the symptoms and signs form the bridge that enables this leap between the Western and Chinese medical interpretations of disease.

Western medical diagnoses are, in keeping with their reductionist roots, based on detailed analyses of symptoms and signs, as well as pathological changes and test results. For example, an early diagnosis of rheumatoid arthritis is hinted at by hot symmetrically swollen joints, characteristic deformity and fever. This may then be confirmed by blood tests that demonstrate the measurable presence of specific auto-antibodies and inflammatory markers. These features distinguish this inflammatory polyarthritis from a number of conditions presenting with similar symptoms and signs. Western diagnoses describe physical conditions, the features of which can be measured objectively, akin to the way in which a geographer might describe mountains, rivers and forests in a landscape.

Chinese medicine diagnoses, however, may be based on broad sweeps of clinical information, which are qualitatively rather than quantitatively assessed. Chinese diagnosis describes a state that is reflected in the whole person. The person *is* the diagnosis rather than *has* the diagnosis, and cannot be separated from it. In geographical terms, a Chinese medicine diagnosis is more comparable to an ever shifting climate or to an environment, rather than to a fixed feature such as a mountain or a forest. The diagnosis is based on the answers to questions such as "is the patient hot?," "is there dryness?," "is there swelling?" and "is the pain fixed and boring, or dull and improved by movement?" The answers to these questions are supported by characteristic changes in the pulse and tongue that can only be subjectively assessed. The fine distinctions made within Western diagnoses may not be so apparent in Chinese diagnoses. A case of early rheumatoid arthritis is likely to be described on the basis of hot swollen painful joints and fever as a form of "Heat Bi" syndrome (pattern) in which it is understood that pathogenic factors have transformed to Heat with resulting Blood and Qi Stagnation in the Channels and Collaterals.[1, 2] These descriptions may also be applied to any number of forms of polyarthritis that involve hot, swollen and painful joints.

In Chinese medicine the very subtle distinctions in diagnosis will emerge as a consequence of the uniqueness of the patient who is displaying the symptoms. While all patients with a symmetrical hot polyarthritis may readily be described as manifesting the imbalances of Heat with Blood and Qi Stagnation in the Channels and Collaterals, this tells us nothing about the cause of the Heat and the Stagnation, or indeed if these need to be treated directly. It may be more important in such a case to assess the degree of underlying deficiency (e.g. of Heart Qi or Kidney Yin), which could be a more appropriate focus of treatment.

In this text, attempts to make linguistic links between Western and Chinese medicine have been made using the consistent constellation of symptoms and signs as an enabling bridge between the two. There is nothing either remarkable or controversial about this. Once symptoms and signs are clearly described by Western medicine (e.g. fever, constipation, depression, rash, etc.), then Chinese theory very readily allows for a range of possible energetic diagnoses to be suggested. It is important to emphasize, however, that these "translations" are intended to enrich understanding of how Western and Chinese medicine diagnoses may co-exist. They are not intended as guides to treatment.

A perhaps more controversial aspect of this mapping process is the attempt to make statements about Chinese energetic interpretations on the basis of internal or microscopic changes in the body that would not have been directly observed in the patient by the ancient practitioners of Chinese medicine. For example, a pathological process that involves blood clotting might in this text be equated to Qi and Blood Stagnation, or inflammation to Heat and Stagnation, even if the process is going on deep within the body rather than on the surface. A process involving withering and loss of vitality of tissues, such as the degenerative changes seen in the lung in emphysema, might suggest that Yin Deficiency is an underlying imbalance, and a process in which the dynamic function of a body structure is compromised, such as inefficient pumping of the failing heart could be a manifestation of Qi or Yang Deficiency.

The compelling factor about assumptions that Western pathology can be equated to Chinese descriptions is that — very often — what can be assumed about what is happening at a microscopic level in a disease from a Chinese medicine perspective is made manifest in the symptoms and signs commonly associated with that disease. For example, on the basis of there being a blood clot in a coronary artery, a coronary thrombosis might suggest the syndrome of Heart Blood Stagnation. This conjecture is then corroborated by the fact that the common symptoms and signs of coronary thrombosis of intense fixed central chest pain and irregular pulse rate that are indeed consistent with those described in the Chinese medicine syndrome of Heart Blood Stagnation. This of course fits with the understanding that Chinese syndromes are holistic in nature; always in Chinese medicine the energetics of the part will reflect that of the whole. This should apply at the microscopic and even subatomic level as well as at a humanly observable level.

Again it must be emphasized that statements linking Western pathology with Chinese descriptions of disease process (such as "a blood clot suggests the presence of Blood Stagnation," "an accumulation of fluid suggests the Accumulation of Damp") are not intended to be guides for treatment, and are certainly not intended to represent exact equivalences. However, knowledge about how the symptoms and signs of known diseases relate to the syndromes will inform us about what sort of patients are likely to develop these conditions, and what sort of treatment principles might be considered for them. However, it should be repeated that treatment always needs to be planned in the light of the unique constellation of symptoms and signs with which an individual patient presents.

A similar process has been undertaken in this book with regard to the Chinese medicine interpretation of the actions of medical treatments. The Chinese medicine descriptions of drug actions are drawn from what is known in conventional medicine about how those drugs relieve symptoms and signs together with their side effects. It must also be taken into consideration that drugs tend not to directly nourish or replenish the body (nutritional supplements and replacement hormones being possible exceptions), but instead often inhibit or stimulate bodily processes, be they physiological or pathological. For example, the oral contraceptive pill inhibits the natural bodily process of ovulation and the ovulatory drug Clomiphene stimulates ovulation which would not have happened without medical assistance. Beta blockers (such as Propranolol) inhibit the action of the heart and result in slowed heart rate and reduced blood pressure. Beta agonists (such as adrenaline and salbutamol) stimulate the action of the heart and lead to increased heart rate and blood pressure.

Manufactured drugs differ from herbal products in that, with the exception of some binding agents or liquid substrates, they essentially contain the active molecules known to effect the desired changes. Herbal products, when naturally processed, and particularly when prescribed in combination, contain a complex range of natural substances, and are understood in Chinese medicine ideally to have nourishing as well as moving or clearing qualities. If herbal combinations are prescribed appropriately, any potential depletion effected by moving Qi will be ideally supported by simultaneously treating any root deficiency.

What the text postulates is that such interruption of bodily processes by manufactured chemicals, even if they are pathological processes, carries an energetic cost, simply because a root imbalance has not been treated. This could mean that the original imbalance that was manifesting, such as the Stagnation of Qi or Heat, might then become expressed at another level in the body. This has some resonance with the classical homeopathic concept of suppression of symptoms where, as a result of the suppression, the imbalance becomes manifest at a deeper level in the body. Similarly, in Chinese medicine theory pathological bodily processes (e.g. a tension headache) may be the result of a deeper energetic imbalance (e.g. Ascent of Liver Yang resulting from sustained high levels of stress-related emotions such as anger). Simply inhibiting an outer expression of the imbalance (by taking a painkiller) will not necessarily allow the deeper imbalance to be resolved.

Moreover, it is suggested that while stimulating bodily functions by a medical treatment might be beneficial in the short term, ultimately it might be draining for the body. For example, the stimulation of heart rate and blood pressure by beta agonists may in the short term profoundly benefit a bodily system in which these functions might be failing to rally round, and can literally be life-saving. From an energetic perspective, a system that was deficient in Yang has been stimulated. But this is not the same as the Chinese medical concept of "nourishing" Yang, as might be the consequence of careful attention to diet, sleep and exercise. This sudden stimulation of heart rate may well be at the cost of drawing on deep bodily reserves, and so ultimately draining. At a deep level this stimulating of functions that might equate to healthy Yang possibly contributes to the opposite situation, as the deep reserves of Yang are depleted. It makes sense that in this situation the patient will also benefit from some additional treatment approaches to nourish the depleted reserves in the long term.

This theory fits with the common experience of using any of the stimulatory substances in the diet, such as sugar, caffeine or chocolate. After a temporary high, overuse of these substances may leave a person feeling even more drained and out of balance than before (and indeed, all these substances are recognized to exhaust Kidney Qi; Flaws and Wolfe 1983[3]). These effects are all the more pronounced with some of the commonly abused drugs increasingly accessible to all in modern culture, such as nicotine, alcohol, cannabis, cocaine, opiates, and mental stimulants such as methylphenidate.

In this text, these ideas have been drawn into the interpretation of drug energetics. Because of inattention to the root cause of illness, what is happening on the surface as a result of drug treatment may be accompanied by a paradoxical effect at a deeper level. A drug that clearly seems to be Cooling in nature according to Chinese medicine (e.g. an anti-inflammatory medication that palliates red angry joints) may also demonstrate a range of side effects

that are Hot in nature (e.g. rash, fever, inflammation of the stomach). Some of these may be a consequence of the toxic nature of the drug to body tissues, evidenced by the fact that the effects may be experienced by people taking these medications irrespective of the nature of the underlying disease. However, it is worthy of note that many drugs do seem to generate side effects that have an energetic expression that is the opposite of that of their therapeutic action. This might be considered an indication that forcing the expression of the original symptoms to a different level of the organism might partly explain the energetic mechanism of their action.

Again the point needs to be made that these interpretations of drug energetics are intended to enrich the diagnostic process. They are not intended as guides to Chinese medicine treatment, which always needs to be based on the outcome of the Chinese medicine diagnostic process. Drugs may cause dramatic symptoms and signs in a patient, but often it is careful attention to the individual's root imbalance, and the one that probably preceded any drug treatment, which can lead to the most profound shifts in the patient's health.

In summary, the meeting of two independent systems of medicine is a great opportunity to enrich and develop each of them. It is hoped that the interpretations offered in the Chinese medicine sections may deepen the Chinese medicine practitioner's understanding of the patient with a Western diagnosis from a Chinese medicine perspective. Moreover, a Western medical doctor who has begun to embrace the Chinese medicine understanding of the grouping and interrelationship of signs and symptoms may do well to add to their medical diagnostic framework the sophisticated understanding of the environmental, emotional and spiritual correlates of physiological and pathological processes that are at the heart of all the systems of Chinese medicine, and in so doing enrich their conventional medical practice.

Notes

1   Throughout the text the convention will be used to capitalise all terms that relate to Chinese medical diagnoses. This is intended to help distinguish those English words commonly employed when Chinese medical descriptions are translated that actually have a unique meaning which is distinct from the common usage. For example, the Chinese medical terms Heart, Phlegm, Wind and Triple Heater all have unique Chinese medical meanings that bear no correlation to the common usage of the English words heart, phlegm, wind, triple and heater.

2   Deng, L. *et al.* (1987) *Chinese Acupuncture and Moxibustion.* Beijing: Foreign Languages Press.

3   Flaws, B. and Wolfe, H. (1983) *Prince Wen Hui's Cook: Chinese Dietary Therapy.* Brookline, MA: Paradigm Publications.

INTRODUCTION TO MEDICAL SCIENCES

1.1 Introduction to Medical Sciences

1.1a Introduction to physiology: systems of the body

The term physiology,[1] derived from the Greek meaning study of nature, is used to describe how all living organisms work or function. An understanding of physiology has to underpin the study of clinical medicine, as it is only through knowledge of how biological processes function in health that the mechanisms and outcomes of disease may be understood. Throughout this text, physiological descriptions of the body systems will precede the descriptions of how disease manifests in those systems. The introduction and explanation of the key concepts necessary to understand these descriptions is the purpose of this first section.

The study of physiology offers more to the Chinese medical practitioner than simply providing building blocks for the further study of medical sciences. Central to all healing modalities is the development of an understanding and respect for the human body in health and disease. This respect enriches the way in which the practitioner communicates with patients and handles their bodies. It may well, indeed, add to the healing potential of the encounter, as through this respect the patient will feel recognized and understood. Respect comes with knowledge, and although the perspective of Chinese medicine is that the body is a manifestation of a rich interplay of energetic functions, it is nevertheless also very helpful for practitioners to acquire a sound understanding of the structure and normal functions of the physical parts as recognized by the patient and by their medical doctors, which is, of course, the physical manifestation of the energetic foundation.

And so, a physiological understanding of the body will enhance the understanding of the energetic nature of the body parts, as understood in Chinese medicine. Bodily functions are described in diverse ways, but some elements remain constant. All medical systems recognize major functional details – the lungs take in air, the heart pumps blood, the blood clots and the skin produces sweat. Although the processes of these various functions may be described very differently, awareness that all disciplines recognize the same summary descriptions can help when translating from the language of one medical discipline to another.

As an illustration of this, in this text physiological concepts are, from time to time, translated into the language of Chinese medicine. In Chinese medicine the body is understood in terms of constantly interchanging and interdependent forms of Qi, the underlying energetic principle on which that system of medicine is founded. The comparisons with Chinese medical physiology described in this text clearly illustrate not only the internal consistency of thought in Chinese medicine, but also the possibility of translation. This process of translation has the potential to promote increased understanding and respect between conventionally trained practitioners and those Chinese medical practitioners who use the language of energetics to describe the philosophical basis of their practice. It is important that, when translating in this way, we recognize we are not comparing "like for like." The Western descriptors are used to relate to measurable physical forms and functions; the Chinese medical terms relate to energetic processes that cannot be bounded in the same way (for more on this topic, see "Note to the Reader" at the beginning of this book). Whilst the translation process can be deeply informative, the practitioner must avoid the temptation to consider Chinese medicine in a reductionist building block fashion. Concepts such as Liver

Qi Stagnant or Stomach Yin Deficient apply to the whole system and not to a precisely defined body part. Whilst a diseased body part might point to Kidney Qi Deficiency, the converse is not true; Kidney Qi Deficiency will manifest in the whole system and can become apparent physically (and emotionally) in a multiplicity of ways.

Systems of the body

Physiologists consider the human body to be a collection of functionally integrated systems. Although these systems cannot work in isolation, each can be defined in terms of its structure (anatomy) and function (physiology).

The physiological systems of the body are listed in Table 1.1a-I. Most conventional general medical textbooks are subdivided according to these systems. This makes sense because conventional practitioners have learned to classify diseases as they affect each system. The in-depth study of diseases according to a physiological system is known as a medical specialty. Usually, the term for the specialty is the name of the system together with the suffix "-ology." For example, the medical specialty devoted to diseases of the endocrine system is known as "endocrinology."

Table 1.1a-I The 12 physiological systems of the body

- Integumentary (skin)
- Muscular
- Skeletal (bone)
- Neurological (nervous)
- Endocrine (hormone secreting)
- Cardiovascular/circulatory (heart and blood vessels)
- Respiratory (breathing)
- Gastrointestinal (digestive)
- Lymphatic (immune)
- Hematological (blood)
- Urological/renal/urinary (kidneys and bladder)
- Reproductive

Sometimes two or more systems are considered together because their functions are related. For example, the urinary and reproductive systems may be considered together as the urogenital system, and the blood and cardiovascular system can be considered together as the circulatory system.

Conversely, a system can be broken down into component subsystems for study in depth. This leads to terms such as ophthalmology (the study of the eye), otorhinolaryngology (the study of the ear, nose and throat), hepatology (the study of the liver) and cardiology (the study of the heart).

Each system in the body comprises organs that work together to enable the system to perform its role in the physiology of the whole body.

Physiological levels

The distinct systems of the body described earlier can in turn be broken down into subsystems, each of which represents a collection of interrelated organs (see Figure 1.1a-I). The concept of levels of organization can be applied here. The most complex level of organization is the body itself. The next level consists of the 12 systems and their subsystems. The various organs that make up the systems form the next level of organization.

At the next level, organs can be considered in terms of the different tissues out of which they are made. Tissues, of which there are four main types, comprise the range of basic living materials with which organs can be built.

Finally, the simplest level of organization that can be considered a living unit is the cell. This is the single living building block out of which all tissues, and therefore all organs, systems and the body itself, are made, and it is, of course, the original first component part of the human body formed at conception.

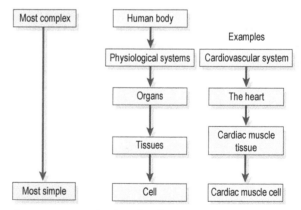

Figure 1.1a-I The levels of organization of the body

Information box 1.1a-I

The organs: comments from a Chinese medicine perspective

Chinese medicine describes 12 Organs, all but one of which is given the same name as the solid organs that are described in physiology. However, these Organs, such as the Heart, Lung and Kidneys, do not correspond to the physiological structures after which all but the San Jiao (Triple Heater) are named. The organs in physiology are defined primarily in terms of their structure and location, and also by their function. In contrast, the Organs in Chinese medicine are not recognized to have a physical structure. They are defined in terms of the functions that they have in the body and these include emotional or spiritual aspects as well as physical ones. They are recognized to have a dominant, but not exclusive, influence over the physical organ after which they are named, but will actually have an influence over every part of the body.

The physiologist is talking about a physically tangible reality when discussing organs, but a Chinese medicine practitioner is describing energetics when using the same term.[2] In Chinese medicine, this energetic body may be defined in terms of Yin and Yang, the Five Elements and the Vital Substances of Qi, Blood, Essence (Jing) and also the Pathogenic Factors (such as Cold and Damp) that may impact upon it.

In this text, to minimize possible confusion between terms used differently in Chinese and Western medicine, all Chinese medicine terms that have a meaning which is particular to Chinese medicine theory are ascribed an upper-case initial letter.

The differences may be briefly summarized as in the table on the right.

Whilst it is tempting to do so, it is important never to presume that the physiological and Chinese medicine use of a term might correspond. It is also important to explain this to patients, who might otherwise make very incorrect assumptions about what their Chinese medical diagnoses might mean for them. Although there are some similarities (e.g. the function of the stomach is to store food both in physiological and in Chinese medicine), there are many more differences (e.g. the physiological spleen has nothing to do with the digestion of food, whereas this is a significant function of the Spleen in Chinese medicine).

The organ correspondence tables in Appendix I demonstrate in more detail the nature of the differences between the functions of the physiological and Chinese medicine Organs. Each table relates to a particular organ, and illustrates how the various functions of the physiological and Chinese medicine Organs can be mapped onto one another.

Physiological organs	Organs in Chinese medicine
Solid physical structures	Terms to describe a collection of functions
The structure and function of the organs can be assessed by scientific means: dissection, physical examination, blood tests, ultrasound, X-ray imaging, etc.	The functions of the Chinese medicine Organs are assessed subjectively by checking the state of the Qi using techniques such as pulse and tongue diagnosis
The function of the organ can be related to the structure of the organ (e.g. the pumping action of the heart organ can be related to its muscular shape, electrical activity and valves)	The function of the Chinese medicine Organs is not related to any structure, although the Chinese medicine Organ may dominate the function of a physiological organ (e.g. the Qi of the Heart Organ as interpreted in Chinese medicine supports the physiological heart organ)
For any one organ there is not necessarily a counterpart Chinese medicine Organ (e.g. pituitary)	For any one Chinese medicine Organ there is not necessarily a counterpart physiological organ (e.g. Triple Burner)

1.1b The cell: composition, respiration and division

At the most basic of the levels of organization of all plants and animals lays the living building block known as the cell. An understanding of how the cell functions will form a basis for the study of those more complex organizational levels of the body, the tissues, the organs and the physiological systems.

Most cells are too small to be seen with the naked eye, but a simple microscope can reveal certain details of their structure, including the boundaries between cells.

Figures 1.1b-I to 1.1b-IV are diagrammatic representations of how cells in different tissues can appear under the light microscope. These indicate the wide variety of cell shape seen in different tissues, and also that each cell contains a large central structure known as the nucleus.

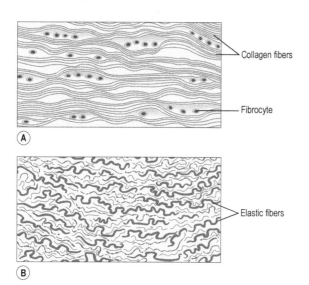

(A)

(B)

Figure 1.1b-I Fibrous tissue, illustrating fiber-generating cells (fibrocytes) and collagen fibers

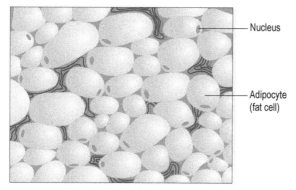

Figure 1.1b-II Adipose (fat) tissue, illustrating fat-filled adipose cells and minimal connective fibers

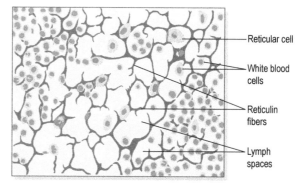

Figure 1.1b-III Tissue from a lymph node, illustrating immune cells (white blood cells and reticular cells) and supportive reticulin fibers

Figure 1.1b-IV Cardiac muscle tissue, illustrating the fiber-like cardiac muscle cells linked by connecting "intercalating discs"

The more powerful electron microscope is required to reveal more detail in cell structure. Although the precise structure of each cell is different, depending on the tissue in which it is found and the role it has to play, all cells in the human body share some basic features.

It is helpful to consider a "generalized cell" to study how all cells are made up and function. No single cell will be *exactly* like this diagram, but most cells will have the features portrayed in the generalized cell, as depicted in Figure 1.1b-V.

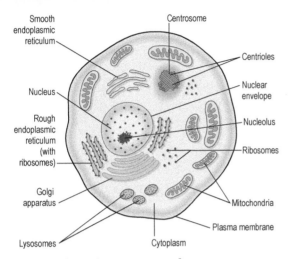

Figure 1.1b-V The structure of a generalized animal cell

Structure of the cell

Each cell contains a plasma membrane and a number of internal structures known as organelles. This terminology reflects the fact that a single cell can be seen as a living unit in isolation, with the organelles corresponding to the organs of the body. The organelles are fluid in nature, being bound by oily fluid membranes and suspended within a fluid matrix known as the cytosol. Together, the cytosol and organelles are called cytoplasm, and this is bounded by an oily fluid plasma membrane.

The plasma membrane acts as the link between the cell and the outside world. Large molecules made of protein in this membrane make the cell unique and structurally respond to various chemicals in the cellular environment to bring about changes within the cytoplasm. In addition, the plasma membrane allows the passage of nutrients into the cell and waste out of the cell, but able to retain essential substances within the cell. This important feature of cell membranes, known as semi-permeability, is described in Section 1.1c.

The nucleus is the largest structure found within the cell. It contains genetic material in the form of chromosomes. These consist of strands of a very complex molecule called DNA (deoxyribonucleic acid). DNA is the template for the synthesis of proteins building materials in the cell. Another complex molecule with a similar structure, RNA (ribonucleic acid), takes the role of the messenger. Messenger RNA transfers the information coded on DNA out to the cytosol and to the ribosomes, where the proteins are actually made.

The other large round structures in the cytosol are the numerous cigar-shaped mitochondria, which utilize oxygen to break down the basic nutrients obtained from carbohydrates and fats (and sometimes proteins) to form an energized compound called ATP (adenosine triphosphate). ATP can be likened to a battery as it holds a readily available store of energy to "power" all processes of the cell. This process of using oxygen and nutrients to form energy is called cellular respiration. The waste product of respiration is carbon dioxide.

A large part of the remaining cytosol consists of many layers of oily membrane called the endoplasmic reticulum (ER), on which the dense ribosomes are situated. Where the ribosomes are numerous the ER is described as rough (rough ER), and where they are less numerous it is described as smooth (smooth ER). Ribosomes are the site at which the long molecule of RNA is used as a template to guide the production of proteins from simple chemicals called amino acids, out of which all proteins are made. Proteins made on the rough ER pass into the space between its membranes in preparation for transport out of the cell.

The Golgi apparatus is an extension of the ER. It takes the proteins made on the ribosomes and covers them with a membrane coating to make "vesicles" (also known as secretory granules). These can travel to the plasma membrane, so that proteins can be released into the outside environment when necessary.

Microfilaments and microtubules are fibers that can contract and cause the movement of substances from one part of the cell to another. These fibers, also known as the cytoskeleton, maintain the structure of the cell and link the various organelles.

The features of the "generalized cell" are summarized in Table 1.1b-I.

Table 1.1b-I The important characteristics of the cell

- The cell is a self-contained living unit
- It is bounded by a "membrane," which is studded with characteristic proteins
- The membrane allows communication with the outside world
- The cell takes in nutrients and oxygen to produce energy to "power" its activities
- It contains genetic material in its nucleus, which allows the manufacture of specific cellular building materials, the proteins
- These proteins can be "exported" out of the cell to the outside environment

---

Information box 1.1b-I

The production of cellular energy: comments from a Chinese medicine perspective

Just as the cell can be compared to a body with the organelles as small organs, it is also reasonable to attempt to describe cellular function in terms of the Organ systems of Chinese medicine. For example, one interesting parallel between the Chinese description and the physiological insight is that of the production of cellular energy. According to Chinese medicine as described by Maciocia (1989),[3] the formation of True (Zhen) Qi is derived from Gathering (Zong) Qi, which, in turn, is a product of Food Qi and Air. According to Chinese medicine theory, vitality from the food, Food Qi, is transported by the Spleen to the Lungs, where it is combined with vitality from the air to form Zong Qi. It is under the catalytic action of Original Qi that the Zong Qi is transformed into Zhen Qi, which then circulates in the Channels and nourishes the Organs in the form of Nutritive (Ying) Qi and Protective (Wei) Qi.

Physiologists recognize that cellular energy is similarly derived from a catalytic process involving food (which is broken down into the essential components of simple sugars and amino acids) and oxygen drawn into the body from the air breathed into the lungs. When explained in this way, there is clearly an interesting parallel with the production of cellular energy, stored in the form of energized ATP as the source of energy for all tissues, and the Chinese description of the production of True (Zhen) Qi, which also outlines food and air as basic substrates.

Cell replication

The replication of cells is a fundamental process within the body that begins with the first division of the fertilized egg (zygote). It is essential both for growth and for the repair of aging and damaged tissues. There are two ways in which cells can divide, known as mitosis and meiosis. Mitosis is the process whereby a single cell divides into two identical cells following the replication and separation of the chromosomes in the nucleus. Meiosis is the process whereby a single cell divides into daughter cells, each of which carries exactly half of the genetic material of the parent cell.

The stages of mitosis are illustrated in Figure 1.1b-VI. In this diagram, for the sake of clarity, only a single pair of the human complement of 23 chromosomal pairs is illustrated. The diagram shows how mitosis results in two identical daughter cells, whereas meiosis results in the production of four genetically unique daughter "half-cells" or gametes.

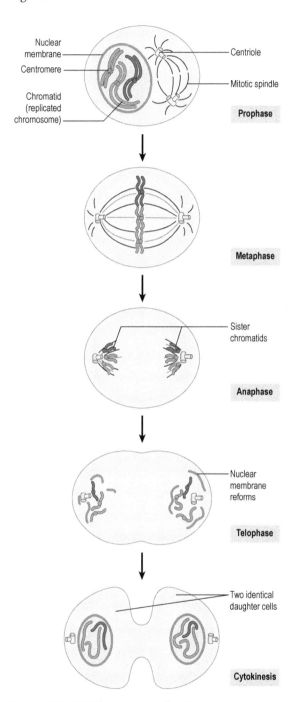

Figure 1.1b-VI The stages of mitosis

Mitosis reproduces the parent cell for the purposes of the growth of the tissue or the repair of damaged tissue, while meiosis produces the reproductive cells (spermatozoa and ova), also known as gametes. When the gamete is fertilized, the resulting zygote (the very first cell, which will later divide to form the embryo) will have a unique combination of genetic material, half from the mother and half from the father. It is the process of meiosis that is fundamental to the uniqueness of every human being.

Both meiosis and mitosis are involved in the development of the fertilized egg (zygote) into an adult human being. Meiosis in the sex organs of the parents leads to the production of the gametes. When a male gamete (spermatozoon) and female gamete (egg or ovum) meet, they fuse through the process of fertilization. The resulting zygote divides and grows by the process of mitosis.

Mutation

When the genetic material of the daughter cells from mitosis and meiosis has become damaged during the process of cell division, this is referred to as a mutation. There are three possible consequences of this. First, the mutation is so minor that the resulting cell is very similar in function to its parent. Second, the mutation disturbs the function of the daughter cells so much that they die. Third, and most significantly, the mutation may lead to disturbed function in the daughter cells, although these cells continue to live and replicate. This may or may not have a significant effect on the tissue of which the parent cell is a part.

If the parent cell is one of the cells in an embryo, a single mutation can have devastating effects, as the daughter cells may have been destined to develop into major body parts. One example of the consequences of mutation occurring during the process of mitosis is the effects of the drug thalidomide, which was developed in the early 1960s as an anti-nausea medication in early pregnancy. It was later discovered that significant limb development mutations had developed in the embryos carried by pregnant mothers using the medication.

A mutation in mitosis can also lead to cancerous change in the daughter cells. Cancer is always the consequence of a mutation that has led to impairment in growth regulation and cell survival in the mutated cells. The affected cells have abnormal and uncontrolled growth patterns, and this is how cancerous change leads to disease.

Mutation in meiosis will also lead to a defect in the genetic code in the gametes. Sometimes this means that affected gametes cannot be fertilized. However, in other cases, fertilization is possible, and the genetic code of the resulting zygote will then carry the defect. This means that every cell of the developing embryo will be affected by the mutation. This may lead to an insignificant or minor change in the function of the adult, such as color blindness, but can also result in severe inherited diseases, such as sickle cell anemia or hemophilia.

Mutation is an important process to understand in the study of pathology. Mutation in mitosis can cause certain physically based congenital diseases and cancer, and mutation of the gametes in meiosis can lead to genetic congenital diseases.

1.1c Cell transport and homeostasis

Cellular transport processes

As previously described, the cell membrane has the property of semi-permeability in which it can allow the passage of some substances but not of others. By this mechanism, the cell takes in nutrients and expels wastes. The membrane can also permit the cell to respond to changes in the outside world. An example of this is the nerve cell, which picks up information from one part of the body (e.g. an image in the eye) and relays this to another part of the body (e.g. to the brain, for recognition of the image). This property of "response to stimuli" is also dependent on the passage of substances across the cell membrane.

The cell membrane is both fluid and oily in nature, and may be pictured as a mobile, slippery and very thin layer surrounding the cell, rather like the wall of a soap bubble. The oily nature means that substances that are soluble in oils, such as gases (oxygen and carbon dioxide) and steroids, can pass through the membrane by first dissolving in it. This oily (phospholipid) layer also contains pathways made through the membrane by large protein molecules embedded within it. These pathways are of a sufficient size to allow the slow, but free, passage of small molecules such as water and salt (see Figure 1.1c-I).

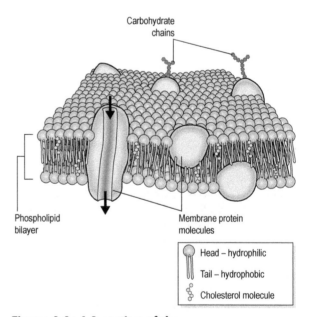

Figure 1.1c-I A section of the fluid plasma membrane

Simple diffusion

Movement of substances within the body, whether inside cells, outside cells or across cell membranes, always involves movement through body fluids. When substances are dissolved or suspended in water they tend to move from an area of high concentration to one of low concentration, and the movement continues until the differences in concentration are evened out as much as is physically possible. This form of movement of substances dissolved or suspended within water is called "diffusion." For example, when orange squash concentrate is poured into a glass of water, the eventual even mix of orange and water occurs as a result of diffusion.

When a semi-permeable membrane such as the cell membrane separates two regions of fluid of different concentrations, the process of diffusion for small molecules is slowed down but not prevented. For example, if there is a strong salt solution on one side of a membrane and water on the other, the water molecules will cross the membrane via the protein channels to mix with the salt solution. The larger salt molecules cannot use the tiny pathways in the membrane proteins and so cannot make this transition. However, because the water molecules can move, over time the concentrated salt solution will become much more dilute. The process may take some time, but even despite this membrane barrier, as with the orange squash, the result is a much more even concentration of solution on either side of it. This movement of water across a semi-permeable membrane into a region of more concentrated solution is called osmosis (see below).

Diffusion of certain fat-soluble substances can actually occur through the membrane itself rather than through the protein membrane channels. This is because the membrane is made up of an oily substance and permits the free passage of molecules that can dissolve in it. Therefore, because of diffusion, a difference in concentration of oxygen on either side of a semi-permeable membrane will eventually become evened out. This will be as a result of the movement of oxygen between the oily molecules, which make up the membrane, from the more concentrated to the less concentrated side.

Facilitated diffusion

In addition to the protein channels (holes), there are also gates (also made of protein) that allow the passage of slightly larger substances such as glucose and amino acids. Movement of larger molecules via these gates is known as facilitated diffusion. The gates restrict the free passage of these substances, so that this form of diffusion is extremely slow. This means that, if one of these specialized gates is present in a membrane, only a small amount of a large molecule such as glucose dissolved within the cytoplasm of a cell will be able to pass through.

Some molecules, such as proteins, are so large that they cannot pass across the membrane by the process of diffusion. This means that any large molecules contained within a membrane, such as proteins forming the microfilaments in the cytoplasm, will be unable to leave.

In summary, the membrane is permeable to water and fat-soluble molecules, slightly permeable to glucose, and impermeable to large molecules. This illustrates the meaning of "semi-permeable." Understanding the concept of semi-permeability is a prerequisite for making sense of the process of osmosis.

Osmosis

The process of osmosis in action is evident when limp flowers are placed in some water and the floppy stems become, after a length of time, much sturdier. What is happening in this example is that the water in the vase is moving across the plasma membranes of the plant cells into the cells themselves. This causes the cells to swell, and then the whole stem to regain its firmness. The water is moving into the cells by diffusion, because the cytoplasm contains a concentrated solution of glucose and large molecules. These larger molecules have a tendency to move in the opposite direction out of the cells, but they are unable to do this because of the barrier of the semi-permeable membrane. Therefore, most of the movement is of water passing one way across the membrane, and this, of course, benefits the plant.

In physiology, the term "osmosis" refers to the process of the transfer of water molecules from within a dilute solution with the result that a more concentrated solution on the other side of a semi-permeable membrane is made more dilute.

Osmotic pressure

In osmosis, the tendency of the water is to continue moving until the solutions on each side of a membrane are of equal strength. However, the movement of water into a concentrated solution of large molecules does not always occur indefinitely. Otherwise, in the example of limp flowers placed in water, the cells in the stems of the flowers would eventually burst. What happens is that, eventually, the process slows down to reach a stable state; the plant cells are firm, but not over-full.

This example illustrates the idea of osmotic pressure. The tendency of the water to dilute the solution on the other side of the membrane can be likened to it being moved under pressure. However, there are opposing pressures to this movement. In the case of the plant cell, the opposing pressure is the tautness of the fibrous skin of the stem. Eventually, the osmotic pressure is matched by opposing pressures, and the one-way movement stops at a "steady state." This explains how plant cells in a stem can contain a concentrated solution of large molecules, but do not burst when placed in water.

The force of osmotic pressure can, in some situations, be strong enough to rupture cells. For example, red blood cells are not supported by fibrous tissue. If a drop of blood is placed in pure water (which is much more dilute than the plasma in which these cells normally circulate), the red blood cells will swell as water molecules move by osmosis into their cytoplasm. Eventually, these cells will burst under the force of the osmotic pressure.

Figure 1.1c-II illustrates what could happen to a red blood cell if it is placed into (a) a solution of the same strength (isotonic) as the fluid in its cytosol, (b) a much more dilute (hypotonic) solution, and (c) a more concentrated (hypertonic) solution. In (a) the movement of water across the cell membrane (indicated by the arrows) is balanced inwards and outwards, and the cell remains the same size. In (b) there is a tendency of a larger volume of the more dilute solution to move into the red blood cell than there is for water to move out. This will cause it to swell; if the solution is very dilute, the red cell might even burst. In (c), the tendency is for more fluid to move out of the cytosol, across the cell membrane and into the surrounding solution; the red blood cell will tend to shrivel as a result.

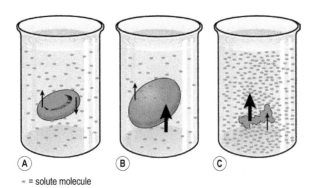

● = solute molecule

Figure 1.1c-II The process of osmosis

This powerful effect of osmosis explains why hospital patients are given intravenous saline solution in a drip rather than pure water. Saline is a salt solution made to be precisely the concentration of the cytoplasm of all cells, and thus the cells will neither burst nor shrivel when mixed with it.

Osmosis also explains why the bouncy and firm quality of the skin is lost in cases of dehydration. Lack of water means the blood becomes more concentrated. The cells are bathed in the fluid derived from blood. Therefore, when the body is in a state of dehydration, the fluid within the cells will be less concentrated than the surrounding fluid. Water will then move out of the cells by osmosis. This leaves the whole tissue limp, as each cell has slightly shriveled due to the cellular dehydration caused by the osmosis.

Active transport

Larger molecules, such as complex proteins and glucose, cannot pass readily through the holes and gates formed by membrane proteins (see Figure 1.1c-I). Instead, for rapid movement, these large molecules rely on a "pump," in the form of a specialized membrane carrier protein powered by the energy stored by the chemical ATP, to permit them to pass. The energy released by the ATP powers a change in the shape of the pump proteins, and this change allows the carriage of the large molecule from one side of the membrane to the other, rather akin to a turnstile that can take a person from one side of a gateway to the other once the entry fee has been inserted (see Figure 1.1c-III). Osmosis and diffusion are known as "passive transport" because they require no added input of energy to take place. In these processes, the movement of molecules occurs simply as a result of the natural tendency of these molecules to be in movement. When added power in the form of ATP is required to move substances from one side of a membrane to another, this is known as active transport.

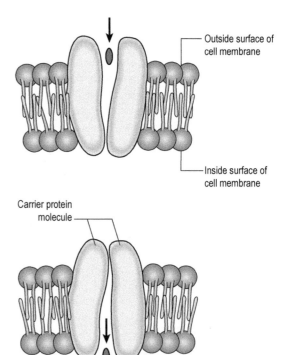

Outside surface of cell membrane

Inside surface of cell membrane

Carrier protein molecule

Figure 1.1c-III The role of the carrier protein in active transport and facilitated diffusion across membranes

Bulk transport

The term phagocytosis (literally "cell-eating") describes the process whereby the cell membrane forms arm-like projections that can reach out and engulf external substances so that they can be drawn into the cell. Exocytosis is the process whereby an intracellular vesicle containing complex substances can fuse with the external membrane of the cell so that those substances can be released. Both are forms of active transport, because the movements of the vesicles in both are enabled by the contraction of ATP-powered microfilaments and tubules.

These simple processes are at the foundation of all that enables a cell to work as part of a living organism. Transport across membranes is what allows a cell to take in nutrients and excrete waste. It also permits a response to changes in the environment, and therefore communication between cells and the ability of one cell to alter the behavior of another.

Homeostasis

Homeostasis (meaning staying the same) refers to the body's ability to maintain a state of balance despite changing external circumstances.

Two important concepts in physiology that relate to homeostasis are those of the internal environment and the external environment. The internal environment describes all parts of the body that are contained by a tissue layer, the outside surface of which has a direct connection with the external environment. The external environment includes those parts of the body connected to the outside by orifices. Therefore, parts of the body such as the air passages leading to the lungs, the long space enclosed by the tube of the gut, and the inside of the bladder are all part of the external environment. The external environment is, of course, unpredictable and prone to change in temperature, composition of the air and the presence of other substances such as food and liquids.

The principle of homeostasis is that the internal environment is always maintained at a steady state despite changes in the external environment. For example, our body temperature remains the same whatever the outside weather through homeostasis (except in the case of illness). Homeostatic processes ensure that diverse variables, including the concentration of the blood, the levels of hormones, oxygen, carbon dioxide, blood sugar and mineral salts, the density of the bone and the muscle tone remain controlled within very narrow limits that maximize function and health.

The process of homeostasis is underpinned by a system of negative feedback loops, which involve changes to re-establish balance occurring in response to changes in the internal balance. Such a system requires a "detector" to recognize a move away from balance, a "control center" that recognizes when the move has been so great that something has to be done about it, and an "effector" that brings about a change in the body to reverse the imbalance. A thermostat is a mechanical example of a negative feedback loop in action. The detector in this case is a thermometer. The control center is the mechanism that is set to recognize when the temperature falls outside a desired range. The negative feedback loop is based on the maximum desired temperature. When the temperature becomes higher than this maximum, the effector, in this case the heating element, is switched off until the time when the temperature drops within the desired range once again.

It is clear that in chronic (long-term) illness, and also in aging, these feedback systems no longer work as effectively. In chronic illness the body never quite achieves the ideal internal environment for optimal function. For example, the blood glucose concentration of a person with untreated diabetes is at a level that is too high for the cells to remain undamaged, and in chronic rheumatoid arthritis the inflammatory processes of the body are always too overactive to be wholly beneficial, and damage to cells will also be the result. With this perspective, it becomes easy to understand how being in a state of ill health can lead to progressively worsening ill health. The way to stop this would be to reset in some way the "thermostat" of the feedback loop. However, many conventional treatments for chronic illness cannot do this. Most conventional medicines tend to act on the consequences of the imbalance in homeostasis, and not its underlying cause (which often has its root in chronic exposure of the body to unhealthy lifestyle patterns or adverse environmental influences).

In conclusion, the physiological view is that health depends on a natural tendency of the body to remain in balance. Illness is the result of a failure in this delicate system.

1.1d The tissue types

Specialization

This section explores in more detail how individual cells are specialized to perform different roles, and how specialized cells form the different tissue types.

Single-cell organisms, such as the amoeba, can survive without specialization because all parts of the cell membrane are in contact with the external environment. It is possible for a single-cell organism to obtain the food and oxygen it needs, to excrete waste and to respond to other changes in the environment, simply because all of its boundaries are in touch with the outside world. Specialization is necessary in larger organisms because most cells are not in contact with the external environment. Cells buried deep within a large organism are unable on their own to obtain nutrients and oxygen, or to excrete their waste. Likewise they will be unable to detect changes in the external environment and to respond appropriately.

Specialization is necessary in larger organisms to overcome this problem of the internally situated cells being unable to "fend for themselves." In larger organisms, specialized organs take over the role of functions such as nutrition, respiration, excretion and sensing the environment. In this way they support all the other cells in the body. For example:

- the digestive tract is specialized to obtain food for all cells in the body

- the lungs are specialized to obtain oxygen and excrete carbon dioxide for all cells in the body

- the liver and kidney are specialized to excrete other waste for all cells in the body

- the nervous system is specialized to sense changes in the environment for all cells in the body.

Tissue types

There are four recognized categories of specialized tissues – epithelial, connective, muscle and nervous tissue. All these can be subdivided into different tissue subtypes within each category, but this section focuses only on the main characteristics of the four types.

Epithelial tissue

All parts of the body that are in direct contact with the external environment are epithelial in nature, whether they are on the outside surface of the body or form the linings of the cavities and passageways of internal organs, such as the lung. Epithelial cells are specialized to protect, secrete and absorb. These are the functions that would be required of an external lining to the body, which has to perform the role of protection, taking in nutrients from the environment and the excretion of waste.

Epithelial cells are also found lining the heart, blood and lymph vessels. Here they are known as the endothelium, reflecting the fact that these epithelial cells are deep within the body rather than on the surface.

Epithelial cells develop from a connective tissue basement membrane that overlies connective tissue underneath. They usually form a single layer of cells, akin to paving stones, but in some regions and organs, including the skin, they develop in layers. These cells tend to multiply rapidly, as they are easily damaged through wear and tear. Figure 1.1d-I illustrates five different forms of epithelium that are found throughout the body.

Simple squamous epithelium

Simple cuboidal epithelium

Simple columnar epithelium

Stratified squamous epithelium

Transitional epithelium

Figure 1.1d-I The five important categories of epithelium found in the body

Connective tissue

Connective tissue is specialized to have a structural role in the body. In its various forms it supports and protects the organs both from within and without. It is characterized by cells supported within a non-cellular substance and supportive non-cellular fibers. Connective tissue has structural and protective roles. The types of connective tissue with obvious structural roles include areolar (loosely structured) tissue, adipose (fat) tissue, fibrous tissue, elastic tissue, cartilage and bone. All these tissues surround, support and protect the muscles and organs, and together form a structural network throughout the body. There are two types of connective tissue that are less to do with structure, and instead comprise the organs of the blood and the lymphatic systems. These have been classed as connective tissue, because the cells found in the blood and lymphoid tissues have similarities with the macrophages, plasma cells and mast cells found in structural connective tissue. All these blood and lymphatic cells, which include the red and white blood cells, have originated from one common type of immature cell found in the bone marrow.

Connective tissue usually underlies all epithelial tissue. In general, it consists of living cells embedded in a "matrix" consisting of structural strand-like proteins and a semi-solid or solid ground material (which together confer both strength and flexibility akin to reinforced concrete). This complex range of tissues forms the padding and support that separates the internal organs from the epithelial linings. This tissue is the next line in defense if the epithelium fails to prevent a wound or the entry of infection. The presence of the immune cells, such as the macrophages, plasma cells and mast cells, whose functions are to work in the processes both of wound healing and fighting infection, makes structural connective tissue a very important aspect of the body's defense mechanisms. Figure 1.1d-II illustrates the diversity of the structure of connective tissues.

Figure 1.1d-II Six examples of connective tissue found in the body

Muscle tissue

Muscle cells are characterized by the fact they all contain protein fibers that can contract. The energy for contraction comes from the cellular energy-storing molecule ATP. Muscle cells also contain another sort of protein, called myoglobin, which is specialized to store the large amount of oxygen required to produce sufficient quantities of energy-charged ATP in the muscle cell. There are three types of muscle tissue: striated, smooth and cardiac. Each is specialized for different roles.

Striated muscle tissue (see Figure 1.1d-III) is primarily found in skeletal muscle. It has cells in the form of long fibers and responds only to impulses from motor nerves. The cells are bound together in parallel, and can contract together as a unit to increase the available power.

Figure 1.1d-III Skeletal (striated) muscle fibers

Smooth muscle tissue (see Figure 1.1d-IV) is mainly found in the hollow organs and consists of sheets of spindle-like cells that have a natural tendency to contract. Although not dependent on motor impulses, smooth muscle can contract in response to the autonomic nerves that supply the hollow organs. The contraction of smooth muscle is slow and sustained.

Figure 1.1d-IV Smooth muscle fibers

Cardiac muscle tissue (see Figure 1.1d-V) is specially adapted for the heart wall, with fibers arranged in sheets, and the cells arranged with intercellular joints. This structure allows for a wave-like contraction across the sheet rather than a single contraction as a unit. Heart muscle tissue also has a natural tendency to contract and is not dependent on motor impulses.

Figure 1.1d-V Cardiac muscle fibers

Nervous tissue

Unlike the other physiological systems that, with the exception of blood, are composed of more than one of the first three tissue types, the nervous system is composed entirely of nervous tissue.

The tissue of the nervous system is made up of two types of cells:

- excitable cells (ordinarily called nerve cells, or neurons)

- non-excitable cells (supportive cells), which can be likened to a specialized form of structural connective tissue. The structure of this tissue is described in detail in Chapter 4.1.

Membranes and glands

The membranes and glands are specialized forms of epithelial tissue.

There are three main types of membrane – mucous, serous and synovial – each of which has an important structural role in the body in that they line and protect the organs.

Mucous membranes are characterized by the presence of mucus-secreting cells, which provide the lining of the mouth and digestive tract, the nose and respiratory tract and genitourinary tracts with a protective coating. They are, therefore, in contact with the external environment.

In contrast, serous membranes are deep within the internal environment. They both surround the body of organs and line the cavities in which they sit. They provide a fluid-filled space to separate the organ from the wall of its cavity.

The synovial membrane is the layer that separates the cartilage-covered ends of bone from the space in the joint. It secretes the fluid that nourishes the cartilage and lubricates the joint.

Glands fall into two broad categories: endocrine and exocrine. Endocrine glands are collections of epithelial cells that secrete hormones. Endocrine glands have no ducts; instead, their secretions are released directly into the fluid surrounding the cells (lymph), and from there to the bloodstream. Exocrine glands secrete specialized substances that are discharged towards the epithelium of the organs via a duct. The secretion therefore ends up in the external environment (e.g. on the skin, or in the gut, respiratory passages or genitourinary tract).

Process of differentiation

The various manifestations of the tissue types illustrate the diversity of ways in which the few identical cells of the very early embryo become differentiated into cells with unique and enduring characteristics. Once a cell of an embryo starts to develop into a squamous epithelial cell or a striated muscle fiber, this is the form in which its daughter cells will continue to appear as long as health is maintained.

Although each cell that is produced by mitosis in the embryo contains the same genetic code, through the process of differentiation parts of the genetic code are "switched off" and other parts are activated. A cell destined to develop into nerve tissue will have the genetic code relevant to the structure of nerve tissue "switched on" and all of that part of the code relevant to other types of tissue "switched off." Nevertheless, underlying the diversity of all the differentiated cells of the body a lifelong unity is preserved. All nucleated cells that develop throughout the lifetime of an individual will carry within them the unique DNA blueprint that defined that individual from the point of conception onwards.

1.1e Introduction to pathology and pharmacology

Pathology

The word pathology is derived from the Greek words for disease and study. The word pathogenic has the same root, meaning disease causing. The science of pathology involves understanding the various ways in which the homeostasis of the perfectly functioning body can fall out of balance.

Conventional pathologists understand that disease arises in the body either as a result of endogenous factors or because of adverse environmental conditions.

From a medical perspective, the internal causes of disease include:

- constitutional weakness (inherited disease)

- autoimmune disease

- cancerous change (although some cancers are understood to be triggered by external causes)

- degeneration of age

- negative emotions (the relation of chronic anger, depression and stress to ill health have all been studied in detail).

The external causes of disease include:

- infections

- inadequate diet

- overeating/obesity

- under-exercise

- physical trauma

- excessive heat or cold and dampness

- chemical damage/poisoning (including dietary and recreational factors such as caffeine, tobacco and alcohol) and radiation

- stressful living and working conditions.

Medical approaches to the management of disease

The full breadth of the role of a medical professional is not easily appreciated by a layperson, as certain very technical aspects of medical care, such as drug treatment and surgery, tend to stand out as the most prominent and memorable defining features. However, it has been argued that it is the more simple or mundane aspects of medical care that have had the most profound effects in terms of improving the health of individuals or populations.[4] To help with understanding the breadth of medical approaches, these are now considered within three categories: prevention of disease, cure of disease and treatment of symptoms in chronic disease.

Prevention of disease

Preventive medicine is an essential aspect of any medical care provided by a doctor, irrespective of the medical specialty in which the doctor has trained. At the foundation of any medical approach to preventive medicine is an ever-expanding evidence-based wealth of knowledge of the diverse determinants of disease listed above. In preventive medicine, the physician is concerned with developing this knowledge base and developing effective methods of influencing medical practice and, at a wider level, national and international health and economic policy, so that the important causes of disease are readily recognized and managed appropriately.

Methods of prevention include:

- social change (e.g. banning tobacco advertising and improved sanitation)

- education and advice to the public (e.g. healthy eating)

- use of medications (e.g. vaccination and antibiotics during surgery)

- surgery (e.g. removal of breast tissue in someone considered to be at high risk of cancer)

- routine screening for treatable risk factors for disease (e.g. tests performed in antenatal care).

Prevention can be focused at the level of stopping a disease event from developing (e.g. preventing heart attacks by focusing on exercise and smoking cessation), in which case it may be termed primary prevention. Alternatively, efforts to prevent disease may be concentrated on a patient who has suffered from a disease so that progression of the disease is minimized (e.g. the prescription of aspirin to someone who has suffered from a heart attack), in which case it may be known as secondary prevention.

Confusingly, the medical profession also uses the terms primary, secondary and tertiary prevention in a slightly different way, and it is important to be clear about this, as both forms of nomenclature appear in current respected texts. Some medical authors use the term primary prevention to mean the practice of preventing any aspect of a disease from developing. An example of primary prevention used in this sense is the recent UK policy of administering the human papilloma virus (HPV) vaccine to young teenage girls. This practice has the aim of preventing wart virus infection, now strongly associated with cervical cancer, from taking hold with the onset of sexual activity in later teenage years. Secondary prevention is the practice of detecting early treatable markers of disease so that early curative treatment can be instigated. The national cervical screening program in the UK is an example of this, in which all women aged between 25 and 60 are offered regular cervical smear tests to look for early precancerous changes, which can then be treated to prevent the development of cervical cancer. In this form of naming of disease prevention, tertiary prevention refers to the approaches used to deal with established disease. Following on from the earlier examples, tertiary prevention would include the surgical and medical treatment of established cervical cancer.

According to this nomenclature, many of the approaches used by doctors to screen for disease, such as a mammography for breast cancer, blood tests for markers of prostate and ovarian cancer, and examination of the testicles for testicular cancer, are all examples of secondary prevention of disease.

It is currently generally accepted that the greatest impact that modern medicine may have on health is in the realm of the promotion of the general health of a population and the prevention of disease.

Cure of disease

Although prevention of disease may have the most significant impact on health, it is the doctor's ability to cure diseases that can engender the greatest respect. Moreover, while medical and surgical approaches often have the most dramatic results in terms of cure, it is important to remember that healing modalities requiring less technical expertise, such as the giving of simple advice or the administration of basic nursing care, may be all that is needed to effect a full return to health.

Methods of cure include:

- medication that reverses the process of disease

- physical therapies (e.g. physiotherapy)

- lifestyle advice

- talking therapies (i.e. psychotherapy)

- surgery

- basic needs supplied through hospital care

- treatment of distressing symptoms or disability resulting from disease.

Treatment of symptoms in chronic disease

Most diseases that impact on the health of Western populations are chronic conditions such as coronary heart disease, diabetes, depression, cancer and dementia. These sorts of conditions are not necessarily amenable to cure. In a developed country, the bulk of the cost of medical care is devoted to the management of these chronic conditions and preventing their progression as far as possible. The financial burden on healthcare systems becomes ever greater as the number of people suffering from chronic disease continues to increase (matching growth in population size, adoption of unhealthy lifestyles and longevity), and as the range of evidence-based medical treatments becomes increasingly complex and "high tech."

Methods of treatment of the symptoms of chronic disease include:

- medication that alleviates symptoms or hinders progression of disease

- surgery

- physical therapies (e.g. physiotherapy)

- advice

- talking therapies (e.g. psychotherapy)

- occupational therapy and rehabilitation

- nursing home/hospital care

- referral to other support agencies (e.g. social services).

Pharmacology

The term pharmacology is derived from the Greek meaning medicine and study. Pharmacology embraces the study of the drugs that may be prescribed for each disease. In addition, it involves understanding the complex way in which each drug interacts with the chemical and cellular processes of the body. As well as defining when a drug might be perceived to be of benefit in the treatment of disease, pharmacologists are interested in predicting possible side effects and contraindications (the situations when a drug should not be prescribed).

Accessing information in medical textbooks

This text is written with the aim of making medical information more accessible to health practitioners with a non-medical background or focus. An important skill to acquire is a facility for using medical texts and online resources and for interpreting the language used within them. Very often the information presented by medical textbooks and on websites is organized in a way that follows a predictable pattern. Familiarity with this pattern can greatly assist in the process of extracting important information.

Texts on physiology and pathology

Medical textbooks are generally structured around the physiological systems, and this will also apply to texts on physiology and the pathology of disease. Physiology and pathology are descriptive subjects, and the information found in pathology texts can generally be trusted as established fact derived from scientific observation. For example, a phrase from a pathology textbook such as "…bone is a connective tissue with cells (osteocytes) surrounded by a matrix of collagen fibers…" has its origins in the scientific observation of the microscopic structure of bone. Most readers would probably not dispute such facts, even though they might hold an alternative view of the body based on an energetic foundation of bone. This technical description is simply a way to describe the material nature of healthy bone.

Similarly, most statements about pathology in medical texts are also facts based on the observation of diseased tissue. For example, the sentence, "In Paget's disease overactive osteoblasts deposit abnormal new bone that is thickened or enlarged or structurally weak," reflects a process that has been observed using scientific methods, including microscopy.

Texts on clinical medicine

Clinical medicine is the term used to describe the real-life practice of medicine on patients in the setting of the clinic or hospital. Texts on clinical medicine are also generally structured around the physiological systems, and may include some introductory physiology and pathology to introduce the description of clinical medical approaches system by system.

Doctors may use the term general (or internal) medicine more specifically to describe the discipline that aims to treat diseases by means of non-surgical techniques. Drug treatments are a principal therapy in the practice of general medicine defined in this way. For mainly historical reasons, the practice of surgery is considered to be a separate, albeit complementary, discipline to general medicine. Textbooks of general clinical medicine do not, therefore, describe in detail those conditions that are primarily managed by surgeons, for example, orthopedics (surgical conditions of the bones and joints), otorhinolaryngology (ear, nose and throat diseases), obstetrics and gynecology (diseases of pregnancy and women's health), urology (diseases of the urinary tract) and plastic surgery.

 Information box 1.1e-I

Western descriptions of pathology: comments from a Chinese medicine perspective

Facts concerning pathological processes can be surprisingly relevant and helpful to the Chinese medicine practitioner. Understanding pathology can help with communicating the conventional view of disease to patients, and can also provide valuable information about a possible energetic interpretation of a particular condition.

For example, consider the sentence about Paget's disease quoted in this chapter: "overactive osteoblasts deposit abnormal new bone that is thickened or enlarged or structurally weak." It is feasible that a Chinese medicine energetic interpretation be inferred from such a description. Overactive cells might suggest the presence of Heat. Structural weakness suggests Deficiency of Yin or Jing. A rapid growth of irregular bone suggests an Accumulation that in Chinese medicine is described in terms of Phlegm. Paget's disease is, in fact, a condition of aging bones. It presents with deformed hot areas of bone, and these areas carry a risk of undergoing cancerous change. This suggests that it is presumably a condition of Phlegm/Heat, with underlying Kidney Yin Deficiency of old age as one possible progenitor of the Heat. Here it can be seen that the detail of the pathology may be reflected in the energetic understanding of the symptoms and signs of this condition.

This process of learning the descriptions of pathological processes as aids to the energetic interpretation of disease is explored further in Stage 2.

The information relating to each disease in medical texts, be they medical or surgical in bias, is ordered according to a structure that is familiar to conventional health practitioners. This method relies on classifying information about the disease under the following categories:

- Disease name

- Definition

- Epidemiology: the study of the causes and manifestations of disease within populations

(as distinct from individuals, e.g. "rheumatoid arthritis affects 2% of the UK population" is a statement about the epidemiology of the disease)

- Etiology: the causation of disease (e.g. "chicken pox is caused by infection with the varicella zoster virus")

- Screening: the approaches used for the prevention of disease (e.g. the cervical smear test and mammography are used in two national screening programs to detect early treatable cervical and breast cancer respectively)

- Pathogenesis: the processes that have instigated the development of disease

- Pathology/pathophysiology: the processes that maintain the disease

- Clinical features: the experience of the patient (the symptoms), and features that can be found on medical examination (the signs)

- Investigations: the tests that might reveal abnormalities

- Differential diagnoses: the range of conditions that might present with similar symptoms, signs and test results (e.g. central crushing chest pain suggests a heart attack, but the differential diagnoses include angina, severe indigestion, bronchial infection, broken rib, etc.)

- Treatment/management

In terms of reliability of information, in contrast to the relatively reliable and slow-to-change information that can be found in texts on physiology and pathology, the information on approaches to the management of disease given in clinical textbooks is based on theories and practice that are in a constant state of evolution. The understanding of how to investigate and treat disease will always be subject to debate. Increasingly the recommended treatment of disease is supported by a range of clinical studies that together will constitute an evidence base. In many cases, however, there is a relative lack of high-quality supporting evidence to distinguish the benefits and harms of the various treatments that may be recommended for a particular disease. If a solid evidence base is lacking, recommended medical treatments may be those that have been advised by expert medical panels.

For the sake of simplicity, many clinical texts, particularly those aimed at medical students or the general public, frequently present the information on diagnosis and treatment as if they are undisputed facts. They may occasionally open a discussion on how beneficial a particular treatment is likely to be. In reality, there is a wide variation in clinical practice, and not all doctors will manage their patients in the way described in respected texts.

Increasingly, the cost implications of medical treatments will influence how their benefits are described, and this is understandable, as the escalating costs of healthcare will necessitate its rationing. The UK National Institute for Health and Care Excellence (NICE) is an example of a body of experts that analyzes medical treatments, both in terms of clinical outcomes and medical economics. (There is a similar body, more recently established in the US, called the Medicare Evidence Development & Coverage Advisory Committee (MEDCAC).[5]) NICE has published a wide range of statements on evidence-based treatment guidelines for various diseases in which the cost-effectiveness of treatments are summarized. The recommendations in the NICE guidelines are intended to encourage medical practice that is both effective, and proportionate, bearing in mind that there is a limited health budget.[6] This approach will inevitably mean that some effective treatments are not recommended, simply because there are much cheaper and nearly good enough alternatives available.

It is also important to be aware that information in texts on clinical medicine, including this one, is likely to become out of date very rapidly. For this reason, new editions of popular clinical medical texts are produced every three to four years.

Conventional Clinical Practice

1.2a The conventional medicine approach

Conventional medical training

Conventional training in medicine (and also the paramedical professions such as nursing, physiotherapy and occupational therapy) is based largely on teaching scientific method and how this applies to health.

The early years of medical school training are focused on the sciences of anatomy, biochemistry, physiology, pathology, pharmacology and psychology. From the outset of the training, medical knowledge in these areas tends to be taught as accepted fact, and there is relatively little emphasis on the history of medicine or on the philosophy that underlies current medical thought. The medical student will, through study, become very familiar with the biomedical model that recognizes the physical basis of the body and its complex physiological processes as measurable domains. Health will be primarily described in the early stages of training in terms of absence of illness or injury,[7] although there will also be recognition that health is better described in terms of mental and social functioning as well as parameters of physical health. This is in keeping with the, at the time groundbreaking, broader definition of health first adopted by the World Health Organization (WHO) in 1946 as "a state of complete physical, mental and social well-being and not merely the absence of disease or infirmity."[8] However, there will be little introduction, if any, in the training to contrasting medical philosophies such as those that underpin Chinese medicine, Ayurvedic medicine or homeopathy, or to the idea supported within these healing traditions that health might relate to the energetic balance of the human being within the wider energetic system of the universe. The concept, sometimes described as vitalism, which links these alternative medical disciplines (defined as "the theory that the origin and phenomena of life are dependent on a force or principle distinct from purely chemical or physical forces"[9]), is not embraced within modern biomedical training courses.

As the training progresses, medical students are given increasing contact with patients in a hospital setting. It is in this clinical setting that the skills of case history taking, clinical examination, diagnosis and treatment are taught. Much of the learning is by example, as students accompany doctors in their practice in the clinic or on the ward.

In the clinical setting the patient is the stimulus for the teaching, which is often in the form of encouraging rapid recall of relevant facts about the case in question. For example, the teaching doctor might ask of a student: "This patient has renal failure. What are the causes of renal failure?" The student is expected to reply with a systematic and complete list of causes of the condition in question. In this way, the diagnostic process becomes ingrained as a reflex in which, with the presentation of characteristic symptoms and signs in a patient, appropriate diagnoses can be made and treatment selected.

Medical training emphasizes the development of skills in eliciting the symptoms and signs of disease through sensitive questioning and physical examination of the patient, and also in-depth knowledge of all possible biomedical diagnoses and treatment options. At the end of their training, clinicians should have developed an ability to put their patients at ease, finely tuned examination skills, a facility in recalling and structuring facts in a rigorous way, and they will also become adept at accessing the ever-changing current medical literature.

Development of a doctor–patient rapport to enable the eliciting of symptoms from a patient is considered essential, and so the foundations of skills in communication are laid down in the early years of medical training. These skills are further honed in later aspects of medical training, particularly in the more person-centered specialties of general practice and psychiatry.

How disease is defined in conventional medicine

As described in Chapter 1.1, medical textbooks describe the defining characteristics of a disease within a series of categories. For example, the characteristics of chickenpox could be presented as shown in Box 1.2a-I. This systematic ordering of information encourages comparison between different diseases, and is a prerequisite for the formation of a differential diagnosis of all the diseases that might be affecting a patient with certain features.

In forming a definition such as this one for chickenpox, the focus is on the characteristic pattern of the disease as it might affect any person, and not on the individual characteristics of the patient.

This model of disease might be described as "reductionist," a term that describes the analysis of a complex system in terms of how it is made up of its more simple constituent parts. The reductionist aspects of modern medicine are explored in more detail in Chapter 1.3.

Box 1.2a-I Defining characteristics of chickenpox

Name: Primary herpes zoster (chickenpox).

Epidemiology: Universal; 95 percent of people in metropolitan communities have had the infection by adulthood.

Etiology/cause: Herpes zoster virus infection. Droplet spread of vesicle fluid.

Symptoms and signs: 13- to 17-day incubation period followed by sudden onset of fever, mild constitutional malaise and, after two days, a widespread vesicular rash with lesions appearing in crops, mainly on the trunk. Lesions leave a scab after rupturing in 3–4 days. Symptoms can be more severe in adults. Complications include bacterial infection of lesions, pneumonia and encephalitis. Can manifest later in life as secondary herpes zoster (shingles).

Investigations: Can be diagnosed by clinical features alone. Rising antibodies can be assayed after 3–4 days (blood test).

Treatment: Usually for symptoms only. In severe cases or vulnerable individuals, treat as soon as possible with oral or intravenous antiviral medication such as acyclovir. Treat infected lesions with oral flucloxacillin or alternative antibacterial medication.

Prognosis: Usually mild and self-limiting. Case fatality: 2/100,000 in children, 30/100,000 in adults.

Prevention: Live attenuated vaccine available for susceptible children in UK and part of usual program in US. Varicella zoster immune globulin can be given within four days of exposure to reduce risk of contracting severe disease in those who are immunocompromised (e.g. patients with leukemia or acquired immune deficiency syndrome, AIDS).

Differential diagnosis: No other illnesses present in this way, but other infectious diseases such as measles, rubella and scarlet fever may be considered in the differential diagnosis.

The stages of disease diagnosis

Disease is diagnosed in three stages that enable the doctor to match the individual patient with the descriptions of diseases that become so familiar through the course of medical training. These stages are: questioning for the presence of symptoms, examining the body for signs, and checking the results of tests. Although a great deal of emphasis can be placed on the results of tests, it is recognized that over 70 percent of diagnoses can be made with skillful questioning of the patient alone.[10] Adding in the results of physical examination can bring this diagnosis rate up to about 90 percent.

Thus, together, symptoms and signs will offer the necessary information for making a firm diagnosis in the large majority of situations. Doctors have been trained to respond to characteristic symptoms and signs (e.g. central chest pain or a painless red rash) by generating a mental list of possible causes. This is the beginning of forming a differential diagnosis. As an aide-memoire, a systematic approach is applied, and diseases that might originate in each of the circulatory, respiratory, digestive, urinary, nervous, endocrine, musculoskeletal and reproductive systems may be considered to start building up this list. Possible infective, inflammatory, degenerative, malignant, social and psychological causes are also brought to mind. This systematic technique for differential diagnosis relies very much on the prior memorization of many medical facts.

With a list of possible diagnoses to hand, the doctor is then ready to ask more questions to narrow down the diagnosis, to examine the patient further, and also to consider whether any investigations might provide further diagnostic information.

Medical tests are thus most often employed to confirm the most likely underlying condition, and to exclude less likely diagnoses. Tests are also used for monitoring treatment. An example would be a blood test for the thyroid-stimulating hormone (TSH) to confirm hypothyroidism in somebody with tiredness, weight gain and a slow pulse. An initial measurement that is well above the normal range would help confirm the diagnosis. TSH levels would be retested after treatment has been instated, and would be expected to drop, thus indicating a good response.

For the practitioner of Chinese medicine, the same three steps of questioning to elicit symptoms, physical examination to elicit signs and, to a lesser extent, performing tests (investigations) are, of course, also used in the diagnostic process.

Questioning for symptoms

The approach to the questioning of the patient in conventional medicine is very similar to the approach taught in the practice of Chinese medicine. Doctors will rely on an internal checklist to guide them through the questioning of patients about their symptoms. The nature of the symptoms can be clarified by the use of nine questions. These relate to the site of the symptom, to where it might radiate, its character, its severity, the time of its onset, its frequency, its duration and any accompanying symptoms. Finally, the patient is asked what factors make the symptom better or worse. In this way the patient is encouraged to give far more information about their experience than they might have naturally expressed. As already explained, the level of detail that is generated by questioning in this way is very often sufficient to suggest the correct diagnosis.

Examination for signs

A medical doctor will take a systematic approach to the physical examination of the body. This is intended to reveal any bodily changes that might indicate the presence of physical disease. The systematic approach involves examining the different systems of the body in turn, and when done thoroughly can take up to many minutes. When there is pressure of time doctors will narrow down this approach to examination of just those areas of the body that appear to be relevant after questioning for symptoms.

Box 1.2a-II illustrates these first two stages of the diagnostic process.

However, it is a rather unsatisfactory aspect of clinical medicine that not all symptoms and signs fit easily into diagnostic categories. Many patients suffer from functional symptoms that may be unique to their individual situation, and there may be no measurable pathological disease process to explain them. For example, syndromes such as chronic fatigue syndrome, panic disorder and irritable bowel syndrome may present with a constellation of physical symptoms and signs, none of which can be clearly attributed to underlying physical disease.

Performing tests

Medical investigations or tests are performed to narrow down a diagnosis and also to monitor the progress of treatment.

The diagnostic aspect of tests can be illustrated by continuing with the case scenario given in Box 1.2a-II, as described in Box 1.2a-III. This illustrates the process of diagnosis and choice of treatment. When this process leads to a clear diagnosis, it becomes a very satisfying aspect of the practice of medicine. The diagnosis is made by a logical process of elimination, and the treatment for a clear diagnosis is usually obvious from the current medical literature.

In practice, refining the diagnosis on the basis of tests may not always be that straightforward. There can be uncertainty around the reliability of characteristic diagnostic signs as indicators of disease. Not all symptoms, signs and positive test results indicate the disease to which they seem to point, in which case they are known as false-positive findings.

Similarly, not all normal measurements are indicative of health; in some people with disease, tests results are within the normal range, and this would be described as a false-negative result. Some of the uncertainty in diagnosis stems from limitations in the measurability of bodily functions.

Box 1.2a-II Questioning and examining

Ian, a 63-year-old man, has noticed that he has started to get up at night to urinate, and goes to see his doctor.

This symptom is known as nocturia. The checklist for the possible causes of nocturia includes:

- endocrine causes such as diabetes

- urinary causes such as chronic renal failure

- degenerative change leading to benign enlargement of the prostate gland

- malignant causes such as prostate cancer

- social causes such as drinking too much alcohol or caffeine late at night

- psychological causes such as anxiety with insomnia.

Ian's doctor uses questioning and examination to find out more about the nocturia. In response to her questions, Ian tells her that he has had the problem for some months, when it started with having to get up just once in the night. Now he gets up three or more times, but more often than not just passes a few dribbles of water, and he usually has to wait at the toilet for some time. Otherwise he is well, so there are no accompanying symptoms. He finds that cutting down on all fluids in the evening improves his chances of a less disturbed night.

The doctor performs a physical examination, which involves examination of the prostate gland. This can be felt just inside the anus. Ian's prostate gland feels smooth but significantly enlarged, and has a rubbery texture. There are no other physical abnormalities.

The task of Ian's doctor is to start to match the symptoms and signs of Ian's condition with the conditions that she knows can cause nocturia. The physical findings, together with a characteristic history, alert her to the possibility that constriction of the urethra by an enlarged prostate gland might be the cause of the problem. She reaches this conclusion because she knows that a common cause of nocturia in men of Ian's age group is benign enlargement of the prostate gland, also known as benign prostatic hyperplasia (BPH). BPH results in gradual obstruction of the urethra, which is the tube that leads from the bladder to the penis. This means that efficient emptying of the bladder is no longer possible, and this leads to a frequent urge to pass small amounts of urine.

An important diagnosis to exclude is prostate cancer, which can also cause symptoms of lower urinary tract obstruction. Both prostate cancer and BPH tend to occur in older men, although BPH is more likely to first present at an earlier age than cancer. Another similarity is that a sign of prostate cancer is an enlarged prostate gland, but the prostate is often irregular and hard. In contrast, in BPH, it is smooth and rubbery. This finding cannot be relied on as prostate cancer can be located deep in the gland and may not produce a perceptible change to the feel of the exterior of the gland on physical examination.

A medical textbook might systematically define BPH as follows:

Name: Benign prostatic hyperplasia (BPH).

Etiology/ cause: Degenerative (aging) disease of unknown cause (a change in balance in the proportion of the hormones testosterone and estrogen is thought to be contributory).

Incidence: In most men over 60 years of age (and 90 percent of those over 90).

Symptoms: Nocturia, difficulty in urination, dribbling, poor stream.

Signs: Smooth, enlarged prostate gland felt on rectal examination.

Investigations: Test urine for infection (culture), blood test to exclude diabetes and kidney disease and assessment of prostate-specific antigen (PSA) to exclude cancer. Detailed imaging of the kidneys and bladder (X-ray and ultrasound) to exclude the kidney problems that can result from prolonged BPH.

Treatment: Drug treatment if mild; surgical resection of the prostate gland if severe.

Differential diagnosis: Prostatic cancer.

It is clear that Ian's doctor needs first to eliminate the diagnosis of prostate cancer before treating Ian for BPH.

Box 1.2a-III Diagnosis and treatment

It is clear that Ian's doctor needs first to eliminate the diagnosis of prostate cancer before treating Ian for BPH, and so she arranges for some tests to be performed, including blood tests for PSA and markers of renal function, and an ultrasound scan of Ian's bladder and kidneys.

On completion of the investigations, Ian's bladder and kidneys do not appear to be damaged, and the PSA test is negative.

The doctor can then explain to Ian that it appears that it is most likely he has a mild form of BPH, which is part of the normal aging process for many men. She might then explain the current treatments for BPH, according to current professional guidelines, which include drug treatments or surgery. She might discuss the pros and cons of these options. This is intended to leave Ian with sufficient information to make a decision about which treatment options he might follow.

Measurability in medicine

According to a reductionist view of a physical system, all functions of the parts of the system should be measurable, because these parts are believed to stem from something that is physical in nature. This perspective is manifest in conventional medicine in the form of a pervasive fundamental belief that, in the course of time, and with the results of high-quality research, all aspects of the body are potentially quantifiable and all diseases treatable. One criticism of the 1946 World Health Organization (WHO) definition of health is that it suggests that the complete cure of ills, be they physical, mental or social, is indeed a possibility.[11] Current news articles frequently describe new treatments as a step towards the goal of the cure for cancer,[12] despite the fact that cancer remains the most significant broad cause of death (just under 30 percent of death certificates in the UK in 2014 attributed cancer as the first cause[13]) in the developed world.

The use of symptoms and signs is a form of measurement. For some symptoms and signs, the measurement is crude and rather subjective, as, for example, in the visual assessment of the redness of a sore throat. For other signs, however, such as pulse rate or temperature, the measurement can be more precisely recorded and then expressed in comparison to a normal range. Normal ranges are derived by taking measurements of a variable – height, for example – from a large population. For many variables, the measurements are found to cluster around the most common, or mean, value.

An example of this is shown in Figure 1.2a-I, which illustrates how the birth weight of babies varies according to the week of pregnancy in which they were born. It shows three almost parallel curves. The central 50th centile curve indicates the average or mean birth weight at any length of gestation. For example, an average baby born at the normal time (the 40th week of gestation) will have a birth weight of about 3.5kg. The 90th and 10th centile curves are an indication of the range of birth weights of most babies born at a particular time. For example, at 40 weeks of gestation, 90 percent of babies will have a birth weight less than

4.0kg, and only 10 percent will have a birth weight less than 2.75kg, and thus, 80 percent of babies have a birth weight between 2.75 and 4.0kg. This can also be expressed in terms of a reference range of 80 percent, and the inference is that babies born within this range can be considered to have "normal" weights for their age.

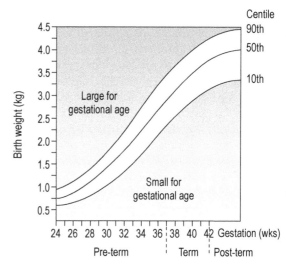

Figure 1.2a-I Mean birth weight according to stage of pregnancy at delivery
Derived from Lissauer and Clayden (1997, p.78), with permission[14]

It follows that 20 percent of babies born at the normal time will, according to their birth weight, fall outside this reference range, and so may be considered unusual in terms of weight. Of course, it does not follow that these babies are unhealthy in any way. Some might be, but others might be small or large because of a familial tendency to be of a small or large build. The important point to draw from this example is that "not usual" as defined by a measurement that falls outside a reference range does not necessarily mean "unhealthy."

In medical practice, most reference ranges express the range of values into which 95 percent of a population might fall for any one variable. This is known as the standard reference range and, by definition, all measurements that fall within the 95 percent range are described as normal. This means that, for every possible variable, 5 percent of the population will be, by definition, abnormal. It follows mathematically that the more tests that are done, the greater the chance that a healthy person falls outside the normal range for at least one of the test results.

To summarize, this approach to defining statistical normality has consequences that are not always appreciated by either the patient or the doctor. These are that some healthy people will, as a consequence of chance, fall outside the normal range for a particular measurement, but also unhealthy people can fall within the normal range. Moreover, if the population from which the normal range is derived is unhealthy, it can be argued that normality does not automatically equate to health.

The issue of the definition of normality is relevant when a seemingly well patient undergoes a health check that includes some routine blood tests of bodily functions. Often a panel consisting of blood tests for many variables is performed, and a long list of results may be generated. As explained above, it is unlikely in such a case, even in a healthy person, for all these results to fall in the normal range. Such tests raise problems. An abnormal test that is a false-positive will tend to be a cause for concern, despite the fact that there may be no actual abnormality in terms of disease. Conversely, a false-negative test will give false reassurance as, despite a value in the normal range, the disease may still be present. The PSA blood test when used to detect prostate cancer is a good example of these points. If the PSA test is positive, this suggests a cancer is present, but it can very commonly be positive in some cases of BPH (i.e. a false-positive result). The PSA test can also be negative in some cases of cancer (i.e. a false-negative result), so giving a false sense of reassurance.[15]

Also, negative tests, even if representative of the medical variables they have been measuring, are not necessarily indicative of full health. A person who feels very unwell, for example, someone with recurrent migraine, may fall within the normal range for all the tested variables. A doctor might reassure such a person with a "clean bill of health" on the basis of blood tests being normal. The problem here is that what is being measured is not necessarily related to any disease that the person may be experiencing.

To return to the scenario of Ian, the 63-year-old man with nocturia, although he may feel that he has been given the "all clear" from cancer, Ian's doctor cannot be totally sure that the smooth prostate is not hiding a small cancer, and that the PSA result is not a false-negative. Given Ian's age, together with the signs and test results, cancer would seem unlikely, but remains possible. The doctor has a dilemma whether or not to discuss this small possibility with Ian. It would actually be a very difficult discussion, because it is not always easy for a non-specialist to track down the most current and accurate information on the certainty of symptoms, signs and test results as predictors of disease. It is clear that this aspect of the diagnostic process is not completely satisfactory, a result of the uncertainty inherent in the diagnostic process.

The problem of functional disease

It is common in medical practice for an unwell patient to be told that all their test results are in the normal range, and so the cause of their malaise remains unexplained. In this situation the patient's condition is described as functional, a term indicating that the problem is linked somehow to the function of the body parts affected, but that there is no actual pathological disease process to be identified and quantified. Because the underlying disease process in functional syndromes is poorly understood, medical treatments for such conditions can only be targeted at relieving symptoms. The term syndrome is applied in these cases to denote a characteristic collection of symptoms and signs, whereas disease is more correctly applied to a condition when pathological changes can be demonstrated. Another term used commonly in medicine to describe functional conditions is medically unexplained symptoms (MUS).

Functional syndromes include irritable bowel syndrome, migraine, low back strain, fibromyalgia and chronic fatigue syndrome. Although most doctors do not interpret such conditions to be serious, in that they are not a threat to life, functional conditions can have a great negative impact in terms of the degree to which they impair a person's well-being and ability to function in day-to-day life.

Functional diseases are a problem for the medical profession because they are poorly understood, difficult to categorize and do not often respond well to treatment. Doctors often find them less satisfying to treat. Patients learn, sometimes only after a long delay whilst tests are being carried out, that they cannot expect to achieve a cure for their condition from their doctor. Functional diseases often result in the patient being referred from one specialist to another to exclude serious disease. Many patients who turn away from conventional medicine to seek benefit from complementary medical therapies could be classified as suffering from functional disease.

1.2b Conventional medical prescribing

It is a common experience in Chinese medical practice to be working with patients who are concurrently taking prescribed conventional drug therapy. This adds the complication of considering the energetic nature of a prescribed drug, and how this might impact on the state of a patient who is already likely to be out of balance in some way. Further challenge comes with the patient's attitude to the medication. Some patients who seek Chinese medical treatment may not be happy about their medications and may wish to stop them. Others, however, may believe, like their doctors, that in taking the medication they are following the best course of action for their health, and had not considered that a response to Chinese medicine might permit a reduction in medication.

It is helpful in such situations for the practitioner first to understand clearly not only the medical reasons behind a prescription choice, but also what other factors might have prompted a doctor to consider giving a prescription. This can help prepare the ground for a discussion with the patient of the benefits and risks associated with their medication, from both the conventional and Chinese medical viewpoints. In some cases, a clear understanding of why the drug has been prescribed may lead to the conclusion that, for that patient, the possible negative energetic side effects are far outweighed by the benefits of the medication. Conversely, a clear understanding might bring the confidence that to withdraw the drug is the best thing to do.

Why conventional practitioners prescribe medication

Prescribing as good practice

The factors that influence medical prescribing are complex. In the case of an ethically motivated physician, the overriding influential factor is the commitment to follow what is currently recognized as good medical practice. Every medical diagnosis will be associated with one or more "textbook" methods of treatment. Increasingly, many of these methods will have been rigorously assessed in clinical trials, and there will be a strong evidence base supporting the fact that they are likely to offer benefit in a significant proportion of patients. For other treatments, although the evidence is less strong, there is at least a clear consensus from expert panels on the correct approach to treatment (e.g. an expert panel of specialists supported by the British Thoracic Society and Scottish Intercollegiate Guidelines Network has produced highly regarded evidence-based guidelines on the management of asthma[16]). A practitioner who chooses a treatment on the basis of either high-quality research evidence or expert guidelines would be considered to be working according to good practice.

There are many other treatments for which there is only poor evidence of effectiveness, and often less agreement on the best approach to management (e.g. a sore throat may lead to a prescription of linctus, soluble aspirin, antibiotics or nothing at all). In a situation in which the value of a particular treatment choice is uncertain, the prescribing doctor may have developed a personal preference for one approach for a variety of reasons. As long as the treatment is one of the range recognized in textbooks for use in that clinical situation, this, too, would be considered good practice, even though the treatment may be of uncertain benefit to the patient.

The case scenario presented in Box 1.2a-II illustrates well some problems that can arise from prescribing as part of good practice. Ian is the 63-year-old man who has been diagnosed with BPH after telling his doctor that he had to get up at night to pass urine. The doctor is thinking about starting Ian on treatment with a drug called finasteride. This counteracts the effect of the male hormone testosterone, and can lead to a reduction in prostate size. Current guidance[17] suggests that this drug may have advantages in the early stages of prostatic enlargement over the surgical option of transurethral resection. The medicines formulary gives Ian's doctor information about the potential side effects of the drug, which includes impotence and breast swelling in 7 and 14 percent of men respectively who take the medication.

With this information to hand, the doctor decides to prescribe the drug and explains to Ian that there is a low risk of side effects as described in the medicines information sheet that is supplied with the prescribed medication. In doing this, she is behaving entirely correctly according to her professional norms. Ian experiences a slight improvement in his symptoms. Over the next few months he becomes affected by impotence. Despite side effects being mentioned at the time of prescription, Ian does not initially link the impotence to his treatment, and so does not mention this to his doctor.

Medical treatments are chosen because they are known to benefit the majority of people. However, there may be a significant minority who do not do so well with the treatment. Side effects are seen as an unavoidable consequence of the risk that has to be accepted when taking a recommended treatment. The treatment has been recommended because it is believed professionally that the benefits to most patients outweigh the risk of side effects in the few.

Good practice includes counseling a patient about a prescription. Doctors should prepare a patient for the possibility of common side effects. The dilemma for the doctor is which side effects, if any, should be discussed. There is a tendency in both doctors and patients to conceptually minimize the potential impact of a possible side effect whilst focusing on the hoped-for benefits of the treatment that has been planned.

To summarize, prescribing according to good practice always means that the majority of patients have been shown to benefit from the treatment and/or the practice is consistent with professional norms. Nevertheless, as is well known, many patients experience less than positive consequences from treatments prescribed according to best practice guidelines. Unwanted outcomes that involve an impact on health and well-being are described as iatrogenic, a term that describes a disease that has been caused by a healthcare provider or institution.

Another factor has crept in to influence best practice prescribing. Increasingly, the concept of cost-effectiveness will influence prescribing decisions. A cost-effective treatment is one that has evidence-based proof of effectiveness and that offers benefit at relatively little cost. Consideration of cost-effectiveness would lead a prescriber to prefer a treatment that might be marginally less effective than another treatment that costs twice the amount. In this case the choice takes a whole population into account as well as the individual, as saving money in one prescribing decision will mean that resources are preserved to fund other treatments in the health service. This influence on prescribing is particularly prominent in state-funded health services such as in the UK.

In the case of Ian above, his medical practitioner in the UK would be more inclined to prescribe finasteride for his symptoms rather than the newer, possibly more effective, but certainly more costly variant of this medication, dutasteride.

Increasingly hospitals and general practices have developed local formularies that ensure only the cheapest of the effective drugs can be prescribed by their practitioners. Cost-effectiveness does not necessarily mean poor practice, although the media and public may interpret this as a form of short-changing patients. Often, cheap therapies are perfectly adequate and comparable to more expensive recently developed drugs. The cost-effectiveness approach is intended to redirect limited resources to those therapies that can achieve the most overall benefit for the whole population.

Some very expensive therapies may be overtly rationed for financial reasons, particularly in state-funded health services. This means that they are either unavailable for prescription, or available only in special clinical circumstances. Rationing is intended to direct limited resources to those treatments that are most likely to bring the most benefit to the most people. Rationed treatments are often of uncertain benefit. The principle of rationing is fraught with ethical dilemmas, as it is often someone who is disadvantaged because of serious illness who misses out on the opportunity of treatment.

Prescribing in response to pressure to do something positive

Conventional medicine deals best with clear diagnoses with explainable pathology. However, many conditions are functional. As described in Section 1.2a, functional conditions have no clearly understood physical cause. They give rise to symptoms, rarely have objective signs, and test results come back showing no abnormalities. In

these conditions a specific therapy cannot be directed towards the causative process, as the cause is unclear.

Examples of functional conditions commonly encountered in general practice are chronic fatigue syndrome, recurrent sore throats and colds, irritable bowel syndrome and many cases of low back pain. In these cases the patient often hopes for treatment to ameliorate symptoms, and the doctor naturally wants to be of some help. As there are no clearly understood disease processes in functional disease, a prescription for a palliative or poorly evidence-based treatment may follow. For example, the doctor might recommend vitamin C to treat recurrent colds, when in fact, current analysis of clinical studies has suggested that this is not likely to be effective.[18] This could be an example of doctors prescribing because of a perceived pressure to do something positive for the patient.

In situations where the cause of the disease is uncertain, a treatment may be prescribed that might benefit one of the possible causes. The response of the patient to the medication might have the additional potentially beneficial outcome of confirming a diagnosis. For example, a doctor might prescribe an antiviral cream for a sore spot on a patient's lip in case this should be an early manifestation of herpes simplex (cold sore). This is considered preferable to arranging a viral test (which takes time to process) in the case of a potentially rapidly evolving condition. This is an example of test by treatment. In some patients the treatment will not have influenced the course of disease, but the cost of this (often borne by the patient) is considered worth the potential benefit of preventing an outbreak of herpes in the minority for whom this treatment was the correct choice.

Prescribing as part of clinical research

A doctor may, from time to time, be involved in clinical research investigating a treatment of as yet unproven benefit to patients. This may be offered to patients ideally within a framework of strict ethical guidelines that protect patients' rights. There should be no situation in which a patient is prescribed a treatment that is still undergoing clinical trials of effectiveness without their express consent. Ethical guidelines also ensure that patients involved in a research project should never be denied any treatment that is known to be more beneficial than the experimental therapy.

The more serious a disease, the more likely it is that new therapies will be part of current treatment for that disease. All new therapies are initially introduced within controlled research programs. This means that many patients with conditions such as the human immunodeficiency virus (HIV) or cancer may receive therapy that is the subject of research.

Prescribing in response to advertising

Advertising by pharmaceutical companies has an insidious and immeasurable influence on prescribing. The pharmaceutical industry makes an enormous financial investment in advertising drug products to the medical profession. There is strict legislation in the UK to control how drug companies are allowed to influence practitioners. This is intended to inhibit overt bribery. Nevertheless, it is very common for free samples and equipment to be supplied by companies to medical practitioners. Ostensibly these gifts come with "no strings attached," but can range from customized ballpoint pens to state-of-the-art operating equipment. The promotion of brand names may well encourage doctors to prescribe the advertised product in a situation in which there are a number of possible treatment options, and in which there is little evidence to suggest that one option is superior to all the others (e.g. in the prescription of emollient creams for eczema, for which there are many formulations available).

Perhaps more importantly, pharmaceutical companies fund most research on new drug therapies. Often the research is of a high standard, and this is a result in part of the fact that reputable publications and medical guidelines will not accept the results from any research from pharmaceutical companies that demonstrates bias in methodology. However, bias is evident in the choice of research topic, which is bound to have been stimulated by potential financial gain rather than clinical need. This means that the range of drugs available for prescription is very much influenced by the choices made for research topics by pharmaceutical companies, and naturally this will influence prescribing decisions.

Financial or material incentives are likely to carry much more weight in prescribing decisions in countries in which the doctor receives some remuneration for each treatment given, or in which the rewards offered by pharmaceutical companies are less tightly regulated.

1.2c Introduction to conventional drugs

A formulary (or pharmacopoeia) is a book or document that categorizes and summarizes the characteristics of all drugs used in a certain setting. This section focuses on the way drugs are categorized in conventional medicine, and specifically, on how they are listed and described in the medical formularies. The *British National Formulary* (BNF)[19] is used in this text as an example of a good quality medical formulary. However, principles explored here will be applicable to the structure of any formulary. At the time of writing the BNF, together with information on cost-effectiveness, could be accessed online via NICE's website.[20] This is an amazingly rich resource of information for health practitioners, and it is well worth taking the time to understand how it systematically presents information about all the drugs that can be prescribed in the UK. In the BNF the WHO-endorsed INN (International Nonproprietary Names) system is followed for the naming of generic (non-branded) medication. Because of its constitutional mandate to "develop, establish and promote international standards with respect to biological, pharmaceutical and similar products,"[21] the WHO has recommended that all newly manufactured drugs worldwide are given an INN generic name. However, older drugs across the world will continue to be named according to systems unique to their country of origin, for example, the USAN (United States Adopted Name) and JAN (Japanese Accepted Name) systems. Despite this confusing proliferation of names for the same drug, a translation from INN to any of the standard naming systems can be easily performed using online tools such as the Drugs.com International Drug Name Database.[22]

Description of drugs

When the characteristics of a particular drug or class of drug are described in a formulary, they are often structured under the following headings: indications, cautions, contraindications, side effects, dose and nomenclature.

Indications

The term indications describes the medical conditions for which a drug preparation may be prescribed. For example, the BNF lists the indications for the antibiotic benzylpenicillin sodium in a list that includes throat infections, otitis media and endocarditis.

Cautions

Cautions describes those situations in which the drug needs to be prescribed with caution as there is an increased risk of adverse reaction.

Contraindications

Contraindications describes those situations in which it is advisable not to prescribe the drug because of a very high risk of adverse reaction.

Side effects

Side effects are unwanted additional effects of the drug on the body that will affect some but not necessarily all people. For example, the BNF lists one side effect of benzylpenicillin as hypersensitivity reactions including urticaria, fever and joint pain.

Dose

The dose is the recommended amount and frequency for taking the drug. This is usually expressed in terms of metric weight and daily regimen, for example, 500 milligrams every eight hours (three times a day).

Nomenclature

In formularies drugs may be named in three ways. First, the drug may be described by means of its chemical name, and this would be an internationally recognized term that indicates the structure of the compound that is the active part of the drug. For example, salicylic acid, sodium bicarbonate and lithium carbonate are all chemical names for commonly prescribed drugs.

Second, drugs are always also known by a generic name, which is an often less complicated term than the chemical name, and is assigned to the drug for ease of reference. For example, aspirin is the INN generic name recognized in the UK for salicylic acid.

The third way in which a drug may be named is by a proprietary name. This is a name chosen by the pharmaceutical manufacturer for the purposes of branding and marketing the drug. The proprietary name is chosen to appeal to the ears of the culture to which it is intended to be sold, and so may be unique to a single country. For example, Disprin, Amoxil, Remegel, Zantac, Prozac and Ibuleve are proprietary names used in the UK for the commonly used medications soluble aspirin, amoxicillin, calcium carbonate, ranitidine, fluoxetine and ibuprofen gel, respectively. Drugs are marketed under their proprietary name and often cost a lot more than the same drug sold under the generic name.

For example, one proprietary name for amoxicillin is Amoxil. According to the BNF (April 2016), 21 capsules of 500mg Amoxil cost £6.77, whereas the same quantity of the same drug sold under the generic name of amoxicillin cost £1.57. The proprietary drug Amoxil therefore costs over five times the price of the non-proprietary (generic) version of the same antibiotic. The prescribing of marketed drugs can obviously be a major source of expense to the prescriber, but generally offers no added benefit to the patient.

Origins of conventional drugs

Some drugs have their origins in antiquity, and are derived directly from herbal preparations or other natural sources. Contrasting examples of prescribed drugs originally derived from natural substances are oil of evening primrose (gamma linoleic acid), derived from the seeds of the evening primrose plant, penicillin, derived from mold, and insulin, extracted from a dog's pancreas. However, the majority of drugs can now be manufactured synthetically, so that the natural source is no longer necessary to produce the same product. For example, injectable insulin used for the treatment of diabetes is now largely manufactured by recombinant genetic technology.

Some drugs are modifications of the original naturally derived substance. The modifications are an attempt to make the drug more suited to its role. It may be found that a natural substance, although effective, has very severe side effects. Modification, which is the work of research chemists, may give rise to a substance that is as effective, but has fewer side effects. Nowadays, many drugs are modifications of natural substances. Amoxicillin, for example, is chemically derived from the naturally occurring substance penicillin. Natural penicillin can only be taken by injection, and is effective against a narrow range of bacteria. Amoxicillin has activity against a broad spectrum of bacteria and can be taken by mouth. This is obviously preferable for both the patient and the prescribing doctor.

Increasingly, new drugs are being developed for which there are no natural predecessors. Popularly known as designer drugs, these formulations have been be tailor-made to suit a particular requirement. For example, the development of the antidepressant fluoxetine (Prozac) was based on the knowledge that the neurochemical in the brain called serotonin (5HT) is important in depression. Fluoxetine was designed to inhibit uptake of serotonin into surrounding nerve cells via membrane-based protein channels, by developing a molecule that had structural similarities to 5HT.[23] The resulting higher concentrations of serotonin are manifest in a measurable improvement in mood (amongst a range of less desirable side effects) in people who take fluoxetine.

Whether natural or synthetic, all drugs have to go through a very rigorous testing process before being released for public use. This invariably requires multiple testing on animals, many of which die in the process. If animal testing reveals no problems, the drug is then tested on humans within clinical trials. These trials have to conform to a rigorous ethical framework, so that the participants are protected as much as possible from unintended harm. However, sometimes serious side effects are not revealed by this testing process, as was the case in the development of Vioxx (rofecoxib), an anti-inflammatory drug developed by the company Merck. Rofecoxib was withdrawn from public use in 2004 as an ongoing clinical trial revealed an increased incidence of cardiovascular side effects, including heart attacks, in people taking this drug for more than 18 months. This outcome was not revealed by the results of earlier trials conducted over a shorter timescale by the company, which had seemed to suggest that the drug would be safe for public use.[24] Subsequent lawsuits claiming Merck had not revealed the outcome of less favorable studies resulted in the company agreeing to settle 35,000 claims in 2007 without admitting fault.

A system for classification of conventional drugs

The vast range of drug types presented in formularies such as the BNF is structured in a complex system of nested medical categories. However, for the purposes of considering the energetics of conventional medication, it is helpful to simplify the way in which drugs are categorized by grouping them into eight categories according to the way in which they are conventionally seen to act in the body.

The information provided by a formulary such as the BNF about any one drug will be all that is required to decide the category in which that drug can be placed.

The categorization of drugs according to mode of action in the body is shown in Table 1.2c-I.

Table 1.2c-I Categorization of drugs according to mode of action in the body

Mode of action of drug	Examples of drugs
1. Replaces a deficient substance that is normally obtained from the diet	Iron (ferrous sulfate) in iron-deficiency anemia
2. Kills or suppresses the growth of infectious agents (microbes and other life forms that cause infection)	Benzylpenicillin sodium in meningitis
3. Toxic to rapidly dividing human cells, in particular, cancer cells	Vincristine in cancer chemotherapy
4. Replaces a substance that is normally produced by the body	Insulin in diabetes mellitus
5. Specifically stimulates the immune response by the introduction of an antigen	Polio vaccine
6. Other drugs that artificially stimulate natural bodily functions	Clomifene to stimulate ovulation
7. Suppresses natural bodily functions	Corticosteroids used to suppress the immune response in autoimmune disease
8. Counteracts the damage caused by toxins	Acetylcysteine in paracetamol overdose

Each of the categories listed will now be explored in more detail.

1. Drugs that replace a deficient substance that is normally obtained from the diet

These drugs are synthetic forms of the nutrients, vitamins and minerals that the body requires for full health, and which for dietary and other reasons (e.g. impaired digestion) are not available to the patient in sufficient quantities to meet their needs.

Examples include iron, vitamin C and fluid replacement.

2. Drugs that kill or suppress the growth of infectious agents (microbes and other life forms that cause infection)

This category includes all drugs that work against microbes and life forms that are foreign to a normally healthy body. They are listed together in Section 5 of the BNF, "Infections."

Examples include antibiotics such as amoxicillin. Some antibiotics are known only to suppress the growth of some infectious agents rather than kill them outright. This is true for the antiviral drugs such as oseltamivir (Tamiflu).

3. Drugs that are toxic to rapidly dividing human cells, in particular, cancer cells

This category includes the cytotoxic anticancer drugs. When human cells are recognized to have become diseased, particularly in the case of cancer, the conventional response is to remove them. This can either involve the surgical removal of a lump, or the use of radiation or drugs that are chemically designed to attack cells with the particular properties of cancer cells. One important characteristic of the cytotoxic drugs used to kill cancer cells is that they are also toxic, to some extent, to all other human cells in the body.

For example, vincristine is a cytotoxic drug that is commonly used in chemotherapy. It works by blocking the physiological process of cell division, and so rapidly dividing cancer cells will be most affected. However, hair loss and diarrhea are signs that rapidly dividing hair and gut cells have also been damaged by the drug. The development of numbness and weakness in a patient on vincristine is a sign that vital nerve cells are being damaged. In such a case the drug treatment will be stopped.

4. Drugs that replace a substance that is normally produced by the body

These drugs are used to treat disorders in which the body fails to manufacture the basic chemicals (including hormones) that are essential for healthy homeostasis.

One example is thyroxine replacement in thyroid deficiency. The thyroid gland in this condition is diseased and no longer able to produce thyroxine, which is essential for life. The drug is chemically synthesized to be exactly the same as, or very similar to, the natural hormone.

5. Drugs that specifically stimulate the immune response by introduction of an antigen

This category of drugs includes all the vaccines. Vaccines are designed to mimic natural infections, and so stimulate a natural bodily process. In this way the action of the vaccine can be compared to that of an infectious agent.

6. Other drugs that artificially stimulate natural bodily processes

Drugs in this category are used to bring about a recognized bodily process that is not occurring naturally, usually because of underlying disease. This category actually also embraces drugs in categories 4 and 5. However, the drugs in these categories have been separated from category 6 because they have additional unique energetic characteristics.

Examples of drugs that artificially stimulate natural bodily functions include drugs such as clomifene, which are used in infertility to stimulate ovulation. Other examples include oxytocin, which is used to stimulate labor, and hormone replacement therapy (HRT), which is given to delay a natural menopause (this "stimulates" the continued maintenance of the female secondary sexual characteristics, including pubic hair growth, vaginal moistness and fleshiness of breast tissue).

Other examples of drugs in this broad category include fluoxetine for depression (these prolong the effect of 5HT in the brain and thus stimulate neural pathways known to be involved in control of mood), salbutamol inhaled in asthma (this stimulates the opening of the airways usually induced by the natural hormone adrenaline) and sildenafil (Viagra) (enables erection by prolonging the effect of local hormones that are released during sexual activity, and so stimulates dilation of penile blood vessels).

7. Drugs that suppress natural bodily or disease processes

This huge category includes a wide range of drugs that suppress natural bodily processes. In some cases the bodily function (e.g. ovulation or menstruation) is simply not wanted because it interferes with the person's perceived needs. In other cases the bodily function is a natural response to disease (e.g. the pain of a fractured leg) and leads to unpleasant symptoms.

Examples include the contraceptive pill, which suppresses ovulation, corticosteroids, which suppress the immune response, anesthetics in surgery, which suppress consciousness, painkillers, which suppress the pain of injury, and anti-sickness medication given with chemotherapy.

Other examples of drugs in this category include omeprazole for duodenal ulcer (suppresses the release of digestive acid in the stomach) and lamotrigine for epilepsy (suppresses seizure activity by stabilizing the chemical reactivity of nerve cells in the brain).

8. Drugs that counteract the damage caused by toxins

This is a category of drugs that are generally used in the emergency treatment of poisoning or overdose. They are not, therefore, likely to be encountered in usual complementary medical practice. The category is included here for completeness.

In general, these drugs prevent the absorption of drugs and poisons from the digestive tract (e.g. charcoal given by mouth), or enable the transformation of the drug within the body to a less toxic form (e.g. acetylcysteine given by intravenous injection in paracetamol overdose).

Chapter 1.3 now explores in more depth how this categorization can be used to help develop an energetic perspective of the action of drugs.

Comparisons with Alternative Medical Viewpoints

1.3

1.3a Contrasting philosophies of health

This section is intended to promote the recognition that different health systems may be built on contrasting philosophical perspectives of the physiology of the body and pathology of disease. These perspectives can be broadly categorized as reductionist and holistic. There are crucial differences between these two approaches, and without asserting that either has greater or lesser value, these differences need to be clarified before the work of trying to compare one discipline with another can begin.

The term reductionist refers to the principle of analyzing complex things by considering them in terms of a collection of parts. Simply speaking, a reductionist view of the body will tend to examine and describe the workings of individual parts, without necessarily having to draw on an understanding of the workings of the body as an integrated whole. From a mechanistic perspective, this is similar to the approach of the engineer who, simply by identifying and replacing a faulty part, such as a distributor or fuel pump, can transform a faltering vehicle into an adequately working model. The process involves testing clearly defined systems within the malfunctioning vehicle, and then identifying and making good the faulty part.

From a reductionist perspective, the body may be described as a wonderfully intricate machine. In this model, illness or disease in one part of the body will not necessarily be manifest in or experienced by other parts. The faulty part will, as in the vehicle, display malfunction in the form of signs and symptoms, and the diagnosis of disease is then made by a thorough examination of all the body parts and systems. From this sort of viewpoint,

the whole assembly is just a collection of individual parts, no more and no less.

By contrast, the term holistic is used to refer to a view that sees each part of a complex system as being inextricably linked with all other parts of the system, and the whole system being more than just the sum of its parts. A problem in one part will resonate widely throughout the system. Furthermore, this immediately brings the non-material aspects of life into the equation, the thoughts and emotions that form part of the whole person, as well as the environmental milieu in which the person is located. Some medical systems that might be described as holistic according to this definition are underpinned by the idea that the individual parts are linked and vivified by an underlying non-measurable energetic state. This is made manifest in the material body, but is more than just the physical body. This understanding of an underlying state, sometimes described as the vitalistic principle, is a concept now largely considered to be discredited, albeit not disproved, by the Western scientific community.[25] Terms such as life force, Qi, Ki and Prana are used to describe this energetic state in different health disciplines.

With a holistic model of health, the body, the emotions, the mind and the spirit are seen as interdependent and intercommunicating. An illness of the body will impact on the function of the emotions, the mind and the spirit, and, conversely, a sickness of the spirit or mind will have repercussions that become immediately manifest in the physical body on examination.

This belief underpins diagnostic systems that focus on just one body part such as the pulse, tongue, iris, sole of the foot or abdomen (Hara). The interconnections within the body, mind and spirit will result in every illness being reflected throughout all parts of the system. By following diagnostic systems such as these, the focus of a skilled practitioner on a single body part could be expected to reveal information not just about the health of the body, but also about the state of the mind and spirit.

One important corollary of this holistic view of health is that symptoms of a disease may become manifest in a different body part, or indeed, at a different bodily level, from that in which a disease first developed. For example, the grief following a bereavement, which might be expected to be experienced at an emotional or spiritual level, may instead also become manifest in the body in the form of an asthma attack or skin rash. These emotional or spiritual correlates of physical disease are of great interest to many holistic practitioners. Some go as far as to suggest that most physical diseases have emotional or spiritual roots, and that some diseases consistently reflect specific emotional or spiritual blocks. A pain in the shoulders, for example, may be considered to represent a difficulty in shouldering the burdens imposed by a busy and complicated lifestyle.[26]

The idea that symptoms are expressions of imbalances throughout all the levels of the body, emotions, mind and spirit has implications when symptoms are treated medically. From a holistic perspective, if symptoms are not treated at their root origin, any other treatment of them may be considered to be potentially harmful. If the root imbalance persists, it makes sense to a holistic practitioner that it will find an outlet at another body site or within another level of the body. This idea, that symptoms treated in this way might re-emerge in a different form at a different body site or level, is a concept that is not tenable within a purely reductionist philosophy of health.

Conventional medicine as a reductionist system

It would be simplistic to state that conventional medicine is a purely reductionist health system. It is true that many of the ideas of modern medicine have sprung from the reductionist view of the world that dominated scientific thought in the 18th to 20th centuries. The Linnaean approach to classification of illness,[27] which modern doctors use to define disease according to body system, is one good example. The tendency of doctors to specialize so that their focus is directed at single body systems or subsystems is also evidence of this approach. Medical training largely focuses on the diseases of body parts and of the mind, and categorizes them as distinct entities that merit defined and agreed treatment approaches.

However, an ever-deepening scientific understanding of the workings of the body and the mind over the latter part of the 20th century has begun to erode the more simplistic reductionist approach to disease. Increasingly, conventional practitioners recognize that the different

body parts and the workings of the brain are inextricably interrelated and interdependent. Moreover, factors such as social class and standing, education, ability to deal with stress and general levels of happiness are now known to have very powerful effects on health and well-being. The healthy human being is no longer seen as a well-oiled machine that responds to a regular service of all parts. Instead, it is seen as a complex entity, the health of which depends on delicate physiological internal relationships and on relationships that exist within the context of the community in which the individual is placed.

This more holistic perspective of health is expressed clearly in the aforementioned World Health Organization (WHO) 1948 constitution, where health is defined as a "state of physical, mental and social well-being and not merely the absence of disease or infirmity." The modern medical model has now more accurately been described as a biopsychosocial model[28] in which biological, psychological and social determinants are readily recognized as contributing to the development of disease. It is also now accepted that treatment focused on a body symptom in isolation may not deal fully with the real root of the problem.

However, there remain important differences, and these can lead to misunderstandings between practitioners of conventional medicine and practitioners of those complementary health disciplines that hold to a more holistic perspective. One author and alternative medicine practitioner, Stephen Gascoigne,[29] has summarized the differences between alternative medicine and conventional medicine, as shown in Table 1.3a-I.

Table 1.3a-I A comparison between alternative and conventional medicine

Alternative medicine	Conventional medicine
Energetic	Physical
Holistic	Separatist/reductionist
Transforms	Eliminates
Cures	Suppresses
Patient-centered	Disease-centered
Symptoms are useful pointers	Symptoms are to be removed
Disease is a group of symptoms (a syndrome)	Disease is a fixed entity
Cure is a move towards balance	Cure is removal of symptoms

This rather stark comparison perhaps unfairly places conventional medicine firmly in the reductionist camp. However, the comparison does illustrate some key differences between the conventional medical view of health and healing and those of medical disciplines such as Chinese medicine, Ayurvedic medicine, homeopathy and craniosacral therapy. All these disciplines adhere to concepts that suggest an underlying vitalistic principle and the interrelationship of the physical with spiritual as well as emotional and mental levels of health, and this is perhaps the most significant difference.

While modern medicine understands that the mind can affect the body, and vice versa, it attempts to explain this in terms of neural and endocrine connections rather than by means of a non-measurable energetic principle.

A discipline such as Chinese medicine, for example, recognizes that when one system is imbalanced, symptoms will always manifest in the physical, emotional, mental and spiritual realms. For example, the symptoms and signs of Heart Qi Deficiency include palpitations, shortness of breath on exertion, a thready pulse, listlessness, lassitude and mental cloudiness.[30] A conventional practitioner will be less ready to make this claim that any disease that involves the heart inevitably includes mental and emotional imbalance. Whilst they may be ready to accept that heart disease can lead to low mood and troubled thoughts, the conceptual link made between the two will be less immediate. For the conventional medical doctor, the low mood of a patient with heart disease will be more a result of having to deal with the pain and disability that accompany heart disease and of carrying the weight of a poor prognosis. This contrasts with the holistic practitioner's expectations that a disease in the system that influences the heart organ will also manifest naturally in the realms of emotions, mind and spirit.

However, while the stereotypical conventional and alternative practitioner may practice within very different conceptual frameworks, this does not necessarily mean that either has a more accurate grasp of an absolute truth. It is blindness to the possibility that there might be alternative ways of describing and treating the patient's disease that arguably might contribute to limiting the potential for cure in the widest possible form. This book has been written from the perspective that conventional and complementary practitioners are working with different aspects of the same essential truth, and with the ultimate aim that practitioners from either perspective become more open to embracing the beneficial aspects of all forms of healthcare.

A helpful analogy can be found in the scenario of a concert violinist and a sound engineer who are both listening to a performance of a violin concerto. The concert violinist may be attentive to the sensitivity of the interpretation of the music, and may be deeply moved as he listens. The sound engineer may recognize the physical characteristics of the harmonics she hears and can comment on the acoustics of the concert hall. No one can deny that they have both been listening to the same piece of music. However, their philosophies for interpreting the music will shape their individual perceptions, and the result will be that what they actually hear can differ markedly.

Similarly, a complementary and a conventional practitioner can both offer valid insights about the health and need for treatment of an individual patient, although it is not always the case that either comprehends or can appreciate the view of the other.

It is also important to recognize that no practitioner, nor indeed medical practice, is wholly reductionist or holistic in focus, although the conventional/reductionist, complementary/holistic labels are frequently misused in this way. Many conventional practitioners adhere strongly to the holistic management of their patients, and are very responsive to individual need when counseling patients and selecting treatments. Conversely, the structured format of some complementary medicine texts and training courses might, through systematization of syndromes and treatment schedules, encourage a practice that is arguably highly reductionist in its nature.

For the patient seeking appropriate healthcare, it is important to recognize that the philosophical framework of any medical practitioner will have both strengths and weaknesses. Just as the violinist and the sound engineer both have a great deal to contribute to the production of a beautiful musical performance, so practitioners with different medical and philosophical frameworks can have truly complementary insights and skills to offer in promoting healing. Clarity about where these strengths and weaknesses lie will enable a patient to make an informed choice between which medical treatment is appropriate to their specific needs at any particular time.

The understanding of the way health and illness manifests in the body will, of course, influence the choice of treatment. A reductionist understanding of physiology and pathology will lead to the choice of allopathic treatments, that is, those that oppose the processes that are considered, after questioning, physical examination and tests, to be going wrong in some way. If the heart is pumping too fast, treatment will be targeted at slowing it down, if there is pain, an analgesic will be prescribed, and if there is spreading infection, an antibiotic. Allopathic treatments are largely understood to have a physical basis to their action, and this could range from a delicate biochemical change, to a macroscopic transformation such as a hip joint replacement. Many medical treatments in the psychological domain are also perceived to have a physical basis, for example, the neurochemical changes that are known to result from antidepressants, hypnotics and electroconvulsive therapy. Even counseling approaches such as the very popular cognitive behavioral therapy

(CBT) might be interpreted as allopathic in that unhelpful thought patterns are identified and then helpful thought patterns are practiced.

A holistic approach will require the practitioner to seek the root cause of the health problem, and with those disciplines that have an underlying vitalistic principle, the root cause will lie within the energetic balance of the patient, and this balance is inextricably linked with the patient's environment. Whilst it may be recognized that difficult or dangerous symptoms need to be controlled promptly, the fundamental task of the holistic practitioner is to work with the patient to engender change at a deep level. This is less likely to involve techniques that have easily measurable physical effects, and more likely to include healing modalities that might appear thoroughly unscientific to the skeptical. Chinese medicine tends to treat illness by means of a combination of lifestyle advice, and herbal and dietary therapy and physical therapy including acupuncture, massage and exercise programs designed to improve energetic balance and flow. Non-material factors such as environmental setting (the focus of Feng Shui), ancestral bequests and spirit-based influences may also be considered to impact on health, and so can be taken into account, particularly in the forms of Chinese medicine that predate the systematization of Traditional Chinese Medicine that occurred under Mao Zedong in the 1950s. The healthy lifestyle recognized by Chinese medicine is characterized by moderation, respect for ancestral values, virtue and spiritual practice, and there is great emphasis placed on living in accord with the seasons and not striving or desiring for much.[31] Chinese therapies have been described as heteropathic rather than allopathic, a term intended to denote the fact that rather than opposing physical symptoms, they attempt to counter unhelpful imbalances in the flow of Qi.[32]

It might be appreciated that the essentially preventative and restorative nature of holistic therapy might be most effective in the early stages of disease. When disease has progressed to the level when there is marked structural bodily damage or change, it is accepted by many holistic therapists that invasive allopathic treatment could be needed in addition to holistic care. Obvious examples include emergency surgery for a ruptured appendix, cardioversion for ventricular fibrillation (heart attack) or intravenous fluid replacement in severe dehydration.

Tables 1.3a-II and 1.3a-III summarize some of the potential advantages and disadvantages of seeking treatment from complementary and conventional medical practices.

These have been drawn up as if from a patient's perspective. Not all patients want to be actively involved in their treatment, or wish to have their world view challenged, and both these things are integral to some complementary therapeutic approaches. This explains why a statement such as "Requires the patient to be active in changing their lifestyle to enable healing" is listed as a possible disadvantage of complementary therapy, and "Treatment is not expected to challenge the patient at a deep level" as a possible advantage of conventional medical treatment.

Being clear about the distinctions between the philosophical foundations of conventional and complementary thought, and how these are likely to influence diagnosis and treatment, is essential when practitioners of different medical disciplines hope to develop a meaningful dialogue. It is important to be both clear and respectful of essential differences, and to avoid the tendency to over-generalize. This clarity becomes perhaps most useful in building up relationships with patients who have complex and enduring health needs, many of whom are likely to benefit by receiving the best aspects of treatment from contrasting medical perspectives.

Table 1.3a-II Advantages and disadvantages of complementary medical treatment

Advantages	Disadvantages
In-depth consultation	Seems expensive
Recognizes and will treat a wide range of contributory factors in the disease process – holistic approach	May not recognize features of serious disease
Will be open to the patient's point of view	Difficult to find out whether therapy is appropriate or if the therapist is adequately qualified
Will clarify to the patient how their lifestyle may have contributed to the problem	Makes the patient responsible in part for the cause of the problem
Empowers the patient to be involved in their own healing	Requires the patient to be active in changing their lifestyle to enable healing
Unlikely to harm	May not be powerful enough to cure advanced disease
Should result in a change at a deep personal level	

Table 1.3a-III Advantages and disadvantages of conventional medical treatment

Advantages	Disadvantages
Usually available as part of a nationally or insurance-funded health service	May not be the time or willingness to allow the patient to be listened to or valued
Directed towards excluding serious disease	Minor functional symptoms may be ignored
The practitioner is likely to be following the recognized approach as accepted by the medical profession	The practitioner may be inflexible if the patient requires an approach that is contrary to the medically accepted view
Will often be consistent with the patient's expectations	May not be tailored to the complex needs of the individual patient
Will often focus on the disease rather than causation, and so the patient need not change lifestyle	Lifestyle factors are not addressed adequately, and so the root of the problem is perpetuated
The practitioner takes responsibility for the healing process	The patient may feel out of control within the healing process
Powerful treatments are available	The risk of iatrogenic disease (disease resulting from side effects of treatment) is high
Not expected to challenge the patient at a deep level	May ignore the need for deep personal change, which could be ultimately the most health-giving

1.3b Drugs from a complementary medical viewpoint

Section 1.2c introduced a method of categorizing drugs by mode of therapeutic action and the concept of iatrogenic disease (illness as a result of medical treatment). This section presents some complementary perspectives on the beneficial and adverse effects of drugs in the body. It also describes some principles of mapping Chinese medicine concepts to Western medical theory. These are introduced in some detail in the "Note to the Reader" at the beginning of this book. It might help to turn now to these pages by way of introduction to the rest of this section.

Suppression of symptoms

The concept of suppression of symptoms in homeopathic theory refers to the idea that the disappearance of symptoms or signs of a disease may not necessarily mean cure, but instead may be a consequence of the disease moving to a deeper, less immediately manifest level.[33] This concept has a parallel with the Chinese medicine idea of disease having a manifestation (Biao) and a root (Ben). According to Chinese medicine theory, treatment that is targeted at the level of the manifestation, and which does not simultaneously attend to the root causes, may actually lead to a worsening of the root imbalance. This concept is expressed in texts as ancient as the *Neijing Suwen* (which presents diverse ideas from Chinese philosophical thought that were drawn together as early as 150 BCE). In the *Neijing Suwen*, the 65th chapter is dedicated to a discourse on when to treat the root and when to treat the manifestation of a disease process.[34] The *Yixue Rumen* (*Introduction to Medicine*, written in 1575 by Li Chan) explains, "In general, to treat disease, first the Ben is treated and then the Biao is treated. If the Biao is treated first and the Ben is treated later, the pathogenic influence becomes stronger and that disease goes even deeper."[35] It is noteworthy that both these texts also emphasize that there are situations when the manifestation (Biao) needs to be treated as a priority, including those cases when life-threatening symptoms are present.

The Chinese medicine description of treating the manifestation (Biao) might be seen as analogous to the homeopathic idea of suppression. In both there is a suggestion that, although treatment may cause an alleviation of symptoms, without treatment of the root (Ben) there may be a worsening of disease at a deeper level. In Chinese medicine, however, the texts imply that in treating the manifestation and not attending to the factors that cause the root imbalance, the root imbalance will become more pronounced and may generate further symptoms. Homeopaths take this a stage further, and argue that the symptom may actually serve a useful purpose by providing some sort of release for the deeper root imbalance. When it is prevented from serving this purpose, it may directly cause the root imbalance to deepen and be expressed in a different and potentially more damaging form. According to both theories, the unattended root imbalance is believed to create more serious problems.

Figure 1.3b-I illustrates this concept of suppression. The bathtub with a running tap has a problem – it is leading to a dripping overflow pipe, thus causing damp to the exterior wall. This would ideally be fixed by turning off the taps, the root of the problem. However, someone outside the house might be tempted to deal with the manifestation of the problem. They could stop the dripping overflow and allow the wall to dry out by blocking the overflow pipe with a cork. This treatment would indeed solve the problem of the dripping pipe, but would, of course, result in a more catastrophic problem inside the house as the bath then proceeds to overflow on to the bathroom floor.

Root of the problem: dripping tap

Treating the root (turning off the tap) cures the problem

Manifestation of problem: overflowing pipe and damp wall

Treating the manifestation (stopping the pipe) suppresses the problem and may cause a worse problem at a deep level

Figure 1.3b-I An illustration of the concept of suppression

Consider the case of an overworked businesswoman who has been self-medicating every day with paracetamol for recurrent tension headaches; this provides us with an example of suppression of symptoms by medication. When questioned, the woman readily admits that she feels dependent on her painkillers. She explains that if she cannot take one for any reason, she suffers with an unusually intense headache.

This patient's underlying condition might have been diagnosed in Chinese medicine in various ways according to more detailed questioning and examination that includes pulse and tongue diagnosis. In this case, let us assume the diagnosis is Liver Yang Rising resulting from a state of Deficiency (Kidney Yin Deficiency). Treatment of the Ben (root) with acupuncture, by Tonification of the Kidneys, would be considered to be beneficial, but alongside this an appropriate treatment of the root of the problem might also include a re-evaluation of working habits, the taking of appropriate rest, and ensuring a diet containing appropriately nourishing foods. All these treatments target the root problem and not the symptom.

However, the painkiller does not work in this way. Although it removes the symptoms (i.e. it subdues the painful headache, a symptom of Liver Yang Rising), it does not deal with the root problem of Depleted Kidney Yin. Its recurrent use may lead the businesswoman to ignore the reasons why her headache might have developed. In her case, one reason is very probably her stress-inducing

lifestyle, which is likely to be Depleting of Kidney Yin. The headache symptoms could be likened to an alarm bell, alerting this patient to the fact something is going wrong for her. However, by taking the painkiller, the alarm bell has been temporarily silenced, and the underlying disease possibly allowed to progress.

The concept of suppression suggests that by taking a painkiller, the underlying imbalance that has led to the headache may now become more pronounced. One obvious reason for this is that the root cause, the pressured lifestyle, is left untreated. A further reason, in line with the homeopaths' beliefs, is that the excess Heat that was being expressed in the symptom of a headache is still held within the energetic system, and instead has to be expressed in a different form such as, for example, agitated anxiety. As this symptom is understood in Chinese medicine to be at the level of the spirit rather than the body, this would suggest progression of the imbalance to a deeper energetic level.

In Chinese medical terms the mechanism for this might be that the painkiller has an energetic property that allows the movement of Stagnant Qi. Many painkillers have side effects (such as rash and gastritis) which suggest they are Heating according to Chinese medicine. This property will move Stuck Qi and release the Exterior, so pacifying Yang Rising, but the cost of this is Wasting of Yang and also toxic damage to Yin by the Hot medicinal. Thus the root problem has been exacerbated not healed, and the body has been energetically depleted overall.

The recognition that allopathic treatment may have deleterious effects, and also possibly lead to dependency, pervades complementary medical practice. Complementary medicine practitioners may support the ideal of patients withdrawing from suppressive medical treatment so that deep imbalance can be exposed and treated appropriately. As the healing of suppressed disease might also be associated with the emergence of suppressed symptoms, the patient might be expected to get worse before getting better. Suppressed disease, although pervasive in nature, is often thought to be subtle, and therefore very difficult to assess or quantify. It could simply manifest in a general sense of malaise or lack of vitality rather than in symptoms and signs that can be studied objectively using the scientific method, and so arguably may not be recognized as significant by conventional physicians.

The use of treatment to palliate the uncomfortable or dangerous symptoms and signs of disease is very commonplace in conventional medical pharmacology. Conventional medicine practitioners do not, in general, recognize that the removal of symptoms of an underlying disease could be harmful. This view is reinforced by the fact that there is no obvious physiological or pathological theory to explain why preventing the expression of a symptom such as a headache or a sign such as high blood pressure would be harmful. In fact, in many cases of acute and chronic disease, symptoms themselves are potentially very damaging. Examples include the swelling of the brain in meningitis, recurrent seizures in children with high fever, escalating blood pressure, unstable angina, and emergence of cancerous tumors threatening the function of vital organs. Very few would debate the need for urgent allopathic treatment as a priority in such situations.

No conventional doctor would deny that allopathic treatments such as paracetamol for chronic pain or atenolol for high blood pressure are actually suppressing these symptoms and signs. These treatments do indeed suppress symptoms, as is evidenced by the fact that when they are withdrawn in chronic disease, the original condition tends to recur. However, the fact that drugs are available that can suppress unpleasant symptoms of chronic disease tends to be seen as largely positive (or at least the best choice out of all possible therapeutic options) from a conventional viewpoint. Moreover, without any physiological or pharmacological proof that suppression of symptoms might be harmful, the homeopathic understanding of the potentially deleterious effects of suppressive medication is incomprehensible to a conventional physician whose beliefs rest on scientifically proven certainties.

Conventional practitioners do, of course, recognize that drug treatment is not without risks, but they see these risks in entirely physical terms – as the harm that a drug may do because it is in some way toxic to the body. The likely benefits and risks of harm caused by a drug can be studied by means of observations of how the drug affects the physiology of the body and also by observing populations of patients who have been given the drug. In these ways the effects of drugs can be evaluated quantitatively. The risks and benefits associated with a particular drug treatment can thus be predicted, and the patient counseled accordingly.

The concept of suppression can be expanded further to help explore the different effects that a drug might have on the body in energetic terms. The term energetics is used in this text to describe the interpretation within certain complementary medicine disciplines of the action of a drug on the energetic body. In Chinese medicine, for example, the energetic body may be defined in terms of Yin and Yang, the Five Elements and the Vital Substances of Qi, Blood, Essence (Jing), and also the Pathogenic Factors (such as Cold or Damp) which may impact upon it.

The energetic effects that may result from any form of treatment may be one or more of the following:

- cure (treatment of the root imbalance)

- suppression (deepening of the root imbalance)

- drug-induced disease (addition of pathogenic factors to the root imbalance)

- placebo (promotion of self-healing of the root imbalance).

Cure

Within holistic complementary medical thought, when a treatment leads to cure, it is the appropriate remedy for the condition. The curative treatment deals with the root of the problem, and so leads to a move towards energetic balance, and an overall improvement in health.

In conventional medical treatment, replacement of iron in certain cases of anemia (i.e. those cases that are due to lack of iron in the diet) is an example of cure. Other examples of medical treatments that are aimed at restoring the body to balance by reversing the effects of an external cause of disease include the setting of a fractured bone, the surgical repair of a road traffic injury, the treatment of burns, the administration of fluids in dehydration and the treatment of poisoning. All these are treating the root problem and are examples of curative approaches.

In some cases, the appropriate treatment of an acute infection with antibiotics will restore the body to balance and might also be interpreted as curative.

Many forms of health promotion are potentially curative in their nature when successful, for example, stop smoking campaigns, weight loss clinics, exercise on prescription schemes and clean water provision in developing countries.

Suppression

In suppression (illustrated earlier with the analogy of the overflowing bath), the treatment causes the disappearance of symptoms, but the underlying imbalance, the root of the symptoms, has not been rectified. As already described, within many holistic medicine systems, symptoms may even be seen as a natural expression of a particular energetic imbalance, and one through which the imbalance may be healed, or at least stabilized.

Suppression can be illustrated in a diagrammatic way in the form of a negative cycle of events, in which suppression of symptoms leads to worsening of the root imbalance (see Figure 1.3b-II).

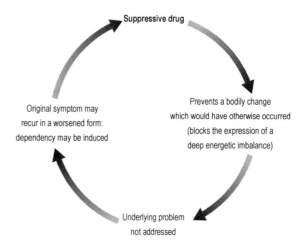

Figure 1.3b-II The negative cycle of suppression

To the holistically minded complementary therapist, one marker of suppression would be that if a drug is withdrawn, the original symptoms can reappear and may be even worse than before treatment because the underlying imbalance has worsened. This, in some circumstances, may lead the patient to have to rely on the drug to feel well; in other words, they have become dependent on the drug.

Suppression of symptoms can be supported with curative treatment. For example, antibiotics may be given for an episode of bronchitis in a smoker, but the smoker is then encouraged to stop smoking and take care of their health in terms of improved diet. The antibiotics do not deal with the underlying vulnerability to infection, but the cessation of smoking will permit a natural recovery, and will likely be accompanied by excessive phlegm production for a while as toxins held in the lungs are cleared by the recovering lining cells of the airways.

According to Chinese medicine bronchitis might represent Phlegm Heat Obstructing the Lungs resulting from a combination of the Heating effect of smoking and also poor diet together with a possible aggravation by an Invasion of Exterior Wind Heat.[36] Antibiotics will directly halt the inflammation induced by bacterial multiplication, and so will minimize acute damage to the material substance of the lungs. In Chinese medicine terms antibiotics are Cooling in nature and this explains their action in Clearing Heat. However, they do not have properties that can ameliorate the underlying profound energetic imbalances. Paradoxically, perhaps, their side effects (of rash, hypersensitivity and anaphylaxis) suggest that they might even introduce Toxic Heat into the system. As is well recognized, the health of the lungs will deteriorate steadily with the persistence of smoking. It is only the cessation of smoking and the change to a nourishing diet that will allow the natural balance of the Lung Qi to tend to reassert itself.

Introduction of drug-induced disease

When considering the energetic effects of medication, as hinted above, not all the harmful effects of a drug can be attributed to suppression. Few drugs target a particular symptom alone; they will often have other effects on the body. Aspirin, for example, recognized in conventional medicine to alleviate headaches because of its anti-inflammatory properties, also has an adverse effect on the lining of the stomach. In most people aspirin will cause inflammation and some degree of bleeding of the stomach lining. This effect is a direct result of the action of aspirin on the function of inflammatory chemicals (the prostaglandins) in the stomach lining. This might be described in Chinese medical terms as the introduction of the Pathogenic Factor (Evil Qi) of Heat into the Interior.[37]

There are some general effects of Western medications that might be recognized in Chinese medication to be relevant in many cases, and particularly with regard to the very powerful medications. The tendency for strong medications to be Cooling in nature whilst at the same time leading to invasion of Pathogenic Heat has been described. They can therefore be damaging to the Blood and Yang and also to the Yin in vulnerable individuals. Many drugs have side effects that include rash, fever, nausea and headache, damage to the blood cells, and damage to the hair listed in their side effects. Qi Stagnation with Damp or Heat are also common sequelae of Western medical treatment evidenced by patients commonly reporting headache, muscle aches and depression with diverse medications. The many hepatotoxic drugs seem to manifest in a syndrome akin to Damp Heat.[38]

The latter two categories of suppression and drug-induced disease will be difficult to distinguish in practice. In both situations the symptoms of the original condition have been improved, but at the cost of the appearance of other, newer symptoms. These other symptoms may either be a consequence of suppression (an old imbalance expressed at a deeper energetic level) or a drug-induced disease, or both.

One important distinguishing characteristic of drug-induced disease is that it will affect even a person who has no disease to suppress. If a well person were to take a high-dose aspirin on a regular basis, they would be very likely to experience symptoms of irritation of the stomach lining after some time, a consequence of the Heating properties of this medication (properties that also confer on it the beneficial aspects of being about to Disperse the Qi and Move the Blood).

Placebo

The placebo effect that results from the giving of either medication or physical treatments is well recognized in conventional medicine. Defined as "a beneficial effect... which cannot be attributed to the properties of the placebo itself, and must therefore be due to the patient's belief in that treatment,"[39] the placebo effect is classically recognized to occur when symptoms improve even when a prescription contains no active ingredient (such as sugar pills). However, the placebo effect may actually play a significant role in the healing response to even highly active medical treatments. It is known to powerfully influence the response to medications, but will also be active as part of the response to physical treatments such as physiotherapeutic manipulation or even surgical operations. It seems to be very much influenced by the packaging of a treatment, so a wide range of factors, from the name of the medication, to the way it is marketed, and the way the physician describes and prescribes it, are known to influence the outcomes in terms of a placebo response. These properties can be manipulated consciously (pharmaceutical companies are masters at this art), but are also influenced by factors that might be largely unconscious, including qualities relating to the physician such as confidence, ability to maintain rapport and intention.

Whilst the placebo effect is often described in scientific literature in a pejorative sense, with the implication that it indicates a treatment that has no medical value, actually the effect, by definition, is that the patient gets better. It is possible that what has been described as a placebo effect can indeed include the truly long-term healing response experienced by many patients who receive energetic-based complementary therapies. By describing genuine healing as a placebo effect the positive changes that result from the non-specific actions of healers are counted as unhelpful noise in scientific studies, and so may remain under-reported and under-investigated.

When is suppression of symptoms acceptable?

Sometimes suppressive treatment is the only option available to enable a person to cope with intolerable circumstances. Conventional medicine has adopted many suppressive treatments where there appears to be no available alternative to improve an intolerable or rapidly deteriorating situation.

Examples of this sort of necessary suppression include:

- chemotherapy in childhood leukemia (now known to save lives in a high proportion of cases)

- strong pain relief and other palliative measures in terminal cancer

- antidepressants or tranquillizers in an acutely suicidal person

- clot-busting medication to reverse the blockage in an artery that is causing an acute heart attack (also known to be life-saving).

Less extreme, and therefore more controversial, examples include:

- antidepressants prescribed to an overburdened single parent, who lives in a district in which social care is underfunded and waiting lists for supportive counseling are full – the prescription has undoubtedly helped the parent cope when no other care was available

- a contraceptive injection for someone who would be physically or emotionally traumatized by pregnancy

- antibiotics to reduce the disfigurement of acne in an under-confident and bullied teenager.

Many conventional medical treatments can be classed as suppressive in nature, but this may be true for many natural or alternative treatments, or for the substances with which many of us choose to self-medicate. In many cases the physician will also recognize these treatments as suppressive, and so will not necessarily consider them as the ideal treatment, but instead the best treatment when choices are limited. It might be considered, in view of their broad use in all cultures, that suppressive treatments are a necessary aspect of coping with the human condition, and because of this the therapist needs to work creatively with this aspect of human nature. The challenge for a Chinese medicine practitioner will often be not "how can I support the patient to stop taking suppressive treatments?" but instead, "how can I offer treatment which helps to treat the root problem in this case for as long as the patient continues to rely on suppressive treatments?"

Energetic effects of the eight categories of drugs

The categorization of conventional drugs introduced in Chapter 1.2 can help with interpreting whether or not a medical treatment is likely to be curative or suppressive in action. Table 1.3b-I demonstrates how an energetic interpretation can be matched to each of the eight categories of mode of drug action, as described in Chapter 1.2.

It is noteworthy that stimulant drugs are also categorized as suppressive according to this interpretation of drug energetics. Although the term suppression evokes pictures of damping something down rather than stimulating it, the stimulant drugs do, in fact, also suppress a more natural state of events. For example, the stimulant drug caffeine suppresses tiredness, the stimulant drug salbutamol suppresses constricted breathing when inhaled, and ovulatory stimulants suppress the state of infertility.

The difference with stimulants is that these drugs force, or boost, a bodily state that would not otherwise have occurred. As drugs carry no nutritive value, they do not actually introduce materials to support growth into the body. Because of this, any boosting of a bodily state is very likely to be at the expense of reserves of the energy that would be described as Qi in Chinese medicine.

Table 1.3b-I Energetic interpretation of each of the eight categories of mode of drug action

Mode of action of drug	Energetic interpretation
1. Replaces a deficient substance that is normally obtained from the diet	Usually returns the body to a state of more balance: energetic cure
	However, if given without attention to a deeper underlying cause of deficiency, e.g. iron replacement given to treat anemia due to ongoing heavy menstrual blood loss: suppression
2. Kills or suppresses the growth of infectious agents (microbes and other life forms that cause infection)	In infections that are a manifestation of strong Evil (Xie Qi) Pathogenic Factor (in Chinese medicine terms) in a healthy individual, the drug may enable full clearance of the bacteria that are causing the manifestation of the infection, and so will enable the restoration of balance as the healthy body can then easily recover naturally: energetic cure
	In infections that have occurred as a result of an underlying imbalance in the individual, the treatment does not target the root cause, and so tends to be suppressive, even with full clearance of the bacterial overgrowth: suppression
	In some cases the end result is one of Residual Pathogenic Factor, and this means that symptoms will continue to present at a deeper energetic level: suppression
3. Toxic to rapidly dividing human cells	These treatments always target the manifestation (a tumor) of a deep underlying imbalance: suppression
	They are also very toxic to a wide range of healthy bodily tissues and are characterized by: marked drug-induced disease
4. Replaces a substance that is normally produced by the body	In cases in which the body will never be able to produce the essential substance ever again, the replacement treatment moves the body towards a state of more balance (e.g. insulin replacement in type 1 diabetes mellitus or chronic pancreatitis, both of which are due to total failure of the insulin cells of the pancreas): energetic cure
	In cases when the body is under-producing an essential substance as a result of an ongoing deeper disease process, the replacement of that substance is suppressive (e.g. thyroxine replacement in mild hypothyroidism): suppression
5. Specifically stimulates the immune response by introduction of an antigen	Vaccines are given to well people. They involve the administration of a foreign substance, which primarily stimulates a natural immune response. In some cases this disease leads to serious symptoms, but in other cases, the individual regains a healthy state of balance as the artificial infection is overcome. This has to be classed as: drug-induced disease
6. Other drugs that stimulate natural bodily functions	These drugs may first stimulate a bodily function that perhaps should be occurring (e.g. lack of ovulation in female infertility) but is not due to an underlying imbalance. By ignoring the underlying imbalance and treating the symptom, these treatments will be depleting. Also, any drug that causes an increase in a natural bodily response (e.g. alertness induced by caffeine, or relaxation of the airways by inhaled salbutamol in asthma) could also be described as a stimulant. If stimulants mask the symptoms of an imbalance then this is: suppression
	Stimulants can be used when there is no medical disease (e.g. in the case of recreational drug use). In this case their immediate effects might be classed as: drug-induced disease
7. Suppresses natural bodily functions	The suppression of a natural bodily function, either in a well or an unwell person, is, of course, classed as suppression as it is not targeting the root cause of the problem: suppression
8. Counteracts the damage caused by toxins	These treatments reverse the damage that would have been caused by an external toxic substance: energetic cure

Figure 1.3b-III illustrates the effect of stimulant drugs in the form of a negative cycle.

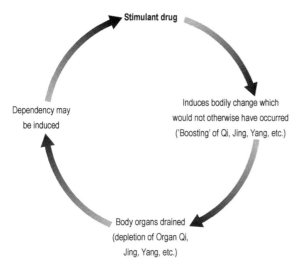

Figure 1.3b-III The negative cycle of stimulant drugs

Figure 1.3b-III illustrates how, from a Chinese medicine perspective, a stimulant drug may actually cause an impression of improving the energetic state of the body by the Moving of substances (such as Qi or Yang), a change apparent in the immediate improved functioning of an organ. One example might be the action of salbutamol, which reduces the wheeze of asthma. This action might be described as the Moving and Descending of Lung Qi despite the underlying condition of Deficient Lung and/or Kidney Qi. However, this drug does not cure asthma, except in the short term. The theory of suppression would suggest that repeated use might actually tend to deplete reserves of Lung and Kidney Qi, as its moving action is unadulterated and is not accompanied, as it would be in an herbal formula, with nourishing herbs. If Lung and Kidney Qi is depleted by this powerful action, in this way, the patient can become dependent on the medication.

It is important to clarify at this point that describing salbutamol as suppressive is not to say that this drug is always harmful. There is no doubt that, in severe asthma, drugs such as salbutamol are potentially life-saving, and are a good example of how suppressive treatment may be the best option for some patients. It is also noteworthy to explain that the Chinese herb ma huang has a very similar effect to salbutamol, and has been shown to contain comparable active chemical constituents (including ephedrine). It, too, is recognized to Move and Descend Lung Qi, but as part of Chinese herbal formulae tends to be prescribed concurrently with warming herbs.[40] With this understanding, it would make sense to support a patient who is reliant on salbutamol with treatment and advice focused on nourishing and conserving Lung and Kidney Yin.

In a similar way, other stimulant drugs can be described as Moving of substances. Caffeine could be described as

Moving of Heart Qi, and ovulatory stimulants could be thought of as Moving of Blood and Essence, and in the same way it would make sense that all stimulant drugs are ultimately depleting to the body's energies.

Energetic action of drugs: from theory to practice

Some fictional case histories from conventional medicine will help these theories of the energetics of drug action come to life. These present different examples of drugs leading to cure, drug-induced disease and suppression. Each is followed by a brief discussion of the energetic interpretations of the action of the drugs described.

Box 1.3b-I Case history 1

Joe, a previously fit teenager, rapidly becomes very unwell after developing a flu-like illness and is rushed to hospital in a nearly unconscious state. Bacterial meningitis is suspected and later confirmed. Joe makes a dramatic recovery after five days of treatment with intravenous antibiotics. He is tired for a few days following his illness, but after two weeks of resting at home he is back to playing football for the school within three weeks. Six months later, he appears to be fully back to his previous level of fitness.

This is a case describing the use of antibiotics. Antibiotics are believed to be Cold in nature, according to Chinese medicine.[41] Evidence for this is that they can Cool the Heat of bacterial infections and may lead to loose stools or profuse white vaginal discharge (thrush) as unwanted side effects. They also can have side effects that suggest Pathogenic Heat Invasion and Depletion of Yin (including rashes and anaphylaxis).

Meningitis is a condition of Strong Wind and Heat, and so requires a strong treatment for the Pathogens to be cleared. Joe was basically healthy and so has good Upright Qi. With antibiotic treatment the acute manifestation of Heat on the Exterior appears to have been cleared and Wind obstructing the Orifices is pacified. In the next few weeks, as a result of resilient Upright Qi and taking care during convalescence, he was able to recover from any negative aspects of the drugs and fully recover from the original acute illness.

As the Pathogen is cleared and there is no feature to suggest suppression, this does seem to be an example of cure that has been helped by treatment of the Biao (manifestation) with antibiotics and the Ben (root) with rest and nourishment. In Joe's case this is a case when the Biao (manifestation) of the illness is the invasion of a strong Pathogenic Factor in someone with good Upright

Qi, and so the Cooling antibiotic could even be interpreted as an appropriate remedy.

Box 1.3b-II Case history 2

Alf, the elderly grandfather of the teenager in Case history 1, also contracts the infection. He presents first with symptoms of a cold and then becomes increasingly confused for five days before the condition is recognized. With the same treatment, the older man makes a much slower recovery and has to be nursed in hospital for three weeks. He develops a prolonged case of diarrhea following the antibiotics, and even when this is better after three weeks, he is never quite as sprightly again.

Alf is an elderly man and his Upright Qi is not as strong as that of his grandson. He will also be in a state of Yin Deficiency as a result of his advanced years. For this reason, Alf's body does not respond as suddenly to the infection as his grandson's body, and so the diagnosis is delayed. Because of his deficiency the Pathogenic Heat is more likely to progress to the Interior to induce further Deficiency of Blood and Yin, and so affect the function of all the Organ systems. Diarrhea is a common side effect of antibiotics and in Alf's case may be a consequence of having weak Spleen Qi. For all these reasons he takes much longer to recover, and never fully regains his previous level of health.

However, without the treatment Alf is likely to have died. This is, therefore, an example of partial cure, but with drug-induced disease complicating the older man's recovery.

The depletion following the illness (possibly a result of Full Heat consuming Yin) is more likely mostly due to the effect of the meningitis than the antibiotics. However, in view of the prolonged diarrhea, the antibiotics may possibly have contributed to Alf's reduction in overall health. A possible Chinese description for this is that the illness has caused Deficiency of Yin and impaired the function of the Spleen, and antibiotics have led to the accumulation of Damp. In Western medical terms the antibiotics will have caused a long-term unhelpful imbalance in the natural bacteria (the microbiome) resident in the gut.

Box 1.3b-III Case history 3

Joe's sister Sue is worrying about school examinations, and has a distracting sore throat. She receives a prescription for a broad-spectrum antibiotic (amoxicillin) from her doctor. Her sore throat gets better, but she develops vaginal thrush (profuse white discharge with an itch), and is very uncomfortable. She buys some antifungal medication for this (clotrimazole cream and a fluconazole tablet) from the chemist. Although her vaginal infection gets better in two days, it recurs just before the exams, and continues to do so for the next few months. Each time it responds less well to the chemist's treatment. A year into the sixth form she goes to her doctor feeling depressed and exhausted. She doesn't think to mention the thrush. All her blood tests come back within the normal range, but she is worried that she is developing chronic fatigue syndrome.

Sue has been studying hard for school examinations. She developed a sore throat just before her examinations and was prescribed antibiotics with the intention of shortening the course of her symptoms. Unfortunately, she has now developed a well-recognized side effect of antibiotics, vaginal thrush. From a conventional perspective, this is understood to occur because the antibiotic destroys natural protective bacteria (lactobacilli and bifidobacteria) in the vagina as well as those thought to have contributed to the chesty cough. From a Chinese medicine perspective, the Cooling action of the antibiotics has impaired the function of the Spleen Qi, and led to the formation of a discharge with characteristics of Cold and Damp (but possibly some local Blood Deficiency also evidenced by the itch). This can be interpreted as drug-induced disease resulting from the energetic effect of the antibiotic. In this case, Sue might have been predisposed to a Spleen-related pattern as her studying for exams could have also compromised the function of this Organ system.

The fact that the symptoms persisted, and only temporarily responded to antifungal treatment, suggests that suppression is also part of the picture. The antifungal treatment has appeared to clear the symptoms that were a manifestation of Pathogenic Cold and Damp, but as this imbalance becomes apparent again within a short time, this suggests it was never fully resolved in the first place. As time goes on Sue develops more symptoms, but this time at a deeper physical and also emotional level, and this could be evidence of the original imbalance having progressed and presenting in a different, more complex form (e.g. Spleen Qi Deficiency with Damp Heat and Liver Depression with Qi Stagnation). The interrelationship between Spleen Qi Deficiency and the development of chronic patterns involving Stasis of the substances known as the Yin Evils and Heat is explained with wonderful clarity by Flaws and Sionneau (2001).[42]

Looking back, it may have been the stress of Sue's exams that led to an energetic imbalance such as Spleen Qi Deficiency and consequent Wei Qi Deficiency, which was then followed by Wind Heat Invasion. The medication just treated the manifestation of the imbalance, so possibly allowing the root cause to worsen, but there was also in this case incomplete clearance of the Pathogenic Factor and the emergence of the syndrome of Residual Pathogenic Factor. The treatment also introduced additional imbalance resulting from Cold and Damp (drug-induced disease). The Cold in the Lower Jiao in time later led to Heat in the Middle Jiao as a result of Chronic Stagnation.

Box 1.3b-IV Case history 4

Meanwhile, Sue's best friend Ann had been experiencing similar symptoms of exhaustion, and also night sweats. She had also been putting these symptoms down to stress in the sixth form, but one evening she felt a firm swelling on one side of her neck. Her doctor was concerned to discover that Ann had markedly swollen lymph nodes on that side. After referral to a specialist, urgent investigations revealed that Ann had developed a rare form of tumor of the lymph glands called Hodgkin's disease. She was told she had "early stage disease", which has a good prognosis, but requires intensive treatment to maximize the chances of this good outcome.[43] She was started on a regime of chemotherapy, which made her feel nauseous and caused her hair to fall out. She then also had to undergo a program of radiotherapy to certain groups of lymph nodes in her body. Ann felt awful on this regimen and had to drop behind a year at school.

After the course of treatments the doctor said that she was in remission. This meant there was no evidence of any tumor in any of her glands, but cure could not be proven. Ann would have to return for yearly check-ups. Nevertheless, she was determined to fight against a possible recurrence, and paid careful attention to eating a diet free of any processed food or addictive substances. Within two years she had raised money for a cancer charity by taking part in a marathon cycle ride.

Now, five years later, she is completing her training at medical school, feeling well, still clear of disease, and keen to be an oncologist. Ann now says that her current problems are that her teeth need frequent dental attention, and that she is worried that she may be infertile. She knows she will be under medical review by the specialists for the next five years at least, and will have an increased risk of additional cancer as a result of her treatment compared to her peers for years to come.

Ann has received chemotherapy and radiotherapy for lymphoma. Radiotherapy and chemotherapy are toxic to dividing cells, and so fit into category 3 of drug action, as summarized in Table 1.3b-I. Therefore, it can be assumed that the action of the treatment is suppressive. The fact that the treatment caused severe side effects at the time is an indication of additional significant drug-induced disease.

There is no doubt, from the historical understanding of the prognosis of lymphoma before treatment, that Ann would have died without therapy. Therefore, this case is an example of how a powerfully suppressive treatment, and one that also causes marked drug-induced disease, has prevented death and given a person the opportunity to continue to live life to the full.

A lymphoma is an initially painless mass, which might be considered as Phlegm (or possibly Blood Stagnation) in Chinese medicine. In Chinese medicine the etiology of cancer would be that there must have also been a pre-existing Deficiency in terms of Yin and/or Yang to allow such a substantial mass to develop. Flaws (2002)[44] argues that a range of deficiency states can lead to the formation of Phlegm in lymphoma, and these include External Wind Heat invading to Dry the Blood and Congeal the Fluids. For this to happens there needs to be a Vacuity resulting from chronic over-taxation. The combination of Heat, Congealed Fluids and Deficiency all facilitate the engenderment of Phlegm Damp development. In his view, chronic Deficiency of Spleen and/or Kidney Yang are the basis of the accumulation of Evil Dampness, which is a precursor to the development of tumors. Flaws goes on to explain that Liver Pathology is also often causative as it can both promote Spleen Vacuity and also lead to the Stagnation that allows the accumulation of Damp.

Chemotherapy has a range of side effects, which suggests that it is energetically Heating: it causes angry inflamed tissue if it leaks out of the infusion needle, it leads to a painful sore tongue and mucous membranes, and also increases the risk of bleeding. From a Chinese medicine perspective, chemotherapy (and radiotherapy) is seen as a form of Heat toxin that combats the Pathogen that is manifesting as the tumor. Because it is hot and attacking, it is also recognized to deplete Righteous Qi and also lead to Qi and Yin Depletion.[45]

Depletion of Spleen Qi and Liver Qi Stagnation is manifest in the very common side effects of chemotherapy – vomiting and diarrhea. The known complication of infertility and impairment of the immune system and long-term cancer risk are features of Depletion of Kidney Qi or Jing. Here is the evidence for additional drug-induced disease.

Chemotherapy attends only to the manifestation of Ann's underlying imbalance, but does not treat the root deficiency. The additional drug-induced disease can clearly actually compound the root deficiency, which, as we have seen, is one of deficiency or vacuity. This is the nature of suppressive treatment.

However, in Ann's case, although drug-induced disease and suppression are not in themselves desirable, it is clear they were a price worth paying in the face of a rapidly progressive disease process. Flaws (2002)[46] explains that in Chinese medicine it is clearly understood that cancer chemotherapy, whilst necessary, does not treat the root. The saying "supporting the righteous and banking the root" relates to the principle of combining aggressive Western medication with protective and nourishing herbs with the intention that the patient gets the best of both worlds of medicine.

This case history also illustrates the strong tendency of the human body/spirit to be healed despite the presence of suppressed symptoms. Ann's determination to continue to live life in as full a way as possible, and also her subsequent attention to her health, are both likely to have enabled her body to resolve the original deficiency that had led to the cancer (although she must take care not to continue to deplete her vitality further whilst she is still recovering from the double onslaught of illness and treatment).

Systematic interpretation of the energetics of individual drugs

The case histories have provided examples of the energetic effects of the eight broad categories of drugs, and have illustrated how their effects can fall into one or more of the four categories of cure, placebo effect, suppression or drug-induced disease. It is possible to work through cases such as these in a systematic way in order to arrive confidently at a basic interpretation of the energetics of the drugs being used.

A method for interpreting the action of individual drugs will now be introduced, drawing on the Chinese medicine language of energetics. By way of illustration, the energetic properties of two common drugs are explored. This method involves gathering information about the action of a drug in six steps. Each step involves a question, the answer to which will contribute towards a final energetic interpretation. As Case histories 1–3 illustrate, the energetic interpretation of the same drug might be different according to the clinical setting of its use (e.g. antibiotics may either be curative or suppressive in action), so it is important when using this method to first be clear about the clinical setting.

The six steps relate to the following aspects of treatment:

1. *How does the drug give relief of symptoms?* First describe how the drug gives relief of symptoms.

2. *What is the Chinese medicine interpretation of the disease?* Give a simple Chinese medicine interpretation of the disease being treated.

3. *How does the drug alleviate disease in Chinese medicine terms?* Explain the alleviation of this disease in Chinese medicine terms.

4. *What are the common side effects of this drug?* List the common side effects of the medication (use a formulary such as the British National Formulary, BNF[47]).

5. *What is a simple Chinese medicine interpretation of the side effects?* Explain side effects in Chinese medicine terms.

6. *Into what category of mode of action does the drug fit?* Decide if the drug might have caused suppressed symptoms in addition to drug-induced disease.

To help illustrate this process, it will now be followed for a commonly taken painkiller, ibuprofen, which is classed as a non-steroidal anti-inflammatory drug (NSAID). The name NSAID describes the fact that, even though it is not a corticosteroid preparation, ibuprofen will act to calm down the natural process of inflammation in the body. It does this by chemically interfering with the natural production of inflammatory substances called prostaglandins in the body. Ibuprofen gives relief for swollen painful joints, but is also very effective in headache and period pain. All this information can be gleaned from a formulary such as the BNF.[48] Each of the six questions will now be answered for ibuprofen in the clinical setting of it being used to relieve pain and inflammation.

1. *How does ibuprofen give relief of symptoms?* The answer to this question need only be given in the simplest descriptive terms, and will be obvious as long as it is understood why the drug has been prescribed.

Ibuprofen in this clinical setting relieves pain, stiffness and dysmenorrhea.

2. *What is the Chinese medicine interpretation of the disease?* In this case the disease that ibuprofen treats is pain and inflammation. The answer to this question requires some understanding of how symptoms relate to Chinese medicine syndromes.

In Chinese medicine, the pain and inflammation for which ibuprofen may be prescribed is generally described in terms of Stagnant Qi and Blood (pain). Inflammation may represent (Wind) Heat.

3. *How does ibuprofen alleviate pain and inflammation in Chinese medicine terms?* The answer to this question relates to the alleviation of the syndromes, given as the answer to question 2.

A simple answer in this clinical setting would be that ibuprofen alleviates pain by Moving Qi and Blood and Clearing Heat.

4. *What are the common side effects of ibuprofen?* To answer this question requires access to a formulary.

The most common side effect for ibuprofen listed in the BNF is inflammation of the stomach lining, which can, in turn, lead to indigestion, slight oozing of blood, and occasionally a stomach ulcer. Rare side effects that can affect susceptible people include headache, tinnitus (ringing in the ears), dizziness, liver and kidney damage and asthma.

5. *What is a possible simple Chinese medicine interpretation of the side effects?* Like the answer to question 3, to answer this question requires some basic knowledge of how Chinese medicine syndromes relate to symptoms. However, this is a more difficult question to answer because the information given in the BNF is not presented in the detail with which a complementary medical practitioner might describe symptoms. Because of the paucity of details of symptoms, often only a guess at the most likely possible syndrome can be made on the basis of a few key symptoms such as headache, depression and abdominal disturbance. Sometimes, knowledge of the pathological process at play can offer helpful additional information; for example, local inflammation and bleeding suggests Heat, painless overgrowth of tissues suggests Phlegm, degeneration of the substance of tissues suggests Yin Deficiency, and impairment of function might suggest Qi or Yang Deficiency. The rationale for these assumptions is explained in more detail in the "Note to the Reader" at the beginning of this book.

The common gastric side effects of ibuprofen imply impairment of Stomach Yin, a key symptom of which is epigastric discomfort. If a painful stomach ulcer develops, the more intense fixed pain characteristic of this condition implies the development of Blood Stagnation. Bleeding from the stomach suggests Heat, presumably as a result of prolonged Blood Stagnation. Headaches, dizziness and tinnitus may imply Stagnation of Liver Qi and Liver Yang Rising and/or impairment of Kidney Qi. Deep organ damage to the kidneys and liver also suggest that the drug in some way has the potential to damage Liver and Kidney Qi and Yin.

6. *Into what category of mode of action does ibuprofen fall?* This question relates to the eight categories of modes of action listed in Table 1.3b-I.

As the pain is always the symptom of some other underlying condition, such as arthritis or injury, ibuprofen fits into category 7. Its action is therefore suppressive. As the condition being treated is one of Heat and Stagnation, the two common side effects (digestive disorder resulting from impairment of Stomach Yin and headaches resulting from Liver Qi Stagnation and impairment of Kidney Yin) may also be exacerbated as a result of not fully attending to these Pathogenic Factors.

Summary: We can say that ibuprofen is a drug with properties of Moving Qi and Blood and is able to Dispel Heat. However, its side effects indicate Toxic Heat: it may damage Stomach Yin, and also the Liver and Kidney Yin and Qi in susceptible people. These side effects may be the result of direct damage from the drug itself, but may also be contributed to by the fact this medication acts in a suppressive rather than curative way, so leaving the root imbalances untouched.

Because it is possible to make only very general energetic interpretations from the limited information given in the BNF, one key way of keeping this approach a manageable tool is to aim for the Chinese energetic interpretations to be as simple as possible.

A similar process is now followed for caffeine, a drug that is commonly included in cold and pain remedies, but is much more familiar as a prominent component of the Western diet.

Caffeine is a bitter tasting white chemical originally obtained from the seeds, nuts or leaves of a number of tropical plants, of which coffee and tea are the most well known. It is considered to be a mild stimulant that acts by blocking the action of a chemical called adenosine in the brain that would otherwise lead to drowsiness. It improves reaction time and arousal in sleep-deprived people. Caffeine slightly speeds up the pulse and metabolic rate, and is recognized to help move the bowels and promote urination. It is claimed to have slight painkilling properties, although this is disputed in the BNF. When present in tea or coffee, it appears to lift the mood (the poet William Cowper described tea as the cup that "cheer[s] but not inebriates"[49]). Caffeine may cause bronchodilation in some people, so relieving asthma symptoms. For some people caffeine can cause indigestion, a migraine-type headache or palpitations. Caffeine has a known withdrawal syndrome of severe headaches and reduced mood for days after suddenly stopping intake. In Chinese medicine, coffee is not a herb that has traditionally been part of the pharmacopeia. It has been described as a bitter-sweet bean, having properties that include the Moving of Liver Qi, Purging of Gallbladder, aiding of assimilation and digestion and also Opening the Orifices of the Heart. Side effects are attributed to the strength of the Moving effect on Liver Qi compared to the Tonifying effect on the Spleen, so leading it to be ultimately Depleting of Qi and Blood if used in excess.[50]

Each of the six questions is now answered for caffeine in the clinical setting of it being used in tablet form as a "pick me up" at a time of lethargy and lack of enthusiasm.

1. *How does caffeine give relief of symptoms?* In this setting caffeine lifts the mood and induces wakefulness.

2. *What is a possible Chinese medicine interpretation of lethargy and lack of enthusiasm?* Caffeine may be taken in times of lethargy, and also may lift the spirits. Lethargy could have a range of causes, but at its simplest could be accounted for by Qi Deficiency or Stagnation. Likewise, low spirits could be attributed to Heart Qi Deficiency or Qi Stagnation.

3. *How does caffeine alleviate lethargy and lack of enthusiasm in Chinese medicine terms?* Caffeine therefore acts possibly by Moving and Boosting of Qi, and in particular, of the Liver and Heart.

4. *What are the common side effects of caffeine?* In susceptible people caffeine can cause indigestion, headaches, palpitations and chronic tiredness.

5. *What is a possible simple Chinese medicine interpretation of the side effects?* Indigestion suggests impairment of Stomach Yin or Spleen Qi, headaches could result from a wide range of Deficiency and Excess Syndromes including Blood Deficiency, Qi Deficiency and Liver Qi Stagnation. Tiredness might suggest Stagnation of Qi and/or impairment of Qi (of Heart, Spleen or Kidneys).

6. *Into what category of mode of action does caffeine fall?* Caffeine primarily masks the natural bodily response of tiredness. This fits into category 7. In those who are dependent on caffeine, it relieves a craving for caffeine, headaches and low mood, which are all symptoms of a deeper imbalance. The energetic action is therefore suppressive.

Summary: Caffeine is a substance that has primarily Moving properties, and seems to result in Moving of Qi, in particular, Heart and Liver Qi. It might also benefit Spleen Qi if taken in moderation. The side effects of indigestion, palpitation and chronic tiredness are signs of drug-induced disease that might involve Liver Qi Stagnation, Stomach Yin Deficiency and Heart Yin Deficiency. The presence of a marked withdrawal syndrome tells us it has a suppressive action. In this case, caffeine can mask the features of an underlying condition of Stagnation of Liver Qi and Depletion of Blood and Qi.

These two summaries of the six-step approach to summarizing the energetic action of drugs illustrate that this simple process can be applied to two very different treatments. To further illustrate the simplicity and flexibility of this approach, some more worked examples of energetic interpretations of drug actions are given in Appendix II.

Notes

1   Waugh, A. and Grant, A (2014) *Ross and Wilson: Anatomy and Physiology in Health and Illness.* Twelfth Edition. Edinburgh: Elsevier, Chapters 1–3.

2   The term "energetics" is used in this text to refer to any description of a manifestation of the Chinese concept of the energetic body, and also the action of a drug on this body in Chinese medical terms.

3   Maciocia, G. (1989) *The Foundations of Chinese Medicine.* Edinburgh: Churchill Livingstone.

4   Illich, I. (1976) *Limits to Medicine: Medical Nemesis – The Expropriation of Health.* London: Calder & Boyars.

5   For more information on this, see www.cms.gov/Regulations-and-Guidance/Guidance/FACA/MEDCAC.html

6   NICE (National Institute for Health and Care Excellence) (2016) 'NICE guidance.' Available at www.nice.org.uk/guidance, accessed on 5 May 2016.

7   English Oxford Living Dictionaries (2016) 'Health.' Available at www.oxforddictionaries.com/definition/english/health, accessed on 6 June 2016.

8   WHO (World Health Organization) (2016) 'Trade, foreign policy, diplomacy and health.' Available at www.who.int/about/mission/en, accessed on 6 June 2016.

9   English Oxford Living Dictionaries (2016) 'Vitalism.' Available at https://en.oxforddictionaries.com/definition/vitalism, accessed on 6 June 2016.

10 Gruppen, L.D., Woolliscroft, J.O. and Wolf, F.M. (1988) 'The contribution of different components of the clinical encounter in generating and eliminating diagnostic hypotheses.' *Research in Medical Education 27*, 242–247.

11 Huber, M. (2011) 'How should we define health?' *British Medical Journal 343*, d4163.

12 Boseley, S. (2016) 'The closest thing yet to a cure for terminal cancer?' *The Guardian*, 4 February. Available at www.theguardian.com/science/2016/feb/04/revolutionary-drug-immune-system-advanced-cancer, accessed on 6 June 2016.

13 ONS (Office for National Statistics) (2015) 'Deaths registered in England and Wales: 2014.' Available at www.ons.gov.uk/peoplepopulationandcommunity/birthsdeathsandmarriages/deaths/bulletins/deathsregistrationsummarytables/2015-07-15, accessed on 6 June 2016.

14 Lissauer, T. and Clayden, G. (1997) *Illustrated Textbook of Paediatrics.* Maryland Heights, MO: Mosby.

15 Prostate Cancer UK (2016) 'The PSA test.' Available at http://prostatecanceruk.org/prostate-information/getting-diagnosed/psa-test, accessed on 6 June 2016.

16 British Thoracic Society and Scottish Intercollegiate Guidelines Network (2014) *British Guideline on the Management of Asthma: A National Clinical Guideline.* Available at www.brit-thoracic.org.uk/document-library/clinical-information/asthma/btssign-asthma-guideline-2014, accessed on 6 June 2016.

17 NICE (National Institute for Health and Care Excellence) (2015) *Lower Urinary Tract Symptoms in Men: Management.* Clinical Guideline CG97. Available at www.nice.org.uk/guidance/cg97/chapter/1-Recommendations#drug-treatment, accessed on 6 June 2016.

18 Cochrane Library (2013) 'Vitamin C for preventing and treating the common cold.' Available at http://onlinelibrary.wiley.com/doi/10.1002/14651858.CD000980.pub4/abstract, accessed on 6 June 2016.

19 British Medical Association and Royal Pharmaceutical Society (2016) *British National Formulary 71.* London: BMJ Group and Pharmaceutical Press.

20 NICE (National Institute for Health and Care Excellence) (2015) 'British National Formulary.' Available at www.evidence.nhs.uk/formulary/bnf/current, accessed on 30 August 2015.

21 WHO (World Health Organization) (2015) 'International Nonproprietary Names.' Available at www.who.int/medicines/services/inn/en, accessed on 30 August 2015.

22 Drugs.com (2016) 'International Drug Names.' Available at www.drugs.com/international, accessed on 6 June 2016.

23 Wong, D.T., Perry, K.W. and Bymaster, F.P. (2005) 'Case history: The discovery of fluoxetine hydrochloride (Prozac).' *National Review of Drug Discoveries*, September, 4(9), 764–774.

24 Drugwatch (2016) 'Vioxx, what is it? Its uses and interactions.' Available at drugwatch.com/vioxx, accessed on 6 June 2016.

25 Bechtel, W. and Richardson, R.C. (1998) 'Vitalism.' In E. Craig, *Routledge Encyclopedia of Philosophy.* London: Routledge. Available at https://mechanism.ucsd.edu/teaching/philbio/vitalism.htm, accessed on 29 June 2016.

26 Northrupp, C. (2012) *The Wisdom of Menopause.* Carlsbad, CA: Hay House, p.491.

27 Moriyama, I.M., Loy, R.M. and Robb-Smith, A.H.T. (2011) *History of the Statistical Classification and Causes of Death.* Washington, DC: US Government Printing Office, p.9.

28 Engel, G. (1977) 'The need for a new medical model: A challenge for biomedicine.' *Science 196*, 129–136.

29 Gascoigne, S. (2001) *The Clinical Medicine Guide: A Holistic Perspective.* Clonakilty, Ireland: Jigme Press.

30 Xinnong, C. (1990) *Chinese Acupuncture and Moxibustion.* Beijing: Foreign Languages Press, p.289.

31 Maoshing, N. (1995) *The Yellow Emperor's Classic of Medicine: A New Translation of the Neijing Suwen with Commentary.* Boston, MA: Shambhala.

32 Flaws, B. and Wolfe, H. (1993) *Prince Wen Hui's Cook: Chinese Dietary Therapy.* Brookline, MA: Paradigm Publications, p.19.

33 Little, D. (2007) 'Hering's Preface to *The Chronic Diseases* (1845).' Available at www.simillimum.com/education/little-library/homoeopathic-philosophy/hpcd/article.php, accessed on 9 June 2016.

34 Maoshing, N. (1995) *The Yellow Emperor's Classic of Medicine: A New Translation of the Neijing Suwen with Commentary.* Boston, MA: Shambhala, Chapter 65: 'Biao and Ben and the Transmission of Disease.'

35 Matsumoto, H. (1997) 'Thoughts on Ben and Biao.' *North American Journal of Oriental Medicine 3*, 7, 5–8.

36 Maciocia, G. (1989) *The Foundations of Chinese Medicine: A Comprehensive Text for Acupuncturists and Herbalists.* Edinburgh: Churchill Livingstone, p.238.

37 Legge, D. (2010) 'Xie Qi or pathogenic energies.' Accessed on 10 May 2016 at www.sydneycollegepress.com.au/articlesXQPE.html.

38 Dharmananda, S. (1998) 'Countering the toxic effects of modern medicines with Chinese herbs.' Available at www.itmonline.org/arts/sidefx.htm, accessed on 9 May 2016.

39 English Oxford Living Dictionaries (2016) 'Placebo effect.' Available at www.oxforddictionaries.com/definition/english/placebo-effect, accessed on 10 May 2016.

40 Dharmananda, S. (2000) 'Safety issues affecting Chinese herbs: The case of ma-huang.' Available at www.itmonline.org/arts/mahuang.htm, accessed on 9 May 2016.

41 Dharmananda, S. (1998) 'Countering the toxic effects of modern medicines with Chinese herbs.' Available at www.itmonline.org/arts/sidefx.htm, accessed on 9 May 2016.

42 Flaws, B. and Sionneau, P. (2001) *Treatment of Modern Western Diseases.* Boulder, CO: Blue Poppy Press, pp.1–39.

43 Tidy, C. (2014) 'Hodgkin's lymphoma.' Available at http://patient.info/doctor/hodgkins-lymphoma-pro, accessed on 11 May 2016.

44 Flaws, B. (2002) 'Chinese medical treatment of malignant lymphoma.' Available at www.acupuncturetoday.com/mpacms/at/article.php?id=28009, accessed on 16 May 2016.

45 Flaws, B. (2002) 'Chinese medical treatment of malignant lymphoma.' Available at www.acupuncturetoday.com/mpacms/at/article.php?id=28009, accessed on 16 May 2016.

46 Flaws, B. (2002) 'Chinese medical treatment of malignant lymphoma.' Available at www.acupuncturetoday.com/mpacms/at/article.php?id=28009, accessed on 16 May 2016.

47 NICE (National Institute for Health and Care Excellence) (2016) 'British National Formulary.' Available at www.evidence.nhs.uk/formulary/bnf/current, accessed on 16 May 2016.

48 NICE (National Institute for Health and Care Excellence) (2016) 'British National Formulary.' Available at www.evidence.nhs.uk/formulary/bnf/current, accessed on 16 May 2016.

49 Cowper, W. (1794) 'The Task, Book IV.' Available at www.poetryfoundation.org/poems-and-poets/poems/detail/44037, accessed on 18 May 2016. The quote is found in the following paragraph of this poem: "Now stir the fire, and close the shutters fast, Let fall the curtains, wheel the sofa round, And, while the bubbling and loud-hissing urn Throws up a steamy column, and the cups, That cheer but not inebriate, wait on each, So let us welcome peaceful ev'ning in."

50 Dharmananda, S. (2003) 'Coffee in China.' Available at www.itmonline.org/arts/coffee.htm, accessed on 18 May 2016.

INTRODUCTION TO PROCESSES OF DISEASE

2.1

Barriers to Disease and Susceptibility

2.1a Health and susceptibility: what makes us vulnerable to disease?

In this first half of Stage 2 there is a progression from the introductory topics of Stage 1 to an exploration of the foundations of pathology, the study of how the body responds to disease. We begin with a discussion of the concept of susceptibility to disease.

Susceptibility as vulnerability to disease

In Section 1.1e the basic causes of disease from the perspective of both conventional and more holistic approaches to medicine were introduced. This section explores the topic of causation of disease in more detail, and in particular, which factors influence susceptibility to disease. Susceptibility is used commonly in conventional medicine to refer to vulnerability to disease. From a holistic perspective, susceptibility might more accurately be defined as vulnerability to imbalance, as within a holistic paradigm, including that of Chinese medicine, reduced health tends to be considered in terms of patterns of imbalance rather than as disease.

Conventional view of barriers to disease

Conventional medicine considers susceptibility in terms of weakness of one or more of a series of levels of defenses, or barriers to disease. This concept is highly suggestive of the prevailing view that the body is a fortress and disease an invading enemy. The body is understood to have several methods of protection against disease. Some of these are located in the superficial layers of the body, within the skin and mucous membranes, and others offer their protective action from within the deeper levels of the tissues beneath the skin and also from within the organs themselves.

Conventional medicine recognizes mechanical and immune barriers to disease. Mechanical barriers are those that confer protection as a result of the physical structure of the barrier (e.g. the keratinized squamous epithelium of the skin). Immune barriers are those that protect by means of a complex interaction of the immune cells and proteins (including antibodies) that circulate in the body fluids and can move into tissues when required. Table 2.1a-I summarizes those parts or functions of the body that have a protective role.

Table 2.1a-I Examples of barriers to disease

Depth	Name of barrier	Type
Superficial protective barriers	Skin, and body hair	Mechanical
	Oily secretion of skin (sebum)	Mechanical
	Antibodies in sweat	Immune
	The structures that protect the orifices (e.g. eyelids, nostrils, urethra)	Mechanical
	Mucous membranes	Mechanical
	Mucus secreted from mucous membranes	Mechanical
	Antibodies in mucus and tears	Immune
	Ability of wounds to heal	Mechanical
	Ability of blood to clot	Mechanical
Deep protective barriers	Cushioning of subcutaneous tissues (fat)	Mechanical
	Supportive and protective nature of other types of connective tissue in all parts of the body	Mechanical
	Bony skeleton	Mechanical
	Ability of wounds to heal	Mechanical
	Ability of blood to clot	Mechanical
	Immune cells and antibodies in the blood and lymph	Immune

Most of the mechanical barriers serve as a protective method for the body literally by providing physical protection against damage. For this reason healing of wounds and the blood-clotting mechanism have been classified as a mechanical barrier, even though a chain of physiological and chemical responses has to be set in action for them to exert their protective effect. The role of the immune system in protection is even more complex, as it involves the interaction of specialized white blood and other immune cells with substances identified as foreign that are located in the fluid components of the body. Wound healing, blood clotting and the immune system are each discussed in more detail in the following sections.

Health and susceptibility

Overarching the specific protection that the deep and superficial barriers to disease provide is the protection conferred by the general health of the body. Healthy function of any organ or body part will in itself provide a barrier against disease. For example, a perfectly structured heart organ will be less susceptible to heart disease than one with damaged heart valves or a weakness in the heart muscle. A failing organ will be more susceptible to further damage, and this is more likely to become a negative cycle of increasing disease.

In ill health susceptibility is increased because one or more of the barriers to disease will not be functioning as they should. The susceptibility that results from ill health can be categorized as either congenital (dating from the time of birth) or acquired (developing at a later stage in life as a result of deficiency, disease or injury).

Congenital susceptibility

Examples of congenital disease conferring susceptibility to progressive disease include albinism, hemophilia and congenital heart disease. In albinism an inability to produce the skin pigment melanin leads to vulnerability to sunburn and skin cancer and visual impairment. In hemophilia an inability to produce sufficient blood-clotting proteins leads to vulnerability to bleeding into joints and muscles. In congenital heart disease poorly formed heart valves and gaps in the internal muscle wall of the heart lead to vulnerability to poor heart pumping action, breathlessness and, over time, lung damage. The important congenital diseases are described in more detail in Section 5.4c.

Some forms of congenital susceptibility are more subtle. Although a named inherited condition, such as cystic fibrosis, may not be present, it is clear that some people fall ill more often than others, and for some, this has been the case since infancy. The term weak constitution might be applied in such a situation. This will be because the inherited barriers to disease are not as strong as they could be, but the impairment is not so specific as to constitute a named disease.

Acquired susceptibility

Acquired susceptibility is the consequence of a weakening of the barriers to disease after birth. Any one of the conventionally accepted causes of disease (Section 1.1e), such as poor diet, lack of exercise, obesity and smoking, will contribute to increased susceptibility well before disease has developed. For example, a long-term smoker may appear to be very fit but is, in fact, very likely to have sustained damage to a number of the barriers to disease, meaning that they have a higher risk of succumbing to disease. Reasons for this include the fact that smoking damages the protective lining of the lungs, so lung infections are more likely to take hold, and also that it impairs the free circulation of blood and increases the tendency of the blood to clot, which means that diseases of the cardiovascular system such as heart attack are more likely to occur. However, the fact that some smokers do not develop smoking-related diseases tells us that susceptibility is not the same as disease.

A smoker will always increase their risk of developing smoking-related disease by smoking because cigarette smoke invariably damages the lungs and circulation to some degree. If the smoker's constitution is strong, the damage from smoking may not be so severe as to lead to a very high risk of disease, even though the personal risk of disease has undoubtedly increased. A person with an established impairment of the function of the lungs or circulation (e.g. someone with asthma or diabetes) already has an increased risk of developing lung and heart disease. The risk of these diseases therefore becomes even higher if such a person smokes.

Nevertheless, both types of smoker may avoid disease as other factors may be present that reduce susceptibility. For example, in the case of smokers, living in a warm, dry climate may reduce the risk of bronchitis, and eating a healthy, low-fat diet may reduce the risk of circulatory problems. Such factors are known as protective factors. Some protective factors may be far less easy to assess clinically than others – for example, personality traits such as a generally positive attitude or a calm approach to the vicissitudes of life may well be protective against illness.

Periods of naturally increased susceptibility

There are also times within a healthy lifespan when the barriers to disease are less effective. These can be seen as periods of naturally increased susceptibility to disease. Three significant periods when a healthy individual is more than usually susceptible to disease are infancy, pregnancy and old age. In infancy the barriers to disease such as the immune system or the ability to maintain a steady body temperature are not fully mature. In pregnancy the vitality required to maintain the healthy barriers to disease is diverted to the growing fetus (e.g. calcium is diverted to the fetus and the mother's teeth become more vulnerable to decay) and also the rapid and significant changes to the structure and function of a pregnant woman's body can in themselves lead to disease (e.g. hypertension of pregnancy, gestational diabetes, varicose veins and low back pain). In old age, all barriers to disease are in a state of degeneration (e.g. the skin and bones become less strong and are more vulnerable to damage by trauma).

Risk factors

The term risk factor is used medically to describe anything that increases the risk of disease. For example, high blood pressure is a risk factor for stroke, and unprotected sex is a risk factor for developing human immunodeficiency virus (HIV) infection.

Therefore, the presence of a risk factor means that the susceptibility to disease is increased. In fact, any of the conventional external causes of disease (e.g. inadequate diet, insufficient exercise, exposure to radiation and smoking) can also be seen as risk factors for disease.

Preventive medicine

Conventional doctors aim to reduce risk factors in order to prevent disease. Preventive medicine therefore aims to decrease susceptibility to disease.

Disease prevention may be directed at an individual patient, in the form of personalized health education advice, screening for early signs of preventable disease, or by prescribing medication to reduce the impact of risk factors such as high blood pressure. Alternatively, changes can be instituted at a community-based, national or even international level to prevent disease. Such changes may require political reform. The advances in sanitation in the UK made in the 19th century are an example of this sort of wide-scale public health measure. Other examples include legislation concerning the advertising of tobacco products, and supplementation of foods with nutrients, such as folic acid in breakfast cereals. Table 2.1a-II lists some more examples of approaches to the prevention of disease.

Table 2.1a-II Examples of preventive measures against known risk factors for disease

Risk factor	Preventive measure
Meningitis outbreak	Information to the public about warning signs of meningitis to enable early recognition of cases
	Antibiotics prescribed to close contacts of the person with the disease
Unprotected sex	Education campaign about safe sex
	Free condoms at family planning clinics
	Chlamydia infection screening programs
High-fat diet	Education about healthy eating
	Provision of healthy foods in schools
	Government subsidies of healthy foods
Sedentary lifestyle	Encouragement to exercise by providing cheap access to leisure centers, cycle tracks, etc.
	Workplace policies to encourage staff to exercise
Tendency to accidents in childhood	Education of parents about risks
	Safe play area and school environments
	Promotion of safety measures in the home: smoke alarms, stairgates, etc.

Smoking tobacco	Stop smoking campaigns
	Prescription of nicotine patches
	Legislation to control tobacco advertising and packaging
	Taxation of tobacco products
	Smoke-free areas
Alcohol	Restriction on the sale of alcohol to children
	Taxation of alcohol

2.1b Barriers to disease: wound healing

The role of wound healing and clotting[1]

The processes of wound healing and clotting were introduced in Section 2.1a as two of the mechanical barriers to disease. Unlike more structural barriers such as the skin or bony skeleton, these are both dynamic processes that are set in motion after injury has occurred. They prevent the damage from worsening, and enable

repair to take place. In this way, their role is similar to that of the immune system.

The physiology of wound healing[2]

A description of the mechanism of wound healing is fundamental to a full understanding of how the body responds to disease. There are many situations in disease when the healthy structure of the body tissues is damaged and has to be repaired by means of this delicate process. The formation of a blood clot is the first stage of wound healing, and this is described in more detail in Section 2.1c.

Wound healing is least complicated when the injury is clean and there has been a simple cut or puncture to the tissue rather than a loss of tissue. With a clean cut or a puncture the edges of the wound can stay in alignment with each other, and if this ideal is enabled (e.g. by sutures or sterile adhesive tape strips), this provides the conditions for the process known as primary wound healing (or healing by first intention). If there has been loss of skin and underlying tissue, the wound healing has to fill and repair a gaping hole. The reparative process is more complex, takes longer and is prone to complications resulting from trauma and infection. This is known as secondary wound healing (or healing by second intention).

Primary wound healing

Primary wound healing can take place when the edges of a cut or puncture are in close opposition (see Figure 2.1b-I).

	Fibroblast
	Phagocyte

Formation of blood clot   Proliferation   Maturation

Figure 2.1b-I The stages of primary wound healing (healing by first intention)

Figure 2.1b-I illustrates the three stages of primary wound healing after a neat laceration to the skin. The laceration in this image only just penetrates the dermis of the skin, which means it is very superficial. The edges of the wound ooze blood from the broken capillaries, and the blood rapidly

forms into a clot in the confined space. The blood clot releases messenger chemicals that stimulate the process of chemotaxis, the attraction of the cells of the immune system (the leukocytes) and the fibroblasts (the connective tissue repair cells) into the region of the clot. The phagocytic (engulfing) leukocytes move into the clot and absorb and remove cell debris, dirt and bacteria. Fibroblasts lay down a delicate network of fibrous strands that begin to bridge the gap formed by the wound. Into this meshwork the broken ends of the capillaries start to grow a new network of tiny vessels so that this developing scar tissue has a rich blood supply. At the same time, the deepest layer of the epithelium of the broken skin grows through the upper regions of the blood clot to close the breach formed by the injury. This stage is one of proliferation, and when the fibrous and capillary network is sufficiently strong, it causes the scab, the dried blood clot overlying the wound, to drop away, leaving the pink and delicate scar tissue protected by a layer of new epithelium beneath. The proliferative stage takes between 5 and 30 days depending on the size of the wound and the health of the patient. Over the next few days to weeks (the maturation phase) the delicate scar tissue becomes strengthened and more organized as a result of increasing amounts of fibrous tissue. The initially complex network of tiny capillaries is simplified in this phase. At the end of this phase what remains is a stronger, more densely structured and pale tissue than the newly formed scar.

Secondary wound healing

Secondary wound healing is the process that takes place when the wound leaves a gap in both the skin and the underlying connective tissue. Figure 2.1b-II illustrates the three stages of secondary wound healing. As is the case with primary wound healing, the first stage is the lining of this breach with a blood clot originating from blood that has oozed from the remaining damaged tissue. The clot encourages the ingrowth of new fibrous tissue and capillaries and the appearance of phagocytic cells to remove debris and bacteria. This delicate new tissue is known as granulation tissue. This proliferative stage takes longer than the corresponding stage in primary wound healing, the time to healing being dependent on the size of the breach in the tissue, and the health and quality of blood supply to the underlying tissue. If foreign bodies (dirt) and bacteria are present they can be the focus for ongoing damage, and will further slow this stage of the healing process. The initially shallow layer of proliferating new tissue cannot yet be lined by the epithelium and, once the scab drops away, it is covered by a moist yellowing layer of dead cells called slough. Like the old blood clot, slough continues to be a stimulus for the chemotaxis of fibroblasts, leukocytes and new capillaries. Once the new scar tissue reaches the level of the edges of the broken skin epithelium, the new epithelium can grow inwards, closing the breach by degrees. Any breach in an epithelium is called an ulcer, which means that secondary wound healing always involves the formation of an ulcer. Ideally, the ulcer is gradually reduced in size until it is has been closed over entirely by new epithelium. Following the closure of the ulcer the maturation phase continues to strengthen and

organize the new fibrous tissue until the healed wound eventually appears as a pale, shiny patch of tough new scar.

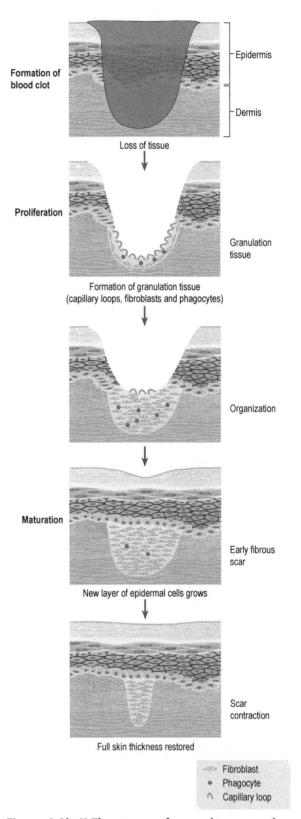

Figure 2.1b-II The stages of secondary wound healing (healing by second intention)

The pathology of wound healing

In general, secondary wound healing is more likely to become problematic than primary wound healing. This is because, in the former, the area of exposed wound is larger, and the new delicate granulation tissue is therefore more likely to become damaged or infected.

There are a number of factors that can negatively affect the healthy course of wound healing. These include the state of nutrition of the body, the richness of the blood supply to the damaged tissue, the presence of infectious organisms or foreign bodies in the wound, and the age of the person.

In malnutrition the response of both the immune system and tissue healing is less efficient. Scurvy, the disease resulting from vitamin C deficiency, is particularly associated with poor wound healing.

In old age, the connective tissue supporting the skin is less vital and more easily damaged, and the healing response is less rapid. A compromised blood supply, such as occurs in the degenerative condition of arteriosclerosis, will also reduce the speed and effectiveness of healing, as this will impair the delivery of the blood that is the source of nutrients and immune cells to the tissues.

Diabetes mellitus is another condition in which the blood supply to the tissues may be compromised. The nerve supply to the tissues may be deficient, meaning that injuries are more easily sustained, and there is an increased risk of minor infections taking hold – this means that wound healing can be very problematic.

Finally, a wound may not heal if it becomes infected or if it becomes repeatedly damaged. This is why such careful attention is given to the application of sterile, strong and breathable dressings in the surgical management of wounds.

Chronic skin ulcer

If a patient has a condition that leads to impaired wound healing, a wound may reach a state of becoming resistant to becoming fully healed. This is particularly likely if it is secondary rather than primary wound healing that is taking place. In such patients, the granulation tissue can easily become infected or damaged, and the wound repeatedly oozes or bleeds. This prevents new skin from growing to close the gap. Such a condition is known as a chronic skin ulcer.

The term chronic refers to the fact that a condition is long-standing. The opposite of the term chronic is acute, meaning short-lived. Contrary to popular understanding, the medical use of these terms does not tell us anything about the severity of a condition. A minor condition can be chronic (e.g. athlete's foot) and a life-threatening condition can be acute (e.g. heart attack).

A chronic skin ulcer is a condition that can be a cause of great disability as a continually discharging wound is both exhausting and painful. Ulcers also carry a long-term risk as a focus for infectious organisms, and for this reason may result in the need for amputation. Patients with diabetes, poor circulation, immobility or malnutrition are particularly at risk of developing a chronic ulcer. The lower legs and areas in which there is repeated damage (e.g. the feet) or pressure (e.g. the buttocks) are the most common sites for ulcers to develop.

Keloid scars

In some people, scars can heal in an abnormal way, with an excessive production of fibrous tissue. This poorly understood condition leads to raised lumps of scar tissue at the site of even minor wounds. These overgrown areas of scarring are known as keloid scars. These can be a cause of distress for the patient, because they may be cosmetically unsightly. Keloid formation appears to be more common in certain individuals and, in particular, in black skin.

Keloid scars are considered very difficult to treat, as simple surgical removal may lead to a scar that produces another keloid. Injection of a corticosteroid preparation into the scar may reduce the swelling in some people.

Conventional treatment of wounds

There are some basic principles that are conventionally followed to enable wounds to heal. These include:

- preventing infection by removing any foreign matter or dead or dying tissue

- encouraging primary wound healing if possible by opposing and stitching the sides of a clean wound

- protecting the healing area with a sterile, breathable, dry dressing

- treating any infection rapidly by cleaning and the use of antibiotics, which are either applied to the wound or taken orally.

Prevention and treatment of poor wound healing and ulcers

In general, there are four broad approaches to someone who is at risk of poor wound healing:

- Preventing injury, for example, attentiveness to skin care in diabetes, and prevention of falls in elderly people.

- Treating the underlying cause, for example, vitamin supplements and increased carbohydrates and proteins in the diet in malnutrition, and improvement of blood supply by means of vascular surgery or drugs that affect the circulation.

- Attentive care to any wound that occurs – the basic principles of enabling wound healing are essential to support healing in vulnerable groups such as elderly people or those with diabetes.

- A chronic ulcer requires regular sterile dressing and cleansing of the open wound area. There can be increasing problems with recurrent infection as the bacteria become resistant to the repeated use of antibiotics. Methicillin-resistant *Staphylococcus* *aureus* (MRSA) has become a particular problem in chronic wounds in recent years, as this form of the normally harmless skin bacterium is now resistant to all the common antibiotics, and can become a life-threatening condition in the immunocompromised. Ideally, the patient should be under the care of a specialist nursing team – access to expertise in approaches to the healing of ulcers is necessary for complex cases.

 Information box 2.1b-I

Wound healing: comments from a Chinese medicine perspective

The Chinese medicine view is that a wound, by disruption of Qi and Blood flow in local Channels, causes impaired flow of Qi and Blood, and thus local Qi and Blood Stagnation. The pain and formation of the blood clot are physical reflections of this. However, here is an example of when Qi and Blood Stagnation in the Channels perhaps may not necessarily signify a wholly negative energetic state, because in this case, from a conventional perspective, the pain and blood clot are both essential to help the healing process.

The intricate processes of healthy wound healing may be seen as manifestations of strong Upright Qi and Blood, and these permit a return to normal flow of the Vital Substances. In particular, the health of the three Chinese Organs of the Spleen and Lung, which govern the muscles and flesh and the transportation of essence to the skin respectively, and of the Kidney, which is the basis of the Yang functions of the Spleen and also supports the grasping of Lung Qi, will be important foundations for wound healing.[3]

An area of scarring will represent relative Qi and Blood Deficiency in the Channels (indicated by the lack of elasticity and patches of numbness associated with scars), but this will be minimal if healing by first intention is possible. This should make sense from the perspective of Chinese medicine, because if the edges of the wound can be brought together, it will mean that the natural flow of Qi and Blood in the area is less likely to be disrupted.

If the damage to the area is large and the original shape of the tissues cannot be restored, Qi and Blood Stagnation are likely to be prolonged, and long-term Qi and Blood Deficiency in the area more marked. In the case of scars that remain painful, this suggests persisting Qi and Blood Stagnation.[4]

Wound healing is dependent on healthy tissue with a rich blood supply and an ability to fight infection. This would suggest that any conditions that involve poor wound healing might point to either a local or a general Blood and Qi Deficiency, and also healing could be complicated if Pathogenic Factors such as Heat, Damp or Phlegm are part of the energetic pattern, either generally or locally. An inherited tendency to poor healing or the poor wound healing seen in old age could indicate an underlying Jing (Kidney Essence) Deficiency.

Healing wounds that continue to ooze blood and fluid suggest the presence of local Heat and/or Damp. However, in Western medicine people with local problems such as this often manifest a number of other symptoms such as poor circulation and cold extremities. This might suggest that the poor wound healing is connected with wider systemic problems such as Deficiency of Spleen Qi, and Spleen not Holding Blood. This is particularly the case in a chronic ulcer, in which poor healing of the underlying flesh might well point to the involvement of the Spleen, which is responsible for the tone and quality of flesh in general.

By contrast, the lumpiness of keloid scars might be interpreted as a manifestation of Phlegm. Preventing a keloid from forming with steroid injections could be interpreted as Moving local Stagnation and Phlegm, but this might carry energetic costs as these injections will not be treating the root imbalance. Steroid injections are recognized to cause thinning and weakening of tissues, and so the benefits of local improvements may come at the price of subsequent local damage of Qi and Yin.

2.1c Barriers to disease: blood clotting

The physiology of blood clotting[5]

As is common experience, in health, bleeding is rapidly terminated by the process of clotting if the skin or mucous membranes become damaged. Gradually, and particularly if the wound is held closed or is padded, the flow of blood from the wound slows down and is replaced by a dark and rubbery mass of congealed blood.

If a syringe of fresh blood is left untouched at room temperature, within a few minutes the blood within it will have separated into a solid clot and a clear fluid known as serum. The serum is the original fluid component of the blood, whereas the clot contains all the blood cells within its solid mass.

Unclotted blood consists of a clear fluid (plasma) that contains a vast range of nutrients, salt and proteins, and three broad groups of cells: red blood cells (erythrocytes), white blood cells (leukocytes) and much smaller cells called platelets (thrombocytes). The tiny platelets and proteins contained in the plasma together constitute the basis of the clotting reaction.

The role of platelets in clotting

Platelets are tiny fragments of cells that are continually produced from larger parent cells within the bone marrow. Their function is to bind with the clotting-factor proteins in the plasma to enable an efficient and controlled clotting reaction. Platelets circulate for only a few days in the blood before they start aging and are removed and broken down in the spleen. If the platelet level falls too low, the kidneys release a protein hormone called thrombopoietin into the bloodstream. This stimulates the bone marrow to generate more platelets to redress the balance. The spleen serves as a store for platelets and can release these in time of stress, such as during a hemorrhage.

Platelets are very sensitive to changes in the blood vessel walls. If a blood vessel wall becomes damaged in any way, the platelets that move past the damaged area respond by adhering to it and then forming a clump around the damaged area. This change is also accompanied by a release of a hormone called serotonin (5HT), which stimulates the damaged vessel to constrict. The sticky platelets also release a chemical called adenosine diphosphate (ADP), which attracts more platelets to the site of damage so that the platelet clump enlarges. The platelets release chemicals that encourage the damaged blood vessel to constrict, so contributing to the reduction of bleeding.

Both these changes, the platelet clumping and the narrowing of the passage through the blood vessel, serve to block the blood flow and reduce any bleeding that might be occurring at the site of the damage. If the wound is small, the platelet plug may be sufficient to stem the bleeding totally in the short term.

The role of clotting factors in clotting[6]

The platelet plug is not sufficiently strong to stem the bleeding from larger wounds or to be maintained for any length of time. In these situations the clotting proteins, a family of 13 different proteins produced by the liver and dissolved in the plasma of the blood, come into play. These proteins undergo a dramatic series of changes at the site of injury that enable the platelet plug to be strengthened. The clotting factors all have descriptive scientific names but are commonly referred to as factors I–XIII.

There are two stimuli that encourage the clotting factors to undergo change. The first is tissue damage and the release of certain chemicals that result from this. These chemicals react rapidly with some of the clotting factors to result in the change of factor II (prothrombin) into an activated form of this factor known as thrombin. Thrombin then stimulates the change of factor I (a soluble protein called fibrinogen) into the fibrous and insoluble fibrin.

The second stimulus to affect other clotting factors in this way, but less rapidly, is the formation of the platelet plug. The end result of this change in this other group of clotting factors is the same as it leads to the formation of activated thrombin and then insoluble fibrin.

The change of fibrinogen to fibrin can be compared to the change that occurs when heat is applied to the soluble albumin contained in egg white. A small change in the external environment generates an irreversible change in the molecular structure and physical nature of the liquid egg white as it transforms into the solid opaque white interior of the hard-boiled egg. So it is with fibrinogen – a small change induced by thrombin causes the production of insoluble fibers that are deposited as a network at the site of tissue damage. This fibrin network traps blood cells and thereby forms the familiar rubbery mass of a blood clot.

This process would carry on unchecked without an opposing process known as fibrinolysis. In fibrinolysis, chemicals released through the activation of clotting factors and from the lining of blood vessels lead to the activation of a plasma protein called plasmin. Plasmin acts to break down fibrin fibers, and so its production helps to ensure that the clotting process is never excessive.

The balance of clotting is very delicate. It seems that, with these closely opposed mechanisms of clotting and fibrinolysis, it is almost as if the body can sense when a clot is of sufficient size for the positive feedback process of its formation to stop, and for the opposing process of fibrinolysis to begin.

The miraculous nature of this degree of sensitivity and balance in the control of clotting becomes apparent when the balance is lost in certain disease states. In some conditions the blood does not clot sufficiently, and this results in excessive bleeding and bruising. In other conditions, excessive blood clot formation is the problem, as it impairs the free circulation of blood in the vessels.

The pathology of insufficient clotting

The speed and efficiency of blood clotting will be impaired if either the number of platelets or the amount of blood clotting factors is insufficient.

Insufficient platelets (thrombocytopenia)[7]

The condition wherein there are insufficient platelets is known as thrombocytopenia (literally meaning too few thrombocytes). This can be the result of a poorly understood immune reaction, when it is called autoimmune idiopathic thrombocytopenic purpura (AITP), or can be a rare side effect of some drug treatments. As platelets are formed in the bone marrow, any condition that damages the bone marrow will also reduce the platelet numbers, as well as the numbers of all the other types of blood cells. Thrombocytopenia therefore also occurs in bone marrow failure. The causes of bone marrow failure include cancer spreading in the bone marrow, and toxic reactions to drugs and radiation. An enlarged spleen can also cause thrombocytopenia. This is because one of the roles of the spleen in health is to store excess platelets, and when the size of the spleen is excessive, too many platelets become hidden from the circulation within the spleen.

The main symptoms and signs of thrombocytopenia are those that result from insufficient stemming of bleeding from broken blood vessels. These include easy bruising, nosebleeds and heavy periods in women. Petechiae are clusters of tiny pinpoint bruises (less than 2mm in diameter) that are a characteristic of thrombocytopenia, and can appear in clusters on areas of skin that are exposed to minor trauma. Purpura refers to slightly larger bruises of 2–10mm in diameter. Purpura and larger bruises will also be seen in this condition.

The treatment of thrombocytopenia is dependent in part on the underlying cause. In AITP and drug-related thrombocytopenia, mild cases may settle naturally or may respond to oral corticosteroid medication (prednisolone tablets). In severe, long-standing (chronic) cases, a surgical option is the removal of the spleen (splenectomy) so that the reduced numbers of platelets are not reduced further by this organ (this operation is described in Section 3.4d). In cases when the numbers of platelets are so low as to lead to a risk of life-threatening bleeding, platelets that have been extracted from donated blood are given by transfusion.

Clotting (coagulation) disorders[8]

Diseases involving insufficiency of one or more of the 13 clotting factors are known as coagulation (clotting) disorders. Hemophilia is a term used to describe the range of disorders of blood coagulation that result from defective production of clotting factors. The three most common forms of hemophilia are hemophilia A, hemophilia B (Christmas disease) and von Willebrand's disease.

Hemophilia A[9] is an X-linked recessive condition, affecting 1 in 5000 of the male population in the developed world. X-linked recessive inheritance means that the gene defect is carried in the X chromosome, and so is rarely expressed in girls because a defective gene from both parents is required for this to happen. As boys only have one X-chromosome, they need inherit the defect from only one parent or have a single spontaneous mutation to develop the condition. The disorder results from defective production of clotting factor VIII. The gene that codes for the production of this factor is found on the X chromosome. Some gene defects lead to more severe forms of the disease than others.

Hemophilia A can become apparent after minor procedures such as circumcision or venepuncture when bleeding is slow to stop naturally. It can lead to life-threatening situations with major surgery if not previously diagnosed. Bleeding associated with factor VIII deficiency tends to manifest in the joints and within muscles much more than is the case in thrombocytopenia. This means that a person with hemophilia might suddenly experience an acutely hot swollen joint (hemarthrosis) or a painful swelling in a muscle (hematoma). As free blood stimulates a powerful reaction from the immune system, it can cause damage and scarring when confined within a joint capsule or in the body of the muscle. Serious long-term complications include joint deformity and contracted muscles. Some patients become wheelchair bound as a result of disability resulting from the scarring from multiple internal bleeds.

The bleeding in hemophilia A is treated by means of replacement of factor VIII. This has to be given intravenously (by means of injection into a vein). Recombinant factor VIII is now manufactured using genetic engineering techniques, but can also be obtained from the plasma of pooled donated blood.

In severe cases when the risk of bleeding is high, regular recombinant factor VIII injections are administered up to three times a week to prevent bruising from occurring.

In the 1980s and 1990s it became clear that thousands of people with hemophilia had contracted HIV and hepatitis C infections through receiving contaminated factor VIII from donated blood. Many people died, or are continuing to suffer from the consequences of these infections. The treatment was given before these diseases were recognized or their mode of transmission was clearly understood. Although blood products are now screened and treated for these viruses, there is still a possibility that they contain as yet uncharacterized transmissible agents, and so the ideal treatment is recombinant factor VIII.

Hemophilia B (Christmas disease) is clinically very similar to hemophilia A. It, too, is an X-linked recessive condition, but results from the absence of clotting factor IX. It affects 1 in 30,000 males.

Von Willebrand's disease (VWD) results from a deficiency of a protein factor that aids in both platelet adherence and the action of factor VIII. This common but usually mild form of hemophilia affects up to 2 percent of the general population. It has various causes, but its most frequent form is as a recessive condition because the

defective gene is found on chromosome pair 12 rather than on an X chromosome. VWD can present with spontaneous bleeding of the gums, excessive bleeding during dental work or heavy menstrual bleeding. It only rarely has more serious presentations, but patients will need specialist preventative treatment to allow them to have surgery.

In all three of the above-described conditions, the severity of the condition depends on the precise nature of the genetic defect.

 Information box 2.1c-I

Insufficient clotting: comments from a Chinese medicine perspective

In Chinese medicine, abnormal bleeding may be described in terms of four Syndromes. These are Spleen Qi Deficiency with Spleen not holding Blood (bleeding tends to be in lower parts of the body), Full Heat (causing profuse bleeds), Yin Deficiency with Empty Heat (less profuse blood; can be a cause of purpura) and Blood Stagnation (dark blood with pain).[10]

Thus the characteristics of these syndromes may be observed in varying degrees in different patients with problems in blood clotting. It would make sense that Yin Deficiency underlies the bleeding in both thrombocytopenia and hemophilia, as the cause of both is a deficiency in the components of the blood. Blood as a body substance carries many of the properties that the Chinese equate with Yin (being, for example, Fluid in nature and Nourishing in action).

The Chinese medical causation of petechiae and purpura in thrombocytopenia is understood in terms of diverse patterns including Wind Invasion, Empty Heat causing blood to leave the blood vessels, Full Heat, Qi Deficiency with Spleen failing to Hold Blood and also Blood Stagnation,[11] whereas profuse bleeds are more in keeping with a diagnosis of Full Heat. It is interesting to note that the site of the destruction of the platelets is the spleen. It would make sense from

this observation that Spleen not holding Blood may also be an aspect of the diagnostic picture in clotting disorders. The purple fixed nature of bruises of all sizes would suggest that local Blood Stagnation is a feature of all forms of thrombocytopenic purpura.

Hemophilia, being a congenital condition, would be understood primarily in terms of an underlying Deficiency in Kidney Essence (Jing). It is this deficiency that engenders Deficiency of Spleen Qi and the inability to Hold Blood. The clotting factors are manufactured in the liver, and this would support a suggestion that Qi Stagnation could be part of the diagnostic picture in the consequences of bleeding in hemophilia. Hemophilia can lead to painful joint bleeds and fixed deformities and contractures of the muscles, which, in Chinese medicine, are most likely to be attributed to Stagnation of Liver Qi and Blood.[12]

Treatment of both involves replacing the missing blood components with a transfusion of concentrates from donated blood. This could be described as a form of Nourishing Yin. Transfusion, however, has a wide range of possible side effects, including allergic reactions, suggesting that there is a risk that Pathogenic Factors, and in particular, Toxic Heat, may be introduced at the same time.

Disorders of excessive clotting

Disorders of excessive or inappropriate clotting are thrombosis, embolism and infarction. These are classed together as one of the seven basic processes of disease, and are introduced in Section 2.2a and discussed in detail in Section 2.2d.

2.1d Barriers to disease: the immune system

A healthy immune system protects against diverse infectious diseases and the development of cancer. It also plays a vital role in the removal of dead or damaged tissues. If it is out of balance, intractable infections, allergies, autoimmune disease and cancer can result.

This section explores the physiology of the immune system and immunity in health. The consequences of deficiency in the immune system, including infections, cancer, allergies and autoimmune disease, are described in Chapter 2.2.

The physiology of the immune system[13, 14]

A crucial difference between the immune system and the other physical barriers to disease is that it is able specifically to distinguish foreign material (e.g. a microbe) within the body and initiate a series of events to neutralize and remove that foreign material.

The structure and function of the immune system can be summarized very broadly as follows:

- the immune system is made up of various different types of white blood cells (leukocytes) that work together to perform the role of protection

- the immune system is able to recognize foreign material

- recognition of foreign material enables the immune cells to make the foreign material harmless to the body through a series of events known as the immune response.

The lymphatic system can be considered to be the home of the immune system.

The lymphatic system

All tissues are bathed in fluid that originates from blood capillaries. This tissue fluid is drained away via vessels called lymphatic vessels. The lymphatic vessels are a complex network of streams that eventually converge to return 3 liters of fluid a day back to the blood circulation at a meeting with the major veins deep in the thorax. As they start to converge, the lymphatic vessels pass through lumps of tissue called lymph nodes. The lymph nodes act as filters for this fluid, and their role is to cleanse the lymph of any foreign matter such as microbes, cancer cells and cell debris.

The network of lymphatics approximately follows the course of the arteries and veins in the body. Like the arteries and veins, the lymphatic system consists of larger vessels deep within the body, which branch repeatedly outwards to form tiny networks of vessels lined only with a single layer of flattened epithelial cells at the periphery of each of the organs and other body parts. Figure 2.1d-I illustrates the distribution of the lymphatic vessels and the lymph nodes in the body, and the way in which the lymphatic system drains into the subclavian veins within the upper thorax.

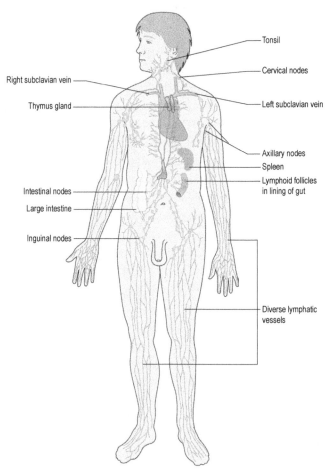

Right subclavian vein

Thymus gland

Intestinal nodes

Large intestine

Inguinal nodes

Tonsil

Cervical nodes

Left subclavian vein

Axillary nodes
Spleen
Lymphoid follicles in lining of gut

Diverse lymphatic vessels

Figure 2.1d-I The lymphatic system

Apart from the lymphatic vessels, the bulk of lymphatic tissue is in the form of lymph nodes, which can be found in deep and superficial groups throughout the body. The large superficial nodes cluster in groups that, when enlarged, can be felt through the skin in the neck (cervical nodes), the elbow and the armpit (trochlear and axillary nodes), at the back of the knee (popliteal nodes) and in the groin (inguinal nodes). There are other important lymph node groups deep within the chest (thoracic cavity), abdomen and pelvis. The structure of a typical lymph node is illustrated in Figure 2.1d-II. This demonstrates the fact that the lymphatic vessels contain valves that enable a one-way circulation of fluid throughout the lymphatic system and the nodes. It also shows that a lymph node consists of islands of dense lymphoid tissue supported by looser (reticular) connective tissue. This lymphoid tissue is the site of maturation of some of the white blood cells (leukocytes).

Figure 2.1d-II Section through a lymph node

In addition to these nodes, lymphatic tissue is found in the form of the tonsils, appendix, spleen and thymus gland, as well as in clusters of cells, called follicles, distributed under the mucous lining of the respiratory and gastrointestinal tracts (known as mucosa-associated lymphoid tissue, or MALT). Each of these regions of the lymphatic system contains islands of lymphoid tissue similar to that found in the lymph nodes. The lymphatic system is structured in such a way that all fluid from the tissues drains through a series of nodes containing lymphoid and reticular tissue before being returned to the bloodstream.

The leukocytes (white blood cells)

The three types of blood cells, red cells, white cells and platelets, are derived from a parent blood cell line that is continually dividing and maturing in the bone marrow. Various subtypes of immature white blood cells emerge from the bone marrow to enter the bloodstream. Some of these subtypes that are important in the immune response

are the T-lymphocytes, B-lymphocytes and phagocytes (e.g. the macrophages and neutrophils). Phagocytes are cells that have the amoeba-like ability to engulf and digest debris and other cells.

T-lymphocytes

The T-lymphocytes are so called because they undergo further maturation in the thymus gland, situated deep in the thorax (see Figure 2.1d-I). While still in the bone marrow, each T-lymphocyte acquires an ability to recognize a very specific molecular shape (known as an antigen). Myriad variations of the T-lymphocyte are formed at this stage in development, each with the ability to recognize a different antigen. It is understood that any T-lymphocytes that develop an ability to recognize a molecular shape that is found in healthy body tissue (i.e. a self antigen) are rapidly inactivated, so that only those that recognize non-self antigens (e.g. proteins on viruses, bacteria, cancer cells and foreign cells) remain to emerge from the thymus gland and to re-enter the circulation.

B-lymphocytes

The B-lymphocytes develop in a similar fashion in the bone marrow, so that myriad subtypes develop. The B-lymphocytes are not just able to recognize foreign antigens, but can also produce and export a protein with a precise structure that enables it to adhere to particular non-self antigens, and so is specifically targeted, rather like a guided missile. The protein manufactured by B-lymphocytes is called immunoglobulin. The individual, specifically shaped immunoglobulin structures that the B-lymphocytes produce are known as antibodies. The molecular shape of the antibody is such that it fits the shape of the antigen rather like a lock fits around a key.

The response of lymphocytes to antigens

When both B- and T-lymphocytes first meet up with a foreign antigen that they have a specific ability to recognize, they become sensitized to it and are stimulated to multiply so that, in time, large numbers of antibodies and T-lymphocytes specific to that foreign antigen are produced. The immune system has a memory for foreign antigens, which is reflected in the fact that if an antigen should be encountered a second time, this response of the sensitized immune cells to multiply and produce antibodies is much more rapid. For T-lymphocytes sensitization occurs in the thymus gland, and for B-lymphocytes it occurs in the lymphoid tissue of the lymph nodes.

When the antigen key fits the lock of the T-lymphocyte surface or the circulating antibody produced by B-lymphocytes, a chain of events, known as the immune response, is triggered (see below).

In the case of a T-lymphocyte, the connection with an antigen may first require the antigen to be presented to the T-lymphocyte by means of one other immune cell, the macrophage. This intermediary role of the macrophage is not necessary for antigens on the surface of large cells, such as cancer cells. The recognition and connection with the non-self antigen triggers a change within the T-lymphocyte so that it will then act in diverse ways to enable the removal of the foreign matter. Subtypes of T-lymphocytes act in different ways to do this. Cytotoxic T-lymphocytes (CTL) recognize and respond to foreign, cancerous and infected cells, and inject toxins to destroy them. Helper T-lymphocytes (TH) multiply to produce chemicals to support the other immune cells. These cytokines, which include interleukins and interferons, stimulate the action of cytotoxic T-lymphocytes and macrophages. Helper T-lymphocytes also appear to be important in enabling the role of the B-lymphocytes in the production of antibody in the lymph nodes. Again, the cytokines are important in this role. A third category, the suppressor T-lymphocyte, is important in modulating the immune response so that it is not too excessive and is not directed towards self antigens. Finally, the memory T-lymphocyte persists to stimulate the production of specific cytotoxic, helper and suppressor T-lymphocytes when the need arises. The different roles of the T-lymphocytes are illustrated in Figure 2.1d-III.

The B-lymphocytes that leave the bone marrow migrate and lodge in lymphoid tissue, and here they stay. In the presence of foreign antigens, sensitized helper T-lymphocytes drawn from the circulation encourage the expansion of specific B-lymphocytes into specific antibody-producing plasma cells. The plasma cell has a very short life of less than a day, but in this time produces an antibody that can circulate in the bloodstream and target the foreign antigens. The short life of the plasma cell means that, once the antigen has been removed, the antibody response ceases. Memory B-lymphocytes persist to stimulate the production of more plasma cells should the need for more antibodies continue. The production of the two forms of B-lymphocytes is illustrated in Figure 2.1d-IV.

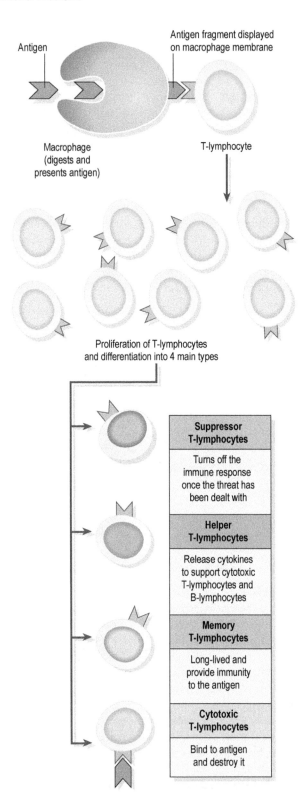

Figure 2.1d-III The four types of T-lymphocyte

Antigen

Receptor for antigen

+

Sensitized
T-lymphocyte

**T-B lymphocyte
co-operation**

B-lymphocyte in
lymphoid tissue

Proliferation of B-lymphocytes
and differentiation into 2 main types

Antibodies

Antigen

Plasma cells	Memory B-lymphocytes
Produce and release antibodies that bind to the antigen and cause its destruction	Long-lived and provide immunity to the antigen

Figure 2.1d-IV The two types of B-lymphocyte

The immune complex and activation of complement

When an antigen-specific antibody is circulating in the bloodstream, the connection of antibody with the antigen on the surface of the foreign matter forms a structure called an immune complex. The characteristic shapes of immune complexes are recognized by phagocytic (cell-engulfing) leukocytes such as neutrophils and macrophages, which are then stimulated to surround and digest the foreign matter. The antibody-antigen immune complex is also a trigger for the activation of a group of proteins in the bloodstream called complement. Activated complement protein is toxic to cells that are bound by antibodies, and it also stimulates the healing response of inflammation, another very important aspect of the healing response to foreign material (described later in this section).

Different forms of antibodies

Different forms of antibodies are recognized, although each has a similar immunoglobulin (Ig) structure.

Immunoglobulin M (IgM) is the antibody produced when a foreign antigen is first encountered by B-lymphocytes. A raised level of specific IgM detected by a blood test tells the doctor that the patient is showing a first response to an infection. IgM is a particular trigger for the activation of the complement proteins that enable destruction of foreign organisms and stimulate inflammation.

IgG is the antibody that is produced once B-lymphocytes have been sensitized, and this will persist after an infection has settled down. If specific IgG levels are raised, this tells a doctor that a person has immunity to a condition.

IgA is a particular form of antibody produced in body fluids such as tears and saliva and is also found in breast milk. IgA forms one of the first lines of defense for the body as well as the newborn baby.

IgE is present on the surface of other leukocytes called basophils, eosinophils and mast cells, which, when they encounter antigens, release chemicals that also stimulate inflammation.

The effect of the immune response

The immune response is a chain of reactions that culminates in the removal of the foreign material. To summarize, the aspects of the immune response that enable the foreign material to be removed include:

- Release of chemicals to attract more immune cells around the foreign material (complement and cytokines from helper T-lymphocytes).

- Release of chemicals in response to immune complexes, which can break down and digest foreign material that has been bound by antibodies (complement).

- Direct killing of foreign or damaged human cells (cytotoxic T-lymphocytes).

- Phagocytosis of microbes and particles of other foreign material that have been bound by antibodies (neutrophils and macrophages).

- Stimulation of the production of more antibodies (helper T-lymphocytes and plasma cells).

- Release of chemicals (complement, basophils, eosinophils and mast cells) to stimulate inflammation (a process that provides the best possible environment for the immune response to take place).

These reactions have the following effects that are experienced by a patient suffering a microbial infection:

- The attraction of more immune cells and inflammation at the lymph nodes leads to swollen and tender lymph nodes (glands). In a generalized infection, all nodes can be affected. If the infection is in only one part of the body, for example, in the thigh, only the local lymph glands, in this case, the inguinal nodes, will be affected.

- Release of various chemicals by the leukocytes into the bloodstream can lead to the symptoms of fever and malaise. These may have a protective function in that they cause the patient to rest while the infection is being dealt with.

Immunity

Immunity describes the ability of the immune system to recognize foreign material, such as a microbe, and to produce an effective immune response. Immunity is the consequence of the B- and T-lymphocytes being able to become sensitized to foreign antigens and thereafter develop a memory to a specific infectious agent. Immunity enables a rapid immune response to an infection. In an immune person large quantities of IgG antibody can be produced so quickly that the infection may not be allowed to take hold. This ability of the immune system to respond tends to wear off with time, but the memory can be reinforced if the body has repeated encounters with a microbe in a short period of time.

The development of immunity explains why there are certain illnesses, such as chickenpox, which are usually experienced only once in a lifetime. During the initial infection, the immune system learns to develop very effective antibodies to the chickenpox virus. When the body next encounters chickenpox, these antibodies are reproduced so rapidly that the virus is destroyed and removed from the body before the infection can take hold.

Active immunization

Active immunization (vaccination) is a process through which the tendency of the body to develop a memory to foreign antigens is encouraged. The aim of active immunization is to induce immunity to a certain disease, but without the risks inherent in first developing that disease.

Active immunization involves exposing the patient to a foreign material (a vaccine) that is very like a particular infectious agent or a toxic product of that agent. However, the ideal vaccine contains an infectious agent that has been altered so that it no longer has the properties that cause the original disease, and thus carries no risk of disease. The ideal vaccine still retains the antigens of the original infectious agent, so that the immune response is stimulated. In most cases the vaccine is administered by injection into a muscle or just under the skin. One exception to this rule is the live poliovirus vaccine (Sabin vaccine), which is administered by mouth, although this is no longer the usual form of this vaccine used in childhood vaccine programs in many developed countries.

Vaccines usually need to be given more than once, as they are unlikely to stimulate as strong an immune response as the infectious disease itself. For example, in the UK the combination vaccine containing diphtheria, tetanus, pertussis, inactivated polio and *Haemophilus influenzae* type b (DTaP-IPV-Hib vaccine) is given to infants in a course of three successive injections separated by four weeks. All but the Hib component are then repeated at the preschool entry, and the DTa-IPV is then offered to teenagers as a booster. A final DTa booster is recommended to complete protection for tetanus a further ten years later.[15]

Vaccines may come in the form of live, but attenuated, strains of the original infectious agent. The measles, mumps and rubella (MMR) vaccine contains three live attenuated viruses. These all induce an immune response, and can cause fever and even a rash in the recipient, but have been modified in a way that means a dangerous contagious infectious disease will not develop. Nevertheless, each of the three strains is sufficiently similar to measles, mumps and rubella that immunity to the diseases will result in 91–95 percent of those who receive the vaccination (this involves giving two doses separated by a minimum of three months).[16]

Alternatively, some vaccines consist of agents that have been treated so that they no longer have infectious potential. For example, the tetanus immunization carries no risk of causing infectious disease. This is because it contains formaldehyde-modified tetanus toxin (toxoid), which is sufficiently like the tetanus toxin to stimulate immunity, but modified so as to no longer be toxic.

Passive immunization

Passive immunization is a term used to describe the administration of antibodies that confer immunity but do not stimulate an immune response or an immunological memory. Passive immunization is achieved by preparing concentrates of immunoglobulin from the plasma of donated blood. Passive immunization is useful when the risk of infection is high and there is no time to stimulate immunity by means of a course of vaccination, for example, the use of rabies-specific immunoglobulin to prevent rabies after a bite from an infected dog.[17]

Babies are born in a state of passive immunization, as their mother's IgG antibodies remain circulating in their bloodstream for a few weeks after birth. The protection these offer is reinforced by IgA antibodies present in breast milk.

Information box 2.1d-I

The immune system: comments from a Chinese medicine perspective

A healthy immune system protects against diverse infectious diseases and the development of cancer. If it is out of balance it can lead to infections, cancer, allergy and autoimmune disease. According to Chinese medicine theory, healthy Wei (Defensive) Qi and its foundation, Kidney Yang, are required to protect against invasions of External Pathogenic Factors, so it might be an easy assertion to make that a healthy immune system suggests flourishing Wei Qi and Kidney Yang. The foundation of Wei Qi and Kidney Yang is healthy Kidney Essence (Jing), which, according to Chinese theory, is the basis of constitutional strength.[18]

However, from a broader perspective, the health of the Qi of all the Organs, and in particular, Zheng (Upright) Qi, is necessary for good health. As Maciocia comments, "If Qi is flourishing, there is health, if it is weak there is disease, if it is balanced there is quiet, if it moves in the wrong direction there is disease."[19] It is therefore reasonable to suggest that there is no one Substance or Organ in Chinese medicine that directly corresponds to the immune system. A healthy immune system corresponds to a body with good Upright Qi and healthy Organ functions.

According to Chinese medicine, the coarse form of Qi known as Wei Qi is the superficial defense against invasion of Pathogenic Factors. If strong invasions of Pathogenic Factors, then in particular, Exterior Wind, cannot penetrate, and the person is protected from coughs, colds, chills and fevers. As defenses from coughs and colds are considered to reside in the immune cells of the circulation and lymph nodes, as well as the integrity of the defenses of the respiratory system, a physiological counterpart to the defensive Wei Qi might be the leukocytes of the immune system and the health of the tissues of the nose, throat and the respiratory tree and the subcutaneous tissues.

With regard to the protection against autoimmune disease and cancer, from a Chinese medicine viewpoint, both conditions occur on a background of long-standing Deficiency of Blood, Kidney Yang and/or Yin. These two complex diseases are manifestations of the additional presence of Pathogenic Factors, including Heat, Damp, and accumulations such as Blood Stagnation or Phlegm, which have developed as a consequence of the long-standing background deficiency.

With this understanding we can also see that the healthy immune system depends not only on healthy Wei Qi and Jing, but also healthy Vital Substances, Yin and Yang. This would fit with the general observation that any form of slight imbalance (e.g. feeling stressed or run down) can increase susceptibility to infections, irrespective of the nature of the imbalance.

The concept of acquired immunity following an infectious disease is also difficult to describe in Chinese medicine terms. On that basis it would have to be asserted that, following an infection, defensive Wei Qi is actually strengthened. As a febrile disease is perceived as an invasion of an External Pathogenic Factor like Wind Heat, it appears that, when immunity is strengthened as a result of an infectious disease, this infection has, in the long term, had a beneficial outcome. It has been suggested, for example, by Gascoigne (2001),[20] that in some infectious diseases the appearance of a Pathogenic Factor on the Exterior is potentially beneficial because it represents the release of deeply rooted Heat Toxins. In this way minor infectious disease is seen as a potentially beneficial experience, through which deeper Pathogenic Factors can be expelled and Upright Qi strengthened.

2.2 Processes of Disease

2.2a Introduction to processes of disease

Classification of disease

Within conventional medical thought, diseases can be classified according to specific, clearly defined criteria. There are various methods of classification that all share the potential benefit of clarifying those features that disparate diseases may have in common, thus aiding communication about these diseases.

Diseases may be classified according to cause, and this is known as classification by etiology. Understanding the language of etiology is essential for the discussion of prevention of disease. A classification system that focuses on the disease mechanisms (pathogenesis of disease) is a prerequisite for beginning to understand which treatments may be most effective for different diseases and also for predicting outcome (prognosis).

All systems of medicine, be they holistic or conventional, have their own systems of classification of etiology and pathogenesis.

Etiology of disease

Etiology, literally meaning the study of causes, is the term used to describe the causation of disease. From a conventional medical viewpoint, the cause of disease can be simplified into a few distinct categories, including:

- congenital defects (acquired between the time of conception and birth)

- infectious agents

- physical trauma (including extremes of temperature and radiation)

- effects of drugs, chemicals and toxins

- degeneration (resulting from overuse and aging)

- psychological stressors

- iatrogenic condition (caused by medical treatment) – this category will, of course, overlap with any one of the others

- unknown cause – the terms idiopathic and essential may be ascribed to diseases of unknown cause (e.g. idiopathic thrombocytopenic purpura and essential thrombocythemia).

The seven processes of disease

Pathogenesis (literally, the birth of disease) is the term used to describe the physical basis of how disease develops in terms of the basic biological processes of disease. The diverse forms of the disease process can be grouped into seven broad categories:

- inflammation (redness, swelling, heat, pain or loss of function of tissues)

- tumors (excessive or inappropriate growth of cells)

- abnormal immune mechanisms (either under- or overactive immune responses)

- thrombosis, embolism and infarction (excessive or inappropriate clotting)

- degeneration (wearing out of tissues through aging or trauma)

- metabolic abnormalities (homeostatic biochemical functions of the cells become imbalanced)

- genetic abnormalities (the cells carry defective genetic material that means they function in a less than healthy way).

From the perspective of the study of clinical medicine, classification of the processes of disease is important because it generates principles of causation of disease that can then be applied to all diseases. For example, if the process of inflammation is understood, this will aid in the study of any one of the diseases that involves inflammation, such as arthritis, dermatitis, meningitis and pneumonia. Because the understanding of the first four basic processes of disease is fundamental to the study of the pathology of all diseases, they are explored in some depth in this text, in Sections 2.2b, 2.2c, 2.2d and Chapter 2.3.

The remaining three processes of disease – degeneration, metabolic disease and genetic disease – are now briefly attended to.

Degeneration is the result of aging. In general, aging (senescence) involves cell loss and atrophy of tissues. Rapidly regenerating active tissue may, through the process of senescence, become replaced with tough, fibrous, less active tissue, and organs may cease to function as effectively. Deformities (e.g. of skin, joints or bones) become commonplace. Degenerative diseases are discussed later, according to the physiological system that they affect.

The category of metabolic abnormality embraces all diseases that result from imbalance in the homeostatic function for metabolism (the chemical processes that go on continuously in living cells). These include common diseases such as diabetes, and hypothyroidism. Again, the metabolic disorders are discussed throughout the text according to the physiological system that they affect.

The principles of genetic (congenital) abnormalities have been discussed in Section 1.1b, under the heading "Mutation."

An understanding of the processes of disease can aid thinking about disease from the perspective of another medical system. If it is possible to consider each process of disease in terms of corresponding pathological descriptions described in another medical system, it is possible to take these correspondences and use them to help describe pathological processes in all manner of diseases. For example, inflammation always involves the generation of redness and heat in tissues. According to Chinese medicine, redness and local heat always corresponds to the Pathogenic Factor of Heat. Therefore, it would be reasonable to conclude that all inflammatory diseases will be described, amongst other things, in terms of Heat in Chinese medicine. In this section, all the processes of disease are also interpreted in terms of Chinese medicine, and this will provide the foundation for the Chinese medicine interpretations of all the individual diseases described later in the text.

In summary, it cannot be overstated how much the understanding of the basic processes of disease can enrich the understanding of conventional pathology. An added benefit is that processes of disease can also inform us about Chinese medical pathology and so help us to understand what sort of Chinese medical disease descriptions (syndromes) might be relevant in the diseases described by Western medicine.

 Information box 2.2a-I

Processes of disease: comments from a Chinese medicine perspective

As a general introduction, it is important to explain the rationale for comparing the conventional view of the processes of diseases with a Chinese medicine understanding of pathology. As stated in the text, in the study of clinical medicine classification of the processes of disease is important because it generates principles of causation of disease that can then be applied to all diseases. For example, an understanding of the process of inflammation will aid in the study of any disease that involves inflammation, such as arthritis, dermatitis, meningitis and pneumonia.

An important aspect of this system of classification from our point of view is that, although the understanding of conventional processes would have involved knowledge that would not have been familiar to the ancient Chinese, the manifestations of the processes in signs and symptoms are consistent within each process. It is these that are the bridge between the two systems of medicine.

Inflammation will always have characteristics of heat and swelling, and degeneration will always involve a drying and withering of tissue. As observable phenomena, these would form the basis for making a diagnosis in Chinese medicine. However, the way in which the heat and swelling is generated in each individual case does not share the same consistent internal process as understood in the conventional view, and looking for parallels of process is a trap for the unwary.

When a patient presents with a condition that results from one or more of the seven processes of disease, it can reasonably be expected that the symptoms and signs normally associated with those processes are evident. The meaning and importance of the signs and symptoms can then be assessed within the entirely different understanding of the manifestation of symptoms and signs described in Chinese medicine. What this means is that the symptoms and signs of the conventionally described processes of disease will help point to the Chinese medicine syndromes that might be expected to be discerned in any medical condition, first assuming the underlying process of disease is recognized.

A Chinese energetic interpretation of inflammation

Inflammation is a basic response to tissue damage that results in increased blood flow to the tissues, swelling from increased tissue fluid, pain as a result of the release of irritant cell contents and loss of function of the body part as a result of pain and swelling. Together these factors result in the five characteristics of inflamed tissue described in medicine as redness, swelling, heat and pain (or in Latin, as "rubor, tumor, dolor, calor"), and loss of function.

In Chinese medicine the characteristics of redness and heat would point to Heat, either locally or generally. The excess tissue fluid would often be associated with an underlying Pathogenic Factor such as Damp, especially if there was any oozing of liquids or the swelling was considerable. The swelling in a clearly defined area would itself point to local Stagnation, usually of Qi or Blood, and the character of the pain would indicate which. If inflammation is confined to one peripheral body part, the term Bi Syndrome may be applied in Chinese medicine, as this describes localized manifestations of Pathogenic Factors in the Channels, particularly in the region of the joints.

In conclusion, inflammation in the body might be described as evidence of localized or generalized Heat with Qi or Blood Stagnation, often with underlying Damp.

A Chinese energetic interpretation of tumors

Tumors result from excessive and inappropriate overgrowth of tissue cells. The underlying problem from a conventional medicine perspective is that the genetic control of cell multiplication has become disordered, and the immune system has failed to recognize and control the growth of these disordered cells.

In Chinese medicine, substantial masses that do not move easily are often regarded as manifestations of either Phlegm or Blood Stagnation (or sometimes a combination of both). Blood Stagnation is characterized by hardness and intense boring pain with violaceous color changes. Phlegm is more often associated with numbness, and will usually develop against a backdrop of Heat and Damp, which will manifest in other signs and symptoms. For long-standing masses to develop there has to be a pre-existing state of Stagnation of Qi, as it is only healthy Qi moving freely that prevents the development of Stagnation and Phlegm. Usually this means there has been underlying Deficiency of Qi together with chronic emotional factors causing the Stagnation of Qi. However, some masses can manifest against a background of good Upright Qi, the strength of which ideally should be considered when determining priorities in treatment.

Chinese medicine recognizes that in addition to Qi Stagnation and the ensuing Accumulation and Blood Stagnation that a cancerous lump may also be manifesting the presence of a Heat Toxin that could well be environmental in origin, and so Chinese medical treatments for cancer would include herbs for clearing Toxins.[21, 22]

In conclusion, tumors in the body might be described as evidence of Phlegm and/or Blood Stagnation (with possible additional Heat Toxins) having developed on an underlying background of Stagnation of Qi with likely Qi Deficiency.

A Chinese energetic interpretation of abnormal immune mechanisms

Abnormal immune mechanisms fall into two broad categories: those involving an insufficient response to infection, and those involving inappropriate responses, where there is hypersensitivity to specific stimuli or the misrecognition of the body's own cells as a threat.

In Chinese medicine, the functions of a healthy immune system are reflected in the concept of healthy Upright Qi. The foundation of healthy Upright Qi lies in Kidney Essence and also Spleen Qi, and both are the basis of healthy Wei Qi.

Some of the patterns of abnormal immune responses, for example, type I allergic hypersensitivity, which manifest features of acute invasion of Pathogenic Factors, are reflected in recognized patterns of disruption of Wei Qi, and suggest deficiencies either in Wei Qi or in the underlying Kidney Essence itself. The allergen is seen in Chinese medicine as a Toxic Pathogenic Factor, to which healthy people are resistant. In the case of allergy, it is usually chronic Spleen Qi that leads to Wei Qi insufficiency and allows for invasion of Pathogenic Wind Cold (causing rhinitis, for instance) or Wind Heat (urticarial itch). Susceptible individuals may also be susceptible because of chronic Phlegm or Heat affecting their system. These Pathogenic Factors may then become manifest following exposure to the environmental trigger.[23]

Others, for example, in multisystem autoimmune disease, present much more of a pattern of Toxic Pathogenic Factors against a background of long-term chronic deficiency that very often appears to be rooted in Spleen Qi Deficiency with Liver Qi Stagnation and resulting Deficiencies of Liver Blood, Kidney Yin and Yang.[24]

In conclusion, inappropriate immune responses might be described as evidence of Chronic Deficiency of Qi and, in particular, Spleen Qi leading to Deficiency of Wei Qi in the case of allergy, and a wider pattern of mixed chronic Deficiency and Excess in multisystem autoimmune disease. Deficiency of Kidney Essence may well, of course, be at the root of either condition.

A Chinese energetic interpretation of thrombosis, embolism and infarction

Excessive blood clotting in the peripheral parts of the body is characterized by intense pain, coldness, violaceous coloration and loss of function if severe (e.g. arterial blood flow restriction in the lower leg) or by swelling, less intense pain and local inflammation (venous thrombosis) if less severe. Thrombosis in the brain can lead to stroke and, of the other internal organs including the heart, severe life-threatening illness.

The former symptoms of pain, coldness and purple coloration are all associated with what is described in Chinese medicine as Stasis of the flow of Blood, and there are numerous factors, including the Deficient states of Qi, Blood and Yang Deficiency, and also the more Full conditions of Qi Stagnation and Cold that can predispose to Blood Stasis. In most cases of Stasis unrelated to trauma, the patient will be depleted in some way. Causative patterns include Depleted Blood, Qi and Yang Deficiency, which all predispose to invasion of factors that can impair the flow of Blood and Qi, such as Toxic Cold, Heat and Phlegm. Dietary and lifestyle factors as well as emotional imbalance will all contribute to Blood Stasis. Blood Stasis can then also in itself engender Heat, Phlegm, and also Wind.

Peripheral venous thrombosis results from a significant region of blood clot in a deep vein, often resulting from sustained inactivity. The substantial accumulation of solid mass is suggestive of the concept of Phlegm resulting from Blood Stasis in Chinese medicine, and indeed, the symptom of swelling with less intense pain in venous thrombosis is consistent with this. The inflammation seen with venous thrombosis is also suggestive of Heat. Peripheral venous thrombosis can dramatically extend and progress to pulmonary embolus, which, if mild, leads to severe localized chest pain and, if severe, collapse and death. These suggest Blood Stagnation and Phlegm misting the Orifices of the Heart respectively. Again, the severe Phlegm-related Syndrome seems to be a progression from Blood Stasis in pulmonary embolus.

In angina there is restriction of blood flow to the heart. This manifests as severe stabbing pain in the chest and in Chinese medicine this is understood as Blood Stasis resulting from various factors including severe Deficiency of Blood and Qi (such as occurs in old age) and with invasion of Cold or Phlegm Heat blocking the Channels leading to Blood Stasis and pain. If severe, there can be coronary thrombosis, a result of total blockage of coronary arteries. There are life-threatening arrhythmias that might relate in Chinese medicine to extreme Heart Qi/Yang Depletion due to the Heart lacking in nourishment from Blood and Qi. These may cause loss of consciousness, again, a manifestation of Phlegm misting the Orifices of the Heart.[25]

A stroke also suggests Phlegm misting the Orifices of the Heart.

In conclusion, thrombosis, embolism and infarction might be described as evidence of Blood Stasis and Qi Stagnation and resulting from prior Deficiency, and with subsequent invasion of Pathogenic Factors that contribute to formation of Phlegm. In severe cases, Yin and Yang may be consumed, and this will manifest in severe life-threatening illness.

A Chinese energetic interpretation of degeneration

In conventional medicine, degeneration of tissues involves excessive cell death, poor healing responses and the formation of less vital tissues, with excessive fibrous tissue and deposits of substances such as calcium salts that impede healthy function. The resulting tissues tend to be less springy and soft and resilient, and may also manifest with deformities (lumps and bumps).

In Chinese medicine language, all these changes, if seen across large areas of the body, would be primarily described in terms of broad deficiencies of Yin and Yang, as these substances are expressed in the vitality and healthy function of the tissues respectively. More particularly, they are linked with a deficiency rooted in the Kidneys, and are characteristic of the aging process as Kidney Essence becomes depleted. The deposits and deformities are evidence of a widespread impairment in flow of Qi, leading to an accumulation of Pathogenic Factors such as Phlegm and Damp and Blood Stagnation. If these are localized, there may be evidence of local Qi or Blood Stagnation impairing the flow of Qi to part of the body, in which case there may be pain and purplish discoloration.

In conclusion, degeneration of a body part might be described as evidence of Deficiency or Yin and/or Yang, in particular, of Kidney Qi/Essence, leading to a tendency to Qi and Blood Stagnation and an accumulation of Phlegm/Damp and other Pathogenic Factors.

A Chinese energetic interpretation of metabolic abnormalities

The metabolic diseases are complex and have diverse symptoms depending on the fundamental abnormality. Most metabolic diseases will be manifest in the function of all the body tissues and so reflect a fundamental and profound state of imbalance.

Chinese interpretations of metabolic disease will be equally complex, and are likely to describe deep deficiency. Often these conditions will fit in to the category of "Knotty Disease"[26] in Chinese medicine. This is because a profound and prolonged deficiency will often result in full Pathogenic Factors, which create complex patterns of signs and symptoms. As in conventional medicine, the effects are likely to be widespread in the energetic system rather than confined just to Channels.

A Chinese energetic interpretation of genetic abnormalities

A genetic abnormality may affect every cell in the body (if present from the time of conception), or may be the result of a developmental problem in the womb and thus affect some body parts and not others. From a conventional medicine perspective, there is no doubt that a congenital abnormality will compromise the health of the child and, unless carefully managed, is likely to affect the growth and development of the affected child.

The ancient Chinese interpreted congenital disease (i.e. a condition present from the time of birth) as a Deficiency of Kidney Essence (Jing). Zhang Jing Yue (c.1563–1640; original name, Zhang Jie Bin) described the Ming Men (which he associated with both kidneys) as the source of Essence and the foundation of full health: "Ming Men is the mansion of both water and fire, the house of Yin and Yang, the sea of Essence and Blood, the nest of Life and Death. If the Ming Men is depleted and damaged, the five Zang and six Fu lose their sustenance, and the Yin and Yang will become sick, causing all types of disorders."[27]

To the Chinese, Kidney Essence was passed to the fetus from the parents at the time of conception. It was what determined a person's constitutional strength and vitality, and is fundamental to healthy growth and development.[28, 29] Kidney Essence underlies the health of all the organs, and so more specific imbalances will often be present as the visible sequelae of the congenital disorder (e.g. of Spleen and Lung Qi in cystic fibrosis).

In conclusion, a congenital problem might be described as evidence of primarily Jing Deficiency, but may be described as a specific Organ Deficiency, depending on where the underlying genetic defect manifests.

2.2b Inflammation

The physiology of acute inflammation

Inflammation is the term used to describe a complex bodily response to damage. It is derived from the Latin, meaning to set on fire, reflecting the fact that two manifestations of inflammation are heat and redness. Two other important features are swelling and pain. These characteristics of inflammation have been familiar to doctors over many centuries. They were noted by the 1st-century Roman medical encyclopedist Celsus as calor (heat), tumor (swelling), rubor (redness) and dolor (pain).[30]

Inflammation has one other major characteristic in that it leads to loss of function of the affected body part. Swelling and pain largely contribute to this loss of function. In mild disease, loss of function can be beneficial, as it encourages the patient to rest the inflamed area, and this should promote healing. For example, inflammation of the voice box (laryngitis) may give rise to discomfort and malaise. This means that the patient avoids talking, and may wish to rest in bed. Both these responses will promote healing.

In severe disease, the loss of function can jeopardize the health of the whole body, and is not beneficial. For example, inflammation of the lining of the brain resulting from bacterial infection (meningitis) leads to swelling of the brain and carries the risk of coma and death.

The five characteristics of inflammation are listed in Table 2.2b-I.

Table 2.2b-I The characteristics of inflammation

Redness
Heat
Swelling
Pain or tenderness
Loss of function

When a body part is inflamed, it is often medically described by the suffix "-itis." This may be added on to the common name for the affected organ or, more usually, to the Latin term for the organ. Hence in tonsillitis, dermatitis, laryngitis, osteomyelitis and tendonitis we would expect to find inflammation of the tonsils, skin, larynx, bone marrow and tendons, respectively.

The trigger for inflammation is tissue damage. When tissues are damaged, cells are ruptured and release their contents. The presence of cell contents in the extracellular space has a powerful effect on the immune system and the capillary cells. The released chemical contents of cells signal to the immune system and capillary cells that there is cell debris that needs removing, that repairs may need to be performed, and that there might be foreign bodies and infectious organisms to be eradicated. Their presence induces responses in immune and epithelial cells that bring about the inflammatory response, and thus begins the process of healing. The chemicals released include the inflammatory mediators including prostaglandins, histamine, serotonin (5HT) and bradykinin.

The purpose of inflammation in health is protective. It enables isolation and inactivation of foreign material and damaged tissue, and leads to its removal from the body.

Some of the key players in the inflammatory response to tissue damage (described below) are illustrated in Figure 2.2b-I.

Hyperemia

A cardinal response in inflammation is that blood flow to the damaged area increases, a result of widening of the small blood vessels (vasodilatation). This response is termed hyperemia (literally meaning more blood). Hyperemia leads to the increased warmth and redness that are characteristic of inflammation. Hyperemia also contributes to tissue swelling.

Exudation

Another response of the blood vessels to inflammatory chemicals is that gaps form between the epithelial cells of the vessels so that molecules and fluids move out of capillaries into the fluid surrounding the tissue cells. In this way important proteins such as antibodies and fibrinogen enter the site of the damage. This reaction, known as exudation, leads to the swelling that is characteristic of

inflammation. Fibrinogen, one of the 12 clotting factors in the blood, is converted to fibrin once it enters tissue fluid, and in this way it forms a meshwork that contains the inflamed area and thus prevents the spread of any infection that may be present. Antibodies bind to foreign antigens at the site of the inflammation and so form immune complexes that are then engulfed by phagocytic cells such as neutrophils.

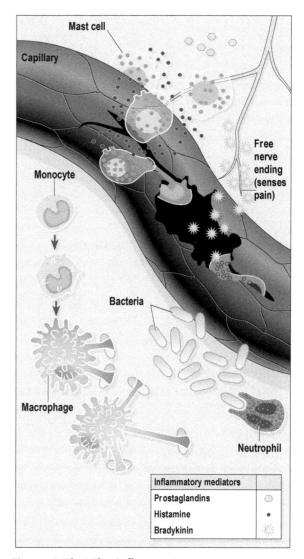

Figure 2.2b-I The inflammatory response

Migration of leukocytes

Various forms of leukocytes, which are the basis of the immune system, are attracted from the blood and the tissue fluid to the site of the damage by the chemicals (chemotaxins) that have been released as a consequence of the damage. Neutrophils are amoeba-like white cells that appear rapidly at the site of inflammation. These have the capacity to engulf and digest any material that presents foreign antigens in the form of an immune complex. In this process, the phagocytic cells may die, releasing their greenish cell contents. It is these discharged cell contents that contribute to the green color of pus, which is usually only formed as a consequence of a heavily infected wound. Macrophages are slower moving, larger phagocytic cells, which, after a few hours, also enter the site of inflammation to engulf and digest cell debris, microbes and dead neutrophils.

Increased body temperature

If the bodily response of inflammation is sufficiently large, interleukin-1, a chemical released by macrophages, can lead to an increase in the core temperature of the body. The fever that results leads to more efficient activity of phagocytes and also encourages the patient to rest. Fever is thus understood to be beneficial to the healing process in inflammation.

Pain

The chemicals released by damaged and inflammatory cells tend to irritate the local nerve endings, so leading to the acute pain and intense tenderness associated with inflammation.

Resolution of acute inflammation

In uncomplicated situations, the inflammatory process leads to removal of damaged cells, dirt and infectious organisms, and provides a clean environment for the process of wound healing. The redness, swelling, pain and heat resolve, the function of the area is restored and healing is complete, with or without scar formation.

Chronic inflammation

The resolution of inflammation may be hindered by a poor blood supply, the presence of a foreign body or as a response to certain organisms. In the case of chronic inflammation, after a time increasing numbers of lymphocytes get attracted to the area and the scar tissue-forming cells, the fibroblasts, are continually activated, meaning excess scar tissue may be formed. The chronic skin ulcer described in Section 2.1b is an example of chronic inflammation.

Tuberculosis is an example of an infection in which the slow-growing infectious organism *Mycobacterium tuberculosis* encourages a chronic inflammatory response and the formation of clusters of immune cells around foci of infection known as granulomas. These tiny clusters of immune cells are characteristic of this disease, and are evidence to the pathologist of its ability to induce damaging chronic inflammation.

Information box 2.2b-I

Inflammation: comments from a Chinese medicine perspective

Redness and warmth signify the presence of Heat in Chinese medicine. The characteristics of pain, with aversion to pressure, and a purplish discoloration suggest a degree of Blood Stagnation. In Chinese medicine, Blood Stagnation can lead to Heat, and Heat can be a cause of Blood Stagnation. Therefore, these Pathogenic Factors are inextricably interrelated in inflammation.

Excess tissue fluid and the swelling and oozing that result could be equated with the Pathogenic Factor of Damp. This may be localized or systemic, in which case there may well be underlying patterns of Spleen Deficiency.

The pathology of inflammation

Boils and abscesses

Boils and abscesses result from excess pus collecting within the tissues at a site of inflammation. Abscesses are simply big boils; there is no clear-cut difference between the two. Pus is more likely to collect if a foreign body is present at the site of inflammation and also if certain pyogenic organisms are present. The most common pyogenic organism to cause medical problems is *Staphylococcus aureus*, one of the many normal and healthy (commensal) skin bacteria.

A collection of pus is a problem because it is a reservoir of microbes that are not in close contact with a blood supply. Because of this it inhibits full resolution of the inflammation. It is also a source of chemicals that act as pyrogens (i.e. lead to fever and malaise).

A boil or abscess ideally heals by means of discharge of pus to the surface. For example, a stye (a boil on the edge of the eyelid) will ideally come to a point after a few days, which then breaks open to release the pus and allow healing.

This ideal outcome is not always achieved. In some cases the pus does not discharge fully, and the channel leading from the pus to the skin does not heal fully, remaining as a sinus that discharges pus in the long term. This can lead to long-term ill health, as the body is always in a state of dealing with infection. An infection in the bone (osteomyelitis) can easily lead to sinus formation, because the bone is relatively protected from the immune system, and thus chronic inflammation can readily develop in bone. This is a particular problem with shrapnel wounds in combat-related injuries, in which case there may be a continual discharge of pus from the bone through a sinus to the skin.

When a sinus is formed, the discharge of pus can go two ways: the first is into closely apposed organs (e.g. stomach and bowel, or bladder and bowel) so that a permanent channel known as a fistula is formed between them. This can have severe consequences. One common cause of a fistula is Crohn's disease, a form of inflammatory bowel disease. Diverticulitis of the bowel is another cause of fistula.

If the pus is not discharged at all, it is eventually phagocytosed. This is a common occurrence with small boils (pustules) such as occur in severe acne. Instead of discharging fully, these form tender lumps that gradually become less painful. This form of healing is more likely to lead to scarring resulting from chronic inflammation, as fibrous tissue is formed to fill the cavity formed by the pus, and this can have severe cosmetic consequences.

The most appropriate medical treatment of boils and abscesses promotes natural resolution. Astringent medication in the form of hot packs (poultices) can be applied to the site of a superficial abscess to encourage the pus to discharge outwards.

Resolution can be assisted surgically by lancing, where a clean wound is made in the skin to allow natural drainage of the pus. A larger abscess may be drained by inserting a sterile tube to connect with the outside for a few days. When the pus has drained, the tube is removed and, ideally, the cavity will then heal by the process of primary wound healing.

Antibiotics are often given to prevent spread of infection whilst the abscess is healing, although in some cases this treatment may be inappropriate. With adequate drainage, most abscesses will resolve without the need for antibiotics. Paradoxically, antibiotics can prevent full drainage of an abscess, as they may inhibit the process of pointing of the abscess to the surface, thus leading to a more chronic situation.

Fibrosis (scar tissue formation)

Chronic inflammation may be characterized by excessive scar tissue formation (fibrosis). This can be damaging, as scar tissue can cause shrinkage of tissues and damage to the integrity of organs. Cirrhosis is an example of the result of chronic inflammation of the liver. In cirrhosis, scar tissue takes over the space of the healthy liver cells and may result eventually in liver failure. Scar tissue in the abdominal or pelvic cavity can cause adhesions between organs, and may promote obstruction of organs and infertility.

The main treatment for fibrosis is surgical removal of scar tissue, in as much as this is possible. Physiotherapy and massage may be used to encourage the stretching of contracted areas of skin and muscle.

Information box 2.2b-II

Boils and abscesses: comments from a Chinese medicine perspective

In Chinese medicine, boils and abscesses are manifestations of Damp and Heat with Blood Stagnation and Heat Toxin in severe cases. Full resolution represents clearance of these Pathogens; therefore, poultices, lancing and drainage are energetically appropriate treatments that can facilitate full cure.

Antibiotics may actually suppress full cure in the conventional sense of the term, as the causative microorganisms may remain relatively protected from the drug deep within the walled-off center of the abscess. From a Chinese medical perspective antibiotics are Cold and Toxic in nature, and so may actually exacerbate the root cause of the problem that is likely to include Spleen Qi Deficiency (leading to poor health of the tissues). Nevertheless, there are situations in which antibiotic treatment is necessary to prevent the dangerous spread of infection from an abscess (e.g. in a brain abscess).

A discharging sinus or fistula suggests Chronic Damp Heat, usually on a background of marked deficiency such as Qi or Yin Deficiency.[31]

An abscess that does not discharge, but instead resolves to form a hard painless or painful lump under the surface of the skin, might be described in Chinese medicine in terms of Accumulation of Phlegm, which may be the consequence of the action of Heat on Damp, with underlying stasis of Blood and Qi.

Information box 2.2b-III

Fibrosis: comments from a Chinese medicine perspective

Scar tissue is unyielding and relatively dry in contrast to the springy, moist nature of healthy tissue. For this reason, scars are often described in terms of local Qi and Yin Deficiency. If the scar tissue is more bulky than the healthy tissue would have been, this could be interpreted as an Accumulation of Phlegm. If purplish, Blood Stagnation would be described.

A more detailed Chinese medicine interpretation would also depend on the site and on the consequences of the fibrosis. For example, intra-abdominal adhesions may lead to intermittent griping abdominal pain, suggesting Stagnation of Blood and Qi in Middle and Lower Jiao, while fibrosis of the heart muscle may lead to inefficient pumping of the heart and accumulation of fluid in the lower body (edema), suggesting Heart and Kidney Yang Deficiency.

Generalized inflammation

A generalized tendency to inflammation is currently often cited as the underlying basis of chronic debilitating disease as varied as diabetes mellitus, coronary heart disease, rheumatoid disease and Alzheimer's disease. This association is more likely to be found in alternative literature than medical textbooks. According to this theory, the generalized tendency to inflammation leads to over-activity of the inflammatory response with excessive production of potentially damaging inflammatory mediators. The causes of this state include stress, lack of sleep, exposure to environmental toxins and the standard Western diet that is high in processed carbohydrate, saturated fat and processed sugar. As Edwards (2005) states, "Inflammation is now recognized as an overwhelming burden to the healthcare status of our population and the underlying basis of a significant number of diseases. The elderly generally bear the burden of morbidity and mortality, which may be reflective of elevated markers of inflammation resulting from decades of lifestyle choices."[32]

According to these theories certain foodstuffs are considered to be "pro-inflammatory" and these include processed foods, sugar, alcohol, coffee and saturated fats and omega-6 fatty acids in unsaturated fats. Foods that are not inflammatory are advised, and include green leafy vegetables, colorful fruit and vegetables, soy, seeds and nuts, fermented foods, garlic, fish, non-wheat grains, olive oil and rapeseed oil. Weil (2011) has published a visual diagram of how these foods might be incorporated into a healthy diet in his "anti-inflammatory food pyramid."[33]

The recommendations for healthy living cited by authors such as Edwards and Weil have some striking correspondences with advice on lifestyle and diet that are enshrined in Chinese medicine. This perspective on the causation of chronic disease is only slowly permeating into mainstream medicine, but has an increasing body of scientific evidence supporting its recommendations for a long and disease-free life.[34]

2.2c Disorders of the immune system

Immune-related disease can be grouped into two broad categories:

- disease resulting from an insufficient immune response – immunodeficiency (also termed immune deficiency) syndromes

- disease resulting from an inappropriate immune response – allergy or autoimmune disease.

These broad categories of immune-related disease are discussed in turn.

The pathology of immunodeficiency syndromes

An insufficient immune response occurs when the complex interaction between the various types of lymphocyte fails to function in a balanced way. A person with immunodeficiency will therefore be less able to fight off infection.

Immunodeficiency may be a congenital condition, and if so, results from specific problems in the function of the leukocytes, the production of antibodies or deficiencies in the complement proteins. The severity of inherited immunodeficiency can vary. In severe forms, a patient may be susceptible to life-threatening infections. In milder forms, the patient may just experience a few more colds and other minor infections than the average person.

Immunodeficiency can also be the result of illness acquired in later life. Illness affecting the ability of the bone marrow to produce white blood cells (bone marrow failure) can become manifest in devastating immunodeficiency. This state can become apparent in conditions such as leukemia and secondary bone cancer. Acquired immunodeficiency syndrome (AIDS) is a particular form of immunodeficiency that is the result of infection with the human immunodeficiency virus (HIV). HIV targets T-lymphocytes and impairs their action in the immune response, and the result is a characteristic pattern of opportunistic infections and vulnerability to tumors (see below), including pneumocystis pneumonia, *candida* fungal infections and Kaposi's sarcoma.

A patient with immunodeficiency can develop unusual infections that most healthy people would be able to resist. Often these opportunistic infections do not present in a dramatic way. Instead, there may be a gradual development of symptoms that are not very specific, such as mild fever or slight sweats. Also characteristic of immunodeficiency are low-grade fungal infections of the skin and the mouth lining, and long-standing but slight diarrhea. The vagueness of the symptoms and signs of opportunistic infections means that there can be a delay in their diagnosis. However, even though symptoms of opportunistic infections may not be marked, the infection can take hold and rapidly become life-threatening. The infectious agents that cause opportunistic infections are often resistant to common antibiotics. This can further complicate their treatment.

The other major health risk that faces a person with an immunodeficiency syndrome is cancerous change, as new cancerous cells are usually destroyed by a healthy immune system.

Information box 2.2c-I

Immunodeficiency: comments from a Chinese medicine perspective

A patient with an immunodeficiency syndrome does not have a strong response to pathogens. From the perspective of Chinese medicine, this suggests that the Upright Qi is weak. More specifically, as many of these infections manifest on the Exterior, with skin rashes and sweats, it points in these cases to the Wei Qi, and its foundation, Kidney Essence, being deficient.

The symptoms of immunodeficiency can also include low-grade fever, night sweats, enlarged lymph nodes, a tendency to diarrhea and fungal skin problems such as athlete's foot and thrush. There is a tendency to develop cancer. Taken together, the wide range of potential symptoms usually reflects an underlying Kidney Qi Deficiency, with a consequent effect on many of the other Organs. Spleen Qi Deficiency, Damp and Phlegm are all possible outcomes, as are specific symptoms arising from Kidney Yin and Yang Deficiency.

Although it is likely that each of these components is present to some degree in a case of immunodeficiency, the symptom picture in each patient will be unique, and it is the skill of the practitioner in tracing the complex etiology of the patterns that will point to a more precise Chinese diagnosis.

The pathology of allergy

Allergy (also termed hypersensitivity) is seen to occur when there is an excessive immune response to a substance that does not normally provoke such a reaction in healthy people. Allergies are common, with up to one-third of people experiencing one at some point in their lives. The substance that provokes the allergic response is called the allergen. The allergic response may be localized to the part of the body that has been exposed to the allergen (e.g. in contact allergic eczema or hay fever), or it may be a generalized response to an allergic trigger (e.g. an anaphylactic response to a bee sting or a penicillin-induced rash).

The incidence of food allergy and also to environmental allergens is known to be increasing, but the reasons for this are scientifically unclear.[35]

Many people commonly use the term allergy to mean that they do not react well to certain substances, and will complain of symptoms such as fluctuating digestive or respiratory disturbances or headaches. However, conventional medicine tends to recognize only those situations in which a definite abnormality of the immune system can be detected. This is why doctors may deny that there is an allergic component to conditions such as chronic tiredness and irritable bowel syndrome. Nevertheless, many patients with these conditions will notice a consistent adverse relationship between their symptoms and coming into contact with substances to which they feel they are allergic. It is perhaps more appropriate in terms of medical language to use the term intolerance rather than allergy in these cases.

Examples of diseases that doctors would agree are the result of allergic reactions are listed in Table 2.2c-I. It is clear from the information presented in the table that allergic reactions can have very different presentations. This is because for each type of allergic reaction, different aspects of the immune system may be over-reacting. The two broad ways in which the immune response can result in allergic disease are termed type I and type IV hypersensitivity.

Table 2.2c-I Allergic conditions recognized by conventional medicine

Condition	Symptoms	Allergen
Anaphylactic shock	Extreme bodily reaction, including severe asthma, and swelling and rash of skin	Can be various; common ones include bee stings, peanuts, egg, antibiotics
Worsening of childhood eczema and asthma	Symmetrical itchy rash distributed all over the body	Various, including dairy products, egg, wheat and oranges; sometimes no allergen is found
Hay fever	Streaming eyes and nose, sneezing, itchy throat	Grass and tree pollen
Contact eczema	Rash on the skin at the site of contact with the allergen	Metals, including nickel, detergents, garden plants, sticking plaster
Perennial rhinitis and chronic sinusitis	Blocked and runny nose, sneezing, facial pain	House dust and molds
Urticaria (nettle rash)	Blotchy, raised rash widely distributed over the skin	Dietary allergens such as shellfish and eggs are common triggers
Migraine	Unilateral headache, nausea and neurological symptoms and signs	Cheese, chocolate and red wine are common triggers

Type I hypersensitivity

In some people the white blood cells that release histamine in the inflammatory response, the mast cells and basophils, react excessively to the antigens on certain trigger substances such as house dust, pollen, animal dander, bee stings and specific dietary components (commonly eggs, peanuts and fish). Histamine in excess causes itching, exudation of fluid into tissues and constriction of the airways of the lungs. If extreme, the result is anaphylactic shock, in which the dramatic exudation of fluid causes a drop in blood pressure, and life-threatening asthma can develop within a matter of minutes of exposure to the allergen. In less severe reactions the person might just experience temporary itching, sneezing or breathlessness. This histamine-mediated allergy is known as type I hypersensitivity. Hay fever, rhinitis, urticaria (hives or nettle rash) from eating shellfish and bee sting allergy are all examples of type I hypersensitivity.

Type IV hypersensitivity

Another form of allergy involves the T-lymphocytes reacting excessively to externally originating antigens. The antigens cause a delayed reaction, as lymphocytes are slow to accumulate at the site of injury. Over time, this sort of allergic reaction will cause a local area of inflammation, with itching. The skin can react in this way to contact with substances such as latex, nickel, leather and certain plants. The result is a localized area of skin irritation, with itch and thickening of the skin (contact allergic eczema). This is also the allergic reaction that can cause some forms of transplant operation to fail (e.g. skin graft). This form of T-lymphocyte-mediated allergy is known as type IV delayed-type hypersensitivity.

Type III (immune-complex-mediated) hypersensitivity

Type III hypersensitivity is a less common mechanism for an allergic reaction. It describes the excessive formation of immune complexes (antibody-antigen complexes), which can circulate in the bloodstream before becoming deposited in the kidneys, skin and joints. They then trigger inflammatory damage in these tissues, leading to symptoms and signs such as blood in the urine, a bruising rash and joint aches. The allergic response to penicillin is understood to be a type III response.

Treatment of allergy

It is helpful before treating allergies to diagnose the cause. In some cases this is obvious, but certain hospital tests can clarify a range of potential allergens that might cause reactions in an individual. Skin prick tests involve the injection of tiny amounts of allergen under the surface of the skin, and monitoring for a wheal response. These tests are used to diagnose type I hypersensitivity. It is also possible to test whether or not a patient is sensitive to particular antigens in type I allergic conditions by means of a specific immunoglobulin E (IgE) blood test.

Skin patch tests involve holding an allergen against the skin by means of an adhesive plaster, and assessing the reaction over the next few days. These test for type IV hypersensitivity. Skin prick and skin patch tests are usually designed to test for sensitivity to a battery of potential antigens at the same time.

The first principle in treatment is to avoid the offending allergen, or to protect the skin if avoidance is not possible. This is often very difficult to do, as many allergens, such as pollen and house dust mites, are impossible to remove totally from the environment.

Antihistamines, anti-inflammatories and corticosteroids are all drugs that reduce the effect of the overactive immune and inflammatory responses.

Antihistamines (e.g. cetirizine and loratadine) counteract the effect of the excessive release of histamine that occurs in type I allergic reactions. Side effects include dry mouth, rashes and palpitations in some people. The more sedating, older antihistamines (e.g. promethazine) can also reduce nausea, and may be prescribed to prevent travel sickness and for sedation in children.

There is a wide range of anti-inflammatory drugs, many of which are used to reduce pain. Those that are used in allergy and asthma (e.g. sodium cromoglicate) appear to reduce the release of histamine from the mast cells.

Corticosteroids (commonly described by patients as steroids) can be taken by mouth, applied to the skin or inhaled into the nose according to the type of allergy. These are known to suppress the function of immune cells (in particular, the T-lymphocytes) and also the inflammatory response by reducing the production of pro-inflammatory chemical mediators such as interleukin-2. They are, therefore, both anti-inflammatory and immunosuppressant. Whilst very effective, they tend not to be used in non-life-threatening allergies as their long-term use leads to serious physical side effects including weight gain, increased blood pressure, thinning of the skin and vulnerability to serious infections.

Decongestants (such as oxymetalozine, the active constituent of Afrin and Vicks Sinex nasal sprays) are available in the West in various forms "over the counter" from pharmacists. Because of the ease of their availability they are commonly used preparations. They act by causing constriction of blood vessels in the nose that, in the case of runny nose, reduces the amount of fluid that can ooze out. The main problem with these drugs is that, when they wear off, the nasal drip can be worse than before, so that people can become dependent on using them. Constriction of blood vessels in the head can cause headache, and may increase blood pressure in some people.

Desensitization injections may be administered in hospital settings to help overcome grass pollen or wasp sting allergies. These carry a risk of severe allergic reactions so are only offered in severe cases and always in settings where resuscitation can be performed rapidly.

Information box 2.2c-II

Allergy: comments from a Chinese medicine perspective

Most true allergic reactions have characteristics of what is described in Chinese medicine as Wind Invasion. The runny nose, itchy eyes, itchy skin and rashes characteristic of many allergies often come on suddenly, and change rapidly. The rash of urticaria can move across the body from site to site dramatically. This suggests that the allergic person has a specific Deficiency of Wei Qi, which in some way is exacerbated by contact with the particular allergen.

The allergen has been described as a form of Toxic Xie (Pathogenic) Qi to which only certain people are susceptible. It is thought that vulnerable individuals may have deep lying Phlegm or Heat that only becomes apparent through contact with the trigger. Flaws (2001) explains this in his description of the mechanism of chronic rhinitis,[36] which he attributes to Chronic Spleen Qi and Kidney Yang Deficiency leading to Phlegm and also Wei Qi Deficiency. Liver Qi Stagnation will predispose to vulnerability by making Spleen weak as well as promoting upward flow of Qi, thus explaining the often noticed emotional causation to allergic reactions.

Chronic allergic reactions that affect the skin often manifest as pallor and dryness, symptoms usually ascribed to Blood Deficiency. This, in turn, may also predispose the sufferer to Wind Invasions.

Antihistamines reduce the response to the allergen, although this sensitivity returns when the drug is stopped. The usual medical view is that there are usually no obvious long-term side effects or worsening of the condition if these drugs are taken for a long time, but it is clear that many patients become dependent on taking them. As the allergy is usually in the form of acute Invasion of Wind Heat/Cold, this suggests that the drugs in some way prevent the invasion (i.e. expression) of the Pathogen. Subduing the Pathogenic Factor in the Interior is a possible energetic mechanism. If this is the case, then in theory, the root imbalance will have not been attended to as a result of the suppression of symptoms, but this might not become immediately apparent in symptoms that are significant medically. Subdued Heat or Phlegm, for example, may just become apparent in the form of mental agitation or restlessness, which may not be attributed directly to the drug treatment. It is of note that recent research has placed antihistamines in a wider list of anticholinergic drugs that have been associated with dementia in the long term.[37] This would be in keeping with the theory that their action might be Phlegm-forming in nature.

Possibly more marked drug-induced disease is occurring with the older forms of antihistamine. These often cause drowsiness and are chemically related to the stronger first-generation major tranquillizers, such as chlorpromazine used to sedate and suppress thought in severe mental illness. This effect suggests a tendency to promote Non-Substantial Phlegm and thus Obstruct the Shen.

Although newer forms of antihistamine do not have this property, both types can cause dryness of the mouth and difficulty urinating. These both suggest damage to Kidney Yin. The palpitations that can be caused by the newer antihistamines also suggest damage of Heart Blood/Yin, and both these side effects also suggest that antihistamines are Hot in nature as well as Phlegm-forming.

Decongestants are chemically related to the ephedrine in the Chinese medicine herb ma huang (*Ephedra sinica*). Ma huang is understood to be able to Release the Exterior, Resolve Wind Cold and help Move Lung Qi, and has been widely used over the centuries in Chinese medicine. Medically it is recognized to open the bronchial tubes, stimulate the heart and nervous system and increase blood pressure. It became popular in the West in the 1970s as a weight loss medication and also as a mental stimulant. Misuse is associated with serious side effects including skin reactions, irritability, trembling, headache, profuse perspiration, dehydration, irregular heartbeat, seizures, heart attack, stroke and even death. These side effects suggest additional Chinese medical effects when used in excess indicating damage to the Liver and Heart Yin and generation of Liver Yang Rising and Liver Wind, presumably a consequence of its powerfully Dispersing effect on Qi.[38]

Decongestants are medically recognized to have a suppressive action, as the runny nose that they help to resolve returns in a more pronounced form on withdrawal. The headache and hypertension that they can cause suggests that they might also lead to the expression of the syndrome of Liver Yang Rising in susceptible people.

Food intolerances are not considered to be true allergies according to conventional medicine. However, many patients report that certain foods will worsen conditions such as bloating and irritable bowel syndrome. From a Chinese medicine perspective, conditions that manifest in bloating, abdominal discomfort and unstable bowel habit often have Spleen Qi Deficiency with Liver Qi Stagnation as their foundation. In these conditions it would appear that the symptoms brought about by the offending dietary substance (e.g. wheat, citrus or dairy products) are characteristic of weakened Spleen Qi and Stagnated Liver Qi. These syndromes also can permit the generation of a Pathogen such as Heat or Damp, and so the process by which the patient manifests symptoms such as flushing or vaginal discharge.

In contrast to most patients with true allergies, patients with food intolerances may notice that their sensitivity to certain foods fluctuates significantly over time and often in relationship to stress. This is presumably a reflection of the quality and harmony of their Spleen and Liver Qi at a given point in time.

The pathology of autoimmune disease

Autoimmune disease is the result of antibodies that bind to antigens that are part of the body itself. These antibodies are called autoantibodies. This means that the immune response, which leads to inflammation, is directed toward normal body tissue, and causes damage that includes swelling, pain, heat and loss of function. Fibrosis (scarring) of the affected tissue can also occur. There are more than 80 autoimmune diseases that affect a wide range of organs and bodily systems.

Type II (cytotoxic) hypersensitivity

Strictly speaking, autoimmunity is viewed from a conventional perspective as another manifestation of hypersensitivity. Much autoimmune disease is the consequence of type II (cytotoxic) hypersensitivity, in which there is a deleterious immune response to the self-antigens present on tissue cells. This results in the death of the cells that carry the antigens. The T-lymphocytes are the cytotoxic cells in this disease process, but their action in cell damage is supported by the helper B-lymphocytes (see Section 2.1d).

In some autoimmune diseases there is further tissue damage resulting from circulating antibody-antigen immune complexes (e.g. this type III hypersensitivity is the cause of kidney damage in systemic lupus erythematosus (SLE)).

Organ-specific autoimmune diseases

In organ-specific autoimmune diseases, the autoantibodies are usually targeted at only one type of tissue cell, and so the damage is located within a single organ. Table 2.2c-II illustrates the diversity of some of the common organ-specific autoimmune diseases.

People with one organ-specific autoimmune disease are more likely than an average person to develop another one. It is not uncommon that a person with diabetes, for example, may also develop hypothyroidism. In general, the damage in organ-specific autoimmune disease is mediated by type II (cytotoxic) hypersensitivity.

Table 2.2c-II Some of the organ-specific autoimmune diseases

Autoimmune disease	Tissue affected
Diabetes mellitus	Insulin-producing cells of the pancreas gland (endocrine tissue)
Thyrotoxicosis (Graves' disease) and hypothyroidism (some antibodies stimulate the gland, and some cause destruction of the gland)	Thyroxine-producing cells of the thyroid gland (endocrine tissue)
Pernicious anemia (anemia due to vitamin B12 deficiency)	Cells in the stomach that secrete a chemical called intrinsic factor, essential for the absorption of vitamin B12
Vitiligo	The cells in the skin that produce melanin; vitiligo leaves symmetrical pale patches of unpigmented skin
Addison's disease (a deficiency of cortisol, a natural corticosteroid)	Cells in the adrenal gland that secrete a steroid hormone called cortisol

Multisystem autoimmune diseases

In multisystem autoimmune diseases, a wider range of tissues are damaged as a result of excessive immune reactions, which means that the symptoms are much more diverse. Multisystem autoimmune disease is also termed rheumatic autoimmune disease, because in many of these conditions, the joints are affected, leading to joint pain and swelling (arthritis). Another commonly applied term for a subclass of these conditions is connective tissue diseases.[39]

Other tissues commonly affected in the multisystem autoimmune diseases include the arteries, the kidney and the skin. This can lead to the development of thrombosis, kidney failure and rashes, respectively.

These conditions are often progressive and debilitating, and can lead to death from kidney failure. Rheumatoid arthritis is the most common multisystem autoimmune disease. Systemic lupus erythematosus (lupus or SLE) is another important multisystem disorder. The immune damage in the multisystem disorders is mediated by a combination of type II (cytotoxic) and type III (immune complex-mediated) hypersensitivity.

Treatment of autoimmune disease

In organ-specific autoimmune diseases the damage done to an organ may be irreversible. The treatment in these conditions tends not to be targeted at the autoimmune process. Instead, the important aspect of treatment is to deal with the imbalance resulting from the loss of organ function. For example, in type 1 diabetes mellitus an autoimmune process has caused irreversible damage to the insulin-producing beta cells of the pancreas. The treatment is insulin, given to replace the deficiency resulting from damage to the insulin-producing cells of the pancreas.

In the multisystem autoimmune diseases, significant damage to widespread tissues is ongoing and progressive, and disease processes include tissue inflammation, scarring and increased tendency to thrombosis in small, medium and large vessels.

In multisystem autoimmune diseases treatment is targeted towards the overactive immune system. Drugs are used that inhibit the immune response. These are known as immunosuppressants. Immunosuppressant drugs are also used commonly as part of cancer chemotherapy as they seem to inhibit the multiplication of cancer cells. They are also essential for preventing the rejection of an organ that has been transplanted. This rejection is the result of a normal immune response to the foreign tissue, but has to be suppressed to ensure the viability of the transplanted tissue.

Corticosteroids

Corticosteroids are a commonly prescribed class of immunosuppressant drugs that also have the property of inhibiting inflammation. They are, therefore, doubly effective in autoimmune disease. They act by reducing the production of the chemical mediators that promote the immune response, and this has a particular impact on the phagocytic neutrophil leukocytes. In this way they can slow down the damage caused by autoantibodies throughout the tissues of the body, and can prevent the development of life-threatening conditions such as kidney failure and thrombosis.

Corticosteroids can be given by mouth or by intravenous injection. The two most commonly prescribed oral preparations are dexamethasone and prednisolone.

Corticosteroids are closely related to a natural hormone called cortisol, which is produced by the cells of the cortex (outer layer) of the adrenal gland. Cortisol is essential for life, demonstrated by the fact that people with the organ-specific immune condition Addison's disease will die if their deficient cortisol is not replaced by synthetic corticosteroids. It is known that under conditions of stress cortisol is released in increased amounts by the adrenal gland. Its role includes ensuring that the body cells can have ready access to the sugar that is present in the diet and stored in the liver, and also that extra sugar is manufactured (by breaking down proteins) if necessary. Cortisol also acts at the kidney to ensure that sufficient salts and water are maintained in the circulation to keep blood pressure at an adequate level. These responses are essential in the short term, but may contribute to the development of diseases such as diabetes and hypertension in people who are continually under stress.

Cortisol also influences diverse inflammatory mediator chemicals and also the response leukocytes, which bring about a normal immune response and assist in wound healing. However, when in excess, cortisol leads to a suppressed immune response and poor wound healing. This effect could offer one reason why stressed people with chronically raised cortisol levels tend to succumb to illness more often, and also may not recover from injury so rapidly.

Patients on corticosteroids prescribed to suppress immune responses will experience problems consistent with the physiological effects of cortisol in excess. These include:

- high blood sugar (can lead to diabetes mellitus)

- high blood pressure and fluid retention due to the effects on the kidney

- excessive loss of muscle because muscle protein is broken down to make sugar

- impaired generalized immune response leading to increased risk of infection and poor wound healing.

Other important side effects of corticosteroids include:

- alteration of mood (they can cause depression and manic states)

- impaired growth in children

- thinning of tissue under the skin leading to easy bruising, stretch marks and damage to skin

- thinning of the bones (osteoporosis) in adults

- weight gain, particularly around the face, on the shoulders and over the abdomen.

One important side effect of synthetic corticosteroids is that they suppress the body's natural production of cortisol. For this reason corticosteroids should never be withdrawn suddenly, because their sudden removal can lead to a condition similar to Addison's disease, and there is a risk that the patient may collapse and die.

The constellation of serious side effects of corticosteroids was first described by a doctor called Cushing, and so is called Cushing's syndrome (see Figure 2.2c-1). Cushing's syndrome will only become apparent after weeks of treatment with high-dose corticosteroids.

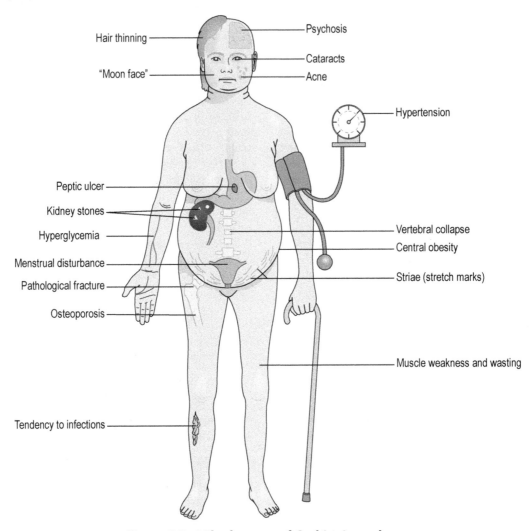

Hair thinning

"Moon face"

Psychosis

Cataracts

Acne

Hypertension

Peptic ulcer

Kidney stones

Hyperglycemia

Menstrual disturbance

Pathological fracture

Osteoporosis

Vertebral collapse

Central obesity

Striae (stretch marks)

Muscle weakness and wasting

Tendency to infections

Figure 2.2c-I The features of Cushing's syndrome

When corticosteroids are being considered for treatment of an allergic or autoimmune disease, the potential benefits will always be weighed against the risks of Cushing's syndrome. Patients on corticosteroid therapy should be clearly warned about the side effect of an impaired response to infection, as a minor infection can lead to a life-threatening situation in a person on this form of steroid treatment. They should also be warned never to stop their medication suddenly.

Other immunosuppressant drugs

Immunosuppressant drugs are a diverse group of drugs that act by inhibiting various aspects of the immune response. They may be prescribed to reduce the need for high doses of corticosteroid (so-called steroid-sparing effects). In severe autoimmune disease they are often used in combination with corticosteroids. Some of the more commonly used immunosuppressant drugs include methotrexate, cyclophosphamide and azathioprine. These cytostatic agents act by inhibiting the production and action of the lymphocytes. They are also used in higher doses for their cytotoxic effects in cancer chemotherapy. Because they cause a degree of damage to healthy cells, they have a wide range of toxic side effects.

Ciclosporin and tacrolimus are immunosuppressants that have a more powerful effect on lymphocyte function (by inhibiting cytokine production) and are commonly used to prevent transplant reactions. Both are associated with an impressively long list of potentially serious side effects.

More recently introduced immunosuppressants include immunologically derived products such as monoclonal antibodies that target specific sites on leukocyte membranes (e.g. basiliximab and daclizumab) or circulating inflammatory mediators such as tumor necrosis factor (TNF) (inflizimab, etanercept, adalimumab).

TNF is also inhibited by curcumin in turmeric and catechins in green tea, which accounts for their possible anti-inflammatory effects.

Information box 2.2c-III

Autoimmune disease and its treatment: comments from a Chinese medicine perspective

In organ-specific autoimmune diseases, the main symptoms come from the reduced function of the affected organ. The syndromes that result are diverse. The Chinese medicine view of the main organ-specific autoimmune conditions such as diabetes and thyroid disease is discussed later.

The multisystem autoimmune diseases (such as rheumatoid arthritis, Sjögren's syndrome and SLE) have some common energetic features. In these diseases, the common primary causes of damage to the body tissues are inflammation, fibrosis and thrombosis. Inflammation suggests Heat as an important common Pathogenic Factor. Fibrosis suggests Phlegm formation and damage to the Yin and Thrombosis, Blood Stagnation and Phlegm formation.

In many of these conditions there is also a degree of painful joint swelling and deformity, as well as thickening of the tissues or formation of nodules. These also suggest Damp and Phlegm and Blood Stagnation.

Such profound energetic disturbance would not occur without there being a background history of marked depletion. Autoimmune disease does run in families, and this suggests that an inherited Jing Deficiency plays a part in the susceptibility to autoimmune disease. If this is the case, imbalances such as Kidney Yin Deficiency and Spleen Qi Deficiency are also likely to be evident, and these in turn may create a susceptibility to Pathogenic Factors such as Heat, Damp and Phlegm. Lifestyle factors that are causative for Depletion, Stagnation and Phlegm formation will very likely play a part in the etiology of such profound disturbance. These might include physical inactivity, dietary indiscretion, excessive work and emotional strain over many years.

The energetic interpretation of the action of corticosteroids (steroids) is very complex. When the treatment of keloid scars was described in Section 2.1b, the local action of injected steroids was interpreted as clearing of Heat, Phlegm and Stagnation. This would also be a reasonable interpretation of the effect when steroids are injected into inflamed and swollen joints.

The action of corticosteroids taken into the whole body by tablet or intravenous injection might also, at one level, be described in terms of subduing these Pathogenic Factors, as inflammation, swelling and pain are ameliorated. However, the side effects embraced by Cushing's syndrome suggest there is a range of less beneficial energetic effects. Possible energetic interpretations of these side effects are summarized in the following table:

Side effect of corticosteroid drugs	Possible Chinese medicine energetic interpretation
High blood sugar/diabetes (leads to excessive thirst and urination and damage to blood vessels)	Internal Heat leading to Kidney Yin Deficiency
High blood pressure	Kidney Yang and Yin Deficiency (leading to water retention and Accumulation of Damp and Phlegm)
Retention of fluids	Kidney Yang Deficiency
Muscle wastage and thinning of flesh beneath the skin	Spleen Qi Deficiency
Poor growth in children	Jing Deficiency
Thinning of the bones	Kidney Deficiency
Acne	Damp Heat
Elevated mood, mania, depression	Phlegm/Heat obstructing Heart Orifices
Weight gain	Damp
Poor wound healing	Blood and Qi Deficiency
Poor response to infection	Wei Qi and Jing Deficiency

In summary, the symptomatic benefit of corticosteroids may come at a cost of serious side effects. Many of these may be described in terms of damage to the Kidney Qi and Kidney Essence from a Chinese medicine perspective. The corticosteroids also have side effects that would suggest accumulation of Heat, Damp and Phlegm. It is noteworthy that these are the Pathogenic Factors that appear to be cleared when corticosteroids have a therapeutic effect. According to the theory of suppression introduced in Section 1.3b, this might point to the possibility that the apparent clearance of Pathogenic Factors is actually suppression of imbalance to deeper levels in the body.

The energetic effects of cytostatic immuno-suppressant medication have to be considered in a similar light as they subdue manifest symptoms but have a wide range of potentially dangerous side effects that include vulnerability to infections and cancers. Again, the pacifying of Pathogenic Factors would appear to come at the cost of damage to Blood and Qi and Yin. In Chinese medicine such powerfully acting drugs would be seen in terms of acting as Heat Toxins (as are other forms of cancer treatments).

2.2d Thrombosis, embolism and infarction

In Section 2.1c clotting was described as a barrier to disease. This section focuses on what happens when clotting is excessive to bodily requirements. When this happens, the conditions of thrombosis, embolism and infarction may be the result. In conventional pathology, these together are considered as one of the basic processes of disease.

Causation of thrombosis, embolism and infarction

The term thrombosis describes a blood clot (thrombus) that forms within a blood vessel, and which then stops the usual flow of blood within that vessel.

Embolism is a term used to describe the situation when any substance (known as an embolus; plural emboli) is transported within the bloodstream until it wedges in a narrow artery from where it can then stop the flow of blood. The most usual cause of an embolus is a piece of clot that has broken away from the site of a thrombosis.

Infarction describes what happens to tissue that is damaged as a result of the blockage caused by a thrombosis or the lodging of an embolus in an artery. The tissue normally nourished by the blocked blood vessel becomes suddenly deprived of nutrients, most importantly oxygen. Sensitive tissues such as the brain or the heart muscle can only survive for a short amount of time without these essential nutrients. If the blockage is prolonged, the tissue cells die, release their contents and the process of inflammation is triggered. Infarcted tissues become acutely painful and swollen. However, if infarction occurs in an external part of the body, in the first instance the body part (e.g. a limb) becomes cold and purplish rather than hot and red, because its blood supply has been cut off.

Together, these disease processes account for more than half of all adult deaths, as they are the cause of conditions such as heart attacks (myocardial infarction), strokes (cerebral infarction) and blood clots in the lung (pulmonary embolism). These conditions are explored in more detail later, while this section focuses on the general features of these disorders of excessive clotting.

Thrombosis and embolism occur for four main reasons:

- damage to a vessel wall
- damage to the heart and the disturbance in blood flow resulting from atrial fibrillation (AF)
- increased platelet adherence
- thrombophilia, an inherited tendency to increased blood clotting.

Thrombosis resulting from damage to a vessel wall

As described in Section 2.1c, damage to a vessel wall stimulates the formation of a blood clot. Usually this is a useful bodily response, as the blood clot will stem bleeding from a damaged vessel. However, the lining of the vessel can be damaged not just by traumatic injury but also by deposits of fatty atheroma (one of the causes of hardening of the arteries) or by external compression, such as might occur in an injury. In these cases, a blood clot forms in the region of the damaged vessel, even though there is no bleeding.

Embolism resulting from damage to the heart or atrial fibrillation (AF)

Like the blood vessels, the heart is lined with smooth epithelial tissue. Compromise of this tissue by disease, which most commonly occurs as a result of a heart attack (coronary thrombosis), may stimulate the formation of a blood clot within one of the chambers of the heart. The pumping action can then cause particles of blood clot to dislodge and form emboli, which are ejected into the circulation. Similarly, irregular or artificial heart valves cause abnormal turbulence in the jets of blood that are pumped through the heart, and this can also, through damage to the platelets, stimulate the clotting cascade and lead to embolism. Finally, AF, a condition in which the wall of the heart muscle of the atria pumps irregularly, can also stimulate the formation of small clots within the chambers of the heart.

Thrombosis resulting from increased platelet adherence

In certain bodily states, the platelets tend to adhere to each other and the vessel wall more readily than they should. Platelets become stickier in many conditions of serious ill health, such as cancer and systemic infection, as a result of increased levels of inflammatory chemicals in the circulation. This is also the cause of increased platelet adherence after major surgery and trauma.

Pregnancy is another condition in which this can occur. The use of hormone-containing drugs such as the contraceptive pill also carries a risk of thrombosis because of increased platelet adherence.

Smoking increases platelet adherence and is often contributory in a case of thrombosis.

Platelets are more likely to adhere in cases of dehydration, when the proteins and cells in the plasma become more concentrated.

All these factors may become more significant in a situation in which there is physical immobility, which is, of course, more likely in serious illness, after surgery or trauma, and during pregnancy. If there is physical immobility, the circulation in the peripheries of the body may become sluggish and there is an increased risk of thrombosis.

Thrombophilia

Thrombophilia is a term used to describe any condition in which there is an increased susceptibility to thrombosis and embolism. There are several inherited forms of thrombophilia, in which gene defects lead to abnormalities in the function of the clotting factors. The most common mild form, which may affect up to 5 percent of the population to some degree, is an inherited tendency for the clotting factor V (Leiden) to persist in the circulation longer than it normally should. Protein C and S mutations hinder the clearance of factors V and VIII from the circulation, and a prothrombin (factor II) mutation leads to abnormally high levels of this clotting factor. Antithrombin deficiency is a rare but serious genetic abnormality of a protein that aids in the breakdown of thrombin (activated factor II).

Thrombophilia can result from the development of autoantibodies. Antiphospholipid syndrome is a condition characterized by thrombosis and recurrent miscarriage, which is sometimes associated with the multisystem autoimmune disease SLE. In this condition autoantibodies are directed towards anticoagulant proteins present both in the general circulation and the placenta.

Thrombophilia is also more likely in certain other disease states including cancer and nephrotic syndrome of the kidneys. It is more likely in pregnancy and in women who take hormone-related contraception. A combination of these factors might increase thrombotic risk (e.g. factor V Leiden disease and concurrent use of the contraceptive pill).

The consequences of thrombosis and embolism

The consequences of thrombosis and embolism depend very much on the site of the blood clot. Thrombosis may occur either in arteries, which bring blood to tissues, or veins, which drain blood away from the tissues. Because of the way in which they are transported in the bloodstream, which is from the location of a thrombus and thence to the heart through large veins, emboli tend to lodge within a vessel in the narrowing network of the arterial tree.

Arterial thrombosis or embolism has serious and immediate consequences because it suddenly cuts off the blood supply to tissues. It is blockage of an artery that causes infarction. The bigger the artery that is blocked, the greater the amount of tissue that is deprived of its blood supply. Ischemia is the term given to a poor blood supply. Ischemic tissue is at risk of infarction unless the blood supply is regained rapidly. Infarction is more likely to occur in areas of tissue that are dependent on a single blood vessel for their supply of oxygen and nutrients.

Arterial thrombosis can occur anywhere in the body. The most common sites for severe arterial thrombosis are the vessels supplying the heart muscle (coronary arteries) and the vessels supplying parts of the brain (cerebral arteries). The consequences of these are heart attack (myocardial infarction) and stroke (cerebral infarction), respectively. These are particularly serious occurrences, because both the brain and the myocardial tissues have high demands for oxygen and nutrients, and so suffer rapidly when deprived of these. Significant arterial thrombosis can also occur in the main vessel supplying a limb or in a vessel supplying a segment of the bowel. If the blood supply to a limb is suddenly compromised, the limb becomes cold and acutely painful. Thrombosis of the bowel will lead to acute abdominal pain and collapse (the syndrome of acute abdomen).

Deep venous (vein) thrombosis (DVT) is a term given to a thrombosis of a deep vein, which usually occurs in the deep veins of the calf, thigh or pelvis. DVT prevents the free drainage of blood from the tissues, and leads to swelling and discomfort behind the thrombosis. The discomfort is not as severe as the intense pain that results from an arterial thrombosis. It is particularly likely to occur in veins where the blood flow is sluggish. DVT most commonly occurs in the calf muscle vein after long periods of inactivity or ill health.

The acute serious problem that results from DVT is that the obstructing thrombus can enlarge and clot particles can break off to become emboli. These are then carried through the large veins in the blood supply towards the heart. Because the chambers in the heart are relatively large, the emboli are pumped through the heart and end up lodging in the blood vessels of the lungs. This is called pulmonary embolism (a term derived from the Latin *pulmo*, meaning lung).

Treatment of thrombosis and embolism

The treatment of thrombosis and embolism depends on whether the event has just happened (acute thrombosis or embolism) or whether treatment is required to prevent the formation of a blood clot in someone at high risk.

Treatment of acute thrombosis or embolism

Acute (sudden) thrombosis or embolism in a major artery is a serious threat to the life of the tissue supplied by that artery. If the artery is accessible, the first choice of treatment is surgery, in which the artery is opened, the thrombosis or embolus removed, and the cut in the artery repaired.

Another less invasive surgical approach is angioplasty. In this case a tube is passed into the blocked artery via the large artery in the groin or the neck (a bit like rodding a blocked drain), and with the help of X-ray imaging, guided into the clot. The end of the tube is then expanded, which compresses the clot against the wall of the vessel, ideally leaving a passage through which the blood circulation can continue. This procedure is used most commonly in heart disease, to open up narrowed coronary vessels that have become blocked with thrombus, but may also be employed if there has been thrombosis of a major limb artery. Angioplasty can also involve leaving a metal tube behind, known as a stent, to keep the vessel patent. In some cases this tube may be impregnated with medication intended to prevent the proliferation of cells that might tend to block the newly formed channel in the blood vessels (drug-eluting stent). The patient will need to take some form of anticoagulation medication for some time after a stent has been inserted to prevent new thrombosis forming in the bare metal-lined channel.

If the clot is large and has occurred within 24 hours of access to treatment, patients may be given a clot-busting (thrombolytic) drug by intravenous injection. The most commonly used of these are streptokinase (derived from streptococcal bacteria) and genetically engineered recombinant tissue plasminogen activator (tPA). These drugs act in the same way as the body's natural process of fibrinolysis. They activate plasminogen to form plasmin, and so can cause fresh clots to dissolve. The thrombolytic drugs carry the risk of causing embolism as the clot breaks up, and sometimes lead to life-threatening bleeding at other sites in the body.

In the case of DVT and pulmonary embolism, rapid anticoagulation is achieved by means of a drug called low-molecular-weight heparin (LMWH), which has to be given by daily injection. This drug may also be used to prevent thrombosis in patients who are in high-risk situations.

In the long term, almost all patients who have experienced thrombosis or embolism will receive treatment with either aspirin, an ADP (adenosine diphosphate) receptor inhibitor (such as clopidogrel or ticagrelor), warfarin or one of the novel oral anticoagulant drugs (NOACs) such as dabigatran or apixaban. These drugs are commonly said to thin the blood. This is not exactly the case, as it is not the blood cells but rather the platelets and clotting mechanism that are affected in various ways by these medications.

Aspirin acts by reducing the adherence of platelets, and is known to be effective at a daily dose of 75mg (one-quarter of a proprietary aspirin tablet). It has a moderate effect on reducing clotting, without a markedly increased risk of bleeding. It is generally given in a dose of 300mg in acute cases such as heart attack and stroke, both to treat the acute event by prevention of the spread of the clot, and to prevent future events. At the low dose, aspirin has few side effects. Its most common side effect is inflammation/bleeding of the stomach lining.

Clopidogrel and ticagrelor both act, like aspirin, to reduce platelet adherence. Both are taken on a daily basis. Clopidogrel is the most commonly prescribed, sometimes in combination with aspirin, to prevent stroke and heart attack, and commonly ticagrelor is prescribed (always in combination with aspirin) to be taken in the year following a heart attack to prevent recurrence.

Warfarin (a drug infamous first, having been developed in the US from fermented red clover to produce agricultural rat poison) acts by inhibiting the manufacture of four of the clotting factors in the liver. This reduces the effectiveness of the clotting cascade, and therefore reduces the formation of clots. Patients with thrombosis or embolism may be started on this drug in hospital. As warfarin takes a few days to reach therapeutic levels in the blood, the patient is treated with injections of LMWH until this time. The dose of warfarin is adjusted in accordance with the results of regular blood tests (the international normalized ratio (INR) test is used) to check that the clotting time of the blood has been increased, but not by too much.

Patients remain on warfarin for six weeks to six months in the case of a single episode of thrombosis/embolism, but may have to be on lifelong treatment if the problem recurs, or if there is a long-term risk such as from a damaged heart valve or a severe form of inherited thrombophilia. The main problem with warfarin is difficulty in achieving ideal levels of the drug in the blood, and thus an increased risk of severe bleeding. In overdose, vitamin K acts as an antidote for warfarin as it promotes the formation of the clotting factors that warfarin inhibits. Patients are advised to avoid alcohol and drugs that can affect the liver and alter the effect of warfarin. Other rare side effects of warfarin include rashes, nausea and jaundice.

NOACs such as apixaban and rivaroxaban act by inhibiting factor 10a in the clotting cascade, and dabigatran is a direct thrombin inhibitor. They all have the effect of inhibiting the action of thrombin and thus the formation of fibrin from fibrinogen. They are all more rapid in action than warfarin and also have a shorter half-life, meaning that they are metabolized more quickly. Their dosage does not need to be controlled in the same way as warfarin, and regular blood tests are not needed. In many ways these medications are more user friendly than warfarin, although the lack of an antidote in the case of severe bleeding is a concern. Their side effects include rashes, anemia and digestive symptoms such as dyspepsia and abdominal pain.

Prevention of thrombosis and embolism

Lifestyle factors that may be discussed with a patient with regard to prevention of thrombosis and embolism include:

- weight loss
- avoidance of long periods of immobility
- smoking cessation

- stopping the combined oral contraceptive pill

- strict attention to control of blood lipids and diabetes.

Aspirin and warfarin are both used for the long-term prevention of thrombosis in patients who are more susceptible to thrombosis and embolism. Low-dose aspirin is advised for patients with angina, some patients with AF, and for patients who have had a heart attack or stroke.

Clopidogrel is commonly prescribed to prevent stroke and heart attack, and ticagrelor in particular for the vulnerable year after a heart attack.

Warfarin is advised for patients who have had recurrent DVT/embolism, patients with damaged or replacement heart valves and most patients with AF.

NOACs are recommended for prevention of stroke in AF and also for prevention of incidence or recurrence of DVT.

LMWH is given by injection to some patients who are undergoing surgery. This acts in a similar way to warfarin, but is rapid acting and the effects wear off quickly. Heparin cannot be given by mouth, so is generally confined to hospital use, but is prescribed in a form that makes injections possible for self-administration at home by patients.

 Information box 2.2d-I

Thrombosis, embolism and infarction: comments from a Chinese medicine perspective

In Chinese medicine inappropriate clotting could be described in terms of Blood Stagnation and Phlegm formation. Blood Stagnation is described by Chinese medicine in terms of severe stabbing pain, fixed masses and purple discoloration, all of which may commonly accompany thrombosis or embolism. The congealed clot is a manifestation of Phlegm, and associated symptoms may include local swelling and collapse with loss of consciousness.

The recognized causes of Blood Stagnation in Chinese medicine include Liver Qi Stagnation, Blood and Qi Deficiency, Interior Cold and Heat in the Blood. It is therefore likely that one or more of these patterns will be apparent in the case of an individual patient who is at risk of thrombosis or embolism. Additional factors that promote Phlegm formation such as Spleen Qi Deficiency and poor diet will also contribute to the risk of thrombosis, embolism or infarction.

Aspirin relieves symptoms by reducing platelet stickiness, and common side effects include bleeding from the stomach lining, asthma and allergic reactions. By preventing the blood from clotting, the action of aspirin might be described as Moving Blood and Qi. The movement of Blood and Qi has been interpreted as resulting from the Warming action of aspirin. Aspirin is also recognized to play a role in releasing the Exterior in the treatment of febrile disease.

The side effect of gastrointestinal bleeding, however, suggests that aspirin causes Stomach Heat. The other recognized side effect of aspirin, asthma, has associations with an allergic response. As noted above, this suggests that aspirin might also have a depressive effect on Wei Qi in susceptible people, and so permit the Invasion of Wind.

In summary, broad statements about aspirin in terms of Chinese energetics are that it is Warming in nature and that it also seems to cause Heat in the Stomach. In susceptible people it may result in depression of Wei Qi (leading to allergic asthma).

Warfarin relieves symptoms by increasing the clotting time of blood. This is through the action it has on the liver in which it inhibits the formation of clotting factors. Side effects listed in the *British National Formulary* (BNF) include bleeding, rash, hair loss, low red blood cell count (hematocrit), diarrhea, purple toes and death (necrosis) of skin, and liver and pancreatic disorders.

In Chinese medicine, the syndromes related to an increased tendency to bleed include Full Heat, Yin Deficiency with Empty Heat, Spleen not holding Blood and Blood Stagnation.

Bleeding resulting from warfarin anticoagulation can be profuse. Profuse bleeding would be in keeping with the Chinese medicine description of Heating the Blood. The purple toes and skin necrosis suggest that warfarin can also cause Blood Stagnation. This may be a consequence of Liver Qi Stagnation, and thus it is of interest that this drug acts directly on the liver, and can cause liver disorders. The remaining side effects imply that the function of the Spleen is also affected, explaining, for example, the diarrhea.

In summary, broad statements about warfarin in terms of Chinese energetics are that it is Heating in nature and that it also seems to cause Disharmony of the Liver and Spleen. The energetic effects of NOACs are very similar to those of warfarin.

2.3

Cancer

In developed countries the impact of cancer on health is enormous. The lifetime risk of developing cancer in the US is 42 percent for men and 38 percent for women.[40] The statistics are comparable in the UK for which, according to Cancer Research UK (2016), one in two people born after 1960 will be diagnosed with some form of cancer during their lifetime.[41] Not all of these people will die from cancer, however. In terms of mortality, in 2015 cancer accounted for approximately 22.5 percent of all deaths in the US, second only to cardiovascular disease. The proportion of total mortality attributable to cancer was calculated to be 29 percent for the UK based on 2011 data.[42] The worldwide percentage figure for cancer deaths is 13 percent, only lower because in developing countries diseases relating to malnutrition and infection significantly contribute to premature non-cancer-related mortality.

The commonest forms of cancer worldwide are of the lung, stomach, liver, bowel and breast. At least a third of cancers are known to be associated with potentially modifiable risk factors of which smoking, physical inactivity, alcohol, diet, obesity and exposure to the human papilloma virus (HPV) (through sexual activity) are the most significant in terms of numbers of people affected.

Many people who have been offered conventional therapy for cancer will also seek complementary medical treatment. Increasingly, and perhaps more so for cancer than for other chronic diseases, the conventional medical approach in Western countries is embracing complementary treatments such as acupuncture, reflexology and visualization as part of the normal provision of care for a patient with cancer. This is very common in the context of cancer care centers or hospices. It is particularly important that those practitioners of complementary medicine who may be working in a conventional medical setting have a clear understanding of the conventional understanding of the causation of cancer and how it can be treated.

This chapter focuses on the broad principles of pathology and treatment that apply to all forms of cancer. Each type of cancer has its own particular features. More details about the most important types of cancer can be found in those later sections in which the diseases of the physiological systems in which they arise are discussed.

The pathology of cancer

The initiation of cancer

As explained in Section 1.1b, cancer is the result of cumulative mutation in mitosis (leading to genetic change of the DNA) and also additional damage to the way in which the DNA in a cell functions (epigenetic change). A cancer cell develops when this cumulative damage leads to increasingly poorly controlled growth in the daughter cell lines.

A healthy cell responds to the cells around it such that it only self-replicates in a controlled way. There are many proteins produced within the cell that control its replication. These are coded for by genes called proto-oncogenes located within the chromosomes of the cell's nucleus. The delicate function of these replication proteins within the cell becomes disordered if the proto-oncogene becomes mutated or moved during mitosis, or if it loses its relationship to another controlling gene on a chromosome as a result of insertion of the genetic material from a virus. When the function of a proto-oncogene is altered so that cell replication is no longer so well controlled, it is then known as an oncogene.

It is increasingly recognized that epigenetic processes are key to the evolution of a cancer cell line.

These processes do not involve change to the genetic code embodied by the DNA, but instead affect the way by which the DNA is repaired or replicates. Some of these involve the control of genes that provide the information that directs the manufacture of the cell tumor-suppressor proteins. Tumor-suppressor proteins have diverse roles, including the recognition and repair of damaged DNA in the nucleus (over 150 different forms of these protein enzymes have been identified). Others activate the process of apoptosis (programmed cell death) in cells that have sustained too much damage. Apoptosis is a controlled form of cellular suicide that does not involve an inflammation-inducing release of cell contents.

If tumor-suppressor genes lose their function through mutation, or the proteins they code for are inhibited in some way, cancerous multiplication of cells is more likely. One tumor-suppressor mutation in the gene coding for the protein known as p53 has been identified in up to 50 percent of all forms of human tumor, depending on type of cancer. In health p53 is activated by damaged DNA, and when activated it halts the normal process of mitosis to allow for DNA repair. It also initiates apoptosis if the DNA damage is too extensive.[43]

Carcinogens and viruses can inactivate tumor-suppressor proteins, and this is an example of an epigenetic change that can promote cancerous growth.

In summary, cancer cells have lost the ability for ordered growth because of changes such as the presence of oncogenes and the production of ineffective tumor-suppressor proteins. The generation of an established cancer is called carcinogenesis (literally meaning the creation of cancer). For carcinogenesis to occur, a complex series of mutations must have occurred in proto-oncogenes and the genes that code for the manufacture of tumor-suppressor proteins. These mutations and alteration in DNA control proteins may have developed over many cycles of cell division, sometimes taking years, until they eventually give rise to a cancerous growth. As cancer cells continue to multiply, more mutations may arise, and the growth can become inexorably chaotic. The cancer may eventually invade neighboring tissues. The result is an irregular mass of cells called a tumor (meaning swelling) or neoplasm (meaning new growth).

In order to sustain continued growth, tumors require a blood supply. Invasive tumors do this by secreting proteins that promote the ingrowth of new blood vessels, a process known as angiogenesis. These proteins are also the by-product of cancerous mutations.

Most mutated cells are recognized by the immune system as abnormal because they present unfamiliar patterns of proteins in their cell membranes. As a result

they are removed by cytotoxic T-lymphocytes as part of the immune response. It is only those cells that slip through this protective net that develop into tumors. Some tumors effectively paralyze this protective action of the immune system by secreting immunosuppressive proteins. These contribute to the general immunodeficiency seen in some patients with cancer.

The newly mutated cancer cells need to bypass the safety net provided by the immune system. Cancer is, therefore, more likely in those people who have impaired immune systems, in those in whom the rate of spontaneous mutation of the genetic material in certain cells is higher than normal, or in those who have inherited or acquired less efficient tumor-suppressive mechanisms.

The cause of increased mutation: carcinogens

It is known that mutation occurs frequently simply as a result of natural error. Cells are dividing all the time, and some of these divisions are not perfect, resulting in a mutation in the genetic material of the daughter cells. In most cases all these defective cells are removed either by the action of diverse tumor-suppressor proteins or by the cytotoxic cells of the immune system.

However, under certain conditions the number of mutations arising in a tissue will increase, and the risk of the formation of cancerous cells will also increase. The effectiveness of the tumor-suppressive mechanisms can also be impaired by external factors impacting on the health of the DNA and the tumor-suppressor proteins. When this happens there is an increased susceptibility to the development of established cancer, as the sheer numbers of cancer cells being produced increases the risk of failure of the tumor-suppressor and immune mechanisms to eliminate every single abnormal cell.

Diverse environmental factors, including tobacco smoke, alcohol, dietary factors, ultraviolet light, chemicals in the environment, infectious microbes and drugs, have all been shown to be carcinogenic. Most of these are carcinogenic because they tend to promote mutations, either of proto-oncogenes or of tumor-suppressor protein genes, or because they impair tumor suppression directly. Also, certain viruses can insert cancer-promoting sections of DNA into the chromosome or, as described earlier, can inhibit the action of tumor-suppressor proteins. Other carcinogens, such as X-radiation and cancer chemotherapeutic agents, impair the protective action of the immune system. Table 2.3-I summarizes some of the common carcinogens and the diverse forms of cancer that can result from exposure to them.

Table 2.3-I Some common carcinogens and the cancers they cause

Carcinogen	Cancer caused
Tobacco smoke	Mouth, esophagus, larynx, lung, bladder
Alcohol	Mouth, esophagus, larynx, colon, rectum
High-fat diet	Colon, rectum
Naturally occurring environmental factors, e.g. ultraviolet light	Skin
Naturally occurring environmental factors, e.g. radon gas	Lung
Industrial exposure: asbestos	Lung
Industrial exposure: vinyl chloride	Liver
Industrial exposure: radiation	Leukemia, thyroid
Infectious agents: hepatitis B and C infection	Liver
Infectious agents: Helicobacter pylori	Stomach
Infectious agents: human papilloma virus (HPV)	Cervix
Infectious agents: human immunodeficiency virus	Kaposi's sarcoma, lymphoma
Medications: estrogens	Endometrial, breast
Medications: androgens	Prostate
Medications: cytotoxic drugs	Bladder, bone marrow

Congenital susceptibility to cancer

It is recognized that a tendency to develop cancers may be inherited. In some cases the tendency to suffer from particular cancers can run very strongly in families. For example, there is one rare form of breast cancer that will develop in over 80 percent of the daughters of women who have been diagnosed with that cancer. This cancer develops as a result of the transmission of the *BRCA1* and *BRCA2* gene defects. These defects result in inefficient DNA repair mechanisms in breast and ovarian tissues. Inherited defects in the aforementioned p52 tumor-suppressor gene are also well researched and correlate with increased incidence of cancer.

In such inherited cases, there is increased susceptibility to cancer, either because of an inherited relative deficiency of the immune system, or because the cells of certain tissues are genetically more prone to mutation.

Acquired susceptibility to cancer

The susceptibility to the effect of carcinogens also depends on the health of the immune system. This is impaired in conditions that cause immunodeficiency, as described in Section 2.2c. In addition, factors such as stress and aging will also contribute to impaired immune responses, and may permit a mutated cell to continue to divide and form a malignant tumor.

The development and spread of cancer

Tumors may be considered as benign or malignant. Benign growths are areas of overgrowth of normal tissue in which the replication of the individual cells remains orderly. Common benign growths include fatty subcutaneous lumps, lipomas and leiomyomas (the muscular fibroid commonly found in the womb). Benign growths tend to be very slow growing and, because they are non-invasive, have a smooth distinct boundary that separates them from neighboring tissue. They do not spread to distant sites.

In general, the term cancer is only used to describe malignant tumors. Malignant tumors demonstrate much more chaotic growth and may contain a number of different cell lines (a state described as pleomorphic) as a result of repeated mutations. The spread of the primary malignant tumor tends to be invasive and irregular as it finds its way through the normal tissues from which it has arisen. The name cancer is derived from the Latin word for crab. This term expressed for early pathologists the claw-like growth of the cancer tissue into neighboring tissues.

The term primary cancer describes a malignant growth that is the result of local spread at the site of the original cancer cell.

Secondary, or metastatic, cancer describes new cancerous growths that have spread to other sites from the original location of the primary cancer. Secondary spread can occur by seeding of malignant cells via the lymphatic system, the circulation or across the body cavities such as the intra-abdominal space. For example, a primary lung cancer is situated within the lung, but secondary lung cancer might develop in the thoracic lymph nodes, the brain and the adrenal glands as a result of spread via the lymphatic and circulatory systems.

The effects of malignant tumors

As malignant tumors continue to grow they can exert a diverse range of symptoms. Pain is a much feared symptom of cancer, although it is not necessarily a significant cause of distress in many cases. Pain can result from the pressure of a tumor in an enclosed space, blockage of a hollow organ causing the organ to distend, and also from invasion of or pressure on nerves.

Cachexia is the term used to describe loss of appetite, weight loss and general feeling of malaise that affects many patients with advanced cancer. Nausea and constipation can also be very distressing symptoms of advanced cancer.

The immune system is often depressed in advanced cancer, partly because of the malnutrition that accompanies cachexia, and partly because of the tumor's ability to produce immunosuppressant proteins. Moreover, if the cancer invades the bone marrow (leading to bone marrow failure), the production of leukocytes will be impaired. Immune deficiency leaves the body open to infectious diseases that may give rise to symptoms such as cough, fever and cloudy urine. These symptoms may have the characteristics of opportunistic infections.

Additional consequences of bone marrow failure are anemia and bleeding from thrombocytopenia. Organ failure (e.g. failure of parts of the brain, kidney or liver) can lead to severe life-threatening symptoms.

Bleeding resulting from damage to blood vessels is a common first symptom of cancer, and can be so severe as to be life-threatening.

 Information box 2.3-1

Cancer: comments from a Chinese medicine perspective

From a conventional medicine perspective, tumors result from excessive and inappropriate overgrowth of tissue cells. The underlying problem is that the genetic control of cell multiplication has become disordered, and the immune system has failed to recognize and control the growth of these disordered cells.

The category of cancer was not one recognized in ancient Chinese medicine. Instead, the various manifestations were described according to the individual constellation of symptoms and signs presented. For example, the symptomatic description used in the *Jia Yi Jing* written by Huang-Fu Mi in the 3rd century CE, for the External Cold-induced Intestinal Mushroom, would appear to relate to colon cancer.[44]

Modern Chinese medicine oncology dates only from the 20th century, and recognizes diverse etiological factors including disordered emotions, poor diet and external attack by Pathogens (Toxins) and weakened Zang-Fu organs.[45] There are diverse names for the different sorts of tumors (e.g. fan wei, gastric regurgitation due to obstruction, and xuan pi, a cord-like swelling). The etiology of each is different and suggestive of a chain of events and cumulative damage over a long period of time. Important Syndromes predisposing to cancer include Stagnation of Qi and Deficient Spleen and Kidney Qi. These contribute to Accumulation and Stasis of Blood, Generation of Heat and Congealing of Blood and Fluids into Phlegm Cold or Phlegm Heat. Heat Toxins and other Pathogenic Factors may complicate this process. This process will be manifest in tumors, and is in keeping with the understanding that any substantial masses that do not easily move are regarded as Accumulations of either Phlegm or Blood Stagnation or a combination of both. Blood Stagnation is characterized by hardness and intense boring pain, with violaceous color changes. Phlegm is more often associated with numbness, and will usually develop against a backdrop of Heat and Damp, which will manifest in other signs and symptoms. For long-standing masses to develop there will be a pre-existing state of Deficiency of Qi, either locally or generally, as it is only healthy Qi moving freely that prevents the development of Stagnation and Phlegm.

In contrast to the Western medical approach, which is to remove the tumors, the focus of treatment in Chinese medicine oncology is generally a combination of strengthening the root by nourishing Upright Qi and supporting the Spirit (a treatment approach known as Fu Zheng Qu Xie) and also moving of Blood and Dispelling Stasis (Huo Xue Qu Yu) and also expelling Toxins. It would be usual in modern Chinese oncology, if Chinese medicine is to be used, for it to be combined with conventional medicine as it is recognized that once a tumor had developed, a powerful treatment is required to dissolve the mass.[46]

The conventional treatment of cancer

From a conventional medical viewpoint the ideal cancer treatment would relieve symptoms by total removal of the cancerous growth and elimination of any remaining cancer cells.

However, when the cancer is so advanced that cure is not possible, the main aim of treatment is symptom relief. Treatment that is directed at symptom relief is called palliative care. The provision of palliative care is now considered to be a medical specialty in itself.

Treatment of the cancerous growth

There are three broad approaches to treatment aimed at removing or inhibiting the cancerous growth:

- surgery (removal of cancerous tissue)

- chemotherapy (treatment by means of drugs)

- radiotherapy (treatment by substances that emit radiation).

SURGERY

The main principle underlying the surgical treatment of cancer is to remove all the cancer cells or, if this ideal is not attainable, to remove as much cancer tissue as possible. Even if total cure is not possible, debulking surgical treatment may be performed to mitigate the deleterious pressure effects of tumors.

Cure may be possible if a malignant growth is diagnosed before secondary spread has occurred. The surgical ideal is to cut out (excise) the growth and the normal tissue surrounding it to a certain depth. This may mean that a lot of normal tissue is removed, such as the whole breast in a mastectomy for breast cancer, or a large circle of skin and underlying flesh when a melanoma is excised. The tissue that has been removed can then be examined under the microscope to ensure that all the apparent boundaries of the cancer have been completely excised.

In practice it is never possible to be absolutely sure that an excised malignant growth has not already led to tiny secondary metastases. For tumors that are known to spread easily, such as breast, cervical and bowel cancer, a patient who has had surgery may also be offered treatment with radiotherapy and chemotherapy, which is intended to shrink tumors and kill or hinder the growth of any possible remaining cancer cells. This additional supportive treatment is called neoadjuvant therapy if used prior to surgery and adjuvant therapy if used after surgery.

If a cancer is in such a location that it cannot be removed fully by surgery, it is described as inoperable. This term applies to very large spreading tumors, or those that are growing into vital structures such as the major blood vessels.

CHEMOTHERAPY

Chemotherapy in its broadest sense literally refers to any form of medical treatment that employs chemical substances (drugs). However, the term is most commonly used to describe the drug treatments used in cases of cancer. Chemotherapy in cancer can involve treatments that are intended to target and kill all cancer cells. This is known as cytotoxic treatment. Other forms of chemotherapy have been introduced that aim either to modulate the immune response to the tumor or to affect the way in which it responds to hormones.

One major problem with chemotherapy is that all classes of cancer drug have powerful side effects (drug-induced disease). The science of cancer chemotherapy is very complex and continually changing in response to the rapidly increasing understanding of the genetics and pathology of cancer. For this reason, its use is usually overseen in clinical practice by hospital specialists known as oncologists.

CYTOTOXIC DRUGS

Cytotoxic drugs are the group of drugs most commonly used to inhibit the growth of cancer cells. These drugs are preferentially absorbed by rapidly growing cells and lead to their death by inhibiting the replication of the DNA within them. Because of their rapid growth, cancer cells in particular are affected by cytotoxic drugs. However, normal tissues are also affected, largely depending on how rapidly the cells divide in those tissues. The rapidly dividing cells of the lining of the bowel, bladder and lungs, the sex organs, bone marrow and hair are particularly affected by cytotoxics. Common side effects include inflammation of tissues around the site of injection, sore mouth, nausea and vomiting, hair loss, suppression of blood cell production in the bone marrow and impaired fertility.

Different cytotoxic drugs affect different aspects of cancer growth, and so are commonly given in combination. This practice also reduces the risk of the tumor developing resistance to the chemotherapeutic agents, an unfortunate consequence of ongoing mutations in cancer tissue.

The alkylating cytotoxics include drugs such as cyclophosphamide, chlorambucil, busulfan and carmustine. These all act by causing damage to DNA. With prolonged use they are very toxic to sex cells (in particular, sperm), and also carry a risk of causing a form of leukemia.

Anthracyclines, which include doxorubicin, daunorubicin, bleomycin and mitomycin, are antibiotic-like drugs. These tend to inhibit DNA repair in multiplying cells and so lead to cell damage. Their effects seem to be similar to those of radiotherapy, and some of the side effects include strong inflammatory reactions, including inflammation of tissues at the site of infusion and red skin eruptions.

Antimetabolites, including methotrexate, cytarabine and fluorouracil, block the synthesis of DNA in dividing cells.

Topoisomerase inhibitors such as etoposide work by inducing breaks in the cell DNA during cell replication, so hastening cell death.

Vinca alkaloids, originally derived from the periwinkle plant, block the action of the spindle that separates the two nuclei in dividing cells, and so inhibit cell division. This class of drugs includes vincristine and vinblastine.

Taxanes, such as paclitaxel, are derived from the bark of the yew tree, and these also interfere with the formation of the spindle in mitosis.

Finally, the platinum-containing cytotoxic drugs tend to cause damaging cross-links between strands of DNA, and so impair cell reproduction. Drugs of this type include cisplatin and carboplatin.

CORTICOSTEROIDS

Corticosteroids are commonly used in cancer chemotherapy for their anti-inflammatory effects. They have antitumor effects in leukemia and lymphoma, and are frequently included as part of the treatment regimens for these conditions. They are also used to minimize the effects of inflammation, and improve appetite and well-being in advanced malignant disease.

BIOLOGICAL THERAPY

Biological agents are all complex protein compounds that are designed to interfere with the growth and development of the cancer tissue. Some of these act as immunotherapy. For example, interferon alpha (IFA) and interleukin-2 (IL-2) are genetically engineered copies of naturally occurring substances that are central to the control of the immune response. In cancer therapy both IFA and IL-2 hinder cell proliferation and promote the action of the lymphocytes. Other forms of cancer immunotherapy include using cultures of the patient's own lymphocytes to target cancer cells, and bacteria to stimulate a cancer-specific immune response (e.g. the tuberculosis vaccine, Bacillus Calmette-Guérin (BCG), has been used to stimulate an immune response to bladder cancer).

An increasing number of genetically engineered antibodies are available that target and cause the destruction of the protein growth factors produced by tumors. These include trastuzumab (Herceptin), which was designed to counteract a growth factor known as *Her2*. *Her2* plays a role in the maintenance of metastatic breast cancer.

Other antibody products have been designed to target cancer cells directly, for example, rituximab, which can cause the death of cells in B-cell lymphoma.

ENDOCRINE THERAPY

Some breast, prostate and womb (endometrial) cancers are dependent on sex hormones for their continued growth. In these cases, if the hormones are prevented from exerting their effects, the cancer will shrink and may even disappear. Endocrine therapy involves treatments that affect the balance of the sex hormones for those forms of cancer that are recognized to be hormone dependent.

Approximately one-third of breast cancers will grow more rapidly in the presence of the female sex hormone, estrogen, as a result of protein estrogen receptors within the cytoplasm of the cancer cells. The male sex hormone, testosterone, likewise stimulates the growth of prostate cancer.

The growth of hormone-dependent tumors may therefore be hindered by means of drugs that counteract the effect of the hormones, drugs that inhibit the release of these hormones, or by surgical removal of the ovaries (oophorectomy) or testes (orchiectomy).

Drugs that counteract the effect of estrogen are commonly used in the treatment of breast cancers. Tamoxifen and raloxifene partially block estrogen receptors, and so prevent circulating estrogen from having

such a marked effect on breast cancer cells. Tamoxifen is prescribed in the form of a tablet to be taken daily for at least five years. Anastrozole is an example of a drug that prevents the manufacture of estrogen in cancer cells from other steroid hormones, and is considered more useful in the treatment of hormone-dependent breast cancer in postmenopausal women. Goserelin is an example of a drug that acts at the pituitary gland to reduce the release of a hormone (known as luteinizing hormone (LH)), the function of which is to stimulate hormone production by the ovaries and testes. This drug may be prescribed in both breast cancer and prostate cancer.

THE PRINCIPLES OF CHEMOTHERAPY

The smaller the tumor, the more likely it is that cytotoxic drugs can cause sufficient damage to the cancer cells to completely eliminate the tumor. The dose of the cytotoxic drug has to be moderated by the potential damage it may cause to normal tissues. This is one reason why cytotoxic drugs are given in combination with immunosuppressant drugs and in repeated cycles over the course of a few days or weeks. The immunosuppressant drugs hinder the growth of the tumor, and so keep it small during the course of the treatment. The time allowed between repeated cycles is intended to permit normal tissues to recover before another dose of cytotoxic drugs is given to target the cancer cells.

If, after a course of chemotherapy, all cancer cells seem to have disappeared, the patient is said to be in remission. This is not the same as cure, as there may still be a few tiny clusters of cancer cells remaining that may lead to recurrent tumors in the future. However, the longer patients are in remission, the greater the likelihood is that they have achieved full cure.

RADIOTHERAPY

Certain tumors appear to shrink rapidly in response to radiation treatment. This can be given to the patient either in the form of concentrated X-radiation or gamma radiation emitted by an external machine (external beam radiotherapy), or from an implant of a radioactive substance surgically inserted or injected into the body close to the tumor for a short period of time (brachytherapy). The effect of the radiation is to induce breaks in the DNA and to induce apoptosis (programmed cell death) of dividing cells.

The principles of treatment and risks of radiotherapy are remarkably similar to those of chemotherapy. The aim is to kill all rapidly dividing cells, but normal dividing cells can be damaged at the same time. Radiotherapy, therefore, is also given in cycles of treatment over the course of a few weeks. The primary tumors that may respond well to radiotherapy include brain tumors and tumors of the eye, skin cancer, cancers of the mouth, larynx and esophagus, cancer of the cervix and vagina, and cancer of the prostate and lymphoma. Radiotherapy can also be used as an adjuvant therapy after surgical removal of a primary tumor. For example, patients with cancer of the breast, lung, uterus, bladder, rectum or testis may be treated with radiotherapy after the cancer has been excised.

The risks of radiotherapy are of inflammation and long-term scarring of normal tissue in the area exposed to the radiation, and also of future cancers as a result of the carcinogenic effects of the treatment.

Staging and prediction of benefit

In general, the chances of cure are considered greater when treatment is given to cancer at an earlier stage of progression than one that is more advanced. Complex systems of quantifying exactly how advanced a cancer has become have been developed for most cancer types. This quantification is called staging. It is considered important to stage a cancer accurately before a prediction of outcome can be made. This is why patients with cancer may have to undergo many tests such as biopsies and scans before they begin treatment. Patients may then be given statistical figures to express the chances they have of cure with a particular treatment. These figures will have been derived from clinical studies of the treatment given to patients with the same type of cancer at the same stage of progression.

For example, a patient with a form of testicular cancer may be told that they have a 90 percent chance of survival. This means that nine in every ten people who received the treatment for that sort of cancer at the same stage of progression in clinical studies recovered completely. Another example is that a patient with esophageal cancer may be told that they can expect to live for 12 months. This means that in studies of that form of cancer at the same stage the average length of time from diagnosis to death was 12 months.

Another way of expressing outcome is in terms of years of survival. The chemotherapy used for a form of cancer of the ovary may be said to lead to a 70 percent five-year survival rate, and a 10 percent ten-year survival rate. This means that at five years after the treatment 70 percent of patients are still alive, but after ten years many more have died, leaving only 10 percent of the original patients alive.

The challenge for patients in making sense of these figures is that they are derived statistically from clinical studies involving large groups of people. The patient with cancer is an individual and may or may not be typical of the majority of people in the experimental group. It is impossible to be confident that the statistics are relevant to an individual person. There may be a number of variables, including positive outlook, lifestyle change and use of complementary therapies, which may alter dramatically the outcome of that individual's treatment, and so make the statistics meaningless in the context of their particular situation. Nevertheless they are always very useful figures for comparing treatments.

Ideally these data should be considered to help inform any decision about what forms of cancer treatment might be the best choice for an individual patient.

Palliative treatments in cancer

Surgery, chemotherapy and radiotherapy

The three treatment modalities of surgery, chemotherapy and radiotherapy may also be used in advanced cancer to alleviate symptoms, even when there is no hope of cure. This is because they all tend to remove the bulk of the tumor, and so can temporarily alleviate distressing symptoms.

In palliative treatment, the discomfort of the side effects has always to be balanced against the amount of relief that can be expected to result from the treatment. This is not always easy to do, and often the patient is left with a difficult decision about whether or not to accept treatment. In recent years the most debilitating side effect of nausea has been treated effectively with powerful medications (e.g. ondansetron) in 75 percent of patients on chemotherapy. Advances such as this are likely to increase the proportion of patients with an incurable cancer who are offered chemotherapy or radiotherapy.

It is recognized that many patients may not fully realize that such invasive treatment is not intended to produce cure, even when every attempt has been made to explain the reality of their poor prognosis. This may lead them to accept treatment while holding false hopes that their cancer will be cured.

Painkillers

Painkilling (analgesic) medication may be prescribed liberally in cases of advanced cancer. If pain starts to become chronic, it is considered good practice to encourage the patient to maintain a steady dose of analgesic so that distressing pain never breaks through. Ideally, combinations of different classes of painkilling drugs are prescribed that may act in different and complementary ways to reduce pain. These include the simple painkillers (anti-inflammatory drugs, such as ibuprofen and paracetamol) and opiate drugs, which are related to morphine. The most important classes of painkillers are discussed in detail in Section 4.2c later.

Opiate drugs

Opiate drugs fall into a class of medication used widely for symptom relief in serious disease in conventional medicine. The most commonly used opiate medications include morphine, diamorphine (heroin), oxycodone and pethidine. Small amounts of opiate drugs are found in combination with simple painkillers in preparations such as co-codamol and co-dydramol.

Opiates are the most powerful painkillers available. Their side effects include drowsiness, suppressed respiration, constipation and nausea. They can also promote a sense of profound well-being, thus explaining why they are also commonly used as illegal recreational drugs. The effects of opiate drugs wear off rapidly, however, and this can lead to recurrence of symptoms and a drop in mood. They induce dependency because they reduce the body's response to its naturally produced opiates.

Patients using opiates for pain relief often require gradually increasing doses to keep their symptoms under control. It is not uncommon for a cancer patient eventually to be able to tolerate a dose of opiates that would be lethal to a healthy person.

Constipation almost always complicates the prescription of strong opiates such as morphine or diamorphine. Therefore, most patients will be prescribed a stimulant laxative such as dantron when initiating opiate treatment.

Non-steroidal anti-inflammatory drugs (NSAIDs)
Non-steroidal anti-inflammatory drugs (NSAIDs) are very effective painkillers for pain that has inflammation or bone disease as its cause. Very often, NSAIDs may be prescribed in combination with opiates in the treatment of chronic pain. As NSAIDs carry a high risk of inducing irritation and bleeding of the stomach lining, they are often prescribed together with a proton pump inhibitor (PPI) acid-suppressing medication such as omeprazole.

Tricyclic antidepressants for pain
Antidepressants such as amitriptyline may be prescribed for their ability to alleviate certain types of chronic pain. They have the additional benefits of mood elevation and sleep promotion.

Drugs for nausea
Nausea is a common side effect of chemotherapy and painkillers, and can also occur as a result of the cancer alone. It can be a very debilitating side effect, and affects over 60 percent of terminally ill cancer patients.

Antinausea drugs include metoclopramide, which is most effective if the cause of the nausea is gastrointestinal in origin. If the cause is more likely to be a result of some sort of central brain disturbance (as a consequence of metabolic imbalance), cyclizine, which is also used for travel sickness, may be more effective. Major tranquillizer drugs such as prochlorperazine and haloperidol are also effective in reducing central nausea.

To prevent the nausea that results from cancer chemotherapy the 5-HT3 antagonists such as ondansetron and intravenous corticosteroids may be prescribed in the hospital ward prior to and during treatment. Some centers recommend that during chemotherapy their patients wear Sea-Bands, which put pressure at the wrist on the acupoint Nei Guan (PC-6).

Treatment for depression
The emotional burden on a patient with cancer has many components. Factors such as fear of dying, regrets about past events, inability to express negative emotions, discomfort from side effects, changing body image and disempowerment in hospital can all contribute to the development of a disabling depression. It is now recognized that patients require support to enable them to express these issues, and to be given as much dignity and freedom as possible. The ideal is to enable a cancer patient to remain at home for as long as possible.

The more holistic approach to palliative care, which involves counseling, alternative therapies, spiritual support and support of relatives, is intended to help patients deal with the development of distressing symptoms and to reduce depression.

The SSRI (selective serotonin reuptake inhibitor) antidepressants, such as paroxetine and sertraline, are also prescribed very readily in palliative care. They take two to four weeks to exert a therapeutic effect.

Red flags of cancer

The red flag syndromes that might indicate the presence of cancer are summarized in Table 2.3-II, the first of the red flag tables. A summary of the red flags in a format designed for quick reference in clinical practice can be found in Appendix III. This summary also gives advice on the degree of urgency of referral for each of the red flag conditions listed.

Table 2.3-II A1: Red flags of cancer

Cancer is characterized by progressive growth of diseased tissue over the course of weeks to months and the loss of function that can result from the damage caused by this growth. The patient may therefore experience deterioration in function that may either be gradual or may appear with the sudden development of new symptoms that do not go away. The red flags of cancer include any progressive unexplained symptoms that persist over the course of weeks to months without resolution. Unexplained sizeable lumps and lymph nodes may also be indicative of cancerous change.

Red flag	Description	Reasoning
A1.1	Progressive unexplained symptoms over weeks to months: e.g. weight loss, recurrent sweats (especially at night), fevers and poor appetite	Symptoms that progress (i.e. gradually worsen rather than fluctuate in intensity) over this sort of time period are strongly suggestive of cancer Note: There is usually no need to request a high-priority referral when wanting to exclude a diagnosis of cancer, as this might increase rather than allay anxiety. Only consider high-priority referral if you suspect rapidly progressive disease, or if the patient is already very anxious
A1.2	An unexplained lump >1cm in diameter: characteristically hard, irregular, fixed and painless	Cancerous lumps are usually irregular, may be fixed to associated tissues, and are often painless unless they obstruct viscera, cause pressure on other structures, grow into bone or grow into nerve roots Soft, round mobile lumps are more likely to be benign tumors. Painful lumps are more characteristic of inflammation or infection than cancer
A1.3	Unexplained bleeding: either from the surface of the skin, or emerging from an internal organ such as the bowel, bladder or uterus (e.g. blood in vomit, blood in urine, rectal bleeding or vaginal bleeding)	Cancerous tissue is poorly organized, and bleeding may easily be provoked from the surface of an epithelial tumor (e.g. of breast, skin, lung, mouth, stomach, bowel, bladder or uterus)
A1.4	Features of bone marrow failure: severe progressive anemia (see A18.2), recurrent progressive infections or bruising, purpura and bleeding	Secondary cancer and cancer of the blood cells often infiltrate the bone marrow and prevent it from performing its role of producing healthy red and white blood cells and platelets Purpura is pin-point bruising, which looks like a rash of flat, purplish spots, and is one of the signs of a low platelet count
A1.5	Multiple enlarged lymph nodes (>1cm in diameter): painless, with no other obvious cause (e.g. known glandular fever infection) and lasting for more than two weeks	Groups of lymph nodes can be found in the cervical region, in the armpits (axillary nodes) and in the inguinal creases (groin). In health, lymph nodes are usually soft, impalpable masses of soft tissue, but these can enlarge and become more palpable when the node is active in fighting an infection, or if it is infiltrated by tumor cells. If a number of nodes are enlarged (to >1cm in diameter), this may signify a generalized infectious disease such as glandular fever or human immunodeficiency virus (HIV) infection The other important cause of widespread lymph node enlargement (lymphadenopathy) is disseminated cancer, in particular, cancers of the white blood cells (leukemia and lymphoma) If multiple enlarged lymph nodes are found, it is best to refer for a diagnosis, and as a high priority if the patient is unwell with other symptoms
A1.6	A single, markedly enlarged lymph node (>2cm in diameter) with no other obvious cause	Even in the situation of infection it is unusual for a lymph node to become very enlarged. Cancerous infiltration can lead to a firm enlarged lymph node that may be painless. This is particularly typical of lymphoma

A1.7	Painless abdominal swelling or bloating	Abdominal epithelial malignancies such as colon, stomach and ovarian cancer may lead to the accumulation of fluid within the abdominal cavity, which may initially be painless. This sign is known as ascites. Ascites is a sign that the cancer has metastasized, and so carries a poor prognosis. Other causes of ascites include chronic congestive cardiac failure, liver failure and kidney disease
		Bloating that fluctuates, occurs after meals or at the end of the day is not usually a serious sign, and is more commonly a feature of irritable bowel syndrome. However, progressive abdominal bloating over the course of weeks may indicate tumor bulk (particularly in ovarian cancer), and merits referral

 Information box 2.3-II

Cancer treatments: comments from a Chinese medicine perspective

Surgery will always target the end result of a complex etiological process and cannot completely deal with the whole of the disease process. According to Chinese medical theory, if chronic Deficiency and Stagnation was at the root of carcinogenesis, surgery alone will not treat these, even if a mass has been totally removed. The patient will remain in a vulnerable state and will need supportive treatment, rest and attention to lifestyle change in order to promote full recovery. Surgery will also lead to local Qi and Blood Stagnation as a result of tissue removal and damage, and this will need to be taken into account in order to help the patient heal.

Chemotherapy and radiotherapy tend to cause preferential death of cancerous tissue, but will also lead to damage and inflammation of healthy tissues. Rapidly growing tissues such as hair follicles, mucous linings and sex cells are damaged. The potential adverse effects include redness and heat of tissues in the short term, and dryness, scarring and infertility in the long term. This suggests that these treatments are intensely Heating, and exert their effects in a Toxic way by burning the cancerous mass. The term *Yi Du Gong Du* (using a poison to treat a poison) may be applied. In their toxicity, chemotherapeutic agents risk depleting Yin and Kidney Essence. Other side effects secondary to these Toxic effects suggest Damage to Spleen Qi and Stomach Yin (vomiting and digestive disturbance), Stagnation of Liver Qi (vomiting) and Blood Stagnation (painful syndromes).

Flaws (2002) describes the Chinese medical view of chemotherapy for cancer as follows:

> In Chinese medicine, chemotherapy is regarded as a species of "using toxins to combat toxins." According to Sun Bing-Yan, a famous traditional Chinese medical cancer specialist, although most cancers develop in a cold, damp internal terrain or bodily constitution, most cancers are also a species of localized heat toxins. Because chemotherapeutic agents are strongly "attacking" according to the logic of Chinese medicine, they easily damage the righteous qi. Because they tend to be hot in nature, they also can engender their own evil or pathological heat. Therefore, in terms of Chinese medicine, the side-effects of chemotherapy tend to fall into the categories of qi vacuity; yin vacuity; and heat toxins.[47]

According to Flaws, Qi Vacuity, Yin Vacuity and Heat Toxins are the Chinese medical interpretations of the drug-induced disease that results from chemotherapy.

For this reason, Chinese medical treatments prescribed to support chemotherapy are often focused on Cooling and Nourishing Yin and Essence. Treatments for dealing with the side effects of chemotherapy, such as nausea, vomiting, peripheral neuropathic pain and anemia, may also be used. Herbal therapy and moxibustion is the mainstay of modern Chinese medical treatment for cancer.

More specific interpretations of individual anticancer medications will be addressed later, when individual cancers are discussed.

2.4

Infectious Disease

2.4a Principles of infectious disease

Introduction to the systematic study of disease

The principles of susceptibility to disease and the pathological processes of disease were introduced in Chapters 2.1, 2.2 and 2.3, where it was explained how some of the processes of disease, such as the disorders of excessive clotting and cancer, are considered as diseases in their own right. However, in most diseases, the name of the condition does not necessarily indicate the underlying processes of disease. From this point onwards, the information given about diseases is structured according to either the pathological agent (e.g. infectious diseases), the physiological system affected (e.g. diseases of the cardiovascular system) or the type of patients affected (e.g. child) rather than according to the process of disease.

As practitioners of acupuncture, it is not necessary, of course, to be fully conversant with all the different conventionally described diseases and their treatments. However, when it becomes relevant to the management of a particular clinical case, it is of great value to be practiced in researching information about a disease and its treatments. This approach first requires a basic understanding of the physiology of the various systems of the body and the processes of disease as described in earlier sections. It is also important to be familiar with how information about diseases is presented systematically in medical texts and websites. For this reason, the disease-specific information presented in the following sections is written in language chosen to be accessible to non-medically trained practitioners, but ordered in the way that information is structured in conventional texts. It is intended that these sections of the book will provide a conceptual bridge for the understanding of more in-depth descriptions of disease and therapeutics found in other more technically detailed sources of medical information.

Introduction to the study of infectious disease (communicable diseases)

Diseases can be broadly classified as infectious and non-infectious. According to conventional medicine, infectious diseases result from damage to the body following infection or infestation by an external infectious agent. Infection may lead to a range of processes of disease and may affect one or more of the physiological systems.

The infectious agents are summarized in Table 2.4a-I. They may be microscopic, in which case they are called microbes. If a microbe is a bacterium or a single-celled animal such as an amoeba, the term microorganism may also be used, denoting that the microbe is a life form. Viruses are non-living microbes. Most infectious diseases are caused by microbes, but larger creatures such as worms can also cause infectious diseases. When the infectious agents are arthropods (insects and mites), the term infestation may be used to describe the disease process.

Table 2.4a-I Different types of infectious agent

Agent	Description
Microbes	
Viruses and prions	Non-living particles capable of replication; prions are made of protein alone, and viruses of a combination of protein and genetic material
Bacteria	The smallest life form; bacteria consist of single cells, but are more simple in structure than the generalized cell described in Section 1.1b
Fungi	Yeasts and molds; like bacteria, these are composed of very simple cellular units
Protozoa	Single-celled animals such as the amoeba; the cells of protozoa contain all the organelles of the simple cell described in Section 1.1b
Larger organisms	
Roundworms, flukes and tapeworms	E.g. threadworm
Mites	E.g. head and body lice
Insects	E.g. fleas

The definition of infectious disease

Infectious diseases are so termed because they are contracted by transmission of the infectious agent from a person, animal or even an inanimate object (termed the carrier). This also explains the use of the term communicable.

Not all infections can be classified as infectious diseases. For example, an infection can arise when a person succumbs to microorganisms that naturally live within the body, but which do not usually cause disease in a state of healthy balance. A bladder infection, also called cystitis, is an example of such a disease, in that the bacteria that cause a person to develop cystitis usually originate from the person's own natural perineal and bowel bacteria.

The impact of infectious disease

The description of infectious disease is often the subject of one of the first chapters in general textbooks about pathology and clinical medicine. This is a reflection of its clinical significance. In terms of causation of disability and death, infections are the single most important cause of disease worldwide. However, in developed countries, infections do not have quite the overwhelming impact as they do in developing countries. In the developed world the most important causes of death and disability are now the non-communicable diseases, and most importantly, disease of the cardiovascular system, cancer and, in young people, accidents.

The modern developments of vaccination and drug treatment for infections are widely acknowledged in conventional medicine to have led to the decline in infectious disease in developed populations. However, it is increasingly understood that the provision of basic needs, such as clean water and the removal of sewage (sanitation), good housing and adequate diet, are also important factors that account for the reduction in infection-related morbidity. The provision of these basic needs contributes to the attainment of a basic level of health, and in health, the body is better able both to withstand contracting some infections, and also to overcome those infections that do develop.

The study of the epidemiology of diseases such as tuberculosis (TB), rheumatic fever and diphtheria supports this theory that healthy populations resist infectious disease. All these diseases have declined dramatically in well-nourished Western populations, and yet are major causes of ill health in developing countries. For all three, the decline preceded the introduction of vaccinations or antibiotic treatment, and this is understood to relate to improvements in nourishment and sanitation. The reports that TB is on the increase again in Western countries reflect an increase largely confined to marginalized groups, such as those people who are homeless, who do not have access to good nutrition and housing, to those who have recently emigrated from developing countries, or those with HIV (human immunodeficiency virus) infection/AIDS (acquired immune deficiency syndrome).

Measles is an infectious disease from which most well-nourished children make a full recovery, with less than 0.1 percent developing long-term serious consequences. However, measles is still one of the major causes of infant death and blindness in developing countries, causing death in up to 30 percent of infants who contract it in some impoverished localities. This modern statistic illustrates the fact that infectious disease still has much more impact in populations that are more susceptible as a result of malnutrition and poor living conditions.

Nevertheless, there are many infections that cause serious disease within healthy populations. Examples of such diseases include bacterial meningitis, certain types of pneumonia, certain types of food poisoning (including *Escherichia (E.) coli* serotype O157), HIV infection and many of the tropical diseases (e.g. malaria and typhoid). Although it is true that these diseases often tend to have a greater impact on those who are more susceptible, such as the very young and elderly people, they are also well recognized to be the cause of significant ill health and mortality in previously fit young people. This is an indication that some infections can take hold and cause damage even when the individual does not obviously appear to be particularly susceptible to a severe illness.

Immunity and infectious disease

The topic of immunity was introduced in Section 2.1d. The general level of immunity to a disease in a population is another major factor that affects the impact of the disease. Diseases that are very common in a population are termed endemic. Chickenpox and the common cold are diseases that are endemic in the UK, whereas malaria is endemic in a tropical country such as Uganda. It is common for a population in a locality that has been exposed from birth to an endemic disease to have less marked reactions to that disease than visitors to that locality. This is why travelers to foreign countries frequently succumb to infections that do not seem to affect the locals, leading to symptoms such as fevers, diarrhea and vomiting.

The resistance of a population to an endemic disease is attributed in part to herd immunity. This term describes the immunity that results from the fact that a large proportion of the population has already encountered that infection, often in infancy. For this reason, they will not thereafter easily contract the disease. If herd immunity exists, the disease is less likely to take hold in the population because there are fewer people to whom it can be passed on. This is one of the principles of vaccination campaigns that aim to ensure that a large proportion of the population is immune. The end result of a successful vaccination campaign is an increase in the herd immunity to a specific disease such as measles.

However, acquired herd immunity is not the whole story. Local people who have not yet experienced endemic diseases still generally appear to be able to fight off these infections when they do experience them more efficiently than travelers to the area. A striking example of this is the impact that was made by minor infections taken by the first explorers to the New World. Diseases such as the common cold and chickenpox caused serious consequences in communities to whom they were totally new infections. It seems as if the immune system of a person in a locality is prepared in some way to deal with an endemic disease, but is seriously challenged by one that is not a normal part of the local pattern of infections. This extra level of protection may possibly be the result of a genetic adaptation of the local population over generations of exposure to endemic diseases.

If a disease suddenly appears to be on the increase in a population, the term epidemic is used. An epidemic disease is not necessarily severe, but occurs much more often than expected. Epidemics occur either because a new type of infectious agent has emerged for which there is no pre-existing herd immunity, or because over the course of time the herd immunity has diminished so that the disease can rapidly take hold once again.

The pathology of infectious disease

There are two properties of infectious agents that result in them being able to cause harm. The first is that they have the ability to penetrate the normal barriers to disease, and the second is that, having penetrated, they are able to damage the body tissues.

An example of these two stages is the damage caused as a result of flea infestation. The flea can penetrate the barrier of the skin because it is able to puncture it by biting. Damage is due to substances in the flea's saliva that enter the deep layers (dermis) of the skin. These substances are irritating to the cells in the dermis, and so cause inflammation at the site of the puncture. This leads to the small red and itchy bump of the flea bite. In some people these chemicals behave as antigens and provoke a pronounced immune response. This leads to the site of the bite becoming firmer and larger and even blistered over the course of a few days.

Infectious diseases can lead to damage as a result of one or more of the seven processes of disease described in Section 2.2a. The flea bite is an example of how an infectious agent can give rise to inflammation, which is the most common disease process to result from infectious disease. However, infectious agents can also lead to disease by causing problems in the immune system, causing cancerous change, and also by causing degeneration.

The following descriptions of infectious diseases illustrate the diversity of the disease processes involved.

TONSILLITIS

The tonsils are masses of lymphoid tissue (like lymph nodes) that sit at the entrance to the pharynx (they can be seen in most people at the back of the mouth, just behind the arch formed by the palate). Tonsillitis can be passed on from one person to another by the inhalation of droplets of infected fluid, following a cough, for example. However, tonsillitis is not always contagious. It can also occur when a person becomes susceptible to relatively harmless bacteria that they have been harboring in their tonsils for some time. This might explain how some people get recurrent bouts of tonsillitis whenever they are run down.

The symptoms of tonsillitis are primarily due to inflammation of the tonsils. The bacteria and viruses that cause tonsillitis are able to attach to the epithelial cells of the surface of the tonsil by means of chemicals (proteins) on their coating. Damage is caused partly because the microbes can kill tonsil cells by first attaching to them, and as a result they stimulate inflammation. Some bacteria encourage the excessive production of pus, consisting of dead phagocytic leukocytes. The chemicals released during the immune response and inflammation give rise to the general feelings of malaise that are common in tonsillitis. In most cases the immune response is sufficient to hinder the spread of infection so that it settles down within a few days.

The rare complications of glomerulonephritis and rheumatic fever can follow tonsillitis resulting from a bacterium called *Streptococcus*. In these conditions, the antibodies that develop in the immune response to the bacteria do not just target the bacteria, but also proteins in the kidney and heart valves, respectively. This is a type II hypersensitivity reaction. The kidney and valvular diseases that result are, therefore, autoimmune diseases, but ones that are triggered by an infection.

COLD SORES (HERPES LABIALIS)

The herpes simplex virus is transmitted through intimate contact such as kissing. The virus is present in the saliva of the carrier, and from there penetrates into the cells of the lining of the partner's mouth, where it initially, in a quasi-parasitic way, uses the supply of nutrients within the mouth's lining cells to replicate itself. It also penetrates the ends of nerve cells in the connective tissue of the lining of the mouth, and this leads to the characteristic tingling sensation. Eventually, the infected cells will rupture and die, and cause inflammation, which is the cause of the redness and scabbing. Each ruptured cell will release thousands of new viruses into the saliva of the person with the cold sore.

Intense pain can result as an effect of the infection of the nerve cells. When the infection has healed, some viruses remain latent within some of the nerve cells, but these are prevented from replicating by the immune system. When the person becomes run down, this hidden source of infection can emerge as another cold sore.

ACQUIRED IMMUNE DEFICIENCY SYNDROME (AIDS)

HIV is carried in body fluids. Close contact with infected body fluids together with a break in the normal barrier of the skin is necessary for HIV to be transmitted. Sexual contact and childbirth provide these conditions, as does transmission of human fluids by a hypodermic needle.

The presence of the virus in the bloodstream leads to an immune response that then causes the flu-like syndrome characteristic of many viral infections. Although antibodies are formed, they are most often unable to clear the HIV from the body. This is because the virus is able to penetrate into leukocytes via the CD4 protein receptor, and in this way hide from the immune response. In this intracellular state the HIV remains and multiplies, dividing with the leukocytes over a period of years, until gradually the function of those cells becomes impaired. The presence of the virus leads to gradually reduced numbers of lymphocytes over time as their early death is promoted by the presence of the virus. Therefore, the major consequences of HIV infection are not primarily due to inflammation, but instead to a disorder of the immune system. This disorder leads to the combined problems of opportunistic infections and cancer.

In advanced disease, the nerve cells of the brain may also be damaged by cytokines produced by virus-infected immune cells, leading to a form of dementia. AIDS is, therefore, an example of an infection causing degeneration as well as inflammation and a disorder of the immune system.

These diverse examples illustrate how infections cause disease by various mechanisms. Although inflammation is the most common damaging consequence of infections, autoimmune disease, immunodeficiency, cancer and degeneration can also be caused by them. Infections can also cause congenital disease in the embryo and fetus if contracted during pregnancy, such as congenital rubella syndrome, which results from a rubella (German measles) infection during the first trimester of pregnancy.

Transmission of disease

The three examples of infectious diseases described above also illustrate the diversity of ways in which infections can be transmitted. Tonsillitis is transmitted by inhalation of droplets, the cold sore virus through infected saliva penetrating the mucous membranes of the mouth, and HIV is transmitted via infected body fluids penetrating the usual skin barriers.

There are an enormous number of possible routes of infection, illustrating the complex ways by which infectious agents have adapted themselves to find their way into their human hosts. Modes of transmission can be broadly considered in two categories: person-to-person and animal-to-person spread. Examples of these are listed in Table 2.4a-II.

Table 2.4a-II Different modes of transmission of infectious agents

Person-to-person spread

Infection in the gastrointestinal tract passed on through contact with human feces (usually indirectly by eating contaminated food or water), e.g. typhoid and cholera

Infestations passed on through clothing and bedding, e.g. body lice

Animal-to-person spread

Infection carried by insects and mites passed on through bites, e.g. malaria

Infection passed on through contact with animal feces, e.g. food poisoning due to bacteria such as *Salmonella* and *E. coli* originating from poorly cooked contaminated meat and eggs

Infection passed on through eating meat containing parasites, e.g. tapeworm

Infection carried in rat urine that penetrates the skin via contaminated water, e.g. Weil's disease

Emerging infections

For each of the known infections, the causative infectious agent has adapted to target particular human tissues and causes damage in a characteristic way. The conventional view is that such adaptation is the consequence of evolution over the course of many years. Evolution is believed to be the result of mutation that is beneficial to the infectious agent. As a species of microbe replicates, mutation occasionally leads to daughter microbes that are better able to reproduce than their parents. In the case of infectious disease, this successful adaptation is often one that leads the daughter microbes to be more efficient at infecting human cells. This is because it is through infection that microbes obtain the nutrients necessary for survival and replication.

Evolution in complex species such as humans is believed to occur very gradually over many thousands of years. However, evolution of simple species such as viruses and other microbes may lead to a dramatic change in a species over a much shorter time. This is because the microbes replicate at a very rapid rate.

HIV is an example of an infection that seemed to emerge, probably originally in Africa, within the last 50 years, before which time it was completely unknown. HIV currently appears to be perfectly adapted to thrive in the human body through having a protein on its coat that connects exactly with the CD4 proteins found on various leukocytes of the immune system. One theory is that HIV previously existed as a monkey virus,[48] and through chance mutation acquired this protein that enables it to survive and replicate in humans.

New microbes are emerging in this way all the time, as they change in form through replication. Over the past quarter of a century, more than 30 new or newly recognized infections have been identified around the world. The newly emerging infectious diseases include hepatitis C and E viruses, Lyme disease, staphylococcal toxic shock syndrome, H5N1 pandemic influenza, SARS (Severe Acute Respiratory Syndrome) virus and nvCJD (new variant Creutzfeldt-Jakob disease) virus.

Mutation not only gives rise to new species of infectious organism; it can also lead to subtle changes in existing organisms. These changes, which lead to new strains, can lead to organisms no longer being recognized by the immune system of someone who previously had immunity to that disease.

This type of mutation appears to occur more readily in some infectious organisms than others. For example, the influenza virus rapidly changes its characteristic coat through mutation. This gives rise to the frequent epidemics of influenza that are experienced in the UK. Each influenza epidemic reflects a wave of infections by a new strain of the virus. This explains why people can contract influenza repeatedly during their life, and why a new vaccine for influenza needs to be developed on an annual basis.

In contrast, the chickenpox virus appears not to mutate significantly, reflected in the fact that most people retain their immunity to chickenpox for life.

2.4b The different types of infectious disease

Infectious organisms

The main groups of infectious agents were introduced in the last section and summarized in Table 2.4a-I. Each one of these groups is now considered in turn, together with some of the diseases that these diverse agents can cause.

Diseases caused by viruses

Unlike bacteria and human cells, viruses and prions are so small that they cannot be seen using a simple microscope. Instead, the more powerful electron microscope is used to produce images of these particles. Figures 2.4b-I and 2.4b-II show electron micrographs of two different viruses: the envelope-bounded DNA of the herpes simplex virus, and the icosohedral (20-sided) RNA of the rotavirus. The size of these viruses is measured in nanometers (nm), which is an unimaginable one-billionth of a meter (1×10^{-9} m) in size. These viruses are 160 and 80nm in diameter, respectively. By way of comparison, a human red blood cell is 6000–8000nm in diameter, so up to 100 times larger than these tiny infectious particles.

Figure 2.4b-I Electron micrograph of the herpes simplex virus

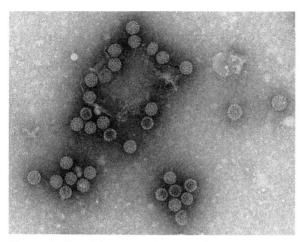

Figure 2.4b-II Electron micrograph of the human rotavirus

Viruses contain some genetic material that is similar in structure to that found within human chromosomes, together with additional proteins that form a surrounding coat. Prions are composed of a single complex protein alone. Because of their simplicity, viruses and prions often have a structure that resembles a geometric crystal. This is in contrast to the complex and unique rounded structures found in each living cell.

Viruses cause damage because they have adapted to be able to penetrate living cells, and then to utilize the nutrients within those cells to replicate. Viruses cannot replicate, obtain nutrients or respond to environmental changes without living cells and so cannot, by definition, be considered a life form.

Viruses cause disease both because they damage living cells, and also because they trigger an immune response. The high temperature, rash, aches and malaise characteristic of many viral infections are manifestations of the immune response generated against viruses circulating in the bloodstream.

Viruses can damage human cells in different ways: some simply cause cell death, as, for example, does the cold sore virus. This can have many consequences, depending on which tissue is affected. The death of human cells and release of cellular contents leads to inflammation, so the familiar features of redness, heat, swelling and pain are commonly found when part of the body is affected by a virus.

Other consequences include:

- disturbance of cell replication, leading to benign growths (e.g. wart virus)

- cancer, as a result of interfering with the proto-oncogene function in a cell (e.g. genital wart virus, which can be a trigger for cervical cancer)

- disturbance of the development of the fetus, leading to congenital malformation (e.g. rubella virus) if the infection occurs in pregnancy.

An excessive immune response to viruses can also be damaging. Possible consequences include:

- bleeding within tissues (e.g. the viral hemorrhagic disease Lassa fever)

- delayed immune damage to the nervous system, which can manifest as numbness, weakness and mood changes (e.g. Guillain-Barré syndrome).

The poorly understood post viral fatigue syndrome (PVFS), which describes depression and exhaustion following a viral infection, has also been attributed to delayed immune damage to the nervous system following a viral infection.

Viruses are classified into groups (families and subfamilies) according to their structure. Some of the major families of viruses are listed in Table 2.4b-I, and some of the diverse diseases that result from viral infections are listed in Table 2.4b-II.

Table 2.4b-I Some different families of virus

Class of virus	Description
Adenoviruses	A large group of DNA-containing viruses that commonly cause minor upper respiratory infections
Herpesviruses	DNA viruses responsible for cold sores, chickenpox and glandular fever. All are capable of causing latent infections that can reappear at a later date
Poxviruses	DNA viruses causing crusting diseases such as smallpox, cowpox, monkey pox and orf
Picornaviruses	Small RNA viruses causing diseases including poliomyelitis, viral meningitis and the common cold
Reoviruses	Small RNA viruses responsible for epidemics of infectious diarrhea and mild respiratory symptoms
Retroviruses	Viruses that are able to replicate by inserting a protein called reverse transcriptase into a cell. Includes HIV

Table 2.4b-II Various viral diseases

Disease	Causative virus
Pharyngitis (sore throat)	Adenovirus
Cold sores	Herpes simplex
Genital herpes	Herpes simplex
Chickenpox	Varicella zoster
Viral encephalitis	Measles, mumps, herpes simplex
Viral meningitis	Coxsackie virus, measles, mumps
Rabies	Rabies
Croup	Respiratory syncytial virus
Glandular fever	Epstein-Barr virus
Kaposi's sarcoma	Epstein-Barr virus
Smallpox	Variola
Poliomyelitis	Poliovirus
Mumps	Mumps virus
Lassa fever	Lassa virus
Viral pneumonia	Measles, varicella zoster
Diarrhea	Rotavirus, norovirus, adenovirus
Rubella (German measles)	Rubella
Yellow fever	Yellow fever
Influenza	Influenza
Measles	Measles
Common cold	Rhinovirus

Diseases caused by prions

Prions have only recently been discovered and described as infectious agents. They have a very simple structure consisting of a single folded protein, making them the only infectious agent that doesn't contain the self-replicating material DNA or RNA. Prions are believed to cause disease by inducing prion-like folds in the structure of essential proteins in the nervous system of their animal hosts. This leads to an irreversible change into useless complex protein structures. This leads the host cells to degenerate, and enables the prion to increase in quantity. Creutzfeldt-Jakob disease (CJD) and the new variant form (nvCJD) are two prion diseases that have been shown to affect humans. As far as it is known, prion diseases can only be transmitted when infected animal tissue or blood enters the body of another animal, either by the ingestion of infected flesh, or through surgery and possibly through blood transfusion.

Diseases caused by bacteria

Bacteria (singular bacterium) are microorganisms that consist of a single simple cell. The structure is far less complex than the typical animal cell described in Section 1.1b. Bacteria do not have nuclei or mitochondria, for example, but instead, the copying of genetic material and the energy-generating processes all take place around large molecules that are situated free within the cell cytoplasm. Nevertheless, the bacterium still uses basic nutrients and reproduces in a similar way, and for this reason, a bacterium is considered a life form. Bacteria are, on average, about one-tenth of the size of human cells, but can be seen through a simple microscope.

Figure 2.4b-III shows a simplified drawing of a rod-shaped bacterium, *Escherichia (E.) coli*. The size of bacteria is generally measured in micrometers (μm), which are one-millionth of a meter (1×10^{-6}m) in size. An *E. coli* bacterium is 3μm in length (3000nm), which is 20 times wider than the diameter of the complex herpes simplex virus, and half the diameter of a red blood cell.

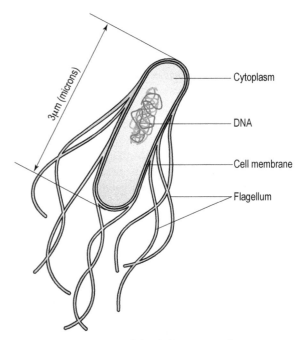

Figure 2.4b-III Simplified diagram of a coliform bacterium (Escherichia coli)

If a bacterial disease is suspected, a doctor might take a swab of the infected site, for example, an inflamed tonsil. The swab is taken to the laboratory, where it is swept across a glass slide, stained with a dye that is absorbed by bacteria, and the smear then viewed through a microscope. In the examination of a smear from an inflamed tonsil resulting, for example, from infection by the *Streptococcus* bacterium, the microscope might reveal clumps of large epithelial cells from the tonsil, and chains of tiny darkly stained circular forms, the streptococcal bacteria (also known as streptococci).

Bacteria are classified according to their shape, ability to absorb stains and other properties that can be tested in the laboratory, and have been given Latin names that often reflect these characteristics. Very often bacteria are classified as Gram-negative or Gram-positive. This simply indicates the way that a bacterium reacts to a stain first used by an early Danish pathologist called Hans Christian Gram, and is a reflection of the nature of the protective coat around the bacterium. Bacteria may also be classified according to their morphology. The two broad categories of cocci (spherical cells) and bacilli (rod-shaped cells) are morphological categories.

More recently, bacteria have been classified according to their genetic makeup. This has led to the reclassification of some groups, because genetic analysis reveals similarities and differences that are not apparent from their morphological characteristics.

Important Gram-positive bacteria include species of *Staphylococcus*, *Streptococcus*, *Bacillus*, *Clostridium* (including tetanus), *Mycobacterium* (including tuberculosis), *Corynebacterium* (including diphtheria) and *Listeria*.

Important Gram-negative bacteria include species of *Chlamydia*, *Escherichia* (e.g. *E. coli*), *Salmonella*, *Vibrio* (e.g. cholera), *Helicobacter*, *Neisseria* (e.g. gonorrhea and meningococcus), *Bordetella* (e.g. whooping cough), *Legionella* (e.g. Legionnaires' disease) and *Treponema* (e.g. syphilis).

Some infectious diseases, for example, tonsillitis and pharyngitis, can be caused by both bacteria and viruses. Other examples include meningitis, encephalitis, pericarditis, bronchitis and pneumonia. Although in these conditions there are a range of possible infectious agents, the end result of the infection is similar in terms of the development of inflammation within a particular organ.

Many infectious diseases are described by terms that end with the suffix "-itis." However, this suffix refers only to the fact that an organ is inflamed, but not what the cause might be. This is also true for the term pneumonia that describes inflammation in the lung tissue and not the causative agent. In fact, some inflammatory conditions, including bronchitis, pneumonia, cystitis, pericarditis and meningitis, can also be the result of damage by chemicals, radiation and autoimmune disease. They are, therefore, not always infectious diseases.

Diseases caused by protozoa, flukes and worms

Protozoa are single-celled animals that share all the characteristics of the typical animal cell. They multiply by simple binary fission (mitosis).

Flukes, tapeworms and worms are more complex multicellular animals that possess a rudimentary nervous system and gut. They multiply by producing eggs that develop through an immature stage to the adult form.

Often an additional animal host to the human is required for the life cycle to complete itself. For instance, the eggs of the pork tapeworm have to mature in the flesh of pigs before the parasite can be passed on to humans (as a result of eating infected meat).

Collectively, protozoa, flukes, tapeworms and worms are considered to be parasites when they infect human beings. The scientific definition of a parasite is a plant or an animal that lives in or on another living entity and at the expense of that entity (plant or animal). In medicine this term is not used to describe bacteria or viruses. Nevertheless, the damage wreaked by parasites is similar to that resulting from infection with bacteria and viruses, and includes inflammation and an excessive immune response.

Protozoal diseases include giardiasis and amoebiasis (both causes of diarrhea), malaria and sleeping sickness (tropical disease), and *Trichomonas* infection (a sexually transmitted disease). Most worm and fluke infections are tropical diseases, although threadworms and toxocariasis are worm infections that are commonly contracted in the UK.

Diseases caused by fungi

Fungi are a large class of life forms that includes the familiar mushrooms and toadstools, but also molds and yeasts. Strictly speaking, they are classified as part of the plant kingdom.

Fungi are different from all other plants in that they do not contain the green pigment called chlorophyll. Because of this they cannot use sunlight to manufacture energy. Instead, fungi require living or rotting animal and plant tissue to survive. Therefore, many have evolved to be parasites, obtaining nutrients from other living organisms, including humans.

In general, fungi do not cause serious disease in humans unless there is depletion of the immune system. In people with immunodeficiency, fungal disease can become a significant and sometimes life-threatening problem. However, minor fungal skin and mucous-membrane infections are very common in healthy people. These include athlete's foot, ringworm and thrush.

Athlete's foot is generally a mild fungal infection that targets damp skin. The most common site for the infection to start is the skin between the fourth and fifth toes. It rarely spreads beyond this area, although it can affect the growing nails, resulting in thickening and discoloration.

Ringworm is a fungal skin infection that forms an itchy, spreading ring of redness and scaling on the skin in a way that can be compared to the "fairy ring" produced by some mushrooms. This mild but very contagious rash is often contracted from handling animals.

Thrush is due to a yeast called *Candida albicans*, which is a natural resident (commensal) of the bowel and genital tract of healthy human beings. It becomes problematic when the natural balance of the microorganisms in the body becomes disturbed. The *candida* then becomes too dominant, akin to overgrowth of one plant species in a poorly tended garden. Excessive *candida* leads to thick white patches and discharge, and can cause inflammation of the mucous membranes of the genital tract and the mouth.

Candida syndrome, first widely publicized by William Crook in 1984,[49] is recognized by some complementary health practitioners as a complex constellation of symptoms that include digestive problems, such as diarrhea, irritable bowel syndrome and bloating, other fungal problems, such as athlete's foot, and mental problems, such as exhaustion and depression. Thrush may or may not be present in *candida* syndrome. The symptoms of chronic fatigue syndrome (CFS) (also known as myalgic encephalomyelitis or ME) have also been attributed to *candida*. Excessive sugars and yeasts in the diet are claimed to be one of the causes of the *candida* syndrome, and so the treatment involves a strict diet and the use of antifungal preparations. The use of preparations of the natural bacterium *Lactobacillus acidophilus* is recommended to help regain a healthy natural balance of microorganisms as well as long-term antifungal medication. However, *candida* syndrome is not currently recognized as a disease entity in conventional medicine.[50] For this reason, patients who believe that they have *candida* syndrome will not routinely be offered antifungal treatment by conventional doctors unless they have the white discharge, soreness and itching characteristic of genital or oral thrush. The clinical evidence supporting the benefits of *Lactobacillus* supplementation or long-term antifungal medication in chronic fatigue and minor digestive disturbance is also not believed to be strong. Nevertheless, many doctors will recommend *Lactobacillus* supplementation to treat depletion of these bacteria resulting from antibiotic treatment or for the treatment of thrush.

Fungal infections are very problematic for someone with immunodeficiency. For example, patients with AIDS commonly experience severe thrush outbreaks, which can affect the whole esophagus and mouth as well as the genital mucous membranes. In severe immunodeficiency, *candida* can spread to invade the lining of the bowel and other deep parts of the body, and this can be life-threatening. If HIV progresses to AIDS, then patients may also develop a skin condition called seborrheic dermatitis, which is also due to overgrowth of a usually harmless skin fungus, *Malassezia*. Unusual fungal infections, such as cryptococcosis and pneumocystis pneumonia, are common causes of death in patients with immunodeficiency syndromes such as AIDS. Both these species of fungi are found as commensals in the microbiome of the healthy person (see below).

Infestations

Infestations by arthropods such as lice, scabies and fleas are different in nature to the other infectious diseases, as it is generally only the surface of the body that is affected. Biting and burrowing by these creatures causes damage to skin tissue and allergic responses, which then give rise to itching and discomfort.

Although the itch and discomfort can cause moderate distress, infestations are a cause of serious disease because arthropods can carry other diseases that are transmitted through bites. The Black Death, which caused millions of deaths in Europe in the 14th century CE, is a disease transmitted through the bite of rodent fleas and caused by the Gram-negative cocco-bacillus *Yersinia pestis*. Other arthropod-borne infections include typhus (tick-borne) and malaria (mosquito-borne). Many other tropical diseases are also transmitted via insect bites.

Beneficial (commensal) microorganisms

In the healthy human being, as in all other large animals, there are thousands of bacteria and fungi resident throughout the body, totaling at least the number of human cells that make up that body.[51] Microorganisms can be found on all epithelia that are in contact with the outside world, including the skin and the epithelial linings of the lung, bowel and genital organs. A person starts to inherit these guests from the moment they are born and come into close contact with caregivers. Newborn infants are very prone to episodes of oral thrush and colic, possibly an indication that the delicate balance of fungi and bacteria has yet to become established. It is estimated that a balanced microbiome is not established until one year of life. This population of microorganisms is dynamic and the genetic balance highly responsive to environmental changes. One study showed that exposure to breast milk, fever, baby rice, antibiotics and final adult foods all induced increases in complexity of the microbiome in babies in their first year.

Each human being can be considered as a distinct ecosystem, in which ideally the human host and its microorganisms live in harmony. It is known that the health of the human depends in part on the balance of these microorganisms, also termed the human microbiome. For example, some bacteria in the bowel assist with the digestion of food. It is noteworthy that the medical term for these healthy bacteria is commensal, literally meaning that they share the same dining table as their hosts. Also, a healthy balance of microorganisms is known to prevent the development of infection by less desirable infectious agents. The use of antibiotics and excessive washing (e.g. of the genital areas) can alter this balance, and this is why these practices may lead to problems such as diarrhea, thrush and soreness. Imbalances in the microbiome have been linked with diseases as diverse as obesity, psoriasis, bacterial vaginosis and esophageal cancer, and this is the focus of a burgeoning area of scientific research.

As part of this research the genetic makeup of the biome has been investigated in depth, and a huge range of bacterial species and fungi and viruses have been found to inhabit any one individual. The genetic makeup of the microbiome is extremely complex and may be up to 90 percent different between individuals. Some of these commensals are bacterial species that are associated with known disease, such as *Streptococcus pneumoniae*, *Staphylococcus aureus*, *Haemophilus influenzae*, *Neisseria meningitis* and *E. coli*, and yet they do not cause disease in the healthy individual who lives alongside them.

As a result of this new awareness of the microbiome, there is a rationale for supplementing the friendly commensal bacteria of the body with dietary products containing bacteria such as the *Lactobacillus* species (sp.) (the family of Gram-positive, rod-shaped bacteria, which include those responsible for the conversion of milk to yogurt) and other fermented products such as miso, sauerkraut and tempeh. It is recognized that oral supplementation with preparations of live *Lactobacillus* sp. will not only encourage the colonization of the bowel with these bacteria, but also the external genitalia and the vagina. *Lactobacillus* sp. are recognized to increase the acidity of their environment, and in this way to reduce the overgrowth of yeast-like organisms such as *candida*, the cause of thrush.

The precise balance of the biome is unique to individuals, but similarities are shared between cultural groups. Close contact between individuals will lead to shifts in the balance of microorganisms in the biome, and this is bound to happen to a certain extent between groups of small children and their families.[52]

The long-term consequences of powerful medical treatments including antibiotics and vaccinations on the biome are not by any means fully understood. One study showed that a broad-spectrum antibiotic left the microbiome in the gut markedly denuded of bacterial species, but some individuals recovered their bacterial diversity much more rapidly than others. Some individuals still demonstrated the effects for up to four years following the antibiotic treatment. *Clostridium (C.) difficile* is a bacterium that can overgrow and cause life-threatening chronic diarrhea in vulnerable patients who have been given broad-spectrum antibiotics, presumably because competing bacteria have been eliminated. Ironically the main treatment for this is another very powerful broad-spectrum antibiotic. Novel approaches to this problem are being explored with trials of fecal transplants containing bacteria from donors. These have shown benefits in intractable *C. difficile* infections.[53]

Studying infectious diseases

Knowledge of the classification of infectious agents and their modes of transmission, together with an understanding of how infectious agents can lead to processes of disease, is invaluable in the study of infectious diseases. Moreover, it can help in understanding how the different broad groups of infectious agent can each lead to some characteristic manifestations of disease. Table 2.4b-III illustrates some features of diseases that can point to a particular type of infectious agent, but there are many exceptions to these rules.

Table 2.4b-III Characteristics of disease caused by infectious agents

Infectious agent	Features of disease that are characteristic of the agent
Viruses	Can cause a syndrome of malaise, joint aches, mild fever and slight rash as infection takes hold
	Lead to watery discharges more commonly than pus
	Rarely, can lead to cancerous change or benign tumors
	Infections may be followed by a syndrome of prolonged exhaustion, depression, muscle weakness and numbness
Prions	Transmitted by insertion of infected tissue into the body either by eating or by medical procedures
	Lead to degeneration of nervous tissue
Bacteria	Pus formation, such as abscesses and boils, may occur
	The most common disease process in bacterial disease is inflammation. May also trigger autoimmune responses
Protozoa, flukes and worms	A common cause of tropical intestinal disease. Eggs of parasites often enter the bowel from contaminated food and water
	Allergic reactions, such as itch and cough, may also occur
Fungi	A cause of relatively mild skin problems in healthy people
	A major problem in patients with immune deficiency
Infestations	A cause of irritating skin problems, but do not in themselves affect deeper tissues
	May lead to serious disease by transmission of other infectious agents

Information on infectious diseases is presented in medical textbooks in a structured way, often ordered within the following categories:

- causative agent
- mode of transmission
- clinical features
- complications of infection
- treatment.

For example, a textbook description of the infectious disease measles might give the following information:

- Causative agent: a virus from the family of paramyxoviruses.

- Mode of transmission: the spread is by droplets (infected fluid particles from the nose and throat of a carrier). A person is infectious for a total of six days. The infectious period begins four days before the rash develops to two days after it has appeared.

- Clinical features: these occur after an incubation period of 8–14 days. This means that the disease will only manifest 8–14 days after contact with a carrier. First, malaise, fever, runny nose (rhinorrhea), cough and redness of eyes (conjunctival suffusion) occur. This is when the patient is infectious. After two days of this, gray spots (known as Koplik

spots) develop in the inside of the mouth. These are diagnostic of measles infection. On day four, a rapidly spreading maculopapular (spotty, slightly raised) rash moves from the face to include the whole body.

- Complications: measles is generally a mild infection in well-nourished people. However, complications are common in poorly nourished people, and include pneumonia, bronchitis, ear infection and bowel infections. A serious long-term brain infection is a very rare complication in infections in infants less than 18 months old. Measles, when caught in pregnancy, can lead to loss of the pregnancy, but not to fetal abnormalities.

- Treatment: there is no direct treatment of the infection available. Measles in a healthy person generally requires only supportive treatment. However, if the patient is vulnerable because of immunodeficiency or malnutrition, or if neurological or respiratory signs develop, hospital admission and intravenous nutrition may be necessary.

Information about infectious diseases structured under these five headings encapsulates the essential facts required for medical practitioners to understand how a disease will impact on the life of a patient. Awareness of these headings can help structure information for the purposes of the study of infectious diseases.

 Information box 2.4b-I

Infectious disease: comments from a Chinese medicine perspective

The concept of epidemic disease was well established in China from at least the 3rd century CE. It has been understood for centuries that certain diseases with contagious properties and manifesting with Heat symptoms could progress through deepening levels of the body with more serious consequences. These diseases no doubt included viral upper respiratory illnesses, and also more serious life-threatening diseases such as epidemic influenza, smallpox, plague, typhoid and typhus. These diseases were seen to be more likely to seriously afflict those who had Deficiency. For this reason, prevention by Nourishing Deficiency was fundamental to the management of epidemics. Whilst infectious agents were not recognized, epidemic diseases were understood in terms of Invasion of Wind Heat or Heat Toxins. Theories such as the Four Levels (Wen Bing) and Six Divisions (Shang Hun Lun) explained these diseases. These were the foundation for herbal formulas, the ingredients of some of which in recent times have been found to

have antibacterial and antiviral properties. The classic treatment principles were to Clear Wind Heat, Clear Toxins, Resolve Heat, and very importantly, to Tonify and Nourish Qi and Blood.[54]

However, not all diseases that are described as infectious in conventional medicine will equate to these classically recognized epidemic warm diseases.

To help us to describe conventionally described infectious diseases in Chinese medical terms, two important concepts need to be grasped. These are:

- *The origin of the Pathogenic Factor.* Chinese medicine describes how the Pathogenic Factor that is manifested in a conventionally recognized infectious disease (e.g. Wind Heat) can originate from outside the body (i.e. externally, e.g. climatic Wind Heat) or from within the body (i.e. internally, e.g. Heat from Stagnation of Qi and Blood), or can be a combination of the two.

- *The depth of the Pathogenic Factor.* According to Chinese medicine, the Pathogenic Factor may be situated either on the Exterior of the body or at a deeper level in the Interior. Maciocia (1989)[55] makes the point that, in practice, the origin of the Pathogenic Factor is far less relevant than the depth at which it is located in the body. However, the depth of the Pathogenic Factor does not tell us about its origin. The depth is an important aspect of the identification of patterns according to the Eight Principles, which are described in accessible language by Maciocia (1989).[56]

It is important to be very clear about the distinction between the origin of a Pathogenic Factor (External/Internal) and its location/depth (Exterior/Interior). It is also important not to conclude, because of the poetic nature of Chinese descriptions such as "Wind Heat has invaded the body and caused disease," that the Pathogenic Factor is synonymous with an infectious agent. This is not the case. The Pathogenic Factor is actually a description of the clinical picture (e.g. redness, fever and pain indicate Heat; rapidly changing symptoms indicate Wind).

The reverse is also true; microbes are not synonymous with the Chinese medicine Pathogenic Factors. However, according to an integrated view of infection, microbes can and do give rise to manifestations (Invasion) that are taken to be evidence of Pathogenic Factors. This means that the typical signs and symptoms of infectious diseases from a conventional viewpoint have some close correlations with the Chinese medicine view of Pathogenic Factors, and can inform a Chinese medicine diagnosis.

The origin of the Pathogenic Factor

In the case of an infectious disease interpreted in Chinese medicine terms, the actual origin (cause) of a Pathogenic Factor may be Internal or External, depending on the situation. For example:

- *Pathogenic Factor of External origin.* When the Pathogenic Factor has an External origin, its manifestation can be put down purely to the energetic effects of a factor that is manifest in the external environment. This could be an infectious agent, but could also be an allergen, a carcinogen or other environmental factors such as climate and diet. For example, a virus infection and exposure to a cold wind may together lead to the manifestation of Wind Cold on the Exterior in an otherwise healthy person.

  Another example is a case of vomiting and diarrhea in a healthy person after eating contaminated food. The Chinese medicine interpretation might be Invasion of Damp Heat in the Intestines. This describes the manifestation of the condition. In this case, the origin of the Pathogenic Factor is External, and the development of the syndrome has been triggered by the toxins produced by the bacteria in the contaminated food.

  Finally, one more example of an infectious disease leading to the appearance of a Pathogenic Factor in this way might be any one of the contagious infestations such as scabies and head lice, which can affect very healthy people who come into contact with them. The itch and rash associated with these diseases are symptoms of Heat, but follow the damage to the skin by mites. In both these infestations, the mites are very irritating to the skin, and based on the signs and symptoms it would be appropriate to describe their bites and burrowing as having led to a Channel Invasion of a Pathogenic Factor (in this case, Wind Damp Heat).

- *Pathogenic Factor of Internal origin.* When the Pathogenic Factor has an Internal origin, the manifestation of an illness is an appearance of a deeper imbalance (such as pre-existing Damp Heat). If the illness is considered to be an infectious disease in conventional medical terms, this infection is an expression of a deep imbalance, rather than a new condition. An example of this might be the appearance of cystitis (Damp Heat in the Bladder) in someone who has pre-existing Damp Heat and Kidney Deficiency. In this example, the infectious agent according to conventional medicine terms is usually a microbe that normally forms part of the human ecosystem and which has multiplied out of its usual state of balance to lead to the symptoms of inflammation. If the person regained their healthy state of balance the manifestations would disappear.

The crucial difference between these two categories is that, in the former, an infectious agent (akin to a strong Pathogen) has contributed to the generation of an imbalance, and in the latter the infection appears as a manifestation of an underlying deep imbalance for which the infectious agent is an aspect of its expression. In all probability, the symptoms of many infections are a result of a combination of the two, in that the energetic property of the infectious agent triggers the manifestation of a Pathogenic Factor in a person who already has some degree of underlying imbalance.

An example of this might be the fungal infection known as tinea pedis or athlete's foot. The athlete's foot fungus thrives in damp conditions, and infection often occurs in situations in which external climatic damp is prominent (e.g. swimming pools). This suggests that the Pathogenic Factor in athlete's foot is at least partly of External origin, and many healthy people who visit a pool may suffer a short-term and easily treatable infection. However, it does seem that those people who suffer from persistent attacks of athlete's foot often have a pre-existing internal imbalance such as Spleen Qi Deficiency leading to Damp. In these people it appears that the infection has become a trigger and an outlet for the external and frequent expression of the internal imbalance.

The distinction between these three categories is of fundamental importance in using the classifications of conventional medicine to inform a Chinese medicine diagnosis.

The depth of the Pathogenic Factor

Over the centuries, the Chinese medicine interpretation of those diseases that involve fever evolved into theories that acknowledge that a Pathogenic Factor can manifest at various levels in the energetic body. Three of these theories identify patterns of disease according to "The Six Stages," "The Four Levels" and "The Three Burners," respectively.[57] According to these interpretations, it is possible to be more precise about how deeply the Pathogenic Factor is manifested in the Interior.

These patterns of differentiation often reflect how diseases progress in a conventional medicine perspective.

The energetics of two common infectious diseases

When interpreting the energetics of infectious disease, the important questions that need to be addressed are:

- What Pathogenic Factors are manifesting (consider symptoms and signs)?

- Are the Pathogenic Factors manifesting on the Interior (organs) or Exterior (skin and muscles – the domain of the Jing Luo)?

- What is the origin of the Pathogenic Factor (has it come from without, or has it been generated internally)?

There are several important guidelines to bear in mind. These are:

- Infection will *always* represent the presence of a *Pathogenic Factor*.

- The person who develops the disease may already have a degree of Depletion of *Blood*, *Qi*, *Yin* or *Yang*. An already present Pathogenic Factor such as *Damp* or *Heat* may also be complicating this deficiency. This will affect how the symptoms of disease manifest.

- Characteristics that suggest that the manifestation of the Pathogenic Factor results from an energetic property of the infectious agent (*External origin*) include a *high level of infectiousness* and symptoms that are *strongly characteristic* of a particular type of infectious agent.

- Infections that result from exposure to extremes of climate, or other miscellaneous causes of disease (e.g. unclean food), also suggest a *Pathogenic Factor of External origin*.

- Infections that are not easily contagious but which recur in the same person over and over again suggest a *Pathogenic Factor of Internal origin*.

- *Wind* is often present in infectious disease, and is suggested by any symptoms that change rapidly and move around the body.

- Redness and fever reflect *Heat*.

- Discharges often reflect *Damp* – yellow/green if *Damp Heat* and white/watery if *Damp Cold*.

- Nasal secretions may simply reflect *Wind* preventing the descent of Lung Qi (as in the common cold or allergies).

- Pus and swellings (including lymph nodes) may represent *Phlegm* or *Damp*.

- Susceptibility to infection reflects Depletion of Vital Substances (*Blood*, *Qi*, *Yin* or *Yang*).

- Susceptibility to infections that manifest on the Exterior may reflect depletion of *Wei Qi* in particular (and it is important to remember that the Kidneys (Essence) are the root of Wei Qi[58]).

The common cold

In the case of a familiar example, the common cold, the symptoms are conventionally attributed to infection by any one of a number of viruses. The common cold is unusual in that it is an infectious disease that is neatly described by a basic Organ syndrome, that is, either Wind/Heat or Wind/Cold invading the Lungs. This makes it a good example to use for an interpretation of energetics.

The common cold gives rise to symptoms such as runny nose, cough, sneezing and slight fever. Often it begins with discomfort in the throat or nose, and then the symptoms change over the course of two to five days before the patient gets better.

From a Chinese medicine perspective:

- *Wind* is present because the symptoms start suddenly, change rapidly and move to different parts of the body.

- *Cold* may predominate if secretions are watery and the patient feels cold.

- *Heat* may predominate if secretions are yellowish and fever is marked.

- Profuse secretions suggest impairment of *Descent of Lung Qi* due to *Wind*.

The Pathogenic Factors manifesting in the common cold

The Pathogenic Factors usually manifest on the *Exterior*. Exterior features are slight fever and sweating, headaches, sneezing and runny nose. There are often no features of a deeper Pathogenic Factor in a simple cold.

Occasionally, symptoms such as diarrhea accompany a cold. This might suggest possible involvement of the *Interior* with *Depletion of Spleen Qi* and *Damp Cold* or *Damp Heat*.

The origin of the Pathogenic Factors in the common cold

Most features are suggestive of an *External origin*. The common cold is highly infectious. Often, a particular type of cold that is "going around" will have a characteristic pattern of symptoms that will be experienced by most people who catch it. This suggests that the cold virus contributes a characteristic energetic property, and that the Pathogenic Factor is, at least in part, of External origin.

In addition, many people report that their symptoms follow exposure to particular extremes of climate such as cold wind. This suggests that climatic factors can also contribute to the nature of the Pathogenic Factor that is manifested.

Some features, however, may be suggestive of an *Internal origin*. Some people report that they benefit from having an occasional cold, particularly if the symptoms have been quite pronounced, but short-lived. This suggests that the infection has enabled clearance of existing internal imbalances, which may be seen as contributing to the severity of the symptoms. However, other people suffer from frequent or chronic cold symptoms that they are never able to shake off. They may suffer from colds even

when one is not going around, and in energetic terms, this suggests that it may have become a manifestation of a lingering Pathogenic Factor of Internal origin.

Integrated energetic interpretation of the common cold

The above considerations can be summarized as follows:

- The different strains of the cold virus seem to have a characteristic energetic property that leads to manifestation of Wind/Heat or Wind/Cold on the Exterior and impairment of the Descent of Lung Qi.

- Deficiency of Wei Qi predisposes to development of the common cold. External climatic factors can contribute to the way in which the Pathogenic Factors are manifested.

- In health, the development of a cold may permit clearance of an internal imbalance, leaving the person in a more balanced state on recovery.

- If defenses are less strong, a cold may lead to a deepening imbalance with depletion of substances such as Qi, Yin and Yang, and continued manifestations of Lingering Pathogenic Factors.

Cellulitis

The condition of cellulitis offers a slightly different perspective from that of the common cold. Cellulitis is an infection of the subcutaneous tissues that usually follows a wound to the skin. It can cause a hot, red swelling of the skin, often around an abrasion on the leg or face, and which can spread. The patient feels unwell and feverish. The spread of the infection may be rapid and can lead to a red line tracking up the course of a lymphatic vessel. Lymph nodes draining the infected area can then become swollen and tender.

If untreated, cellulitis can become severe, and in some cases life-threatening, as infection leads to local death of tissues and septicemia (infection in the bloodstream). The cause of cellulitis is most commonly a skin commensal bacterium of either the *Streptococcus* or *Staphylococcus* families.

Cellulitis is more common in older people and in people with chronic conditions such as diabetes.

From a Chinese medicine perspective:

- *Wind* is present because the symptoms start suddenly, change rapidly and move to different parts of the body.

- Redness, tenderness and fever all indicate that *Heat* is present.

The Pathogenic Factors manifesting in cellulitis

In cellulitis *Wind Heat* initially manifests on the *Exterior*, as indicated by an enlarging red area on the skin.

Symptoms such as lymphatic vessel involvement and malaise suggest that the infection has moved to a deeper level. As the cellulitis progresses, this suggests a progressively deeper level of pathology into the *Interior*.

The origin of the Pathogenic Factors in cellulitis

A wound is usually the trigger for cellulitis, and this means there will be local damage and Stagnation of Blood and Qi that might predispose to the generation of *Heat*. Other features of cellulitis are suggestive of *Internal origin*. Cellulitis is not a contagious disease. Even though superficial wounds can introduce germs, many people recover from these without developing cellulitis. Cellulitis is more likely to occur in people with depleted energy, such as elderly people and those with diabetes. It is also more likely to develop in regions of the body where there is poor circulation or local edema. In each of these situations, Deficiency of Qi and Blood, Blood Stagnation and internal Phlegm Damp and Heat are likely to be patterns that are already apparent in the patient.

Integrated energetic interpretation of cellulitis

The above considerations can be summarized as follows:

- Cellulitis is due to a spreading infection by the *Streptococcus* bacterium. It has features of Wind Heat invasion of the Exterior, but can progress to involve deeper levels in some people.

- Its features are predominantly those of a Pathogenic Factor of Internal origin, which suggests that a person who develops cellulitis is susceptible because they already have deficiency of Vital Substances such as Blood and Qi and Yin, together with Internal Heat.

Summary

The Chinese medicine interpretation of what conventional medicine would describe as infectious diseases demonstrates very effectively how the symptoms that form a bridge between the two viewpoints can ultimately enrich an understanding of the pathological processes at play.

2.4c The red flags of serious infectious disease

This section considers some of those general features of infectious diseases that might point to the possibility of serious underlying disease. These red flags should prompt consideration of making a referral to a medical practitioner.

Some of the most important infectious diseases are described in detail later according to the system that they predominantly affect. For example, pneumonia is explored in Chapter 3.3 as it primarily affects the respiratory system. Red flags specific to these important conditions are listed in these later chapters or sections.

Naturally, there will be some overlap between the information given in this section and that in later sections concerning the infections that affect the various systems. All the information about the various red flags of infectious disease is brought together and reviewed in Section 6.3a and summarized in Appendix III.

Table 2.4c-I A2: Red flags of infectious disease: vulnerable groups

Infections are more likely to cause problems in individuals who cannot sustain a strong immune response, either because of immaturity, old age, illness, pregnancy, or because of exposure to unusual organisms (such as occurs during foreign travel).

Treat anyone from the following vulnerable groups with caution if they are displaying features of an infectious disease (e.g. **fever**, **confusion**, **diarrhea and vomiting**, **spreading areas of inflammation** or **yellowish discharges**)

Red flag	Description	Reasoning
A2.1	Infants (especially if <3 months)	Infections in infants can become serious conditions very quickly because of their immature immune system, poor temperature control and small size. They lead easily to high fever and dehydration. Infants are at increased risk of convulsions and circulatory collapse
		Fever of >38.0°C (>100.4°F) in a child of 0–3 months needs to be referred as a high priority
		Fever of >39.0°C (>102.2°F) in a child of 3–6 months needs to be referred as a high priority
		If the child with fever is distressed or shows any other red flags, refer as a high priority
		Otherwise, fever in a small child who is not otherwise distressed may be of no cause for concern, but the child will need vigilant attention to ensure no deterioration
A2.2	Elderly people	Infections can take hold rapidly in elderly people because of a weakened immune system. Serious disease can "hide" behind mild-appearing symptoms
		Always consider referral for same-day medical assessment if high fever >38.0°C (>100.4°F) is apparent
A2.3	Those who are immunocompromised	Those who are immunocompromised are particularly vulnerable to severe overwhelming infections, in particular, of the respiratory and gastrointestinal systems
		Any grade of fever is of concern in those who are immunocompromised
A2.4	In pregnancy	Certain infections can directly damage the embryo/fetus or lead to miscarriage. Others may be transmitted to the baby during labor. Prolonged high fever may induce miscarriage or early labor
A2.5	Anyone with a recent history of travel to a tropical country (within the past month)	Certain tropical diseases (including malaria) can become rapidly overwhelming and may present up to four weeks after return from the tropical country. Always refer for medical assessment if tropical disease is a possibility

Table 2.4c-II A3: Red flags of infectious disease: fever, dehydration and confusion

Definitions
Normal body (tympanic) temperature: 36.8 ± 0.7°C (98.2°F ± 1.3°F)
37.5°C is the upper limit of normal for teenagers and adults
Moderate fever: 37.5–38.0°C (99.5–100.4°F)
High fever: body temperature >38.0°C (>100.4°F)

Red flag	Description	Reasoning
A3.1	Infants (0–6 months)	Infections in infants can become serious conditions very quickly because of their immature immune system, poor temperature control and small size. They lead easily to high fever and dehydration. The infant is at increased risk of convulsions and circulatory collapse
		Fever of >38.0°C (>100.4°F) in a child of 0–3 months needs to be referred as a high priority
		Fever of >39.0°C (>102.2°F) in a child of 3–6 months needs to be referred as a high priority
A3.2	High fever in an older child or adult who does not respond to treatment within five days	Although risk of convulsions is low in this group of patients, a high fever of >38.0°C (>100.4°F) is very depleting and can lead to dehydration. If a high fever is not responding to treatment in five days, this suggests the possibility of a serious condition that merits further investigations
		If a child with fever is distressed or shows any other of the red flags, refer as a high priority
A3.3	Any fever of unknown cause that persists or recurs for >2 weeks	Most mild infectious diseases have run their course within a week; a prolonged fever suggests either a chronic inflammatory or infectious condition, or cancer, all of which merit further investigations
A3.4	Dehydration in a small child (<5 years): signs include dry mouth and skin, cold extremities, gray or mottled complexion, loss of skin turgor (firmness), drowsiness, sunken fontanel (soft spot on the crown of the head in the region of acupoint DU-24, Shen Ting) and dry diapers	A dehydrated infant is at high risk of circulatory collapse because of its small size and immature homeostatic mechanisms. Infants who are dehydrated may lose the desire to drink, and so the condition can rapidly deteriorate. High priority or urgent referral is required
A3.5	Dehydration in older children and adults if severe or prolonged for >48 hours. Signs include: dry mouth and skin, loss of skin turgor, low blood pressure, dizziness on standing and poor urine output	Although not as unstable as an infant, a dehydrated child or adult still needs hydration to prevent damage to the kidneys. Referral should be made if the patient is unable to take fluids or if the dehydration persists for >48 hours. Refer elderly people as a high priority, as the ability to take in fluids is often reduced and the kidneys and brain are more vulnerable to damage
A3.6	Confusion in older children and adults with fever	Temporary confusion is common and benign in young children (<8 years) and older frail people when a fever develops. However, it is not usual in healthy adults, and should be referred to exclude central nervous system involvement (e.g. meningitis, brain abscess). Refer in all cases if the confusion might pose a risk to the patient or to others
A3.7	Febrile convulsion in a child: ongoing	Refer a case in which the convulsion is not settling within 2 minutes as an emergency. Ensure the child is kept in a safe place and in the recovery position while help arrives
A3.8	Febrile convulsion in a child: recovered	Refer all cases in which the child has just suffered a first febrile convulsion (the parents need advice on how to manage future fits, and the child should be examined by a doctor)

Vulnerable groups and infectious disease

Infections presenting with certain features or affecting certain categories of vulnerable patients need to be treated with caution. Although not all infections in the red flag groups listed below will be serious, if there is any uncertainty it is wise to refer for a second opinion.

Fever, dehydration and confusion

Infections may be accompanied by fever, dehydration and confusion. These three complications of infections are not specific to any particular infectious agent. All three can carry the risk of serious consequences to the patient.

FEVER

Fever (by definition, a body core temperature over 37.5°C or 99.5°F) is believed, from a conventional medicine perspective, to have a positive effect on the course of infection. Fever is a result of the inflammatory and immune responses that occur in infections, but potentially dangerous if the body temperature becomes very high, particularly in young children.

The distinction between a moderate and a high fever is somewhat arbitrary, particularly as there is significant variation in the day of up to 0.5°C (0.9°F), and there is also significant variation depending on which sort of measurement is taken. The more reliable rectal measurement of core temperature is neither practical nor safe for day-to-day use. Axillary and ear measurements tend to under-measure the core temperature by up to 0.5°C (0.9°F), and also do not provide consistent readings compared to core readings. However, it is generally accepted that a body temperature measured by axilla (armpit) or by ear (tympanic) of 37.5–38.0°C (99.5–100.4°F) is classified as a moderate fever, and a temperature greater than 38.0°C (100.4°F) is classed as a high fever.

Treatment of all high fevers should start with removal of excess clothing and ensuring the patient maintains hydration levels by drinking water at room temperature. Attempts to cool the patient by sponging, exposure to cold draughts or giving iced drinks are now felt to be unsafe as they can cause a bodily reaction to conserve heat, and so can be counterproductive.

Conventional advice is to give a maximum dose of paracetamol or ibuprofen to adults to reduce fever if it is high, but only if the patient is in distress. Otherwise antipyretics (medications intended to reduce fever) are no longer advised for routine use in the presence of fever. Aspirin is an alternative to paracetamol but should never be given to children under 16. Instead, paracetamol and ibuprofen are available in suspension form for young children. Ibuprofen should not be given to children with chickenpox or with asthma.

High fever >38°C (>100.4°F) is considered a serious warning sign in a child less than 3 months, but after this age is no longer so concerning unless reaching >39°C (>102.2°F) in the 3–6 month age group. Even in this age group antipyretic treatment is now only advised if the feverish child is distressed, as it is no longer believed to prevent febrile convulsion. In older children and adults, fever less than 40°C (104°F) is on its own not a concern unless prolonged for more than five days.[59]

DEHYDRATION

Infectious diseases can lead to dehydration of the body as a result of insufficient intake of fluids and prolonged fever with sweating. Prolonged dehydration and loss of salts can lead to confusion and can be damaging to the kidneys. It should be prevented if at all possible.

Patients suffering from an infectious disease need to be encouraged to drink plenty of fluids. This is particularly important for young children and elderly people. Ideally, salts need to be replaced as well as water. For most illnesses, diluted fruit juices or squash contain sufficient salts to meet the body's needs. If it is not possible to maintain hydration, the patient should be referred to a hospital setting where they can be administered fluids intravenously.

CONFUSION

Confusion is one of the responses of the brain to extreme metabolic disturbance. When exposed to extremes of heat or cold, or imbalances in levels of salts, nutrients and toxins, the function of the brain is impaired and the patient may become confused. Often confusion is accompanied by physical agitation, fearfulness and visual hallucinations.

Extreme fever can induce confusion. However, this is rare in a robust adult, and in this case may indicate a more serious underlying condition such as meningitis. However, children very readily enter a confusional state, and this is not necessarily a serious sign. Similarly, elderly people can easily become confused, even in the situation of a mild illness such as a bladder infection. In themselves, confusional states in children and elderly people are not serious. However, they may need to be treated with seriousness and the patient referred if, as a result of the confused state, they pose a risk to themselves or others.

FEBRILE CONVULSION

High fever can induce a fit in a small child (usually under the age of six), which, if prolonged, can carry the risk of asphyxiation or permanent brain damage. A febrile convulsion is known to occur in 3 percent of children. In 2–4 percent of these cases a febrile convulsion is the first symptom of one of the forms of childhood epilepsy. An ongoing febrile convulsion (lasting more than 5 minutes) requires emergency management. If the convulsion has ceased, for a first seizure the child must be referred as a high priority to exclude serious underlying infectious disease such as meningitis, and to receive advice on how to prevent a recurrence. It is not currently felt that antipyretic treatment such as paracetamol or ibuprofen will prevent convulsions, and so should not be routinely given in fever for this reason.

2.4d Diagnosis, prevention and treatment of infectious disease

Diagnosis of infectious disease

It was explained in Section 1.2a that diagnosis involves the three stages of questioning, examination and investigation. In the diagnosis of infectious disease, questioning and examination are performed to look for characteristic features of the different diseases. Many infectious diseases (e.g. tonsillitis, mumps, threadworm and head lice infestation) have their own distinct pattern of symptoms and signs, and can be diagnosed effectively using these two approaches alone.

Additional information can be provided from investigations, which can be broadly categorized as:

- tests to look for the presence of the infectious agent (examination of body fluids and tissue samples)

- tests to look for evidence of characteristic processes of disease (blood tests and imaging techniques such as X-ray imaging)

- tests to examine for a current or previous immune response to the infectious agent (mostly blood tests looking for antibodies).

Tests to look for the presence of the infectious agent

The most straightforward tests for the presence of an infectious agent involve examining specimens of fluids or tissues taken from the body. The simple microscope is necessary to examine for bacteria, protozoa, fungi and the small immature forms of larger parasites.

The choice of specimen depends on the nature of the disease. If a particular organ is involved, specimens of fluid of tissue from that organ will be sought. Examples include:

- swab from tonsil/throat/nose and sputum sample in upper respiratory infections

- urine sample in urinary infections

- feces sample in gastrointestinal infections

- skin swab in skin infections

- scrapings of skin and nail clippings in fungal skin infections

- swab or sample of pus leaking from an abscess or boil.

Obtaining each of the samples listed above involves a relatively non-invasive procedure, but sometimes the search for infection has to be more penetrating. Examples of invasive investigations include:

- blood samples to look for bacteria in the blood

- surgical removal of a sample of deep organ tissue (biopsy), e.g. liver, bone marrow and even brain.

The samples of body fluid or tissue have to be processed in different ways in order to allow an infectious agent to be diagnosed. Part of the processing often involves allowing the microbe to grow for a few days (culture) before there are sufficient quantities for accurate diagnosis. This is why some tests take some time before the results are ready.

The next stage of processing is to detect the agent in the specimen. This can involve the use of chemical dyes, such as the Gram stain, which show up certain bacteria. More recently, the detection of infection has become an increasingly complex but very precise science with the use of DNA and RNA probes.

Tests to look for evidence of characteristic processes of disease

Some investigations involve examination not for the infectious agent but for the signs that it has caused damage to the body. For example, a sample of the blood can be examined to see if the leukocytes are changed in shape or number in any way. Different diseases lead to different types of change in these white blood cells. The test that is performed is called a full blood count (FBC).

Blood tests called the erythrocyte sedimentation rate (ESR) and C-reactive protein (CRP) are commonly performed when it is uncertain whether or not an infection has occurred. The ESR and CRP are both raised when the inflammatory response has been triggered in the body. A typical example when these tests might be used is when someone complains of feeling tired all the time, a complaint that very often has no measurable physical cause. The doctor might take blood for an ESR or CRP, amongst other tests, to exclude the possibility of an infective or other inflammatory reason for the symptoms.

The following five imaging techniques are also used in the investigation of infectious diseases:

- chest X-ray

- ultrasound scan

- computed axial tomography (CT) scan

- magnetic resonance imaging (MRI)

- radionuclide scan.

The chest X-ray differentiates between dense tissue, such as bone, and air-filled tissue, such as the lungs. Patches of infection (fluid) show up as shadows in the lung area. The X-ray image is not able to show up much detail in most body parts, and is most useful for examining bones and the chest. It is acknowledged that excessive exposure to X-rays may cause cancer, but that the exposure from a single X-ray investigation is very unlikely to be damaging. The additional risk is that 1 in 200,000 patients will develop a cancer as a result of a single X-ray study.[60]

An ultrasound scan utilizes ultrasound waves to produce images of those soft tissue parts of the body that cannot be imaged using X-radiation. The ultrasound scan can show up collections of pus within deep organs. The technique is considered to be very safe compared to X-ray imaging. There is currently no known risk from exposure to ultrasonic waves.

The CT scan uses computer processing of a series of X-ray images to produce an image of a "slice" of the body. The image produced by a CT scan gives far more detail than an X-ray image, but involves the patient in a prolonged and uncomfortable procedure, and also exposes the patient to more radiation. In infectious disease the CT scan can expose collections of pus in body spaces and patches of infection in the lungs. The additional significant risk is that 1 in 2000 patients will develop a cancer after a single abdominal CT study.[61]

The MRI scan produces similar images to the CT scan, although it seems to give better definition of nervous tissue. MRI involves the use of a powerful magnetic field, and is thought to be less harmful than X-radiation. There are currently no known additional risks from exposure to the magnetic field in MRI scans.

Radionuclide scanning involves first giving the patient a radioactive substance, either by mouth or by injection, and then scanning the body to see the location of the substance in the body. In an infection of unknown source, radioactive leukocytes or antibiotics may be given to the patient. These will concentrate at the site of infection, and a scan will therefore show up the site as an area of increased radioactivity. The radioactivity wears off very rapidly, and the procedure, like X-ray imaging, is considered to be relatively safe to the patient. Nevertheless, the risk is that 1 in 3000 patients might develop cancer as a result of a radionuclide white blood cell study.

Tests to examine for a current or previous immune response to the infectious agent

The use of tests to examine for a current or previous immune response is also known as immunodiagnosis. This group of investigations focuses on testing for whether the body has started to produce antibodies to a particular infection. The presence of the antibody shows that the body has encountered that infection. The type of antibody found will indicate whether or not the infection is current

or whether it occurred in the past. The same tests are performed to check whether somebody is already resistant to a disease, whether they require a vaccination, and also whether a vaccination has induced a sufficient immune response to protect against disease.

Prevention of infectious disease

Prevention of death and disability from infection is arguably the area in which conventional medicine has had the most impact on health. The death rates from many of the infectious diseases, which were major killers in the past (e.g. diphtheria, tuberculosis, poliomyelitis, cholera, typhoid, leprosy, the plague, smallpox), have declined so dramatically that these diseases have been virtually eradicated in developed countries – indeed, smallpox is believed to have been entirely eradicated worldwide, with the last case recorded in 1977. The increase in life expectancy that has occurred over the past two centuries can be largely attributed to the reduction in deaths from infections. Although much of this reduction in death and disability from infectious disease can be attributed to improvements in the general health and well-being of the populations of developed countries, undoubtedly medical approaches to the prevention of infectious disease have also had a significant impact.

In conventional medicine there are four main aspects to the prevention of disease:

- maximizing hygiene and the health of the population
- immunization (vaccination)
- having an active approach to detecting and monitoring new cases of disease (surveillance)
- rapid isolation and treatment of new cases of disease so that spread is reduced.

Maximizing hygiene and the health of the population

There is no doubt that the largest part of the change in life expectancy can be attributed to improved hygiene and health of the population. The beneficial effects of good nutrition, housing and sanitation were introduced in Section 2.4a. Many of the world's most deadly diseases cannot take hold in a population that has a good basic level of health and sanitation. Nevertheless, as described in Section 2.4a, some diseases (e.g. meningitis) can have devastating effects, even in a seemingly healthy population.

Immunization

Conventional medicine recognizes immunization as a very powerful weapon in its armory for the prevention of disease. The principles of immunization were described in Section 2.1d.

There are two main strategies behind the practice of immunization. The first is to target a vaccine at "at-risk individuals" so that the personal risk of developing disease is reduced. A well-known example of this approach is the use of certain vaccines for the protection of travelers against tropical diseases such as hepatitis A, typhoid and yellow fever. Another example is the use of vaccine against influenza in elderly people and those who have particular health problems such as heart disease.

The second strategy is to eradicate or significantly reduce the occurrence of a disease in a population. For this an organized immunization program is necessary, because a sufficiently large proportion of the population has to be immunized to mimic the situation of herd immunity. It is known that if a large proportion of the population is immune to a disease, epidemics of that disease are unlikely to occur, and the disease may even die out.

This is the rationale behind childhood programs of immunizations, which involve giving vaccines and booster doses for some of the childhood diseases. The UK childhood immunization schedule aims to protect all children against the following infectious organisms:

- diphtheria

- tetanus

- pertussis (whooping cough)

- *Haemophilus influenzae* type b (Hib)

- poliomyelitis

- *Meningococcus* serogroups ACWY

- *Meningococcus* serogroup B

- rotavirus

- pneumococcus (*Streptococcus pneumoniae*)

- measles

- mumps

- rubella

- human papilloma virus (HPV).

The timing of the vaccinations in the UK immunization schedule is summarized in Table 2.4d-I.

In addition to the immunizations listed in the table, the immunization against tuberculosis (TB), known as the BCG (Bacillus Calmette-Guérin), is now offered as part of a risk-based program. This means it is targeted at those individuals most at risk of exposure to TB, such as newborns from immigrant families and people recently emigrated from at-risk countries. However, the national schools program that offered BCG to all 14-year-old children in the UK was stopped in 2005 because of the declining incidence of the disease in the general population, but diphtheria and tetanus, HPV and meningitis vaccines are still offered to teenage school children.

Table 2.4d-I Timing of the vaccinations in the UK immunization schedule

Age at immunization	Vaccines given	Mode of administration
2 months	Five-in-one vaccine: diphtheria, tetanus, pertussis (whooping cough), polio and Hib (DTP-Hib)	One combined injection
	Pneumococcus (PCV)	One injection
	Meningitis B (Men B)	One injection
	Rotavirus	Oral vaccine
3 months	Five-in-one vaccine: diphtheria, tetanus, pertussis (whooping cough), polio and Hib (DTP-Hib)	One combined injection
	Meningitis C (Men C)	One injection
	Rotavirus	Oral vaccine
4 months	Five-in-one vaccine: diphtheria, tetanus, pertussis (whooping cough), polio and Hib (DTP-Hib)	One combined injection
	Pneumococcus (PCV)	One injection
	Meningitis B (Men B)	One injection
12 months	Hib and Meningitis C	One combined injection
	Measles, mumps, rubella (MMR)	One injection
	Pneumococcus (PCV)	One injection
	Meningitis B (Men B)	One injection
All children aged 2–6 on annual basis	Influenza	Nasal vaccine
3–5 years (preschool)	Four-in-one vaccine: diphtheria, tetanus and pertussis and polio (DTP/polio)	One combined injection
	Measles, mumps and rubella (MMR)	One combined injection

12–13 years for girls only	Human papilloma virus (HPV)	Two injections given over the course of six months
14 years	Three-in-one vaccine: tetanus and diphtheria (Td) and polio	One combined injection
	Meningitis ACWY	One combined injection

The immunization strategy requires a high coverage of the population to be successful. This is considered to be important because most vaccinations have an efficacy of only 90–95 percent and thus leave 5–10 percent of those vaccinated still vulnerable to disease. If more than 10 percent of a population remains unvaccinated, this could mean that 20 percent of the population is unprotected, giving a herd immunity of less than 80 percent. The lower the herd immunity is, the greater the risk that an epidemic of the disease could spread within the unprotected minority. The risks of epidemics are greatly reduced if herd immunity can be raised to above 80 percent. In the UK, the Department of Health coordinates a process of public health education to encourage uptake of vaccination, including internet-based information such as the National Health Service (NHS) Choices web resource.[62] In addition, the provision of childhood immunization is a required service as part of the General Medical Services contract for provision of care by general practices. This means that UK general practices need to have rigorous reminder-and-recall systems to ensure children do not slip through the immunization net. As a result of these factors, in recent years national vaccine coverage has been well over 90 percent of eligible children.

There is very good statistical evidence to show that immunization does reduce the incidence of immunizable diseases. Although health and hygiene have had by far the most powerful impact in reducing the number of cases for most diseases, including TB and diphtheria, immunizations have been clearly shown to contribute to this reduction.

The statistics that the medical establishment use to support the use of immunization to prevent disease are the result of long-term, well-conducted studies of immunized and non-immunized populations. It is difficult to refute the results of such high-quality studies and to argue against the suggestion that immunization reduces the risk of an individual contracting a particular disease and reduces the incidence of the disease in the population.

There is an energetic and multifaceted anti-vaccination movement, which tends to place value on diverse methods of natural approaches to healthcare over and above invasive medical interventions.[63] The diverse expressions of the anti-vaccination groups are easily found through an internet search, together with evidence of a more recent phenomenon, the numerous articulate and pro-vaccination arguments that have been written and posted in response to this movement. The concerns expressed by anti-vaccinationists range from possible long-term damage to the immune system of the child by the altered infectious agent, the induction of long-term chronic disease and also toxic damage by the constituents of the vaccines.

However, anti-vaccinationist claims that vaccinations have led to an increase in diseases such as diabetes, inflammatory bowel disease, multiple sclerosis, asthma and autism have not been proven by the medical studies that have been performed to date, and the medical establishment strongly refute links to these serious conditions.[64] A very clear and systematic medical argument against the diverse alternative medical concerns about vaccination has been published by the US pediatrician Paul Offit (2009, with Charlotte Moser) in the journal *Pediatrics*.[65] This was made in response to the best-selling book written by Dr Robert Sears in 2007 entitled *The Vaccine Book: Making the Right Decision for Your Child*.[66] Offit and Moser's highly referenced article illustrates both the breadth of concerns about the practice of vaccination and also the medical evidence that can be used to counter these concerns, and is worth reading to get a succinct overview of the debate, albeit written from a medical viewpoint.

What long-term medical studies on the effects of vaccination are less able to demonstrate for sure is whether or not a vaccination may have caused subtle but significant changes in health and well-being. Studies generally look for clear and measurable outcome measures (such as death, or rashes, or clear diagnoses of disease or fevers), and may not pick up more generalized and non-specific symptoms such as tiredness, digestive upset, recurrent minor respiratory infections and low mood.

In conventional medicine terms it is appreciated that vaccinations carry risks of adverse reactions in a small number of people who receive them. However, for any medically recommended immunization, the respected medical evidence shows that the risks to the population as a whole from having the vaccine are far less than the risks to the population as a whole of contracting the disease.

It is not commonly appreciated that vaccines are available for only a few diseases. To date, vaccines have been developed for some viral and bacterial infections, but not for fungal or parasitic diseases or infestations. Despite much research, it has not yet been possible to mimic successfully some diseases, such as the common cold, malaria and HIV, in the form of a vaccine. Vaccines, therefore, can form only part of the approach to the prevention of infectious diseases.

Information box 2.4d-I

Vaccination: comments from a Chinese medicine perspective

Written records of "variation" in China exist from the 18th century describing various practices, including nasal inoculation of powdered smallpox scabs and encouraging children to wear clothes from infected children, which dated from at least the 16th century CE.[67] This suggests that the underlying principle of vaccination, possibly based on an archaic principle of "poison attacked by poison," was not at odds with the Chinese medical theory of the time.[68] The current term for vaccination, Zhong Dou, means "planting pox" and dates from this ancient practice. Evidence that the Chinese medical energetic effect of vaccination has been historically considered comes in the *Yi Lin Gai Cuo* (1830) by Wang Qing-Ren. In this classic text the Chinese physician is expressing his view in the debate about whether or not smallpox was entirely due to the external manifestation of "Fetal Toxin," which was believed to be a lingering Heat Toxin that entered the child in utero, and that could lead to chronic illness in later life if not cleared.

Wang Qing-Ren notes that smallpox has epidemic qualities and affects regions at a time, and argues that if the pox were due to Fetal Toxin alone, it would not behave in this way. He uses the practice of vaccination in his argument. He questions, if the disease was due to Fetal Toxin alone, how could vaccination lead to a disease with a "favorable course" in all cases? Instead he proposes that there are toxins of varying severity, and these could explain the wide range of presentation of the disease from severe to the most mild. Here he is suggesting that vaccination is the introduction of a "favorable toxin,"[69] thus showing that vaccination was recognized as having a disease-like property, and that it engendered symptoms akin to the infectious disease it was intended to prevent.

The theory of Fetal Toxin being central to the mechanism of childhood infections has persisted in Chinese medicine, and generally nowadays the infectious diseases such as measles and mumps are seen as "a combination of fetal toxins plus invasion by external pathogen."[70] This view explains the epidemic properties of these diseases, but still maintains the idea that some of the imbalance expressed in these diseases was already present in a latent form in the child prior to the infection.

Fetal toxins are understood to be allowed to emerge and dissipate through the experience of the childhood infections such as measles, mumps and rubella that present with a red rash and fever, and so this means that, according to Chinese medical theory, a well-managed childhood infection can actually leave the child in a better state on recovery. It is understood that Fetal Toxins persisting until adulthood might be the cause of chronic internal disease.

And so, according to the Chinese medical perspective, a vaccine is a form of Heat Toxin. However, when given in most cases it leads to apparently mild disease. Thus it apparently does not permit the expression of Internal imbalance that may be present in the form of Fetal Toxins. Nevertheless, vaccination was seen to be beneficial, and this suggests it was recognized to Tonify the Upright Qi. As vaccination is known to work by stimulating the immune system, it is noteworthy that many Chinese herbs that have actions described as Tonifying Qi are also now known to have immunomodulatory action.[71] Vaccination can thus be compared to the administration of a Qi Tonifying medicinal, albeit one with Toxic properties.

One of the concerns expressed by Western-trained practitioners of Chinese medicine about vaccines is that they might prevent the emergence of Fetal Toxins by preventing the occurrence of common and usually mild childhood infections at the time in early childhood at which they most usually would have occurred.

Moreover, there is a concern that the toxin introduced by the vaccine may not be fully cleared, particularly if introduced in early infancy when the immune system is immature. Instead the toxin persists in the system as a Latent Pathogenic Factor, and, rather like a Fetal Toxin, this may be the cause of chronic internal disease.[72]

Both these concerns are based on observation of patients and are not proven by scientific study. However, they both make entire sense in terms of Chinese medical theory and observation of patients.

In summary, the history of Chinese medicine suggests that vaccination was recognized as a therapeutic procedure and that it could Tonify Upright Qi, but current Chinese medical theory supports the case that vaccination could in itself cause severe disease, either immediately by introducing Toxic Heat or chronically via Latent Heat.

Ideally vaccination will prevent deaths from overwhelming serious disease. However, in some cases prevention of mild disease by vaccination might well have deleterious effects, particularly in those individuals who are unable, because of Kidney Deficiency, to clear its Toxic Heat. In all cases of vaccination it would be prudent to ensure that it was given at a time when the immune system was not compromised, and also to offer supportive treatment to enable the clearance of Toxic Heat.

Surveillance

Most developed countries have a system of disease surveillance in place. Through these systems, cases of important diseases are reported by health professionals, and are recorded and monitored by means of a central database.

The surveillance system in the UK relies largely on notifications of disease from doctors. It is one of the duties of doctors in the UK to submit a notification in writing of every case of a "notifiable disease" that they treat. Notifiable diseases are those infections that are considered to have the potential to impact significantly on the health of the community (see Table 2.4d-II). The list of notifiable diseases includes conditions such as food poisoning, meningitis, most tropical diseases and all the immunizable diseases. HIV infection is not a notifiable disease.

Table 2.4d-II Notifiable diseases in the UK

Notification of a number of specified infectious diseases is required of doctors in the UK as a "statutory duty" under the UK Public Health (Infectious Diseases) 1988 Act and the Public Health (Control of Diseases) 1988 Act.

Public Health England (PHE) collates details of each case of each disease that has been notified. This allows analyses of local and national trends.

This is one example of a situation in which there is a statutory requirement for a doctor to breach patient confidentiality.

Diseases that are notifiable include:[73]

Acute encephalitis
Acute infectious hepatitis
Acute meningitis
Acute poliomyelitis
Anthrax
Botulism
Brucellosis
Cholera
Diphtheria
Enteric fever (typhoid or paratyphoid fever)
Food poisoning
Hemolytic uremic syndrome (HUS)
Infectious bloody diarrhea
Invasive group A streptococcal disease
Legionnaires' disease
Leprosy

Malaria
Measles
Meningococcal septicemia
Mumps
Plague
Rabies
Rubella
Scarlet fever
Severe Acute Respiratory Syndrome (SARS)
Smallpox
Tetanus
Tuberculosis (TB)
Typhus
Viral hemorrhagic fever (VHF)
Whooping cough
Yellow fever

Surveillance depends on the accurate and complete notification of disease. This can, of course, never be fully attained, as doctors are busy, and may fail to notify or accurately diagnose many cases of infectious disease. Nevertheless, the figures on notified diseases are of sufficiently good quality to produce useful local and national reports of the incidence of these diseases. These reports can demonstrate whether the disease is on the increase, or whether it is declining.

It is this information that has shown the marked reduction in diseases such as measles following the institution of immunization campaigns. This evidence is the basis on which conventional medicine argues for the continuation of immunization programs or for the cessation of an immunization program (e.g. the school BCG vaccination program for TB was stopped in the UK in 2005 on this basis). Surveillance can lead to a campaign being stepped up (e.g. the preschool booster dose of MMR vaccine was introduced in 1996 in the UK when it was found that too many children who had only a single dose of vaccine were developing measles). Surveillance can also detect a cluster of cases of an unusual disease (e.g. meningitis or food poisoning), which may highlight the need for a focused local campaign of treatment. This is relevant to the final aspect of prevention of disease – isolation and treatment.

Rapid isolation and treatment of new cases

It is accepted within conventional medicine that improved health and hygiene and a thorough vaccination campaign contributed to the eradication of smallpox.

However, there was a fourth approach to prevention that was a vital additional factor. This approach was a worldwide surveillance program, which involved the rapid reporting and treatment of any patient who developed smallpox. Patients with the disease were nursed in isolation so that the disease could not spread. This program prevented the development of epidemics of the disease, and gradually the disease became extinct.

This approach of rapid isolation and treatment is considered essential in cases such as bacterial meningitis and food poisoning. In these cases, patients are treated rapidly and possible contacts are actively traced and advised on how to recognize symptoms of the condition, and what to do if they occur. This is a powerful approach to minimizing the spread of the disease. A recent example of this is the worldwide program that has resulted in the containment and control of the outbreak of Ebola hemorrhagic fever that emerged in West Africa in 2014.

Prevention can, of course, be seen to overlap with treatment, particularly when treatment involves isolation of cases of a disease and treatment of contacts who have not yet developed the disease.

Treatment of infectious disease

The ideal treatment option for infectious disease is the use of a therapy that targets the infectious agent, but which has a minimal effect on the person with the infection. This can be compared to the action of a weed killer used on a lawn that is specific in its action on the unwanted weeds, while leaving the grass unharmed.

In conventional medicine the main therapy used to treat infections is chemical medicine, either taken internally or applied externally. It is in the drug therapy for infections that the distinction between the different types of infectious agent becomes relevant, as a drug that will damage a bacterium will not necessarily damage a flea, and vice versa. Drugs are developed to target weak spots in the defenses of the particular infectious agent.

Historically, the first drug to target bacterial infections was discovered by serendipity by a scientist called Alexander Fleming. In 1928, Fleming discovered that the seemingly harmless *Penicillium notatum* mold, an accidental contaminant of one of his experiments, caused the death of the bacterial cultures that he was trying to grow in his laboratory. In this discovery was the potential for an ideal therapy. This particular mold killed bacteria but was relatively non-toxic to humans. Since Fleming's discovery, a rapidly increasing number of drugs have been developed that have this selective property of targeting an infectious agent. Many of these are closely related in chemical structure to natural substances such as molds.

With the advent of modern pharmacology over the last few decades, completely novel "designer" drugs have been created using the detailed knowledge that there now is about the life cycle of the various infectious agents. The new drugs used to slow down the progression of HIV infection (the highly active antiretroviral therapy (HAART) drugs) are an example of this. These are compounds that have been structurally designed to interfere specifically with the replication of the HIV virus.

In formularies of prescription medications such as the *British National Formulary* (BNF) or the United States *Pharmacopoeia – National Formulary* (USP-NF), drugs intended to target infections are usually categorized under the following five headings:

- antibacterial drugs (counteract bacteria)

- antifungal drugs (counteract fungi)

- antiviral drugs (counteract viruses)

- antiprotozoal drugs (counteract single-celled animals)

- anthelmintic drugs (counteract worms, tapeworms and flukes, collectively known as "helminthes").

Within these five categories, drugs are then sub-classified according to their chemical nature and the specific type of bacterium, virus, fungus or animal parasite that they affect.

Side effects

The ideal antimicrobial drug targets the microbe but leaves the human host untouched. Unfortunately, this ideal is never perfectly attained. All antimicrobials can result in side effects in the person taking them, as well as damage to the infectious agent. Serious side effects for most antibiotics are not common, but they can be very severe in a small, often unpredictable, proportion of people. The most common side effects of antimicrobial treatment are allergic reactions such as rash and itch, and gastrointestinal disturbance. The latter often occur because the drug affects the healthy commensal bacteria in the bowel.

Drug formularies usually list side effects in an order that reflects their frequency, with the most common being listed first. For example, the side effects of a commonly prescribed antibiotic, tetracycline, are listed in the BNF as nausea, vomiting, diarrhea (antibiotic-associated colitis reported occasionally), dysphagia and esophageal irritation. Other rare side effects are also listed as including hepatotoxicity, pancreatitis, blood disorders, light sensitivity of the skin and hypersensitivity reactions (including rash, exfoliative dermatitis, Stevens-Johnson syndrome, urticaria, angioedema, anaphylaxis and pericarditis). In addition, benign intracranial hypertension in adults and bulging fontanels in infants have been reported.

In the case of tetracycline, even the common side effects of nausea, vomiting and diarrhea will not affect the majority of people using the drug, and more rare side effects such as hepatotoxicity are uncommon, affecting one in 10,000 patients who take the medication.

Most people who take a drug such as tetracycline will not experience any side effects, but doctors need to bear the potential risks in mind when prescribing drugs such as this. Some antibiotics may be prescribed for up to a few months at a time for relatively minor health problems. This is the case with tetracycline, a commonly prescribed treatment for acne, so doctors need to warn patients to be vigilant about the emergence of side effects.

The conventional view is that antimicrobials are harmless to the individual except in the few cases in which side effects develop. A medical practitioner who prescribes repeated doses of antibiotics to a young child with eczema and asthma will not consider that the antibiotics will have caused any harm to that child if the child recovers from the acute infection. Likewise, a prolonged course of tetracycline might be prescribed to a fit teenager with acne without any concern that there might be any problem in taking these drugs for such a long time. In cases such as this, the doctor is prescribing in a way that is in keeping with the values and beliefs of the medical profession. In contrast to the concern with which antibiotics may be held within some complementary health disciplines, in conventional medicine it is simply not recognized that antimicrobials, if apparently well tolerated, could, in the majority of cases, be the cause of long-term problems for the individual.

However, it is certainly the conventional medical view that inappropriate prescribing of antimicrobial drugs can be very harmful to the health of the population, in that it might lead to the development of drug resistance in the microbes endemic in the community. This important concept of drug resistance is discussed in the following section.

Principles of treatment with antimicrobials

There is increasing professional concern about the levels of prescribing of antimicrobial drugs. In the UK in 1998, a House of Lords Select Committee produced a detailed report on how the use of antimicrobials in agriculture, as well as in healthcare, should be controlled.[74] The major concern that promoted this inquiry was the development of antimicrobial resistance. In 2014 the World Health Organization (WHO) produced a report that confirmed that microbial resistance is a current and very significant global concern.[75]

Section 2.4a introduced the concept of emerging infections, and how "beneficial mutations" can allow microbes to adapt to their environment. Since the widespread use of penicillin, new strains of bacteria have emerged that are no longer killed by penicillin. Some particularly common strains of bacteria have now adapted to produce substances called "beta lactamases" (including penicillinase), which can destroy penicillin.

It is now widely appreciated that the more an antibiotic is used, the more likely it is that these "resistant" strains will develop. This is not only a product of excessive prescribing for health reasons; there is increasing concern that drug-resistant microbes are developing in farm animals, which are given high doses of antibiotics to promote growth. These bacteria then get passed on to humans through the food chain.

It is also known that an infection that is treated inadequately may also encourage the expansion of drug-resistant mutations. This is particularly likely to occur if the dose of antibiotic is too low to kill the microbe completely, or if the drug is taken on an irregular basis, thus allowing a few remaining bacteria to multiply in the presence of low concentrations of the drug.

The current advice to doctors in choosing a drug to prescribe is as follows.

DO NOT PRESCRIBE IN MINOR INFECTIONS

It is recognized that in minor infections the majority of prescriptions of antibiotics do not lead to any significant health benefit. In some infections, such as acute sore throat, bacterial otitis media (infection of the middle ear) and tonsillitis, the most an antibiotic seems to do is reduce the length of the infection by one to two days. It is probably true that for many prescriptions in the community the patient might well have got better without the prescription. Doctors are now being encouraged to think very carefully before prescribing in such cases.

MAKE SURE THE CORRECT TYPE AND DOSE OF ANTIBIOTIC IS CHOSEN

The best way to ensure that the correct antibiotic is chosen is to take a specimen for diagnosis before treatment is started. This might be a urine sample in a urinary infection or a throat swab in tonsillitis. This specimen has to be cultured in the laboratory. The pathologist dealing with the specimen can then test to see which antibiotics are best to target that particular infection. Often it is necessary to "treat blind," which means choosing an antibiotic without knowing for sure that the infection is sensitive to that drug. Ideally, the specimen should still be tested, so that if after two to three days the result shows that the antibiotic should be changed, this can be done.

In reality, in general practice this process is rarely followed through. Often prescriptions are for minor illness and for short periods (three to five days). Doctors in these circumstances may choose to treat blind and use an antibiotic that has a very broad action rather than one that targets the particular infection. However, the use of broad-spectrum antibiotics, such as amoxicillin, is known to be more likely to promote the development of drug resistance. For this reason, local formularies will give advice on the best narrow-spectrum antibiotic to choose for each sort of illness based on local prevalence of microbial resistance.

COMPLETE THE FULL COURSE OF TREATMENT, WITHOUT SKIPPING DOSES

For the reasons mentioned earlier, it is important to maintain a high concentration of antibiotic in the bloodstream throughout the time required to kill the infectious agent. Some infections are very sensitive and require only a single dose of antibiotic, but others may require months of continuous therapy (e.g. TB, fungal nail infections, HIV).

It proves very difficult for most people to maintain a strict regimen of tablet taking when it is required that one dose be taken three times a day for more than two to three days. It is no wonder that some of the conditions that require such a regimen to be successful are very difficult to treat.

This problem of poor compliance or concordance with the demands of a prescription can have severe consequences. For example, it is believed that the haphazard use of therapy for TB is one of the contributory factors leading to the appearance of a multiple drug-resistant strain. As a result there are increasing cases of untreatable, and therefore fatal, TB in the developing world.

Nevertheless, despite the problems of side effects and drug resistance, there is no doubt that antimicrobial drugs do play an important part in the reduction of disability and death from serious infectious disease. Although it is increasingly clear that many prescriptions of antibiotics for minor conditions are not justifiable clinically, antimicrobial therapy plays a vital role in the prevention of and recovery from serious infectious disease.

 Information box 2.4d-II

Antimicrobials: comments from a Chinese medicine perspective

According to Chinese medicine, antimicrobials will appear to clear the superficial symptoms and signs of infections, and may introduce symptoms including, most commonly, diarrhea, digestive disturbance and rashes. They are understood to be Cold and Bitter medicinals that Cool the Heat symptoms of infectious disease, but that may injure the Spleen and engender Dampness.

In some cases antibiotics can also trigger anaphylactoid allergic reactions, suggesting that they act like a Heat Toxin in some individuals.

Dampness can impede the free flow of Yang Qi and lead to Heat resulting from Stagnation, and this can combine with Dampness to form Chronic Damp Heat. According to Flaws,[76] the presence of "Heat Evils" resulting from antibiotics might become apparent from time to time in the form of "infections," and so the patient is treated again with antibiotics. A negative spiral of increasing Spleen Qi Deficiency and Damp Heat is engendered.

Maciocia notes that antibiotics can cause peeled patches on the tongue, a sign of Stomach Yin Deficiency.[77]

It would make sense that if antibiotics are absolutely necessary, supportive treatment and diet to Nourish the Spleen and Stomach and Clear Damp might also be recommended.

Notes

1 Waugh, A. and Grant, A. (2014) *Ross and Wilson: Anatomy and Physiology in Health and Illness.* Twelfth Edition. Edinburgh: Elsevier, Chapter 14.

2 Guo, S. and DePietro, L.A. (2010) 'Factors affecting wound healing.' *Journal of Dental Research 89*(3), 219–229.

3 Flaws, B., Johnstone, M. and Rogers, T. (1994) *Statements of Fact in Traditional Chinese Medicine.* Boulder, CO: Blue Poppy Press.

4 Abbate, S. (2001) 'A simplified approach to the treatment of scars with Oriental Medicine.' Available at www.acupuncturetoday.com/mpacms/at/article.php?id=27842, accessed on 20 May 2016.

5 Waugh, A. and Grant, A. (2014) *Ross and Wilson: Anatomy and Physiology in Health and Illness.* Twelfth Edition. Edinburgh: Elsevier, Chapter 4.

6 Knott, L. (2014) 'Bleeding disorders.' Available at http://patient.info/doctor/bleeding-disorders, accessed on 20 May 2016.

7 Tidy, C. (2015) 'Thrombocytopenia and platelet disorders.' Available at http://patient.info/doctor/thrombocytopenia-and-platelet-function-disorders, accessed on 20 May 2016.

8 Knott, L. (2014) 'Bleeding disorders.' Available at http://patient.info/doctor/bleeding-disorders, accessed on 20 May 2016.

9 Knott, L. (2014) 'Haemophilia A (factor VII deficiency).' Available at http://patient.info/doctor/haemophilia-a-factor-viii-deficiency, accessed on 20 May 2016.

10 Maciocia, G. (1994) *The Practice of Chinese Medicine.* Edinburgh: Churchill Livingstone, p.710.

11 Shen-Nong Limited (2016) 'Bleeding under the skin and Chinese medicine.' Available at www.shen-nong.com/eng/exam/bleeding_symptoms_bleeding_under_the_skin.html, accessed on 20 May 2016.

12 Becker, S. (2000) *A Handbook of Chinese Hematology.* Boulder, CO: Blue Poppy Press, p.213.

13 US Department of Health and Human Services and National Institutes of Health (National Institute of Allergy and Infectious Diseases and National Cancer Institute) (2003) *Understanding the Immune System: How it Works.* Available at www.imgt.org/IMGTeducation/Tutorials/ImmuneSystem/UK/the_immune_system.pdf, accessed on 20 May 2016.

14 Waugh, A. and Grant, A. (2014) *Ross and Wilson: Anatomy and Physiology in Health and Illness.* Twelfth Edition. Edinburgh: Elsevier, Chapter 15.

15 NHS Choices (2016) 'When to have vaccinations.' Available at www.nhs.uk/conditions/vaccinations/pages/vaccination-schedule-age-checklist.aspx, accessed on 20 May 2016.

16 Public Health England (2013) *The Green Book.* Chapter 21: 'Measles.' Available at www.gov.uk/government/uploads/system/uploads/attachment_data/file/147968/Green-Book-Chapter-21-v2_0.pdf, accessed on 20 May 2016.

17 Public Health England (2013) *The Green Book.* Chapter 27: 'Rabies.' Available at www.gov.uk/government/uploads/system/uploads/attachment_data/file/85762/Green-Book-Chapter-27-v3_0.pdf, accessed on 20 May 2016.

18 Maciocia, G. (1989) *The Foundations of Chinese Medicine.* Edinburgh: Churchill Livingstone, pp.44–46.

19 Maciocia, G. (1989) *The Foundations of Chinese Medicine.* Edinburgh: Churchill Livingstone, p.59.

20 Gascoigne, S. (2001) *The Clinical Medicine Guide – A Holistic Perspective.* Clonakilty, Ireland: Jigme Press.

21 Dharmananda, S. (1997) 'Oriental perspectives on cancer and its treatment.' Available at www.itmonline.org/arts/cancer.htm, accessed on 24 May 2016.

22 Flaws, B. (2002) 'Chinese medical treatment of malignant lymphoma.' *Acupuncture Today 3*, 7. Available at www.acupuncturetoday.com/mpacms/at/article.php?id=28009, accessed on 24 May 2016.

23 Flaws, B. (2001) *The Treatment of Modern Western Medical Diseases.* Boulder, CO: Blue Poppy Press, Chapter 2, 'Allergic Rhinitis', p.47.

24 Flaws, B. (2001) *The Treatment of Modern Western Medical Diseases.* Boulder, CO: Blue Poppy Press, Chapter 62, 'Polymyositis/Dermatomyositis', p.455.

25 Flaws, B. (2001) *The Treatment of Modern Western Medical Diseases.* Boulder, CO: Blue Poppy Press, Chapter 22, 'Coronary Artery Disease', p.193.

26 Shao, N.-F. (1990) *The Treatment of Knotty Diseases with Chinese Acupuncture and Chinese Herbal Medicine.* Jinan, Shandong: Shandong Science and Technology Press.

27 Unschuld, P. (1998) *Medicine in China: A History of Ideas.* Berkeley, CA: University of California Press.

28 Sionneau, P. (2014) 'The concept of constitution in Chinese medicine.' Available at http://sionneau.com/medecine-chinoise/articles/the-concept-of-constitution-in-chinese-medicine, accessed on 29 May 2016.

29 Cheng, X.-N. (1987) *Chinese Acupuncture and Moxibustion.* Beijing: Foreign Languages Press.

30 Scott, A., Khan, K., Cook, J. and Durinio, V. (2003) 'What is "inflammation"? Are we ready to move beyond Celsus?' *British Journal of Sports Medicine 38*, 248–249.

31 Flaws, B. (2001) *The Treatment of Modern Western Medical Diseases.* Boulder, CO: Blue Poppy Press, Chapter 24, 'Crohn's Disease', p.210.

32 Edwards, T. (2005) 'Inflammation, pain, and chronic disease: An integrative approach.' *Alternative Therapies 11*(6), 20–27.

33 Weil, A. (2011) 'Reducing whole body inflammation.' Available at www.drweil.com/drw/u/QAA401013/Reducing-Whole-Body-Inflammation.html#_ga=1.202052305.1351492746.1464258316, accessed on 29 May 2016.

34 Manohar, G. and Wood, L. (2013) *Nutrition and Physical Activity in Inflammatory Diseases.* Wallingford: CABI Publishing.

35 Knott, L. (2014) 'Allergic phenomena.' Available at http://patient.info/doctor/allergic-phenomena, accessed on 29 May 2016.

36 Flaws, B. (2001) *The Treatment of Modern Western Medical Diseases.* Boulder, CO: Blue Poppy Press, Chapter 2, 'Allergic Rhinitis', p.47.

37 Gray, S.L. (2015) 'Cumulative use of strong anticholinergics and incident dementia: A prospective cohort study.' *Journal of American Medical Association 175*(3), 401–407.

38 Dharmananda, S. (2000) 'Safety issues affecting Chinese herbs: The case of ma huang.' Available at www.itmonline.org/arts/mahuang.htm, accessed on 29 May 2016.

39 Ahmad, Y. and Bruce, I. (2005) 'Connective Tissue Disease and the General Practitioner.' In A. Adebajo and J. Dickson (eds) *Collected Reports on the Rheumatic Diseases*, Series 4. Arthritis Research Council. Available at www.arthritisresearchuk.org/external-resources/2012/09/17/15/21/connective-tissue-diseases-and-the-role-of-the-general-practitioner.aspx, accessed on 29 May 2016.

40 American Cancer Society (2016) 'Cancer facts & figures 2016.' Available at www.cancer.org/research/cancerfactsstatistics/cancerfactsfigures2016/index, accessed on 3 August 2016.

41 Cancer Research UK (2016) 'Lifetime risk of cancer.' Available at www.cancerresearchuk.org/health-professional/cancer-statistics/risk/lifetime-risk#mlktqlRKcYLyx2Wa.99, accessed on 12 December 2016.

42 Cancer Research UK (2016) 'Cancer mortality statistics.' Available at www.cancerresearchuk.org/health-professional/cancer-statistics/mortality, accessed on 12 December 2016.

43 Olivier, M., Hollstein, M. and Hainaut, P. (2010) 'TP53 mutations in human cancers: Origins, consequences and clinical use.' *Cold Spring Harbor Perspectives on Biology*, January, 2(1), a001008. Available at www.ncbi.nlm.nih.gov/pmc/articles/PMC2827900, accessed on 1 June 2016.

44 Yang, S.-Z. and Chase, C. (translators) (1994) *The Systematic Classic of Acupuncture and Moxibustion by Huang-Fu Mi: A Translation of the Jia Yi Jing*. Boulder, CO: Blue Poppy Press, p.309.

45 Lahans, T. (2007) *Integrating Conventional and Chinese Medicine in Cancer Care: A Clinical Guide*. Philadelphia, PA: Churchill Livingstone.

46 Dharmananda, S. (1997) 'Oriental perspectives on cancer and its treatment.' Available at www.itmonline.org/arts/cancer.htm, accessed on 1 June 2016.

47 Flaws, B. (2002) 'Chinese medical treatment of malignant lymphoma.' *Acupuncture Today 3*, 7. Available at www.acupuncturetoday.com/mpacms/at/article.php?id=28009, accessed on 16 May 2016.

48 Sharp, P. and Hahn, B. (2010) 'The evolution of HIV-1 and the origin of AIDS.' *Philosophical Transactions of the Royal Society of London. Series B: Biological Sciences*, 27 August, 365(1552), 2487–2494. Available at www.ncbi.nlm.nih.gov/pmc/articles/PMC2935100, accessed on 1 June 2016.

49 Crook, W. (1984) *The Yeast Connection: A Medical Breakthrough*. Jackson, TN: Professional Books.

50 American Academy of Asthma, Allergy and Immunology (2001) 'Position Statement on Candida Hypersensitivity Syndrome.' Available at http://web.archive.org/web/20010609033347/http://www.aaaai.org/professional/physicianreference/positionstatements/ps14.stm#Candidiasis, accessed on 2 June 2016.

51 The NIH Human Microbiome Project Working Group (2009) 'The NIH Human Microbiome Project.' *Genome Research 19*(12), 2317–2323. Available at www.ncbi.nlm.nih.gov/pmc/articles/PMC2792171, accessed on 2 June 2016.

52 Leung, M. *et al.* (2015) 'Insights into the pan-microbiome: Skin microbial communities of Chinese individuals differ from other racial groups.' *Scientific Reports 5*. Available at www.nature.com/articles/srep11845, accessed on 18 August 2016.

53 Ursell, L. *et al.* (2012) 'Defining the human microbiome.' *Nutrition Reviews*, August, 70, S38–S44. Available at www.ncbi.nlm.nih.gov/pmc/articles/PMC3426293, accessed on 12 August 2016.

54 Fratkin, J.P. (2010) 'Treating acute and chronic viral disease with Chinese herbal products.' Available at http://drjakefratkin.com/articles/health-and-disease-articles/treating-acute-and-chronic-viral-infections-with-chinese-herbal-products, accessed on 6 June 2016.

55 Maciocia, G. (1989) *The Foundations of Chinese Medicine*. Edinburgh: Churchill Livingstone, p.293.

56 Maciocia, G. (1989) *The Foundations of Chinese Medicine*. Edinburgh: Churchill Livingstone, p.176.

57 Maciocia, G. (1989) *The Foundations of Chinese Medicine*. Edinburgh: Churchill Livingstone, pp.177–178, 479–483.

58 Maciocia, G. (1989) *The Foundations of Chinese Medicine*. Edinburgh: Churchill Livingstone, p.40.

59 NICE (National Institute for Health and Care Excellence) (2013) Clinical Knowledge Summaries: 'Feverish children – Management.' Available at http://cks.nice.org.uk/feverish-children-management#!scenario, accessed on 2 June 2016.

60 X-rayrisk.com (2016) *Risk Calculator*. Available at www.xrayrisk.com/calculator/calculator-normal-studies.php, accessed on 2 June 2016.

61 X-rayrisk.com (2016) *Risk Calculator*. Available at www.xrayrisk.com/calculator/calculator-normal-studies.php, accessed on 2 June 2016.

62 NHS Choices (2016) 'Vaccinations.' Available at www.nhs.uk/conditions/vaccinations/pages/vaccination-schedule-age-checklist.aspx, accessed on 2 June 2016.

63 RationalWiki.org (2016) 'Anti-vaccination movement.' Available at http://rationalwiki.org/wiki/Anti-vaccination_movement, accessed on 16 August 2016.

64 WHO (World Health Organization) (2016) 'What are some of the myths – and facts – about vaccination?' Available at www.who.int/features/qa/84/en, accessed on 16 August 2016.

65 Offit, P. and Moser, C. (2009) 'The problem with Dr Bob's alternative vaccine schedule.' *Pediatrics 123*(1). Available at http://pediatrics.aappublications.org/content/123/1/e164, accessed on 16 August 2016.

66 Sears, R.W. (2007) *The Vaccine Book: Making the Right Decision for Your Child*. New York: Little, Brown & Co.

67 Shen Nong (2006) 'The Qing Dynasty.' Available at www.shen-nong.com/eng/history/qing.html#small, accessed on 17 August 2016.

68 Plotkin, S., Orenstein, W. and Offit, P. (2008) *Vaccines*. Philadelphia, PA: Saunders Elsevier.

69 Chung, Y., Oving, H. and Becker, S. (2007) *Correcting the Errors in the Forest of Medicine by Yi Lin Gai Cuo*. Boulder, CO: Blue Poppy Press.

70 Flaws, B. (2006) *A Handbook of TCM Pediatrics*. Boulder, CO: Blue Poppy Press, p.244.

71 Li, W. (2006) 'The modulation effect of Chinese medicines.' Available at www.shen-nong.com/eng/principles/modulationeffectimmune.html, accessed on 17 August 2016.

72 Maciocia, G. (2012) 'Latent heat.' Available at http://maciociaonline.blogspot.co.uk/2012/07/latent-heat.html, accessed on 16 August 2016.

73 PHE (Public Health England) (2010) 'List of notifiable diseases.' Available at www.gov.uk/guidance/notifiable-diseases-and-causative-organisms-how-to-report#list-of-notifiable-diseases, accessed on 6 June 2016.

74 House of Lords (1998) *House of Lords Science and Technology – Seventh Report*. Available at www.publications.parliament.uk/pa/ld199798/ldselect/ldsctech/081vii/st0701.htm, accessed on 6 June 2016.

75 WHO (World Health Organization) (2014) *Antimicrobial Resistance: Global Report on Surveillance 2014*. Available at www.who.int/drugresistance/documents/surveillancereport/en, accessed on 6 June 2016.

76 Flaws, B. (2016) 'Intestinal dysbiosis, leaky gut syndrome, candidiasis and Yin Fire.' Available at www.craneherb.com/shared/articles/9_Intestinal_Dysbiosis.aspx, accessed on 16 August 2016.

77 Maciocia, G. (2015) *The Foundations of Chinese Medicine: A Comprehensive Text*. Edinburgh: Churchill Livingstone, p.293.

THE GASTROINTESTINAL, CARDIOVASCULAR AND RESPIRATORY SYSTEMS

3.1

The Gastrointestinal System

3.1a The physiology of the gastrointestinal system

In this chapter we examine the physiology and diseases of a particular physiological system, in this case, the digestive or gastrointestinal system. This section is concerned with the function of the digestive system in health, and provides a foundation for the study of the investigation and treatment of digestive diseases that is described in the successive four sections.

Because of its length, this section is divided into two parts. If you are using this book as a study course, you are advised to work through the two parts of this section in separate study sessions.

Part I: From our food to the stomach[1]

The digestive system and digestion

The function of the digestive system is to ensure that the water and nutrients present in the diet are absorbed adequately by the body and extraneous waste products are eliminated effectively. It also has a protective function in that it minimizes damage from toxins and microbes in the diet. Digestion takes place along the length of a tube known variously as the gastrointestinal or digestive tract, the gut or the alimentary canal. All these terms are used in medical language and are interchangeable.

Through the process of digestion, the complex contents of food are broken down to release nutrients in a form that can pass easily through the lining of the digestive tract and thence into the bloodstream. Water taken in with the diet is

absorbed into the bloodstream at the same time. Not all of our food has value as a source of nutrients, and not all the water within it is absorbed. Some is left within the digestive tract to become waste material. This waste food material and water travels down the length of the digestive tract to be expelled in the form of feces.

The nutrients in our diet

A nutrient is any substance that can be used by the body either to produce energy or to enable other vital chemical processes to take place. There are six classes of nutrients: carbohydrates, fats, proteins, mineral salts, vitamins and water. A healthy diet should contain an ideal balance of these. In addition to these nutrients, a healthy diet should also provide fiber. Fiber is a medical term used to describe indigestible cellulose from plant-derived foods. Fiber enables healthy transit and elimination of waste, as it provides bulk and water-retaining properties to the feces. Dietary fiber may also encourage a healthy balance of bacteria in the colon that are associated with beneficial anti-inflammatory benefits.

A healthy diet will consist largely of starchy foods such as bread, rice, pasta and cereals, and fruit and vegetables. Current UK guidelines for the public are that over one-third of our diet should consist of starchy foods, and that additional nutrients should come from at least five portions of fruit or vegetables a day. In addition, there should be some food containing protein, either from the meat/ eggs/pulses food group or from the milk/cheese food group. Foods containing fats and sugars should be kept to a minimum. The UK Food Standards Agency "eat well plate" summarizes this advice in pictorial form, as shown in Figure 3.1a-I.[2]

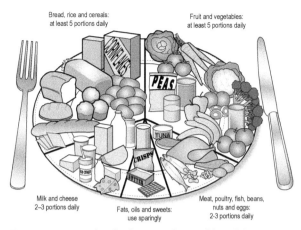

Bread, rice and cereals:
at least 5 portions daily

Fruit and vegetables:
at least 5 portions daily

Milk and cheese
2–3 portions daily

Fats, oils and sweets:
use sparingly

Meat, poultry, fish, beans,
nuts and eggs:
2-3 portions daily

Figure 3.1a-I The balance of good health

CARBOHYDRATES

Starchy foods and fruit and vegetables together provide the carbohydrates that the body needs. Carbohydrates contain the elements carbon, hydrogen and oxygen. These are the foods that, once broken down, provide the basic fuel for the energy-producing process of internal respiration (see Section 1.1b). Internal respiration takes place in the mitochondria of all living cells, where simple sugars and other small molecules derived from fats and proteins react with oxygen to produce cellular energy. Carbon dioxide and water are the waste products. The energy produced is stored partly in the form of the charged molecule adenosine triphosphate (ATP), and is partly released as heat.

The simplest carbohydrates are the monosaccharides, or simple sugars, such as glucose and fructose. These are in a perfect form to be utilized by the mitochondria, and so provide the most rapidly accessible form of energy. Monosaccharides taste sweet.

The molecules of the monosaccharides are also found linked together in pairs in our food in the form of sweet-tasting disaccharides, such as sucrose and lactose (the sugar in milk). Monosaccharides are also found in the form of chains known as polysaccharides, of which starch is an example. These do not immediately taste sweet, but can be broken down in the digestive tract to release the monosaccharides. Starches are therefore a form of slow-release energy for the body. Cellulose, which forms the fibrous parts of fruit and vegetables, is also a polysaccharide, but cannot be readily utilized by the human digestive tract. This is why it can perform its role as fiber. Grass-eating animals, however, have the capability of breaking down cellulose and extracting its valuable food energy.

If carbohydrates are in excess in the diet, superfluous monosaccharides can be converted within the liver to a polysaccharide called glycogen. Glycogen is held in the liver so that when blood sugar levels are low it can readily be converted back to accessible glucose. Any excess carbohydrate after this process has taken place is converted to fat for long-term energy storage.

FATS

Fats (lipids) are non-soluble oily substances found in diverse foods in our diet, including meat, nuts, eggs, milk and some vegetables. Most fats consist of two components joined together, a fatty acid and glycerol. When broken down by the body, the fatty acids and glycerol are released to provide energy for the bodily processes.

Saturated fat is so called because of the nature of the chemical bonds in the fat molecules. Saturated fat molecules contain more hydrogen than unsaturated fat molecules and this property causes saturated fat to tend to form into a solid more readily than unsaturated fat. Lard from meat and butter are both largely saturated fats. Saturated fat is a good source of energy for the body, but an excess in the diet is known to cause the lipids in the bloodstream to be carried in the more unhealthy form of low-density lipoprotein and triglycerides (LDL and TGs). It is believed that LDL is more likely to contribute to the formation of atheroma that leads to cardiovascular disease than another main category of lipoprotein, HDL (high density lipoprotein), which is considered to have a more protective role in this regard.

Unsaturated fat is generally derived from vegetable matter, and tends to form clear oil rather than a solid fat. It consists of molecules containing an unsaturated fatty acid and a glycerol. The omega-3, omega-6 and omega-9 fatty acids are all unsaturated fatty acids derived from unsaturated fats. These polyunsaturated fatty acids are essential components for cellular and intercellular communication processes and the building of cellular structures.

Vegetable, nut and olive oils contain unsaturated fat that provides largely omega-6 and omega-9 fatty acids. Fish oils contain unsaturated fat that provides omega-3 fatty acids. Most vegetable oils are made of polyunsaturated fats, but olive oil, canola oil and avocados contain a particular form of unsaturated fat known as a monounsaturated fat (this contains omega-9 fatty acids).

Unsaturated fats and monosaturated fats in particular seem to have the property of reducing the amount of more unhealthy LDL in the bloodstream. For this reason, it is now considered important for a healthy diet that these forms of fats predominate over saturated fats, and that monounsaturated fats predominate over polyunsaturated fats (as is found in the Mediterranean diet).

Unsaturated fats may protect against cardiovascular disease by providing more membrane fluidity than the more solid saturated fats.

Moreover, a current dietary theory is that some oils and fats are less likely to contribute to unhealthy inflammation in the body. The omega-3 fatty acid-containing oils that are present in fish oils are meant to be most beneficial in this regard. Whilst all vegetable oils contain omega-3 fatty acids, rapeseed oil and flax seed oil carry the highest percentage of these potentially beneficial components (found in the form of EPA and DHA in fish and ALA in nuts and vegetable seeds).

It is possible that the Western diet which contains much more omega-6 oils than omega-3-containing oils (over ten times omega-6 to omega-3 on average) is not presenting these vital molecules in a healthy ratio. Current evidence suggests that this is one of the many factors in the Western diet that promotes disease, in this case, by promoting inflammatory processes.[3]

Cholesterol is another oily substance that is particularly important as a component of cell membranes, supporting nerve cells and also for making hormones and other essential molecules, including the steroids and vitamin D. Cholesterol is found in dairy products, meat and eggs, but for use in the body it is largely synthesized in the body itself, particularly in the liver, where it is built up from more simple molecules. Cholesterol is carried in the blood in the form of the complex compound molecules of LDL, very low-density lipoprotein (VLDL) and HDL. These structures package the cholesterol so that it is readily accessible to the cells. As mentioned, LDL (and VLDL) is associated with vascular ill health, but HDL appears to be protective against vascular damage. All these components of the blood are measured in the frequently performed fasting lipids blood test, and the figures are often described in terms of high or low cholesterol. However, the balance of these lipid structures in the blood seems to be less affected by the amount of cholesterol in the diet than by the relative amounts of saturated and unsaturated fats, and so cholesterol in the diet is no longer considered to be unhealthy. This is in direct contrast to the health advice given freely by doctors at the end of the 20th century. Nevertheless, dietary cholesterol's falsely attributed bad reputation persists in the public consciousness. In fact, it is now saturated fats and trans fatty acids that are thought to be most deleterious to health.

Trans fatty acids are only found in traces in a natural diet. However, they have made up a significant proportion of many Western diets because they are found in vegetable oils that have been processed forming partially hydrogenated oils (PHOs) to preserve their longevity for foods such as margarines, cakes and biscuits. The United States Food and Drug Administration (FDA) stated that, according to recent estimates, the average American was eating 5.8g of trans fatty acids a day. It is known that trans fatty acids alter the balance of cholesterol in the blood to an unhealthy state (they increase levels of LDL at the expense of the more healthy HDL). For this reason, in some European states (e.g. Denmark and Switzerland) the use of trans fatty acids in food manufacturing has been banned. In 2015 the FDA passed legislation limiting the manufacture of foods containing PHOs, which will be enforceable by 2018. This is predicted to have a large health benefit in terms of reduction of deaths from cardiovascular disease,[4] although this would be even more marked if the foods that currently contain trans fats (processed cakes, biscuits and pastries) were a far less prominent component of most Western people's diet altogether.

PROTEINS

Proteins are complex chain-like structures that are made up of simple molecules called amino acids. All amino acids contain the element nitrogen as well as carbon, hydrogen and oxygen. Some also contain trace minerals such as zinc, iron and copper. There are just over 20 different amino acids, which can be combined in potentially infinite permutations to form protein chains. Proteins are made in animal and plant cells in the location of the ribosomes as a result of decoding instructions held on the cellular DNA (see Section 1.1b). The ribosome is the site at which amino acids are linked together to form a unique and characteristic protein chain, after which the particular makeup of the protein chain encourages the structure to fold in a characteristic way. Proteins are large molecules that have a unique three-dimensional shape. The shape and form of a particular protein might give it special structural properties (e.g. the flexible protein collagen found in skin and hair) or make it soluble in water (e.g. the albumen found in blood and in egg white). In other proteins the shape is essential for communication, and this is the basis of how cell membrane proteins recognize the external stimulants, such as hormones, that bring about internal change in the cell itself. Antibody-antigen recognition also depends on the protein antibody having a unique shape that fits the shape of the antigen.

Protein in food is found in meat, eggs, fish, cereals, nuts and pulses. All the essential amino acids can be derived from the complete proteins in meat, fish, eggs, milk and soya. Without soya products, a vegetarian will need to eat combinations of nuts, cereals and pulses to ensure that all amino acids are obtained from the diet.

Protein is broken down to soluble amino acids in the body, and these circulate dissolved in the blood so that they reach all the tissues. The ribosomes of the cells utilize amino acids to produce their own proteins so that they can reproduce and continue performing their unique functions. Proteins are used to make cellular and extracellular structures (such as the contractile fibers in muscle cells and the connective tissue fibers in cartilage), plasma proteins (such as the clotting factors and albumen), antibodies, enzymes and also some hormones.

In a state of starvation, proteins are broken down by the cellular mitochondria to produce energy. The by-products of this process include chemicals called ketones. When excess ketones are produced, the body is said to be in a state of ketosis.

MINERAL SALTS

Mineral salts are simple inorganic substances that are required in small quantities to maintain bodily processes. Unlike carbohydrates, fats and proteins, they are not a source of energy. Essential minerals include calcium, sodium, potassium, iodine, phosphate, iron, chromium, zinc, selenium, magnesium and manganese. Certain minerals, such as calcium and phosphate (in bone) and sodium (as dissolved salt in the body fluids), constitute a significant proportion of the body mass, whereas others are required only in trace amounts.

VITAMINS

Vitamins are more complex compounds than minerals, and are also essential for bodily processes. They are essential dietary components because either they cannot be made by the body at all, or they cannot be made in sufficient quantities to sustain health. Vitamins are now broadly grouped into the four fat-soluble vitamins A, D, E and K, and the nine water-soluble vitamins B1–B8 and C. The lettering system approximately relates to the order in which the vitamins were discovered (beginning with vitamin A in 1909). Those substances initially called F–J were either reclassified as B vitamins or were subsequently deemed not to qualify as vitamins at all. The B vitamins are now grouped together because they are all vital in the production of energy from nutrients by the mitochondria. The food sources and the functions of the 13 vitamins are summarized in Table 3.1a-I.

Table 3.1a-I The 13 vitamins, their main food sources and their functions in the body

Vitamin	Food sources	Use in the body
A (retinol)	Green vegetables, milk, liver	Pigments in the eye and health of the skin
D (calciferol)	Milk, eggs, cod liver oil; ultraviolet light	Calcium absorption and bone formation
E (tocopherol)	Margarine, seeds, green leafy vegetables	Antioxidant: protects fatty acids and cell membranes from damaging oxidation
K (phylloquinone)	Green leafy vegetables	Formation of certain clotting factors
B1 (thiamine)	Meats (pork), grains, legumes	Carbohydrate metabolism; also nerve and heart function
B2 (riboflavin)	Milk, liver, eggs, grains, legumes	Energy metabolism
B3 (niacin or nicotinic acid)	Liver, lean meats, grains, legumes	Energy metabolism
B5 (pantothenic acid)	Milk, liver, eggs, grains, legumes	Energy metabolism
B6 (pyridoxine)	Wholegrain cereals, vegetables, meats	Amino acid metabolism
B7 (biotin)	Meats, vegetables, legumes	Fat synthesis and amino acid metabolism
B9 (folic acid)	Whole wheat foods, green vegetables, legumes	Nucleic acid metabolism
B12 (cobalamin)	Red meats, eggs, dairy products	Nucleic acid production
C (ascorbic acid)	Citrus fruits, green leafy vegetables, tomatoes	Collagen formation in the teeth, bone, and connective tissue of blood vessels; may help in resisting infection

WATER

Water is an essential part of the diet because the body is continually losing water through urine, feces, sweat and in exhaled air. About 60 percent of the adult body mass is water, and all the essential bodily processes take place in a watery milieu. Water has to be lost as it is the vehicle through which waste chemicals (in urine and sweat) and also waste food materials (in the feces) are carried for expulsion from the body. It is also lost through the breath and sweat to aid with cooling of the body.

On average, about 2.5 liters of water need to be replaced by the diet every day. Much of this is contained in food, and so a human being can survive on about 1.5 liters of water in drinks per day. Any water that is excess to requirements is passed out of the body in the form of dilute urine. If insufficient water is drunk, the kidneys make dark concentrated urine from the fluid in the plasma. In this case the water required for excretion of wastes is drawn from the tissues, which then become dehydrated. A significant state of dehydration will be reflected in a loss of body weight of more than 2–3 percent. Because the sensitive tissues of the body are not able to withstand the state of dehydration for more than a few days, water is essential for life. Loss of more than 10 percent of the body weight through dehydration is usually not compatible with life.

Information box 3.1a-I

The nutrients: comments from a Chinese medicine perspective

In Chinese medicine, each food has a characteristic energetic property and also a tendency to affect a particular bodily substance or organ. For this reason, food can be used as medicine, and a diet can be recommended to suit the needs of the patient. The taste and consistency of the food bear an important relationship to its energetic properties. Moreover, the freshness and the method of cooking can have a bearing on the value of the food.

For example, fresh grapes are recognized to Tonify the Qi and Blood, and affect the Lungs, Spleen and Kidneys. Beef is recognized to Tonify Yin and Qi and Blood, and affect the Large Intestine, Stomach and Spleen. Some foods, such as pears, are Cool, and so may be useful in moderation in Hot conditions, and some are Warm in nature, such as chicken liver, and so are used to treat Cold conditions.

Foods contain a complex array and unique balance of nutrients that contribute to their characteristic taste and consistency as recognized in Chinese medicine. For example, a wide range of aromatic substances gives herbs and spices their characteristic flavors, and would result in a Pungent or Bitter nature as recognized by Chinese medicine. Acids in foods such as fruit and vinegar cause the Sour flavor, and salts the Salty flavor. The Sweet flavor is more likely to come from starch, fat or protein. There is an increasingly large body of knowledge about what chemical constituents of individual foods (and herbs) give

them their characteristic health-giving properties, so providing a scientific foundation for the centuries-old dietary wisdom of Chinese medicine. For example, cardamom, widely used in Chinese formulas for relief of congested Qi and Blood, contains 11 different aromatic terpenoids that give it its unique flavor.[5]

However, the distinctions on the basis of flavor and organ and direction are not usually made in conventional medicine when dietary advice is given. Instead, rather broad statements are made about the six types of nutrients found in food groups and how to aim for a balance of these.[6] Furthermore, very little emphasis is placed on how the food is prepared, apart from avoidance of overcooking, as this might inactivate the vitamin C in fruits and vegetables. There is also little recognition that cold or raw food might be deleterious for the digestion.

The preparation of dietary supplements (such as vitamin pills, minerals such as zinc and isolated food components such as curcumin from turmeric), which are chemically derived key ingredients, makes total sense to a scientific nutritionist. However, these supplements would not be recognized by a Chinese medicine practitioner to have the complex beneficial properties of the foods in which these nutrients can be naturally found. Instead, it is fresh food, carefully prepared and combined with other foods, which would be considered to be alive and most nourishing for the Qi, Blood, Yin and Yang.[7, 8]

The structure of the digestive tract

The digestive tract is a tube that begins at the mouth and ends at the anus. At both these orifices there is a junction between the tough and dry keratinized epithelium of the skin and the soft and moist mucous epithelium that lines the whole of the digestive tract. This junction can be easily examined in the mouth where the two lips meet. At the junction, the dry, slightly ridged keratinized skin of the external lip becomes moist and smooth mucous epithelium on the inside of the lip.

The tube of the digestive tract has a basic structure that can be found in slightly different forms along its length. The tube has four distinct layers (see Figure 3.1a-II):

- The adventitia is the outer layer of the digestive tract. Below the diaphragm, the adventitia forms the peritoneum that is a serous membrane (i.e. it secretes watery fluid). This protects and lubricates the digestive tract so that it can move easily within the abdominal cavity.

Mucosa
Submucosa
Circular muscle layer
Longitudinal muscle layer
Peritoneum (adventitia)

Fine layers of nerve fibers

Figure 3.1a-II The general structure of the digestive tract

- The muscle layer consists of two layers of smooth muscle. The longitudinal and circular fibers contract in coordinated waves to propel the contents of the food down the length of the tract. This motion is called peristalsis.

- The submucous layer is a layer of connective tissue that contains blood vessels, collections of lymph nodes, lymphatic vessels and networks (plexuses) of nerves.

- The mucosa consists of a mucous (epithelial) membrane (see Section 1.1d), with its combined functions of protection, secretion and absorption, and two supportive connective tissue layers beneath this. The mucous membrane secretes mucus for further protection and lubrication. Other specialized cells in the mucous epithelium are sensitive to changes in the contents of the digestive tract. These secrete hormones into the bloodstream within the submucous layer.

The mouth is the only section of the digestive tract that does not have this general structure.

The tube of the digestive tract has accessory organs, which open out or project into the hollow of the tube. These organs are the tongue, salivary glands, liver, gallbladder, pancreas and appendix.

The salivary glands open via tubes (ducts) into the mouth; the pancreas, liver and gallbladder all open via ducts into the duodenum; and the appendix opens directly into the beginning of the colon. Figure 3.1a-III illustrates the position of the organs associated with the digestive tract, and how, with the exception of the mouth and the esophagus, the main part of the digestive tract is situated below the diaphragm.

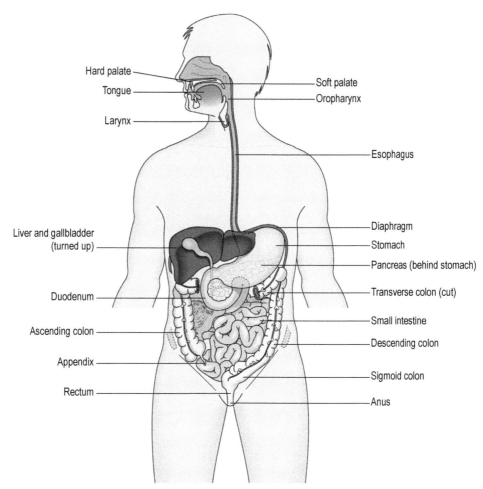

Figure 3.1a-III The organs of the digestive system

THE MOUTH

The mouth is where the process of digestion begins. The teeth, tongue and the muscles of chewing are adapted to grind up food into a paste with saliva.

Saliva is produced by six exocrine salivary glands that open into the mouth. The size and extent of these important glands is illustrated in Figure 3.1a-IV.

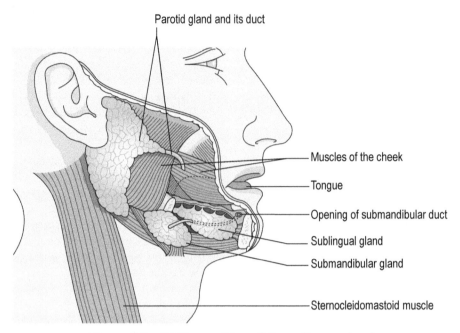

Parotid gland and its duct

Muscles of the cheek

Tongue

Opening of submandibular duct

Sublingual gland

Submandibular gland

Sternocleidomastoid muscle

Figure 3.1a-IV The position of the salivary glands

Saliva is produced in response to the action of eating, and also in response to the anticipation of food. Certain flavors, such as the sourness of lemons, are particularly powerful in inducing a good flow of saliva. About 1.5 liters of saliva is produced a day, and the moisture is very important to help maintain the health of the mouth and to assist with chewing. The moisture is also essential for enjoyment of food, as it enables food to be tasted. Saliva also contains protective substances such as mucus and antibodies, together with the protein lysozyme, all of which protect the digestive tract from damage by microorganisms and toxins.

The salivary glands also produce the first digestive enzyme that the eaten food will encounter, and thus begins the breakdown of the nutrients into the building blocks that are absorbed into the bloodstream. An enzyme is a biological substance that encourages a chemical reaction. In this case the enzyme is called salivary amylase, and in its presence the chains of complex polysaccharides in carbohydrate come apart to form disaccharides. This reaction only occurs in the mouth, as the acid contents of the stomach stop the amylase from working. This is one reason why it is important to chew thoroughly.

The tongue is a muscular structure adapted for two distinct functions: eating (taste, chewing and swallowing) and speech. It is covered with little bumps called papillae, which are sensitive to the four main tastes: salt, sweet, sour and bitter. The subtleties of taste are also dependent on a healthy sense of smell, as anyone who has a heavy cold will recognize. Figure 3.1a-V illustrates the position of the different sorts of papillae.

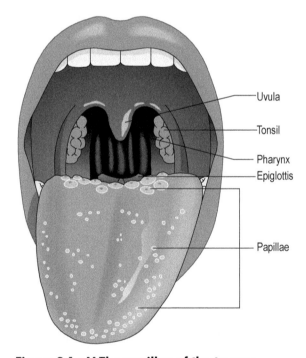

Uvula

Tonsil

Pharynx

Epiglottis

Papillae

Figure 3.1a-V The papillae of the tongue

THE ESOPHAGUS

The esophagus runs from the pharynx at the back of the mouth to the opening of the stomach. As it descends the thorax it runs posterior to the airways that lead to the lungs. A muscle ring (sphincter) at the end of the pharynx prevents air entering the esophagus during breathing in. The opening of the stomach coincides with the position where the esophagus passes through the diaphragm.

The muscles of the diaphragm act as a sphincter to prevent stomach contents from returning into the esophagus. This muscle ring is also known as the cardiac sphincter, because it lies just below the heart. The cardiac sphincter is situated at the level of the xiphisternal joint (the location of acupoint REN-16, Zhong Ting[9]).

THE STOMACH

The stomach is a stretchy expansion of the tube of the digestive tract, but still retains the four layers of mucosa, submucosa, muscle and adventitia. Figure 3.1a-VI illustrates that the stomach is bounded by the cardiac sphincter above and the pyloric sphincter below. These muscle rings keep food contents within the stomach for up to six hours to enable the beginning of a thorough digestion process. The stomach muscles enable the muscle to churn the food contents stored within it to aid digestion.

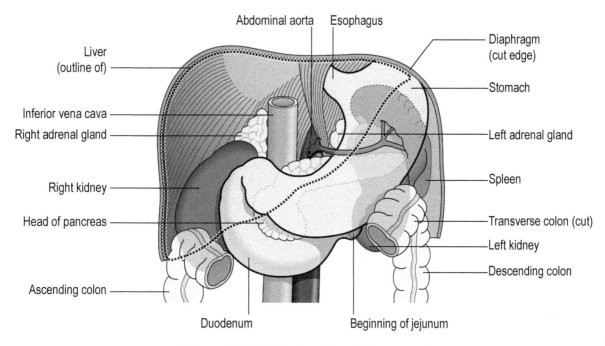

Figure 3.1a-VI The location of the stomach

Gastric (the term coming from the Greek for stomach) juices are secreted by specialized glands that open into the stomach. These juices consist of water, acid and an enzyme called pepsin, which enables the breakdown of protein into amino acids. The acid is generated by specialized proteins in the cell walls of the gastric glandular cells known as proton pumps. The stomach lining also secretes copious mucus to protect its own cells from the acid produced by the proton pump cells.

In the stomach, the food is churned with the fluid of the gastric juice to form a liquid soup known as chyme. Pepsin and acid work together, breaking down the protein in the food into amino acids. The smell of this process is the familiar smell of vomit. Very little of the diet is absorbed through the lining of the stomach, but water and alcohol are two exceptions. This explains why drinking alcohol on an empty stomach can have such a rapid effect.

The stomach is also the source of a protein called intrinsic factor, which has an attraction for vitamin B12 (cobalamin). This is important, as each molecule of this essential vitamin can only be later absorbed if it is bound to a molecule of intrinsic factor.

Part II: From the duodenum to the outside world

The duodenum (the first part of the small intestine)

The duodenum is the first 12 inches of small intestine that receives the partly digested food that descends from the stomach. It is into the duodenum that bile from the gallbladder and pancreatic juices from the pancreas enter the digestive tract and mix with the food. Both these fluids are extremely important in the final stages of the digestion of food.

Information box 3.1a-II

The duodenum: comments from a Chinese medicine perspective

It is interesting to note that the duodenum, the entry point for the pancreatic digestive juices as well as the bile duct leading from the liver and gallbladder, is situated at the level of the origin of 12th thoracic vertebra, the level of the Back-Shu point of the Spleen (BL-20, Pi Shu). This point function has the profound role of regulation and harmonization of the Qi of the Middle Jiao.[10] This first 12 inches of small intestine is linked by the ligament of Treitz to the aorta. This is the major vessel leading down from the heart at this level in the abdomen that is responsible for blood flow to the digestive organs and kidneys as well as to the rest of the body. In this way, Keown (2014)[11] points out there is an anatomical link which mirrors the link recognized in Chinese medicine between Small Intestine and Heart. At this level the spleen and the pancreas are anatomically linked with both the duodenum and also the splenic artery that branches away from the aorta at this level.

The pancreas

The pancreas is a gland with two distinct roles – one is endocrine and the other is exocrine. (For a reminder of the difference between these two categories of epithelial structure, see Section 1.1d.)

One of the endocrine roles of the pancreas is to secrete the hormones insulin and glucagon directly into the bloodstream. Both these hormones are important for ensuring that the concentration of glucose in the blood remains at the optimum level for the function of the cells of the body.

The exocrine role of the pancreas is to secrete a diverse array of digestive enzymes into the duodenum via the pancreatic duct. The enzymes can digest all three of the complex food components (carbohydrates, proteins and fats), and therefore complete the work started by the salivary glands and the gastric juices.

Figure 3.1a-VII illustrates how the C-shaped loop of the duodenum hugs the pancreas. The spleen, kidneys, liver and transverse colon are all situated at this level of the abdomen. This diagram also illustrates the closely located aorta descending posteriorly, and some of the blood vessels that lead away from the aorta to nourish all the aforementioned organs.

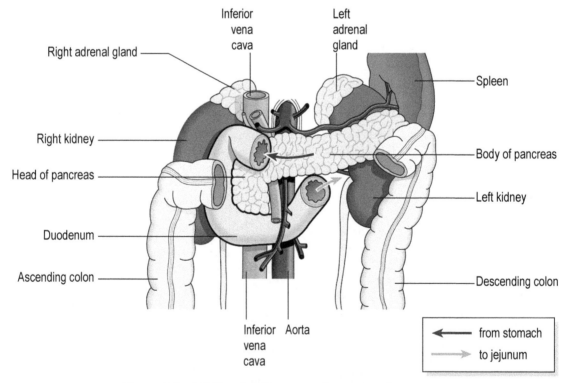

Figure 3.1a-VII The duodenum and associated structures

Information box 3.1a-III

The pancreas: comments from a Chinese medicine perspective

It is generally understood that the Ancient Chinese considered the pancreas and spleen as one anatomical organ as the pancreas is never directly referred to in the classics of Chinese medicine. The Chinese medical organ of the Spleen embraces, amongst all its other functions, the health and tissue functions of both these structures, as the deep branch of the meridian runs through the spleen and stomach (and therefore must also affect the adjacent pancreas).

It is of note that the endocrine role of the pancreas is to allow the accessibility of glucose to the cells, an essential prerequisite for the production of cellular energy in the process of internal respiration. This could be interpreted as broadly parallel with the wider Transforming and Transporting function that the Spleen Organ has according to Chinese medicine on Gu (food) Qi.

The exocrine role of the pancreas is directly to do with digestion and breaking food into an accessible form for entry into the bloodstream. In this way it contributes to the function of digestion that is described as "rotting and ripening" and "transportation of food essences," and attributed to the Stomach in Chinese medicine.[12]

The gallbladder

This hollow organ is a store for the dark green and bitter tasting fluid called bile, which is manufactured in the liver. Bile contains substances called bile salts that aid the digestion of fats. It also contains some of the body's waste products that have been processed by the liver. These will pass eventually into the feces. These by-products of the liver's detoxification include a deeply hued chemical called stercobilin (derived from the breakdown of hemoglobin), which gives the feces their characteristic brown color.

When food enters the duodenum, the cells of its lining respond to the change by releasing hormones, including a substance called cholecystokinin (CCK) into the bloodstream. These messengers travel to the gallbladder and stimulate it to contract and release bile when it is most needed. Similarly, other duodenal hormones stimulate the pancreas to release pancreatic juices.

The small intestine

The small intestine is simply a continuation of the duodenum. It receives the fluid mixture of partly digested food and digestive enzymes from the duodenum, powered by the wave-like muscular contractions of peristalsis.

The small intestine is about 5 meters long, and its lining is thrown into folds. Microscopic peaks of mucosa project from these folds, and appear, when greatly magnified, like a vast mountain range. These peaks are called villi. Each cell of the mucosa has tiny projections called microvilli. This unique structure greatly increases the area of the mucosa that is in contact with the fluid contents of the digestive tract, an adaptation that maximizes absorption. Figure 3.1a-VIII illustrates the microscopic structure of a villus, including the tiny microvilli on each cell, and also the way the blood and lymph supply of the digestive tract lining project into the center of the villus.

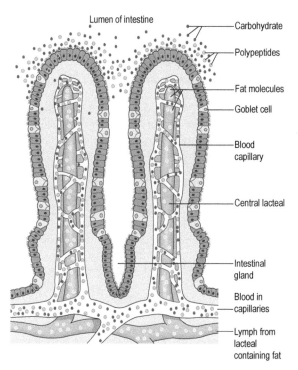

Lumen of intestine — Carbohydrate
— Polypeptides
— Fat molecules
— Goblet cell
— Blood capillary
— Central lacteal
— Intestinal gland
— Blood in capillaries
— Lymph from lacteal containing fat

Figure 3.1a-VIII One complete villus in the small intestine

As the digestive process continues along the length of the small intestine, the saccharides, amino acids, glycerol, water-soluble vitamins and salts resulting from digestion are taken up (usually by facilitated diffusion) into the mucosal cells. From here they pass into the bloodstream. Numerous collections of tiny lymph nodes in the submucosal tissues protect the bloodstream from any infectious agents that may have been present in the diet.

Fatty acids and the vitamin B12 intrinsic factor complex are absorbed by the very end segment of the small intestine (known as the terminal ileum). The bile acids, which aid the digestion of fats, are also reabsorbed here and circulate in the bloodstream back to the liver, from where they can be used again in the bile. Vitamins A, D, E and K are soluble in fats, and so are also absorbed at this end of the small intestine. Fatty acids, glycerol and these vitamins pass directly into the lymphatic system rather than the bloodstream. The small intestine also reabsorbs over 8 liters of water a day from the fluid contents that initially enter the duodenum. This leaves a semi-solid residue to enter the large intestine. This residue consists of fiber, waste from the bile, and many thousands of dead mucosal cells and intestinal bacteria that have been shed along the digestive journey.

Information box 3.1a-IV

The anatomy of the organs associated with the duodenum: comments from a Chinese medicine perspective

Note from Figure 3.1a-VII that the spleen lies at the same level as the pancreas. As mentioned previously, these organs share a common embryological root and blood supply. The spleen is conventionally considered to have its main role in the lymphatic system, with absolutely no part to play in the digestion of food. However, in keeping with its embryological roots, it has been found to contain pancreatic stem cells, and its absence is associated with an increased risk of developing diabetes, thus demonstrating it may have more of a directly digestive role than previously understood.[13]

It is interesting to see that the kidneys are also at this level in the body, and very close by are the liver, gallbladder and loops of the large and small intestines, all clustering around the C-shaped loop of the duodenum.

Keown (2014) also explains that the duodenum shares a fascial (connective tissue) plane with the right kidney, so speculating that, again, there is a direct anatomical correspondence in this powerful region of the body that mirrors the link recognized between Ming Men and Spleen and Stomach, in that one function of the Ming Men is to provide warmth for the Spleen and Stomach in the function of digestion.[14]

As well as its function in digestion, Yuan Qi from the Kidneys in Chinese medicine is also the motive force for all the Organs. In light of this, it is interesting that the physiological kidneys, recognized to be influenced by the deep branch of the Kidney meridian in Chinese medicine, sit at the center of a cluster of so many other organs, and in particular the kidneys are located very close to those that deal with digestion.

The large intestine

The large intestine, or colon, receives the residue of digestion from the small intestine. The first few centimeters of the colon is called the cecum, which literally means blind ending. This is because it is above the cecum that the end of the small intestine opens into the colon, with the result that the cecum is like a cul-de-sac opening out from the passage. At the end of this cul-de-sac is the narrow tube of the appendix. The parts of the large intestine are illustrated in Figure 3.1a-IX. Note how the horizontal stretch of the transverse colon overlies the duodenum and pancreas at the level of the T12 thoracic vertebra. This is one more organ to traverse this remarkable part of the body, described by the ancient Chinese as the Middle Jiao.

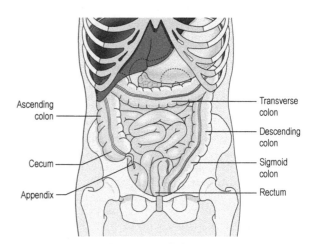

Figure 3.1a-IX The parts of the large intestine

The large intestine is home for most of the healthy commensal bacteria and yeasts described in Section 2.4b. The food residue that enters the large intestine is digested further by these organisms. The by-product of this digestion is gas, which is eventually passed out of the anus. Amongst the by-products of this process are some necessary vitamins, which are absorbed from the large intestine into the bloodstream.

In animals that live on a diet of grass, such as sheep, the cecum and appendix are much longer than those in humans and contain many bacteria. Here, the bacteria can further digest the cellulose fiber in grass to release more saccharides, which can be used by the sheep. It is believed that the appendix in humans is simply a vestige of this larger organ found in vegetarian animals. Cellulose cannot be digested by humans, and instead provides an important role as dietary fiber.

The muscular contractions of the colon are slow and infrequent. The contractions cause the food residue to move gradually along the length of the colon before entering a storage region called the rectum. The rectum is closed at its bottom end by the muscular sphincter of the anus. When the rectum is filled, there is the sensation of needing to open the bowels. However, the act of emptying the rectum is voluntary, and can usually be delayed to a convenient time. About two-thirds of the fluid that enters the large intestine is reabsorbed, so that the substance that enters the rectum has the familiar consistency of feces. Mucus secreted along the length of the colon lubricates the passage of the semi-solid feces.

The liver

The structure and function of this important organ have been left to last because many of the functions of the liver are less directly related to the process of breakdown of food into basic nutrients. Instead, most of the important functions of the liver are about the processing of these nutrients to make them useful to the cells of the body.

The liver is the largest organ in the body and sits under the diaphragm on the right-hand side. If the palm of the right hand is rested on the lower section of the front of the right-hand half of the rib cage so that the little finger runs along the bottom edge of the rib cage, the hand will be resting over the liver.

The liver receives all the blood that has passed through the digestive tract, so that it is the first stop for all the nutrients, and also toxins, that have been absorbed during the process of digestion. This nutrient-rich blood passes through tiny channels in the liver called sinusoids, so that all the liver cells can come into close contact with it. This means that at any one time the liver is holding a large volume of blood within its tissue. This link between the blood leaving the digestive tract and the tissue of the liver is the physical basis for the liver's two distinct roles in the digestive process.

The first role is to act as a filter for toxins and other harmful substances such as drugs and alcohol. The liver cells are able to first absorb and then destroy or change some of these substances that have entered the bloodstream from the diet before they can affect other tissues of the body. This is why many drugs and toxins, if in excess, may damage the liver (e.g. paracetamol and alcohol). There are also many phagocytic white cells (macrophages) lining the sinusoids. One of their functions is to clear away any microbes that may have entered the bloodstream from the diet.

The second role is to begin processing some of the nutrients into a useful form for the cells, or into a form in which they can be stored for later use. Glucose, for example, is stored in the stable form of glycogen within the liver, from which it can be obtained at a later time if sugar supplies are needed quickly. Amino acids are processed so that they can be used by the cells to build new proteins. A similar process occurs for fats. Many vitamins and iron are also stored for later use in the liver. This is why animal liver is such a nutritious source of food.

Other roles of the liver include:

- The use of amino acids to make the proteins carried within the plasma (including the clotting factors).

- The removal of worn-out red blood cells. The spleen has the main responsibility for this function (see Section 3.4a), but is assisted in this task by the liver. Phagocytic white blood cells in the spleen and the liver digest the old red blood cells and then release many of the by-products of digestion into the blood for reuse by the body. The waste product of this process is bilirubin, the green-yellow colored substance that is excreted into the bile.

- To be a source of heat. The liver is such an active organ that it is one of the most important sources of heat for the body.

- To secrete bile. All the liver cells are able to produce bile that contains bile salts and bilirubin. This is secreted into tiny tubules in the liver. From here, the bile drains into a duct that leaves the liver and enters the duodenum. The gallbladder also opens into this duct, so that the bile collects here rather than passing directly into the duodenum.

Figure 3.1a-X helps to illustrate how the gallbladder can be surgically removed without disturbing the free flow of bile from the liver. The function of the gallbladder is simply to delay the entry of bile into the duodenum until the best time for digestion of fats. Removal of the gallbladder results in a constant trickle of bile into the duodenum. This is not ideal for perfect digestion of fats, but is not conventionally considered to be a problem for over-nourished Western people.

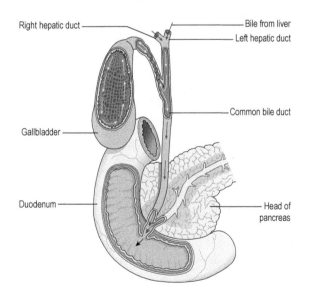

Figure 3.1a-X The direction of the flow of bile from the liver to the duodenum

Information box 3.1a-V

The liver: comments from a Chinese medicine perspective

The vascular spaces formed by the liver sinusoids are receptacles for all the blood that drains from the digestive tract. Here, the blood is cleansed and refreshed before traveling on to nourish other tissues. This is in keeping with the Chinese medicine observation that the Liver stores Blood, and that this function is necessary for replenishing the Qi.

The liver is also responsible for receiving nutrients via the digestive venous system, and ensuring that a steady clean supply of useful nutrients is available to the cells. This would very much be in accord with the Chinese medicine function of the Liver of ensuring the smooth flow of Qi. It would also suggest that the liver plays a part in the processes attributed in Chinese medicine to the Spleen: the Transformation and Transportation of Gu (food) Qi.

Keown (2014) postulates that the liver's role in the metabolism of the allergy hormone histamine may provide an explanation for the Chinese association of the Liver with irritability, allergies and menstrual problems, all of which can be associated with raised levels of histamine.[15]

However, there is no obvious conventional link between the function of the liver and the function of tendons and the sinews (although Keown cites a study that links tendon rupture with high cholesterol levels), or indeed in the ability to plan, which are other functions of the Liver Organ in Chinese medicine. The concept of the Hun, or the ethereal soul, has no counterpart in conventional medicine.

Interestingly, however, chronic liver disease can be conventionally recognized to cause changes in the nails, as the deficiency of plasma protein that results leads to characteristically white nails. Similarly, although there is no conventional link between the liver and the eyes in conventional medicine, in chronic liver disease the white of the eyes is the first place in which jaundice becomes apparent.

For more details on the correspondences between the functions of the liver and gallbladder as described in conventional medicine and the Liver and Gallbladder Organs in Chinese medicine, see Appendix I.

The metabolism

This last section touches on the metabolism, which can be seen as the end result of the digestive process. Metabolism simply means all the chemical processes that take place in the body. These processes require basic nutrients, oxygen and water to occur.

Metabolism can be broadly considered in two categories:

- Anabolism includes all those reactions that lead to the building up of new substances for cellular growth or function (this might be described as a Yin process in Chinese medicine language).

- Catabolism includes all those reactions that lead to the breakdown of the complex structures of the cell, and often leads to the release of energy (this might be described as a Yang process in Chinese medicine language).

In health, the anabolic and catabolic processes generally balance each other. This leads to a constant process of turnover of the old substances in the body for replacement with the new. It is this balance that allows for adaptation to change. In times of growth and development the anabolic processes are more prominent, and in times of illness and aging the catabolic processes are more prominent.

Healthy metabolism is dependent on an adequate supply of fuel – the basic nutrients and oxygen. If either of these is lacking, fuel has to be obtained from within the body. Initially, the glucose store in the liver is drawn upon, but very soon after this body fat and muscle protein is broken down. This is a state in which catabolism is in excess, and is not a healthy state if prolonged. Nevertheless, it is the state that people who diet successfully put themselves into by choice. Conversely, if there is excess fuel, or if the metabolism is sluggish, a state in which anabolism is in excess results. If there are no demands for the body to grow or develop, the excess nutrients are laid down as fat.

 Information box 3.1a-VI

The metabolism: comments from a Chinese medicine perspective

Signs and symptoms of disorders of metabolism suggest that the overall control of the metabolism might be broadly equated with the Spleen Organ, as Spleen Deficiency can lead to both weakness and inability to gain weight, and conversely to Accumulation of Damp and weight gain. The function of the Liver and Kidneys are intimately intertwined with that of the Spleen, so it would make sense that all three of these Organs might be expected to be out of balance in disorders of metabolism.

3.1b The investigation of the gastrointestinal system

Patients with suspected disease of the gastrointestinal system may be referred for further investigation by their doctor either to a gastroenterologist (a hospital physician who specializes in the medical management of digestive disease) or to a surgeon who specializes in surgery of the bowel.

Investigation of the gastrointestinal system

Once referred to any hospital specialist, patients may be offered a series of tests chosen to exclude a wide range of possible diagnoses that may affect the gastrointestinal system. Some tests might involve the patient in considerable inconvenience or discomfort, but are performed because it is believed that it is best to be as informed as possible about the health of the system before treatment is chosen.

The investigations that are most likely to reveal information about the digestive tract include:

- a thorough physical examination including abdominal palpation and per rectum examination

- blood tests

- examination of feces

- tests to visualize the inside of the gastrointestinal tract and the accessory organs, including endoscopy, X-ray studies with barium contrast, and ultrasound and computed tomography (CT) scans

- tests to remove samples of tissue for examination (biopsy).

These tests are considered briefly below in turn.

Physical examination of the gastrointestinal system

Physical examination of the gastrointestinal system involves the stages listed in Table 3.1b-I. For the purposes of physical examination of a supine patient, the accessible region of the abdomen is considered to occupy the approximately hexagonal region that is bounded by the ribs above and the inguinal ligaments and pubic bone below.

As Figure 3.1b-I illustrates, many important organs are situated underneath the nine named regions of the abdomen. A lump felt in the suprapubic area, for example, might suggest a problem of the bladder or the uterus, whereas pain in the left iliac fossa would suggest a problem of the colon or left ureter. The names for these nine regions of the abdomen are frequently used in medical texts for the description of abdominal conditions, so it is useful to be familiar with them.

Table 3.1b-I The stages of physical examination of the gastrointestinal system

General examination for signs of severe disease of the gastrointestinal system, such as pale nails, pallor, wasting and edema

Visual examination of the lips, mouth and tongue for features of gastrointestinal disease

Palpation of the cervical (neck) lymph nodes (indicating disease in the mouth and upper esophagus)

Palpation of the supraclavicular lymph nodes (indicating disease, in particular, cancer, of the lower esophagus, stomach and duodenum)

General palpation of the abdomen for tenderness and masses

Examination of the lower rectum and anal canal by means of insertion of a gloved finger

Blood tests

The two most common tests are:

- Full blood count (FBC) (see Section 2.4d). This is the test used to exclude the anemia that can result from long-term bleeding in conditions such as a chronic stomach ulcer, and also will reveal a rise in white cell count that might be indicative of infection or inflammation of the digestive system.

- Serum sample. Proteins in the serum of the blood are examined to look for features of liver disease (a test known as the liver function test (LFT)). In addition to the LFT there is a wide range of other less commonly performed serum tests that are used to help diagnose particular digestive diseases.

Examination of feces (stool sample)

Examination of the feces may reveal the presence of blood. Culture of the stool is performed to look for infectious agents. The presence of undigested nutrients in the stool, such as fat or sugars, may indicate a problem with digestion known as malabsorption.

Visualization of the digestive tract

The most precise way of visualizing the esophagus, stomach and duodenum is by means of a slim, flexible tubular telescope called an endoscope. In upper gastrointestinal endoscopy a sedated patient is encouraged to swallow the tube. As the fiber-optic end of the endoscope descends, images of the lining of the upper digestive tract can be seen by the examining doctor on a screen. This procedure does not use X-rays.

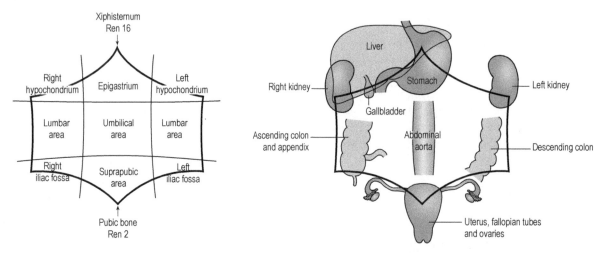

Figure 3.1b-I The regions of the abdomen and the underlying major organs

X-ray studies are also used in the investigation of digestive disease. Because the soft tissue of the bowel is not clearly exposed by X-ray imaging, a liquid mixture containing the salt barium sulfate is used to provide contrast between the hollow space within the bowel and the surrounding soft tissues (as the metal of barium shows up as white on X-ray images). In barium studies, the patient is requested to drink a liquid containing barium sulfate. As the liquid lines the upper digestive tract, X-ray images will reveal its outline and show up areas of muscle spasm, ulcers or tumors. Figure 3.1b-II is a clear barium-swallow X-ray image, in this case depicting an esophageal cancer. The white area shows the internal shape of the esophagus, and the arrows indicate the irregular narrowing caused by the tumor.

The endoscope can also be used to pass a fine tube into the pancreatic duct and bile ducts. Barium can be injected up this tube so that X-ray images can show up the delicate internal structure of the pancreas and the gallbladder. This procedure is known as endoscopic retrograde cholangiopancreatography (ERCP). Figure 3.1b-III illustrates an image taken during an ERCP. The thick white curved tube in this image is the end of the endoscope.

Figure 3.1b-III An ERCP image from a patient with gallstones

To investigate the lower digestive tract, a form of endoscope called a colonoscope is directed into the anal canal and thence into the rectum and colon. To investigate the lower part of the colon (sigmoid colon) and the rectum, a rigid telescope-like instrument called a sigmoidoscope may be used. This is slightly less invasive than a colonoscopy. Both ideally require a "prepared bowel," which means that the

Figure 3.1b-II A barium-swallow image, showing a carcinoma of the esophagus (narrowing by tumor indicated by arrows)

Barium X-ray studies are also useful for producing images of the colon and the rectum, this time by instilling barium liquid or paste by means of an enema into these spaces.

patient needs to have taken powerful laxatives prior to the examination.

Ultrasound scans, magnetic resonance imaging (MRI) and computed tomography (CT) scans are all useful investigations for diseases of the digestive tract, as these all can reveal the presence of soft-tissue masses, fluid and stones. Ultrasound is the least invasive of these investigations. MRI exposes the patient to strong magnetic and radiofrequency fields, but these are currently considered to carry little risk.

An MRCP is an MRI scan used to expose the bile ducts, and is a far less risky procedure than the invasive ERCP. An abdominal CT scan gives better overall information than the MRI in the abdomen, but exposes the patient to over 50 times the amount of radiation associated with a chest X-ray. Its use has to be guided on the basis that the potential benefits of the information outweigh the significant risks of carcinogenesis (cancer formation) from radiation exposure.[16]

Biopsy of the gastrointestinal tract

Biopsy literally means visual examination of a living sample. In the investigation of digestive disorders, a sample of the bowel lining can be obtained by use of the endoscope tube. Delicate instruments at the end of the tube can be manipulated to pinch off a section of tissue, which can then be removed and examined under a microscope.

Biopsy is a very informative investigation in liver disease. The biopsy of the liver is taken through a small incision in the skin overlying the ribs.

3.1c Diseases of the mouth, esophagus, stomach and duodenum

This section looks at the most important diseases of the upper digestive tract. The diseases described are those that are important either because they are common, or because they have serious consequences for the patient. These are:

- Diseases of the mouth and salivary glands:
  - mouth ulcers
  - cold sores
  - oral thrush (candidiasis)
  - leukoplakia
  - gingivitis
  - salivary gland infection
  - salivary gland stones
  - salivary gland tumors

- Diseases of the esophagus:
  - hiatus hernia and gastro-esophageal reflux disease (GERD)
  - esophagitis and esophageal stricture
  - globus sensation (hystericus)
  - cancer of the esophagus

- Diseases of the stomach and duodenum:
  - gastroenteritis
  - dyspepsia, gastritis and peptic ulcers
  - pyloric stenosis
  - pernicious anemia
  - cancer of the stomach.

To help with progression along this journey of diseases of each part of the gastrointestinal tract, it may be useful to be reminded first of the physiological descriptions to be found in the relevant parts in Section 3.1a.

Important diseases of the mouth and salivary glands

Mouth ulcers

The term ulcer describes a break in the epithelium. This term is used for conditions of the gastrointestinal system in which the protective mucosal layer has become damaged for some reason.

Mouth ulcers are usually isolated, small, painful, whitened breaches in the mouth lining, and often have no obvious precipitating cause. They tend to be more common in some people than others. In most cases the sufferer is otherwise well, although occasionally a vitamin deficiency might be found. False or sharp teeth occasionally trigger ulcers. A small mouth ulcer will usually heal within one to three days.

A crop of very painful reddened ulcers points to a viral infection. The very first encounter with the cold sore virus (herpes simplex) can cause such a condition. This is most common in young children, and can be so severe that hospital admission is necessary to give fluids by intravenous drip, as severe inflammation of the mouth prevents eating and drinking for a few days.

Less commonly, mouth ulcers may be part of a more severe digestive condition. The lower gastrointestinal diseases of Crohn's disease, ulcerative colitis and celiac disease are all associated with mouth ulceration. These conditions are studied in more detail in Section 3.1e.

Non-healing painless or painful mouth ulcers are always a cause for concern and may indicate early mouth cancer.

Information box 3.1c-I

Mouth ulcers: comments from a Chinese medicine perspective

In Chinese medicine, ulcers in the mouth suggest Heat in the Stomach, whereas ulcers on the tongue suggest Heat in the organ suggested by the site of the ulcer on the tongue (commonly Liver and Heart). A white base to the ulcer might reflect Phlegm and a purplish color Blood Stagnation.

Cold sores

The nature of infection by the herpes simplex virus (HSV) in the causation of cold sores was introduced in Section 2.4a by means of an example of the pathology of infectious diseases. Primary infection by HSV may cause a crop of painful ulcers. After this the virus remains latent in a nerve cell, and characteristic symptoms of the painful crusting and weeping cold sore may reoccur at times of stress or exposure to extreme sunlight.

The same virus may also cause genital herpes infections. Oral sex can lead to the transmission of an oral cold sore to the genitalia of the sexual partner (for more detail on genital herpes, see Section 5.2d).

Patients may be recommended by their doctor or pharmacist to apply an antiviral drug called aciclovir in the form of a cream to the affected area at the onset of a cold sore. Aciclovir prevents the replication of viruses and does seem to shorten or abort the attack, although it does not prevent future recurrences. In patients with recurrent cold sores a daily low dose of oral antiviral medication may be recommended.

Information box 3.1c-II

Cold sores: comments from a Chinese medicine perspective

In Chinese medicine, the appearance of a cold sore would be described as an invasion of Wind Heat and Damp. Aciclovir, which reduces the inflammation and crusting, is therefore Cooling in its action. As aciclovir does not treat any underlying Heat and Damp that may have been expressed in the form of the cold sore, it may be described as energetically suppressive in its action, and this means the Heat and Damp may continue to be an energetic pattern expressed in some way for the patient.

Oral thrush (candidiasis)

Overgrowth of the candida yeast (thrush) is described in Section 2.4b. Overgrowth of the candida yeast in the mouth (oral thrush) appears as white patches on the tongue and lining of the mouth, and may or may not be painful. Thrush of the esophagus can result in difficult and painful swallowing. It is a common first feature of the progression of human immunodeficiency virus (HIV) infection to acquired immune deficiency syndrome (AIDS).

Except in the case of newborns, in whom oral thrush is common, thrush in the mouth should be taken as an indication of possible depletion of the immune system. It is seen most commonly in frail elderly people, people with diabetes and people with advanced cancer and immune suppression.

The medical treatment of thrush is by means of antifungal drugs in the form of drops or lozenges to suck. Nystatin and amphotericin are the two most common preparations. A course of oral treatment with an antifungal drug such as fluconazole may also be used for intractable cases.

Information box 3.1c-III

Oral thrush: comments from a Chinese medicine perspective

In Chinese medicine, thrush would be viewed as a sign of internal Damp or Damp Heat. Nystatin, amphotericin and fluconazole appear to clear Damp. Their action is likely to be suppressive in nature, dealing as they do with only the outward expression of a deeper internal weakness.

Leukoplakia

Leukoplakia literally means white plaques, and appears as a dense, painless, immovable white area on the side of the tongue or inside of the mouth.

Leukoplakia is important as it may reflect early cancerous changes. It is more common in smokers and those who drink alcohol in excess. A patient with leukoplakia should be referred, because an early diagnosis of cancer of the tongue can be life-saving.

Information box 3.1c-IV

Leukoplakia: comments from a Chinese medicine perspective

In Chinese medicine, the signs and symptoms of leukoplakia would be interpreted in terms of Damp Cold or Phlegm, and the location on the sides of the tongue would indicate Liver pathology.

Gingivitis

Gingivitis literally means inflammation of the gums, and is the common condition that causes bleeding of the gums on brushing. Gingivitis is due to inflammation of the gum in contact with plaque on the teeth, and is encouraged by poor dental hygiene. Gingivitis results from an overgrowth of the commensal bacteria, which normally reside harmlessly in the mouth. It is very common in pregnancy and is more common in smokers.

Occasionally, gingivitis will flare up to lead to an acutely painful ulcerated gum and tenderness in the associated teeth. This is a common reason for an urgent visit to the dentist. The treatment of this condition that may or may not involve a collection of pus around the roots of teeth (dental abscess) is a three to seven day course of an antibiotic (usually metronidazole or amoxicillin) and antiseptic mouthwashes. This acute form of severe gingivitis is much more common in smokers. The conventional explanation for the vulnerability to gum disease in smokers is that the toxins in smoke impair the natural immune barriers to infection in the mouth (the mucosa and saliva).

Information box 3.1c-V

Gingivitis: comments from a Chinese medicine perspective

In Chinese medicine, the signs and symptoms of gingivitis would be described as Full Heat in the Stomach. Antibiotics in this case are therefore Cooling in their action.

Salivary gland infection (sialadenitis)

There are three pairs of major salivary glands (see Section 3.1a). The parotid glands hug the posterior border of the masseter muscle on the face, the submandibular glands sit under the inferior edge of the lower jaw bone (mandible), and the sublingual glands sit under the tongue. All are exocrine glands and release their secretions via ducts into the mouth cavity.

These glands can become inflamed as a result of infection. The mumps virus is probably the most common infectious cause of this in otherwise healthy people, although this disease is much less common since the introduction of widespread vaccination of children. The hamster face seen in children with mumps is due to inflammation and swelling of the parotid glands.

Bacteria can cause infections in the salivary glands, although this should be seen, like thrush, as a sign of immune depletion. Underlying causes can include dehydration, alcoholism and diabetes. The symptoms include tender painful swollen salivary glands and fever. Eating, which causes salivation, is painful. The cause is

an overgrowth of healthy oral bacteria. This would be an indication for prompt oral antibiotic treatment.

Information box 3.1c-VI

Salivary gland infection: comments from a Chinese medicine perspective

In Chinese medicine, swelling of glands from infection commonly reflects Damp Heat. Salivary gland infections might reflect Damp Heat on a background of Stomach Yin Deficiency, as they do not tend to occur in healthy people.

In Chinese medicine, the rapid development of the symptoms of mumps is consistent with its description of Invasion of Wind Heat and blocking of the Shao Yang meridians. Deeper penetration of Heat and Toxic Heat Stagnation is the cause of the painful swellings.

Salivary gland stones

A stone (calculus) forms in a salivary gland when secretions dry up and accumulate to form a hard solid mass. If a stone develops it may periodically block the flow of saliva, most commonly in a single parotid gland. The patient might complain of pain and swelling of the cheek after eating, and may be more at risk of bacterial infections of the salivary glands.

Salivary gland stones that cause persistent problems can be removed by means of a minor surgical procedure.

Information box 3.1c-VII

Salivary gland stones: comments from a Chinese medicine perspective

In Chinese medicine, the drying of secretions to form a mass suggests Phlegm. Salivary gland stones could be seen as a manifestation of Phlegm in the Stomach on a background of Stomach Yin Deficiency.

Salivary gland tumors

Salivary gland tumors are not uncommon. They are most frequently found in the parotid glands of elderly people. They usually give rise to a firm, irregular painless swelling of one cheek. Eighty-five percent of these tumors are benign and can be removed by surgery. Features that suggest a malignant tumor include rapid irregular growth, lymph node involvement and weakness of the muscles of the mouth on the same side as the swelling (a result of cancerous infiltration of the facial nerve).

Information box 3.1c-VIII

Salivary gland tumors: comments from a Chinese medicine perspective

The Chinese medicine interpretation of all tumors includes Phlegm and/or Blood Stagnation on a background of severe depletion; in this case, as the tumors are in the region of the salivary glands, deep imbalance of the Stomach Qi amongst other imbalances is likely to play a part in carcinogenesis.

The red flags of diseases of the mouth

Some patients with diseases of the mouth will benefit from referral to a conventional doctor for assessment and/or treatment. Red flags are those symptoms and signs that indicate that referral is to be considered. The red flags of the diseases of the mouth are described in Table 3.1c-I. A summary of the red flags in a format designed for quick reference in clinical practice can be found in Appendix III. This gives advice on the degree of urgency of referral for each of the red flag conditions listed.

Table 3.1c-I A4: Red flags of diseases of the mouth

Red flag	Description	Reasoning
A4.1	Persistent oral thrush (candidiasis) (appearing as a thick white coating on tongue or palate)	Although common in the newborn, oral thrush in children and adults is not a normal finding, and merits referral to exclude an underlying cause. Common causes include corticosteroid use (including asthma inhalers), diabetes, immunodeficiency (including HIV/AIDS) and cancer. Dentures in elderly people can also predispose to oral thrush
A4.2	Persistent painless white plaque (leukoplakia) (appearing as a coating that appears to sit on the surface of the sides of the tongue)	Leukoplakia is a precancerous change that signifies an increased risk of mouth cancer. It is more common in smokers and in those with a high alcohol intake. A particular form of leukoplakia is also associated with HIV/AIDS Early treatment of leukoplakia can prevent invasive mouth cancer, so referral is merited
A4.3	Painless enlargement of a salivary gland over weeks to months	This needs referral to exclude salivary gland cancer, which is most common in people >60
A4.4	Painful or painless enlargement of salivary gland immediately after eating	This suggests a salivary gland stone or obstruction from dried secretions. Early treatment is to maximize hydration by encouraging drinking, and to encourage salivation (e.g. with lemon juice). If the problem is persistent, referral is recommended, as surgical removal of the stone may be necessary
A4.5	Tender or inflamed gums or salivary glands that do not respond within days to treatment	May be accompanied by fever or malaise. These symptoms suggest chronic gingivitis, dental abscess or infection of the salivary gland, and if they persist, indicate a need for referral for antibiotic treatment to prevent inflammatory damage to dental roots or salivary glands
A4.6	Ulceration of mouth if persistent (>1 week) or if preventing proper hydration	The most common cause of painful ulceration of the mouth is herpes simplex virus (HSV) infection. This can be so severe as to inhibit drinking in a child. If this is the case, the child may need to be hospitalized for rehydration If ulceration persists for >2 weeks it might suggest an underlying inflammatory condition (e.g. Crohn's disease) or mouth cancer, which will require further investigation Rarely, severe mouth ulceration can be the first sign of bone marrow failure (see Table A1: Red flags of cancer), and in this case results from a very low white blood cell count

Important diseases of the esophagus

Hiatus hernia and gastro-esophageal reflux disease (GERD)

The hiatus is the medical name for the gap in the diaphragm through which the esophagus passes to meet the stomach. The cardiac sphincter of the stomach is situated at the hiatus of the diaphragm.

Hernia is the medical term used to describe the movement of an internal organ outside its usual anatomical position through an area of weakness of the surrounding supportive tissue. A hiatus hernia is, therefore, a condition in which part of the stomach has moved upwards through the hiatus so that it sits in the cavity above the diaphragm. This means that the cardiac sphincter has been stretched to permit the stomach to move upwards.

A hiatus hernia is in itself a very common occurrence, and is known to be present in about one-third of people aged over 50. In most cases a hiatus hernia is a consequence of a Western sedentary lifestyle. In such cases, long-term obesity or habitual straining to open the bowels gives rise to years of increased pressure below the diaphragm. This puts strain on the muscles of the diaphragm that form the cardiac sphincter at the top of the stomach. Gradually, this sphincter is stretched and the top of the stomach is pushed up above the diaphragm. The tight sphincter is then no longer there to prevent stomach contents from refluxing back up into the bottom end of the esophagus.

It should be easy to understand how pregnancy may cause a temporary hiatus hernia, as the enlarging uterus pushes the abdominal contents up against the diaphragm. This physical effect is compounded by the fact that the hormone of pregnancy, progesterone, exerts a softening and relaxing effect on muscles and ligaments, and likewise affects the cardiac sphincter.

Even if a hiatus hernia is not physically manifested, the function of the cardiac sphincter in containing the stomach contents may be relatively weak. The incompetence of a weak sphincter has the same effect as a hiatus hernia in allowing upwards reflux of the stomach contents. Reflux of acid above the level of the cardiac sphincter can lead to a cluster of symptoms collectively known as gastro-esophageal reflux disease (GERD).

The most distressing symptom of a hiatus hernia or incompetent cardiac sphincter is heartburn. It is estimated that up to 25 percent of Western adults have experienced heartburn and 5 percent experience this daily. Heartburn is a sensation that ranges from mild burning to intense crushing pain felt in the area of the epigastrium. The pain or burning may also be experienced rising up the sternum from this site towards the middle of the chest, and may even lead to discomfort in the throat area.[17]

Heartburn is a result of the acidic stomach contents passing through the overly lax cardiac sphincter and then irritating the lining of the esophagus. If prolonged, the lining of the esophagus can become permanently inflamed, leading to redness, swelling and pain. This is called esophagitis.

Heartburn may be triggered by leaning forward or lying down, and by anything that makes the stomach contents more irritating, such as alcohol, spicy food, chocolate and coffee. Overeating, smoking and stress are all exacerbating factors, and certain medications can also promote reflux of acid or esophagitis (e.g. non-steroidal anti-inflammatory drugs (NSAIDs), doxycycline and bisphosphonate medication).

The pain of heartburn can be so severe that it mimics the pain of a heart attack. Sometimes the only way to distinguish between the two is for the patient to undergo urgent hospital tests. All patients who suffer severe, crushing central chest pain should be referred to a hospital emergency department as a matter of urgency.

Another common unpleasant symptom is for the patient to belch acid fluid into the mouth. This is known as water brash.

It has also been increasingly recognized that reflux of tiny amounts of acid, particularly at night, may irritate the vocal cords and respiratory pathways, and result in hoarseness, chronic cough and asthma. These symptoms may develop in the absence of significant heartburn. It has been estimated that up to 10 percent of chronic unexplained cough is due to reflux of acid and inhalation into the respiratory tree. These respiratory symptoms will improve as the reflux is treated.

In terms of treatment of the symptoms of hiatus hernia and reflux, the best treatment approach is prevention. Weight loss, treatment of constipation and dietary moderation can reverse the problem entirely in some people. Cutting down on smoking, hot foods and alcohol can markedly reduce symptoms. Simple advice, such as raising the head of the bed, can help night-time symptoms.

Antacid medication (to reduce the acidity of the stomach) is commonly prescribed, and this primarily means the proton pump inhibitor (PPI) group of medications such as omeprazole and lansoprazole. Alginates in suspension form may also be prescribed in cases of unexplained hoarseness, chronic cough and asthma to deal with the possibility that acid reflux may be the cause of the condition. Both these types of preparation are described in more detail, in relation to the treatment of stomach and duodenal ulcers, at the end of this section.

Drugs that promote the downward movement of peristalsis can also help in GERD. These include metoclopramide and domperidone, although there are now concerns that these medications have an association with adverse cardiac events if used on a regular basis.

In severe cases, surgery to tighten the hiatus can be performed.

 Information box 3.1c-IX

Hiatus hernia and gastro-esophageal reflux disease: comments from a Chinese medicine perspective

In Chinese medicine, a hiatus hernia and GERD could be seen as the result of a long-term deficiency of the holding power of Spleen Qi. The rising burning sensation and acid in the mouth could be attributed to Heat in the Stomach, with Stomach Qi rebelling upwards. Intense pain would suggest additional Liver Qi and Blood Stagnation.

Most drug treatments for reflux reduce the intensity of the acidity. In this way they are energetically Cooling. However, none of them address the root cause of the problem, and therefore they are suppressive in action.

The treatments to enhance peristalsis appear to promote the descent of Stomach Qi and move Stagnation.

Esophagitis and esophageal stricture

If the esophagus becomes very inflamed by refluxed stomach contents, the pain that results locates behind the sternum and can be intense and crushing in nature. This condition is called esophagitis. Long-term inflammation of any body part may lead to scarring. Scarring resulting from esophagitis can lead to narrowing of the width of the lumen (stricture). This is most common in older people.

A stricture can lead to a sensation of difficulty in swallowing, known as dysphagia. The term dysphagia comes from the Greek meaning difficulty in eating. (Note that this is different to the term dysphasia, which comes from the Greek for difficulty in speaking. Dysphasia describes any problem in producing clear speech. These terms are commonly confused with each other, but mean very different things.)

Dysphagia can have a range of causes, but the characteristic that suggests a problem of a physical blockage is that solid foods are much harder to swallow than liquids. A patient with a stricture might locate the problem by placing a hand over the lower aspect of the sternum.

A stricture is treated by surgery to stretch the scarred area.

 Information box 3.1c-X

Esophageal stricture: comments from a Chinese medicine perspective

In Chinese medicine, the symptoms of a stricture could be attributed to Liver Qi Stagnation, giving rise to Qi Phlegm (plum stone in the throat), although if a stricture were to lead to weight loss and malaise, additional more severe imbalances would also be part of the diagnostic picture.

Globus sensation (hystericus)

This Latin term means imagined lump, and is the name used for the very common functional symptom described by the ancient Chinese as "plum stone in the throat." There is a sensation of a blockage, often at the level of the voice box, and a perception of difficulty in swallowing. Formerly termed globus hystericus, this symptom used to be considered an emotional problem in conventional medicine, but it is now increasingly recognized in some cases to be a symptom of GERD.

The key difference between the dysphagia in this condition and between that due to physical obstruction is that the difficulty usually affects liquids and solids equally, and the discomfort is present even when not swallowing. There will be no associated weight loss in globus hystericus.

The main medical treatment is primarily explanation and reassurance. However, globus accounts for 4 percent of referrals to UK Ear, Nose and Throat (ENT) hospital departments after which physical abnormalities can be excluded. If GERD is suspected, alginates or PPIs such as omeprazole may be prescribed. Alternatively, speech therapy or psychological support may be considered.

 Information box 3.1c-XI

Globus sensation: comments from a Chinese medicine perspective

In Chinese medicine, the symptoms of globus may readily be attributed to Stagnation of Liver Qi or Qi Phlegm (plum stone in the throat).

Cancer of the esophagus

Esophageal cancer most commonly develops in the lower two-thirds of the esophagus and is usually seen in people over 60. In many cases, cancer of the esophagus has been preceded by long-term acid reflux and esophagitis, as cancerous change is another complication of chronic inflammation. As well as reflux, obesity, heavy alcohol intake and smoking increase the risk of this fairly common cancer.

The first symptom is almost always dysphagia for solids, which becomes increasingly worse over a period of weeks to months. This symptom means that the cancer is quite advanced. By the time of diagnosis about half of all patients have cancerous spread to their lymph nodes.

The treatment for early disease is surgical removal of the tumor, and this might be attempted endoscopically. Light, laser and radiofrequency ablation may also be used for early tumors. If the tumor is more advanced but localized, a length of the affected esophagus may be removed surgically. This is a major operation with a 4 percent mortality rate, and is only offered to those without lymph node spread. One study shows that cure may be as high as 48 percent in this group of patients if chemotherapy is also used before surgery. However, overall, over seven out of ten patients with this cancer will have died of the disease within five years of diagnosis.[18]

Palliative treatment involves the passage of a firm tube into the blocked esophagus to permit swallowing to continue. This can relieve the distressing dysphagia in terminally ill patients. In selected patients chemotherapy might be offered to help control symptoms.

Information box 3.1c-XII

Cancer of the esophagus: comments from a Chinese medicine perspective

The Chinese medicine interpretation of cancer is Phlegm with Qi and Blood Stagnation on a long-term background of depletion of Yin or Yang. Heat toxins may or may not be part of the diagnostic picture. In the case of esophageal cancer, the long-term depletion is likely to be of Stomach and Spleen Yin, a resulting buildup of Heat and Liver Qi and Blood Stagnation. Heat toxins from dietary sources may play a part in the etiology of this aggressive disease.

The red flags of diseases of the esophagus

Some patients with diseases of the esophagus will benefit from referral to a conventional doctor for assessment and/or treatment. Red flags are those symptoms and signs that indicate that referral is to be considered. The red flags of diseases of the esophagus are described in Table 3.1c-II. A summary of the red flags in a format designed for quick reference in clinical practice can be found in Appendix III. This gives advice on the degree of urgency of referral for each of the red flag conditions listed.

Table 3.1c-II A5: Red flags of diseases of the esophagus

Red flag	Description	Reasoning
A5.1	Difficulty swallowing (dysphagia), which is worse with solids (in particular, if progressive over days to weeks)	A sensation of difficulty in swallowing or a lump in the throat is a common and often benign symptom, which may fluctuate with emotional stress (the syndrome known as globus pharyngeus). Usually, swallowing of food is still possible with this form of dysphagia However, if there is a physical obstruction in the esophagus, which may be the result of cancer or stricture (scarring), there may be progressive difficulty in swallowing stiff foods, and this will be accompanied by a loss of weight. This needs prompt referral
A5.2	Difficulty swallowing (dysphagia) associated with enlarged lymph nodes in the neck	See A5.1. Dysphagia that is also associated with enlarged lymph nodes raises the possibility of a malignant or inflammatory cause, and merits referral
A5.3	Swallowing associated with central chest pain (behind the sternum)	Swallowing that is associated with a delayed pain behind the sternum suggests esophagitis or structural damage to the esophagus (e.g. a tear or puncture by a fishbone). Refer if symptoms are not settling within 24 hours, or sooner if pain is severe

Important diseases of the stomach and duodenum

Gastroenteritis

The term gastroenteritis literally means inflammation of the stomach and intestines. In practice, this description is given to infections of the digestive tract that lead to symptoms that include nausea, vomiting, diarrhea, blood in the stools and abdominal pain. The inflammation of the digestive lining prevents absorption of fluid, and excess fluid in the bowel is what leads to the diarrhea and vomiting.

A common serious consequence of gastroenteritis is dehydration, which can be life-threatening, particularly in vulnerable individuals such as infants and frail elderly people. The symptoms of early dehydration are dry mouth, and sparse and concentrated urine. Later on the patient may feel faint and confused, the eyes appear sunken, and the skin lacks its usual bouncy quality and will appear dry. In infants, the fontanel, which is the soft spot in the skull, sinks inwards, and the child becomes floppy and listless. This state can develop alarmingly quickly in vulnerable individuals, and there is a risk of kidney failure. The treatment is urgent administration of fluids, and by intravenous drip if fluids cannot be tolerated by mouth.

Most causes of gastroenteritis in the UK are due to infection and, in particular, viral infection. Many cases are caught from contact with another person who is excreting the infectious agent in their stools. Bacterially contaminated food causes the form of gastroenteritis commonly referred to as food poisoning. Protozoa such as amoeba and *Giardia* are additional causes of cases contracted from infected water, more commonly in less developed countries. Food poisoning is a notifiable disease in the UK, so patients should be advised to report any suspected case to their GP.

Escherichia (E.) coli and *Salmonella*, *Cholera*, *Campylobacter* and *Giardia* species are some of the bacterial organisms that can cause gastroenteritis. Norovirus (Norwalk virus) and rotavirus are the most common viral causes, and these often become apparent in winter epidemics. The Ebola virus is a cause of a very severe form of gastroenteritis that caused many deaths in 2014–15 in West Africa.

The best treatment is prevention of infection. In addition to provision of clean water and efficient sanitation, personal hygiene practice such as scrupulous hand washing after going to the toilet or contacting patients is important to minimize spread of infectious viruses and bacteria. This is of particular importance in food handlers.

As bacteria are commonly found on raw meat and in raw eggs, insufficient cooking can lead to contaminated food. Contaminated food left at room temperature is even more risky, as this provides ideal conditions for bacteria to multiply. Any food that has been in contact with raw meat or eggs (such as might occur when using a common chopping board) should also be treated as contaminated.

In established infections, the best treatment is to avoid eating heavy spicy food and to drink plenty of fluids, and allow the infection to take its course. In healthy people most cases, although unpleasant, get better on their own in two to five days. Even alarming symptoms such as blood in the stools should settle down naturally.

Doctors might prescribe a sugar and salt preparation known as oral rehydration therapy or ORT to dissolve in water. This replaces mineral salts that are lost through vomiting and diarrhea, but the evidence to support its benefit in healthy people is not convincing.

Antibiotics are usually used only in those cases in which the symptoms are proven to be the result of bacterial infection and which are not settling in five to seven days. It is not considered good practice to prescribe antibiotics in simple cases of gastroenteritis.

Frail patients with dehydration and anyone with severe dehydration should be nursed in hospital.

Antibiotic use can induce a form of gastroenteritis, partly as a result of reducing the healthy commensal bacteria of the bowel. In most cases this gives rise to mild self-limiting diarrhea, and recovery may be aided by supplementing the diet with live yogurt (to restore the balance of healthy bacteria). In vulnerable people, and particularly in a hospital setting where this infection is more likely to be contracted, the bacterium Clostridium (C.) difficile can take hold in the digestive system. This can lead to a potentially devastating form of gastroenteritis. The treatment for this antibiotic-induced infection is administration of even more powerful antibiotics. This treatment is problematic, as antibiotic resistance is increasingly prevalent.[19]

Information box 3.1c-XIII

Gastroenteritis: comments from a Chinese medicine perspective

A Chinese medicine interpretation of gastroenteritis depends very much on the symptom picture. Diarrhea and blood suggest Damp Heat in the Intestines, whereas the other symptoms of nausea, vomiting and cramps suggest Liver Qi Stagnation invading the Stomach and Spleen with Stomach Qi rebelling upwards. Dehydration could be described as Stomach Yin Deficiency leading to Kidney Yin Deficiency.

Dyspepsia, gastritis and peptic ulcers

Indigestion is a commonly used term that may be applied to the symptoms of any one of the three conditions of dyspepsia, gastritis and peptic ulcer. The prescribing to treat these three conditions accounts for one of the heaviest cost burdens on the UK National Health Service (NHS) budget.

This is because most people will have at some point experienced indigestion (it is very common), and many will seek prescribed medication for their symptoms. One study showed that one in five people suffer from dyspepsia and one in four of these people will consult a doctor for this, so this suggests over 6 percent of the population seek prescribed medication for this symptom, and many, many more will turn to over-the-counter medications such as antacids.

Dyspepsia, like dysphagia, is a symptom and not a disease. The term, which is derived from the Greek meaning bad digestion, is used to describe any discomfort arising from the process of digestion in the stomach. The common equivalent of this term is indigestion, although patients may use this non-specific word to describe any sort of discomfort from the chest to the groin. It is important that practitioners obtain a precise description of symptoms from their patients rather than simply accepting a complaint of indigestion to be the same as their own medical understanding of the term.

Typically, dyspepsia involves discomfort in the epigastric region, which often has a burning or gripy quality. It is usually related to eating, being triggered either by hot, spicy foods, alcohol and caffeine, or by leaving too long a space between meals. The symptoms of dyspepsia and heartburn can overlap. It is now understood that dyspepsia has a range of possible causes including esophagitis (described above), gastritis, peptic ulcer disease and irritable bowel disease. Although mostly resulting from benign conditions, dyspepsia should not be ignored as it could signify a malignancy, and so needs to be carefully monitored and appropriately investigated.

Gastritis is inflammation of the stomach lining. The lining becomes reddened and thickened, and may bleed in places. It can only be definitely diagnosed by using an endoscope. The symptoms are of a mild to severe dyspepsia. Gastritis can be caused by overeating, spicy foods, alcohol and coffee or tea. Aspirin, and the painkillers known as non-steroidal anti-inflammatory drugs (NSAIDs) (e.g. ibuprofen or diclofenac), are known to cause slight gastritis in most people who take them. In some people this can become a severe situation.

Stress is a known cause of inflammation of the stomach lining. A shock resulting from a car accident or a surgical operation can cause sufficient stress to lead to an acute flare up of gastritis.

Mild gastritis may have no symptoms or may give rise to dyspepsia. Severe gastritis may lead to epigastric pain and vomiting, and at worst, bleeding into the stomach. The patient may vomit blood, which appears like black gravel (due to the action of the stomach acid on the blood), or may pass altered blood in stools, which then look like black tar. A severe gastric hemorrhage can be life-threatening and so is a medical emergency.

It is now known that many people who suffer with gastritis have the *Helicobacter (H.) pylori* bacterium in their stomach. This is an initially silent infection, which is contracted in early adult life and which in some people gives rise to long-term inflammation of the stomach. In fact, over 60 percent of the population may be carrying this organism, many of whom contracted it during childhood, but not all of these will develop symptoms.

The presence of *H. pylori* can be diagnosed by means of a breath test in which the patient blows a breath sample after drinking a formulated drink. Alternatively, it can be diagnosed by means of a blood test that looks for antibodies to the bacterium. It is now considered good practice to aim to eradicate *H. pylori* by means of a short-term course of two high-dose antibiotics combined with a PPI (triple therapy), because chronic infection with this bacterium is associated with an increased risk of stomach cancer.

Peptic ulcer is the term used to describe a breakdown of the mucosal lining of either the stomach or the duodenum. The terms gastric ulcer and duodenal ulcer are used to describe the site of the peptic ulcer. Peptic ulcer disease (PUD) can be seen as a progression of gastritis or inflammation of the duodenum (duodenitis). The causation of a peptic ulcer is generally the same as that for gastritis, and it tends to run in families. The *H. pylori* bacterium is strongly linked to PUD.

Gastric and duodenal ulcers tend to have slightly different characteristics in terms of causation and symptoms, but in practice are often difficult to distinguish without performing an endoscopy.

Dyspepsia is the main symptom of peptic ulcer, and pain is often present. The patient may describe a gnawing hunger pain, but sometimes the pain can be intense and stabbing. Often the patient can point to a particular site in the epigastrium where they locate the pain. This pointing sign is believed to be highly suggestive of an ulcer. If the ulcer is on the posterior wall of the stomach or the duodenum, the pain may also be felt in the mid-back.

A gastric ulcer is more likely to lead to nausea and loss of appetite. Eating makes the symptoms worse, so the patient may lose weight. It is less common than duodenal ulcer.

A duodenal ulcer is more likely to lead to hunger pains, and certain foods such as milk may relieve the discomfort. The pain is worse when the duodenum is empty, and it may therefore occur at night. The patient may put on weight. Duodenal ulcer is common. It is estimated that about 15 percent of the population may suffer from a duodenal ulcer at some point in their lives.

Many peptic ulcers will heal spontaneously, like mouth ulcers, although there may well be a recurrence when the person is exposed to a trigger such as overeating, an alcohol binge or stress. Some ulcers become chronic, meaning that the patient suffers from long-term digestive discomfort and recurrent pain. The two serious, but rare, complications are hemorrhage and perforation.

Hemorrhage results from stomach acid eroding the exposed area of stomach lining and damaging the blood vessels in the deeper layers. A slight, but persistent, hemorrhage can lead to loss of iron and the development of anemia. The patient might not notice the blood, as it can be hidden in the stools. However, a severe hemorrhage can be life-threatening and can lead to shock (for more explanation of the syndrome of shock, see Section 3.4d).

Perforation means that the full thickness of the stomach wall has been breached so that the stomach contents leak out into the surrounding peritoneal cavity. This situation leads to acute abdominal pain resulting from an inflammation of the peritoneum (peritonitis). This is almost invariably fatal unless treated as a surgical emergency. The symptoms are those of the acute abdomen. This important syndrome is described in detail in Section 3.1d.

Dyspepsia, gastritis and PUD should all respond dramatically to lifestyle changes, and these are similar to those recommended for gastro-esophageal reflux disease (GERD). However, many Western patients find these changes hard to make.

Nowadays, the main treatment of these conditions is by means of drugs rather than surgery.

Self-medication with antacids is extremely common. Drugs such as Rennie and Remegel counteract the acid in the stomach and can relieve the burning discomfort of dyspepsia and heartburn. Patients can buy a wide range of antacid medications over the counter at a pharmacy. As a result of powerful advertising, many of these brands are household names. Patients may even forget that these are medications, and this is worth bearing in mind when taking a medication history to ask specifically about antacid use.

The UK National Institute for Health and Care Excellence (NICE) guideline on dyspepsia[20] suggests that, in most cases, medical treatment can be instituted without the need for diagnostic endoscopy. The exceptions are those cases in which there might be alarm symptoms of progressive disease (cancer) or of imminent or ongoing bleeding or perforation. These alarm symptoms include new onset of symptoms after the age of 55, weight loss, unexplained iron deficiency anemia and severe pain.

If there are no alarm symptoms, the recommended medical approach is first to test for H. pylori infection, and if this is present, to treat the infection with triple therapy. This might be sufficient to resolve the symptoms. If H. pylori infection is not present, the patient may be prescribed a simple antacid or a PPI (such as omeprazole). These drugs prevent the formation of gastric acid by the parietal cells in the stomach lining. In the majority of patients, one of these two medical approaches will resolve the symptoms. The H2 blockers (e.g. ranitidine or cimetidine) are a less commonly prescribed alternative to the PPIs. These also reduce gastric acid secretion, but seem to be less effective than the PPIs. Because of recurrence of symptoms on withdrawal from H2 blockers or PPIs, some patients remain on a regular dose of these drugs for months to years. It is recognized that withdrawal from these medications results in a temporary state of excessive acid production, which means that it is all the more likely that a patient will be reluctant to withdraw from them.

Even in the case of hemorrhage, most bleeding peptic ulcers respond to drug treatment alone. It is only in rare cases that patients who suffer from either a severe hemorrhage or perforation will require emergency surgery.

Information box 3.1c-XIV

Dyspepsia, gastritis and peptic ulcers: comments from a Chinese medicine perspective

In Chinese medicine, the symptoms of dyspepsia, gastritis and PUD might be classified as manifestations of a range of Stomach and Spleen-related patterns, including Stomach and Spleen Deficiency, and full conditions of the Stomach such as Retention of Food, Stomach Heat, Stomach Fire, Stomach and Liver Heat and Liver Qi Stagnation invading the Stomach. The pain of an ulcer signifies Liver Qi invading the Stomach and/or Stagnation of Blood in the Stomach.

The antacids and anti-ulcer drugs are Cooling. They do not cure the underlying condition, and are therefore suppressive. Anti-ulcer drugs are powerful in their action and have many possible side effects, which include gastrointestinal and liver disturbance. This implies that they tend to deplete the Spleen Qi and Stagnate Liver Qi.

Antibiotic treatment has a more long-term effect. The clearance of H. pylori suggests that this treatment can actually clear a Heat Toxin from the stomach. The antibiotics themselves are energetically Cold and Damp, and so side effects such as thrush and loose stools may occur.

Pyloric stenosis

Pyloric stenosis is a condition in which there is a stricture of the outflow of the stomach, the pyloric sphincter. In adults, just as in esophageal stricture, the cause is usually scarring following the inflammation of an ulcer or gastritis. Occasionally, cancer is a cause.

The main symptom of pyloric stenosis is vomiting without pain. Often the vomiting is forceful or projectile. The patient can rapidly develop dehydration.

Pyloric stenosis can be an inherited condition, in which case it becomes apparent in the first few weeks of life.

The newborn infant will also develop projectile vomiting and is at great risk of dehydration. The only treatment for this congenital condition is surgery.

Pernicious anemia

This is a type of anemia that results from an inability to absorb vitamin B12 from the diet. Before it can be absorbed from the small intestine, vitamin B12 needs to be linked with a bodily-produced substance called intrinsic factor (see Section 3.1a). Intrinsic factor is manufactured by cells in the stomach lining. In pernicious anemia these cells are progressively destroyed by an autoimmune process, and the person is no longer able to absorb vitamin B12.

Vitamin B12 is necessary for the healthy formation of red blood cells, and also for the functioning of the nervous system. Therefore, in untreated pernicious anemia the patient both gradually develops anemia and also a severe form of irreversible disease that eventually leads to paralysis and dementia.

This autoimmune condition is not uncommon in older women, affecting about 1 in 8000 of the population over the age of 60. It used to be fatal, hence the term pernicious. Nowadays, if the condition is diagnosed and treated early with regular vitamin B12 injections, the symptoms disappear totally.

Pernicious anemia is associated with other autoimmune conditions such as thyroid disease, Addison's disease and vitiligo (patchy depigmentation of the skin), and so these conditions may coexist in the same patient.

Information box 3.1c-XV

Pernicious anemia: comments from a Chinese medicine perspective

In Chinese medicine, the impaired digestive function in pernicious anemia, in which there is insufficient production of gastric acid, sore mouth and lemon-yellow skin coloration, might be described in terms of depletion of Stomach and Spleen Qi. Anemia is a manifestation of Blood and Qi Deficiency. The development of the paralysis and dementia is due to malnourishment of the nervous system. These symptoms suggest that vitamin B12 also nourishes Kidney Essence (Jing), so untreated pernicious anemia can accelerate Jing Deficiency.

Vitamin B12 injections could, therefore, be seen as a replacement treatment that nourishes Blood, Qi and Jing. The treatment does not address the underlying Stomach and Spleen imbalances, but is not, according to the definition made in this text, suppressive, because the underlying imbalances are irreversible and supplementation brings the body to an improved state of balance.

Cancer of the stomach (gastric carcinoma)

Stomach cancer is a common form of cancer in the West. It now seems to be strongly linked with *H. pylori* infection, presumably as a result of the long-term inflammation that this infection causes. It is also believed that components of the Western diet (e.g. salt and nitrates, and nitrosamines from overcooked meat) may also increase the risk of cancer.

The main symptoms of stomach cancer are pain and dyspepsia. As the cancer may have developed in someone who has tended to experience indigestion for years, the early symptoms may be ignored. For this reason stomach cancer is often diagnosed late, with up to 30 percent of people having metastases (usually in the liver) at the time of diagnosis. If pain and dyspepsia develop for the first time in someone over the age of 55 it is important to consider referral for investigations to exclude stomach cancer.

A minority of patients are diagnosed when the tumor is sufficiently small for it to be totally removed with surgery, but in most cases this cancer is inoperable. For these patients chemotherapy may be offered, to prolong life but not to cure. Only one in ten of people diagnosed with stomach cancer will be alive five years after diagnosis.

Information box 3.1c-XVI

Cancer of the stomach: comments from a Chinese medicine perspective

In Chinese medicine, cancer is understood to be the result of Phlegm and Blood Stagnation. These, together, account for the mass and the pain. These effects often develop on a background of long-term depletion of Stomach Qi or Yin.

The red flags of diseases of the stomach

Some patients with diseases of the stomach will benefit from referral to a conventional doctor for assessment or treatment. Red flags are those symptoms and signs that indicate that referral should be considered. The red flags of diseases of the stomach are described in Table 3.1c-III. A summary of the red flags in a format designed for quick reference in clinical practice can be found in Appendix III. This gives advice on the degree of urgency of referral for each of the red flag conditions listed.

Table 3.1c-III A6: Red flags of diseases of the stomach

Red flag	Description	Reasoning
A6.1	Severe diarrhea and vomiting if lasting >24 hours in infants or elderly people	In most cases diarrhea and vomiting is self-limiting and will need no medical intervention. However, infants and elderly people are vulnerable to dehydration (see A3.4) and should be referred for assessment if symptoms continue for >24 hours
A6.2	Diarrhea and vomiting if continuing for >5 days in otherwise healthy adults	See A6.1. If symptoms persist for >5 days this is unusual and merits referral for investigation of infectious or inflammatory causes Food poisoning (diarrhea and vomiting from contaminated food) and infectious bloody diarrhea are notifiable diseases.* If a notifiable disease is a possibility, the patient should be advised to consult their doctor so that the disease can be reported for the benefit of public health
A6.3	Diarrhea and vomiting associated with features of dehydration (see Table A3: A3.4 and A3.5)	If features of dehydration (low blood pressure, dry mouth, concentrated urine, poor skin turgor and confusion) are apparent, refer as a matter of high priority, and urgently in infants and elderly people. In these cases continuing vomiting will exacerbate an already unstable situation Food poisoning and infectious bloody diarrhea are notifiable diseases (see A6.2)
A6.4	Vomiting of fresh blood or altered blood (looks like dark gravel or coffee grounds)	The appearance of blood in the vomit is always of concern as it is not possible to gauge the severity of bleeding and whether or not the internal bleeding is continuing Refer if more than about a tablespoon of blood appears in the vomit (small amounts may simply be the result of a tear of the esophagus lining during vomiting) The blood may originate from the stomach or the duodenum and may indicate peptic ulcer disease (PUD) or stomach cancer Refer urgently if there are any signs of shock (see A19.3). Signs of shock indicate that there could be dangerous levels of internal blood loss
A6.5	Projectile vomiting persisting for >2 days	Projectile vomiting (vomit appears at a much higher speed than usual) suggests high obstruction to the outflow of the stomach, and should be referred as there is high risk of loss of fluids and salts Refer as a high priority if this is suspected in a newborn baby (a sign of the congenital deformity of pyloric stenosis)
A6.6	Epigastric pain or dyspepsia for the first time in someone over the age of 40 or in anyone if resistant to treatment after six weeks	Pain from the stomach or duodenum typically radiates to the epigastric region (between acupoints REN-12 and REN-14). If the stomach is inflamed, this area can be tender on palpation, and there may be a sensation of acidity or fullness (dyspepsia). However, these symptoms are very common and can respond well to dietary modification and complementary medicine. Only refer if not responding to treatment within six weeks or if presenting for the first time in someone over 40 (as the risk of cancer is more common in older age groups) Persistent dyspeptic symptoms may result from *Helicobacter (H.) pylori* infection, and may respond well to antibiotic eradication treatment. Chronic *H. pylori* infection is associated with an increased risk of stomach cancer as well as peptic ulceration, so it is good medical practice for this infection to be treated
A6.7	Altered blood in stools (melena): stools look like black tar	Altered blood in stools (stools look tarry and have an unusual metallic smell) indicates bleeding from the more proximal aspects of the digestive tract, including the stomach. If melena is apparent in the stools, bleeding is significant and merits prompt referral

A6.8	Onset of severe abdominal pain with collapse (the acute abdomen): the pain can be constant or colicky (coming in waves); rigidity, guarding and rebound tenderness are serious signs	The acute abdomen refers to the combination of severe abdominal pain together with an inability to continue with day-to-day activities (collapse). This syndrome can have benign causes, such as irritable bowel syndrome, dysmenorrhea and ovulation pain, but needs high priority or urgent referral to exclude more serious conditions including appendicitis, perforated ulcer, peritonitis, obstructed bowel, pelvic inflammatory disease and gallstones
		Colicky pain indicates obstruction of a viscus (hollow organ)
		Rigidity of the abdomen, guarding (a reflex protective spasm of the abdominal muscles) and rebound tenderness (pain felt elsewhere in the abdomen when the pressure of palpating hand is released) all suggest inflammation or perforation of a viscus

* Notifiable diseases: notification of a number of specified infectious diseases is required of doctors in the UK as a statutory duty under the Public Health (Infectious Diseases) 1988 Act and the Public Health (Control of Diseases) 1988 Act, and, more recently, the Health Protection (Notification) Regulations 2010. The UK Health Protection Agency (HPA) Centre for Infections collates details of each case of each disease that has been notified. This allows analyses of local and national trends. This is one example of a situation in which there is a legal requirement for a doctor to breach patient confidentiality.

Diseases that are notifiable include: acute encephalitis, acute infectious hepatitis, acute poliomyelitis, anthrax, cholera, diphtheria, enteric fevers (typhoid and paratyphoid), food poisoning, infectious bloody diarrhea, leprosy, malaria, measles, meningitis (bacterial and viral forms), meningococcal septicemia (without meningitis), mumps, plague, rabies, rubella, scarlet fever, severe acute respiratory syndrome (SARS), smallpox, tetanus, tuberculosis, typhus, viral hemorrhagic fever, whooping cough, yellow fever.

3.1d Diseases of the pancreas, liver and gallbladder

This section focuses on the important diseases of the main accessory organs of the gastrointestinal tract: the pancreas, liver and gallbladder. These are:

- Diseases of the pancreas:
  - acute pancreatitis
  - chronic pancreatitis
  - cancer of the pancreas
  - cystic fibrosis (studied in Section 3.3d)
  - diabetes mellitus (studied in Section 5.1d)
- Diseases of the liver:
  - acute hepatitis
  - chronic hepatitis
  - cirrhosis of the liver
  - primary biliary cirrhosis (PBC)
  - cancer of the liver
- Diseases of the gallbladder:
  - gallstones
  - biliary colic and acute cholecystitis
  - chronic cholecystitis.

Before the individual diseases are described in turn, it is important to first introduce a syndrome (i.e. a condition with a characteristic constellation of symptoms and signs) that can result from a number of severe intra-abdominal diseases, the acute abdomen.

Acute abdomen

The acute abdomen is the general term used to describe a syndrome in which a patient becomes acutely ill and has symptoms and signs that are related to the abdomen. It can be caused by severe disease of any of the abdominal organs. The patient characteristically has severe abdominal pain, which has come on rapidly, and may be unable to move easily because of pain. The pain may be constant or intermittent. The syndrome is important as it is a common reason for an urgent admission to a hospital emergency department.

Not all diseases that cause an acute abdomen are serious (e.g. constipation and ovulation pain can occasionally lead to this syndrome), but if it occurs it should be taken seriously as it can be caused by some life-threatening conditions.

Any patient with this syndrome is usually assessed in a hospital emergency department by a surgeon, who will make an examination and perform tests to exclude any serious causes that may need urgent surgery.

Tables 3.1d-I and 3.1d-II list the important causes of an acute abdomen, and illustrate that not all the conditions are gastrointestinal. All these conditions are studied in detail in this and later sections.

Table 3.1d-I Serious causes of an acute abdomen

Perforation of the stomach, and small and large intestines

Rupture of a major organ (e.g. spleen, or fallopian tube in ectopic pregnancy)

Inflammation of an organ (e.g. pancreas, appendix, gallbladder)

Inflammation of the outer lining of the bowel (peritonitis)

Obstruction of the bowel

Stones in the bile ducts or ureter

Table 3.1d-II Less serious causes of an acute abdomen

Menorrhagia, ovulation pain and infections of the womb

Inflammatory bowel disease

Irritable bowel disease

Constipation

The acute abdomen has some characteristic signs that can be assessed by an examining doctor. These are rigidity, guarding and rebound tenderness, which develop because a serious problem in the abdominal cavity has caused the abdominal muscles and the bowel to go into spasm. The abdomen feels rock hard or rigid. The patient involuntarily protects the area by further muscle tension (guarding), and pain is particularly severe when an examining hand is lifted suddenly from the skin (rebound tenderness).

Sometimes these features are found only in a localized area. For example, in the womb infections known as pelvic inflammatory disease, rigidity, guarding and rebound tenderness may be found in the suprapubic area and right and left iliac fossae only. If the features are more generalized and the pain is worse centrally, this implies a more generalized problem such as peritonitis.

If a patient is developing the features of an acute abdomen, they require urgent medical assessment, or direct admission to a hospital emergency department if very unwell or frail.

Information box 3.1d-I

The acute abdomen: comments from a Chinese medicine perspective

In Chinese medicine, the acute abdomen would be viewed as a Full Condition (aggravated by pressure), which could be attributed to a range of syndromes according to the site of pain and exact pattern of symptoms.

These include Stasis of Blood in the Stomach, Liver Qi Stagnation invading the Spleen, Small Intestine Qi Pain, Small Intestine Qi Tied, Cold in the Intestines, Damp Heat in the Liver and Gallbladder, Damp Heat in the Intestines, Heat obstructing the Large Intestine, and Blood and Qi Stagnation in the Lower Jiao. Sometimes it is difficult to distinguish between these syndromes, but this may not be so important in practice as the treatment principles and points used for treatment of acute pain often overlap.

The diseases of the three major accessory organs are now considered. For a reminder of the physiology of these organs, see Section 3.1a.

Important diseases of the pancreas

Acute pancreatitis

As described in Section 3.1a, one important function of the pancreas is to release powerful enzymes of digestion via the pancreatic duct into the duodenum. In acute pancreatitis the pancreas is inflamed, and this inflammation causes the enzymes to be released within the pancreas tissue. This leads to a vicious cycle, in which the enzymes start digesting the pancreas itself, which in turn becomes more inflamed.

The most common known causes of acute pancreatitis are acute alcohol abuse, blockage of the pancreatic duct by a gallstone and infection by the mumps virus. However, in many cases no obvious cause can be found.

The condition of acute pancreatitis may be extremely severe. The inflammation of the pancreas leads to intense abdominal pain, nausea and vomiting, and fever. The pain also tends to be felt in the center of the back.

The pancreatic enzymes can penetrate into the peritoneal cavity, which causes generalized inflammation of the peritoneum, the lining of all the organs of the gastrointestinal tract. This condition is peritonitis, which has already been introduced as a possible outcome of perforation of a peptic ulcer. Pancreatitis is therefore a cause of the acute abdomen syndrome.

The treatment of pancreatitis involves urgent admission to hospital where the severity of the condition can be formally assessed. The digestive system is rested by ensuring the patient stays "nil by mouth," and fluids are given to the patient by intravenous drip. Mild cases can respond very quickly to this treatment, and many patients with pancreatitis (80 percent) achieve full recovery.

However, in the 20 percent of severe cases many patients may die (the mortality from severe acute pancreatitis is up to 30 percent) because the damage to the important organs of the gastrointestinal tract is too great to allow recovery. In those who recover, the pancreas may be permanently damaged, leading to the condition of chronic pancreatitis.[21]

Chronic pancreatitis

Chronic pancreatitis can result from the permanent damage resulting from an acute attack, or may develop gradually over the course of a few years. In this condition the pancreas is damaged and is unable to produce sufficient digestive enzymes (exocrine function), and in some cases may not be able to produce sufficient insulin (endocrine function).

The most common cause of chronic pancreatitis is long-term (ten years or more) high alcohol intake, but there are other rare causes, including cystic fibrosis and congenital susceptibility.

Initially, the main symptom is abdominal pain, which can be severe and may be felt in the epigastrium and the center of the back. Patients may need to take regular doses of very strong morphine-related painkillers. This can lead to problems with addiction.

 Information box 3.1d-II

Pancreatitis: comments from a Chinese medicine perspective

In Chinese medicine, the intense acute symptoms of pancreatitis might correspond to syndromes that include Small Intestine Qi Tied and Stagnation of Blood in the Intestines.

The chronic severe pain of pancreatitis suggests Blood Stagnation. The failure of digestion, with loose, foul-smelling stools, suggests Spleen Qi Deficiency and possibly Damp Heat invading the Spleen. This would fit with a history of alcohol abuse. Diabetes is called the Thirsting and Wasting Disease and corresponds to Internal Heat leading to Yin Deficiency.

Because pancreatic enzymes support the digestive process, and treat the diarrhea resulting from malabsorption, their action in Chinese medicine might be described in terms of nourishing Spleen Qi.

The lack of digestive enzymes will lead to the nutrients in the diet not being adequately absorbed. Instead, they are left in the bowel to become part of the stools, which become loose and foul smelling. This state is called malabsorption, and the patient will lose weight and suffer from vitamin deficiencies. If insulin production is affected, diabetes may develop (see Chapter 5.1).

The treatment of this condition is usually supportive only. The patient is urged to stop drinking alcohol and is given drugs for the pain. Synthetic pancreatic enzymes can be taken by mouth with meals for those with malabsorption. These assist in the digestion of food. Patients with diabetes are treated with insulin to control their blood sugar level. Occasionally, surgery to remove part of the damaged pancreas may be performed for pain relief. This is a major operation, and does not always make a great difference to the symptoms, particularly if the patient continues to drink alcohol.

Cancer of the pancreas

Pancreatic cancer is usually a disease of elderly people. As the pancreas is not contained in a tight anatomical space, this means that significant growth can occur before symptoms become apparent. Common first symptoms include back and abdominal pain, as the mass extends backwards to infiltrate local tissues, or jaundice, as the mass obstructs the flow of bile into the duodenum. Jaundice is a condition in which there is a yellow discoloration of the skin, and particularly the whites of the eyes. The backlog of bile caused by pancreatic cancer invading the bile duct leads to jaundice because the breakdown product of red blood cells, bilirubin, starts to build up in the bloodstream (for an explanation of the physiology, see Section 3.1a). Bilirubin in the skin causes itch, which can be extremely distressing. Excess bilirubin in the urine turns the urine dark, whereas the lack of bile in the stools means that stools become pale. Other symptoms include loss of appetite and loss of weight. Very rarely, the first symptoms will be those of the acute abdomen, as the tumor can rarely trigger an episode of acute pancreatitis.

The diagnosis of pancreatic cancer is a very serious one, as very few patients with this diagnosis (less than 2 percent) survive for more than two years. This is because by the time the tumor is detected it has usually grown to such a size as to be inoperable. Pancreatic cancer does not respond well to chemotherapy or radiotherapy. Very rarely, a major operation can be performed on small tumors, and this can improve the chances of survival.

The treatment is therefore usually palliative. Morphine-based painkillers are generally considered essential in advanced disease because the cancer invading backwards leads to severe abdominal and back pain. As jaundice can lead to uncomfortable itch and malaise, the blocked bile duct can be unblocked by inserting a thin tube, known as a stent, by means of an endoscope.

Information box 3.1d-III

Cancer of the pancreas: comments from a Chinese medicine perspective

In Chinese medicine, the type of pain associated with pancreatic cancer is usually a feature of Blood Stagnation. The growing mass suggests Phlegm. This fits with the fact that this cancer is considered more likely in those who smoke and have a high-fat diet. As always in cancer, there is an underlying severe deficiency, which in this case would most likely embrace Spleen Qi Deficiency and Stomach Yin Deficiency.

The red flags of diseases of the pancreas

Some patients with diseases of the pancreas will benefit from referral to a conventional doctor for assessment or treatment. Red flags are those symptoms and signs that indicate that referral should be considered. The red flags of diseases of the pancreas are described in Table 3.1d-III. A summary of the red flags in a format designed for quick reference in clinical practice can be found in Appendix III. This gives advice on the degree of urgency of referral for each of the red flag conditions listed.

Table 3.1d-III A7: Red flags of diseases of the pancreas

Red flag	Description	Reasoning
A7.1	Symptoms of acute pancreatitis: presents as acute abdomen (see A6.8) with severe central abdominal and back pain, vomiting and dehydration	Pancreatitis is a serious inflammatory condition of the pancreas that may develop for no obvious reason, but can be associated with high alcohol consumption or gallstone obstruction. The patient needs to be nil by mouth and urgently referred for supportive hospital care
A7.2	Symptoms of chronic pancreatitis: central abdominal and back pain, weight loss and loose stools over weeks to months	Chronic pancreatitis may result from long-term alcohol abuse, episodes of acute pancreatitis or be due to inherited tendency. The scarred pancreas can generate deep chronic pain, and the lack of digestive enzymes can lead to the syndrome of malabsorption (see A7.3). There is a risk of diabetes
A7.3	Malabsorption syndrome: loose pale stools and malnutrition; weight loss, thin hair, dry skin, cracked lips and peeled tongue	Malabsorption syndrome develops when there is an inability to absorb the nutrients in the diet, and weight loss and mineral and vitamin deficiencies result. Loose stools are the result of the presence of unabsorbed fat
	Will present as failure to thrive in children	Chronic pancreatitis (see A7.2) is one of the causes of the malabsorption syndrome. Other causes include celiac disease, Crohn's disease and intestinal lymphoma
A7.4	Jaundice: yellowish skin, yellow whites of the eyes, and possibly dark urine and pale stools; itch may be a prominent symptom	Jaundice results from a problem in the production of the bile by the liver or an obstruction to its outflow via the gallbladder into the duodenum. Pancreatic cancer may cause jaundice by growing to obstruct the outflow of the bile via the bile duct. Jaundice always merits referral for investigation of its cause

Important diseases of the liver

Acute hepatitis

Hepatitis literally means inflammation of the liver. The acute form of hepatitis has a wide range of possible causes. The most well-known cause is infection by the hepatitis virus, of which there are a number of types. Hepatitis A, B and C are the most important in terms of rates of significant infections. These viruses result in distinct disease syndromes, which will be summarized in more detail presently.

Other common causes of inflammation of the liver are other types of infectious agents, alcohol abuse and reactions to prescribed drugs. Many drugs in overdose, most notoriously paracetamol (acetaminophen), can cause severe inflammation of the liver.

Hepatitis has characteristic symptoms, irrespective of the cause. The inflamed liver leads to pain under the right side of the ribs (right hypochondrium). The inflammation affects the ability of the liver to clear toxins and also to clear the bilirubin from the bloodstream to make bile. The consequences of this are that the patient with hepatitis feels very unwell. The buildup of bilirubin in the bloodstream leads to jaundice that is indicated by the signs of yellow skin discoloration, dark urine and pale stools.

If the inflammation is very severe, acute hepatitis can lead to acute liver failure, which is life-threatening because the essential functions of maintaining adequate blood sugar levels and clearing toxins are totally lost. A patient with acute liver failure will rapidly fall into a coma if the condition is not reversed.

Treatment of hepatitis primarily involves the removal of any factors that may be causing further liver damage (e.g. prescription drugs), and to support the patient through recovery. In the case of paracetamol overdose, medication (acetylcysteine) can be given that reverses the toxic effect of the paracetamol if the patient can be treated early enough. Patients with acute liver failure will need specialized nursing, with administration of intravenous fluids and nutrients. In rare cases, liver transplantation can save the life of a patient with acute liver failure (see later for more detail on liver transplantation).

Viral hepatitis

The three most common hepatitis viruses each lead to a form of hepatitis with characteristic features.

Hepatitis A (infectious hepatitis) is the commonest form of hepatitis worldwide, and is contracted from contaminated food and water. Jaundice develops within two to six weeks of initial infection, during which time the patient is infectious. In most cases, after two to three weeks of feeling unwell, the patient makes a recovery. Most patients feel unwell for some time after this, and may remain unable to tolerate alcohol and fatty food for many months afterwards. Acute liver failure and death are very rare complications of hepatitis A, and this is more likely in elderly people. Hepatitis A vaccine that is offered to many travelers abroad offers good protection from contracting hepatitis A. A single dose gives immunity for one year, which is increased to ten years if a booster dose is given six months later.

Hepatitis B is a very different condition to hepatitis A, although it also leads to acute hepatitis. One major difference is that, even after recovery, the virus can persist in the blood of some people. These carriers of hepatitis B remain in a lifelong infectious state. Infection with the virus does not necessarily lead to inflammation of the liver, and may pass unnoticed. Therefore, not all carriers will be aware that they have had hepatitis. This is in contrast to hepatitis A, in which patients are no longer infectious after recovery.

The hepatitis B virus (HBV) can only be transmitted through infected body fluids such as semen or blood. In this way it is comparable to human immunodeficiency virus (HIV) infection. People at risk of contracting hepatitis B include healthcare workers who deal with body fluids,

drug users who share needles, those who have unprotected sex with virus carriers and babies born to mothers who carry the virus. Hepatitis B carriage is rare in Western populations, but in parts of Africa and the Far East up to 10–15 percent of the population may carry the virus. It is very important to make travelers to these parts of the world aware of this fact.

In those people who develop acute hepatitis, the disease is more severe than for hepatitis A. The incubation period is longer, with symptoms appearing one to six months after exposure. The hepatitis lasts for longer, and requires a longer recovery period. About 1 percent of patients with hepatitis B die from acute liver failure. A further 10 percent never fully recover, and instead develop a long-term condition called chronic hepatitis. In this condition the function of the liver gradually deteriorates until the terminal condition of cirrhosis develops (see later). These patients are also at particular risk of developing liver cancer. It is these long-term problems that make hepatitis B such a dreaded disease. Figure 3.1d-I illustrates the possible outcomes of acute hepatitis B infection.

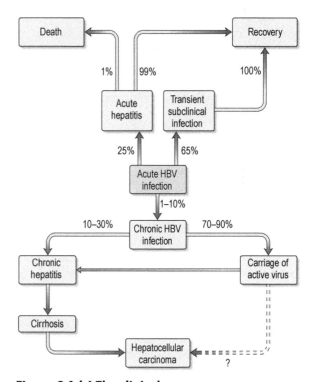

Figure 3.1d-I The clinical course of hepatitis B infection

Treatment for acute hepatitis B is generally supportive, although interferon-alfa 2b and other antiviral drugs may be prescribed in cases of chronic disease in which progressive liver damage and high levels of virus activity can be detected. This treatment is known to reduce the risk of the condition progressing to cirrhosis.

The vaccine for hepatitis B is usually only offered in the UK to healthcare workers, newborn babies of mothers who carry the virus and those who have close contact with at-risk people (e.g. prison officers). It is increasingly being offered in sexual health clinics to those who might be considered to have high-risk sexual behavior.

Hepatitis C causes a condition in which most patients do not develop the symptoms of acute hepatitis, but many continue to carry the virus. This has the serious long-term consequence of chronic hepatitis in up to 85 percent of those infected. In these patients there is particular risk of cirrhosis (develops in 20–30 percent) and liver cancer.

Hepatitis C was only identified in 1988, and it has been discovered to be the cause of thousands of cases of hepatitis resulting from blood transfusion prior to that date. Up to 80 percent of hemophiliacs are estimated to have been infected with hepatitis C prior to 1988. Nowadays, donated blood is tested for hepatitis C.

Hepatitis C is very common in the intravenous drug-using community, and is particularly virulent in those who have untreated HIV infection.

If hepatitis C is demonstrated by liver biopsy to be causing a moderate to severe form of liver fibrosis, long-term treatment with interferon-alfa and the antiviral drug ribavirin is recommended. This treatment needs to be maintained for at least 24 weeks, and is a cause of malaise and depression whilst it is ongoing. Nevertheless, this therapy gives a good chance of total clearance of infection in certain patient groups, depending particularly on the subtype of virus. In the UK, the decision to treat a case of hepatitis C in this way is always made by a specialist.

Chronic hepatitis

This long-term condition of inflammation of the liver has already been mentioned as a possible outcome of infection with hepatitis B and C. It can also be an outcome of an autoimmune process (see Section 2.2c).

The initial changes of chronic hepatitis will only be revealed by means of the liver function serum blood test. Over the course of time, damage to the liver cells revealed by this test worsens. An inexorable rise in the serum levels of liver enzymes such as aspartate transaminase signifies progressive damage to liver cells.

Corticosteroid drugs and immunosuppressant medication (such as azathioprine) are given to slow the progression of autoimmune chronic hepatitis. These drugs often have to be maintained long term to keep the disease at bay, and therefore patients will suffer from the side effects of long-term steroid treatment (see Section 2.2c). However, drug treatment is successful in inducing remission in 80 percent of cases.

Untreated or unresponsive chronic hepatitis eventually leads to damage of a substantial proportion of the liver cells, with areas of scarring within the liver substance.

When scarring has occurred, there is little hope of recovery of the function of the organ. This condition is called cirrhosis of the liver. If the disease progresses to cirrhosis, this means irreversible damage has occurred, and in the long term the only option the patient has for survival is liver transplantation.

Cirrhosis of the liver

The term cirrhosis is derived from the Greek word for yellow, a reflection of the jaundice that can develop in advanced cases. The most common causes of this state of cell damage and scarring to the liver are long-term alcohol abuse and viral hepatitis (B and C) infections. There are a number of much less common causes, including autoimmune hepatitis (described above) and biliary cirrhosis (described below). The conditions hemochromatosis, Wilson's disease and alpha-1-antitrypsin deficiency are rare genetically transmitted causes.

Serious chronic damage to the liver has a number of long-term effects. There are two main consequences of severe liver damage:

- gradual loss of the important functions of the liver due to loss of the liver cells

- increasing restriction of the usually free flow of blood through the liver due to the scarring.

These consequences are described below.

Loss of liver functions

Progressive damage to the liver cells means that the manufacture of sex hormones and blood proteins (including clotting factors) is impaired. In addition, bilirubin builds up in the bloodstream, toxins are not cleared from the body and the blood sugar level becomes unstable. This can lead to progressive symptoms and signs of bruising and bleeding, jaundice, itching, illness and confusion. The nails become pale because of reduced proteins in the bloodstream. Pubic hair can become thin, and men may develop breast tissue and shrunken testicles due to problems in the manufacture of the sex hormones. Increasing confusion and the onset of a coma resulting from accumulated toxins is the most common cause of death in cirrhosis.

Another characteristic feature of chronic liver disease that can be found on examination of the skin is the presence of more than five small (2–6mm diameter) stars of broken veins on the face, arms or hands. These are known as spider nevi because of their shape.

Restriction of blood flow through the liver

Scarring around the blood vessels that drain blood from the digestive tract through the liver leads to a buildup of pressure within the blood vessels of the digestive tract. This can lead to stretching of these veins under pressure, which then become dilated (varicose). The most serious consequence of this is that varicose veins in the esophagus can spontaneously rupture, leading to severe hemorrhage into the stomach. This often comes without any warning symptoms or signs. The patient will suddenly start to vomit darkened blood, and may collapse due to extreme blood loss. This is also a common cause of death in cirrhosis.

A combination of increased pressure in the digestive circulation and low blood protein leads to the movement of fluid from the bloodstream out into the tissues (edema). This occurs particularly in the peritoneal area surrounding the lower digestive organs, so that the abdomen noticeably swells with the fluid. Fluid accumulating in the peritoneal space is called ascites. Ankles and calves may also become swollen.

A final complication of cirrhosis is that it increases the risk of liver cancer, presumably as a result of chronic damage to the liver tissue.

A sinister aspect of cirrhosis is that it tends to develop silently, and symptoms generally only become apparent once the disease process is very advanced. The complexity of the features of chronic liver disease/cirrhosis is illustrated in Figure 3.1d-II.

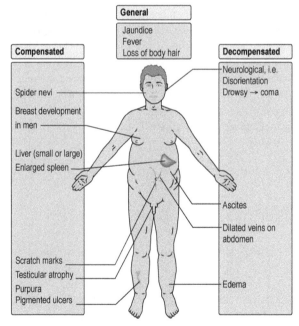

Figure 3.1d-II The physical signs seen in cirrhosis of the liver

Treatment for cirrhosis is limited. Patients with cirrhosis from alcohol abuse are urged strongly to stop drinking, but for those with an alcohol problem, this often comes much too late in their habit to be able to make changes. If ascites has developed, a low-salt diet may be recommended and diuretics prescribed.

Esophageal hemorrhage is a medical emergency from which one in five patients dies. The endoscope is used to visualize and treat the bleeding veins. However, for those who survive this, the risk of a repeat bleed within the next two years is very high.

The only potential cure for cirrhosis is to transplant the liver. Patients receive a liver from a donor who has died no more than 20 hours earlier. The recipient has to remain on lifelong immunosuppressant drug treatment (see Section 2.2c) to suppress the immune system and prevent the body from rejecting the foreign liver. This means that the patient will suffer from the side effects of these powerful drugs, and will be at increased risk of opportunistic infections. The immunosuppressants are commonly prescribed in combination, and include tacrolimus, ciclosporin, azathioprine and corticosteroids.

Nevertheless, liver transplantation is one of the most successful transplant procedures, with over 75 percent of recipients surviving to at least five years following the operation. Most centers do not offer the possibility of this operation to those who cannot abstain from alcohol.

 Information box 3.1d-IV

Hepatitis: comments from a Chinese medicine perspective

In Chinese medicine, the symptoms of acute hepatitis correspond to Damp Heat in the Liver and Gallbladder, and possibly the Spleen, depending on the balance of symptoms. The profound condition of acute liver failure might be interpreted as embracing depletion of Liver Yin.

Chronic hepatitis and cirrhosis are the long-term consequence of Damp Heat in the Liver and Gallbladder, which in turn leads to a complex state of energetic depletion. The tendency to profuse bleeds, itching and broken veins on the face reflect the presence of Internal Heat. The loss of the substance of the Liver Organ suggests depletion of Liver Yin, presumably as a consequence of the Heat. Edema in advanced liver disease is a result of low blood albumin and also excessive constriction of the portal venous system. The edema develops slowly, is located in dependent parts of the body and is pitting in nature. In the absence of signs of Heat or Wind, in Chinese medicine all these would be attributed to depletion of either Spleen or Kidney Yang. Tendency to cancer and the end-stage occurrence of confusion and coma may be a reflection of insubstantial Phlegm, a consequence of long-standing Damp Heat and Stagnation.

Primary biliary cirrhosis (PBC)

Primary biliary cirrhosis (PBC) is a rare autoimmune condition in which damage occurs to the tiny bile ducts in the liver. It predominantly affects women around the age of 50, and is commonly associated with other autoimmune conditions such as thyroid disease, rheumatoid arthritis and glomerulonephritis.

The first symptoms include tiredness, itch and malaise and the progressive development of jaundice. Diarrhea can develop because of poor fat absorption. The condition is diagnosed by means of a rise in alkaline phosphatase on serum testing of liver function and the presence of characteristic antimitochondrial antibodies (AMA). Definitive diagnosis is by liver biopsy.

Treatments can be given to relieve itch (cholestyramine) and diarrhea (codeine). One drug, ursodeoxycholic acid, may slow progression of the disease, but in many cases the outlook is very poor, particularly once jaundice has developed. Immune suppressant drugs may be used, but studies suggest not always beneficial effects, and these might therefore readily outweigh the benefits. Approximately 50–70 percent of patients are alive ten years after diagnosis. There is a risk of recurrence of the disease in a transplanted liver, but this is the only treatment that offers any chance of a cure.[22]

Cancer of the liver

Cancer in the liver is very common, but in 90 percent of cases is due to secondary spread of a cancer originating elsewhere. The most common primary sites for secondary liver cancer are the digestive tract, the breast and the lung. Once cancer has spread to the liver it is very rare for the person to be cured.

Primary cancer arising in the liver is much less common. It is most common in those who are carrying the hepatitis B or C virus, or in those who have cirrhosis of the liver. The only possible treatment is surgery, including liver transplantation in certain cases, but the cancer is only rarely operable. Most people with this cancer die within six months of diagnosis.

Both types of cancer can present with symptoms and signs of an enlarged liver, pain in the right hypochondrium, with weight loss and loss of appetite.

Information box 3.1d-V

Cancer of the liver: comments from a Chinese medicine perspective

In Chinese medicine, both primary and secondary cancer of the liver may correspond to Blood Stagnation or Phlegm on a background of long-standing Deficiency of Yin, Yang, Qi or Blood. The pain and swelling in the right hypochondrium is characteristic of Liver Blood and Qi Stagnation.

The red flags of diseases of the liver

Some patients with diseases of the liver will benefit from referral to a conventional doctor for assessment or treatment. Red flags are those symptoms and signs that indicate that referral should be considered. The red flags of diseases of the liver are described in Table 3.1d-IV. A summary of the red flags in a format designed for quick reference in clinical practice can be found in Appendix III. This gives advice on the degree of urgency of referral for each of the red flag conditions listed.

Table 3.1d-IV A8: Red flags of diseases of the liver

Red flag	Description	Reasoning
A8.1	Jaundice: yellowish skin, yellow whites of the eyes, and possibly dark urine and pale stools; itch may be a prominent symptom	Jaundice results from a problem in the production of the bile by the liver or an obstruction to its outflow via the gallbladder into the duodenum
		Jaundice may result from inflammation of the liver (hepatitis) or from liver cancer
		Hepatitis can be a result of infection (e.g. hepatitis A, B or C or glandular fever) and can also result from inflammation caused by certain prescription medications and alcohol
		Jaundice always merits referral for investigation of its cause
		Viral hepatitis of any form is a notifiable disease*
A8.2	Right hypochondriac pain (pain under the right ribs) with malaise for >3 days	This suggests liver or gallbladder pathology and should be considered for investigation, even in the absence of jaundice, if persisting for >3 days

A8.3	Vomiting of fresh blood or altered blood (looks like dark gravel or coffee grounds)	The appearance of blood in the vomit is always of concern as it is not possible to gauge the severity of bleeding and whether or not the bleeding is continuing
		Refer if more than about a tablespoon of blood appears in the vomit (small amounts may simply be the result of a tear of the esophagus lining during vomiting)
		There can be profuse bleeding from the base of the esophagus in chronic liver disease, as distended varicose veins (varices) can rupture in this site. The patient in this situation can easily go into shock (see A19.3) and should be treated as an emergency
A8.4	Known liver disease with the syndrome of edema, bruising and confusion	Liver disease may remain in a stable state for months to years, but the patient may become suddenly much more unwell once the disease has progressed to a certain point. This is the point at which the liver is no longer able to perform its function of the manufacture of blood proteins (including those necessary for blood clotting) and detoxification
		Bruising, edema and confusion can result. This syndrome requires urgent medical management

* Notifiable diseases: notification of a number of specified infectious diseases is required of doctors in the UK as a statutory duty under the Public Health (Infectious Diseases) 1988 Act and the Public Health (Control of Diseases) 1988 Act, and, more recently, the Health Protection (Notification) Regulations 2010. The UK Health Protection Agency (HPA) Centre for Infections collates details of each case of each disease that has been notified. This allows analyses of local and national trends. This is one example of a situation in which there is a legal requirement for a doctor to breach patient confidentiality.

Diseases that are notifiable include: acute encephalitis, acute infectious hepatitis, acute poliomyelitis, anthrax, cholera, diphtheria, enteric fevers (typhoid and paratyphoid), food poisoning, infectious bloody diarrhea, leprosy, malaria, measles, meningitis (bacterial and viral forms), meningococcal septicemia (without meningitis), mumps, plague, rabies, rubella, scarlet fever, severe acute respiratory syndrome (SARS), smallpox, tetanus, tuberculosis, typhus, viral hemorrhagic fever, whooping cough, yellow fever.

Important diseases of the gallbladder

Gallstones

As described in Section 3.1a, the gallbladder is a storage vessel for bile, which is manufactured in the liver. Bile consists of some waste products, including bilirubin, and also chemicals called bile salts, which are essential for the digestion of fats. In addition, bile contains the fatty substance cholesterol.

In some people the composition of this rich mixture in the gallbladder becomes unbalanced, so that some of the substances come out of solution and form solid masses. This is more likely to occur if cholesterol is present in excess in the bloodstream, a result, in part, of the rich Western diet. These masses, which can range in size from that of lead shot to large marbles, are known as gallstones.

Gallstones, which tend to rest in the gallbladder, very often cause no problem. It is estimated that up to one-fifth of adults in the West have gallstones and less than one in five of these will develop any problem from them. They are twice as common a finding in women as in men, and seem particularly common in overweight Western women of late childbearing age.

Information box 3.1d-VI

Gallstones: comments from a Chinese medicine perspective

In Chinese medicine, the condensation of the fluid bile to form masses would be seen as condensation of Phlegm. This fits with the observation that a fatty diet predisposes to gallstones.

Biliary colic and acute cholecystitis

Figure 3.1d-III is a diagrammatic representation of the liver and gallbladder. It illustrates the problems that can result from gallstones: the stones can leave the gallbladder and become lodged in either the neck of the gallbladder or the cystic duct, or in the common bile duct, which leads into the duodenum, or finally in the pancreatic duct.

Stones in the neck of the gallbladder or cystic duct obstruct the outward flow of bile. The gallbladder contracts against a resistance, which causes intense pain often in the left upper abdomen and radiating up the back in between the shoulder blades. Because the contractions occur in waves, the intense pain may also come in waves. At its peak the pain can be so severe as to cause the patient to writhe, sweat and vomit. Pain that fluctuates in intensity like this is conventionally termed colic. This pain is therefore known as biliary colic, but actually in some cases may be constant and severe for a few hours at a time. Biliary colic may be brought on after a fatty meal, because it is the presence of fat in the duodenum that stimulates the contraction of the gallbladder.

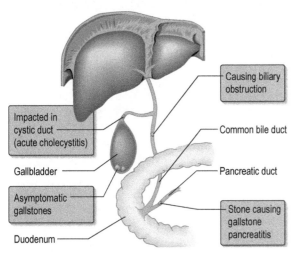

Impacted in cystic duct (acute cholecystitis)

Gallbladder

Asymptomatic gallstones

Duodenum

Causing biliary obstruction

Common bile duct

Pancreatic duct

Stone causing gallstone pancreatitis

Figure 3.1d-III The important clinical outcomes of gallstones

Often the stone drops back into the gallbladder, and the attack will subside. Sometimes the stone becomes impacted. This means that the bile in the gallbladder becomes stagnant, and eventually infection will develop. The gallbladder then becomes very inflamed and the patient becomes acutely unwell, and this is described as acute cholecystitis. The term cholecystitis is derived from the Greek roots *chole* meaning bile and *cystis* meaning bladder. The features of the acute abdomen are part of the clinical picture. The condition needs urgent treatment to relieve the blockage before the infection leads to the patient becoming very unwell with peritonitis.

Stones in the common bile duct will not only cause colic as the fine duct contracts to release bile into the duodenum, but will also prevent the free flow of bile from the liver. This means that, as was described for pancreatic cancer, bilirubin cannot be cleared from the blood by the liver. It therefore starts building up in the blood, and the patient becomes jaundiced.

Sometimes a stone becomes lodged at the far end of the common bile duct at the sphincter of Oddi, where the pancreatic duct opens into the duodenum (see Figure 3.1d-III). This is how gallstones can cause pancreatitis, as a stone at this site will block the free outflow of pancreatic enzymes.

The simple non-invasive ultrasound scan is used to distinguish acute cholecystitis from the other abdominal conditions. In the case of cholecystitis this will reveal gallstones in a thickened and distended gallbladder.

If iagnosis is uncertain, a test called a hepatobiliary imino-diacetic acid (HIDA) scan may be performed; this scan, which involves the injection of a radioactively marked precursor chemical, tracks the flow of bile from the liver and will expose whether or not bile is entering the gallbladder. Increasingly, a non-invasive MRI scan called magnetic resonance cholangiopancreatography (MRCP) may be used, as this produces clear three-dimensional images of the biliary ducts and gallbladder, together with associated structures.

The pain of an acute attack of cholecystitis is treated with powerful opiate painkillers given by injection. These not only relieve the colic, but may also allow the gallbladder and ducts to relax so that the stone either drops back into the gallbladder or is passed into the duodenum. Opiate painkillers are studied in more detail in Section 4.2c. Many patients with an attack settle down if they are kept nil by mouth, as this will remove the stimulation of the gallbladder to contract. Strong antibiotics are given because it is assumed infection of the stagnant bile in the gallbladder is also part of the condition.

Most people who have had an acute attack will be offered a cholecystectomy to remove the gallbladder. This is because it is very common for attacks of acute cholecystitis to recur. This is considered the best treatment for this condition. It is now preferably performed by means of a flexible telescope (laparoscope) through a tiny keyhole incision in the right hypochondrium. Patients tend to recover quickly from this operation. In fit people the operation can be performed whilst they are in hospital within two to three days of the acute attack, while in the less fit the attack is allowed to settle down so that the patient can be in the best possible physical state for a planned (elective) operation.

The conventional understanding is that the loss of the gallbladder has no ill effects in most people. It is recognized, however, that some people suffer from long-term uncomfortable symptoms after surgery. A recurrence of pain similar to biliary colic in the months to years after gallbladder removal is known as the post-cholecystectomy syndrome. In many cases this is attributed to excessive bowel spasm, but in a few the causes may be a retained gallstone or spasm of the sphincter of Oddi, problems that can sometimes be relieved by another minor operation.

If stones are blocked in the common bile duct they can be removed at the same time as a visualization procedure using an endoscope. This is known as endoscopic retrograde cholangiopancreatography (ERCP). The endoscope is passed into the duodenum, from where a fine tube is inserted into the opening of the common bile duct. Contrast medium is injected up the common bile duct so that X-ray images can be taken of the biliary tree. Guided by X-rays, an instrument is passed through this tube to capture the lodged stone and drag it into the duodenum.

If ERCP-guided removal of stones fails, open surgery is necessary.

Patients who opt not to have the operation after their acute attack can help their condition by cutting down on the amount of fats in their diet. Drugs (including the synthetic bile salts, e.g. ursodeoxycholic acid, and statins, e.g. simvastatin) can be prescribed that encourage the gallstones to dissolve back into the bile. Another option is to break up the stones using an ultrasound technique called lithotripsy. This does not require an operation, but is only likely to be successful if the stones are greater than 10mm in diameter.

Although removal of stones by endoscopy, drugs or shock waves can be effective, the stones may recur because the root cause has not been dealt with.[23]

Chronic cholecystitis
Chronic cholecystitis is the term given to a condition in which there are recurrent bouts of griping right-sided hypochondrial pain together with an intolerance of fatty food. The patient may complain of wind or indigestion, and may take antacids in an attempt to relieve the symptoms.

It used to be believed that the symptoms were due to a chronically inflamed gallbladder. This was because in some (but not all) people an ultrasound scan showed a shrunken gallbladder with stones. However, it was found that removal of the gallbladder often did not necessarily remove the symptoms. It is now considered that chronic cholecystitis is a functional condition, in that the symptoms do not seem to be related to a specific gallbladder problem. Chronic cholecystitis is therefore seen as a condition very like irritable bowel syndrome (see Section 3.1e). There is no satisfactory medical treatment for these symptoms.

It is important to recognize that conventional medicine does not readily address the root cause of gallbladder disease. For this reason, lifestyle changes and Chinese medicine may have a lot to offer a patient who suffers from gallstones. It would be reasonable to counsel a patient who suffers from acute cholecystitis to accept urgent pain relief if treatment has not helped, but to consider delaying a decision to have surgery while they see if alternative treatment approaches, addressing emotional factors and dietary change are of benefit.

Information box 3.1d-VII

Cholecystitis: comments from a Chinese medicine perspective

In Chinese medicine, the acute attack of acute cholecystitis corresponds to Damp Heat in the Liver and Gallbladder, with underlying Phlegm. The intense pain of biliary colic suggests that Blood Stagnation is also present, possibly as a consequence of Heat and Qi Stagnation.

Damp Heat in the Liver and Gallbladder can be attributed, in part, to Damp and Hot foods in the diet or climatic factors. In addition, a major factor in its causation is considered to be suppressed frustration, leading to Stagnation of Liver Qi. This emotional component is not recognized in conventional medicine.

The symptoms of chronic cholecystitis fit with Liver Qi Stagnation invading the Spleen, or Damp Heat in the Liver and Gallbladder.

A gallstone may be interpreted as a manifestation of Insubstantial Phlegm, a result of the steaming and brewing of Phlegm by Heat. Therefore, treatments that allow the passage of a stone may be described in terms of expelling this accumulated Phlegm. However, these do not address the root cause of the problem, and thus are energetically suppressive in nature. Likewise, removal of the gallbladder does not address the root cause, and it would make sense that such a procedure would cause further depletion of Liver and Gallbladder Qi. The underlying causes of Damp Heat in the Liver and Gallbladder have not been addressed, and this could explain why some people suffer from persistent symptoms.

The red flags of diseases of the gallbladder
Some patients with diseases of the gallbladder will benefit from referral to a conventional doctor for assessment or treatment. Red flags are those symptoms and signs that indicate that referral should be considered. The red flags of diseases of the gallbladder are described in Table 3.1d-V. A summary of the red flags in a format designed for quick reference in clinical practice can be found in Appendix III. This gives advice on the degree of urgency of referral for each of the red flag conditions listed.

Table 3.1d-V A9: Red flags of diseases of the gallbladder

Red flag	Description	Reasoning
A9.1	Jaundice: yellowish skin, yellow whites of the eyes, and possibly dark urine and pale stools; itch may be a prominent symptom	Jaundice results from a problem in the production of bile by the liver or an obstruction to its outflow via the gallbladder into the duodenum
		Jaundice may result from sudden obstruction of the flow of bile by a gallstone. In this case it is usually accompanied by severe colicky pain (see A6.8)
		Jaundice can also develop slowly as a result of gradual obstruction by a tumor of the outflow of the gallbladder
		Jaundice always merits referral for investigation of its cause
A9.2	Right hypochondriac pain (pain under the right ribs) with malaise for >3 days	This suggests liver or gallbladder pathology and should be considered for investigation, even in the absence of jaundice, if persisting for >3 days
A9.3	Right hypochondriac pain that is very intense and comes in waves. May be associated with fever and vomiting. May be associated with jaundice. This is one of the manifestations of the acute abdomen (see A6.8)	Obstruction of bile ducts by gallstones causes waves of intense pain as the duct attempts to contract against the obstruction. Fever and malaise can develop as the obstructed gallbladder becomes inflamed

3.1e Diseases of the small intestine and large intestine

This section describes the important diseases of the lower digestive tract, that is, the small intestine and colon (including the rectum and anus). These are:

- Diseases of the small intestine:
  - malabsorption syndrome
  - celiac disease
  - inflammatory bowel disease – Crohn's disease
  - intestinal obstruction
  - abdominal hernias
- Diseases of the large intestine:
  - irritable bowel syndrome (IBS)
  - constipation
  - appendicitis
  - diverticulitis
  - inflammatory bowel disease – ulcerative colitis
  - cancer of the colon and rectum
- Diseases of the anus:
  - hemorrhoids
  - anal fissure
  - rectal prolapse.

Important diseases of the small intestine

Malabsorption syndrome

The concept of malabsorption was introduced when chronic pancreatitis was described in Section 3.1d. In chronic pancreatitis, the essential nutrients that should be obtained from the diet cannot be absorbed because the pancreatic enzymes are lacking and so the food cannot be fully digested in the small intestine.

In small intestinal disease, malabsorption occurs for a different reason. In this case, although the pancreatic enzymes have fully digested the food into small molecules, the lining of the intestine is diseased, and this prevents their absorption.

There are a number of intestinal diseases that can lead to malabsorption, the most common being celiac disease and Crohn's disease (discussed below). All these diseases have features in common, all resulting from the fact that lack of absorbed nutrients leads to malnutrition. The patient with malabsorption will lose weight and their muscles will waste. Anemia occurs due to deficiencies of iron, vitamin B12 and folic acid. A wide range of other symptoms can occur due to other vitamin deficiencies.

Excess nutrients, including undigested fat, pass into the colon. These lead to loose, foul-smelling stools with excess gas. The patient may suffer from abdominal distension and vague abdominal pain.

Malabsorption is confirmed by detecting fat and nutrients in the stools. Blood tests will reveal anemia and features of other vitamin deficiencies. Endoscopy, barium contrast X-ray studies, ERCP (endoscopic retrograde cholangiopancreatography) and biopsy are used to examine the lining of the small intestine and pancreas.

The treatment of malabsorption is to treat the cause. Without this, oral vitamin and nutrient supplements cannot be of help because these, too, will not be absorbed. While the cause is being treated, it may be necessary to administer nourishment by means of intravenous drip (total parenteral nutrition) if the patient is extremely undernourished.

Information box 3.1e-I

Malabsorption: comments from a Chinese medicine perspective

In Chinese medicine, the symptoms and signs of malabsorption correspond to Spleen Qi or Yang Deficiency. The anemia corresponds to the Blood Deficiency that occurs as a result.

Celiac disease

This term originates from the Greek word *koelia*, meaning belly. In celiac disease the lining of the small intestine is damaged as a result of sensitivity to gluten, a component of wheat, barley, rye and oats. Gluten sensitivity is relatively common, affecting just less than one in 100 people, although many people are never diagnosed. This appears to run in families.

Celiac disease may never be diagnosed because the sensitivity is not always very severe. In some people, slight digestive problems may be the only consequence of having the condition.

In severe cases the condition becomes apparent in childhood. Affected children will not put on weight or grow adequately after weaning. Sometimes diagnosis is delayed until adulthood, when for some reason the sensitivity worsens and the patient starts to lose weight and develop abdominal discomfort and diarrhea.

Gluten sensitivity can be diagnosed by means of detecting particular antibodies or digestive enzymes that are present in the blood of 95 percent of people with celiac disease. A reversible flattened appearance to the intestinal lining is seen if a biopsy is taken from the duodenum, and this more invasive investigation is the definitive test. Celiac disease has been found to run very significantly in families, with one in ten first-degree relatives of a person with celiac disease sharing the diagnosis. Easy access to accurate blood testing for the condition has led to many children with a parent or sibling with celiac disease being diagnosed before serious malabsorption has become apparent.

The treatment of the condition is total lifelong avoidance of dietary gluten. This leads to a dramatic reversal of symptoms in most people. In some patients any slight lapse, such as eating a piece of cake, can lead to recurrence of symptoms.

Long-term poor control of symptoms is known to carry risks over and above those of malabsorption. Other complications of untreated celiac disease include increased risk of miscarriage and a modestly increased risk of intestinal cancer.

Information box 3.1e-II

Celiac disease: comments from a Chinese medicine perspective

In Chinese medicine, celiac disease corresponds to Spleen Qi or Yang Deficiency. The patients with celiac disease appear to be particularly vulnerable to the Damp nature of gluten-rich foods.

Inflammatory bowel disease – Crohn's disease

The term inflammatory bowel disease is used to embrace two conditions: Crohn's disease and ulcerative colitis. These have some features in common and may be very difficult to distinguish in practice.

Crohn's disease is a condition that can affect any portion of the digestive tract, but most commonly leads to disease of the small intestine and the colon. The cause of Crohn's disease is unknown, although it is recognized to be more common in smokers and those who eat a high-sugar, low-fiber diet. Claims that its incidence has a relationship to measles infection or measles vaccine have not been proven conventionally. The disease does tend to run in families.

Ulcerative colitis is a condition that is confined to the colon. For this reason it is described in more detail later.

In Crohn's disease, the bowel spontaneously becomes inflamed and thickened. In 30 percent of patients only the small bowel is affected and in 30 percent it is the large bowel only that is affected. In the remainder both the small and large bowel are complicated by disease. Deep ulcers form in the lining of the affected bowel. This leads to malabsorption if the small bowel is affected and diarrhea with profuse pus and mucus if the colon is affected. Often blood can be found mixed in the stools. In both cases, the abdominal pain is gripy and can be severe. Commonly mouth ulcers occur, and the patient feels generally unwell.

The inflamed bowel can adhere to other structures in the abdominal cavity, and sometimes the ulcers erode through to another organ forming a fistula (see Section 2.2b).

Feces, pus and mucus can then pass through the fistula to different sites, such as the bladder, or even out onto the skin.

The condition tends to come on for the first time in adulthood, often at a time of stress. Smoking increases the risk of aggressive disease. Symptoms tend to become manifest in bouts called relapses. The diarrhea and pain can be so severe as to fit the syndrome of the acute abdomen, and so can result in emergency hospital admission.

The treatment is to rest the bowel by ensuring the patient remains nil by mouth. Sometimes this is sufficient to allow the attack to settle down and the patient to resume normal life for a while. The anti-inflammatory aspirin-related medication mesalazine may be used to help maintain remission, but there are doubts about its effectiveness for all people. In more severe cases, corticosteroids or other immunosuppressant drugs are given (see Section 2.2c), sometimes for weeks on end. These include azathioprine and methotrexate and also the cytokine modulators infliximab and adalimumab. A very simple diet (elemental diet) can be prescribed, which helps healing, but a return to a normal diet can cause a relapse.

The symptoms in some patients do not settle even with powerful drug treatment. Persistent diarrhea and inflammation can lead to loss of essential nutrients and salts. In these patients emergency surgery is performed to remove the affected length of bowel. The majority of sufferers with Crohn's disease will require abdominal surgery in their lifetime. In some cases the problems caused by the acute attack are so severe that the patient dies.

A relatively minor surgical treatment for Crohn's disease is the formation of a defunctioning ileostomy. In this operation the small intestine is opened out onto the skin of the right iliac fossa. This means that the fluid contents of the small intestine pass out of this opening and allow the colon to be rested. This can help the inflammation to settle down, and immediately relieves the symptom of diarrhea. At a later date the ileostomy is surgically repaired and normal bowel function can be resumed.

Sometimes, because of widespread inflammation, it is necessary to remove the whole of the colon and rectum and a portion of the small intestine. The end of the remaining small intestine is opened to form an ileostomy (from the medical term for the small intestine, the ileum), and in this case the ileostomy is permanent. The feces that normally enter the colon are discharged out of the ileostomy and into a bag placed over the opening. Unlike normal feces, the discharge is much more fluid and continuous, so the bag has to be emptied frequently.

Surgery is also necessary if fistulas form between the digestive tract and another organ or the skin. Fistulas occur in 10 percent of cases.

Crohn's disease is a serious condition, which can seriously affect quality of life. Up to 80 percent of sufferers may require abdominal surgery in their lifetime.[24]

 Information box 3.1e-III

Crohn's disease: comments from a Chinese medicine perspective

In Chinese medicine, the symptoms of Crohn's disease are complex and varied. They could broadly be attributed to Liver Qi Stagnation invading the Spleen, Spleen Yang Deficiency and Damp Heat in the Large Intestines.

Intestinal obstruction

The passage through (the lumen of) the small intestine and colon can become blocked for a variety of reasons. These include the inflammation of Crohn's disease, and diverticulitis and cancerous growths. A loop of the bowel can also become pinched as it penetrates into the small opening of a hernia (see below) or by the scarring that can follow surgery (adhesions).

A blockage of the bowel has comparable effects to the blockage of the bile ducts. As the bowel contracts against the blockage, the patient experiences waves of colicky pain. A blockage in the small intestine will rapidly lead to vomiting and dehydration as the contents of the digestive tract are forced backwards by the contractions. A blockage of the colon is more likely to lead to distension as gas and fluid accumulates in the small intestine. Eventually, vomiting will also occur. If the blockage is persistent, whether in the small intestine or colon, it will lead sooner or later to the acute abdomen syndrome, and require urgent surgical attention.

The patient is treated by being kept nil by mouth, and open surgery is used to excise the affected segment of bowel. The two remaining ends of the bowel are usually sewn back together.

If the colon is obstructed close to the rectum, a colostomy may have to be formed, which may or may not be possible to reverse at a later date. A colostomy looks similar to an ileostomy, but the feces that are passed into the bag have a normal consistency. A colostomy is therefore generally easier for the patient to manage than an ileostomy.

Abdominal hernias

Hernia is the term used to describe the situation when the contents of a body cavity become displaced outside of the cavity through a breach in the fascia of the cavity wall. An example already described in Section 3.1c is the hiatus hernia, where part of the stomach has become displaced above the diaphragm through a breach in the fascia surrounding the muscular cardiac sphincter.

In abdominal hernias some of the soft and moveable intra-abdominal contents of loops of bowel, associated fat and blood vessels become displaced outside the muscular abdominal wall. Breaches can develop in the abdominal wall either as a result of congenital weakness in the fascia, or because of the excessive intra-abdominal pressure that can result from coughing, straining, obesity and pregnancy. Common sites for abdominal hernias to develop include the region of the umbilicus, the linea alba (which separates the two bands of the rectus abdominis muscle), the inguinal canal (through which the spermatic cord passes to reach the testicles), and the femoral canal (through which the femoral artery, vein and nerve pass to reach the front of the thigh). Inguinal and femoral hernias appear as smooth bulges in the groin. In all cases hernias represent a movement of tissue out of its usual fascial compartment.

In their early stages, hernias tend to appear when the person is standing, or when the intra-abdominal pressure is raised, for example, when they cough. The hernia appears as a bulge and may be associated with a dragging discomfort. In most cases the hernia will disappear if the patient lies down. If the hernia does not reduce easily on lying down or with firm pressure, it is said to be incarcerated.

Information box 3.1e-IV

Intestinal obstruction and hernia: comments from a Chinese medicine perspective

In Chinese medicine, the acute pain of obstruction might correspond to Small Intestine Qi Tied and/or Liver Qi Stagnation invading the Spleen. Vomiting in intestinal obstruction is the result of reversed waves of peristalsis. It is vigorous in nature and would be described as a Full condition. Reversed peristalsis might be described in terms of Stomach Qi rebelling upwards, as a result of Stagnation of Liver Qi.

A region of herniation suggests deficiency in the holding power of the Spleen Qi. The hernia is a breach in the fascial boundaries that contain the abdominal contents. This might also suggest a deficiency in the Triple Burner organ, the "Organ with no form" that has been described by Keown (2014) as corresponding to the fascial boundaries of the three major compartments of the torso.[25]

Minor hernias may be simply left untreated if not causing too much discomfort, or alternatively may be made more comfortable by the application of pressure. For example, an inguinal truss may be worn to support the region of an inguinal hernia. However, surgical repair of hernias is usually a straightforward operation and is usually recommended. In many cases it can be performed as a laparoscopic (keyhole) day-case procedure and has a relatively rapid recovery time (return to work and driving in less than two weeks).

The reason why surgical repair of a hernia is often recommended is that a hernia poses a risk that loops of bowel and their associated blood supply can become trapped and pinched in the sac of the hernia. This can then lead to the syndrome of intestinal obstruction or even death of bowel tissue. In this case, the patient will experience the symptoms of intestinal obstruction, including intense colicky abdominal pain, abdominal distension and vomiting. An experienced surgeon may be able to reduce the trapped hernia manually back into its correct compartment of the body, but in most cases emergency surgery will be required to treat an obstructed hernia.

Important diseases of the large intestine

Irritable bowel syndrome (IBS)

Irritable bowel syndrome (IBS), formerly medically described as spastic colon and functional bowel disease, is a very common condition in which it is understood that poorly coordinated muscular contractions of the bowel lead to pain and irregular bowel movements. Over 20 percent of typically young adults in developed countries may suffer from this condition, many of whom do no present to a doctor. The term functional means that the symptoms have no physically measurable cause, and this means treatment can only be targeted at the symptoms. In IBS the bowel tends to contract over-forcefully. This tight contraction of muscle is called a spasm.

Symptoms of IBS include constipation and diarrhea, which can alternate, and gripy abdominal pain. The stools in IBS are often described as like sheep or rabbit droppings or ribbons. Mucus may be passed with the stools. Weight loss, blood in the stools and late age at onset (after the age of 40) are not characteristic features and suggest a more serious progressive cause, such as inflammatory bowel disease or bowel cancer.

The patient with IBS may also experience dyspepsia and symptoms of the formerly commonly diagnosed functional condition of chronic cholecystitis. Bloating and excess wind are common, and symptoms are characteristically brought on by stress or by eating certain foods, and helped by lying down. Unlike the symptoms of Crohn's disease, IBS rarely causes a problem at night-time. Occasionally, an attack of IBS can be so severe as to present in a hospital emergency department as an acute abdomen.

All conventionally performed investigations in IBS have normal results, as is usual for functional conditions. In some clinical studies, up to 80 percent of patients with IBS were found to meet the criteria for a concurrent psychiatric diagnosis such as anxiety or depression.

Conventional treatment is often unsatisfactory. Lifestyle changes focused on stress management may be effective. In some people, dietary changes such as cutting out dairy products or excess dietary fiber can help, but this doesn't always seem to be helpful. There is medical interest in eliminating foods that contain sugars classified as fermentable oligosaccharides, disaccharides, monosaccharides and polyols (FODMAPs), and reports suggesting that a low FODMAP diet can be helpful. However, as well as processed sugars such as sorbitol and corn syrup, foods high in FODMAPs include nutritious fruit and vegetables such as apples, cherries, peaches, nectarines, most lactose-containing foods (dairy products), pulses, peas, onions and garlic and many green vegetables (broccoli, Brussels sprouts, cabbage). The breadth of FODMAPs in an otherwise healthy Western diet makes following the diet a great challenge for patients.

In terms of medication, antispasmodics such as mebeverine, and antidiarrheal medication such as loperamide, may be prescribed. A natural plant fiber preparation made from ispaghula is prescribed with modest benefit for some people with IBS-related constipation. This can help those patients with IBS who tend to constipation. Linseeds may help with excess wind.

Increasingly, doctors are recognizing that targeting mental emotional imbalances may be helpful in IBS, and so may prescribe antidepressants, refer the patient for counseling or psychotherapy, or recommend hypnotherapy.

 Information box 3.1e-V

Irritable bowel syndrome: comments from a Chinese medicine perspective

In Chinese medicine, the symptoms of IBS might correspond to Liver Qi Stagnation invading the Spleen and/or Stomach. Mebeverine would appear to smooth Liver Qi, but is suppressive in nature because it does not attend to the root cause of Spleen Qi Deficiency. Ispaghula fiber preparations would appear also to smooth Liver Qi. It also does not treat the root cause of the problem.

Constipation

Like the term indigestion, constipation describes a symptom and has a very different meaning to different individuals. Many people would say that they were constipated if their bowels did not open every day, but another common use of the term is to describe difficulty opening the bowels irrespective of frequency. This is another example of when it is important to get a very clear description of precise symptoms from the patient. The medical definition of constipation is either in terms of low frequency of opening the bowels (less than three times a week) or the subjective experience of difficulty in passing feces, including the experiencing of straining (this is not a healthy aspect of opening the bowels) or discomfort.

The conventional medicine understanding is that constipation is a result of eating a refined Western diet and a sedentary lifestyle. It is a particular problem for older people. It is known that constipation is not a problem in developing countries in which the diet contains a lot of fiber from vegetables and whole grains.

Some prescribed drugs can cause constipation, in particular those that contain opiates such as morphine, some antidepressants and iron preparations. Occasionally, constipation may be the consequence of a medical condition such as hypothyroidism, spinal nerve injury or high calcium levels, and it is important that these conditions are first excluded before the symptoms are managed.

The initial problem with constipation is that it can cause discomfort and a feeling of ill health. However, persistent straining over the years can lead to conditions such as hiatus hernia, diverticulitis and hemorrhoids (piles).

It is conventionally accepted that medication for constipation can lead to dependence on the prescribed drugs. Therefore, initial medical advice is to supplement the diet with fruit and other sources of fiber, such as bran, and to exercise more often.

Preparations that contain natural fiber (e.g. ispaghula husk) or dietary additions such as oats and linseeds are commonly recommended. If these are not helpful, drugs that stimulate the bowel, such as senna, may be chosen. An alternative approach is to use a preparation that encourages fluid to stay within the feces. These are called osmotic laxatives, and include long chain polyethylene glycol (macrogols) and lactulose. The problem with all these preparations is that the patient commonly becomes reliant on the medication.

In severe cases of constipation, a gradual form of intestinal obstruction can develop. This is most likely in older infirm people, in whom symptoms of bloating, abdominal pain and, eventually, vomiting may develop. Severe chronic constipation is both prevented and treated by means of an enema. This is a technique in which fluid is passed into the colon through a tube passed into the anus. This can have the effect of loosening and flushing out blocked stools. Laxative preparations such as polyethylene glycol can also be inserted in the form of an enema.

 Information box 3.1e-VI

Constipation: comments from a Chinese medicine perspective

In Chinese medicine, constipation can be a Full condition due to Heat in the Large Intestine. It can also be an Empty condition and in this case might be attributed to Dryness of the Large Intestine due to Blood or Yin Deficiency.

All laxatives are suppressive in that they do not attend to the root of the problem, and may even worsen the underlying condition in that when they are withdrawn the bowel may be even more sluggish. It is recognized that bowel movements can become dependent on the action of stimulant laxatives in particular.

Appendicitis

As its name implies, appendicitis is a condition in which the appendix becomes inflamed. It is the most common cause of the acute abdomen that requires surgical attention, affecting 6 percent of the UK population at some point in their lifetime. Despite it commonly being considered a disease of childhood, appendicitis can occur at any age.

The cause generally appears to be blockage of the hollow of the appendix with solidified feces. This means the contents of the blind end of the appendix become stagnant. Just as when the neck of the gallbladder becomes blocked, this stagnation leads to infection, which in turn causes inflammation. The appendix contains a lot of lymphoid (immune) tissue, which readily swells when infection develops, and this contributes to the tendency for the passageway (the lumen) in the appendix to become blocked.

The pain of the appendix starts centrally and is vague. The patient may first lose their appetite, and may occasionally vomit. Over the next few hours, as the outside of the appendix becomes inflamed, the site of the tenderness becomes much more localized at a point in the right iliac fossa. The signs of the acute abdomen including rigidity, guarding and rebound tenderness (see Section 3.1d) will be manifest in this area. If the appendix becomes very inflamed it may perforate, releasing its irritating contents into the peritoneal cavity. If generalized peritonitis occurs, the signs of guarding, rigidity and tenderness spread to include the whole abdomen, and the patient becomes much more unwell. In peritonitis the infection can spread rapidly throughout the whole abdominal cavity, and is a life-threatening condition.

Appendicitis is diagnosed primarily clinically on the basis of the characteristic history with additional features such as migration of pain to the right iliac fossa, guarding, tenderness and rigidity. With these findings, a raised white cell count will be very suggestive of the diagnosis. Ultrasound and computed tomography (CT) scans are increasingly used to refine the diagnostic process, although they may cause a dangerous delay in treatment in a more advanced case, and abdominal CT carries a risk of exposure to carcinogenic X-rays.

It is very common for cases of IBS, dysmenorrhea, ovulation pain, ruptured ovarian cyst and ectopic pregnancy to be misdiagnosed as appendicitis, but medical wisdom is that in a case where there is uncertainty, it is better to operate and find that the working diagnosis was wrong than delay a life-saving operation because of the uncertainty. In 10–20 percent of cases of appendectomy the removed appendix is found to be normal.

There is an increasing move towards conservative treatment of appendicitis with rest and antibiotics, meaning that not all cases need surgery. For those that do, removal of the appendix can be performed through a keyhole incision (laparoscopic appendectomy), so that if appendicitis is diagnosed early there is rapid recovery.

Treatment of established peritonitis involves an open abdominal operation to remove the infected tissue and wash the cavity to remove the pus. The patient is given strong antibiotic injections for at least a week after the operation. Peritonitis carries a risk of inducing infertility in women as the inflammation in the pelvic compartment of the body can lead to long-term scarring affecting the fallopian tubes. This, ideally, is avoided by early referral, diagnosis and treatment.

 Information box 3.1e-VII

Appendicitis: comments from a Chinese medicine perspective

In Chinese medicine, appendicitis is viewed as one or more of Damp Heat in the Large Intestine, Stagnation of Qi and Blood, or Accumulation of Toxic Heat. It can be considered to be a condition treatable by means of Chinese medicine (acupuncture and herbs), which, if mild, need not always require surgery.

Diverticulitis (diverticular disease)

Diverticulitis is a condition of the last stretch of the colon, the sigmoid colon, which is situated in the left iliac fossa.

A diverticulum (plural diverticula) is a little blind-ended pouch extending from the wall of the bowel, like the bulging out of a weak area in an inflated balloon. These pouches can become multiple in elderly people, particularly in those who have been prone to constipation as a result of a refined Western diet. It is estimated that diverticula have developed in 30 percent of Western people by the age of 60. However, in 90 percent of people, they cause no problem at all. The problem for the remaining 10 percent with diverticula is that, like the appendix, they provide a cul-de-sac for the passage of feces. Feces can therefore collect in the pouches and become stagnant. The pouches then become inflamed. This condition is called diverticulitis.

Figure 3.1e-I shows two different images of diverticula. The barium enema (a) shows the lining of the sigmoid colon and the hollows of the pouches coated with barium (black in this image). The colonoscopy (b) shows the shiny healthy interior of the bowel, with the openings of the pouches leading off from this.

If inflammation is mild, diverticulitis can grumble on, with symptoms of bouts of pain in the left iliac fossa, slight fever and occasional blood in the stools. Often there is alternating constipation and diarrhea (the condition can overlap with IBS). These mild attacks can be treated by prescriptions of oral antibiotics such as co-amoxiclav or metronidazole.

Long-term slight blood loss can lead to anemia. Sometimes the bleeding from an inflamed diverticulum can be profuse and require emergency treatment.

Occasionally, the inflammation is severe and the condition becomes very similar to appendicitis. The patient may then require emergency surgery to prevent peritonitis.

The symptoms of diverticulitis are indistinguishable from colon or rectal cancer, and so patients with blood mixed in the stools and pain in the left iliac fossa should always be referred for investigation.

Figure 3.1e-I (a) Barium enema image showing diverticula (arrows). (b) Colonoscopy showing openings to diverticula (arrows)

Information box 3.1e-VIII

Diverticulitis: comments from a Chinese medicine perspective

In Chinese medicine, the symptoms of diverticulitis can be equated with Liver Qi Stagnation invading the Spleen either with Damp Heat in the Large Intestine or Accumulation of Toxic Heat.

Inflammatory bowel disease – ulcerative colitis

Inflammatory bowel disease was introduced earlier in this section with Crohn's disease as one possible manifestation. Ulcerative colitis is in many ways a similar disease, so much so that in about 10 percent of patients with inflammatory bowel disease it is difficult to distinguish between the two. Ulcerative colitis is more common than Crohn's disease, affecting about 2.4 per 1000 people. Current theories consider the possibility that it is an autoimmune condition triggered by bowel bacteria.

There are other important differences, however, which mean that the outcome of the two conditions can be quite different. In ulcerative colitis the inflammation of the bowel is less extensive in that it usually affects only the lining of the colon. However, ulcerative colitis results in much larger bleeding areas of ulceration. In Crohn's disease the inflammation can extend throughout the thickness of the bowel wall and can affect anywhere in the digestive tract.

In contrast to Crohn's disease, in ulcerative colitis malabsorption and fistulas do not occur. The main symptoms in common with Crohn's disease are bouts of profuse diarrhea and mucus with gripy pain, all associated with fever and malaise. Blood in the stools is an additional marked symptom in ulcerative colitis, which is less common in Crohn's disease.

Some people with ulcerative colitis may have rare isolated attacks, but otherwise lead a normal life. In others, life can become dominated by frequent relapses and persistent bowel symptoms. Also, in contrast to Crohn's disease, ulcerative colitis is more common in non-smokers than smokers, and stopping smoking may actually trigger a worsening of symptoms.

As with Crohn's disease, in a severe attack the patient may be very unwell and require hospital admission. There is a small risk of perforation of the bowel in an acute attack, and this can lead to life-threatening peritonitis.

Most patients with ulcerative colitis are prescribed a drug that is known to reduce the risk of relapse. Mesalazine, sulfasalazine and olsalazine are three of the most commonly prescribed preparations. These anti-inflammatory medications are known to be more effective in ulcerative colitis than Crohn's disease. Corticosteroids may be given by mouth and by an enema during an acute attack. The immunosuppressant azathioprine or ciclosporin may also be prescribed. The newer cytokine modulator, infliximab, may also be effective. These are all powerful drugs and have a number of possible serious side effects, including digestive disturbance, kidney damage, hepatitis and bone marrow failure. Nevertheless, they can greatly improve the quality of life for people with ulcerative colitis.

If there is a very severe attack, or the symptoms are very unpleasant and persistent, the surgical option of total removal of the colon may be chosen (a colectomy). It may be possible to do this without the need for a colostomy, although this may be necessary in many cases. If a colostomy is necessary, it may be possible to reverse this at a later date by linking the end of the shortened bowel to the anus (ileo-anal pouch). A colectomy will effectively cure ulcerative colitis, as the condition only affects the colon. In those who do not have this operation there remains an increased risk of colonic cancer that relates to the extent and length of time for which the bowel has been inflamed.

 Information box 3.1e-IX

Ulcerative colitis: comments from a Chinese medicine perspective

In Chinese medicine, the symptoms of ulcerative colitis, like Crohn's disease, would equate to combination of Liver Qi Stagnation invading the Spleen, Spleen Yang Deficiency and Damp Heat in the Large Intestines.

Sulfasalazine, mesalazine and olsalazine would appear to Move Liver Qi and Clear Heat, but the side effect of organ failure suggests that they can severely Deplete Yin in the long term. They are suppressive, as are the corticosteroids and immune suppressant drugs used in ulcerative colitis.

Cancer of the colon and rectum

Tumors developing from the wall of the colon are common in the West. It is estimated that up to one-tenth of the population will develop a benign tumor of the bowel, otherwise known as a polyp, although this is a rare occurrence in people from developing countries. Polyps do not usually cause any problems, and most people are unaware of having them. Occasionally they can bleed and cause anemia.

In some cases polyps can become malignant. The more polyps there are, the more likely this is. There is one condition that runs in families (familial polyposis coli) in which hundreds of polyps develop in the colon in later life. There is definitely an increased risk of colon cancer in this condition. Patients with polyposis coli who have too many polyps to be removed surgically may be advised to have the entire colon removed in order to prevent the risk of developing cancer.

Malignant tumors of the colon and rectum are common. They will affect just under one in 30 of the population, most commonly being diagnosed at age 60–65, and are the third most common cause of death from cancer after breast and lung cancer. It is recognized that there is a link between colon cancer and polyps and also a diet high in meat and animal fat and low in fiber. There is an increased risk of colon cancer in people who have ulcerative colitis, and colon cancer tends to run in families.

Half of the cases of colon cancer occur close to or inside the rectum. These tumors commonly bleed and lead to the warning symptoms of a change in bowel habit and blood mixed in with the stools. If a change in bowel habit occurs anew in someone older than 60, the person should be referred for investigation, and the recommendation is applied to all aged over 40 if there is also persistent bleeding. Blood that is clearly mixed in with the stools should always be referred for further investigation.

Other problems that can lead to the diagnosis of colon cancer include the development of anemia from long-standing, low-grade blood loss, and an acute abdomen syndrome resulting from intestinal obstruction.

If a tumor is found, the affected segment of the bowel and associated lymph nodes is removed and, if possible, the ends stitched back together again. With rectal tumors this is often not possible, and the patient is left with a colostomy.

The outcome of the operation depends on the stage of progression of the tumor. Colonic carcinomas are now graded according to the TNM (tumor, node, metastases) system rather than the older Dukes system. Stage 1 means that the tumor is confined to the lining layer of the bowel, the mucosa. If this is the case, after surgical removal there is a very high cure rate, with no need for chemotherapy or radiotherapy. Stage 2 means that the tumor is confined to the bowel but has penetrated to deeper levels, and lymph nodes are not affected. The risk of recurrence after surgery is moderate, and some doctors prefer to prescribe chemotherapy after surgery to reduce the risk of recurrence. Stage 3 means that the tumor has spread to the lymph nodes, and in this case risk of recurrence is high. Chemotherapy is often used in this situation. Stage 4 cancers are those that have metastasized to other parts of the body. They are unlikely to be cured, but surgery and chemotherapy may be used for palliation.

 Information box 3.1e-X

Bowel polyps and tumors: comments from a Chinese medicine perspective

In Chinese medicine, the development of polyps, and cancer within polyps, suggests Damp and Phlegm. This fits with the link between colon cancer and a high-fat diet. The sluggish bowel movements, which are common in Western people, are a reflection of Stagnation of Qi, which can, of course, promote the accumulation of Phlegm. As is common in cases of cancer, the patient will have some long-term underlying deficiency, such as Deficiency of Qi of the Spleen or Large Intestine.

Important diseases of the anus

Hemorrhoids (piles)

Hemorrhoids are fleshy swellings of the highly vascular mucous lining of the anal canal. Initially, the swellings are hidden in the anal canal (first-degree hemorrhoids), but they can enlarge and start to prolapse outside the anal margin where they are felt as soft painless fleshy protuberances. If these protuberances can easily retract back into the anal canal they are known as second-degree hemorrhoids, and if the patient has to push them back in they are classified as third degree. Fourth-degree hemorrhoids remain permanently prolapsed and are the form most likely to require surgical repair.

Any condition that increases the pressure in the abdomen can lead to the blood vessels in the anal margin becoming distended, and the loose fleshy tissue in this area swelling as a consequence. Obesity, pregnancy and a habit of straining on defecation are all contributory factors in the development of hemorrhoids.

Initially, when the bulging tissue is hidden within the anus it may not cause any problems. The most common complication of this hidden swelling is that defecation can cause the surface of the tissue to bleed, particularly if the stool is hard and difficult to pass. This leads to fresh blood dropping from the anus after a bowel motion, although the stool itself has no blood within it. Although this can be distressing for the patient, this bleeding is not a serious sign, in contrast to the sign of blood mixed in with the stools, which points to more serious diagnoses such as inflammatory bowel disease or cancer.

Prolapsing hemorrhoids (second and third degree) cause problems because they can be difficult to clean, and so itching can be a problematic symptom. Sometimes, small loose flaps of skin known as skin tags develop close to the region of the hemorrhoid, and these can cause the same problems. Anal itch can be a very distressing problem in some patients, and may be relieved by proprietary creams that contain soothing agents, local anesthetics and corticosteroids.

Most hemorrhoids respond to increasing dietary fiber, which ensures that the stools remain soft, and by avoidance of straining. Hemorrhoids of pregnancy usually resolve once the baby is born.

Conventional surgical treatments include injection of sclerosant chemicals to cause the excessive soft tissue to scar and shrivel, freezing and infrared coagulation of the hemorrhoids, and pinching off of regions of the hemorrhoids with rubber bands (banding). A specialist may perform all these treatments as outpatient procedures. In the case of fourth-degree hemorrhoids, excision surgery may be the only effective treatment option.

Occasionally, one of the blood vessels in the hemorrhoids fills with clotted blood, usually as a result of trauma. This appears as a tense, sometimes exquisitely painful purple lump at the anal margin. In most cases the intense pain caused by thrombosed external hemorrhoids (also known as a perianal hematoma) will settle down, with bed rest and application of ice, within two weeks. In severe cases, a minor surgical operation to remove the clot will bring immediate relief.

> ## Information box 3.1e-XI
>
> ### Hemorrhoids: comments from a Chinese medicine perspective
>
> In Chinese medicine, hemorrhoids can be viewed as the consequence of Spleen Qi Sinking. The fleshy swelling and profuse fresh blood and itching also suggest that Phlegm and Heat can be factors contributing to their development.

Anal fissure

In contrast to hemorrhoids, which are usually painless, anal fissure is a very painful and sometimes chronic anal condition. A fissure is a crack in the anal skin that initially forms when the patient strains to pass a bowel motion. Once formed, the crack is very painful, and may not get the chance to heal because the action of opening the bowels tears it open again.

An anal fissure can result in a small amount of blood appearing after the bowel has opened. Again, there is no blood mixed in with the stool.

Many fissures will heal if the patient is encouraged to make sure that the stool is softened. Laxatives can help with healing. A cream containing a nitrate medication applied daily can help the associated local muscle spasm to relax and this can promote healing. Only some people can tolerate this as the nitrate may cause severe headaches. Sometimes a minor surgical operation is required to stretch the anal sphincter muscle, which has the same effect in permitting healing.

> ## Information box 3.1e-XII
>
> ### Anal fissure: comments from a Chinese medicine perspective
>
> The intense pain of a fissure suggests local Blood and Qi Stagnation. Bleeding suggests the presence of Heat. There is the possibility of underlying Blood or Yin Deficiency, which has caused the dry anal skin and constipated bowels.

Rectal prolapse

In rectal prolapse, the mucous lining of the rectum drops out of the anus, causing a soft moist mass to appear at the anus. This is usually a problem of frail elderly people who have poor muscle tone. It can also occur in young children.

The condition is often temporary, but may require surgical repair because of mucus discharge and incontinence, and the tendency of the soft rectal lining to become damaged and ulcerated.

> ## Information box 3.1e-XIII
>
> ### Rectal prolapse: comments from a Chinese medicine perspective
>
> In Chinese medicine, rectal prolapse might be understood to be the result of Spleen Qi Sinking.

Diseases of the small intestine and large intestine

Some patients with diseases of the small and large intestine will benefit from referral to a conventional doctor for assessment or treatment. Red flags are those symptoms and signs that indicate that referral should be considered. The red flags of the diseases of the small and large intestine are described in Table 3.1e-I. A summary of the red flags in a format designed for quick reference in clinical practice can be found in Appendix III. This gives advice on the degree of urgency of referral for each of the red flag conditions listed.

Table 3.1e-I A10: Red flags of diseases of the small intestine and large intestine

Red flag	Description	Reasoning
A10.1	Malabsorption syndrome: loose pale stools and malnutrition; weight loss, thin hair, dry skin, cracked lips and peeled tongue. Will present as failure to thrive in children	Malabsorption syndrome develops when there is an inability to absorb nutrients in the diet, and weight loss and mineral and vitamin deficiencies result. Loose stools are the result of the presence of unabsorbed fat Disease of the small intestine (most commonly celiac disease and Crohn's disease) can result in malabsorption syndrome Chronic pancreatitis (see A7.2) is one of the causes of malabsorption syndrome
A10.2	Severe diarrhea with mucus or gripy pain if not responding to treatment within a week	Persistent severe diarrhea (not simply loose stools) with mucus suggests either a serious episode of bowel infection or an episode of inflammatory bowel disease (Crohn's disease or ulcerative colitis) Both causes merit prompt referral for treatment Food poisoning and dysentery (severe bloody diarrhea) are notifiable diseases (see A6.2)
A10.3	Onset of severe abdominal pain with collapse (the acute abdomen): the pain can be constant or colicky (coming in waves); rigidity, guarding and rebound tenderness are serious signs	The acute abdomen is a term that refers to the combination of severe abdominal pain together with an inability to continue with day-to-day activities (collapse). This syndrome can have benign causes, such as irritable bowel syndrome (IBS), dysmenorrhea and ovulation pain, but needs high priority or urgent referral to exclude more serious conditions including appendicitis, perforated ulcer, peritonitis, obstructed bowel, pelvic inflammatory disease and gallstones Colicky pain indicates obstruction of a viscus (hollow organ) Rigidity of the abdomen, guarding (a reflex protective spasm of the abdominal muscles) and rebound tenderness (pain felt elsewhere in the abdomen when the pressure of a palpating hand is released) all suggest inflammation or perforation of a viscus Features of abdominal pain in children that suggest a more benign (functional) cause include mild pain that is worse in the morning, location of pain around the umbilicus, and pain that is worse with anxiety
A10.4	Any episode of blood mixed in with stools	Red blood mixed in with stools suggests bleeding from the lower part of the small intestine, the large intestine or rectum Possible causes are bowel infections, diverticulitis, inflammatory bowel disease (Crohn's disease or ulcerative colitis) and bowel cancer. All merit non-urgent referral for investigation and treatment if persistent and unexplained This symptom is considered a red flag for bowel cancer if persistent for more than four weeks in someone over 60, and in anyone over 50 if there are other symptoms such as a change in bowel habit or weight loss Acute infectious diarrhea is a notifiable disease (see A6.2) Blood that drips from the anus after defecation is common and is usually the result of hemorrhoids (piles). If the blood is not mixed in with the stools, the cause is likely to be benign

A10.5	Signs of an inguinal hernia: swelling in the groin that is more pronounced on standing, especially if uncomfortable	An inguinal hernia is the result of a weakness in the abdominal wall in the region of the inguinal crease (the groin). The abdominal contents can bulge into a narrow-necked passageway formed by this weakness, and this can be very uncomfortable
		An inguinal hernia carries a risk of being the site at which the loop of bowel can become obstructed, and there is a risk of strangulation of that portion of the bowel. The patient should be referred for a surgical assessment of the risk of complications
		Refer as a high priority only if a hernia has become acutely very painful over the course of a few hours
A10.6	Altered bowel habit lasting for four weeks in someone >60	Most people have a predictable pattern of defecation. If this pattern is broken for >4 weeks it may be a warning sign of inflammatory bowel disease or cancer. Consider referral in all people who develop this symptom over the age of 60. This is a medical red flag because of the high risk of bowel cancer in this age group
		If this symptom occurs together with blood in stools or weight loss in someone >50, this also is a medical red flag for cancer
		In these groups an increased frequency of defecation or increased mucus production are of particular concern
A10.7	Infectious bloody diarrhea or food poisoning: any episode of diarrhea and vomiting in which food is suspected as the origin, or in which blood appears in the stools	Bloody diarrhea that results from bacterial infection may manifest in profuse watery diarrhea, abdominal cramps and blood in the stools. Clusters of related cases or a history of recent travel can suggest an infectious cause
		Food poisoning is the consequence of eating food that is contaminated with infectious organisms; it is commonly a result of poor food hygiene, together with insufficient cooking
		Both infectious bloody diarrhea and food poisoning are notifiable diseases (see A6.2), and as such merit referral so that they can be reported by a medical practitioner
A10.8	Anal discharge/ soiling with stool (in underwear or bed)	Always refer for diagnosis if persistent and appearing in a previously continent child (could signify constipation with fecal overflow, a developmental problem of the bowel or emotional disturbance)
		An anal discharge may result from rectal or anal cancer, and in an elderly person a fecal discharge may result from constipation with overflow of fecal fluid. Both situations require referral
A10.9	Painless lump felt in the anus	This could be a benign skin tag or anal warts, and may possibly be an anal carcinoma. An undiagnosed anal lump needs referral for diagnosis if persisting for >3 weeks
A10.10	Painful lump felt in the anus	A painful anal lump could be a prolapsed hemorrhoid, a perianal hematoma (benign) or an anal carcinoma. It needs referral for diagnosis and as high priority if pain is severe
A10.11	Anal itch	A short history of intense nocturnal anal itch might be the result of threadworm infection
		A more prolonged history is most likely to be the result of hemorrhoids and skin tags. However, itch may result from the more serious conditions of lichen sclerosus or anal carcinoma, so should be referred for examination if not responding to simple treatment within three weeks

3.2

The Cardiovascular System

3.2a The physiology of the cardiovascular system

This chapter focuses on the cardiovascular system, also known as the circulatory system. Like Section 3.1a, this section is divided into two parts. If you are using this book as a study course, then, because of its length, you are advised to work through the two parts in separate study sessions.

Part I: The vessels and the heart organ[26]

The cardiovascular system consists of all those structures that have the role of transporting the blood to all parts of the body. It enables the blood to perform its roles of protection, providing nutrients and removal of toxins for all the body tissues.

The cardiovascular system can be considered as comprising two main components – the blood vessels and the heart – and these are explored in turn in this section. The vessels are the channels through which the blood flows. The three main types of blood vessel are the arteries, veins and capillaries. The heart is the pump that provides the power to create the flow of blood through the vessels.

Sometimes the lymphatic system first referred to in Section 2.1d is also included as part of the cardiovascular system. However, in this book, for the sake of clarity, the lymphatic system is treated as a separate system.

The blood (hematological system) is not conventionally considered to be part of the cardiovascular system. The blood is considered to be connective tissue in nature and originates from the bone marrow. The blood is described in Chapter 3.4.

Very simplistically speaking, a typical conventional practitioner might view the cardiovascular system as a fleshy pump, albeit a rather complex one, which is linked to a series of soft-tissue pipes. Although emotions and stress in particular are recognized in modern medicine to have a bearing on the function of the cardiovascular system, the heart and vessels do not have any of the deep emotional correlations that they are ascribed in Chinese medicine and other holistic complementary medical disciplines. For example, a modern heart surgeon may not necessarily consider the part that love plays in the life of a patient to have anything to do with the task of improving the function of that patient's heart. In contrast, a holistic practitioner is much more likely to be interested in how a person's relationships and zest for life are linked to the health and function of the Heart Organ, the energetic system that is linked most with the heart and circulation in Chinese medicine.

The blood vessels

The vascular system is the term used to describe the vessels alone. It consists of a network of tubes lined with endothelium (a form of epithelial tissue). These tubes are at their widest as they leave the heart, and then divide, like the branches of a tree, to form thousands of tiny capillaries within the tissues. The capillaries then meet up again to form wider and wider tubes, which return the blood back to the heart.

Blood vessels that lead blood away from the heart are called arteries and those that lead blood back again to the heart from the tissues are called veins. Arterioles and venules are the names given to the smallest types of arteries and veins.

ARTERIES

An important characteristic of arteries is that they contain both muscle and an elastic material called elastin in their wall, which means that they have the capacity to contract and expand. This means that arteries can alter the flow of blood to an area of the body by altering in width. This is a very important concept to grasp in preparation for understanding the concept of blood pressure.

The blood in arteries is under high pressure because it has just been pumped from the heart. This is why a severed artery will spurt blood in pulses. It is from the arteries, and not the veins, that a Chinese medical practitioner can sense the state of Blood and Qi when taking the pulse.

One important disease of arteries, arterial thrombosis, has already been described in this text (see Section 2.2d).

VEINS

In contrast to arteries, the blood within the veins is under much lower pressure, and it is necessary for veins to contain valves to ensure that the flow of blood back to the heart remains one-way. Veins rely on the pumping action of the muscles to aid in the movement of blood back to the heart. This is partly why sedentary people may develop swollen ankles at the end of the day. Fluid accumulates in the tissues of the lower parts of the body when there is no motive force to propel it upwards against the force of gravity.

One important potentially life-threatening venous disease, deep vein thrombosis (DVT), has already been described (see Section 2.2d). The more common and benign condition of varicose veins is described later (see Section 3.2c).

CAPILLARIES

Capillaries are minute vessels with walls that are only one cell thick. A significant characteristic of capillaries is that they enable the rapid transfer of nutrients, gases and waste products to and from the blood across their very thin walls.

Capillaries were introduced in Section 2.2b, where inflammation was described. In inflammation, the gaps between the cells in the capillary wall widen, making the capillaries more permeable to tissue fluid.

The transfer of nutrients from the capillaries to the tissues

Healthy blood that has just passed through the digestive system will contain a high concentration of basic nutrients, including simple sugars, cholesterol, triglycerides, fatty acids, amino acids from proteins, vitamins and minerals. Once the blood has passed through the capillaries of the lungs, it will also contain a high concentration of oxygen. Thus the blood transports both the oxygen and glucose and other simple nutrients that will be used by the mitochondria of every cell in the body to produce the energy required for many vital cellular processes.

The body relies on the transport processes of diffusion, osmosis and active transport for nutrients and oxygen to enter the bloodstream from the tissues of the digestive

system and the lung. These processes are described in detail in Section 1.1c.

Oxygen, simple sugars, fatty acids, vitamins and minerals all pass with ease through the single-celled wall of the capillary by diffusion. The movement is particularly rapid when it is from a region in which these nutrients are in high concentration to one in which there is a low concentration. For both oxygen in the lungs and nutrients in the tissues of the digestive system this movement enables these substances to readily enter the circulating fluid component of the blood, the plasma.

Conversely, when the nutrient and oxygen-rich plasma reaches other tissues in which the concentration of nutrients and oxygen may be relatively low, the nutrients and oxygen tend to move out of the blood and into the tissues. This transfer of nutrients from digested food in the intestines and of air from the lungs into the tissues happens within a few seconds. Because diffusion is a spontaneous process, this process is incredibly energy efficient, requiring no extra energy over that required by the heart to pump the blood.

In addition to this energy-efficient transfer of oxygen and nutrients into the tissues, another wonderful aspect of the process of diffusion is that it underpins the movement of waste products out of the tissues. As waste products such as urea from protein metabolism and carbon dioxide from respiration build up in the tissues, the tendency is for them to move back into the bloodstream, where they are kept at a relatively low concentration. The waste products can then be carried to the liver, kidneys, sweat glands and lungs, each of which is specially adapted to remove otherwise toxic by-products from the body.

Similarly, water moves into and out of the plasma with ease. In this case, the process is called osmosis. This term describes the movement of water from a region in which it is part of a dilute solution to one in which it is part of a more concentrated solution. This is the means by which water will move from a vase into a wilted (dehydrated) flower stem. In the same way, by osmosis, water will enter the plasma from the tissues if the plasma is more concentrated than the tissue fluid. Conversely, if the plasma is relatively well hydrated, water will move out of the plasma into the tissues. This is another very energy-efficient mechanism, and it ensures that water is transported from the digestive system to the tissues that need it.

The desire for water to move from a region of low concentration to one of high concentration is described in scientific terms as osmotic pressure. This pressure relates directly to the difference in concentration between two regions, and so to the tendency that water will have to move between these regions. When the osmotic pressure is high (e.g. in a dehydrated plant stem), a lot of water can be encouraged to move (in this case, against the downward pull of gravity and into the stem). Thus, in the body, if a dehydrated person drinks some water, there will be a rapid movement of water from the digestive system, through the plasma and into the dehydrated tissues, all under the pull of the increased osmotic pressure of the concentrated tissue fluids.

One other factor needs to be considered in this description of the movement of nutrients into and out of the bloodstream, and this is the effect of the physical pressure of fluid in the vessels. Just as air in an inflated tire is under a measurable degree of pressure (which is what makes the tire feel inflated), so the blood in a blood vessel is under a degree of pressure. In the blood vessels the internal pressure varies according to the proximity to the heart. Arteries close to the heart contain blood that is being pumped by muscular contractions of the heart, and this blood is therefore under significant pressure. As the arteries branch into more and more numerous smaller vessels, the pressure within them gradually decreases, so that at the start of the capillary bed the pressure is much lower. Nevertheless, at the arterial end of the capillaries the pressure is still sufficient to force some fluid through the gaps between the cells of the capillary walls and into the tissues. This can be compared visually to squeezing an inflated bicycle tube punctured with numerous tiny holes; the greater the pressure applied, the more air that is able to escape through the holes. However, unlike the air escaping from a squeezed and punctured bicycle tube, the tendency for water to move out of the blood vessels by physical pressure is countered by the tendency of fluid to stay in the blood vessels under osmotic pressure. In health, a delicate balance between the two forces is established, ensuring that the tissues remain perfectly hydrated, becoming neither too dry nor too waterlogged.

Just under half of the volume of the blood is made up of blood cells that are too large to move between the gaps in the capillaries. A good proportion of the composition of the remaining plasma consists of dissolved protein molecules, which are also too large to pass through the gaps in the capillaries. Therefore, the movement of fluid across capillary membranes is selective for the remaining small molecules, such as water itself, salt and sugars. This is the property of semi-permeability, as first described in Section 1.1c.

An understanding of these forces that affect the movement of fluid between the blood and the tissues is a helpful foundation for the study of the important condition of edema, described in Section 3.2f.

To summarize, the balance of these forces is such that the net movement of fluid is out of the capillaries at the arterial end and into the capillaries at the venous end. This is ideal to suit the body's needs. It means that nutrients and oxygen tend to move out into the tissue fluid from the arterial end, and wastes and carbon dioxide tend to move into the venous end of the capillaries. This is how the blood deposits its nutrients into the cells that need them, and transports away the wastes from the tissues at the capillaries.

The pathway of the arteries

Figure 3.2a-I illustrates the pathway of the major arteries that lead away from the heart. The diagram shows how the blood is directed from the heart to all parts of the body. The arch of the largest blood vessel in the body, the aorta, is shown leaving the top of the heart and then descending to run deep in the body, through the diaphragm to the pelvis. Here, it splits into two main branches, which supply blood to each leg.

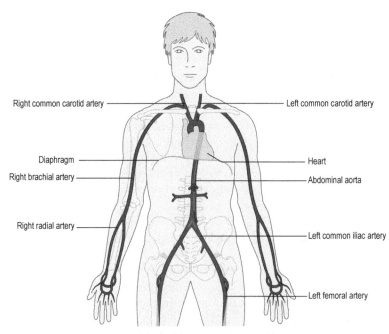

Figure 3.2a-I The pathway of the arteries from the heart

Information box 3.2a-I

The vessels: comments from a Chinese medicine perspective

Maciocia (1989)[27] states that in *The Simple Questions (Suwen)* the vessels are said to be controlled by the Heart, but adds that the Lungs also control circulation of Blood in the vessels because of their role in Governing the circulation of Qi throughout the body.

One of the Chinese medicine functions of the Lungs is to inhale pure Qi and to exhale dirty Qi. The pure Clear Qi (derived from the air we breathe) combines with Gu Qi (derived from food) to form Gathering (Zong) Qi in the chest. True (Zhen) Qi is a further refinement of Gathering Qi and Original Qi, which also arises in the chest. The Lung then enables the dispersion of this Qi in its dual form of Nutritive (Ying) Qi and Defensive (Wei) Qi to the whole of the body. Therefore, the Lungs are important for the generation of essential energy throughout the whole of the body.

This makes an interesting comparison with the conventional medicine interpretation that the vessels permit the transportation of nutrients and oxygen to all the tissues and thus facilitate the production of cellular energy from these ingredients in the mitochondria present in all cells of the body. This is very much in keeping with the Chinese medicine association of the vessels with the Lung Organ.

Figure 3.2a-II shows how the major branches of the aorta in the neck, the common carotid arteries, branch to supply blood to the head. One branch, the internal carotid artery, divides to enter the skull and supply the brain with blood.

Now turn back to Figure 3.2a-I, which shows how arterial branches from the aorta divide down each limb to take blood to the hands and the feet. Compare this with Figure 3.2a-III, which shows the pathways of the veins that return the blood to the heart, ending in two major vessels called the superior vena cava and inferior vena cava. Note how the basic pathways of the veins mirror those of the arteries. This is the pattern for almost all parts of the body, in that an artery delivering blood to a body part runs very close to the vein that is draining the blood away from that part.

A major difference between the position of arteries and veins is that most veins tend to run closer to the surface of the body, whereas arteries generally lie much deeper. The veins that run close to the surface are called superficial veins. All the blue-colored vessels that can be seen through the skin in areas such as the back of the hand, the crooks of the elbows and the neck are superficial veins, not arteries. If these vessels are palpated, no pulse will be felt, and it will be found that they are very easy to compress.

In addition to superficial veins, there is also a system of deep veins. The blood draining from the surface of the body runs first into the superficial veins, and then enters the deep veins through vessels that penetrate the deeper tissues called perforators. It is important to be clear about the distinction between superficial and deep veins in order to understand the pathology of the conditions of varicose veins and also deep venous thrombosis, as described in Section 3.2c.

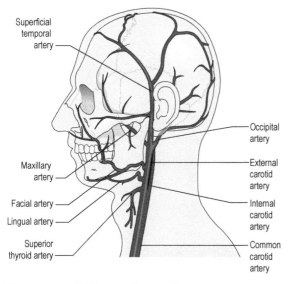

Figure 3.2a-II The pathway of the left common carotid artery

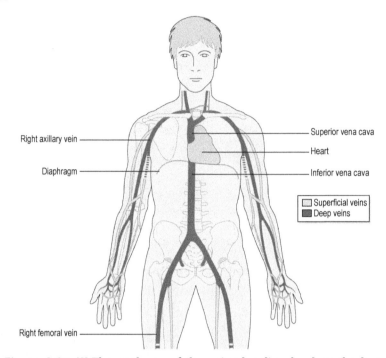

Right axillary vein

Diaphragm

Superior vena cava

Heart

Inferior vena cava

☐ Superficial veins
■ Deep veins

Right femoral vein

Figure 3.2a-III The pathway of the veins leading back to the heart

The structure of the heart

The heart is a fist-sized organ that sits just to the left of midline in the chest. It is situated between the two lungs, and together these organs fill the space that overlies the diaphragm. This space is known as the thoracic cavity, as shown in Figure 3.2a-IV. These organs are so closely related that the inside surfaces of the lungs bear the impression of the shape of the heart on them.

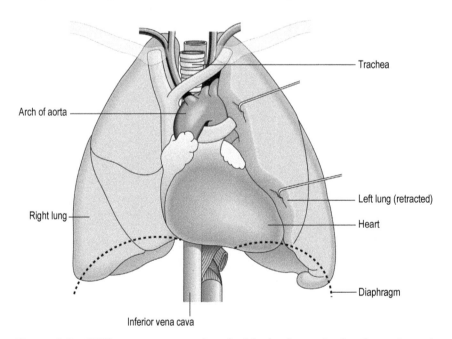

Arch of aorta

Trachea

Right lung

Left lung (retracted)

Heart

Diaphragm

Inferior vena cava

Figure 3.2a-IV The organs associated with the heart in the thoracic cavity

The heart is largely made up of cardiac muscle (the myocardium), and is divided into four chambers. It might be helpful now to turn back to the description of the tissue types given in Section 1.1d for a reminder of the characteristics of cardiac muscle, and how the cardiac muscle cells communicate with each other through specialized joints.

The healthy heart is lined with endocardium, a smooth epithelial tissue lining that is continuous with the lining of the blood vessels. The outside of the heart is protected by a tough fibrous sac called the pericardium. In between the pericardium and the heart organ is a very small space containing fluid. This fluid lubricates the movement between the heart and the pericardium, and contains immune cells. The remainder of the organ consists of the naturally contractile myocardium.

To understand the action and some of the structural disorders of the heart, it is important to understand that the heart is divided into two halves: the right half deals with the flow of the blood from the body and to the lungs, and the left half deals with the flow of the blood from the lungs and to the body. Each half has two chambers known as the atria (singular atrium) and the ventricles, and together these form the four chambers of the heart. There are two valves situated in each half of the heart. Their function is to ensure that the blood flow is always one way. Figure 3.2a-V illustrates the position and shape of the four chambers and the valves of the heart, and the direction of blood flow through the two halves of the heart.

Figure 3.2a-V The interior of the heart and its blood flow

The flow of blood through the heart

The double structure of the heart means that blood can flow through the heart twice in each full circulation of the body. It might help when reading the following description of the flow of the blood to use Figure 3.2a-V to visually trace the pathway the blood takes.

THE FLOW OF BLOOD THROUGH THE RIGHT SIDE OF THE HEART

Blood returning from most of the tissues of the body enters the right atrium of the heart from the two large veins, the superior and inferior vena cavae. This blood has given up its oxygen and is carrying relatively high levels of waste products such as carbon dioxide and urea. The right atrium contracts to force the blood through the tricuspid valve, and thus into the right ventricle. The right ventricle then contracts and this forces the blood through the pulmonary valve into the pulmonary artery. The pressure of blood in the contracting right ventricle closes the tricuspid valve, making a very subtle clapping noise. The blood rushing into the pulmonary artery does not flow back into the right ventricle when it finishes its contraction as the pulmonary valve also closes in turn, making its own clapping noise as it does so. The blood entering the pulmonary artery then passes into a concentrated network of capillaries within the tissue of the lungs.

THE FLOW OF BLOOD THROUGH THE LEFT SIDE OF THE HEART

When blood has passed through the capillary network of the lungs, it has given up its carbon dioxide and is rich in oxygen, all through the effortless process of diffusion (see Section 3.3a for more detail about the structure of the blood vessels in the lungs). This oxygen-rich blood is a brighter shade of red than the darker venous blood. It flows through the pulmonary vein and into the left atrium of the heart. The left atrium contracts to force the blood through the mitral valve, and thus into the muscular left ventricle. The left ventricle then contracts and this forces the blood through the aortic valve into the arch of the aorta, the widest part of the widest blood vessel in the body. The pressure of the blood in the contracting right ventricle closes the mitral valve, also making the valvular clapping noise. Just as was described for blood leaving the right ventricle, blood rushing into the aorta does not flow back into the left ventricle when it finishes its contraction. This is because the aortic valve also closes in turn, again, making its own clapping noise as it does so.

It might be appreciated from this description that the flow of blood in the body can be compared to a figure-of-eight, with the heart situated at the crossing point of the lines of the eight. In this delicate but powerful pumping system, both the right and the left heart contract together in a single heartbeat. This results in a double pumping action, which means that the pulse of flow of blood within the lungs and body occurs at exactly the same time, and the clapping of the four valves closing in turn makes the heart sounds that are audible by means of a stethoscope.

In summary, it is important to understand that the route of the flow of blood through the two halves of the heart is as follows:

- oxygenated blood from the lungs enters the left heart

- the left heart pumps oxygenated blood to all the tissues of the body

- tissues absorb oxygen so that the blood becomes deoxygenated

- deoxygenated blood from the body returns to the right heart

- the right heart pumps deoxygenated blood to the lungs

- blood absorbs oxygen from the lungs so that it becomes oxygenated

- oxygenated blood from the lungs enters the left heart

…and so on.

The blood supply to the heart

It might appear surprising that the heart itself requires a blood supply. However, the heart muscle is working continuously for a full lifetime, and requires a consistent supply of oxygen and nutrients. These high demands cannot be met by the blood flowing through the chambers of the heart alone.

Figure 3.2a-VI illustrates how vessels, known as coronary arteries (derived from *cor*, the Latin root meaning heart), branch from their origin at the aorta to wrap around the heart muscle. An understanding of this blood supply will be good preparation for the study of coronary heart disease (see Section 3.2e), which is the most important cause of death after cancer in developed countries.

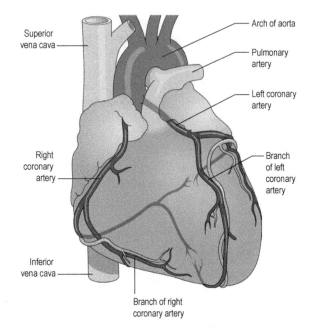

Figure 3.2a-VI The blood supply to the heart

The conduction system of the heart

The conduction system of the heart is what enables the heart to contract in such a way that a wave of contraction moves from the top of the heart to the tip (apex). This means that the blood within the heart is pumped smoothly through the two chambers of the two sides.

The conduction system consists of strands of specialized cardiac muscle cells, which run from an electrically active node situated in the muscular wall between the atria in the upper part of the heart. These cells branch out from this region to connect to all parts of the heart muscle. This node (more specifically known as the sinoatrial node) is the heart's own pacemaker. The cells of this pacemaker have an internal rhythm, giving them the property of being able to contract at a rate of just over once every second. Because of the membranous joints between cardiac cells, the contraction of the cells in the pacemaker can stimulate the contraction of neighboring cells in the conduction system, and so on, until the whole heart muscle has contracted.

Various factors can affect the rate at which the pacemaker cells contract, which explains why people can be aware of changes in their heart rate from time to time. One of these is the nerve supply to the heart. This is part of the autonomic nervous system (described in more detail in Chapter 4.1). The autonomic nervous system plays an essential role in the maintenance of homeostasis in the body, and very probably in the mechanism of many of the effects of acupuncture. For the time being, all that need be understood about this system is that it deals with the control of the involuntary aspects of the function of the body, such as breathing, digestion and sweating. It is conventionally seen as two opposing systems, the sympathetic nervous system (SNS) and the parasympathetic nervous system (PNS). Most parts of the body are under the influence of both these systems.

In the heart, the sympathetic nerves cause the pacemaker to contract more rapidly, and the heart muscle to contract more forcefully (in Chinese medicine this would be interpreted as a Yang response). The parasympathetic nerves cause the pacemaker to contract more slowly, and the heart muscle to contract less forcefully (a Yin response).

Emotional states such as fear and anxiety and also physical exercise all lead to an increased heart rate as a result of activation of the SNS. Other factors that contribute to a relatively increased heart rate include body temperature, being female and young age (infancy and childhood).

The generation of the pulse

The pulse wave, which is of interest to practitioners both of Chinese medicine and conventional medicine, is a direct consequence of the rhythmic pumping of the heart. As blood is forced through the chambers of the heart by the wave of contraction from the base to the apex of the heart, the arteries that leave the heart bulge with the increased amount of blood that has been forced into them, and this distension is propagated down the length of the major arteries. Arteries are elastic vessels that can stretch, but are not flaccid. This bulging is felt on palpation at any artery as a pushing outward of the vessel wall, and this bulge is what is known as the pulse.

When conventional medicine practitioners assess the pulse they use quite firm pressure. In this way they can feel the physical force of the blood in the artery. Practitioners of Chinese medicine apply very little pressure to assess the pulse. This is because they are less concerned with the physical force of the blood and more with the energetics of the vital substances of Blood and Qi, which are believed to move with the physical blood.

The heart sounds

Practitioners of conventional medicine use a stethoscope to listen to the heart sounds. In a healthy person, the heart sounds are like the familiar repeated "lub-dub" used so often to heighten emotion in televised hospital dramas. As mentioned previously, the heart sounds are produced by the heart valves closing as the blood is forced through them. In each chamber, one valve closes before the other, thus producing the "lub-dub" sound.

Different conditions of the heart lead to very subtle changes in these sounds. A valve that does not close properly will give a muffled sound as blood leaks through it, and this is known as a murmur.

Part II: Blood pressure and the Chinese medical view

Blood pressure

Blood pressure is simply a measure of the force that the bulge of blood in the arteries exerts on the walls of the arteries. It can be assessed approximately by palpation of the artery. An artery that feels very tense during the pulse can reflect a high blood pressure, whereas a weak, flaccid pulse can reflect a low blood pressure.

Blood pressure oscillates up and down during the heartbeat. When the heart reaches the peak of contraction, blood pressure also reaches a peak, and this is called systolic blood pressure. When the heart relaxes after its contraction, blood pressure drops down to its lowest point, diastolic blood pressure. When a conventional doctor palpates the force of the pulse, information about the difference between systolic (peak) and diastolic (trough) pressure can also be obtained.

Adequate blood pressure is necessary for ensuring a steady flow of nutrients to all parts of the body. In times of physical stress blood pressure rises, but this is appropriate to the body's needs. It is only if blood pressure remains at too high a level for the body's requirements for too long that long-term damage to the circulatory system can occur. The condition of high blood pressure (hypertension) is explored in more detail in Section 3.2d.

Two important factors combine to affect the blood pressure. The first is the amount of blood being pumped by the heart at any one time. A rapid and forceful heartbeat will lead to a higher blood pressure than a slow and relaxed heartbeat. A frightening experience or strenuous exercise will both temporarily put up blood pressure, as they both lead to an increased and more forceful heart rate.

The second factor that increases blood pressure is the amount of tension in the muscles of the artery walls. If the artery walls are tightly constricted, the pressure of the blood being forced through them will be raised. There are many factors that cause the artery walls to constrict. One familiar cause is extreme cold, which causes the small arteries in the skin to constrict. This leads to cold flesh, numbness and a bluish discoloration. This is an important reflex in the body, because it means that the heat of the blood is not lost so readily from the skin, and is kept deep in the interior where it is vital for the effective function of the organs.

It is important for homeostasis that blood pressure remains generally within a certain range. It has been found that most healthy individuals have comparable ranges of blood pressure. Young people tend to have lower blood pressure than older people, and women tend to have lower blood pressure than men.

Control of blood pressure

It might now be appreciated that blood pressure has to be responsive to a wide range of conditions, which include emotional stress, exercise, pain and blood volume.

As with the heart rate, the autonomic nervous system (ANS) is central in the control of blood pressure. The muscles within the small artery walls are supplied by sympathetic nerves, and thus it is the SNS that deals with increasing the heart rate. In the small blood vessels, activated sympathetic nerves lead to constriction. Conditions such as emotional stress, exercise, pain and loss of blood volume activate the SNS and lead to constriction of the vessels.

Two chemicals that are integral to the activation of the SNS are the hormones adrenaline and noradrenaline. A release of adrenaline from the adrenal glands will lead to an increased heart rate, constriction of the artery walls and an increase in blood pressure. This is explained in more detail in Chapter 5.1.

When the SNS is not activated, the action of the PNS becomes dominant. In this situation, the heart rate slows down, the blood vessels relax and blood pressure drops. A faint often occurs as a result of a strong emotional response to a shock (different to fear) or even to excessive joy. This has the effect of activating the PNS. The result of this is that the heart rate suddenly slows and blood pressure drops. This leads to a sudden drop in the supply of blood and nutrients to the brain, and the person will feel dizzy and may very briefly lose consciousness. However, the act of fainting and the drop in blood pressure that accompanies it then stimulates the SNS, which immediately reverses the situation. A hallmark of a faint is that the person very quickly begins to regain consciousness (within seconds) as the blood pressure rises and the blood supply returns to the brain.

This is also what occurs when a person receiving acupuncture experiences needle shock, which occurs very occasionally, often during a first treatment. Although alarming for the practitioner, this type of faint is usually benign, as long as the patient starts to regain consciousness immediately. It is conventionally believed to be the result of an emotional response to needling, which then leads to over-activation of the PNS. This dramatic response to needling can, however, be framed in terms of a helpful shift in energy, and case studies suggest that if interpreted in this positive light may allow long-term healing from trauma held within the body.[28]

Measurement of blood pressure

Although blood pressure can be roughly assessed by palpation of the pulse, the way to obtain an objective measure of blood pressure is by means of an instrument called the sphygmomanometer. This consists of an inflatable fabric cuff, which is wrapped around a limb, usually the upper arm, and a device to measure the pressure within the cuff.

The pressure can be assessed by a simple manually operated pressure gauge, similar to those used to measure car tire pressure, in which case the equipment is called an aneroid sphygmomanometer. Increasingly, in medical settings, an oscillometric assessment is made, which involves a digitally processed result drawn from the mean arterial pressure. This requires an automated digital sphygmomanometer. The British Hypertension Society (BHS) currently recommends a wide range of oscillometric models for reliable assessment of blood pressure.[29]

The now outmoded mercury-containing sphygmomanometer used to provide the gold standard for measurement. For this reason, the numerical value of blood pressure is conventionally expressed in millimeters of mercury (mmHg). A normal systolic pressure falls within the range 100–140mmHg, and a normal diastolic pressure falls within the range 65–90mmHg. Blood pressure is expressed as a combination of these two values. For example, a blood pressure of 120/80mmHg (described as 120 over 80) would be considered to be a normal blood pressure, and one of 150/99mmHg would be considered to be a high (albeit only classed as Stage 2) blood pressure.

In blood pressure assessment the cuff is inflated to a pressure high enough to totally compress the arteries within the limb. This will be equivalent to a pressure higher than the systolic pressure, and can be in the range of 200–250mmHg. At this pressure the compression of the artery leads to a total cessation of blood flow through the artery, and the pulse can no longer be felt or picked up by an oscillometer. This stage is often uncomfortable for the patient, and this level of pressure should be maintained only for a moment.

In aneroid assessment, a stethoscope is placed over the artery that is distal to the cuff. This is usually at the brachial artery, the pulse of which can be palpated at the elbow (in the region of the acupoint Qu Ze, PC-3). The pressure in the cuff is then gradually reduced. As the pressure in the cuff falls to that of the systolic pressure, squirts of blood can be forced through the now partially compressed artery. This is heard as a pulsatile rushing noise through the stethoscope. The systolic pressure is recorded as the pressure of the cuff when the rushing noises are first heard.

As the pressure in the cuff is reduced further to close the diastolic pressure, more and more blood can pass through the brachial artery. As the blood flows more easily, the rushing noises become increasingly soft. When the pressure in the cuff reaches the diastolic pressure, all the blood can pass freely through the vessel and the sounds disappear altogether. The diastolic pressure is recorded as the pressure of the cuff when the rushing noises stop altogether.

The BHS and National Institute for Clinical Health and Care Excellence (NICE) have collaborated to write guidelines for health professionals on how to take accurate blood pressure measurements and how to treat high blood pressure.[30] These guidelines ask for careful repeated measurements, although this ideal may be rarely achieved in real practice because of time constraints. However, this is not a trivial issue; an inaccurate measurement will lead to a false assumption about the true level of blood pressure, and can lead to inappropriate treatment.

The guidance states that the patient should be seated and should be relaxed. The arm should be resting on a surface so that it is at the level of the heart. The cuff pressure should be deflated very slowly (no more than 2mmHg per second) so that the rushing sounds can be accurately matched with the cuff pressure. The blood pressure should be measured in both arms, and if one of the two readings is consistently higher, this should be considered to be the accurate reading. If the blood pressure measurement is high, it should be repeated after 1–2 minutes and the first reading discarded if the second reading is lower. If more readings are taken, the lowest of these is used to give the final measurement. If the clinic reading is high, the advice is that the doctor should arrange for home readings to be obtained to ensure that a "white-coat effect" (see Section 3.2b) has not raised the blood pressure to higher than its usual level. The gold standard is that the patient is given an automated ambulatory blood pressure monitor to assess blood pressure throughout their day, but the guidelines accept that readings from a simple home monitor may also be valid in the diagnosis of raised blood pressure.

 Information box 3.2a-II

The heart and pericardium: comments from a Chinese medicine perspective

In Chinese medicine, the Heart and Pericardium are Organs to which specific functions are ascribed, and which are manifest on the exterior of the body in the primary Heart and Pericardium Channels respectively.

Maciocia (1989)[31] again quotes *The Simple Questions (Suwen)* when outlining the Chinese medicine view that the Heart is "like the Monarch and it governs the mind." He lists the six functions of the Heart Organ, which are to:

- govern Blood
- control the blood vessels
- manifest in the complexion
- house the mind (Shen)
- open into the tongue
- control sweat.

In order to be clear about how these functions relate to conventional medical understanding, it will help to consider each of these in turn.

First in this categorization, according to Maciocia, government of Blood refers to two aspects: the transformation of food (Gu Qi) into Blood, and also the healthy circulation of Blood. In contrast, in conventional medicine the manufacture of blood from basic nutrients takes place largely in the bone marrow, although the healthy circulation of blood is, of course, recognized as the domain of the cardiovascular system. This is one indication that the Chinese medical description of Blood does not map directly to the Western medical understanding of the blood that flows in the blood vessels. This potential source of confusion is explored in more detail in Chapter 3.4.

The control of the blood vessels is linked to two organs in Chinese medicine, the Heart and the Lungs. This partly refers to maintenance of healthy vessels, and is a reflection of healthy Gathering (Zong) Qi made by the Lung Organ from Gu Qi (from food) and Clear Qi (in air). In conventional medicine terms, the health of the blood vessels results from a healthy cardiovascular system, and does not obviously relate to the lungs. However, it is interesting to reflect that arteriosclerosis, a major cause of vascular (vessel) disease in the Western world, is the result of an activity that directly damages the lungs, namely, smoking. Also, the hormone angiotensin II that is vital for the maintenance and responsiveness of blood pressure is formed in the capillaries of the lungs where the hormone angiotensin-converting enzyme is manufactured.

The complexion is conventionally considered to be a reflection of the health of the skin rather than the heart. However, in conventional medicine it is recognized that certain cardiovascular conditions can cause signs that appear on the face. Malar flush, the pink coloration of the cheekbone area, is one example. This finding, considered an indication of Yin Deficiency in Chinese medicine, is, in a florid form, a medically recognized sign of the valvular heart disease known as mitral stenosis. From a Chinese medical viewpoint a deep branch of the Heart Primary Channel[32] runs up to cross the face and open into the eye, so explaining the link with the complexion of the face.

The mind/spirit is not associated with the cardiovascular system at all in conventional medicine. However, the English language reveals that in Western culture a deep connection has been made between the heart and the emotions. Phrases such as "my heart isn't in it," "to be heartbroken," "he was heartless" and "have a heart!" (to name only a few) are evidence of this connection. In many older cultures the heart is integral to the concept of mind and thought. The spirit of a person is also recognized in the eyes, and these have a direct link with the Heart Primary Channel via its deep branches that course upwards to end in the eyes.

The tongue and speech are also not associated with the cardiovascular system in conventional medicine, although one of the signs of severe heart disease is recognized to be cyanosis, in which a bluish discoloration is seen on the lips and tongue. There is also some recognition that aphasia is a frequent component of shock, which can manifest in other heart-related symptoms. In Chinese medicine the Heart Luo connecting channel connects the Heart Channel with the root of the tongue.

Sweating is not directly linked to the cardiovascular system from a conventional medicine perspective, but is a well-recognized symptom of heart attack.

The functions of the Heart according to a conventional and Chinese perspective can be summarized in the form of a correspondence table (for an introduction to the Organ correspondence tables, see Appendix I). This illustrates the idea that the functions of the fleshy pump, which conventional medicine calls the heart, may be in the domain of not only the Heart Organ in Chinese medicine, but also the Kidney and Liver Organs, and to a lesser extent all the Organ systems. This is because the body is not understood as reduced to its component parts in Chinese medicine. These correspondences are supported by the fact that deep branches of the Kidney and Liver Organs connect either directly or indirectly via the Pericardium with the Heart Organ. It will follow from this that diseases of the conventionally viewed cardiovascular system may manifest in Chinese medicine syndromes involving other Organs, including the Heart, Kidney and Liver.

The Pericardium Organ in the Chinese medicine tradition is loosely associated with the more superficial layers of the heart, the fibrous pericardium and the myocardium. The function of the Pericardium (Heart Protector) is described as similar to that of the Heart, but it also has the particular function of protection of the Heart against external pathogenic influences.[33] This has some overlap with the conventional medicine view in which the pericardium and the fluid that lies between it and the myocardium are very much seen as providing mechanical and immunological protection. In addition, there is the broader role, together with the Kidneys and Triple Burner Organs, of being associated with the Gate of Vitality (Ming Men). This Heart-Master role is as an intermediary within the Heart-Kidney Shaoyin Axis, and locates the Pericardium with the Ming Men at the physical level of the kidneys.[34]

Correspondence table for the functions of the Heart, as described by conventional and Chinese medicine

Functions of the heart
Acts as a pulsatile pump to enable circulation of the blood (Heart and Liver Organs)
The origin of the heart muscle impulse (the pacemaker) (Heart Organ and Kidney Yang)
Contributes to the maintenance of blood pressure (Heart Organ and Kidney Yang)
Will respond to bodily requirements by an alteration in the strength and rate of pumping (Heart Organ and Kidney Yang)

Functions of the Heart Organ
"The Heart is like the Monarch and it governs the mind"
It governs blood (bone marrow, heart, blood vessels)
It controls the blood vessels (blood vessels, adrenal glands, autonomic nervous system)
It manifests in the complexion (heart, blood vessels, blood, skin)
It houses the mind (brain and diverse neurochemical-releasing cells distributed throughout the body)
It opens into the tongue (digestive system)
It controls sweat (skin, autonomic nervous system)

Correspondence table for the functions of the Pericardium, as described by conventional and Chinese medicine

Functions of the pericardium
This is a fibrous membrane that surrounds the heart and allows its free movement. It also protects from mechanical injury. The serous fluid it encloses contains protective antibodies and immune cells (Heart, Liver and Kidney Organs)

Functions of the Pericardium[35]
"The Pericardium is an ambassador and from it joy and happiness derive"
Like the Heart it governs blood (bone marrow, heart, blood vessels)
Like the Heart it houses the mind (brain)
Together with the Kidneys and Triple Burner Organs it has been associated with the Gate of Vitality (Ming Men) (possibly the healthy function of the metabolic processes that go on in all the cells and particularly the sympathetic nervous system and the other diverse cells which derive from the embryonic neural crest[36])

3.2b The investigation of the cardiovascular system

The investigations and treatments for a patient with cardiovascular disease are usually managed within one of three hospital specialties: vascular surgery, cardiology and cardiothoracic surgery.

In the UK, patients who have a problem primarily with their blood vessels will usually be referred by their doctor to a surgeon who specializes in disease of the vessels (a vascular surgeon), because treatments for severe vascular disease very often involve a surgical operation.

In contrast, most patients with a suspected heart problem will be referred in the first instance to a physician who specializes in heart disease (a cardiologist). If the cardiologist decides that the heart requires a surgical operation, the patient will then be referred to a cardiothoracic surgeon.

The investigation of the vessels and circulation

The investigation of the vessels and circulation includes:

- a thorough physical examination

- blood tests

- tests such as a Doppler ultrasound scan and angiography to visualize the vessels in the thorax, abdomen, pelvis and legs.

These investigations are now considered briefly in turn.

Physical examination of the vessels and circulation

Physical examination of the vessels and circulation involves the stages listed in Table 3.2b-I.

Table 3.2b-I The stages of physical examination of the blood vessels and circulation

General examination for signs of poor circulation
Palpation of the pulses (radial, brachial, femoral, popliteal and foot pulses)
Assessment of specific regions of the body for dilated blood vessels (aneurysms)

GENERAL EXAMINATION OF THE SKIN
The examination of the skin is focused on looking for evidence of poor circulation. Signs of this include dry, shiny or itchy skin, reduction in body hair, purplish discoloration and weak or impalpable arterial pulses. If the reduction in circulation is very advanced, areas in which the skin has broken down (ulcers) may be seen. The finding of blackened patches of gangrenous skin is a grave sign of advanced vascular disease.

MEASUREMENT OF BLOOD PRESSURE IN THE UPPER AND LOWER LIMBS
Blood pressure assessment is a central part of the physical examination of the vascular system. A device called a Doppler probe is used to assist this. The same sort of probe is used by midwives to help them assess the heart rate of the fetus through the mother's abdomen. In this case the probe picks up the movement of blood within the fetal circulation, so that the heartbeat is made audible as a rapid pulsatile rushing noise.

The Doppler probe makes use of ultrasound waves to measure the flow rate of blood. A simple hand-held Doppler probe can be placed against a blood vessel, and will produce an audible rushing noise corresponding to the flow in the artery. If an artery is constricted, this sound will be absent.

The Doppler probe is commonly used instead of a stethoscope when measuring blood pressure in the lower limb as it is more sensitive in discerning blood flow, and more convenient to use in this situation. A comparison is made between the pressure measured at the brachial artery and that measured at the ankle artery (assessed using a blood pressure cuff wrapped around the thigh). In health, the ankle artery pressure should be slightly higher than that in the arm. However, in disease of the vessels, the major arteries that lead to the leg from the aorta can become severely constricted, which in turn reduces the pressure of blood within them. In this case, blood pressure measured in the leg will be lower than that measured at the brachial artery. In severe vascular disease the ankle artery measurement can be less than half the brachial artery blood pressure.

PHYSICAL EXAMINATION OF THE DEEP ARTERIES
The examining surgeon will palpate the central abdomen and the pelvis to assess the width of the deep arteries, the aorta and the common iliac arteries. In vascular disease, as the vessel walls become damaged, the major vessels may become distorted and dilated, and be at risk of rupturing. A dilated artery or aneurysm may be felt on abdominal palpation as a pulsatile mass.

Blood tests
Blood tests can be performed to exclude certain conditions that can contribute to disease of the vessels. The most common tests to be performed are serum tests to check for raised blood lipids (such as cholesterol) and glucose (indicative of diabetes). The erythrocyte sedimentation rate (ESR) or C-reactive protein (CRP) may be measured to exclude the rare inflammatory conditions that may affect

the blood vessels. A full blood count (FBC) is performed to exclude anemia in which the oxygen-carrying capacity of the blood is markedly reduced, and this can worsen the symptoms of vascular disease. For this reason, it is important to diagnose and treat anemia in someone with disease of the blood vessels.

Tests to visualize the deep vessels in the thorax, abdomen and pelvis

Non-invasive tests, such as an ultrasound scan or magnetic resonance imaging (MRI), may be performed to examine the structure of the deep arteries such as the aorta and its lower abdominal branches. Ultrasound images that are combined by computer processing with information obtained using a Doppler probe can give good information about the state of the blood flow within these blood vessels.

Increasingly, the Doppler ultrasound scan is taking the place of a more invasive method of investigation called an angiography. The angiogram is a very accurate method for getting good pictorial information about the arteries to the lower limbs, but is more invasive and carries more risks of arterial damage than an ultrasound scan. To obtain an angiogram a fine flexible tube is passed into a limb artery such as the femoral artery at the groin skin crease. The tube is then threaded "upstream," with guidance from X-ray imaging, to the part of the circulation to be studied. A "dye" that shows up on X-ray images (known as a contrast medium) is then released from the tip of the tube, and its flow is captured on X-ray films. These pictures will show the tree-like branching of the blood vessels in the area examined (see Figure 3.2b-I).

An angiogram will demonstrate areas in which the circulation is absent or depleted, and can, as shown in Figure 3.2b-I, expose areas of narrowing in vessels. It will also reveal the dilatation in vessels known as aneurysms.

An angiography carries a small risk of damage to the major blood vessels, which in some cases can have very severe consequences such as hemorrhage, thrombosis or embolism. For this reason, the angiogram is only performed in those situations in which the result of the test is believed to have an important bearing on the subsequent treatment of the patient (e.g. to clarify a decision on whether or not to go ahead with surgery). Increasingly, an angiography is performed in combination with MRI or computed tomography (CT) scanning, and this technique permits a detailed three-dimensional study of the path and patency of the blood vessels.

Figure 3.2b-I An angiogram showing the three major blood vessels of the heart (left coronary angiogram)
The image shows contrast medium filling the coronary vessels. The arrow points to the left anterior descending artery. The path of the artery is partly blocked by an irregular defect. This is a region of atheromatous plaque, and is likely to be the cause of chest pain in this person (see Section 3.2e).

The investigation of the heart

The investigation of the heart includes:

- a thorough physical examination

- blood tests

- electrocardiography (ECG) at rest and during exercise

- chest X-ray

- tests to visualize the heart muscle (in particular, echocardiography, nuclear imaging and CT and MRI studies of the heart)

- tests to assess the pressure of blood within the heart (cardiac catheterization)

- tests to visualize the coronary arteries (angiography).

These are considered briefly in turn below.

Physical examination of the heart

The physical examination of the heart involves the stages listed in Table 3.2b-II.

Table 3.2b-II The stages of physical examination of the heart
General inspection for signs of severe disease of the cardiovascular system, such as cyanosis, edema and enlarged liver
Palpation of the radial pulse (rate, rhythm, volume and shape)
Visual assessment of the pulse wave in the jugular veins at the neck
Palpation of the impulse of the heartbeat at the fifth intercostal space below the left nipple, and at other specific areas over the chest
Auscultation of the heart sounds and murmurs using the stethoscope
Assessment of brachial artery blood pressure

A thorough physical examination of the heart can pick up gross abnormalities of the heart rhythm, strength of heartbeat and integrity of the heart valves. However, physical examination can reveal very little about the health of the coronary arteries, unless coronary artery disease has already caused significant damage to the heart muscle itself. This is important to realize, as a "clean bill of health" on the basis of physical examination by a doctor does not necessarily exclude severe underlying heart disease.

Increasingly, a test known as ambulatory blood pressure monitoring is used in addition to resting brachial blood pressure assessment to give more information about how the blood pressure varies from day to day outside the clinic situation. It is well known that some people find such situations very stressful, which can lead to a marked rise in a usually normal blood pressure to abnormal levels (a phenomenon known as "white coat hypertension"). In ambulatory blood pressure assessment the patient is fitted with an automatic pressure-testing device, which self-inflates to assess blood pressure at intervals during the day and night. Patients are encouraged to record their day-to-day activities to see if there are specific situations that provoke any measured rises in blood pressure (see Figure 3.2b-II).

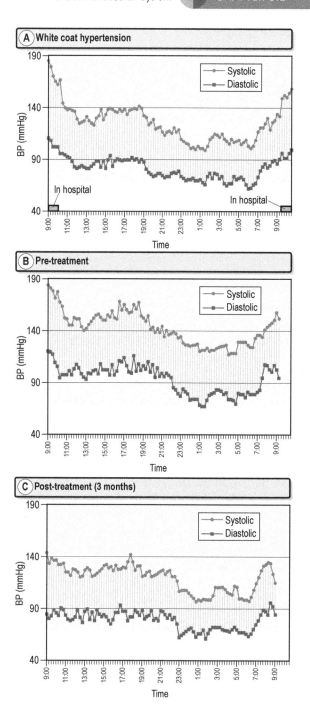

Figure 3.2b-II Results of 24-hour ambulatory blood pressure monitoring

(a) White coat hypertension in one patient (normal blood pressure is 140mmHg systolic and 90mmHg diastolic, indicated by the thin black lines). Note that the blood pressure is in the normal range except for the time during and shortly after the patient is in hospital. (b) The plot for another patient who is hypertensive for most of the day. (c) The plot of the same patient as in (b) after three months on medication for high blood pressure.

Blood tests

Blood tests are used to exclude conditions that may affect the heart, such as high blood cholesterol (hypercholesterolemia) and diabetes. These are also the conditions tested for in the investigation of vascular disease.

When the heart has been acutely damaged by a heart attack, the dying heart muscle cells release substances known as cardiac enzymes into the bloodstream over the next few days. A serum sample can reveal the presence of these enzymes and thus aid the diagnosis of a heart attack. The cardiac enzymes that are currently tested for include troponin, creatinine kinase, aspartate transaminase and lactate dehydrogenase. The levels of these markers all rise and fall at slightly different times in the few days after a heart attack. They are very useful for defining the time and also the severity of the heart attack.

Apart from the situation of a very recent heart attack, blood tests cannot be used to diagnose any of the other common forms of heart disease, such as valvular heart disease, most forms of cardiomyopathy and congenital heart disease.

Electrocardiography (ECG)

Electrocardiography (ECG) is a non-invasive technique that assesses the electrical activity of the heart as measured by electrodes on the surface of the skin. Electrodes are placed on the skin of the wrists, the ankles and at six points on the chest. The electrical activity on the skin originates from the electrical discharge in the conduction system of the heart. The information from these skin sites can be processed to produce a graphical readout that indicates the electrical activity of the heart.

The ECG trace can give information on the health of the conduction system of the heart. As the conduction system consists of cardiac muscle cells, the ECG will also give information on the health of the cardiac muscle. It does not directly assess the health of the coronary arteries, unless this is directly affecting the function of the heart conduction system (such as might occur during an attack of angina). The information from an ECG is often difficult to interpret. Therefore, an ECG recording has to be interpreted in the context of the results of other tests done at the same time.

ECG recording carries absolutely no risk to the patient, as the electrodes are simply detectors of electrical activity, and do not have any influence on the physiology of the patient.

24-HOUR ECG

This is a technique in which the aim is to capture an episode of a heart condition that has not been found on simple ECG testing. In 24-hour ECG recording, the patient is wired up to a small ECG recorder that they carry strapped to their body for the next day. The tape is subsequently removed and analyzed. This is primarily used to investigate episodic irregularities in heart rhythm (arrhythmias).

Like the resting ECG, the 24-hour tape recording carries no risk to the patient.

EXERCISE ECG

In this test, a patient is "wired up" as for an ECG, but is asked to walk on a treadmill while the recording is taken. The work required of the patient is gradually increased while the ECG reading is observed. In some patients, exercise might trigger an episode of an irregular heartbeat or of chest pain, and the ECG in such circumstances can confirm the diagnosis.

Unlike the resting ECG, the exercise ECG carries a risk for some patients. The aim of this test is only to take the patient to a level of exercise that will enable a diagnosis to be made, but not to such a level that might promote a serious attack of their condition. However, very occasionally, an attack of the condition is provoked by the physical exertion. Exercise ECG is, therefore, always performed under medical supervision.

Chest X-ray

Although the chest X-ray is commonly associated with the lungs, it can also be very useful in revealing features of some heart conditions. This is because the X-ray picture gives an outline of the heart and of the major vessels that leave the heart (aorta, vena cavae and pulmonary vessels) (see Figure 3.2b-III).

Figure 3.2b-III Chest X-ray images before and after treatment for pulmonary edema
These images illustrate the value of the chest X-ray in investigating heart disease. In both images the very dark areas with a faint horizontal striping across them are the images of the air-filled lungs and overlying ribs. The white shadow between the lungs is the central mass of soft tissue, which includes the esophagus and trachea. The heart is the lower part of this shadow, which projects slightly more to the right of the picture (to the left side of the patient). (a) The abnormal cloudiness of the lung fields that occurs when fluid accumulates in them as a result of weakened pumping of the heart. (b) The same lungs after medical treatment. The lung fields now appear clear, a sign that treatment has been successful.

A chest X-ray can show up the enlargement of the heart and blood vessels that may occur in heart failure (see Section 3.2f). Valvular disease of the heart can also give a characteristic X-ray picture. X-ray images cannot be used to diagnose coronary artery disease.

Tests to visualize the heart muscle
ECHOCARDIOGRAPHY
Echocardiography is an extremely valuable non-invasive test for looking at the structure of the heart. It uses ultrasound scans to produce images of the heart that not only reveal the outline, but also show the four chambers of the heart, the valves and the speed of flow and pressure of blood within the heart. Blood flow and pressure are assessed using the same principle as with the Doppler probe.

This investigation is considered to be totally harmless. In addition, it does not usually involve the patient in any discomfort, as the probe is placed against the chest wall. Very occasionally it is necessary to place the Doppler probe in the esophagus to obtain a good image of the posterior aspect of the heart. This requires the patient to be sedated, but is nevertheless still a very safe procedure.

Echocardiography has become an essential tool for the precise assessment of valvular conditions, heart muscle problems and heart failure (see Sections 3.2f and 3.2g). However, it cannot give direct information about the condition of the coronary arteries.

NUCLEAR IMAGING
Nuclear imaging describes a number of techniques that involve the intravenous injection of a radioactive "dye," which can then be detected by a machine called a gamma camera. The dyes most commonly used incorporate the radioactive heavy metals technetium and thallium attached to biological compounds that are naturally concentrated in healthy areas of heart muscle and bloodstream, respectively. Images of the healthy parts of the heart and the chambers of the heart can thus be produced.

MAGNETIC RESONANCE IMAGING
The MRI scan is another method for producing a clear image of the structure of the heart. The images can be synchronized with the ECG to provide pictures of the heart during different stages of the pumping cycle (see Figure 3.2b-IV).

Figure 3.2b-IV MRI scan of a cross-section of the lungs and heart at the level of the mid-thorax
These images illustrate the level of detail that can be obtained by means of MRI scanning (compare with the coarse detail seen in the X-rays in Figure 3.2b-III). (a) A computer-generated slice through the chest of a patient, presented as if the patient were lying on his back with his feet pointing in the direction of the observer. The white portions at the periphery of the image represent the bony ribs and scapulae, and the black areas the airspaces of the lungs. In the middle a section through a thoracic vertebra can be seen, and above this the heart. (b) The four chambers of the heart, the right and left atria (RA and LA), and the right and left ventricles (RV and LV). MV indicates the mitral valve that sits between the left atrium and left ventricle.

Tests to assess the pressure of blood within the heart
Although the technique of echocardiography with Doppler can give approximate estimates of the pressure of the blood in the four chambers of the heart, the most accurate method is cardiac catheterization, an invasive investigation. Catheterization of the right side of the heart involves passing a fine tube into a vein (usually the jugular vein of the neck or the femoral vein in the groin) and thence to the vena cava and right atrium. To investigate the left side of the heart, a fine tube is usually inserted into the femoral artery in the groin and then directed via the aorta to the left atrium.

This important test is used to diagnose the seriousness of valvular disease and heart failure. It is uncomfortable and is usually carried out under anesthetic. Catheterization of the heart carries a small risk of thrombosis, embolism and hemorrhage.

Tests to visualize the coronary arteries (angiography)

An angiography is considered to be the most accurate test for visualizing the internal state of the coronary arteries. Coronary angiography involves the same procedure as described for the investigation of vascular disease. It is usually performed as an extension of left-sided cardiac catheterization.

Once the catheter has reached the aorta, its tip is directed into the openings of the three coronary arteries (see Figure 3.2a-VI for a reminder of how the coronary vessels leave the aorta). A contrast medium "dye" is injected into the three arteries. X-ray images can then show up the flow of blood within these vessels, and also any obstructions to the normal pattern of flow. A clear image taken by means of a coronary angiogram is shown in Figure 3.2b-I above.

A coronary angiography is performed in cases of severe angina (see Section 3.2e) to determine whether or not a surgical operation (angioplasty or coronary artery bypass graft) might be of benefit to the patient.

Even more so than for cardiac catheterization, a coronary angiography carries some risk to the patient (just fewer than 1 in 1000 procedures results in a fatal complication).

3.2c Diseases of the blood vessels

This section introduces the most important diseases of the blood vessels. The diseases studied are:

- Diseases of the arteries:
  - arteriosclerosis
  - atherosclerosis
  - ischemia of the legs (peripheral artery disease)
  - aneurysms
  - vasculitis
  - Raynaud's disease
- Diseases of the veins:
  - varicose veins
  - thrombophlebitis (phlebitis)
  - deep vein (venous) thrombosis (DVT).

For a reminder of the physiology of the arteries and veins, see Section 3.2a.

Important diseases of the arteries

Arteriosclerosis (hardening of the arteries)

Arteriosclerosis is the loss of flexible compliance in the vessel walls. A degree of arteriosclerosis is a normal aspect of aging, but in some people this process is accelerated and then becomes an important cause of premature ill health.

As described in Section 3.2a, the arteries normally have an ability to be responsive to the body's needs by expansion or contraction. This responsiveness is a result of the elastic structure of the artery walls. With aging, the elastic tissue is gradually replaced by firmer connective tissue, which in some instances can accumulate calcium. This firm and sometimes calcified connective tissue is unable to contract and expand, and the vessels become hardened.

One of the important causes of premature arteriosclerosis is high blood pressure (hypertension). It is believed that the body responds to the increased pressure within the vessels by laying down more connective tissue in the vessel walls. However, in the larger vessels, the stiffened walls contribute to the further development of hypertension, because the vessels become less compliant. As hypertension is actually a cause of arteriosclerosis, this means a vicious circle is set up in which the arteriosclerosis worsens.

Information box 3.2c-I

Arteriosclerosis: comments from a Chinese medicine perspective

In Chinese medicine hardening and stiffening are generally suggestive of Qi Deficiency and Stagnation, as the responsiveness and springiness characteristic of healthy living tissue is seen as a reflection of freely moving Qi. We might, therefore, expect to see other symptoms and signs of Qi Deficiency and Stagnation when arteriosclerosis has developed.

The fact that vessels are controlled by the Heart and Lungs in Chinese medicine could suggest that it is a Deficiency of the Qi of the chest, Zong Qi in particular, which may underlie the development of arteriosclerosis. This accords with the fact that smoking, a known causative agent in arteriosclerosis, is also recognized in Chinese medicine to damage Zong Qi. Emotional factors impacting on the Heart and Lungs that then lead to Stagnation of Qi in the chest will also be important in pathogenesis.

Smoking is also recognized to lead to arteriosclerosis, because it both reduces the oxygen delivery to the vessel linings and increases the levels of damaging and highly reactive free radicals (chemicals that can damage the lining of the blood vessels, amongst other things) in the body.

The stiffened large vessels are also at risk of becoming distorted, particularly if blood pressure is high. Distorted vessels can suddenly rupture and cause a life-threatening hemorrhage. A distorted and dilated blood vessel is called an aneurysm (see later).

Stiff connective tissue can also cause the inside of smaller arteries to become narrowed. A narrowed and stiff vessel will not permit sufficient blood flow to the organs and to other tissues supplied by the small arteries. Depending on the arteries affected, conditions such as kidney failure, dementia and skin ulcers can be serious consequences of arteriosclerosis.

Atherosclerosis

Atherosclerosis is a condition that can affect the larger arteries in middle to later life. It commonly coexists with the changes of arteriosclerosis.

Atherosclerosis also involves a hardening of the arteries, but in this case the hardening is due to the accumulation of a fatty deposit on the lining of the vessels known as atheroma. Atheroma is recognized to begin to develop in the form of "fatty streaks" on the inner lining of blood vessels from as early as the teenage years. Atheroma contains cholesterol and other fatty substances, and with time can become hardened by connective tissue cells and calcium. In addition to causing stiffening and distortion of the larger vessels, atheroma causes other problems because it narrows the inside of the large vessels and reduces blood flow. It also causes the affected blood vessels to have an irregular and fragile lining (see Figure 3.2c-I).

The irregular lining of vessels affected by atherosclerosis can stimulate the clotting process of the blood, so that small blood clots can develop at sites where atheroma is present. This process will be all the more likely if the fragile lining of the atheromatous plaque ruptures and leaks irritating substances into the affected blood vessel. These processes can lead to the conditions of thrombosis and embolism (see Section 2.2d). Atherosclerosis can therefore lead to infarction of tissues (i.e. tissue death resulting from a suddenly reduced blood supply).

Conditions such as heart attack (myocardial infarction) and stroke (cerebral infarction) are very common severe consequences of atherosclerosis, and it is believed that in many cases it is the rupture of an atheromatous plaque that is a trigger for these devastating conditions.

It is known that low levels of physical exercise, a fatty diet and smoking are all powerful contributors to the development of atheroma. High levels of certain blood lipids (fats) also increase the tendency of atheroma to develop, and current theories focus on saturated fats, trans fatty acids and an unhealthy balance of polyunsaturated fats, together with low levels of protective dietary anti-oxidants, as the main culprits (see Section 3.1a). Diabetes is another cause of long-term adverse changes to the lining of the blood vessels, in this case because raised blood glucose alters the microscopic structure of the lining of the vessels. The causes of atheroma are explored in greater detail in Section 3.2e on coronary heart disease.

A   Normal artery

B   Fatty streak

C   Mature plaque

D   Ruptured plaque with thrombus formation

Key

- Foam cells
- Accumulation of smooth muscle cells
- Cholesterol and other lipids
- Thrombus
- Fibrous cap

Figure 3.2c-I The stages in the development of an atheromatous plaque in an artery

Information box 3.2c-II

Atherosclerosis: comments from a Chinese medicine perspective

The accumulation of a fatty deposit within the vessels is suggestive of the Chinese medicine concept of "Phlegm without a form" or "non-substantial Phlegm." These interchangeable terms are used to describe conditions in which painless lumps and growths develop. Phlegm is usually generated by the action of Heat on Damp, so the lifestyle factors of Damp-forming diet and excess Heat are contributory factors. This again seems to match with the conventional medicine understanding that both a fatty diet (Damp forming) and smoking (Heat inducing) can contribute to atheroma. Cold may also be a factor that leads to congealing and Stagnation of Qi in the Chest in the case of Heart Yang Deficiency of old age, and so can be contributory in atherosclerosis of coronary vessels.[37]

Phlegm may also develop in conditions in which Qi is Stagnant, and treatments to move Qi are usually integral to the treatment of Phlegm. It has already been suggested that Qi Deficiency might underlie hardening of the arteries (arteriosclerosis), and so atherosclerosis, which commonly coexists with arteriosclerosis, may well indicate the same.

Moreover, the impaired blood flow and clotting that can develop from atheroma can easily lead to symptoms of Blood Stagnation (intense fixed pain and purplish discoloration), which, in Chinese medicine, is often seen to result from both Phlegm and Qi Deficiency.

Ischemia of the legs (peripheral artery disease)

As noted in Section 2.2d, ischemia literally means poor blood supply. Ischemia of the legs is a consequence of poor blood supply to the lower half of the body, conventionally known as peripheral artery disease (PAD). Depending on whether or not the reduction of blood flow is of sudden or gradual onset, there are two distinct syndromes relating to leg ischemia. These are known as acute and chronic leg ischemia. PAD can also affect the arms, but this is far less common than leg ischemia, which is known to affect over 15 percent of people over the age of 70 in the UK.

The most common cause of both types of leg ischemia is atherosclerosis of the lower aorta and also of the vessels that branch from the aorta in the lower abdomen to enter the pelvis and to supply the legs. Figure 3.2a-I above illustrates the pathway of the aorta and shows how it divides just above the pelvis to form the common iliac arteries. These are the vessels that in turn provide arterial branches that supply the deep tissues of the pelvis and the legs.

Leg ischemia can also result from atherosclerosis of the vessels of the thigh and lower leg, and predisposing factors include old age, smoking, diabetes, hypertension, obesity and inactivity. Arteriosclerosis in the smaller vessels that supply the skin and muscles of the leg often coexists with atherosclerosis of the larger vessels, and this worsens the condition.

In acute leg ischemia, a major vessel that supplies the leg becomes blocked by thrombosis. The thrombosis is often the consequence of atherosclerosis on the inside of the vessel. The sudden reduction in blood supply leads to a rapid onset of intense cramping pain in the calf, and the limb becomes cold, pale and mottled. This condition is a surgical emergency, and requires removal of the clot before irreparable damage to the tissues of the leg can occur. If the clot is extensive, a surgical operation may be necessary in which the vessel is cut open to remove it. However, some patients can be helped by drug treatment to dissolve the clot. This medical approach, called thrombolysis (in which fibronolytic drugs are given to break up the blood clot), is discussed in more detail within the description of heart attack in Section 3.2e. If the treatment is ineffective or comes too late, amputation may be the only option for the patient.

 Information box 3.2c-III

Acute leg ischemia: comments from a Chinese medicine perspective

A sudden onset of severe pain, with cold and mottling, the consequence of acute leg ischemia, would be indicative in Chinese medicine of Cold Painful Obstruction Syndrome, with predomination of Blood Stagnation. The patient will need urgent conventional medical care, but Chinese medical treatment would be to expel Cold and to Move Stagnant Blood and Qi.

Chronic leg ischemia is another manifestation of PAD resulting from a gradual reduction in the ability of sufficient blood to flow to the lower legs. The main symptom is cramp-like pain (known as claudication, a word derived from the Latin term for limping) in one or both calves. This pain may be provoked by exercise, when there is an increased demand for a good blood supply to the calf muscle. When the condition is advanced, pain can also come on in bed at night, when it can be helped by dropping the lower leg over the side of the bed. This is to be distinguished from the common symptom of benign night-time cramp, which is a much more intense pain associated with contraction of the muscles of the calf, and is not helped by lowering the leg. When chronic leg ischemia becomes as severe as to threaten acute arterial blockage, it is described as critical ischemia.

The physical signs of poor circulation to the legs that can be found by an examining doctor have been described in Section 3.2b. Typically, the feet are cold and without palpable pulses. The skin of the feet may be shiny and purplish, and body hair absent. The blood pressure in the leg will be much lower than expected.

In severe cases of chronic leg ischemia, skin ulcers or patches of blackened skin (gangrene) may be seen on the skin of the heel or toes, a sign that long-term poor circulation has led to the death of these tissues. These areas can be very painful.

A patient with the symptoms of chronic leg ischemia will undergo a Doppler ultrasound scan or an angiogram to visualize the condition of the deep blood vessels in the lower abdomen and leg. In this way the severity of the condition can be assessed.

Some patients may respond rapidly to simple measures such as stopping smoking, treatment of diabetes and hypertension and a gentle exercise program. The antiplatelet drugs aspirin, clopidogrel or dipyridamole will be recommended to continue lifelong, as well as statins and antihypertensive medication if relevant. PAD is often accompanied by vascular disease in the brain and in the heart and kidneys; this means that patients may have serious co-morbidities. Fifty percent of patients diagnosed with PAD will have died within five years of diagnosis.

Those who are found to have only a short region of narrowing of a blood vessel may be treated by means of a balloon angioplasty. In this operation the patient is sedated and a catheter inserted into the affected vessel. The end of the catheter (the "balloon") is then gently inflated when situated in the region of the narrowing. The inflated end compresses the atheroma against the vessel walls, and so, in most cases, widens the narrowing. There is a small risk with this procedure of damage to the vessel or rupture of the atheromatous plaque with further narrowing, but in the majority of patients it provides a relatively non-invasive answer to their symptoms. Alternatively, a surgical operation may be performed to remove the atheroma in the narrowed section of the blood vessel.

Patients with more extensive disease respond very well to surgical bypass of the affected vessels. In this operation the affected aorta and iliac vessels are bypassed by the insertion of either a manmade length of tubing (commonly made from an inert material such as Teflon) or a length of a wide vein taken from the thigh of the patient during the same operation. The blood can then flow freely through this new passageway to the legs. This operation carries a small risk of thrombosis and hemorrhage at the site of the replaced vessel.

Unfortunately, not all patients can benefit from this operation, either because their health is so poor due to atherosclerosis elsewhere, or because the smaller vessels of the legs are so badly affected that the operation would not be of help to them.

In severe inoperable cases, the only answer may be amputation of the affected lower leg. This is always undertaken when gangrene has set in, and when the circulation cannot be improved sufficiently for it to heal. Smokers and people with diabetes are the two categories of patients who are most likely to have to undergo amputation for leg ischemia.

Information box 3.2c-IV

Chronic leg ischemia: comments from a Chinese medicine perspective

The symptoms and signs of ischemia of the lower legs are deep cramping pain on exercise and poorly nourished tissues. These suggest Stagnation of Blood and Qi, with underlying Qi Deficiency. Cold may be a contributory Pathogenic Factor in some cases leading to Congealing of Blood. The presence of atheroma in the vessels suggests that the development of Phlegm may be a contributory factor to the Stagnation. These Pathogenic Factors will be apparent in the pulse and tongue of the patient.

By preventing the clotting of blood, antiplatelet medications would appear to have the energetic effect of Moving Qi and Blood, which could be interpreted as a Warming or Heating action. If so, this is in keeping with the known side effects of these medications that include inflammation of the stomach lining, gastric hemorrhage and rash.

Aneurysms

An aneurysm is a dilated and distorted artery. This is most likely to occur in an artery affected by arteriosclerosis or atherosclerosis, although there are other rare causes.

The aorta is a common site for the development of an aneurysm (see Figure 3.2c-II). This is because the aorta carries blood under high pressure, and is also commonly affected by arteriosclerosis and atherosclerosis.

Lower aortic aneurysms can be detected by abdominal palpation, and their presence confirmed by means of abdominal ultrasound scans. They are a relatively common finding in elderly people, and in men in particular. They are usually relatively small (less than 5cm in diameter) and are unlikely to lead to any immediate problems. However, larger aneurysms can press onto adjacent organs and may lead to back and abdominal pain. The larger the aneurysm, the more likely it is to rupture.

If an aortic aneurysm spontaneously ruptures, the patient is likely to collapse because of severe internal bleeding, and may have intense back and abdominal pain. As this event is most likely to occur in a frail elderly person, there is a high risk of sudden death.

Surgical treatment of an aneurysm involves a bypass of the affected aorta with an artificial length of vessel, by a similar method as described for leg ischemia. This is a major operation, requiring the patient to recover in intensive care, and carries risks. If the operation is carried out as an emergency, the operative mortality is very high (about half of patients who are operated on for a ruptured aortic aneurysm will not survive the operation). However, if the operation is performed as a precaution against rupture in a stable patient, the success rate is far higher. For this reason, if an aneurysm of over 5cm is detected, surgery may be offered even if the patient is otherwise healthy and has no symptoms.

Another fairly common site for aneurysms is around the vessels that enter the base of the brain. Because of their size and shape, these are known as berry aneurysms. In contrast to aortic aneurysms, these are usually present from birth, and are not related to arteriosclerosis or atherosclerosis. However, there is a risk that these, too, will spontaneously rupture, even in young people. If this occurs, a hemorrhage in the area around the base of the brain is the result. This is called a subarachnoid hemorrhage. This life-threatening event is described in more detail in Chapter 4.1.

Figure 3.2c-II X-ray image of the chest, showing an aneurysm of the arch of the aorta
This image demonstrates a sizeable aneurysm of the aorta; compare this with the normal X-ray image shown in Figure 3.2b-III above.

Information box 3.2c-V

Aneurysms: comments from a Chinese medicine perspective

As the health of the vessels in Chinese medicine is underpinned by healthy Zong Qi, this would suggest that the weakness and dilatation of an aneurysm reflects deficiency of Zong Qi.

However, the reported pain and rupture resulting from an abdominal aneurysm is more suggestive of Qi and Blood Stagnation of the Chest or Abdomen, which is presumably a consequence of chronic Deficiency of Qi. The affected patient would be in a state of collapse, with cold extremities and thready pulses, both of which might be described in Chinese medicine as Collapse of Yang.

Vasculitis

Vasculitis is a general term used to describe any inflammation of blood vessels. Most cases of vasculitis are the result of the disordered immune process that occurs in many of the multisystem (rheumatic) autoimmune disorders (see Section 2.2c). The inflammatory diseases that can involve the blood vessels include temporal arteritis (large vessels affected), polyarteritis nodosa, Kawasaki disease (medium-sized vessels affected), systemic lupus erythematosus (SLE), Wegener's granulomatosis and rheumatoid arthritis (small vessels affected).

In many of these disorders, although many tissues may be affected, it is the damage to arteries that leads to the most serious consequences of the disease. In these conditions, antibodies attach to the artery wall, and this leads to inflammation. Long-term inflammation leads to thickening of the artery and thus narrowing of the inside of the vessel. This can result in impaired blood supply. In a few of these conditions, the inflammation can cause an aneurysm and rupture of the vessel.

The consequences of vasculitis depend on the size and site of the vessel involved. Typical features of autoimmune vasculitis are summarized in Table 3.2c-I. No single autoimmune disease will lead to all these features, each type of autoimmune disease having its own characteristic pattern of how the blood vessels are affected. For example, SLE most commonly involves the facial skin and joints, but in severe cases will characteristically involve the brain and kidneys.

Table 3.2c-I The local effects of vasculitis

Site of vasculitis	Possible features
Skin	Red rashes, itchy lumps, purpura and bruises
Brain	Headache, stroke or mental symptoms
Kidney	Kidney failure
Eye	Sudden or gradual loss of sight
Nerves	Numbness and weakness
Gastrointestinal system	Pain and hemorrhage
Cardiovascular system	Angina and heart attack
Joints and muscles	Arthritis, muscular pain and weakness
General features	Fever, malaise and weight loss

 Information box 3.2c-VI

Vasculitis: comments from a Chinese medicine perspective

The inflammation and thickening of vessels and the resulting impaired blood supply in vasculitis might suggest the Chinese Pathogenic Factors of Heat and Phlegm and Stagnation. The involvement of vessels, in particular, suggests a background of Zong Qi Deficiency, and the fact that the immune system is disordered suggests weakness of Kidney Qi. Very often these conditions tend to run in families, which supports the view that the inherited weakness is rooted in weak Kidney Essence (Jing).

Patients with immune-related inflammatory vasculitis may demonstrate symptoms and signs that confirm these imbalances: rashes and fevers suggest Heat, nodules and joint deformities suggest Phlegm, and intense pain from joints or angina would suggest Stagnation. The lungs are frequently involved in these conditions, with breathlessness resulting from fibrosis, which again may suggest Zong Qi Deficiency. The kidneys are also often affected, with kidney failure being a very common cause of serious ill health and death in these patients (Kidney Qi Deficiency).

Some infectious conditions involve vasculitis. For example, the purpuric rash that is found in a severe case of meningococcal meningitis is due to widespread infection in the bloodstream causing patches of vasculitis. The affected small vessels rupture, which leads to a bruising rash that does not fade when pressure is applied to the skin (unlike most skin rashes). Vasculitis is also a recognized consequence of hepatitis B and C.

Raynaud's disease

Raynaud's disease is a common condition in which the muscular wall of the small vessels of the fingers spontaneously tighten (go into spasm), usually in response to cold, anxiety or external vibration. The condition can occasionally also affect the toes. The spasm cuts off the blood supply, with the result that the affected fingers initially go purple or blue, and then white. The fingers feel numb and cold, and can be very painful.

Most people feel more pain as the condition reverses and blood flow is restored. The fingers recovering from such an attack may appear temporarily reddened before returning to normal. An attack can last for up to a few hours.

The cause of uncomplicated Raynaud's disease is unknown, but it is recognized to be more common in slim young women. Under-eating can lead to a propensity to the condition. Smoking very much exacerbates the condition.

If attacks of Raynaud's disease are prolonged and frequent, the impaired blood supply can cause damage to the tissues of the fingers. The skin can become dry and thickened and, in some rare cases, patches of gangrene can develop.

Occasionally, Raynaud's disease has vasculitis as an underlying cause, when it appears as part of a multisystem autoimmune disease. In this case, the impaired blood supply results from inflammation-mediated muscular spasm. Other symptoms of a generalized autoimmune disease may be present, and blood tests such as the ESR (erythrocyte sedimentation rate) and CRP (C-reactive protein) may indicate active inflammation.

Patients with Raynaud's disease are advised to avoid the triggers of attacks by keeping their hands warm and by stopping smoking. In severe cases, the drug nifedipine is prescribed. Nifedipine is one of a family of drugs (calcium channel blockers (CCBs)) that block the entry of calcium into smooth muscle and cardiac muscle cells, and so have the effect of dilating blood vessels. The most common side effects of nifedipine are flushing and headaches, which develop as a result of dilatation of blood vessels in the face, scalp and brain.

Rarely, a surgical approach called sympathectomy may be employed, in which the nerves that cause constriction of blood vessels are intentionally damaged by injection at the site in the neck from where they leave the spinal cord.

Information box 3.2c-VII

Raynaud's disease: comments from a Chinese medicine perspective

The symptoms of cold and poor circulation to the fingers suggest Yang Deficiency and Deficiency of Zong Qi, as it is Zong Qi that is responsible for circulation to the extremities. Flaws and Sionneau (2001) suggests that external Pathogenic Factors such as Cold, Damp and even Heat can enter the Channels at the finger tips and cause obstruction to flow of Blood and Qi.[38] The intense pain and purplish discoloration that can accompany the condition could well be interpreted as Cold and Qi Deficiency leading to Blood Stagnation.

Nifedipine, by relieving these symptoms, could be viewed as Heating in nature, and the facial flushing and headaches that are common side effects support this supposition. The flushing and headaches are commonly full-type symptoms, and this might correspond to Stomach Heat or Liver Fire Blazing. Other side effects include rapid heart rate, rashes, itch, eye pain, muscle aches and jaundice, and together these suggest that the predominant action of nifedipine is one of creating Heat in the Liver and Heart.

Important diseases of the veins

Varicose veins

Varicose veins are those that have become distended and distorted as a consequence of prolonged increased pressure of blood flow within them. The tendency to develop varicose veins runs in families. It is often a combination of congenital susceptibility and increased pressure on the veins that leads to their development.

The most well-recognized site for the development of varicose veins is the lower leg (for a description of the deep and superficial veins in the leg, see Section 3.2a). Varicose veins tend to affect the superficial leg veins only, with the veins that run deep in the leg muscle not affected. In contrast, it is the deep veins and not the superficial veins that are affected by deep vein thrombosis (DVT).

Factors including prolonged standing, obesity and pregnancy contribute to the development of varicose veins in the legs. Standing leads to high pressure in the deep veins of the lower leg as a result of the columns of blood pooling within them. As the superficial veins feed into the deep veins through perforator veins, the pressure in these superficial veins is likewise increased when a person stands. The pressure is increased further if the person is obese and there is excess fatty tissue around the veins. However, when a person walks or runs, the pressure in the leg veins is reduced because the muscular contractions of the calf and thigh help keep the blood flow moving up out of the deep veins and towards the heart, and this can then allow the drainage of the superficial veins. In pregnancy, the enlarged uterus can compress the deep veins in the pelvis, and lead to increased pressure of blood in the deep leg veins.

In prolonged standing, obesity and pregnancy, prolonged increased pressure within the deep veins in the leg can act to distort the structure of the valves in the perforator veins that connect the deep veins to the superficial veins. As the valves distort they can no longer close properly, so that the smooth flow of blood out of the superficial veins is impaired, and the superficial veins become distended with blood.

One common consequence of the distension of blood through superficial varicose veins is an accumulation of fluid in the tissues of the lower leg, which can cause the ankles to swell slightly. The medical term for excess fluid in the tissues is edema. Varicose veins are therefore one of the many causes of edema. In this case it is not usually a serious condition. The edema resulting from varicose veins is generally mild (i.e. it does not extend to above the malleoli of the ankles) and is worse only after standing or at the end of the day.

The most commonly experienced problem of varicose veins is that they are considered unsightly. The poor blood flow to the skin around varicose veins can lead to purplish, thread-like broken veins appearing on the skin, and the edema compounds this problem. This is a cause of distress for many people.

Less commonly, the veins can ache, and this can be to such a degree as to impair a person's quality of life. The skin around the vein can itch, and can develop patches of eczema.

The three serious conditions that can result from varicose veins are ulceration of the skin of the calf, hemorrhage and thrombophlebitis. Skin ulceration can occur near long-standing varicose veins because of the long-term effect that the impaired circulation and buildup of edema has on the skin. The skin becomes thin, dry and vulnerable to injury, and after injury the healing of the skin is impaired due to poor circulation. The most common sites for a varicose skin ulcer to develop are on the inside aspect of the ankle and the lower calf (see Figure 3.2c-III).

Hemorrhage can occur if an injury breaks the skin and damages the vein. Instead of the usual ooze of blood, a gush of dark blood can occur due to the increased pressure of blood flow within the vein. This will usually settle down with the prompt application of firm pressure, but recovery may be complicated by poor healing.

The complication of thrombophlebitis is described in the next section.

When assessing a person with varicose veins, a vascular surgeon will check the extent to which the local skin has been compromised by poor circulation, and will assess the back flow of blood through the venous valves by means of Doppler probes. Surgery for varicose veins is usually only medically advised for reasons of bleeding, pain, ulceration, thrombophlebitis or a severe impact on quality of life. However, many people will choose to pay for surgery to correct the cosmetic effects of varicose veins.

Figure 3.2c-III Varicose ulcer of the inner aspect of the lower leg
This picture shows a very severe case of ulceration in which a large area of the skin has lost its integrity as a result of long-term poor venous blood flow.

Before surgery is contemplated, most patients are initially advised to try lifestyle changes such as losing weight, walking more and putting their feet up when resting. Support stockings can improve the return of the blood from the superficial to the deep veins of the leg.

Mildly affected veins, and especially those below the knee, may be injected with a chemical that causes them to close up completely (sclerotherapy). This is considered to be a minor treatment. The remaining superficial veins of the leg readily enlarge to take over the role of the injected veins. One downside of sclerotherapy is that the varicose veins fairly commonly recur sometime after the treatment, particularly if the underlying causes have not been dealt with.

Surgery for varicose veins involves either removing a length of affected vein through a small incision in the skin, or tying off the connections that the superficial vein had with the deep veins via perforating veins with a surgical stitch, or both. These operations carry small risks of infection of the wounds, hemorrhage from the cut veins and thrombophlebitis (see below). The recurrence rate of varicose veins after surgery is high, but not as high as for sclerotherapy. The problem returns in about one in ten people who have the operation. After both these treatments the patient is advised to wear a support bandage for a few weeks, to lose weight if relevant, and to do as much walking as possible.

Thrombophlebitis

Thrombophlebitis literally describes inflammation (phlebitis) and clotting in a vein. It is a condition of the superficial veins in which the blood within the vein forms small clots and the lining of the wall of the vessel becomes inflamed. It is usually a benign self-limiting condition but can extend to involve the deep veins or lead directly to a pulmonary embolus in vulnerable patients.

Thrombophlebitis of the superficial veins in the legs manifests in very painful, hot and red patches on the leg, but this is rarely serious. In contrast to the dangerous condition of thrombosis of the deep veins of the leg (DVT), the blood clots in superficial veins do not usually send emboli to the deep veins of the pelvis and thence to the heart and the lungs.

The most common underlying problem in a case of thrombophlebitis is varicosities of the veins. The distorted lining of varicose veins can stimulate the clotting cascade, and the clotting leads to inflammation of the veins. Other risk factors for phlebitis are obesity, immobility, physical damage to the veins and also states in which the blood has an increased tendency to clot (e.g. advanced cancer).

The advice to the patient with thrombophlebitis is to continue to exercise the limb unless the clotting is very extensive and to take non-steroidal anti-inflammatory drugs (NSAIDs) such as ibuprofen for their painkilling and clot-preventing effects. These different medications should not be taken together, as the risks of dangerous side effects such as kidney damage and bleeding become significant. Increasingly patients with phlebitis are advised to take blood-thinning medication for up to one month to prevent extension to a DVT. This medication has to be given by subcutaneous injection.

 Information box 3.2c-IX

Thrombophlebitis: comments from a Chinese medicine perspective

The localized pain, heat and redness of thrombophlebitis might suggest a Chinese medicine diagnosis of local Blood Stagnation with Heat. In the absence of external injury, these imbalances may be considered to be the result of internal factors. The location of the inflammation in relation to specific channels would be relevant to a Chinese practitioner. For example, thrombophlebitis in the distribution of the Stomach Channel might be a superficial manifestation of Stomach Heat. The symptomatic benefit of aspirin or NSAID medication may point to their ability to move Qi and Blood.

Deep vein (venous) thrombosis (DVT)

DVT was explored briefly in Section 2.2d. The most common site for DVT to occur is within the deep veins of the calf. This is a serious condition, because the deep veins of the calf have a direct communication with the deep veins of the pelvis, and thence to the heart and lungs. A clot (thrombosis) of the deep veins of the leg can, therefore, spread upward to involve the pelvic veins, or can produce fragments (emboli) that can travel up through the right side of the heart to lodge in the arterial tree of lungs (pulmonary embolus).

A clot in the deep vein of the leg is most likely to occur if the circulation is sluggish. This situation can develop from a combination of factors, including inactivity, obesity, old age, recent surgery, pregnancy and factors that lead to an increased tendency for the blood to clot, such as an inherited tendency to clotting, the oral contraceptive pill, smoking or serious illness. A DVT in this region leads to an acutely swollen, purplish, tender and hot calf. The pain is increased if the patient flexes the foot upwards, but they should not be asked to do this because of the risk of dislodging emboli.

Diagnosis of a DVT was formerly made by injecting contrast medium "dye" into the vein, which could then be visualized by means of X-rays (venogram). Increasingly, a confident diagnosis can be made by means of a Doppler ultrasound scan, which can show up clots in the larger vessels of the thigh. A blood test for by-products of clotting (D-dimer test) can also help to confirm the diagnosis in uncertain cases, thus making the more invasive venogram unnecessary.

A patient who has had a DVT is immediately commenced on daily injections of blood-thinning heparin-like medication (e.g. dalteparin). They will also be started on a slower acting oral anticoagulant, either warfarin or a NOAC (novel oral anticoagulant) (see Section 2.2d). Once the oral anticoagulant has reached active levels in the blood, the heparin is stopped and the patient is advised to remain on the oral drug for between 12 weeks and 6 months. Warfarin and NOACs counteract the formation of some of the clotting factors in the liver, and so reduce the tendency of the blood to clot. All these treatments reduce the risk of the development of pulmonary emboli, and can contribute to the dissolution of the clot.

The patient with a DVT is advised to rest the limb totally for the first couple of days. Support stockings that have been designed to keep the deep veins as open as possible are also prescribed for the first few days after the thrombosis.

Even when the risk of emboli has passed (within a few weeks), many patients who have suffered a DVT continue to have problems. These patients are at greater risk of developing edema, varicose veins and varicose ulcers because the free flow of blood through the leg may be permanently impaired.

 Information box 3.2c-X

Deep vein thrombosis: comments from a Chinese medicine perspective

The swollen, purplish, painful and hot leg resulting from a DVT might be diagnosed primarily as Blood and Qi Stagnation with Heat. There is likely to be a background of marked local or generalized Deficiency of Blood or Qi to permit this condition to develop. The Chinese medicine interpretation of the action of warfarin is described more fully in Chapter 2.2.

The red flags of diseases of the blood vessels

Some patients with diseases of the blood vessels will benefit from referral to a conventional doctor for assessment or treatment. Red flags are those symptoms and signs that indicate that referral should be considered. The red flags of the diseases of the blood vessels are described in Table 3.2c-II. A summary of the red flags in a format designed for quick reference in clinical practice can be found in Appendix III. This gives advice on the degree of urgency of referral for each of the red flag conditions listed.

Table 3.2c-II A11: Red flags of diseases of the blood vessels

Red flag	Description	Reasoning
A11.1	Features of limb infarction: suddenly extremely pale, painful, mottled and cold limb; if infarction is severe the limb may feel more numb than painful	Infarction results from the sudden obstruction of arterial blood supply to a limb, usually by a blood clot. The patient requires urgent referral for surgical removal of the obstruction
A11.2	Features of severely compromised circulation to the extremities: • pain in the calf that is related to exercise and relieved by rest • pain in the calf in bed at night, relieved by hanging the leg out of bed (i.e. not cramp) • cold, purplish shiny skin • areas of blackened skin (gangrene)	If obstruction to the arterial circulation is gradual and/or partial, the pain will only appear when oxygen demands are higher than normal. Pain may appear on exercise and in bed, and there will be changes on the skin of the affected limb that suggest chronic (long-standing) poor circulation. There is a high risk of infarction and also of progressive gangrene, which could lead to the need for amputation. These symptoms require referral for assessment, lifestyle advice (especially advice on smoking cessation), medical treatment, and consideration for vascular surgery
A11.3	Features of an aortic aneurysm: pulsatile mass in abdomen >5cm in diameter (usually affects people >50 and is associated with the degenerative changes of atherosclerosis)	The aorta is palpable in the abdomen as a pulsatile tube of about 2cm in diameter. In the case of aneurysm, the width of this tube increases, and a palpable width of >5cm merits assessment by ultrasonography so that the risk of rupture can be formally assessed Early treatment of high-risk cases is life-saving. Refer urgently if abdominal or central back pain develops with a coexistent aortic aneurysm (see A11.4)
A11.4	Features of a ruptured aortic aneurysm: acute abdominal or back pain, with collapse; features of shock may be coexistent. This is one of the manifestations of the acute abdomen (see A6.8)	A rupture of an aortic aneurysm is an emergency situation and the patient needs urgent surgical treatment A rupture may be presaged by abdominal discomfort or back pain, so if these develop in the presence of a suspected aneurysm refer as a matter of high priority/urgency
A11.5	Features of meningococcal septicemia: acute onset of a purpuric rash, possibly accompanied by headache, vomiting and fever	The purpuric rash in meningococcal septicemia is a result of vasculitis (inflammation of the blood vessels). This is a serious warning sign of a devastating disease process, and the patient requires urgent referral for antibiotic treatment Meningococcal septicemia is a notifiable disease (see A6.2)
A11.6	Features of severe consequences of varicose veins: broken or itchy skin close to the veins indicates a risk of a varicose ulcer	Varicose veins are usually benign, but can reduce the effectiveness of drainage of blood from the affected area. This can result in weakened, dry and itchy (eczematous) skin. A break to the skin can easily develop into an ulcer, and in this situation would merit referral for assessment and nursing care Thrombophlebitis (inflammation of a length of a varicose vein) need not be referred if localized and superficial

A11.7	Features of a deep vein thrombosis (DVT): a hot swollen tender calf can be accompanied by fever and malaise. There is an increased risk after air travel and surgery, and in pregnancy, cancer and if on the oral contraceptive pill	DVT develops slowly and needs to be distinguished from gastrocnemius muscle strain (redness would be minimal and no fever) and thrombophlebitis (redness localized to the path of a varicose vein)
		If DVT is suspected, it merits high-priority referral, as without anticoagulant treatment there is a risk of pulmonary embolism (blood clot breaking off to lodge in the arterial circulation of the lungs)
		The patient should be advised to refrain from unnecessary exercise until they have been medically assessed

3.2d Hypertension

What is hypertension and how is it caused?

For a reminder of the physiology of blood pressure and the principles of its measurement, see Section 3.2a. As described in Section 3.2a, hypertension is a state in which the blood pressure is maintained at a level that is too high for the body's requirements. Hypertension, as defined by the World Health Organization/International Society for Hypertension (WHO/ISH), is blood pressure above 140/90mmHg (millimeters of mercury). By this definition, the state of hypertension is extremely common. A 2011 UK study showed hypertension was present in nearly one-third of men and women over the age of 35, and this strikingly high prevalence only increased as older sections of the population were considered, so that, according to this study, over two-thirds of men and women over 75 had hypertension.[39]

Although the upper range of normal for blood pressure is defined in modern medicine as 140/90mmHg, the optimal level of blood pressure is considered by the WHO/ISH to be less than 140/85mmHg.

It is conventionally understood that clinic readings will generally be higher than optimal home readings, so the upper limit of normal for a home blood pressure reading taken in relaxed circumstances is specified by the National Institute for Health and Care Excellence (NICE) (2011)[40] to be 135/85. Any home readings higher than this would indicate a diagnosis of hypertension.

The level of blood pressure is important for health because, as demonstrated from studies of large populations, the higher a person's blood pressure, the greater the risk that the person has of developing cardiovascular conditions such as stroke, heart attack and heart failure.

It is important to recognize that a person with optimal blood pressure is still at risk of these conditions, because they are all a result of the normal process of aging. However, as the blood pressure of an individual increases,

so does the risk of developing these conditions. There is no sudden increase in risk as blood pressure starts to exceed the normal range. Instead, the risk rises gradually. This can be compared to having a motorway speed limit for safe driving set at 70 miles (113 km) per hour. Although it is obvious that driving at 75 miles (121 km) per hour is more risky than driving at 65 miles (105 km) per hour, it does not mean that driving above 70 miles per hour is suddenly much more dangerous. So it is with blood pressure.

Moreover, the risks of having an accident at 75 miles per hour vary from individual to individual, depending on other factors such as driving skills, reaction times, the nature of the road and quality of the car. It might be appreciated that skilled drivers who just exceed the speed limit are unlikely to have an accident, whereas a distracted or inexperienced driver might be at greater risk of an accident even when driving well below the speed limit. The combined effect of other factors on the risk of adverse outcomes is similar with hypertension. Someone whose blood pressure is high at 150/95mmHg, but who has a healthy diet, is a non-smoker and in a physically active occupation, may well have a much lower risk of cardiovascular disease than someone with normal blood pressure who is a smoking and fast food-eating office worker.

The current teaching in medicine is that a diagnosis of hypertension should be put into context with a person's lifestyle. Not all cases of hypertension need be treated with medication. Instead, a change in lifestyle may be sufficient. A diagnosis of hypertension may cause a lot of anxiety for a patient, but actually, in many cases, the patient can be reassured that there is a lot they might be able to do for themselves to ensure their risk of adverse outcomes is reduced to an insignificant level.

Causes of hypertension

Up to nine out of ten people who are diagnosed with hypertension will have no recognized medical cause for this finding. The medical term for high blood pressure of unknown cause is essential hypertension. It is believed that a range of factors act together to give rise to essential hypertension. These include family history, ethnic origin, dietary factors, nicotine and alcohol intake, obesity, levels of activity and emotional factors. Recent studies suggest that the level of nutrition of the fetus in the womb may also have a bearing on the level of blood pressure in later life. Low birth weight appears to be linked with hypertension in adulthood.

A small and incremental rise in blood pressure resulting from arteriosclerosis is a very normal part of aging. However, as discussed earlier, the development of arteriosclerosis can lead to a vicious circle, in which essential hypertension worsens, and so the conventional advice is that control of hypertension in elderly people is also a very important aim.

About 10 percent of people with hypertension have an underlying physical cause. This is known as secondary hypertension. About half of those with secondary hypertension have kidney disease of some sort. In these people the hypertension is a consequence of the fact that the kidney is the source of hormones that are crucial in the control of blood pressure. Hypertension and the kidneys are discussed in more detail later. Other medical conditions that can lead to hypertension include endocrine diseases (such as Cushing's disease) and an inherited narrowing (coarctation) of the aorta. Drugs such as corticosteroids and the contraceptive pill can also lead to a rise in blood pressure.

Hypertension and disease

Hypertension and the circulatory system

It has already been explained how a prolonged state of hypertension leads to arteriosclerosis of the small blood vessels, and how this tends to increase blood pressure further. Arteriosclerosis can also lead to ischemia of essential organs and other body parts, such as the tissues of the lower limbs. This explains why the risk of chronic leg ischemia in a person with hypertension is two times that of a person with normal blood pressure.

Hypertension also appears to contribute to the development of atherosclerosis of the larger vessels. This can also lead to ischemia, and increases the risk of thrombosis, embolism and infarction.

A common serious complication of sustained hypertension is impaired blood supply to the brain. Thrombosis and hemorrhage of the vessels of the brain are two consequences of hypertension, and when significant they manifest in stroke. The risk of a stroke in a person with high blood pressure is six times that of a person with normal blood pressure. This condition is discussed in more detail in Chapter 4.1.

Another common serious complication is impairment of the blood supply to the heart, leading to all the manifestations of coronary heart disease (CHD), including angina and heart attack (coronary thrombosis). The risk of death from CHD, including heart attack and angina, in a person with high blood pressure is three times that of a person with normal blood pressure. CHD is discussed in more detail in Section 3.2e.

Sustained hypertension will also affect the heart muscle. Years of pumping blood within a system at high pressure puts strain on the heart. One response of the heart to this pressure is to enlarge, rather like an exercised biceps muscle. Although this may sound like a healthy response, an enlarged heart above a certain size cannot pump as efficiently, and it simply cannot cope with shifting the volume of blood that is required of it. This means that fluid starts to accumulate at the venous side of the heart, in both the bodily tissues and the lungs. This condition is known as heart failure, which simply means that the heart is failing to pump as efficiently. It can be a mild condition, and does not mean that the heart is going to stop (contrary to a common misunderstanding of the term). Heart failure is discussed in more detail in Section 3.2f.

Hypertension and the kidneys

As stated previously, kidney disease can lead to hypertension. Conversely, sustained hypertension can damage the delicate structure of the kidneys. As a damaged kidney can in itself lead to hypertension, this is another vicious circle in which hypertension leads to a condition that in itself worsens the hypertension. For this reason, control of blood pressure is vital for patients with kidney disease, as high blood pressure can lead to a rapid deterioration of their condition. Kidney disease is explored in more detail in Section 4.3c.

The kidneys are particularly vulnerable to further damage in people with diabetes and those who are pregnant. For this reason a rise in blood pressure is treated with great seriousness in both these conditions, and medical treatment is likely to be commenced at an earlier stage than for other patients (blood pressure in diabetes and pregnancy is explored further in Chapters 5.1 and 5.3).

Malignant (accelerated) hypertension

If the blood pressure becomes very high, the risks of serious complications are much increased. A diastolic pressure of greater than 120–140mmHg may lead to severe damage to small blood vessels in the kidneys, which then rapidly leads to increased blood pressure. This is a vicious circle in which there is a high risk of death due to a stroke. When severe hypertension is accompanied by signs of damage to organs such as the kidneys or brain, this is understandably termed malignant or accelerated hypertension and constitutes a medical emergency.

Although mild hypertension does not usually give rise to symptoms, in malignant hypertension the rapid cycle of progressive damage will lead to symptoms such as severe headache and blurring of vision. This is why this condition requires urgent medical attention, and needs to be treated in hospital with strong antihypertensive medication.

Categorization of severity of blood pressure

The approach to prevention and treatment of hypertension depends very much on the level of the measured hypertension. As mentioned in Section 3.2a, the recommendation is that the lowest of two or three readings are taken when blood pressure is measured to be raised, and, unless very high, the measurement should be repeated on three separate occasions before treatment decisions are made. Once a reliable measurement has been established, the level of hypertension is now graded as Stage 1, Stage 2 and Severe (replacing the former categories of mild, moderate and severe). Table 3.2d-I shows the ranges of systolic and diastolic pressure that fall into these categories.

Table 3.2d-I The categorization of hypertension according to severity

	Stage 1 hypertension*	Stage 2 hypertension**	Severe hypertension
Systolic pressure (mmHg)	140–159	160–179	180 or more
Diastolic pressure (mmHg)	90–99	100–109	110 or more
Malignant hypertension: Blood pressure greater than 180/110 and acute onset of end organ (kidney, brain, lung, blood vessel) damage, e.g. encephalopathy, vascular dissection, pulmonary edema, nephropathy, papilledema and/or hemolytic anemia			

* This relates to clinic-based readings. Stage 1 hypertension is diagnosed if home-based readings are consistently greater than 135 systolic or 85 diastolic.
** This relates to clinic-based readings. Stage 2 hypertension is diagnosed if home-based readings are consistently greater than 150 systolic or 95 diastolic.

If either the systolic or diastolic pressure is in a higher category than the other, the overall category of the blood pressure is given that of the highest reading. For example, a blood pressure of 160/85 is classified as Stage 2 hypertension, even though the diastolic reading is in the normal range. These are the categories that have been used in the guidelines written in 2011 by the National Institute for Health and Care Excellence (NICE) for the treatment of hypertension.[41]

The current advice in these guidelines is that all hypertensive patients (with any level of hypertension) should follow advice about lifestyle changes irrespective of any other treatment that is considered. These lifestyle changes are the same as those that are recommended for the prevention of hypertension.

Prevention of hypertension

In terms of the prevention of hypertension, there are some factors, such as age, family history and ethnic origin, that cannot be changed, but there are many modifiable risk factors. Table 3.2d-II summarizes the various lifestyle changes that can have a positive impact on reducing blood pressure.

Table 3.2d-II Lifestyle factors that have an impact on blood pressure

Lifestyle factor	Explanation for effect on blood pressure
Loss of weight	Blood pressure rises as weight is gained, and drops again if the weight is lost; excess weight puts a strain on the cardiovascular system
Restricting salt	Salt in the diet increases blood pressure. Simply not adding salt to food in cooking or at the table, without making any other dietary changes, can reduce blood pressure by up to 5mmHg
Reduction in alcohol intake	Cutting down to less than 4 units of alcohol a day will lead to a reduction in blood pressure in heavy drinkers
Stopping smoking	Each cigarette causes a temporary rise in blood pressure and contributes to the development of arteriosclerosis. Stopping smoking will halt this process. If stopping occurs early enough in life, the changes of early arteriosclerosis may reverse
Increased physical activity	Although physical exertion temporarily increases blood pressure, the long-term benefit to the circulation is that the blood pressure is reduced, as long as the exercise is regular and not too excessive
Reducing stress	Although the link between chronic stress and hypertension is difficult to study, some studies have shown that practices such as meditation and tai chi can reduce blood pressure in the short term. Although it is not of proven benefit, it would make sense to encourage hypertensive patients to make lifestyle changes that could reduce the stress that they experience in life
Maintaining health in pregnancy	Focusing on a healthy lifestyle during pregnancy with the aim of benefiting the health of the baby in much later life. Hypertension in adult life has been linked to low birth weight

Information box 3.2d-I

The development of hypertension: comments from a Chinese medicine perspective

The main symptoms of hypertension often suggest underlying patterns of either Kidney Yang or Kidney Yin Deficiency in Chinese medicine. The failure of blood vessels to relax, a contributory factor in hypertension, could readily be ascribed to a Deficiency of Kidney Yang allowing Yin Pathogenic Factors such as Phlegm and Damp to accumulate and affect relaxation.

Deficiency of Yin would also fail to nourish Liver Yin, in turn leading to Hyperactivity of Liver Yang. The resulting Rising Liver Yang and Liver Wind are clearly suggested by the more full symptoms and signs of blood pressure, including headaches and stroke.

Hyperactivity of Liver Yang might also be thought of as corresponding to the effects of excessive adrenaline. Although adrenaline originates from the adrenal glands, which sit close to the kidneys, part of its function is to prepare and equip the body for dynamic change, a characteristic of the Liver Organ. Adrenaline is certainly Yang in nature, as it increases heart rate, muscle strength and metabolic rate, and slows down the more Yin functions such as digestion. The bodily changes brought about by adrenaline, if excessively secreted, are indicative of Liver Yang Rising, and eventually of Liver Fire.

The fatty diet, physical inactivity and smoking that contribute to the development of hypertension are conventionally interpreted as the cause of the excessive fatty deposit (atheroma) that coats the inside of the large arteries of some hypertensive people. The coating is suggestive of Phlegm Damp in Chinese medicine. This makes sense, as a fatty diet will contribute to accumulation of Damp, and the Heat from smoking can be interpreted as causing transformation of Damp into Phlegm. Lack of exercise can contribute to Stagnation and accumulation of fluids, and so can exacerbate the development of Phlegm Damp. Yang Deficiency resulting from Spleen Deficiency or old age will mean that Phlegm and Damp are more likely to accumulate.

The conventional medicine observation that hypertension can become more pronounced with age is consistent with the Chinese medicine view that Liver and Kidney Yin Deficiency are a significant part of the depletion that comes with old age. The lack of compliance of the hardened blood vessels in arteriosclerosis, an important precursor to the hypertension of old age, suggests Yin Deficiency, as Yin describes a condition of softness and the ability to yield.

It is interesting to consider that the Depletion of the Kidneys is very much integral to the understanding of hypertension in Chinese medicine, and to compare this with the conventional understanding that kidney function is very closely associated with the control of blood pressure.

Medical treatment of hypertension

Medical treatment involves the use of up to four different classes of drugs to bring blood pressure to the recommended range of less than 140/90 for anyone under 80 and 150/90 for more elderly patients. Targets are lower for patients with kidney disease and diabetes in whom the target blood pressure is less than 130/80.

TREATMENT OF STAGE 1 HYPERTENSION

Patients whose blood pressure is mildly elevated (Stage 1 hypertension) need not be treated with drugs unless other risk factors such as kidney disease, diabetes or damage to organs such as the cardiovascular system or kidney are evident, or if the cardiovascular risk score predicts risk of a cardiovascular event to be greater than 20 percent in the next ten years. For this reason heavy smoking and high blood cholesterol are risk factors that may influence a decision about whether medication is advisable at this level of blood pressure.

There are various formulae that are currently used to calculate the combined effect of risk factors and to produce an estimate of coronary risk. In the UK the coronary risk tends to be calculated by the QRISK®2 formula,[42] and in the US, the ASCVD algorithm is one favored tool.[43] If coronary risk is calculated as low (i.e. less than 20 percent in ten years), treatment is not considered to be necessary for mild hypertension.

It is generally considered safe in Stage 1 hypertension to delay drug treatment to see if the patient can implement an effective lifestyle change. If there is no benefit from this, very often a single antihypertensive medication can be sufficient to bring about effective blood pressure control.

TREATMENT OF STAGE 2 HYPERTENSION

Drug treatment is recommended for all patients with established Stage 2 hypertension. It would be expected that two separate antihypertensive drugs would be required to achieve satisfactory control.

TREATMENT OF SEVERE HYPERTENSION

All patients with severe hypertension will be prescribed medication as a matter of priority, and if there are any features of malignant hypertension, they will be referred for urgent hospital treatment.

Drugs used in hypertension

For those patients who have sustained mild hypertension and other risk factors for disease, and for all patients with Stage 2 or severe hypertension, drug treatment is recommended. There is a wide range of different types of medication that can be used to reduce blood pressure. The most important of these can be found in Sections 2.2, 2.5 and 2.6 of the *British National Formulary* (BNF).

Although patients should initially be started on a single drug, many will require two or more drugs in combination to bring their blood pressure to within the normal range. Because each drug has its action on a different part of the circulatory system, when used in combination, drugs can have a more powerful effect than a double dose of a single drug alone.

The four main categories of drugs used in the treatment of hypertension helpfully begin with the letters A, B, C and D. They are the angiotensin-converting enzyme (ACE) inhibitors and angiotensin II receptor antagonists (A2RAs), the beta blockers, the calcium channel blockers (CCBs) and the diuretics.

The two recommended types of drugs used in the initial treatment of hypertension are the ACE inhibitors and A2RAs (BNF, Section 2.5) and the CCBs (BNF, Section 2.6).

Beta blockers and diuretics used to be widely prescribed for the treatment of hypertension, but these are no longer considered to carry the greatest benefits for patients in terms of overall risk reduction. Nevertheless, they may still be prescribed as an additional drug when the action of one or two others is not sufficient, or if side effects prevent the use of the other three types of medication.

Because these drugs are so commonly prescribed, they are described below in turn.

Angiotensin-converting enzyme (ACE) inhibitors

ACE inhibitors act at the lungs to reduce the production of the hormone angiotensin II. Angiotensin has two main functions. The first is to increase the tone of the blood vessels and thus maintain blood pressure. The second is to stimulate the kidneys to produce the hormone aldosterone, which promotes fluid retention, again, to maintain blood pressure. ACE inhibitors therefore have a double action of causing relaxation of blood vessels and excretion of fluid by the kidneys.

ACE inhibitors are protective in patients with heart failure, and can prevent worsening kidney damage in patients with diabetes. They are therefore the first choice of drug for these groups of people.

Important side effects include fainting or dizziness due to a sudden drop in blood pressure, and this is most likely on initiation of treatment.

ACE inhibitors can lead to reduced blood flow to the kidneys, and so are dangerous in people who have a poor blood supply to their kidneys. As this condition may be undiagnosed, regular blood tests should be done on patients starting on ACE inhibitors to check their kidney function.

Another common, although not serious, side effect is a persistent cough and weak voice. Others include nausea, diarrhea, headache and rashes.

Commonly prescribed ACE inhibitors that are listed in the BNF include lisinopril, ramipril and perindopril.

Angiotensin II receptor antagonists (A2RAs)

A2RAs are newer drugs that have a similar action to ACE inhibitors, but may offer fewer side effects in some people. They have been less widely studied and so are usually reserved for situations in which ACE inhibitors cannot be tolerated.

Commonly prescribed A2RAs that are listed in the BNF include candesartan, losartan and telmisartan.

Calcium channel blockers (CCBs)

CCBs prevent the entry of the mineral calcium into heart muscle and blood vessel cells, and so reduce the strength of the contraction of these tissues. The reduced force of pumping and the relaxation of the blood vessels that results both contribute to a drop in blood pressure.

Side effects of CCBs include flushing and headaches, a result of dilation of blood vessels in the face and scalp, irregularities of the heartbeat and worsening of heart failure, and ankle swelling.

Commonly prescribed CCBs that are listed in the BNF include nifedipine, felodipine, diltiazem and verapamil.

Diuretics

The term diuretic applies to a range of drugs that promote the production of an increased volume of urine by the kidneys. They reduce pressure in the circulatory system by reducing the volume of circulating blood. This could be compared to letting excess air out of an overinflated tire.

A patient on diuretics will have to urinate more frequently, and will feel thirsty. The diuretics will reduce any fluid accumulation in the tissues and can reduce swollen ankles. For the same reason these drugs will also lead to dry skin. A potentially serious but common side effect is that the reduced blood pressure can lead to dizziness on standing (postural hypotension). Falls in elderly people are a known adverse consequence of the prescribing of diuretics.

Most people tolerate the drugs for years on end, but serious side effects are well recognized. These include loss of essential minerals, such as sodium, potassium and magnesium in the urine. These losses can be life-threatening if not detected. Conversely, diuretics can produce an undesirable rise in blood sugar and lipids (including cholesterol), and for this reason their use should be avoided in diabetic people. Rare side effects include gout (an acute condition of hot, swollen joints), rashes and damage to the blood cells.

Commonly prescribed diuretics for hypertension that are listed in the BNF include bendroflumethiazide, cyclopenthiazide and chlortalidone. These are all from the thiazide family of diuretics.

Beta blockers

The term beta blocker applies to drugs that counteract the effect of adrenaline in the body. Adrenaline raises blood pressure by increasing the heart rate and the force of the heartbeat. It also causes an emotional sensation of urgency, anxiety or fear.

Beta blockers reduce blood pressure by slowing down the heart and reducing the strength of its contractions. They also reduce drive and anxiety levels. This effect improves the quality of life for some people, but can manifest as tiredness, depression, coldness and impotence in others.

Other important side effects of beta blockers include worsening of asthma (as adrenaline prevents constriction of the small airways of the lungs) and worsening of heart failure (due to reduced effectiveness of the pumping of the heart). They should therefore be avoided in people with these conditions.

However, beta blockers are now frequently prescribed for people who have suffered from a heart attack, as clinical studies have demonstrated that by reducing the work of the heart they can improve the prognosis for these people.

Commonly prescribed beta blockers that are listed in the BNF include atenolol and propranolol.

 Information box 3.2d-II

The treatment of hypertension: comments from a Chinese medicine perspective

The four main classes of drugs used in the treatment of hypertension have different modes of action and different side effect profiles. This suggests that the interpretations of their actions according to Chinese medicine theory will also be different.

The following interpretations have been made by means of the systematic approach introduced in Section 1.3b.

Diuretics: a Chinese energetic interpretation

Diuretics promote urination and lead to reduced body fluids, dry mouth and thirst. The loss of fluids directly reduces pressure in the circulatory system. This would normally be interpreted in terms of Clearance of Damp (or Transformation of Water, a process that relies on Kidney Yang). However, the side effects include excessive urination, dizziness on standing, a rise in blood lipids and glucose, gout, dry skin, rashes and imbalance in the levels of sodium, potassium and magnesium in the blood. These suggest additional energetic imbalances.

Excessive urination might appear to correspond to Boosting of Kidney Yang, but the depletion of fluids to Subduing of Kidney Yin. As explained in Section 1.3b, it is suggested that drug-induced boosting of a substance such as Kidney Yang will come at the cost of long-term depletion of the same substance, and so Depletion of Kidney Yang also might be expected in the long term. Dizziness on standing might correspond to a Depletion of Kidney Yang. A rise in blood lipids might correspond to Accumulation of Phlegm Damp. An increase of blood sugar might correspond to Subduing of Spleen Yang, as it represents an inability to make full use of the Qi obtained from food. Gout is a deforming inflammatory arthritis, and as such might be diagnosed as a manifestation of Heat and Phlegm (Hot and Bony Bi Syndrome).

Other side effects that might correspond to damage of Yin include dry skin and mouth, rashes and damage to the blood cells. Excessive loss of the minerals magnesium and potassium from the kidneys can lead to irritability, fits and instability of the heartbeat, all suggesting damage to the Yin.

If diuretics are withdrawn, blood pressure will rise again. This suggests that the mode of action is suppressive.

According to this method of energetic interpretation, diuretics appear to Transform Damp but seem to have a deleterious effect on the Kidney in terms of Boosting Kidney Yang at the expense of Depleting deep reserves of Kidney Yin and Yang. The side effects of these drugs also suggest that there may be concomitant accumulation of Phlegm Damp and Heat, together with the Subduing of Spleen Qi/Yang.

Beta blockers: a Chinese energetic interpretation

These slow the heart rate and reduce the force of the heartbeat, both of which reduce blood pressure. The side effects include depression, impotence, feelings of cold, asthma and heart failure.

A slower and less forceful heartbeat could suggest a Subduing of Heart Yang.

The side effects of depression, impotence and feelings of cold all suggest that the depletion caused by beta blockers Subdues Kidney Yang. The accumulation of fluid that can result from worsening of heart failure is perhaps another manifestation of this. The asthma caused by beta blockers could be described in Chinese medicine as failure of the Kidneys to receive Lung Qi, and this would fit with the interpretation of Subduing Kidney Yang.

For the same reason as for diuretics, the mode of action of beta blockers is suppressive.

According to this method of energetic interpretation, beta blockers tend to Subdue the functions of Heart and Kidney Yang. This suggests that they are Cold in nature.

ACE inhibitors: a Chinese energetic interpretation

These act by reducing the action of the hormone angiotensin on the blood vessels and the kidney. Angiotensin is produced in the lungs. The other action of angiotensin is at the kidneys to promote fluid retention. By counteracting this effect, ACE inhibitors promote the excretion of fluid. Postural hypotension is a common side effect of treatment. Other side effects include a cough, weak voice, rashes and kidney damage.

The action of the ACE inhibitors in promoting urination is consistent with Clearance of Damp, and the action on the blood vessels could possibly be associated with Subduing of Zong Qi, the Qi that supports the blood vessels. This fits with the common side effects of persistent dry cough and weak voice.

There is no doubt that in most forms of kidney disease and in diabetes ACE inhibitors have a protective effect on the kidneys, and can arrest or slow down the progressive damage to the kidneys in hypertensive disease. This might be interpreted in terms of Boosting Kidney Yin. Postural hypotension and increased urination suggest, however, that this might be at the expense of Subduing or Depletion of Kidney Yang.

The common side effects of nausea, diarrhea and headache suggest additional drug-induced disease, possibly due to Subduing of Spleen Qi and/or Stagnation of Liver Qi.

The mode of action of ACE inhibitors is suppressive.

According to this method of energetic interpretation, ACE inhibitors tend to Subdue the functions of Kidney Yang and Zong Qi. They also appear to Boost Kidney Qi. Their energetic effects appear to be directed primarily towards the Lungs and Kidneys.

CCBs: a Chinese energetic interpretation

CCBs reduce the force of contraction of the heartbeat and also promote relaxation of the tone of the blood vessels. Their most prominent side effects include flushing and headaches, and heart failure. Other less common symptoms include rash, itching, eye pain and visual disturbances, muscle aches and jaundice.

The effect on the heart and blood vessels suggests Subduing of Heart Yang, together with Subduing of Zong Qi, a component of Heart Yang. The accumulation of fluid that can occur in worsening of heart failure could be seen as a manifestation of Subduing of Kidney Yang.

Flushing and headaches are symptoms of Full Heat, and may suggest Liver Yang Rising or Liver Fire Blazing. The other less common side effects also suggest that these drugs cause Liver Qi Stagnation and/or Heat.

The mode of action of CCBs is suppressive.

CCBs appear to reduce blood pressure by Subduing Heart and Kidney Yang and Zong Qi. They also seem to cause Heat and Liver Disharmony, and appear to act primarily at the Heart, Kidneys and Liver.

Summary of the Chinese energetic interpretation

All these antihypertensive drugs appear to affect the Kidneys, in particular, all Subdue Kidney Yang, in addition to other imbalances characteristic of the type of drug.

However, there seems to be a paradox here. Depletion of the Kidneys, including Depletion of Kidney Yang, is considered in Chinese medicine to be a primary cause of hypertension, and yet drugs that Subdue Kidney Yang seem to reduce hypertension. To understand this it is important to reconsider the factors that contribute to a normal blood pressure level.

Blood pressure is maintained first by a forceful and lively heartbeat, and good tone of the blood vessels. These are all Yang in nature. Adequate retention of fluid in the circulation by the kidneys is also necessary. This is Yin in nature. The drugs tend to counteract these normally healthy aspects of the Yang and Yin in the body. However, in doing so, the suppression that these drugs produce, dealing with the symptoms but not the underlying cause, may lead to a deepening imbalance.

In reaching this conclusion, it is important to emphasize that conventional medication may still be the best possible option for a patient with hypertension. In many situations, suppression of symptoms is literally vital for the patient when their symptoms threaten to bring about a catastrophic event such as a stroke or heart attack. In discerning the true benefit of a medication it is necessary to weigh up the current risk to the patient of deteriorating health from the hypertension against how much and how quickly other, more gentle treatment can redress the energetic imbalance. This is not always an easy assessment to make.

However, if it is clear that the patient's condition is unstable and the risk is high, suppressive medication will be a necessary option to help regain some stability. This will buy time to enable more gentle complementary medical treatment, together with appropriate lifestyle changes, to be directed at the energetic root of the problem.

The red flags of hypertension

Some patients with hypertension will benefit from referral to a conventional doctor for assessment or treatment. Red flags are those symptoms and signs that indicate that referral should be considered. The red flags of hypertension are described in Table 3.2d-III. A summary of the red flags in a format designed for quick reference in clinical practice can be found in Appendix III. This gives advice on the degree of urgency of referral for each of the red flag conditions listed.

Note that referral is not synonymous with asking for medical treatment. The 2011 NICE hypertension guidelines[44] are clear about the fact that, if coronary risk is low, medication is not necessary. Referral in the situation of mild and moderate hypertension is primarily so that the patient's coronary risk can be assessed accurately.

Table 3.2d-III A12: Red flags of hypertension

Red flag	Description	Reasoning
A12.1	Features of malignant hypertension: diastolic pressure >120mmHg with symptoms, including recently worsening headaches, blurred vision, chest pain	At a certain level, hypertension leads to a negative cycle of increasing vascular damage and worsening hypertension. This is malignant hypertension, which carries a high risk of stroke and other cardiovascular events. Visual disturbances and headaches are serious signs
A12.2	Seriously high hypertension: systolic pressure ≥220mmHg diastolic pressure ≥120mmHg no symptoms	Refer as a high priority. Immediate medical management is required to prevent stroke or other cardiovascular events
A12.3	Severe hypertension: systolic pressure ≥180mmHg diastolic pressure ≥110mmHg	Refer all cases for assessment of coronary risk and consideration of medical treatment
A12.4	Stage 2 hypertension: systolic pressure ≥160mmHg and <180mmHg diastolic pressure ≥100mmHg and <110mmHg	Refer all cases for assessment of coronary risk and consideration of medical treatment
A12.5	Mild hypertension: systolic pressure ≥140mmHg and <160mmHg diastolic pressure ≥90mmHg and <100mmHg	Refer for treatment if major risk factors* are present and if there is no improvement within three months If no major risk factors are present, refer only if you suspect that the cardiovascular risk is increased because of the presence of other risk factors, such as smoking or hyperlipidemia or symptoms of diabetes
A12.6	Hypertension of any level with diabetes	Always refer for medical management, as the wisdom is that blood pressure should be maintained below 130/80mmHg in people with diabetes because of the much greater risk of vascular and renal complications

| A12.7 | Hypertension of any level with established kidney disease | Always refer for medical management, as blood pressure should be maintained ideally below 130/80mmHg in people with kidney disease |
| A12.8 | Hypertension of any level in pregnancy (see A37.9–A37.11) | Always refer because of the increased risk of pre-eclampsia and placental damage |

* In this case *major risk factors* are features that are known to be associated with increased risk of a cardiovascular event in the presence of hypertension. These include *diabetes, past history of heart disease, chronic leg ischemia* and *kidney disease*. Medical doctors now use risk factor calculation tables to predict more accurately the statistical risk in an individual case, and this can help with decision-making about whether or not medication is appropriate. *Other risk factors*, such as sex, age, smoking status and lipid levels, will be taken into account in such calculations. Medication is considered advisable in those for whom the ten-year risk of a cardiovascular event is predicted to be more than 20 percent. For this reason, referral is advised for risk assessment if any of the risk factors mentioned above are present or suspected to be present. Therefore, for example, if lipid levels are not known, referral should be considered. Risk calculation can help a patient make a more informed decision about the potential benefits of medication, and may also help them make the decision to adjust their lifestyle to improve their risk status. In line with current medical wisdom, all patients with hypertension may benefit from advice on lifestyle changes to reduce blood pressure or cardiovascular risk. Relevant lifestyle changes include smoking cessation, weight reduction, reduction of excessive alcohol intake, reduction of dietary salt, reduction of total and saturated fat in diet, increasing exercise, and increasing fruit and vegetable intake.

3.2e Coronary heart disease

This section focuses on two of the conditions that can result from disease of the coronary arteries. These conditions are embraced by the term coronary heart disease (CHD). The two other major conditions that can result from CHD are heart failure and irregularities of the heart rhythm (arrhythmias). These have other causes in addition to CHD, and are discussed in Section 3.2f. CHD is also known as ischemic heart disease (IHD) and coronary artery disease (CAD).

The causes of coronary heart disease (CHD)

The study of CHD as described in this section will be supported by turning back to Section 3.2a to revise the physiology of the blood flow to the heart muscle, and also to Section 3.2c to read about the pathology of atheroma and atherosclerosis.

CHD is the term applied to the conditions that can result from the obstruction and distortion of the coronary arteries by atheroma. As described in Section 3.2c, atheroma in the coronary vessels reduces blood flow and increases the risk of thrombosis in these vessels.

A wide range of risk factors and protective factors are known to work together to affect an individual's risk of developing CHD. These can be broadly categorized as unmodifiable risk factors and lifestyle factors (which can be modified).

Unmodifiable risk factors
The most important unmodifiable risk factors are age, gender and family history. Obviously, these risk factors cannot be altered by attention to advice or through medical treatment.

AGE
The risk of developing CHD increases with age, as development of atheroma is part of the aging process.

GENDER
The risk of developing CHD is greater in men, although the difference in the risk between the sexes evens out after the menopause. It is believed that physiological levels of the female hormone estrogen are protective against CHD.

FAMILY HISTORY
The risk of developing CHD in an individual is greater if the person's close relatives have had CHD. The risk is also higher in some ethnic groups, irrespective of lifestyle. This means that susceptibility to the condition can be inherited.

Lifestyle risk factors
The three most important lifestyle factors that contribute to the development of CHD are a high level of blood lipids, smoking and lack of physical exercise.

BLOOD LIPIDS
Blood lipids refer to the fats that circulate in the bloodstream. These lipids are essential for health, but if their levels become too high or out of balance, they can contribute to the fatty deposit of atheroma. The lipids are found in four important forms in the blood known as high-density, low-density and very-low-density lipoprotein (HDL, LDL and VLDL) and triglycerides (TGs).

HDL, LDL and VLDL contain cholesterol and contribute to the total cholesterol level, which is commonly the figure that patients will be told about by their doctor. Ideally, the total cholesterol level should be less than 5.0mmol/l (millimoles per liter), although, as is also the case for blood pressure, it is well known that a significant proportion of people in Western populations (the majority) have a cholesterol level that exceeds this upper limit of normal. For example, recent data show that over half of US citizens between the ages of 44 and 65 have an average cholesterol of 5.4mmol/dl (209mg/dl). This means that over 50 percent of these people have a total cholesterol level that is significantly higher than the recommended healthy upper limit.[45]

HDL is one form of cholesterol that does not seem to contribute to coronary risk, and instead it may even be protective. HDL levels seem to increase with exercise. For this reason the ratio between total cholesterol and HDL is used for the calculation of coronary risk. This ratio will be lower in value the higher the level of HDL, and so it accounts for the protective effect of HDL. TGs are usually not of concern for most people, but may become adversely high in people with diabetes and in certain family groups.

It is known that some people are more prone to developing adversely high blood lipids than others, and this trait runs very strongly in families. If this inherited trait is marked, it is diagnosed as familial hyperlipidemia. CHD is much more common in people with hyperlipidemia than in the general population.

It is now known that certain types of fats in the diet directly increase levels of the unhealthy LDL and VLDL in the bloodstream. For example, the fats known as saturated fats (found in dairy products and meat) and trans fatty acids (found in cheap margarines, biscuits and cakes) appear to increase the levels of undesirable lipids.

In contrast, the fats known as polyunsaturated fats and monounsaturated fats (found in vegetable oils and fish) appear to reduce levels of LDL and VLDL, and may also instead increase levels of the protective HDL.

A typical Western diet, which is high in dairy produce, fatty meats, cakes and biscuits, is therefore a lifestyle factor that can, over the years, contribute to the development of atheroma.

SMOKING
Smoking increases the development of arteriosclerosis and atherosclerosis, and can also increase the tendency of the blood to clot. Contrary to popular understanding, the greatest health impact of smoking comes from the fact that it causes CHD rather than from its undeniably adverse effect on the lungs.

Studies of large populations indicate that the increased risk of CHD in a smoker drops to become the same as that of a non-smoker within five years of stopping smoking.

LACK OF PHYSICAL EXERCISE
Other studies of large populations indicate that those who are physically active are half as likely to develop CHD as those who are inactive. This is comparable to the difference

in risk between smokers and non-smokers. Physical exercise improves the blood supply to the heart and improves the balance of healthy to unhealthy blood lipids. It is now believed that regular moderate exercise such as brisk walking or cycling is possibly more beneficial than less frequent strenuous exercise such as playing squash or running.

Conventional healthy living advice to all people therefore includes attention to fats in the diet, quitting smoking and taking up regular physical activity. If all three of these factors can be attended to, the risk of developing atheroma and CHD drops dramatically. In addition to these three most important lifestyle factors there are numerous other factors that are conventionally believed to affect the development of atheroma.

OTHER DIETARY FACTORS
There are other components of the diet, in addition to the healthy fats such as vegetable, olive and fish oils, which are actually protective against CHD. Foods that provide vitamins A, C and E (antioxidant vitamins), such as fresh fruit and vegetables, and garlic, have been shown in some studies to reduce the risk of CHD. Flavonoids, another component of fruit and vegetables, also appear to be beneficial. These include anthocyanidins, flavan-3-ols, flavanones, flavones, flavonols, proanthocyanidins and isoflavones. According to McCullough (quoted in Siriwardhana 2012):

> Blueberries, red wine, and strawberries are rich sources of anthocyanidins. Apples, black tea, blueberries, chocolate, and red wine are rich sources of flavan-3-ols. Citrus fruit, juices, and herbal teas are rich sources of flavanones. Celery, garlic, green peppers, and herbal tea are rich sources of flavones. Blueberries, garlic, kale, onions, spinach, tea, broccoli, red wine, cherry, and tomatoes are rich sources of flavonols. Apples, black tea, blueberries, chocolate, mixed nuts, peanuts, red wine, strawberries, and walnuts are rich sources of proanthocyanidins. Soy products and peanuts are rich sources of isoflavones.[46]

Alcohol up to an amount of 2–3 units a day also appears to be protective. The risk of CHD in moderate drinkers actually appears to be less than in those who do not drink alcohol at all. Red wine has recently been considered to be of particular benefit, possibly because it contains diverse flavonoids as well as alcohol (see above). However, consumption of more than 3–4 units of alcohol a day is detrimental – above this level the alcohol contributes to hypertension and produces an unhealthy rise in blood lipids.

Salt can be harmful because it increases blood pressure in some people, and this, in turn, promotes the development of atherosclerosis.

All the beneficial dietary factors can be found in the widely acclaimed Mediterranean diet. Populations who eat a diet rich in fresh fruit, vegetables and fish, plenty of garlic and olive oil, moderate amounts of wine and moderate amounts of meat, but little other saturated fat, demonstrate a relatively low prevalence of CHD.[47]

DIABETES

People with diabetes mellitus (see Section 5.1d) and poorly controlled blood sugar levels are more prone to both atherosclerosis and arteriosclerosis. This is, in part, a result of the effect of the high sugar levels on the walls of the blood vessels, and partly due to the fact that people with diabetes are prone to raised blood lipids. For this reason, people with diabetes are advised to be very attentive to modifying their dietary, exercise and smoking habits to minimize their overall risk of CHD.

It has been confirmed by clinical studies that good control of blood sugar through diet and drugs will also reduce the risk of damage to the blood vessels in some people with diabetes.

HYPERLIPIDEMIA

This is the condition in which the blood lipids are raised above a healthy level. It can be assessed by means of the fasting lipids blood test. The term hyperlipidemia is generally reserved for people who have total fasting levels of cholesterol of over 6.5mmol/l or triglycerides greater than 3.0mmol/l. Because of the high risk of CHD, people with hyperlipidemia are advised to be very careful about fat in their diet, and may be prescribed lipid-lowering medication such as a statin or a fibrate.

People who have had symptoms of CHD may be advised to take lipid-lowering medication even if their blood lipids are not very high. This is because clinical studies have shown that such treatment can reduce the risk of subsequent deaths from CHD.

HYPERTENSION

The link between hypertension and CHD has been explored in detail in Section 3.2d.

SOCIAL EFFECTS AND STRESS

There is good evidence to show that people in low socio-economic groups and in populations subjected to great stress have increased rates of CHD. These increased rates cannot be accounted for solely by poor access to good diet, high levels of smoking and alcohol intake. The current theory is that the stress that arises from being in a low social class or in a nation in turmoil directly affects the development of CHD. Although this factor is recognized in conventional medicine, the mechanism of how stress leads to CHD has not yet been fully explained.

OTHER FACTORS

Other factors that have more recently been linked with an increased risk of CHD include increased tendencies to blood clotting, increased levels of an amino acid called homocysteine, and increased bodily inflammatory processes. At present, none of these factors has been sufficiently established by research evidence to be reflected in wide-scale public health advice for the prevention of CHD.

The important factors that are currently considered to affect the development of CHD are summarized in Table 3.2e-I. An awareness of these factors can inform the content of lifestyle advice given to patients with CHD.

Table 3.2e-I Important factors in the etiology of coronary heart disease

Unmodifiable risk factors	Lifestyle risk factors	Lifestyle protective factors
Age	High levels of saturated fats and trans fatty acids in the diet	Polyunsaturated and monounsaturated fats
Gender	Smoking	Fish oils
Family history	Low level of physical activity	Vitamins A, C and E as part of a healthy diet (not in the form of supplements)
	Excess salt in diet	Flavonoids
	Alcohol intake greater than 4 units/day	Garlic
	Diabetes mellitus	Regular moderate physical activity
	Hyperlipidemia	Moderate alcohol intake
	Social causes of stress	Happiness and freedom from stress
	Hypertension	

The manifestations of coronary heart disease

The heart is supplied with blood by means of the coronary arteries. The damage to the blood supply of the heart resulting from coronary atheroma has four major manifestations: angina, heart attack, heart failure and disorders of the heartbeat (arrhythmias). Angina and heart attack are discussed in some detail in this section because of their importance in terms of their frequency and their impact on health.

Angina

ANGINA PECTORIS – STABLE ANGINA

If one or more of the coronary vessels becomes narrowed and distorted by atheroma, the amount of blood that can be supplied to the heart muscle decreases. When the heart muscle is required to do work with an insufficient blood supply, the muscle becomes ischemic. This leads to intense cramping pain, in the same way as is experienced in chronic leg ischemia. Ischemic pain of the heart is called angina pectoris or simply angina.

Initially, angina may come on only in situations of extreme exercise, but as narrowing of the coronary vessels worsens, the pain will occur at progressively lower levels of exertion. It can also occur whilst eating or when the patient is exposed to the cold. Severe angina can be extremely disabling. In stable angina the pain improves if the patient 0rests.

Anginal pain is characteristically described as heavy or tight, and is not usually described as stabbing (contrary to what is frequently said in Chinese medicine textbooks, possibly a result of mistranslation of a Chinese term). The pain is felt in the center of the chest (rather than to the left), and may radiate up to the neck and down one or both arms.

In some people, particularly elderly people, painless angina may occur. Sometimes all the patient experiences is a feeling of tightness in the chest or breathlessness. However, it is important to recognize that in elderly people serious conditions may produce relatively few symptoms.

If the obstruction of the coronary arteries becomes very severe, angina may come on spontaneously when the patient is at rest. This is a serious symptom, and is described as unstable angina. The rest pain of unstable angina is a warning symptom of impending heart attack. Unstable angina is considered an acute coronary syndrome and is now managed in a very similar way to heart attack.

Stable angina is initially diagnosed from the patient's symptoms, but as chest pain can have a wide range of possible causes, the diagnosis is confirmed through hospital investigations. Patients with suspected angina used to undergo a resting electrocardiogram (ECG) and an exercise ECG (treadmill) assessment; however, the variability of results from these tests, as well as the inherent risks of graded exercise on a treadmill, has led to the National Institute for Health and Care Excellence (NICE) (2010)[48] recommending alternative tests to diagnose or exclude angina in a patient with intermittent chest pain. If angina seems very likely and surgery is a possibility, a coronary angiography may be performed (see Section 3.2b). Otherwise non-invasive functional imaging tests of the heart including MPS with SPECT (myocardial perfusion scanning with single photon emission computed tomography (CT) scanning) and stress echocardiography may be used as diagnostic tests.

Treatment of stable angina: prevention of progression
The treatments used to prevent the worsening of stable angina have a lot in common with the treatments used to prevent all types of CHD. First, the patient is encouraged to attend to lifestyle changes, as discussed earlier. Dietary advice is given and the patient is counseled about taking gentle exercise and stopping smoking.

All patients with CHD will be prescribed either low-dose aspirin or clopidogrel to be taken on a daily basis. Both these medications reduce the tendency of the blood to clot, and in this way reduce the risk of a coronary thrombosis (heart attack). If hypertension and diabetes are present they are controlled as much as possible in order to minimize coronary risk.

Many patients will also be prescribed a drug to reduce the level of blood lipids. The most commonly prescribed class of lipid-lowering drugs is the statin group (see the *British National Formulary* (BNF), Chapter 2.12).

Statins

Statins affect the liver to reduce its production of cholesterol. The main side effects are digestive disturbances and headaches, although rarely inflammation of muscles and severe liver disturbance can occur. Commonly prescribed statins include simvastatin and pravastatin.

Treatment of the symptoms of stable angina
The symptoms of angina can be treated by five classes of drugs, which, in severe angina, may be used in combination. The most commonly used of these are the nitrates, calcium channel blockers (CCBs) and beta blockers. Newer drugs that are used when symptoms persist include ivabradine (modifies the action of the sinus pacemaker of the heart) and ranolazine (affects the flow of sodium ions into the contracting heart muscle).

Nitrates

Nitrates are the first type of drug chosen for patients with angina. Glyceryl nitrate (GTN) is a preparation that can be taken under the tongue (sublingually), by tablet or by aerosol spray, from where it is rapidly absorbed to lead to a reduction in symptoms. Other preparations of long-acting nitrates are taken by mouth on a regular basis to prevent symptoms.

Nitrates act by dilating large blood vessels. They therefore dilate the coronary vessels, and in this way counteract the narrowing in these vessels that has led to symptoms of angina. The common side effects of flushing, headache and feeling faint on standing are all results of the dilatation of blood vessels elsewhere in the body.

Commonly prescribed long-acting nitrates include isosorbide dinitrate and isosorbide mononitrate.

Calcium channel blockers (CCBs) and beta blockers

The remaining two classes of drugs used for angina are the same as those used for hypertension (the action of these is described in Section 3.2d).

Surgical treatment of stable angina

If stable angina remains problematic and the angiography shows that surgical procedures might be of benefit, the patient may be considered for one of two surgical approaches to treating obstructed coronary arteries: percutaneous transluminal coronary angioplasty (PTCA) and coronary artery bypass graft (CABG). Ideally, these procedures are performed in a stable patient to prevent worsening of angina. These procedures may also be carried out as an emergency in the case of acute coronary syndrome.

Percutaneous coronary intervention (PCI)

Percutaneous coronary intervention (PCI) (also known as angioplasty) involves widening of a blocked coronary artery from within by means of a catheter tube with an expanding balloon-shaped tip. In most cases a metal tube called a stent is left in place after this procedure to keep the vessel patent. This may be impregnated with a slow-release drug intended to inhibit clotting and occlusion of the channel formed by the stent. Prior to emergency angioplasty, an infusion of a drug that inhibits platelet adhesion may be commenced. This can further reduce the risk of thrombosis while the patient is prepared for the operation, but carries the risk of severe bleeding during the procedure. Angioplasty is always preceded by an angiography (see Section 3.2b). After the angiography has exposed which coronary vessels are most blocked by atheroma, the tube that has been used to perform the angiography is left in place at the entrance to the coronary vessels. A skilled operator can then direct a finer tube from this point to actually enter the coronary vessel. When situated at the point of greatest narrowing, the end of the tube is inflated slightly. This compresses the atheroma flat against the wall of the vessel, and widens the passageway for the flow of blood (see Figure 3.2e-I). It is at this point that the stent may be left situated in the vessel to keep it open. Although angioplasty is a surgical procedure, in the UK it is performed by a physician (i.e. a cardiologist) rather than a surgeon.

Figure 3.2e-I The dilatation of a coronary artery by means of angioplasty (PCI)

(a) A narrowed coronary artery during angiography. (b) The same artery with a tubular balloon inflated in the narrowed portion. (c) The same artery after angioplasty; the narrowing has disappeared.

The advantage of angioplasty is that it can provide immediate relief from the symptoms of angina, and involves the patient in relatively little discomfort. Angioplasty carries a small risk of triggering thrombosis of the coronary vessel at the time of the procedure. In stable angina, although it may relieve symptoms temporarily, it does not seem to significantly affect the long-term prognosis for the patient. After the stent has been inserted the patient will be required to remain on lifelong antiplatelet medication to prevent clotting within the stent.

Because angioplasty may actually damage the coronary vessel rather than clear the blockage, approximately 1 percent of patients have to proceed to emergency heart surgery (see below) after an angioplasty.

Coronary artery bypass graft (CABG)

In this operation one or more of the three coronary arteries are bypassed using either lengths of veins taken from the thigh or lengths of arteries taken from the wall of the chest. This is a major operation, requiring an incision down the midline of the chest and a period of recovery in an intensive care unit. The success rate in terms of symptom relief is higher for some patients than for angioplasty. In some patients CABG may also reduce the risk of future heart attacks or other deaths from CHD.

CABG carries the risks that come with all major operations. In addition, there are risks that the patient can suffer a heart attack or a stroke. For these reasons, the operation is restricted to those people who are relatively fit, and who thus have a good chance of benefiting from the procedure.

ANGINA PECTORIS – UNSTABLE ANGINA

Unstable angina is a form of acute coronary syndrome and clinically may only be distinguished from heart attack (myocardial infarction) by the fact that blood tests reveal no signs of cardiac muscle damage.

In an episode of unstable angina the patient will present usually with severe chest pain at rest, which may be associated with sweating, shortness of breath, fear and collapse. The pain may radiate to the jaw or upper arm or back. In some cases, particularly in elderly people, pain may be less prominent, and instead the patient may simply present with impaired exercise tolerance with shortness of breath.

This is a very serious condition that carries the risk of fatal complications including ventricular arrhythmias and cardiac rupture, and so needs urgent management.

Treatment of unstable angina

If a patient has an acute attack of unstable angina that does not settle rapidly, they are initially treated as an emergency in hospital, with bed rest, opiate painkillers and oral nitrates. The painkillers and nitrates are intended to minimize the stress and anxiety resulting from pain. Oxygen is given if measurement shows the blood oxygen levels to be low. Aspirin and an anticlotting medication called ticagrelor are given by mouth as quickly as possible. An infusion of the anticoagulant fondaparinux or heparin may also be administered. If chest pain continues despite all these treatments, intravenous nitrate drugs are also given.

If pain continues, an emergency angiography will be performed to assess the extent of coronary artery disease, and a PCI or emergency CABG may follow this investigation.

Information box 3.2e-I

The causes of atheroma: comments from a Chinese medicine perspective

As suggested in Section 3.2c, the substantial fatty deposit of atheroma could possibly be an internal manifestation of non-substantial Phlegm. The hardened non-compliant vessels that result from a combination of atheroma deposition and arteriosclerosis suggest that Qi Deficiency, and in particular, Deficiency of Zong Qi, the Qi that supports the health of the vessels, might also be factors.

It was also suggested that high levels of lipids in the bloodstream might be interpreted as a manifestation of Phlegm Damp. In people who have very high-level blood lipid levels, the serum of the blood actually looks cloudy instead of clear, and this fits with the interpretation.

Smoking leads to Zong Qi Deficiency, Heat and Phlegm. Low levels of physical activity can lead to Qi Stagnation. This might explain why these risk factors are so important in the development of atheroma.

The protective effect of vitamins, flavonoids and vegetable and fish oils may be a result of the ways in which these foods can Nourish Blood and Spleen Qi, and so help to transform Damp.

Alcohol in moderate doses is Warming, and therefore can Move Qi and Blood, but in excess is a source of Damp Heat. This may explain why alcohol can be protective, but is damaging when taken in excess.

Garlic is known to be Warming and Pungent, and also helps to Clear Damp and Phlegm through Moving Qi and Warming the Stomach and Spleen. This is in accordance with the conventional medicine observation that garlic can reduce levels of blood lipids.

Social stresses may Deplete and Stagnate Qi. Loss and emotional isolation are two emotional states that may be particularly important. As these emotions tend to affect the Heart and Lungs, these will both tend to Deplete Zong Qi, the Qi of the chest, and so have a negative effect on the health of the vessels.

TREATMENT OF ANGINA: SUMMARY

The treatment for the prevention of worsening of angina involves:

- lifestyle advice

- daily low-dose aspirin or clopidogrel

- a lipid-lowering drug in those with high blood lipids

- medical management of hypertension and diabetes, if present.

The treatment for the symptoms of stable angina involves:

- nitrates
- CCBs
- beta blockers
- angioplasty (PTCA)
- CABG.

Additional treatment for unstable angina involves:

- painkillers
- oxygen
- oral anticoagulants, including aspirin and ticagrelor
- intravenous anticoagulants including fondaparinux or heparin
- angiography leading to PCI or CABG.

 Information box 3.2e-II

Angina: comments from a Chinese medicine perspective

In Chinese medicine, the symptom of the intense pain of angina might be diagnosed as Heart Blood Stagnation. The recognition that atheroma very frequently underlies angina would suggest that the patient would demonstrate other symptoms and signs of Phlegm and Zong Qi Deficiency.

Cold, Phlegm and Heart Blood/Qi Deficiency are the factors that are considered to promote the development of Stagnation of Blood of the Heart. The emotions of sadness and anger would be particularly important in the etiology of this syndrome, in that each can lead to Stagnation of Qi in the chest.

Aspirin is Warming, and in this way is believed to Clear Cold and Move Blood.

By lowering the blood lipid level, the statins appear to Clear Damp Phlegm. However, side effects of muscle aches, headache and digestive disturbance suggest they also cause Disharmony of the Liver and Spleen.

Nitrates increase the blood flow to the heart, and this can be interpreted as Heat Moving Stagnation. The side effects of flushing and throbbing headache suggest Full Heat (Stomach or Liver).

All these treatments are suppressive in nature.

Myocardial infarction (heart attack)

Heart attack (also known as myocardial infarction) is a result of a sudden blockage of the coronary arteries, usually as a result of a blood clot (coronary thrombosis). This leads to infarction of the heart muscle (the myocardium). Although this can occur on a background of a history of worsening angina, it can also occur out of the blue. Clinically the condition may be indistinguishable from unstable angina, and currently the two clinical presentations are considered together as acute coronary syndrome for the purposes of management of a patient with acute chest pain of coronary origin.

The sudden loss of blood supply to part of the heart is a great shock to the muscle cells. Some of these cells will die, and the resulting damage leads to severe pain, which can be described as crushing or like a tight band around the chest. The pain of the heart attack is often associated with a cold sweat and an emotional sense of deep fear, sometimes described as "a sense of impending doom." The patient can be restless and may vomit.

Just as with unstable angina, the symptoms of heart attack may be much less prominent in elderly people. An episode of tiredness, a "funny turn" or some unexplained breathlessness may be all that an elderly person experiences. In fact, ECG tests occasionally demonstrate the changes characteristic of a previous heart attack, but the patient may not remember any past episode that could explain these changes. These painless heart attacks are termed silent infarctions.

Heart attacks can have a number of serious consequences. Up to half of all patients die within the first few hours because damage to the pacemaker cells of the heart causes the heart to stop beating. This is called cardiac arrest, and although this may be reversed by emergency treatment, if it occurs in a situation where there is no experienced first aider on hand, it is rapidly fatal.

After a heart attack, some patients may continue to suffer from instability of the pacemaker system of the heart. This means they are at particular risk of cardiac arrest within the first few days after a heart attack. A patient who has recently had a heart attack may therefore experience palpitations. These irregularities of the heart rhythm are called arrhythmias. This is why patients who have suffered a heart attack are initially nursed under close observation.

In other patients, the damage to the heart muscle recovers to some extent, but the muscle is never as strong as it was. This leads to inefficiency of the pumping action of the heart, which can manifest as the condition of chronic heart (cardiac) failure. In some patients the damage to the heart muscle is so great that the pumping action of the heart suddenly becomes very weak. This results in the condition of acute heart failure, and the patient experiences severe breathlessness. The conditions of arrhythmia, chronic heart failure and acute heart failure are explored in more detail in Section 3.2f.

Some patients make a full recovery from a heart attack as the damaged muscle heals and new blood vessels form. However, the underlying problem of atheroma will not heal unless the factors causing atheroma are removed. This means that these patients are at high risk of a recurrence unless they can attend to making significant changes in their lifestyle. This is the reason why only about half of those patients who survive a heart attack will still be alive ten years later.

TREATMENT OF ACUTE HEART ATTACK
Treatment of cardiac arrest
Cardiac arrest can occur at any time, but is most likely to happen within the first 48 hours of the attack. For this reason, the heart attack patient should be under intensive medical supervision. If cardiac arrest occurs, the circulation should ideally be sustained by cardiopulmonary respiration (CPR) until medical treatment is available.

For those patients who have suffered cardiac arrest, initial medical treatment involves applying an electric shock to the chest (cardioversion), and this can be sufficient to restart the failing pacemaker of the heart. Various drugs, including adrenaline, may be injected to stimulate the heartbeat.

The combination of CPR and cardioversion for cardiac arrest is known to be life-saving. However, access to these treatments is not always available, and without them a cardiac arrest will rapidly become a fatal condition.

Treatment to reduce permanent heart muscle damage
For those patients who have not suffered cardiac arrest, the initial treatment is to encourage the patient to be as calm as possible. As for unstable angina, aspirin is given orally. Nitrates may be given, and a strong opiate painkiller may be injected to reduce the pain and induce calm. Clopidogrel or ticagrelor, both of which prevent the clumping of platelets, will also be given at this stage.

It is important that an acute myocardial infarction is differentiated from unstable angina, as the two conditions require different treatments. An ECG recording and the results of blood tests for the cardiac enzyme troponin are crucial in helping to differentiate between the two syndromes. The ECG recording further allows the diagnosis to be narrowed down to either the more serious segment elevation (ST) elevation myocardial infarction and the less serious non-ST elevation form (STEMI vs NSTEMI).

Once a diagnosis of STEMI has been confirmed, the ideal treatment, if available, is immediate revascularization with an angiography and PCI. This procedure can make a pathway through the recently formed clot and reverse the damage it would have otherwise caused. If this is not available or feasible, the second ideal treatment would be clot-busting fibrinolytic medication given by infusion. This drug reverses the stage in the clotting cascade that involves the formation of fibrin. If given within the first 24 hours, fibrinolytics can totally dissolve, or at least reduce

the size of, some coronary thromboses, and, together with aspirin, are known to be life-saving. Alteplase and streptokinase are commonly used fibrinolytics in the UK.

If the diagnosis is NSTEMI, a scoring system is used to predict risk of future occurrence of chest pain. If the risk is considered to be high, or if ischemia continues over the next few days in hospital, revascularization with PCI or CABG is considered. Otherwise the patient who has survived a NSTEMI but who is considered at low risk may simply be treated with dual antiplatelet medication, often advised to be continued in dual form for a year, and then single dose (usually aspirin) for the long term.

Additional medications that will be commenced before discharge for patients with STEMI or NSTEMI include a beta blocker that is known to reduce the workload on the heart. Clinical studies have demonstrated that beta blockers provide additional survival benefit, although they may not be given if the patient is suffering from severe heart failure or asthma.

An ACE inhibitor will also be given to reduce the workload of the heart. These drugs were described in some detail in Section 3.2d.

Finally, a statin is also prescribed if the total cholesterol is greater than 4.0mmol/l, which it will be in the majority of patients. This, too, is recognized to improve the chances of long-term survival after a heart attack.

All these medications may be prescribed to be taken in the long term and for a year at a minimum.

Long-term treatment of heart attack
A patient who has suffered an uncomplicated heart attack is usually discharged from hospital within three to five days of the attack. Treatment from this stage on is aimed at preventing a recurrence, and the lifestyle aspect of this is similar to what is recommended for patients with angina. However, after a heart attack, a patient will be recommended to continue taking quite a few new medications. The typical cocktail would include aspirin or clopidogrel, ticagrelor, a beta blocker, an ACE inhibitor and a statin. All of these medications are prescribed to reduce the risk of recurrence, and, with the exception of ticagrelor, which is prescribed for one year only, most may be continued for life.

Increasingly, heart attack patients are referred for cardiac rehabilitation sessions in which they are given a structured program of gentle exercises, guidance about lifestyle change and access to a support group. It is believed that the exercise component of these sessions in particular may help to encourage new growth of coronary vessels and so prevent recurrence of the heart attack.

On discharge from hospital, the patient is advised to increase daily activities very gradually. They are advised not to drive for four weeks, during which time the risk of arrhythmias is significant. Most patients can return to normal activities after two months.

217

TREATMENT OF HEART ATTACK: SUMMARY

The treatment for acute heart attack involves:

- emergency management of cardiac arrest
- aspirin or clopidogrel and ticagrelor
- oxygen, if oxygen levels are low
- strong painkillers (diamorphine or morphine) and nitrates.

For STEMI:

- immediate consideration of PCI/CABG
- if PCI is not possible, then immediate fibrinolytic (clot-busting) medication.

For NSTEMI:

- risk assessment and consideration of revascularization.

In the long term after heart attack:

- aspirin or clopidogrel and ticagrelor
- beta blockers
- ACE inhibitors
- statins
- lifestyle advice and a graded return to daily activities
- cardiac rehabilitation.

The red flags of angina and heart attack

All patients with angina and heart attack will benefit from referral to a conventional doctor for assessment or treatment. Red flags are those symptoms and signs that indicate that referral should be considered. The red flags of angina and heart attack are described in Table 3.2e-II. A summary of the red flags in a format designed for quick reference in clinical practice can be found in Appendix III. This gives advice on the degree of urgency of referral for each of the red flag conditions listed.

Table 3.2e-II A13: Red flags of angina and heart attack

Red flag	Description	Reasoning
A13.1	Features of stable angina: central chest pain related to exertion, eating or the cold and that improves with rest. Pain is heavy, gripping (rather than sharp or stabbing). It can radiate down the neck and arms	Chest pain is a common anxiety symptom, and is also a common feature of peptic ulcer disease, hiatus hernia and esophagitis. Stable angina is distinguished from these syndromes by being predictably related to exertion, and generally develops in those over 35. It is far more likely to develop in elderly people and those with cardiovascular risk factors (see notes to Table A12)
	Beware: can present as episodes of breathlessness/chest tightness but without pain in elderly people	It is advisable to refer for assessment, as angina carries a high risk of heart attack and other cardiovascular events
A13.2	Features of unstable angina or heart attack (acute coronary syndrome): sustained intense chest pain associated with fear or dread. Palpitations and breathlessness may be present. The patient may vomit or develop a cold sweat	Very intense and heavy chest pain that tends to radiate to the left shoulder and arm is suggestive of cardiac pain. If sustained, this is a situation in which there is a high risk of cardiac arrest or worsening cardiovascular damage. Keep the patient calm, upright and still while waiting for urgent help to arrive
	Beware: can present as sudden onset of breathlessness, palpitations or confusion but without pain in elderly people	Under UK Health and Safety Executive (HSE) guidance,* qualified first-aiders are permitted to administer aspirin in the situation of suspected heart attack. There is very strong clinical evidence to support the benefits of aspirin in reducing the risk of fatal complications, and this effect is more powerful the sooner the aspirin is given. The patient should be offered one 300mg tablet to be chewed or swallowed. Aspirin is contraindicated in children <12, in pregnancy, if the patient has a bleeding disorder or is on anticoagulant medication, and in cases where there is a known allergy to aspirin or aspirin-induced asthma
		Note: Chest pain is a common anxiety symptom and is also a common feature of peptic ulcer disease, hiatus hernia and esophagitis. If associated with anxiety, it is more likely to be centrally located and be sharp in quality
A13.3	Sudden-onset tearing chest pain with radiation to the back: features of shock may be present (faintness, low blood pressure, rapid pulse)	This intense, acute form of chest pain is suggestive of a dissecting aortic aneurysm. In this case urgent referral is required, but aspirin should not be given, as it promotes bleeding

* Health and Safety Executive (2013) 'Frequently asked questions on First Aid/Employers/Tablets and Medications.' Available at www.hse.gov.uk/firstaid/faqs.htm, accessed on 7 March 2017.

Information box 3.2e-III

Heart attack: comments from a Chinese medicine perspective

In Chinese medicine, the pain of the heart attack would usually be diagnosed, as is the case for angina, as Heart Blood Stagnation. Similarly, a background of Phlegm and Zong Qi Deficiency may be apparent. However, the severity of the condition in some cases, with cold sweating and high risk of cardiac arrest, implies that Heart Yang has been severely damaged, and is at risk of Collapse.

Aspirin and clopidogrel, because they encourage the free movement of blood, may be considered as Warming in nature, and in this way they can move Heart Blood Stagnation.

Cardioversion and adrenaline both strongly stimulate Heart Yang. In doing so these treatments are likely to draw on bodily reserves of Yang and as such are likely to be ultimately depleting. However, these treatments are without a doubt life-saving in the short term.

By dissolving a clot and allowing the clot to move, fibrinolytic drugs can be interpreted as Heating, and so will move Heart Blood Stagnation. However, they can give rise to the side effect of serious hemorrhage, which is an adverse manifestation of Heat.

The energetics of the ACE inhibitors and beta blockers are more complex, as they both have a tendency to deplete Yang (see energetic descriptions in Section 3.2d), which would seem detrimental. What both these drugs do is reduce the immediate workload of the heart, so that the muscle is under less strain and is able to be better nourished by the blood in the coronary arteries. This would imply that they have the ability to Boost Heart Qi and Blood, but this energetic benefit is at the cost of overall depletion. So, in the long term, this action, which is suppressive in nature, is possibly depleting. However, in the short term, they act to prevent further Heart Blood Stagnation, and can therefore be life-saving.

3.2f Heart failure and arrhythmias

This section introduces two other important conditions that can result from CHD: heart failure and abnormalities of the heart rhythm (arrhythmias). Both these conditions can have other causes, which are also described in this section.

The conditions studied in this section are:

- Heart failure:
    - acute heart failure
    - chronic heart failure
- Arrhythmias:
    - benign (sinus) tachycardia
    - benign (sinus) bradycardia
    - ectopic beats
    - atrial fibrillation (AF)
    - ventricular fibrillation (VF)
    - supraventricular tachycardia (SVT)
    - heart block.

Heart failure

Heart failure is the inability of the heart to pump blood efficiently through the circulatory system. It affects about 10 percent of people over the age of 65.

The clinical syndrome of heart failure is characterized by symptoms of breathlessness, fatigue, ankle swelling and signs of rapid heart rate and peripheral edema.

These symptoms and signs develop because the pumping action of the heart is not sufficiently powerful to deal with all the blood arriving at the heart. For this reason, blood accumulates in the vessels that lead to both sides of the heart. These vessels are the pulmonary veins, which transport blood from the lungs into the left side of the heart, and the systemic (bodily) veins, which transport blood from all the other tissues of the body to the right side of the heart. Figure 3.2f-I illustrates how the blood flows in a figure-of-eight pathway between the lungs and the body, and through the two sides of the heart.

In heart failure, the heart is continually under strain. This can cause further weakening of the heart's pumping function, which means that the condition, if left untreated, can deteriorate rapidly. For this reason, only half of those who are diagnosed with heart failure will still be alive after four years. However, in recent years it has been shown that certain medical treatments can prolong life expectancy in heart failure, and for this reason it is important that early stages of heart failure are diagnosed and treated appropriately.

Heart failure can be categorized as acute or chronic, according to the rate at which the condition develops.

Acute heart failure

Acute heart failure is a serious condition. It occurs when the heart suddenly loses its pumping efficiency, for example, as a result of a heart attack. In acute heart failure, the weakened heart muscle is suddenly faced with a large volume of blood that it is unable to pump. This has the most profound effects in the tissue of the lungs.

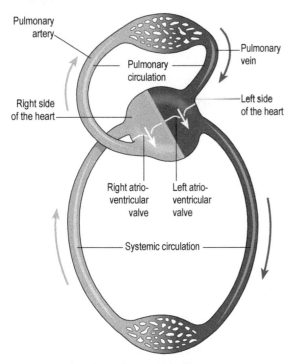

Figure 3.2f-I The relationship between the pulmonary (involving the lungs) and systemic (bodily) circulations

The sudden accumulation of blood in the pulmonary veins in the lungs leads to increased blood pressure within the lung capillaries. The increased pressure forces excess fluid from the capillaries into the tissue of the lungs. This fluid accumulates in the air spaces of the lungs, and severely impairs the ability of the lungs to take in oxygen. Edema is the term given to excessive fluid in the tissues (see Section 3.2a), and this condition is therefore called pulmonary edema.

A patient with acute heart failure will experience a sudden onset of breathlessness. Some patients will cough up frothy fluid in an attempt to clear the air spaces in the lungs. In severe cases, the lips and tongue will appear blue, as oxygen fails to reach the blood because of the fluid in the lungs. The patient has to sit upright and may feel panic stricken. Without medical treatment to reverse the situation many patients with acute heart failure will die.

TREATMENT OF ACUTE HEART FAILURE
Patients with acute heart failure are treated as an emergency. Oxygen is given to assist breathing and to improve the ability of the heart to pump. Diamorphine (heroin), a powerful painkiller, is also given, to relieve the panic and to treat the pulmonary edema, as this drug tends to decrease the blood pressure in the veins of the body.

In addition, a powerful diuretic (furosemide or bumetanide) is given intravenously. This leads to a rapid shift of fluid from the circulation through the kidneys to the bladder. Diuretics are also used in the treatment of hypertension to encourage the kidneys to excrete fluid from the circulation (see Section 3.2d).

 Information box 3.2f-I

Pulmonary edema: comments from a Chinese medicine perspective

In Chinese medicine, the symptoms of the condition of pulmonary edema in acute heart failure could be diagnosed as Kidney Yang Deficiency with Water Overflowing to the Lungs and the Heart. One reason given for the Water Overflowing is that when Kidney Yang is deficient there is insufficient Fire of Ming Men. With insufficient Fire of Ming Men, the Yang of the Heart cannot be warmed, and fluid accumulates in the Lungs and Heart. The condition can progress to Heart Yang Collapse.

Diamorphine relieves pain, relaxes the blood vessels and can induce a state of euphoria and mental detachment. In excessive doses, it can induce confusion, coma and death as a result of depression of breathing. Side effects are nausea, constipation, drowsiness and reduced depth of breathing. It can also cause pinpoint pupils, dry mouth, sweating and difficulty in urination. It is powerfully addictive.

The pain relief, euphoria (joy) and mental detachment caused by diamorphine might be described in terms of Obstruction of the Orifices of the Heart. The Pathological Factors that have this property include Phlegm, Full Heat and Blood Stagnation. Of these three, it would seem most likely that the numbness and later confusion and drowsiness associated with opiates is most fittingly attributed to Phlegm. The nausea could also be attributed to Phlegm obstructing the chest. Therefore, diamorphine might be described as Phlegm Inducing.

The initial beneficial effect on the blood vessels in the lungs could represent Boosting of Lung (or Zong) Qi, but with the long-term consequence of Depletion of Lung Qi, reflected in the long-term effects of depression of breathing and constipation.

Dry mouth, sweating and difficulty in urinating suggest Subduing of Kidney Yin. Kidneys and Lungs are closely related, and it seems that diamorphine exerts much of its influence on the Kidney-Lung Axis. Interestingly, the pupils are related to the Kidneys in Chinese medicine, and so constricted pupils might be seen as a marker of Kidney imbalance.

By stimulating urination, strong diuretics such as furosemide could be described as Clearing Damp (Transformation of Water) by Boosting Kidney Yang. Diuretics like furosemide are conventionally recognized to be toxic to the kidneys, and so their powerful action (Yang in nature) might ultimately be seen as Depleting of Kidney Yin and Yang.

Sometimes nitrates are administered in an emergency situation (see Section 3.2e), as these also have the ability to cause dilatation of blood vessels and so may relieve the strain on the failing heart.

The combination of these treatments, although not always successful, can bring rapid relief to the patient, and can reverse a condition that could otherwise be fatal. After this emergency treatment, the patient requires intensive nursing care and treatment of the underlying cause of the acute heart failure.

Chronic heart failure

Chronic heart failure is the result of a much more gradual deterioration of the heart's ability to pump. A slight degree of heart failure is so common that it can almost be considered to be a normal part of aging.

Coronary heart disease (CHD) is probably the most common cause of chronic heart failure. Other causes include factors that increase the effort required of the heart, such as scarred heart valves, long-standing lung disease or persistent hypertension. Anemia and thyroid disease are conditions in which the heart has to work harder than usual, and this can also lead to heart failure. Irregularities of heart rhythm (arrhythmias) that impair the smooth pumping action of the heart are another common cause.

In contrast to acute heart failure, in chronic heart failure the body has a chance to adapt to the gradual buildup of pressure within the veins leading to the heart. The response to the increased pressure in these veins is that fluid moves out gradually into the tissues of the body as well as into the lung tissue.

Failure of the right side of the heart to pump efficiently leads to a buildup of fluid (edema) in the tissues of the body. This is initially most marked in the areas of the body affected most by gravity, namely, the feet and ankles. However, in severe chronic heart failure, the fluid can accumulate in the thighs and scrotum and also other important tissues, including the liver and the bowel. This can have the serious consequence of damage to the function of these vital organs.

Failure of the left side of the heart to pump efficiently leads to an accumulation of fluid within the lungs. As this process progresses, the patient will experience increasing breathlessness on exertion and possibly a recurrent cough.

A patient with mild chronic heart failure may suffer from slight swelling of the ankles and shortness of breath on exertion, whereas a patient with severe chronic heart failure may have marked leg and ankle swelling, liver and digestive disorders, and experience exhaustion and disabling breathlessness.

Chronic heart failure can be diagnosed by physical examination of the heart, lungs and those areas where edema is likely to develop (e.g. the ankles).

There is a blood test for a hormone that is released from stressed heart muscle called B type natriuretic peptide (BNP). High levels of BNP are highly suggestive of heart failure. A chest X-ray image and an electrocardiogram (ECG) might show characteristic changes of heart failure, but the most informative non-invasive method of investigation of heart failure is recognized to be echocardiography (cardiac ultrasound scan) (see Section 3.2b). Ideally, all patients should receive this test before treatment is started, so that a firm diagnosis can be made.

TREATMENT OF CHRONIC HEART FAILURE

The treatment of chronic heart failure should always include treatment of the underlying cause. If CHD is the cause, reduction of risk factors is essential. Hypertension should be treated (see Section 3.2d), valvular problems corrected by surgery (see Section 3.2g) and arrhythmias treated (see later in this section).

Reduction of dietary salt should be advised, as salt encourages retention of water. Alcohol can impair the pumping action of the heart further, so this should also be avoided.

Recent advances in the drug treatment of chronic heart failure have led to the introduction of a wide range of potentially useful drugs. The most commonly prescribed drugs are the angiotensin-converting enzyme (ACE) inhibitors (e.g. lisinopril) or angiotensin II receptor antagonists (A2RAs) (e.g. candesartan and valsartan), but increasingly patients may be prescribed one or more of the following: beta blockers (e.g. bisoprolol and metoprolol), diuretics of different classes (e.g. bendroflumethiazide, furosemide and spironolactone), ivabradine (affects sinus pacemaker) and digoxin. All these classes of drugs are listed in Chapter 2 of the *British National Formulary* (BNF).

Diuretics include the thiazide diuretics, such as bendroflumethiazide, which are also prescribed for hypertension, and the more powerful loop diuretics, such as furosemide, which are given in acute heart failure. Spironolactone is another form of powerful diuretic that is often used in heart failure. This counteracts the adrenal hormone aldosterone and balances the potassium loss induced by the other classes of diuretics. All these drugs act on the kidney in different ways to promote urination, and therefore help to shift accumulating fluid from the circulation. The patient will notice a reduction in ankle edema and relief of breathlessness within a few days of taking diuretics. However, there is no evidence that diuretics increase life expectancy in heart failure.

The action of ACE inhibitors in hypertension is described in Section 3.2d. ACE inhibitors both reduce the tone of the small arteries and promote urination. The relaxed blood vessels and reduction of fluid in the circulation reduces the load on the heart. Clinical studies have demonstrated that patients with heart failure who are prescribed ACE inhibitors and diuretics have an increased life expectancy compared to those prescribed diuretics alone.

Beta blockers can be helpful in heart failure as they reduce the pressure against which the struggling heart muscle has to work. They are now introduced to patients early in the course of their condition as it has become recognized that, like ACE inhibitors, they appear to reduce mortality in heart failure, possibly by inhibiting fatal arrhythmias, the cause of death in 50 percent of patients.

As fatal arrhythmias are so common in heart failure, an implantable cardioversion device (ICD) is increasingly used. This small subcutaneous device is designed to detect the onset of an arrhythmia and apply an electric shock to the heart muscle to reinstate regular sinus rhythm.

Arrhythmias

Arrhythmia is the medical term used to describe a range of abnormalities of heart rhythm. The basic problem in arrhythmias is either rooted in the function of the pacemaker at the center of the heart, or in that of the conducting fibers that transmit the regular electrical impulse from the pacemaker to the rest of the heart so that it contracts in a controlled and efficient way.

It may help to turn back to Section 3.2a to read about the conduction system of the heart in preparation for the study of arrhythmias.

Causes of arrhythmias

As described above, a heart attack can lead to arrhythmias, as the damage resulting from infarction can involve either the pacemaker or the conducting fibers in the heart. The degeneration resulting from CHD, even without the sudden damage of a heart attack, is probably the most important cause of the arrhythmias found in elderly people. In CHD the pacemaker and conducting fibers of the heart can degenerate as a result of chronic poor blood supply, and so become more vulnerable to triggering arrhythmias.

Arrhythmias can occur for reasons other than CHD. In particular, some can result from a congenital abnormality of the pacemaker system. Other causes of arrhythmias include damage of the heart muscle by drugs (e.g. digoxin) and alcohol, infections of the heart and pericardium (e.g. pericarditis), and strain on the heart muscle, which can result from scarred heart valves. The latter two causes are discussed in Section 3.2g.

Disorders of rate (benign arrhythmias)

Some arrhythmias are classified as benign. This means that the disorder does not indicate a fundamental problem with the pacemaker system of the heart. Benign arrhythmias are always disorders of rate rather than rhythm. In conventional medicine, a rapid pulse (tachycardia) is defined as a rate of

above 100 beats per minute in an adult, and a slow pulse (bradycardia) as a rate of less than 60 beats per minute.

BENIGN (SINUS) TACHYCARDIA

Common non-cardiac causes of a rapid but regular heart rate include anxiety, exercise, pregnancy and fever. Anemia and thyroid disease are two diseases that can lead to a rapid heart rate.

This tachycardia is not always so benign. If very rapid, the racing heart cannot pump efficiently, and heart failure may develop. This is a known consequence of conditions such as severe anemia and an overactive thyroid gland. The tachycardia can lead a patient with coronary atheroma to experience angina because the coronary vessels are unable to meet the heart's increased demand for oxygen and nutrients.

BENIGN (SINUS) BRADYCARDIA

Common non-cardiac causes of a slow pulse rate include cardiovascular fitness (a very common finding in athletes) and extreme cold (hypothermia).

Deficiency of thyroid hormone can also lead to a slow pulse. Some drugs, most commonly beta blockers, can lead to a bradycardia.

Again, this bradycardia is not always so benign. If the pulse rate is very slow, the patient may experience episodes of dizziness or fainting.

Information box 3.2f-II

Benign arrhythmias: comments from a Chinese medicine perspective

In Chinese medicine, a benign tachycardia is experienced as a rapid pulse, indicating Full or Empty Heat, and a benign bradycardia is experienced as a slow pulse, indicating Full or Empty Cold. Although a slow pulse may be interpreted as a marker of fitness from a Western perspective, from a Chinese medicine perspective the low rate would suggest that excessive exercise has led to some depletion of Yang.

All the other arrhythmias to be studied in this section involve a disorder of the conduction system of the heart itself. The investigations and treatment of these arrhythmias have features in common, so these shall be discussed first.

The investigation of arrhythmias

Arrhythmias can, of course, be detected at the pulse, but can only be diagnosed accurately by means of an ECG recording (see Section 3.2b). The ECG can help distinguish between arrhythmias that have similar pulse patterns but different underlying causes. Sometimes a 24-hour ECG is required to capture the irregularity of rhythm when it is intermittent.

Most patients with an arrhythmia will also undergo echocardiography (see Section 3.2b) to exclude valvular and other structural problems, and to assess whether or not there is any degree of heart failure.

Treatment of arrhythmias

Symptomatic or life-threatening arrhythmias are treated medically by a range of different types of drugs collectively termed antiarrhythmic drugs. All these drugs are conventionally recognized as suppressive rather than curative, as withdrawal of the drug usually results in recurrence of the problem.

The drugs include digoxin (see BNF, Chapter 2.1), verapamil, a calcium channel blocker (CCB) (see BNF, Chapter 2.6), beta blockers (see BNF, Chapter 2.4) and a range of drugs listed in the BNF as antiarrhythmic drugs (see BNF, Chapter 2.3). The latter include drugs such as amiodarone and disopyramide.

These drugs each act at different parts of the conducting system of the heart, and so the energetic interpretation of each type is different. Only digoxin, a commonly prescribed antiarrhythmic drug, is discussed in detail in this section. The CCBs and beta blockers have been described in detail in Section 3.2d.

Planned cardioversion by electric shock is a useful technique for some patients. This is described below under the heading "Atrial fibrillation (AF)."

Many patients benefit from the surgical insertion of an artificial pacemaker. This is a small, battery-powered unit that is inserted under the skin of the upper chest. Wires lead from the unit and pass via the blood vessels to rest against the inside wall of the heart. Most pacemakers are dual-chamber units. This means they can stimulate both the atria and the ventricles, and so simulate a natural heartbeat.

The pacemaker unit contains a sensor that can detect deficiencies in the heart rhythm. When an absent or irregular heartbeat is detected, an electrical impulse is sent to the heart to override the failing conducting system, and a regular rhythm is thus reinstated. Some advanced pacemakers can appropriately alter the rate of the heart according to activity or respiration. The programming of the pacemaker can be performed remotely once it has been inserted, so adjustments to its function can be made if necessary.

Some patients may benefit from a surgical operation to remove (by means of radio waves) an abnormal part of the conducting system of the heart. This surgery is called ablation therapy. It is considered a relatively minor intervention, and is performed as part of a cardiac catheterization procedure (see Section 3.2b). Sometimes, if

this involves necessary damage to the natural pacemaker, an artificial pacemaker is inserted to thereafter provide a regular electrical stimulus to the heart (so-called "ablate and pace" treatment).

Implantable defibrillators (ICDs) are increasingly used to prevent sudden death. These devices (see Figure 3.2f-II) are similar in size to a pacemaker, but are programmed to deliver an electric shock to the heart should the sensor detect a burst of chaotic ventricular rhythm. Clinical trials have shown that in certain groups ICDs significantly reduce the risk of sudden cardiac death.

Figure 3.2f-II Chest X-ray image showing the location of an ICD
As with the pacemaker, the ICD is located just superior to the pectoral muscles. The image illustrates the pathway of the leads through the subclavian vein and the superior vena cava, and thence to the right side of the heart.

In summary, the treatment of arrhythmias includes:

- treatment of the underlying cause
- antiarrhythmic drugs
- cardioversion by electric shock
- insertion of an artificial pacemaker
- surgical ablation therapy
- ICDs.

Ectopic beats

The most common disorder of rhythm (rather than rate) is called an ectopic beat. This is felt as a single beat that is out of time with the regular rhythm of the normal heartbeats. The patient may experience a palpitation at the time of the ectopic beat, or may be totally unaware of it.

Ectopic beats are more frequent when the patient is at rest and also in elderly people. On their own, unless very frequent (more than one every ten beats) or accompanied by symptoms, they are not conventionally considered to be a cause for concern.

However, the development of frequent ectopic beats is considered to be a sign of degeneration of the pacemaker system of the heart. A patient with frequent ectopic beats may be investigated for heart disease, and may be offered antiarrhythmic drugs.

 Information box 3.2f-III

Ectopic beats: a Chinese medicine perspective

Ectopic beats would possibly be diagnosed by a Chinese practitioner as a knotted pulse, as the pulse rate is basically regular but has pauses at irregular intervals. However, a knotted pulse is also classically a slow pulse. This is not always the case with ectopic beats, which can occur with a pulse of normal or rapid rate. Nevertheless, whatever the pulse rate, the occasional dropped beats would probably represent a degree of depletion of Heart Qi or Yang, as it is Heart Yang that dominates the rhythmic function of the Heart.

Atrial fibrillation (AF)

Atrial fibrillation (AF) is a very common arrhythmia in old age, and may not be noticed by the patient. Although CHD is the most common cause of AF, other common causes include narrowing of the heart valves, thyroid disease and excessive alcohol intake.

The cause of AF is a degeneration of the pacemaker of the heart, which can no longer transmit a regular impulse to the atria, the upper chambers of the heart. For this reason, the contraction of the atrial muscle fibers is uncoordinated (the fibers are said to be in fibrillation). Heart muscle in fibrillation cannot perform a pumping function.

However, in AF, a second pacemaker deeper in the heart takes over and transmits irregular impulses to the ventricles, the lower chamber of the heart. The ventricles can often take almost the full load of the pumping function of the atria, which is why some patients may be unaware of their AF. However, other patients can suffer palpitations and breathlessness, because the second pacemaker is too fast and irregular, and the inefficient pumping leads to a degree of heart failure.

The pulse of a patient with AF is said to be irregularly irregular in rhythm. This means that there is no pattern to the heartbeat. The pulse varies in both volume and rate from beat to beat. The pulse rate can also be very rapid. In some people, the condition is paroxysmal, meaning that the arrhythmia occurs in episodes separated by periods of normal rhythm.

Apart from causing an inefficient heart pumping action, the fibrillation of the atria has another severe consequence, which is that the turbulent blood within the chambers can clot and form emboli. Although tiny, these particles of clot can travel in the circulation to the brain to cause significant damage. The emboli can lodge in cerebral arteries and lead to areas of infarction. Infarction in the brain leads to the clinical syndrome of stroke.

Sometimes the emboli in the brain are so small that they can break up and the effect on the brain is only temporary. In this case the patient will experience repeated episodes of temporary brain disturbance, such as loss of vision, confusion or dizziness, which typically last for a few minutes only. These episodes are called transient ischemic attacks (TIAs). Although temporary, TIAs should be recognized as red flags that a permanent stroke may follow shortly. For this reason, the treatment of AF, particularly if there is a history of TIAs, is taken very seriously.

There are three considerations in the treatment of AF:

- control of the rate, which is important if the rate is too fast

- control of the rhythm

- prevention of the formation of emboli (anticoagulation).

In elderly people and in those in whom the pacemaker is likely to be permanently damaged, control of rate becomes the most important aspect of treatment. In most people, rate can be controlled by one or more of three types of drug: CCBs and beta blockers and digoxin-like drugs.

Generally rate control is achieved in most cases with beta blockers or CCBs (see Section 3.2d), and these have largely superseded the use of digoxin (also known as digitalis), which is a derivative of the foxglove (*Digitalis lanata*). Digoxin used to be used widely in the management of both AF and heart failure. It is a very toxic substance if taken to excess, which means that the dose has to be controlled very carefully, and may need to be checked by means of blood tests. Digoxin increases the force of the heartbeat and tends to steady the irregularity in AF. In this way it can reverse the heart failure of AF. If digoxin reaches toxic levels, it can cause nausea and vomiting, visual disturbance and severe life-threatening arrhythmias. The actions of CCBs and beta blockers are described in Section 3.2d.

The treatment of choice for rhythm control in AF is controlled administration of an electric shock to the heart in the technique called cardioversion. This can completely reboot the heart's natural rhythm. The shock is administered while the patient is under anesthetic, and in some people can totally reverse the arrhythmia. This process may be supported by prescribing an antiarrhythmic drug to be taken both a short time before and for a few weeks after cardioversion.

Antiarrhythmic medication (including amiodarone and flecainide) may be used to maintain control of rhythm in the long term, although in most cases of resistant AF it is considered more important to control rate and prevent blood clots than control rhythm. These are powerful drugs that can have severe side effects that include corneal, lung and liver damage. They can also adversely affect the blood and nerves, as well as cause unhealthy changes in cardiac function. They need to be carefully monitored and are usually only initiated by a cardiologist.

Whilst control of rhythm will reduce risk of thromboembolism in AF, drug treatment of heart rate does not have this benefit. For this reason, patients with sustained AF are prescribed either a novel oral anticoagulant (NOAC) or warfarin (see Section 2.2d) to reduce the tendency of the blood to clot in the atria. The decision to anticoagulate involves weighing up the risk of stroke in the patient against the risk of severe bleeding side effects from the treatment. Doctors concurrently use risk scores to help them make this difficult decision about whether or not to prescribe what is potentially a dangerous medication. Whilst NOAC treatment requires no monitoring, warfarin treatment requires the clotting ability of the patient's blood to be assessed regularly by means of blood tests. The aim of the warfarin treatment for AF is to increase the time for clotting to fall within the range of between two and three times that of normal clotting (i.e. to have an international normalized ratio (INR) of between 2 and 3). Aspirin is no longer recommended for clot prevention in AF because its effectiveness is significantly less than the NOACs and warfarin.

In special cases, cardiac ablation may be performed to remove the area of the pacemaker system that is considered to be causing the problem, and then an artificial pacemaker is inserted (ablate and pace treatment).

 Information box 3.2f-IV

Atrial fibrillation: a Chinese medicine perspective

Depending on the actual rate and type of irregularity, the pulse in AF might be described as Choppy, Hasty or Knotted by a Chinese medicine practitioner. These pulse findings represent severe Blood Deficiency, Heart Qi or Yin Deficiency with Heat, or Cold with Heart Qi or Yang Deficiency, respectively. All of these suggest severe Depletion of the Heart. In AF, the quivering of the fibrillating atrial muscles, and the paroxysmal nature of the condition, might also suggest the presence of Wind. In keeping with this suggestion is that the most serious consequence of AF, thromboembolic stroke, is a manifestation of upward moving Wind.

The breathlessness and palpitations that can accompany AF also suggest severe Heart Qi/Yang Deficiency. This can progress to a state of heart failure in which fluid accumulates in the lungs and body tissues. This would be described as Kidney and Heart Yang Deficiency, with Water overflowing to the Heart and Lungs.

By improving contractility and normalizing the heart rate, digoxin appears to Clear Heat and boost Heart Yang, but in excess can cause severe and rapid arrhythmias, possibly because this benefit is at the cost of damage to Heart Yin and the Heat that is associated with this. The digestive and visual disturbances that digoxin can cause suggest that in excess it is harmful to the Spleen and Liver.

Antiarrhythmic medications (e.g. amiodarone and flecainide) are powerful drugs that can have severe side effects that include corneal, lung and liver damage. They can also affect the blood and nerves, as well as cause unhealthy changes in cardiac function. These widespread effects suggest toxicity to Blood and Yin, presumably by introduction of Toxic Heat. The Chinese energetic description of cessation of fibrillation might be seen in terms of Clearance of Wind.

The electric shock administered in cardioversion normalizes the heart rate and rhythm and thus boosts Heart Yang and Clears Wind, but is very likely to be depleting of deep reserves of Heart Qi in the process. It would make sense to advise a patient to take time to recover from such a procedure.

Ventricular arrhythmias

In contrast to AF, which may not necessarily seriously impair the pumping action of the heart, if fibrillation of theventricles occurs, the heart cannot pump at all. A patient in ventricular fibrillation (VF) will rapidly lose consciousness and die without emergency treatment. VF is the main cause of cardiac arrest following a heart attack. If an infarcted area of muscle incorporates the conducting system of the heart, the heart muscle fibers go into uncoordinated movement, leading to a quivering mass of tissue that cannot pump.

Ventricular tachycardia describes episodes of a rapid ventricular rate, which in most people leads to dizziness or collapse because of inefficient pumping. Ventricular tachycardia is a red flag for VF, and is thus treated very seriously.

The first emergency treatment that should be given in VF is cardiopulmonary resuscitation (CPR). This does not necessarily reverse the fibrillation, but will provide a temporary pumping action for the body until electric shock treatment (cardioversion) can be given. In some people, simply the physical pressure on the chest can reverse the fibrillation. However, most people require the electric shock of cardioversion, and sometimes intravenous drugs such as adrenaline and amiodarone, to enable a normal pacemaker action to be restored. If the damage to the heart from the infarction is too great, these treatments cannot be successful.

After a successful reversal of VF, an ECG may reveal changes that show bursts of ventricular tachycardia or a continued instability of the heartbeat. This means that a repeated episode of fibrillation is more likely to occur. In this case a powerful antiarrhythmic drug (e.g. amiodarone) is given intravenously to stabilize the pacemaker system. Some people with continued instability of the heartbeat may be prescribed an antiarrhythmic drug in the long term, or alternatively might be offered the implantation of a defibrillator device (ICD, described earlier).

Information box 3.2f-V

Ventricular arrhythmias: a Chinese medicine perspective

In Chinese medicine, the fibrillation of the ventricles again suggests Wind. In the case of heart attack, this Wind has possibly been generated as a response to Heart Blood Stagnation and Phlegm (which were both suggested earlier as components of the etiology of CHD). The consequence of this is Heart Yang Collapse.

Electric shocks, by restoring normal heart function, could be described as Stimulating Heart Yang. A strengthened Heart Yang will permit movement, and thus the clearance of the internally generated Wind.

Supraventricular tachycardia (SVT)

A supraventricular tachycardia (SVT) is a disorder of rapid heart rate. It is not classified as benign, as during the arrhythmia the electric impulse travels to the ventricles either from a site other than the atrioventricular node or via an unusual pathway of the conducting system.

The patient, who is often a young adult on first presentation, experiences a sudden onset of palpitations. This may come on out of the blue, but sometimes is provoked by coffee or exertion. The pulse rate can be very rapid (140–280 beats/minute). Additional symptoms include dizziness, breathlessness and sometimes chest pains. In some cases the episode stops spontaneously within minutes to hours of onset.

The most common condition that can mimic an SVT is a panic attack, in which anxiety causes the heart to race. One differentiating feature, apart from the level of the associated anxiety, is the rate of the pulse. In a panic attack the pulse rarely exceeds 140 beats per minute.

The simplest treatment for an attack of SVT is for the patient or a practitioner to massage the area that overlies the carotid arteries in the neck (in the region of acupoint ST-9, Ren Ying). Ideally, the patient should be lying supine during this maneuver. The pressure in this area sets up a reflex that causes the heart rate to slow down. Other techniques include immersing the face in cold water and rapid squatting. In a significant proportion of episodes these simple techniques will stop the tachycardia.

If non-medical approaches are not successful, antiarrhythmic drugs are given intravenously to stop the SVT. The most common drug now given is adenosine. This is a very rapid-acting drug that can cause a temporary block in the pacemaker and so can abort the arrhythmia. This drug has to be given under medical observation just in case a serious arrhythmia results from treatment.

A long-term prescription of an antiarrhythmic drug may be given to prevent future attacks. Beta blockers or CCBs are commonly prescribed. Currently, many patients with SVT are offered surgical ablation therapy to remove the abnormal part of the conducting system. This is not considered to be a major operation, as it can be performed by a similar approach as used for cardiac catheterization (see earlier). This procedure is successful in over 95 percent of cases.

Information box 3.2f-VI

Supraventricular tachycardia: a Chinese medicine perspective

The very rapid rate of the pulse in SVT suggests Empty or Full Heat. This would accord with the observation that coffee, which is Heating, through depleting the Kidneys and aggravating the Liver, can trigger attacks of SVT. The rapid onset and abrupt end of an episode of SVT suggests that Wind might also be an additional factor.

The physiological cause of SVT is an area of abnormal heart tissue, which in many cases can be successfully ablated to cure the problem. Ablative surgery could possibly enable Clearance of underlying Pathological Factors that may have been present since before birth. Although physically damaging, this treatment might engender an energetic cure.

Heart block

This rather alarming term describes an arrhythmia that results from an impairment of the smooth passage of an electrical impulse through the conducting system of the heart, if there is a literal block in the way. In most cases the block is due to an area of damaged heart muscle resulting from CHD. Like AF, heart block is an arrhythmia that can be a common incidental finding in elderly people.

The result of partial heart block is that one or more impulses fail to "get through" the conduction system, and this can lead to a regular pulse with missed beats at regular intervals. If the pathway from the node to the rest of the heart is completely deficient, a second pacemaker can set up a regular rhythm from the ventricles. This leads to a very slow regular heart rate of about 40–50 beats per minute. This is called complete heart block. Heart block, even when complete, may give rise to no symptoms, but can lead to breathlessness, palpitations and, in the case of complete heart block, blackouts. Blackouts resulting from complete heart block are called Stokes-Adams attacks. A patient recovering from a Stokes-Adams attack may be aware of rapid palpitations and facial flushing in the period as consciousness is regained.

Heart block is of concern in that it may herald a more serious arrhythmia, and so, if diagnosed, it may be treated with insertion of an artificial pacemaker.

From the point of view of a complementary therapist, as a simple rule of thumb, if the presence of either heart failure or the pulse irregularity of a non-benign arrhythmia is suspected, referral should be considered. A medical diagnosis can help with an assessment of the seriousness of the underlying condition.

Information box 3.2f-VII

Heart block: a Chinese medicine perspective

The pulse of partial heart block would be described as Intermittent, signifying in Chinese medicine a serious imbalance of one of the Yin organs. Complete heart block gives rise to a pulse that would be described as Slow. Heart block can be interpreted as a Deficiency of Heart Qi/Yang (with Internal Cold if there is complete heart block).

A pacemaker stimulates Heart Yang, and in this way counteracts the fundamental imbalance of Yang underlying heart block.

The red flags of heart failure and arrhythmias

Most patients with heart failure and arrhythmias will benefit from referral to a conventional doctor for assessment or treatment. Red flags are those symptoms and signs that indicate that referral should be considered. The red flags of heart failure and arrhythmias are described in Table 3.2f-I. A summary of the red flags in a format designed for quick reference in clinical practice can be found in Appendix III. This gives advice on the degree of urgency of referral for each of the red flag conditions listed.

Table 3.2f-I A14: Red flags of heart failure and arrhythmias

Red flag	Description	Reasoning
A14.1	Features of mild, chronic heart failure: slight swelling of the ankles, slight breathlessness on exertion and when lying flat, cough and with no palpitations or chest pain Dry cough may be the only symptom in sedentary elderly people	In chronic heart failure the pumping ability of the heart is reduced, and this results in accumulation of tissue fluid in the lungs (breathlessness) and ankles (edema). It may remain undiagnosed if mild, but it is associated with increased risk of worsening damage to the heart Current medical guidance is that all patients will benefit in terms of reduced symptoms and increased life expectancy from medical treatment of heart failure, and referral is recommended for assessment by electrocardiography (ECG) and echocardiography
A14.2	Features of severe chronic heart failure: marked swelling of the ankles and lower legs, disabling breathlessness and exhaustion	Severe chronic heart failure is a serious condition associated with a high mortality. It will benefit from prompt medical management, and this is associated with an improved life expectancy
A14.3	Features of acute heart failure: sudden onset of disabling breathlessness, and watery cough	Acute heart failure results from a sudden loss in the ability of the heart to pump effectively, and most commonly results from heart attack, arrhythmia or valve damage. The patient requires emergency treatment and needs to be kept calm and sitting upright until help arrives

A14.4	An irregularly irregular pulse (possible atrial fibrillation)	An irregularly irregular (totally unpredictable) pulse is a feature of atrial fibrillation (AF). This arrhythmia carries a risk of the production of tiny blood clots within the chaotically contracting atria of the heart. These clots may then be dispersed (as emboli) to lodge in the circulation of the brain, and so carry a risk of transient ischemic attack and stroke
		Refer in all cases for further assessment, and as a high priority if features of heart failure or angina are also present, or if there is a history of blackouts or neurological symptoms
A14.5	A very rapid pulse of 140–250 beats/minute (most likely to be supraventricular tachycardia or atrial fibrillation)	Episodes of tachycardia (very rapid pulse) can be exhausting for the patient, and may progress to a more serious arrhythmia or lead to the symptoms of acute heart failure. If the attack is not settling in 5 minutes, refer urgently for medical management. If the attack settles, refer as a high priority so that the cause can be investigated
A14.6	A very slow pulse of 40–50 beats/minute (complete heart block), either of recent onset or associated with features such as dizziness, light-headedness or fainting	Some healthy individuals have a naturally slow heart rate, particularly if they have trained as athletes. However, if the rate suddenly drops to 40–50 beats/minute, this is characteristic of an arrhythmia called complete heart block, in which the natural pacemaker of the heart becomes unable to transmit a more frequent impulse to the ventricles. In this case the patient will start to feel dizzy and breathless, and may pass out. Refer urgently if ongoing, and as a high priority if the attack has settled down. The patient will need assessment for the implant of a pacemaker system
A14.7	A pulse that is regular but skips beats at regular intervals (i.e. 1 out of every 3–5 beats is missing) (incomplete heart block)	The occasional missed beat (ventricular ectopic) is not a worrying finding. It is more likely to occur in elderly people. However, if the beat is missed at a regular and frequent rate (more often than 1 in every 5 beats), this suggests a conduction defect called incomplete heart block, which carries a risk of progression to a more serious arrhythmia, and merits referral for cardiological assessment
		If the patient is well and was unaware of the problem until you found it, refer non-urgently
A14.8	Unexplained falls or faints in an elderly person	These may be the result of an arrhythmia (cardiac syncope). A temporary cardiac arrhythmia may result in a dizzy spell or sudden loss of consciousness from which an elderly person may recover very quickly. These episodes may account for unexplained falls. Consider referral if a patient reports a fall but cannot remember how it happened
A14.9	Cardiac arrest: collapse with no palpable pulse	Cardiac arrest results from the arrhythmia known as ventricular fibrillation (VF). The most common cause is heart attack (myocardial infarction), but VF can also occur spontaneously as a result of degenerative damage to the conducting system of the heart. VF may also result from electric shock
		In contrast to AF, in which the heart continues to pump fairly efficiently, when the ventricles of the heart go into chaotic rhythm the pumping function of the heart is totally lost and there is immediate circulatory collapse. Once help has been called, the patient requires urgent cardiopulmonary resuscitation (CPR) from a qualified first-aider

3.2g Diseases of the heart muscle, pericardium and heart valves, and congenital heart disease

This final section on the cardiovascular system focuses on those conditions that affect the structural components of the heart: the heart muscle, the pericardium and the heart valves. The inborn structural problems of the heart, which include "hole in the heart" and "blue baby syndrome," are also described. These problems are collectively termed congenital heart disease. Prior to reading this it might be helpful to turn back to Section 3.2a for a simple reminder of the structure of the heart chambers and valves.

The conditions studied in this section are:

- Diseases of the heart muscle:
  - myocarditis
  - cardiomyopathy
- Diseases of the pericardium:
  - acute and chronic (constrictive) pericarditis
- Diseases of the heart valves:
  - incompetent (leaking) valves
  - stenosed (constricted) valves
  - endocarditis
- Congenital heart disease:
  - hole in the heart
  - narrowing of aorta or aortic valve
  - cyanotic heart disease.

Diseases of the heart muscle

Myocarditis

As might be understood from the name, myocarditis refers to inflammation of the heart muscle (myocardium). The most common causes of this inflammation are infections by viruses, bacteria and protozoa, and adverse reactions to drugs. The viruses that cause myocarditis may be the same as those that usually cause colds and flu in most people, suggesting that the patient with myocarditis has a pre-existing susceptibility. The inflammation may be due in part to direct toxicity of the causative agent or otherwise because the effect of the agent on the cardiac cells is to stimulate an autoimmune response against the myocardium.

The inflammation affects the pumping action of the heart, and so patients will have fever, a rapid pulse and, in severe cases, features of heart failure.

Because of the rapid onset, the inability of the inflamed heart to pump efficiently leads to breathlessness as a result of pulmonary edema (see Section 3.2f). The patient is treated with bed rest to rest the heart, and antimicrobial drugs if appropriate. The heart failure is controlled by means of diuretics, angiotensin-converting enzyme (ACE) inhibitors, beta blockers and/or digoxin until the inflammation settles down.

It is considered important for the patient to refrain from athletic activities for six months to allow full healing after an episode of myocarditis. Most patients who survive the acute inflammation get completely better, although some are left with a permanent impairment of the heart muscle known as cardiomyopathy.

Information box 3.2g-I

Myocarditis: comments from a Chinese medicine perspective

A rapid onset of fever and tachycardia could be diagnosed in Chinese medicine as an invasion of Wind Heat. This would be in keeping with a condition that results commonly from an external agent such as a virus. However, damage to the cardiac muscle cells and the resulting inflammation is suggestive of the more profound imbalance of Heart Yin Deficiency, and this is evidence that the Heat has penetrated to a deep level to cause this imbalance. It would make sense from a Chinese medicine perspective that a pre-existing imbalance of Heart Yin would predispose a person to be vulnerable to this condition. The development of pulmonary edema would be diagnosed as Deficiency of Heart and Kidney Yang, with Water Overflowing to the Heart and Lungs, and this would make sense in that a severe Depletion of Yin (substance) is usually accompanied by a Deficiency of Yang (function).

Cardiomyopathy

Cardiomyopathy is a general term used to describe any impairment in the ability of the heart muscle to perform its pumping action. As stated above, inflammation in myocarditis can leave the patient with a permanent cardiomyopathy. Other causes include long-term damage from drugs and alcohol, and also rare inherited conditions. Coronary heart disease (CHD) can lead to a form of cardiomyopathy that results from the long-standing state of impaired nourishment of the heart muscle.

The major issue in cardiomyopathy is that the heart cannot pump efficiently, and so the state of heart failure develops. In cardiomyopathy the onset is often gradual, in which case the heart failure is chronic in presentation.

The damage to the heart muscle may also affect the pacemaker system and so arrhythmias, which can sometimes be life-threatening, may also develop.

Cardiomyopathy is one possible cause of sudden death in apparently healthy young people. These deaths commonly occur when the person has been engaged in strenuous activity. It seems that in these tragic cases an undiagnosed cardiomyopathy has led to ventricular fibrillation (VF) and thus to cardiac arrest. Another cause of sudden cardiac death is undiagnosed CHD or congenital heart disease (see later).

Information box 3.2g-II

Cardiomyopathy: comments from a Chinese medicine perspective

The reduced ability of the heart to pump efficiently and the resulting edema might be diagnosed as Heart and Kidney Yang with Water Overflowing. However, the fundamental root of the problem is in the substance of the heart muscle, which is impaired due either to a genetic weakness or to damage by toxins or infectious agents. This would constitute Depletion of Heart Yin. Stiffened, dilated or scarred myocardium could be described in terms of Blood Stasis or Phlegm (resulting from Depletion of Yin and Yang). Sudden unexpected death from VF suggests Invasion of Wind and Yang Collapse. In contrast to acute myocarditis, in which Deficient Yin and Heat are the prominent imbalances, in cardiomyopathy it is Deficient Yang that predominates.

By replacing a failing, distorted heart muscle with a healthy functional one, heart transplantation literally replenishes Yin and Yang, but comes at a cost. The foreign antigens (which can possibly be likened to Pathogenic Factors) induce autoimmune damage that has to be kept in check by immunosuppressant medication. Degenerative change suggestive of Blood Stasis and Phlegm (atheroma and hyperlipidemia) is an unfortunate consequence of a partly suppressed immune response to a foreign heart.

In cardiomyopathy, the damage to the heart muscle has been done, and treatment is therefore aimed at reducing heart failure and the risk of arrhythmias by means of the approaches discussed in Section 3.2f. Alcohol is not advised in cases of cardiomyopathy as it has a very deleterious effect on the function of failing heart muscle. In some cases the deterioration in the function of the heart is so severe that life expectancy is assessed to be less than six months. In these cases cardiac transplantation is the only available option.

Heart transplant certainly improves life expectancy in many people; 75 percent of patients who have received a new heart will be alive five years after the operation. However, the risks and complications of this operation, and the lifelong immunosuppressive treatment (see Section 2.2c) that has to follow it, are significant. Atherosclerosis of the coronary arteries in the transplanted heart is a particular problem, which seems to be in part a response of immune rejection of the foreign vascular tissue, and in part a result of the hypertension and hyperlipidemia that can also be a response to transplantation. Nevertheless, the immediate result of a successful cardiac transplantation is a huge improvement in quality of life.

Diseases of the pericardium

Pericarditis

Pericarditis refers to inflammation of the pericardium, the fibrous protective lining of the heart muscle. The condition can be acute or chronic in its development.

Acute pericarditis is usually due to infection or to the inflammation that follows the damage caused by a heart attack. As in myocarditis, the most usual infectious agents are the viruses that cause colds and flu. In the few days after heart attack it is probably inflammatory agents released from infarcted myocardial cells that trigger inflammation. If the pericarditis develops over a week after the heart attack it may be the result of an abnormal immune reaction to the damaged heart muscle lining (Dressler's syndrome).

Acute viral pericarditis commonly affects young adults. It is usually a less severe condition than myocarditis, although it can have severe complications. Nevertheless, from a holistic perspective, the development of pericarditis also suggests that the patient has a pre-existing susceptibility in terms of depletion of heart energy. Pericarditis is increasingly diagnosed in people who have human immunodeficiency virus (HIV) infection.

The symptoms of acute pericarditis include a sharp pain in the center of the chest, which can be felt in the region of acupoint REN-17 (Shan Zhong). The pain can go up to the neck and is worse on movement, lying down and breathing in. Fever and a rapid heart rate are usually present.

The medical treatment is rest in bed and non-steroidal anti-inflammatory drugs (NSAIDs) such as ibuprofen (except in the case of heart attack, when these drugs should be avoided). Most people will fully recover from an episode of pericarditis, although a small proportion may suffer from recurrent episodes.

In more severe cases, the inflammation affects the function of the heart, and arrhythmias or heart failure can develop. In some cases, excess fluid builds up between the two lining layers of the pericardium, forming a pericardial effusion (see Figure 3.2g-I). This can be so extensive as to constrict the heart function and thus lead to heart failure. In these cases, the patient requires more intensive medical observation, as the condition may worsen or life-threatening arrhythmias may occur.

Figure 3.2g-I Chest X-ray image showing the appearance of a large pericardial effusion
The heart appears globular, and the cardiac shadow is almost double the width of that seen in a normal chest X-ray image.

In a minority of cases the inflammation does not settle and a long-standing condition called chronic pericarditis develops. One of the consequences of long-standing inflammation is scarring or fibrosis (see Section 2.2b). The scarred pericardium becomes thickened, irregular and tight, and can physically restrict the pumping of the heart, when it is known as constrictive pericarditis, which can lead to severe chronic heart failure.

Recurrent attacks of pericarditis may be kept at bay by means of immunosuppressant medication (e.g. colchicine and azathioprine).

The main treatment for constrictive pericarditis is surgical removal of a section of the damaged pericardium. This permits the heart to pump more freely. Many patients continue to suffer from impairment of heart function after this operation.

Diseases of the heart valves

The diseases of the heart valves have some features in common – they all tend to lead to a degree of heart failure and also may lead to arrhythmias (see Section 3.2f).

The symptoms can initially be treated with drugs but, if severe, surgical treatment of the damaged valve may be necessary. Patients with valvular disease are susceptible to a very severe infectious condition of the valves called endocarditis (discussed later).

For simplicity, the diverse problems are listed below in two categories: incompetent valves and stenosed valves.

Information box 3.2g-III

Acute pericarditis: comments from a Chinese medicine perspective

The stabbing pain of acute pericarditis might be interpreted as Heart Blood Stagnation. The fever and rapid pulse rate suggest Full or Empty Heat. As is the case with myocarditis, viral infection may have led to an invasion of External Wind Heat, which has penetrated to the interior to damage Heart Yin and thus led to the Blood Stagnation. In other cases (e.g. following a heart attack) the Depleted Heart Yang may have contributed to the development of Blood Stagnation.

The impaired action of the heart in constrictive pericarditis and pericardial effusion suggests that the initial acute condition has led to marked Depletion of the Heart function, in particular, of Heart Yang. The thickened stiff pericardium or fluid-based effusion both suggest that Phlegm or Damp, in addition to Blood Stagnation and Yang Deficiency, are contributing to the symptoms. The patient will develop the features of Heart and Kidney Yang Deficiency with Water Overflowing as heart failure ensues.

Incompetent (leaking) valves

As explained in Section 3.2a, heart valves ensure a one-way flow of blood through the two sides of the heart. Some conditions of the heart valves cause them to become leaky or incompetent. The other term used to describe this phenomenon of leaky valves is regurgitation.

The name given to a particular valve condition relates to the exact site of the leak. For example, mitral incompetence (or regurgitation) refers to a leaky mitral (left atrioventricular) valve.

The main consequence of a leaky valve is that, during contraction of the heart, blood is forced the wrong way, with the result that blood dams up at the venous side of the heart.

Heart failure is an important consequence of valve incompetence. The symptoms of heart failure depend on the side of the heart affected. In mitral incompetence, it is the left side, and so blood dams up in the pulmonary veins of the lung and causes pulmonary edema. This is left-sided heart failure. In tricuspid incompetence it is the right side that is affected, and the symptoms that result from bodily edema and liver and spleen congestion are most prominent. This is right-sided heart failure.

Other symptoms of valve incompetence include arrhythmias and exhaustion.

Incompetent valves in elderly people are commonly the consequence of what used to be a common and severe childhood illness, rheumatic fever. This is a bacterial infection that primarily causes an inflammation of the joints, but can progress to lead to an antibody-mediated inflammation of the heart and valves. The way in which rheumatic fever affects the joints is described in Section 4.2f. People who recover from rheumatic fever are commonly left with scarring or weakening of the heart valves. Sometimes the damage to the valves only becomes apparent in later life. This cause of valve incompetence is much less common in younger people because over the past few decades rheumatic fever has become a very rare disease in developed countries. It is still, however, a significant cause of ill health in the developing world.

Other causes of valve incompetence include damage to the structure of the heart from CHD and myocarditis. It can also be an inherited condition.

Valve incompetence may be diagnosed initially by the detection of a murmur through a stethoscope. The structure of the damaged valve can then be assessed by means of echocardiography (cardiac ultrasound scan). A patient with severe valvular disease may also require cardiac catheterization in order to assess accurately the degree of heart failure.

The initial treatment of valve incompetence depends on the severity of the symptoms. If progressive heart failure is developing and is not responding to drugs, surgical replacement of the heart valve is the best treatment (see below).

Stenosed (constricted) valves

One other major problem that can occur with the heart valves is that they can become scarred and tightened. This is called valve stenosis. A tightened (stenotic) valve will restrict the passage of blood through the heart. This puts the heart muscle under strain, and reduces the amount of blood that can exit the heart to go to the rest of the body. Stenosis will also cause blood to dam up on the venous side of the heart and is thus also a cause of right or left heart failure.

The condition is named after the affected valve. The two most common forms of stenotic valvular disease are mitral stenosis and aortic stenosis.

The symptoms include those of left- or right-sided heart failure. Because of the severely reduced amount of blood leaving the heart, blackouts can occur. The strain on the heart muscle can lead to palpitations due to arrhythmias. Mitral stenosis is particularly associated with atrial fibrillation (AF), and in severe cases there is a risk of sudden death.

The most common cause of valve stenosis in elderly people is childhood rheumatic fever. The tightening can get progressively worse over a period of years. Stenosis can also be due to a congenital defect. In elderly people it can be a degenerative condition, resulting from the gradual deposition of calcium in the valves that causes them to harden and narrow.

The investigations of valve stenosis are the same as those for valve incompetence.

Valve stenosis may be improved by a simple operation (which may be performed as an extension of a cardiac catheterization) to stretch or cut the tightened valve. Otherwise, a valve replacement is necessary.

VALVE REPLACEMENT

This surgical procedure can transform the lives of people who would otherwise be severely disabled by valvular disease. The replaced valve is either a mechanical structure, or is fashioned from a pig valve, or a human valve taken from the body of someone who had chosen to donate organs after death.

Foreign heart valves do not seem to stimulate an immune response and so, unlike the cardiac transplant, the patient does not need to take immunosuppressive medication because there is no risk of rejection of the valve.

The problem with mechanical valves is that their clumsy structure can stimulate clotting and the formation of emboli within the heart. For this reason, the patient with a mechanical valve will have to take a high dose of warfarin continually for the rest of their life.

Both types of valve may wear out and require replacement within about ten years, although a mechanical valve generally has a longer life than a tissue valve.

Implanted valves are at risk of becoming infected, and this leads to the very serious condition of endocarditis (discussed below).

***

Information box 3.2g-IV

Valvular disease: comments from a Chinese medicine perspective

In Chinese medicine, the symptoms of valvular disease suggest a deficiency of Heart Yin. Interestingly, one of the conventionally recognized features of mitral stenosis is a malar flush (reddening of the upper aspect of the cheeks), which in Chinese medicine is a marker for Yin Deficiency. The symptom of palpitations, common in valvular heart disease, is consistent with this interpretation.

The development of heart failure would suggest additional Depletion of Yang, with Water Overflowing to the Heart and the Lungs.

The thickened tightened valves in stenosis and the risk of embolism suggest that Phlegm and Blood Stagnation are also a contributory factor.

***

Endocarditis

Endocarditis is inflammation of the endocardium, the lining epithelium of the heart, and is usually the result of a bacterial infection. Often the infectious agent is found to be one of the healthy types of bacteria that normally reside in the patient's mouth, throat or bowel.

People who have damaged heart valves or a heart valve replacement are more at risk of endocarditis. Any procedure that increases the risk of surface bacteria entering the bloodstream (including dental and surgical operations) may cause endocarditis in at-risk groups. Intravenous drug users are also at high risk from the injection of contaminated material into the bloodstream.

This infection is very relevant to the practice of acupuncture, as endocarditis is one of the serious recognized complications of acupuncture treatment worldwide. However, this complication of acupuncture is very rare in the UK, as a result of good attention to sterile needling procedures.

In endocarditis the infectious agent travels to the heart via the bloodstream, and causes damage after settling on the lining of the heart muscle and valves. The bacteria colonize at the edge of valves and can lead to progressive damage to their structure. The inflammation leads to the formation of clumps of platelets and other debris, which can break off from the valves to form emboli, and thus carries the risk of distant tissue damage and stroke.

A patient with endocarditis will initially suffer from a prolonged state of malaise, with intermittent fever, flitting joint pains, night sweats and tiredness. At this stage it may be difficult to diagnose the cause of the illness. After some weeks the progressive valve damage gives rise to features of heart failure or emboli in the circulation. The patient may develop syndromes of thrombosis and infarction in the diverse tissues of the body, including the kidneys and brain.

 Information box 3.2g-V

Endocarditis: comments from a Chinese medicine perspective

In Chinese medicine, the features of intermittent fever and solid clumps of infection on the heart valves can be interpreted as Wind Damp Heat Invasion. Flitting joint aches and joint swelling reflect Bi Syndrome due to Wind Damp Heat.

The Toxic Heat damages the Yin of the Heart, leading to the night sweats and damaged structure of the valves. Eventually, the Heart and Kidney Yang are also damaged, leading to Water Overflowing to the Heart and Lungs. Thrombosis and embolism would be diagnosed in terms of Blood Stagnation.

The condition is diagnosed by means of echocardiography, and samples of blood are taken to culture the infectious organism. Because diagnosis is often delayed, the patient can become very unwell. Significant damage to the heart may also have occurred before appropriate antimicrobial treatment can be given.

Powerful antibiotics in combination are given intravenously for two weeks. Antibiotics in tablet form are then continued for a few more weeks.

Severe valvular damage requires emergency valve replacement. This operation carries great risks because the patient is already in such an unstable state. Overall, 30 percent of patients who have endocarditis will either die or suffer long-term disability as a result of the condition.

PROPHYLAXIS OF ENDOCARDITIS
Because endocarditis is a particular risk for people with damaged or replaced heart valves, until recently people with those conditions were advised to take precautionary measures whenever there was a high probability of bacterial infection entering the bloodstream. The medical term for precautionary measures is prophylaxis.

In particular, patients with valvular problems and who had to undergo significant dental treatment or invasive medical investigations such as endoscopy were advised to take antibiotics during the course of the procedure. However, in 2008 the National Institute for Health and Care Excellence (NICE) published a guideline and review of evidence for prophylaxis against endocarditis. The conclusion of this guideline is that antibiotic prophylaxis may in fact carry more risks than benefits, and so should no longer be offered to patients. This is, as the guideline states, "a paradigm shift," and as such it may take many years for the advice to filter down to current medical practice.[49]

However, prophylaxis has never been considered necessary for minor procedures such as taking blood, because the risk of infection by the insertion of a sterile needle is considered to be low. Although recent critics of acupuncture have suggested that antibiotic prophylaxis should be given to acupuncture patients with heart valve problems, this is inconsistent with current medical thinking about the risks of introducing infection by means of a needle. Moreover, taking into account the current NICE guidance, it need not be a concern at all, as long as single-use, non-indwelling needles are used.

Having said this, it is the responsibility of acupuncturists to be very familiar with the features of endocarditis, so that if a patient develops early symptoms they can be referred for early treatment. The main red flag of endocarditis is intermittent unexplained fever for more than two weeks.

Congenital heart disease

Congenital heart disease is the term used to describe a range of defects of the heart and valves that may develop in the growing fetus. Some of these defects are minor, but some can be very severe, leading to cyanosis (blue baby syndrome) and heart failure in the first few weeks of life. Others do not seem to produce significant problems in early life (like some of the valvular diseases) but can progress as the child gets older. If undetected, these defects can lead to severe and sometimes fatal heart disease.

The cause of most cases of congenital heart disease is unknown. However, factors that are known to increase the chances of a congenital defect include maternal rubella (German measles) infection, high maternal alcohol intake, and maternal exposure to certain drugs and radiation in pregnancy. There is a slightly increased risk of congenital heart disease in children born to parents who have a heart defect.

Defects of the chromosomes that cause conditions such as Down syndrome also commonly give rise to heart defects in affected babies.

In most cases, the defect only causes a problem after birth; prior to this the oxygenation of the blood takes place via the placenta. However, with the increasing use of ultrasound scanning in mid-pregnancy, the defects are most often detected before birth. This helps prevent the situation of defects only becoming apparent in later life once irreparable damage has been done to the circulatory system.

Congenital heart disease is common, affecting approximately one in 100 babies. In many of these cases, the defect is a minor one, and may be detected at an early health check by means of the characteristic murmur heard via the stethoscope. In such cases, after investigation by echocardiography, parents can be reassured that the defect will resolve itself as the child's heart grows.

Hole in the heart

The most common severe defects involve a gap in the muscle wall that separates the two sides of the heart, which is commonly described as a "hole in the heart." In conventional medicine this problem is termed a septal defect. If a large septal defect is detected early, the gap in the muscle is repaired surgically. The operation is often straightforward and can have very good results.

However, a septal defect is one of the conditions that can go undetected in early childhood, and over the ensuing years can lead to progressive strain on the heart and the circulatory system. Affected adults may develop recurrent chest infections and breathlessness on exertion as first symptoms. If not diagnosed early and surgically repaired, it may not be possible to reverse the damage done to the circulatory system, and so may result in death in early adulthood from heart failure.

Narrowing of the aorta or aortic valve

These defects, also known as aortic coarctation (narrowing of the vessel) or aortic stenosis (narrowing of the valve), severely impair the ability of the heart to pump blood into the bodily circulation. They can lead to heart failure very shortly after birth. The affected baby is breathless and unable to feed. If less severe, the defect may appear only later in childhood, with dizziness, fainting and chest pains.

The treatment is surgical correction of the narrowed valve or aorta.

Cyanotic heart disease

In cyanotic heart disease, a complex defect is present that causes some of the deoxygenated blood arriving at the heart to be redirected straight back into the bodily circulation, without first being oxygenated by the lungs. This means that the body does not receive the full amount of oxygen it requires.

As deoxygenated blood is blue in color, the child will have a bluish tinge to the lips and tongue (cyanosis), particularly after exercise. A characteristic sign is that the child is breathless and may need to squat to rest after exercise. This is another condition that may get diagnosed only later in childhood. The treatment is by means of a complex operation, which should be performed as early as possible.

LONG-TERM CONSEQUENCES OF CORRECTED
CONGENITAL HEART DISEASE[50]

This is still an area in which there is incomplete knowledge, as it is only over the past 40–50 years or so that some of the most complex of the life-preserving surgical techniques have been developed. It is not yet fully known how the history of congenital heart disease and its surgical correction will affect the lives of affected individuals in the future.

The structure of the heart will never be perfect after surgical correction. It is now becoming apparent that some of the young adults who have undergone the more major forms of surgery may suffer from arrhythmias due to impairments in the structure of the heart muscle. They are also at an increased risk of cardiomyopathy and sudden cardiac death.

 Information box 3.2g-VI

Congenital heart disease: comments from a Chinese medicine perspective

According to Chinese medicine, congenital defects are often rooted in a Deficiency of Essence (Jing). The defective heart structure and resulting weakened function correspond to Deficient Heart Yin and Yang. Heart failure corresponds to Water Overflowing to Heart and Lungs secondary to Heart Yang Deficiency. The bluish color seen in children in cyanotic heart disease suggests that Qi or Blood Stagnation has developed as a consequence of severe Heart Deficiency.

The red flags of diseases of the heart muscle, pericardium and heart valves

Red flags are those symptoms and signs that indicate that referral should be considered. The red flags of most of the conditions discussed in this section have already been described, because severe myocarditis, cardiomyopathy and congenital heart disease in adults all present first with symptoms either of arrhythmias or of heart failure (see Table 3.2f-I).

The red flag of endocarditis is intermittent unexplained fever lasting for more than two weeks, which is one of the red flags for infectious diseases in general. The red flags for congenital heart disease in young children have a lot of similarities to those that apply to many childhood chronic illnesses (see Chapter 5.4).

Thus the only additional red flags listed here are those for pericarditis, and these are described in Table 3.2g-I. A summary of the red flags in a format designed for quick reference in clinical practice can be found in Appendix III. This gives advice on the degree of urgency of referral for each of the red flag conditions listed.

Table 3.2g-I A15: Red flags of pericarditis

Red flag	Description	Reasoning
A15.1	Features of uncomplicated pericarditis: sharp central chest pain that is worse on leaning forward and lying down. Fever should be slight and the pulse rate ≤100 beats/minute. Complications include: • features of heart failure (breathlessness and edema) • features of arrhythmia (tachycardia) • symptoms of heart attack/unstable angina	Pericarditis can result from a viral infection or as part of a complex metabolic illness such as renal failure. It can also complicate recovery from a heart attack In its uncomplicated form the patient will have central chest pain that is affected by posture and other chest movements. If pericarditis is suspected, it is advisable to refer for further cardiac investigations in hospital, as the condition can deteriorate and affect the rhythm or pumping capacity of the heart Refer urgently if complications are apparent

3.3

The Respiratory System

3.3a The physiology of the respiratory system

This section concentrates on the physiology and pathology of the respiratory system, looking at the structure and function of the respiratory system in health.

The role of the respiratory system[51]

As described earlier in Section 1.1b, oxygen is one of the essential ingredients for the process of cellular respiration. The respiratory system is specialized to enable an adequate supply of oxygen to the tissues. It is also the role of the respiratory system to allow carbon dioxide, a waste product of respiration, to be removed from the body.

In common usage, the term respiration refers simply to the act of breathing. However, in physiology there are three aspects to respiration that can be clearly defined. These are external, internal and cellular respiration.

The respiratory system is primarily concerned with external respiration, which is indeed the process of breathing. This leads to the exchange of gases between the blood and the lungs.

Internal respiration is the exchange of gases between the blood and the cells of all the body tissues, and is one of the functions performed by the circulatory system.

Cellular respiration is the process (described in Section 1.1b) by which oxygen and nutrients are converted to cellular energy (adenosine triphosphate (ATP)) and carbon dioxide within the cell itself. It is important to be clear about the distinction between these three processes, as these terms help define the precise roles of the respiratory system.

The respiratory system is conventionally divided into two sections, the upper and lower respiratory tract. A simple representation of the organs of the respiratory tract is given in Figure 3.3a-I. The division between the upper and lower parts occurs at the point at which the trachea splits into the two tubes called bronchi.

The diagram illustrates that this division occurs at a deep level in the chest, just above the position of the heart. It also illustrates the close physical relationship between the heart and the lungs. In fact, if the heart is removed through dissection, an imprint of its shape is seen in the tissue of the lungs.

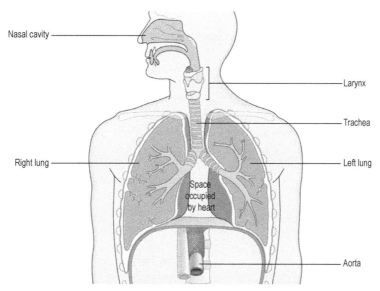

Figure 3.3a-I The organs of respiration

The upper respiratory tract

The upper respiratory tract leads from the entrance of the respiratory system at the nose to the end of the trachea, the tube that directs the inhaled air into the chest cavity (thorax) towards the lungs.

The function of the upper respiratory tract is to provide a plentiful supply of warm, clean and moist air to the lungs. To help it perform this function it consists of wide air spaces and is lined by a specialized form of epithelium. The respiratory epithelium consists largely of ciliated columnar cells, but it also has many mucus-secreting (goblet) cells.

The water-containing mucus moistens the air that rushes through the respiratory tract, and picks up dirt particles and other foreign bodies present in the air. Cilia are structures akin to microscopic hairs on the surface of cells. They are powered by the energetically charged molecule ATP to move in coordinated waves. In the respiratory tract the cilia beat in an upward direction. Their function is to cause an upward movement of the mucus, allowing the foreign material to be moved away from the delicate lung tissue and up to the back of the throat, from where it can be swallowed or expectorated.

The connective tissue layer below the respiratory epithelium has a number of lymphocytes scattered throughout its length. These respond to foreign antigens by producing antibodies and attracting other immune cells. This is an important aspect of the protection of the respiratory tract from infection.

The important parts of the upper respiratory tract are the nose, pharynx, larynx and trachea.

The nose

In the breathing of a healthy person at rest, all air is drawn in through the nostrils into the nasal cavity. This space has a deeply ridged surface that has a rich blood supply. This means that the current of air comes into contact with a large area of warm epithelium before its descent towards the lungs. In addition to the cilia on the epithelial cells, body hairs are present in the opening of the nose to filter out any large foreign particles.

Opening out into the nasal cavity are the sinuses. These are cavities deep within the facial bones that have narrow passageways leading into the nasal cavity. Their function is to give the voice a resonant quality, the loss of which is apparent in anyone who has suffered from a head cold, when the sinuses become filled with thick secretions. A tiny duct leading from each eye also opens into this space. This continually drains away tears from the eyes. The runny nose that accompanies a bout of crying is a result of the excess tears flooding into the nose through this duct.

The nose is the specialized sense organ for smell. To perform this function, delicate nerves originating from the base of the brain penetrate the bone above the nasal cavity to supply the nasal lining. These are sensitive to the chemicals in the incoming air, which become dissolved in the mucus. The sense of smell is also important to enrich the experience of taste. Occasionally, in a head injury, these nerves become permanently severed, even though there may be no other major brain damage. The person may recover fully but be left without a sense of smell and with a highly impaired sense of taste.

Other nerves in the nose are very sensitive to the irritation that can result from foreign particles and from inflammation of the lining of the nose. These nerves can trigger the protective reflex of the sneeze, which is a very effective mechanism for expelling unwanted material from the nasal cavity.

The pharynx

The pharynx is the space at the back of the nose that connects with the throat. The adenoids (nasal tonsils) are two collections of lymph node tissue situated at the back of this space. The tonsils (palatine tonsils), which are similar collections of lymphoid tissue, are situated a little lower down. The palatine tonsils can be seen in most people on either side of the space behind the arch of the palate, as illustrated in Figure 3.3a-II, whereas the adenoids are hidden up behind the palatoglossal arch.

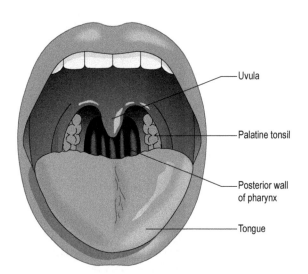

Figure 3.3a-II The location of the palatine tonsils

The function of the tonsils is to complement the protective function of the lymphocytes in the respiratory epithelium. Their presence is an indication of the need for the lungs to be protected from foreign material. The adenoids are most active in early childhood, because this is the time when immunity to a wide range of infections has to be rapidly developed. After reaching five years of age, the adenoids usually shrink to a negligible size, although the palatine tonsils persist into adulthood.

The Eustachian tube opens from the middle ear into the pharynx close to the location of the adenoids. The middle ear is also lined with respiratory epithelium, and the Eustachian tube allows the drainage of mucus from this enclosed space.

The larynx

The larynx, popularly known as the voice box, is the structure that separates the pharynx from the trachea. Although it is primarily associated with voice production, it also plays a very important protective role. Figure 3.3a-III is a diagrammatic representation of the nasal cavity, pharynx and larynx, which illustrates how these structures relate to each other.

Figure 3.3a-III The pathway of the air from the nose to the larynx

The tube-like larynx has stiff cartilage in its walls that enables it to maintain its shape. The cartilage at the front of the larynx is what can be seen and felt as the "Adam's apple." Because the thyroid gland sits close to this structure, the medical term for this is the thyroid cartilage.

The vocal cords are two fine flaps of tissue that are suspended from the surrounding cartilage tube. Figure 3.3a-IV shows a view of the aperture of the larynx. The vocal cords are depicted on either side of the aperture, leaving a triangular space through which the air can pass. Tiny muscles in the larynx contract to change the shape of this triangle between the vocal cords so that the space can vary from being a wide gap to a tiny chink. The tone of the muscles also affects the tightness of the vocal cords. During quiet breathing the gap is wide to allow a free passage of air in and out of the lungs. During speech, the gap narrows and the cords tighten. The expired air causes vibration of the tightened cords, which produces the sound of the voice. The tighter the cords are the higher the pitch of the voice.

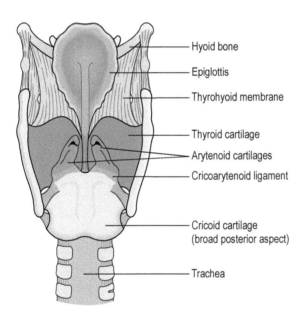

- Hyoid bone
- Epiglottis
- Thyrohyoid membrane
- Thyroid cartilage
- Arytenoid cartilages
- Cricoarytenoid ligament
- Cricoid cartilage (broad posterior aspect)
- Trachea

Figure 3.3a-IV The interior of the larynx, viewed from above

The protective reflex of the cough involves a temporary tightening of the vocal cords so that the gap closes altogether. This occurs during a forced expiration of air. The closed gap means that the pressure of air below the vocal cords is suddenly increased. At this point the muscles relax and the gap widens. This results in a sudden forceful rush of air accompanied by the familiar sound of the cough. Like the sneeze, the cough is stimulated by the irritation of nerves in the larynx and the tubes that branch from the trachea into the lungs. The cough also has the effect of expelling unwanted material from the trachea, larynx and pharynx out through the open mouth.

The other important protective structure in the larynx is a stiff flap of cartilage-containing tissue called the epiglottis, which sits above the larynx. During swallowing this flap descends to completely cover the gap between the vocal cords. This protects against the inhalation of food during swallowing.

The trachea

The trachea is the wide tube that descends from the larynx to the division of the bronchi deep within the thorax. It is held open by rings of cartilage within its walls and is also lined by respiratory epithelium.

The lower respiratory tract

The lower respiratory tract begins where the trachea divides into the two narrower tubes called the bronchi. The bronchi further subdivide, like the branches of a tree, to penetrate the tissue of the two lungs.

The bronchi and bronchioles

The bronchi and the smaller tubes into which they divide (the bronchioles) are structurally similar to the trachea, and are also lined with respiratory epithelium. Therefore, they, too, are concerned with ensuring the air that reaches the depths of the lungs is as warm, moist and as clean as possible.

The width of these air passages varies according to need. During exercise the bronchi and bronchioles widen, so that a large amount of air can enter the lungs in each breath. At rest, they narrow again because the need for a large volume of air is not so necessary, and because the protective mechanism of these tubes is more efficient when they are narrower.

The alveoli

At the end of each of the tiniest branches of the tree-like air passages that penetrate the lung are masses of tiny air sacs only a few cells in diameter. These are known as alveoli (singular alveolus). The lungs are composed of millions of these tiny air spaces packed together, and all connecting with the outside world through the bronchioles and bronchi. The alveoli are lined with only a single layer of flat squamous epithelium, and are supplied by a dense network of fine blood capillaries.

Figure 3.3a-V illustrates how the alveoli branch from the bronchioles, and how a network of capillaries supplies each one.

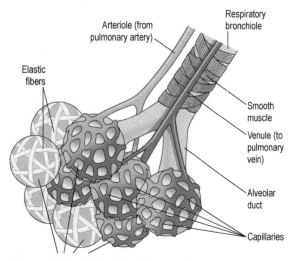

Figure 3.3a-V An alveolus and its capillary network

EXCHANGE OF GASES IN THE ALVEOLI

The blood that enters the capillaries surrounding the alveoli has originated from the pulmonary arteries. These large vessels originate from the right ventricle of the heart and carry deoxygenated blood pumped by the right side of the heart. The blood is deoxygenated because the cells of the body tissues have used up all the oxygen in the process of cellular respiration. As well as being deoxygenated, this blood is also carrying a high concentration of carbon dioxide, the by-product of cellular respiration. In contrast, the air inspired into the alveoli is rich in oxygen from the outside air, and carries very little carbon dioxide. Therefore, there is a tendency for the oxygen in the alveoli to move into the deoxygenated blood in the capillaries. This movement occurs readily, as oxygen can diffuse with no restriction through the cell membranes of the alveolar and capillary walls. At the same time, there is a movement of carbon dioxide out of the capillary blood and into the alveolar air. This exchange of the two gases of respiration occurs very rapidly.

The capillaries that leave the alveoli converge to form the pulmonary veins, which return all this blood to the left side of the heart. This blood is now rich in oxygen, and has been cleared of carbon dioxide. The pulmonary veins are the only veins in the body that carry oxygenated blood. All the other veins carry blood away from the body tissues, and this blood is, of course, deoxygenated.

The air left in the alveolus now contains more carbon dioxide than oxygen, and is expelled to the outside world by the process of expiration, so that the whole process can begin afresh with the next in-breath.

This process of exchange of gases is assisted by the fact that there are millions of alveoli, each with its own rich blood supply. In some conditions, such as emphysema, the delicate structure of the alveoli is damaged and their number is reduced (see Section 3.3e). This severely impairs the process of exchange of gases, so that the blood does not get replenished with an adequate amount of oxygen, and carbon dioxide fails to be fully cleared.

The lungs

The lungs consist of the branching air passages of the bronchi and bronchioles, and the thousands of alveoli clustered around the ends of the bronchioles. The lungs are surrounded and supported by elastic connective tissue, which has the tendency to cause the fully expanded lung to contract. The lungs sit within the thorax, which is protected by the rib cage and its supportive muscles, and they rest on the sheet of muscle below known as the diaphragm.

The lungs are surrounded by a double layer of protective fluid-secreting serous membrane called the pleura. In the pleura the secreted fluid forms a thin lubricating layer between the two pleural membranes akin to the fluid that separates the pericardium from the heart. The outer pleural membrane is attached to the inner surface of the rib cage from above and at the sides, and to the diaphragm below. It is this attachment that prevents the elastic lungs from collapsing. Figure 3.3a-VI illustrates the relationship between the pleura and the lungs.

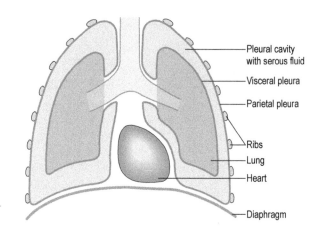

Figure 3.3a-VI The relationship of the pleura with the lungs

External respiration

External respiration is the process whereby air is drawn into the lung tissue through inspiration and is then expelled through expiration. This process permits the exchange of gases to occur.

Inspiration involves the inflation of the lungs. Like an expanded bellows, the inflated lung naturally draws air into itself. The lungs are inflated by a lifting and expansion of the rib cage walls and a descent of the diaphragm. This action occurs as a result of contraction of the diaphragm and of the muscles that link the ribs together.

Expiration involves the deflation of the lungs. This naturally forces air back out of the lungs. In relaxed breathing, expiration requires no muscular effort. A simple relaxation of the rib cage and diaphragm has the effect of reducing the volume of the thorax and thus deflating the lungs.

In normal, quiet breathing the cycle of inspiration and expiration occurs at about 15 times per minute (4 seconds/cycle). There is an automatic reflex that originates from a control center in the base of the brain that sets this regular rhythm. Nerves travel down from this control center to stimulate the synchronized and rhythmic muscular contraction of the rib cage and diaphragm.

All variations in the resting respiratory rate are brought about by changes that take place in the breathing control center in the brain. The breathing control center is essential for maintaining homeostasis of the levels of oxygen and carbon dioxide in the arterial blood. The oxygen level must, of course, be maintained at a high concentration, whereas the level of carbon dioxide must not be allowed to rise too high. To perform this role, the breathing control center contains cells that are very sensitive to the level of carbon dioxide in the blood. A miniscule rise in the level

of carbon dioxide leads to an increase in the breathing rate so that excess carbon dioxide can be breathed out of the body. If the level of carbon dioxide drops, so does the rate of breathing. The levels of carbon dioxide in the blood can then build up again.

The control center in the brain is also sensitive to drops in the concentration of oxygen in the blood. However, the responsiveness of the control center to carbon dioxide also indirectly controls the homeostasis of oxygen in the blood, as increased external respiration will increase oxygen levels, and reduced external respiration will reduce oxygen levels.

Any voluntary wish to modulate the breathing, such as for speech, singing or laughing, generates nerve impulses from other parts of the brain (the cerebral hemispheres) to the control center of breathing, which then alters the breathing rate accordingly. The sneeze and cough reflexes involve a direct link between the irritated nerve endings and the control center.

The way in which the brain is responsible for the voluntary and involuntary control of body functions is described in more detail in Chapter 4.1 on the nervous system.

 Information box 3.3a-I

The lungs: comments from a Chinese medicine perspective

According to the *Simple Questions (Suwen)*,[52] the Lungs are "like a minister from whom policies are issued." The functions of this Organ are to:

- govern Qi and respiration
- control channels and blood vessels
- control dispersing and descending
- regulate the Water passages
- control skin and body hair
- open into the nose
- house the Corporeal Soul (Po).

Government of Qi and respiration refers to two aspects, as described below.

Government of Qi

The Government of Qi refers to the conversion of Gu (food) Qi and Heavenly (Clear) Qi in the Lungs to produce Zong (Gathering) Qi. Zong Qi is important for supporting the Lungs, the Heart and the circulation. It also gives strength to the voice. The Lungs are therefore seen as the site of the combination of Gu Qi and Heavenly Qi into a readily available source of energy (Zong Qi) for the organs of the Upper Jiao, as well as for the circulation and the voice.

In conventional medicine no distinction is made between different sorts of energy as there is in Chinese medicine with the various types of Qi. There is also no idea that the Lungs play any role in the production of energy over and above their function in external respiration, which is to draw oxygen into the body.

However, conventional medicine recognizes that the lungs spring from the voice box region in embryology. A weak or hoarse voice can simply be a product of weak inspiration and expiration, as it is the force of the out-breath that controls the strength of the voice. The recurrent laryngeal nerve that controls the production of speech also runs deep into the thorax. The hoarseness that can characterize a case of lung cancer is a result of damage of this nerve by encroaching cancer.

Government of respiration

Government of respiration refers here to external respiration. This is a direct parallel with the understanding of conventional medicine. Strictly speaking, the role of the breathing control center in the brain would also be seen in Chinese medicine as part of the Lung functions, as it plays an important part of the control of external respiration.

Control of channels and blood vessels

There is no direct correspondence here with conventional medicine, as the channels are not conventional concepts, and the blood vessels are seen as part of the circulatory system. But actually, as Keown (2014)[53] points out, the lungs are actually "more (blood vessel and) blood than lung" in that each tiny alveolus is cradled with a mesh of blood containing capillaries. In fact, the blood in our circulation is within the blood vessels of the lungs for exactly half of the time, and in this time is charged by life-giving oxygen and cleansed of acidic carbon dioxide.

Control of dispersing and descending

The dispersing function refers to the ability of the Lungs to spread Wei Qi and body fluids to all body parts. This protects the body from external pathogens and keeps the skin and muscles moist and warm. It is also important for the control of sweating. The lungs are not seen to have this sort of function in conventional medicine. Instead, the defensive and warming roles would be attributed to the immune system and circulatory system, respectively. Conventionally, the skin is seen as the organ that deals with sweating.

The descending function refers to the Descent of Qi, which is important to enable clearance of fluids via the Kidneys and Bladder, and also for defecation. If impaired, the loss of this function may give rise to edema, retention of urine and constipation.

However, in conventional terms there is no link between the lungs and the kidneys or the large intestine. Although the lungs can become waterlogged in a case of pulmonary edema, this is usually the result of a condition that primarily affects another part of the body, such as heart failure.

Regulation of the Water passages

This is part of the dispersing function of the lungs (see above).

Control of the skin and body hair

Again, there is little correspondence with conventional medicine, as the skin and body hair are not seen as linked to the function of the lungs. Although the common skin condition of eczema is commonly associated in conventional medicine with asthma, these are still seen as separate conditions. The reason they are understood to be linked lies in a deficiency of the immune system, not the lungs.

Opening into the nose

The nose is an organ of the respiratory system, so there is an obvious correspondence here with conventional medicine.

Housing the Corporeal Soul (Po)

The Po is the most physical aspect of the spiritual body and gives rise to clarity of thought and movement. Its health relies on a healthy rhythm of breathing.

In Chinese medicine it is believed that imbalanced emotions, in particular, grief and anxiety, will upset the pulsating rhythm of the Po by constraint of free movement of the chest.

Although conventional medicine makes no explicit link between the lungs and emotions or spirit, it is recognized that emotions have an effect, via the breathing control center in the brain, on the respiratory rate and rhythm, and also that mindful deep breathing can calm the emotions.

The Lungs in Chinese medicine have a much broader role than their purely physical counterpart in conventional medicine. It seems that the role of the Lungs in Chinese medicine also embraces aspects that would be attributed in conventional medicine to the cardiovascular, urinary, gastrointestinal and immune systems as well as the skin.

The functions of the Lung according to a conventional and Chinese perspective can be summarized in the form of a correspondence table. This illustrates the idea that the functions of what conventional medicine calls the lungs, including the air-filled sacs and the blood that circulates perpetually around them, may be the domain not only of the Lung Organ in Chinese medicine, but also of the Kidney and Liver Organs. It will follow from this that diseases of the lungs may manifest in Chinese medicine syndromes involving the Lung, Liver and Kidney Organs.

Correspondence table for the functions of the Lung, as described by conventional and Chinese medicine

Functions of the lung
Involved in the process of external respiration, which enables the exchange of oxygen and carbon dioxide between the circulation and the outside environment (**Lung and Kidney Organs**)
Helps to maintain a healthy balance of oxygen, carbon dioxide and acidity of the blood (**Lung and Liver Organs**)
Helps protect the body from noxious substances in the inhaled air (**Lung and Kidney Organs**)
Enables the production of a hormone (angiotensin) that is important in the maintenance of blood pressure (**Kidney, Spleen and Heart Organs**)
Very closely linked in structure and function to the heart on which they depend for an adequate supply of blood to oxygenate (**Heart, Kidney and Liver Organs**)
Provides a steady flow of air to power the production of speech from the larynx (**Lung, Liver and Heart Organs**)

Functions of the Lung Organ
"The Lungs are like a minister from whom policies are issued"
Governs Qi and respiration (respiratory system, process of cellular respiration that goes on in the mitochondria of all cells, circulatory system)
Controls the channels and the blood vessels (**circulatory system**)
Controls dispersing and descending (**immune system, skin, large intestine, bladder**)
Regulates the Water passages (**circulatory system, kidneys, bladder**)
Controls skin and (body) hair (**skin, immune system**)
Opens into the nose (**nose, upper respiratory system**)
Houses the corporeal soul (**no correspondence to a physiological organ**)

3.3b The investigation of the respiratory system

The bulk of minor respiratory disease, particularly infectious disease affecting the upper respiratory tract, is managed in the UK entirely by the doctor (general practitioner (GP)). More severe problems affecting the nose and throat may be referred for the opinion of a specialist in diseases of the ear, nose and throat (otorhinolaryngologist).

A patient with any other severe respiratory disease will be referred by their GP to a specialist in respiratory medicine. These doctors are commonly known as chest physicians.

If a surgical operation is necessary, the chest physician will refer the patient to a thoracic surgeon. Very often the thoracic surgeon is also skilled in heart surgery, in which case they are more accurately described as a cardiothoracic surgeon.

The most common investigations of the respiratory system include:

- a thorough physical examination
- laryngoscopy to examine the vocal cords
- microscopic examination of the sputum
- pulse oximetry
- lung function tests to assess the mechanics of the breathing
- blood tests relevant to lung function
- chest X-ray imaging, computed tomography (CT) scans and bronchoscopy to visualize the lungs
- biopsy of the lung tissue
- radioisotope scanning.

Physical examination

The physical examination of the respiratory system involves the stages listed in Table 3.3b-I.

Table 3.3b-I The stages of physical examination of the lungs
General examination for signs of poor oxygenation of the blood (seen as the bluish discoloration of the lips and tongue known as cyanosis) and for the swelling of the base of the nails, known as clubbing (this is a sign of severe lung disease such as cancer and bronchiectasis)
Visual assessment of the rate and quality of the breathing
Physical examination of the chest for deformities, with the use of percussion to assess for any abnormal areas of dense tissue (indication of infection, fluid or tumor)
Auscultation of the breath sounds in all parts of the chest

Laryngoscopy

This is an examination performed by an ear, nose and throat specialist to examine the vocal cords. It involves the skilled insertion of an instrument that carries a tiny mirror into the mouth and thence into the pharynx. It is usually painless.

Examination of the sputum

A patient with an infection or a possible tumor may be requested to produce a sample of phlegm. When examined by microscope, this can reveal the presence of infectious organisms, and occasionally, in cancer, will demonstrate cancerous cells. In the case of infection, the sample can be used to test for sensitivity to a range of antibiotics.

Pulse oximetry

This simple non-invasive test involving a probe applied to the finger tips can give a rapid estimation of the blood oxygen levels, and is now an important aspect in the assessment of the severity of lower respiratory disease.

Lung function tests

Lung function tests are performed when disease of the lower respiratory tract is suspected. These tests require the patient to blow into a machine that measures the force and volume of the out-breath, and detects the changes that are characteristic of the diseases that lead to restricted breathing, such as asthma and emphysema. These tests are straightforward and painless for the patient to perform.

The most simple of these tests is the peak expiratory outflow assessment, which is done using a peak flow meter. This is a hand-held tool that the patient can be taught to use at home. Its main purpose is to assess the severity of asthma in a patient on ongoing treatment, although it does not provide as detailed or helpful information as the more complex tests available in a hospital outpatient department. A more complex examination of lung function includes assessment by means of a spirometer. This will provide a graphical computer printout that describes the rate and quantity of air flow throughout a prolonged expiration. Assessment of exhaled nitric oxide, a marker of the inflammation of asthma, and also carbon monoxide, a marker of cigarette smoking and carbon monoxide poisoning, may be performed. Both these tests also require the patient to exhale into a machine.

Blood tests

Serum samples can be used to examine for antigens of infectious agents and for antibodies to confirm the presence of infection. Certain antibodies can also indicate the tendency to allergy, which is common in asthmatics.

Blood tests can also reveal other markers of chronic respiratory disease such as autoantibodies in connective tissue diseases and anticholinesterase levels in sarcoidosis.

In the investigation of lower respiratory tract disease, a sample of arterial blood is drawn from the radial artery to measure the concentration of oxygen and carbon dioxide in the blood.

Chest X-ray imaging

This test is performed on all patients with suspected lower respiratory tract disease. Most serious disease, such as pneumonia, cancer, emphysema and lung fibrosis, will show characteristic changes on a chest X-ray image. However, in asthma, even when severe, the chest X-ray image usually appears normal.

Computed tomography (CT) scan

This test is most commonly used to assess the size and spread of lung cancer. A CT scan will reveal not only the lung tissue, but also the lymph nodes deep within the chest. It can also indicate changes caused by other chronic lung diseases such as pulmonary fibrosis and asbestosis.

Figure 3.3b-I shows a CT scan of the lungs in a patient with advanced lung cancer. This is a slice of the upper chest presented as if the patient is lying on their back with their feet facing the viewer. The white structures are bones, and the sternum, one vertebral body, some ribs and the scapulae are visible. The very black areas are regions of normal air spaces in the lungs. The cancer is clearly seen as a gray shadow invading the normal lung tissue.

Figure 3.3b-I A CT scan of the lung indicating a large area of cancerous tissue (arrow)

The less-invasive technique of magnetic resonance imaging (MRI) is less valuable in imaging of the tissues of the lung because the respiratory movements affect the quality of the images.

Bronchoscopy

This invasive test involves the passage of a flexible telescope into the wider air passages of a sedated patient. The tube can be inserted as far as the larger bronchioles. Tumors can be seen directly by means of this technique.

Alternatively, salt water can be squirted down the tip of the tube to retrieve cells from the deeper parts of the lungs in cases of possible infection or cancer when sputum does not reveal any features of disease. This technique is known as broncho-alveolar lavage.

Biopsy of the lung tissue

Biopsy involves the removal of a piece of lung tissue for examination under the microscope. The biopsy can be taken from the bronchi or bronchioles through the bronchoscope. Biopsy of the pleura can be taken through a small incision in the skin overlying a gap between the ribs. Sometimes a thoracic surgeon is required to open up the chest to remove tissue from deep in the chest.

Biopsy is most commonly used to confirm the diagnosis of cancer, but can also be used when sarcoidosis or infection is suspected, but cannot be detected by any other means.

Fluid can also be drawn from between the pleura by means of a syringe needle inserted between the ribs into the space. This is used only in those conditions that have caused fluid to accumulate in this space, known as pleural effusion. Such conditions include cancer of the bronchus, pneumonia and pulmonary edema.

Radioisotope scanning

Radioisotope scanning may be used to examine for possible blockages to blood flow in the lungs, usually a result of blood clot emboli. The blood is injected with a safe radioactive marker with a very short half-life (i.e. its activity declines to insignificant levels very rapidly). Defects in blood perfusion of the lungs can then be revealed by means of scanning the lungs for radioactivity.

3.3c Diseases of the upper respiratory tract

Minor diseases of the upper parts of the respiratory tract such as coughs, colds and flu are a well-recognized part of normal life. Conditions that affect the structures progressively further down the respiratory tract, such as the tonsils, larynx and trachea, are seen in conventional medicine as more significant conditions. Nevertheless, on the whole, most acute conditions of the upper half of the respiratory tract are relatively benign.

The conditions of the upper respiratory tract studied in this section are:

- Acute infections of the upper respiratory tract:
    - the common cold
    - sinusitis
    - tonsillitis and pharyngitis
    - glandular fever (infectious mononucleosis)
    - laryngitis, tracheitis and croup
    - epiglottitis
    - influenza (flu)
- Allergic rhinitis
- Cancer of the larynx (see also Chapter 2.3).

Acute infections of the upper respiratory tract

With the exception of some forms of tonsillitis and pharyngitis and the childhood infection acute epiglottitis, all the common infections of the upper respiratory tract are initially caused by viruses. A wide range of viruses has been identified to affect the respiratory epithelial cells. Viruses tend to enter the upper respiratory tract through inhalation of infected droplets of moisture. The inhaled virus is able to penetrate and damage the cells, and this leads to inflammation (redness and swelling) and the production of sometimes profuse watery secretions. Fever is a common symptom of these infections, although frequently it is mild in nature. Breathlessness (which is significant if respiration rises to over 30 breaths per minute in adults) is not a feature of upper respiratory conditions. Breathlessness suggests a more serious lower respiratory condition or obstruction to the upper airways, and if severe merits same-day referral for a medical opinion.

The different syndromes that result from upper respiratory infection seem to be dependent on the characteristics of the virus. Some primarily affect the throat and the nasal lining, leading to the symptoms of the common cold, whereas others tend to affect lower structures, causing tonsillitis or laryngitis, for example. The evidence for this is that a virus that is "going around" will tend to cause the same range of symptoms in most people who contract the infection.

Usually, viral infections of the upper respiratory tract are short-lived. In some people the infections can progress to affect further regions of the respiratory system, including the lower respiratory tract. In these cases, it is often believed that a further bacterial infection has arisen in the region of the already damaged respiratory epithelium. It is often the case that it is the healthy bacteria, which usually reside harmlessly in the lining of the upper respiratory tract, that cause these complications. Therefore, these sorts of deeper bacterial infections are not usually contagious. This complication of bacterial infection is recognized to be more likely in people who are susceptible due to some form of chronic ill health. As long as upper respiratory conditions last for less than five days there is usually no need for medical referral, except in the case of infants or frail individuals.

The treatment for all minor viral upper respiratory conditions needs be supportive only, as the antiviral drugs currently available are expensive, carry risks and only shorten rather than eliminate the symptoms of illness in healthy individuals. For this reason, the use of these drugs in the National Health Service (NHS) is restricted according to the UK National Institute for Health and Care Excellence (NICE) guidance (2009),[54] being given only in cases of influenza in vulnerable individuals. Common treatment approaches recommended by doctors include aspirin and paracetamol to reduce pain and fever, plenty of fluids to counteract fluid loss through fever, keeping warm and letting the body rest.

There is no doubt that smokers are more prone to severe forms of upper respiratory tract infections. It is also recognized that atmospheric pollution results in increased rates of severe respiratory infections. Both these factors reduce the health of the respiratory epithelium so that it is less well equipped to deal with minor infections. Smoking, in particular, is known to damage the action of the cilia in the respiratory epithelium and also to cause a change in the production of the mucus so that it becomes much thicker and thus resistant to clearance from the air passages.

The accumulation of thick and sticky mucus that results when a smoker develops a viral respiratory infection is much more likely to become further infected by bacteria and to result in a persistent phlegmy infection.

The cough and profuse phlegm familiar to people who have recently stopped smoking is a healthy sign. It is a result of the recovery of the cilia, which are then able to clear accumulated toxins and mucus from the lower parts of the respiratory tract.

The common cold

The common cold virus affects the nose and pharynx (throat), leading to sore throat, stuffy and runny nose, and watery eyes. The secretions are usually clear. Fever is slight or absent. Simple treatments for the common cold include vitamin C and zinc preparations and steam inhalations to loosen secretions. Eucalyptus and menthol oils can be a helpful addition to a steam inhalation, and these aromatic compounds are also commonly found in proprietary cough sweets and medicines. Aspirin or paracetamol may be taken to relieve the discomfort of sore throat and to reduce fever.

Decongestant preparations that act by constriction of the blood vessels of the nose are not generally considered to be of great benefit. However, they are freely available as proprietary medications in the form of tablets or nasal sprays. Some of these contain drugs similar in action to the chemical ephedrine. Decongestants reduce the swelling of the nasal lining and reduce the secretions. However, these are conventionally recognized to be suppressive, and so the symptoms may recur in a more pronounced form when the drug wears off. Examples of decongestant medication include Vicks Sinex and Sudafed nasal sprays.

Some cold preparations available from the chemist contain mild sedatives, which are intended to help by allowing the person to rest.

A common cold is not seen to be serious in conventional medicine except in people who have a risk of further infection due to ongoing chronic disease or immunodeficiency.

 Information box 3.3c-I

The common cold: comments from a Chinese medicine perspective

In Chinese medicine, the symptoms of the common cold are described as an Invasion of Wind Heat or Wind Cold (and occasionally Wind Damp Heat or Wind Dry Heat) on the Exterior. They are believed to occur because of the relative weakness of Wei Qi compared to the strength of the Pathogenic Factor. As such, if treated in its early stages by releasing the Exterior and Clearing Wind, the development of a common cold is believed to be preventable.

According to the Six Levels theory in the *Shang Han Lun* (On Cold Damage: *Zhang Zhongjing*, circa 200 CE), a common cold due to Wind Cold is at the most superficial Greater Yang (Tai Yang) level. According to the Four Levels theory from the Discussion of Warm Diseases (Ye *Tianshi*, circa 1710 CE), a common cold due to Wind Heat is at the most superficial Defensive (Wei) Qi Level.[55]

In contrast to conventional medicine, an Invasion of Wind Heat or Wind Cold is taken very seriously in Chinese medicine, as there is a risk it may descend to deeper energetic levels and change into Heat unless appropriate care and treatment is given.

From the integrated perspective of infectious disease introduced in Section 2.4d, the infectious viruses might be seen as the source of a Pathogenic Factor of external origin, whereas many bacterial complications of these infections might be interpreted as the result of additional Pathogenic Factors of internal origin. This is comparable to the concept in Chinese medicine that superficial invasions of Wind Heat or Wind Cold can progress to deeper levels in people with Depleted Qi, and so fits in with the idea that in these cases the Pathogenic Factor is of internal origin.

For example, the development of a phlegmy bacterial bronchial infection following a minor viral illness, as is common in heavy smokers, could be interpreted in Chinese medicine as the Accumulation of Heat and Phlegm at a deeper level than the Exterior. These Pathogenic Factors are consequences of long-term damage from smoking, and so would be recognized as internal in origin. The initial assault on the patient would be a pathogen from outside the body, but it is permitted to penetrate to deep levels as a result of Deficiency in Wei Qi. Here it prevents proper descent of Lung Qi and leads to Accumulation of Phlegm, which readily combines with Internal Heat that may be a pre-existing problem as a result of smoking, alcohol, poor diet or emotional factors.

Aspirin may be an appropriate energetic remedy for an Invasion of Wind Cold or Wind Heat, in that it is believed to release the exterior and promote sweating. Aspirin is known to be anti-inflammatory and will temporarily relieve discomfort due to fever, sore throat and aching joints. This suggests a Clearing of Heat from the Exterior level and a moving of Stagnant Qi. However, the tablet preparation of aspirin is also Heating at a deep level, as evidenced by its causing inflammation of the stomach and increasing the tendency to bleed. This may not be desirable in a patient with Wind Heat Invasion. Although aspirin clears Heat at a superficial level, it could also lead to further problems related to internal heat because of its Heating properties.

Paracetamol also temporarily reduces fever, inflammation and pain. Like aspirin, this represents the Clearing of Heat from the Exterior level and moving of Stagnant Qi. Although it does not have the Heating properties of aspirin, in overdose it is known to be toxic, to the liver in particular.

Decongestant drugs reduce secretions from the nose and stuffiness. This would correspond to the Clearing of Wind Cold. Interestingly, these drugs have a very close relation in Chinese medicine known as ma huang (ephedra), which, as a pungent warm herb, is recognized to Clear Wind Cold. However, conventionally, decongestants are known to be suppressive in action. This suggests that if used without simultaneous attention to the root deficiency, the action of ma huang can also be suppressive.

Sinusitis

Sinusitis is the result of infection of the respiratory epithelium that lines the sinus cavities situated in the facial bones. Although it is commonly triggered by a virus infection, it can readily become more persistent due to subsequent bacterial infection. This is because the narrow

opening of the inflamed sinuses into the nasal cavity easily becomes blocked, and the stagnation of the secretions within predispose to further infection, often by the healthy bacteria that usually reside harmlessly in the nose.

Prolonged sinusitis is more likely to occur in certain susceptible people. Susceptibility can be the result of a congenital structural abnormality of the sinuses (and so could run in families), a tendency to produce excessive phlegmy secretions, and smoking.

The symptoms of sinusitis include painful and tender sinuses, with foci of pain over the inner aspect of the eyebrows and in the center of the cheekbones. In a persistent infection the patient may feel very unwell and feverish, and may have a headache over the forehead. Thick green secretions, indicating bacterial infection, may be produced.

 Information box 3.3c-II

Sinusitis: comments from a Chinese medicine perspective

In Chinese medicine, sinusitis may simply be a manifestation of Wind Heat or Wind Cold Invasion, but more severe cases may indicate other full conditions such as Lung Heat, Liver and Gallbladder Fire or Stomach and Spleen Damp Heat.[56] These conditions occur on a pre-existing deficiency, commonly of the Spleen, which predisposes to Accumulation of Damp, Phlegm and Heat, and, as the mother of the Lung, commonly co-exists with Deficiency of Lung Qi.

In sinusitis the tenderness is commonly focused around acupoints Zan Zhu BL-2, Si Bai ST-2 and Ju Liao ST-3.

If, as in most cases, the problem is a result of an internal imbalance, antibiotic treatment will not be treating the root cause, and due to its Cold and Damp nature may be compounding the problem with additional drug-induced disease. Therefore, the main action of antibiotics in this sort of case is suppressive. This explains why sinusitis can often recur after treatment.

Inhalations of steam benefit the Lung in a case of Lung Heat because they provide moisture. It is also possible that pungent aromatic oils stimulate Lung Qi.

Supportive measures include inhalation of aromatic oils, such as Olbas oil, in steam. Saline douches may be recommended. The currently recommended drug treatment for sinusitis is regular use of a corticosteroid nasal inhaler such as beclometasone. Nevertheless, doctors will frequently prescribe antibiotics (most commonly amoxicillin) in a severe case of sinusitis. Other antibiotics such as doxycycline or erythromycin may have to be chosen because of increasing bacterial resistance to amoxicillin.

In susceptible people, sinusitis, even when treated with antibiotics, can become recurrent. Occasionally it can become chronic, with symptoms that never totally go away. In such cases the patient may be referred to an ear, nose and throat specialist for consideration of endoscopic sinus surgery, which is a means of widening and draining the sinus passages.

Tonsillitis and pharyngitis

It is very common for a virus infection to affect the back of the throat and/or the tonsils without also affecting the nasal lining. The inflammation that results from this sort of infection is termed pharyngitis (sore throat) or tonsillitis, depending on the site of the worst symptoms.

Like the common cold, this sort of viral infection, although uncomfortable, should be mild and short-lived. In more severe cases the tonsils can become very inflamed and enlarged, and this can be accompanied by high fever, headache, joint pains and malaise.

Infection with the bacterium *Streptococcus pyogenes* used to be a very common cause of tonsillitis and pharyngitis, although it is now less common. The bacterial tonsillitis is characteristically more severe than that resulting from a viral infection, with yellow areas of pus often seen on the tonsil. However, there is no absolute distinction, as some viral tonsillitis can be very severe, and may also generate pus on the tonsil. Bacterial tonsillitis and pharyngitis can be diagnosed by means of a throat swab, although this takes a few days to process, and so is rarely performed in the UK.

The treatment for bacterial tonsillitis is penicillin (phenoxymethyl) rather than amoxicillin. Often, a doctor might choose to prescribe penicillin in a severe case of tonsillitis, even when it is uncertain that the cause is bacterial. The delays involved in processing a throat swab and the discomfort for the patient deter many doctors from performing this test. This is an example of "treating blind" (see Section 2.4d). In many cases it may never be known whether the antibiotic helped because the tonsillitis naturally gets better in most people by three to seven days of onset.

There are two reasons to prescribe antibiotics in tonsillitis. The first is that the symptoms of bacterial infection may be reduced in severity by penicillin. The second, more important, reason is that in some people the *Streptococcus* infection can have more serious complications. These are scarlet fever, rheumatic fever and glomerulonephritis (also known as acute nephritis). However, for reasons that are unclear, these complications are becoming increasingly uncommon, even when the use of antibiotics is accounted for. For this reason current medical guidelines (NICE 2008)[57] recommend that antibiotics are not prescribed in uncomplicated cases of pharyngitis and tonsillitis.

In rare cases, one tonsil can become very inflamed and full of pus. This condition, which is a tonsillar (quinsy) or peritonsillar abscess, is very debilitating, and is associated with fever. The treatment is with antibiotics and may require urgent surgical drainage of the pus from the tonsil. In some cases the enlarged tonsil may compromise breathing, in which case it becomes a surgical emergency.

In some people, and children in particular, tonsillitis can become recurrent. It used to be common practice to remove the tonsils surgically in such cases. However, surgery is now performed only relatively rarely, as it is recognized to be a risky and traumatic experience for a child, and does not necessarily reduce recurrent attacks of pharyngitis. A tonsillectomy would only currently be considered if attacks of tonsillitis exceeded five a year for at least two years.

Information box 3.3c-III

Tonsillitis: comments from a Chinese medicine perspective

In Chinese medicine, the signs and symptoms of tonsillitis and pharyngitis are usually attributed to Wind Heat Invasion. In children in particular, Stomach Heat may be an additional internal source of the Pathogenic Factor. The symptoms of severe tonsillitis correspond to the Chinese medicine condition of Fire Poison, especially with the accumulation of pus and high fever that can occur in such cases. There may be underlying Kidney or Spleen Deficiency in cases of Fire Poison.

Quinsy is a severe example of Fire Poison, and develops because of underlying deficiency. Antibiotics, although necessary in many cases because of the severity of the condition, are suppressive in action. Surgical drainage is energetically appropriate, as it simply speeds up the body's tendency to discharge pus, and probably acts by enabling clearance of the Pathogenic Factor (extreme Damp Heat).

Antibiotic treatment in tonsillitis may often have either no effect or a simple placebo effect if prescribed in viral infections. However, it may also damage Stomach and Spleen Qi because of its Cold and Damp nature, and so may be less than helpful in the patient with viral tonsillitis. It may, however, be the appropriate energetic remedy in streptococcal infections if the Pathogen is of external origin. This is most likely if the case is one of many "going round." Tonsillitis often has an internal component, and is an external manifestation of internal Stomach Heat. If this is the case, antibiotics will be suppressive, and recurrence of the condition is a possibility.

Recurrent tonsillitis always suggests an internal cause. In such cases, treatment with antibiotics and tonsillectomy are suppressive in nature.

Glandular fever (infectious mononucleosis)

Glandular fever is one of the more severe forms of viral tonsillitis, and is caused by a virus known as the Epstein-Barr virus (EBV). However, most cases of EBV infection are mild. The evidence for this comes from studies of young people, in which blood tests showed that 89 percent of those between 18 and 19 had contracted the infection at some point in their lives.[58] Most of these infections had occurred without the young people having developed the classic symptoms of glandular fever.

However, severe cases can be prolonged and draining. The patient can suffer from marked tonsillitis, with fever and joint aches. The lymph nodes in the neck are enlarged. There may be abdominal pain as other lymph tissue in the body, including the spleen, can become enlarged, and the liver may become inflamed. Occasionally, a red, measles-like rash can develop, particularly in patients who have been mistakenly prescribed amoxicillin because a bacterial tonsillitis was suspected. In very rare cases the virus can affect the lining of the brain and cause meningitis.

EBV infection can be diagnosed by a blood test that detects antibodies to the virus in or after the second week of symptoms. Treatment is supportive only. In severe cases, when there is enlargement of the spleen, corticosteroid tablets may be prescribed.

Information box 3.3c-IV

Glandular fever: comments from a Chinese medicine perspective

In Chinese medicine, most mild cases of glandular fever would have the same diagnosis as tonsillitis.

In severe cases, the swelling of glands, muscle and joint aches, and disturbance of the liver and spleen, suggest that the Pathogenic Factor has penetrated to deeper levels. This suggests either Residual Pathogenic Factor with Damp Heat in the muscles, or the Lesser Yang (Shao Yang) pattern of the Six Levels, or a combination of both.

Laryngitis, tracheitis and croup

Some of the other viral infections primarily affect the larynx and the trachea. The result is inflammation of these tissues, leading to one or more of hoarseness, cough and pain felt beneath the sternum. The pain is related to coughing and deep breathing. Again, these infections may be short-lived except in those who are susceptible, particularly young children and smokers. In susceptible people there is a risk that tracheitis can descend to involve the bronchi and cause a much more severe and prolonged infection.

In children under the age of three the swelling of the vocal cords can be so severe as to lead to difficulty in breathing. The affected child will be hoarse, have a rapid respiratory rate and may have a barking cough. If severe, a rasping noise, known as stridor, is heard as the child breathes in. In very severe cases the child needs to be administered high-dose steroids and may be administered adrenaline via a nebulizer (which forms a mist that the child breathes in via a mask). The barking cough in such cases is called croup, and may persist in a child for weeks. Steam is no longer recommended in the treatment of croup.

In some cases laryngitis may persist to give a syndrome of persistently hoarse voice and thick stringy mucus that is difficult to clear. This is known as chronic laryngitis. The patient is otherwise well. This is more common in people who smoke or in those who overuse their voices, such as singers.

The treatment of chronic laryngitis is to rest the voice and avoid smoking. Steam inhalations can soothe the vocal cords and loosen the mucus. However, if the hoarseness persists for more than three weeks it is considered good practice for the patient to be referred to an ear, nose and throat specialist. The vocal cords can then be examined by laryngoscopy to exclude the unlikely possibility of a tumor of the vocal cords. It is increasingly recognized that poor use and emotional strain can lead to long-standing hoarseness, and so vocal training may be helpful in chronic laryngitis.

Information box 3.3c-V

Laryngitis and tracheitis: comments from a Chinese medicine perspective

In Chinese medicine, the symptom of a hoarse voice is usually associated with Wind Heat or Wind Cold Invasion. However, the pain and depth of tracheitis suggests that the Pathogen has penetrated to a deeper level than the Exterior. The cough and breathlessness that accompany tracheitis in children in particular is suggestive of Lung Heat (Qi Level according to the Four Levels categorization). Chronic laryngitis is also consistent with a diagnosis of Lung Heat, although in these cases the likely origin of the Heat is internal, as the condition affects smokers in particular. Qi Stagnation is likely to play a role in those cases in which poor use of the voice and emotional strain are significant in the etiology of the condition. The dryness resulting from Lung Heat explains why inhalation of steam can be of relief.

Epiglottitis

Acute epiglottitis is a childhood infection caused by the bacterium *Haemophilus influenzae B* (HiB). This infection in most marked in children under five. The infection has a rapid onset, with a high fever and difficulty breathing. Inflammation of the epiglottis narrows the aperture of the larynx, and in severe cases this leads to acute stridor and can cause death by asphyxiation. The same bacterium can also cause a form of meningitis.

A child with stridor must be treated as an emergency and is nursed in an intensive care unit. It is essential in such cases that the child is not asked to open their mouth to show the tongue, as this can precipitate total blockage of the airway. The antibiotics chloramphenicol and cefotaxime are the recommended medical treatments for this infection.

A vaccine is available to protect children against HiB infections, and is given in the first few weeks of life as part of the routine childhood vaccination program in the UK. There is clear evidence that the introduction of this vaccine in the UK was followed by a marked drop in the reported number of cases of HiB infections.

Information box 3.3c-VI

Epiglottitis: comments from a Chinese medicine perspective

In Chinese medicine, the symptoms of epiglottitis would be regarded as an Invasion of Wind Heat that has penetrated to the Qi Level to lead to Lung Heat, as evidenced by the high temperature and the stridor.

Influenza (flu)

Influenza is a result of infection by one of the many strains of the influenza virus. This tends to invade the pharyngeal epithelium, but it also gives rise to a much more severe form of general malaise than the common cold. Symptoms include sore throat, dry cough, muscle aches, headache, vomiting, diarrhea, high fever and exhaustion. A period of up to a few weeks of tiredness and depression is common following recovery.

In susceptible people, particularly the very young and elderly people, the virus can also affect the respiratory epithelium of the lower respiratory tract, and this can lead to bacterial infections in the form of bronchitis and pneumonia. In very weak individuals this can be life-threatening.

As with all viral infections, treatment is supportive. Bed rest is recommended, and the patient is advised to take regular doses of aspirin or paracetamol, with plenty of fluids. If bacterial infection of the lower respiratory tract is suspected, antibiotics will be given and hospital admission may be necessary. In susceptible individuals the antiviral drugs zanamivir and oseltamivir may be prescribed to reduce the severity of complications.

A vaccine is available every autumn/winter that is specific to the currently most virulent and common strain of influenza. This is recommended to be given annually to all elderly people and to any others who may be particularly susceptible because of chronic heart, kidney or lung disease, diabetes or immunosuppression. However, the vaccine is known to protect only about 70 percent of those who receive it, and it does not provide protection from any of the other respiratory viruses. Oseltamivir may be prescribed as a prophylactic medication for individuals at high risk who come into contact with a case of flu because of their susceptibility.

Swine flu was a strain of H1N1 influenza that reached epidemic proportions in 2009. Because of international concerns about a possible high mortality rate, expensive antiviral prescriptions became a routine aspect of treatment for symptoms of infection in many developed countries. It was later shown that this intensive program of antiviral medication for flu was possibly not cost-effective.[59]

Information box 3.3c-VII

Influenza: comments from a Chinese medicine perspective

In Chinese medicine, all cases of influenza would be seen as an invasion on the exterior of Pathogens such as Wind Heat or Wind Cold. In this way, there is no clear distinction made between influenza and the common cold. The severity of the condition in many cases suggests that the Pathogen has descended to the Qi Level to lead to syndromes such as Lung Heat or Stomach Heat. The precise syndrome depends on the symptoms of the patient.

Allergic rhinitis

Rhinitis is the medical term for inflammation of the nose, the symptoms of which are similar to those of the common cold, including a runny and blocked-up nose.

As described in Section 2.2c, there are two main types of allergy that affect the nose – hay fever (seasonal rhinitis) and the more chronic condition of perennial rhinitis. In both, the symptoms include runny nose, sneezing, itchy throat and blocked-up nose. In hay fever, itchy and watery eyes are additional common symptoms. Both forms of rhinitis are the result of excessive sensitivity of the immune cells of the respiratory lining to common substances in the atmosphere, such as pollen, house dust and animal dandruff.

In some cases the sinuses can also become inflamed, and this can predispose to bouts of sinusitis, with tender sinuses, headaches and thick yellow discharge from the nose.

Patients who have a long history of allergic rhinitis may develop permanent fleshy swellings of the nasal lining called nasal polyps. Polyp is the term given to a growth, either benign or malignant, that has a stalk as its attachment to the flesh from which it grows. Nasal polyps are benign swellings but may be the cause of a permanently blocked-up nose.

Medical treatment of rhinitis includes avoidance of the allergen, regular antihistamine medication (including cetirizine, loratadine and fexofenadine) and anti-inflammatory medication (e.g. sodium cromoglicate) in the form of a nasal spray or eye drops. Decongestant medication (e.g. xylometolazine), some formulations of which can be bought without the need for a prescription, may also be used. A corticosteroid nasal spray (beclometasone or fluticasone) may be very effective in suppressing symptoms. In severe cases, oral corticosteroids may be prescribed.

A course of oral corticosteroids may help nasal polyps to subside, but if there is no response to medical treatment, the only satisfactory treatment is surgical removal.

Information box 3.3c-VIII

Allergic rhinitis: comments from a Chinese medicine perspective

In Chinese medicine, both types of allergic rhinitis might be diagnosed as Invasion of Wind Cold on a background of Deficiency of Wei Qi. This will account for the runny nose, sneezing and itching. Flaws and Sionneau (2001)[60] explain that in all cases there is "deep lying or hidden Phlegm" in the lungs. Moreover, they suggest that many patients will have an underlying Spleen-Lung or Spleen-Kidney Deficiency. Phlegm and Liver Qi Stagnation may lead to Blood Stagnation in severe chronic cases when the nostrils are blocked all of the time.

The development of sinusitis suggests a Pathogen at a deeper level, such as Liver and Gallbladder Heat, Lung Heat or Spleen Heat. In these cases, as sinusitis is a chronic condition, the origin of the Pathogen is internal.

Nasal polyps are fleshy swellings that might be interpreted as Accumulations of Phlegm.

Cancer of the larynx

Laryngeal cancer predominantly affects male smokers, and commonly develops between the ages of 55 and 65. The cancer develops on the larynx as a result of long-term irritation from cigarette smoke. The first symptoms often occur early in the disease, as the delicate structure of the vocal cords is frequently first affected and unexplained hoarseness develops. If other parts of the voice box are affected, the tumor may grow for some time until the patient notices symptoms or swollen lymph nodes in the neck.

The diagnosis is made by laryngoscopy and removal of tissue for a biopsy, and a magnetic resonance imaging (MRI) scan is used to stage the progression of the disease. If caught early, there is a high cure rate with radiotherapy to the larynx alone. In these cases, speech is preserved, although the voice may remain hoarse. If the tumor is extensive the whole of the larynx has to be removed, and the trachea is opened into the neck in an operation known as a tracheotomy. An artificial opening with a valve, also known as a tracheostomy, is inserted into the hole in the neck to keep it open and to protect it from foreign bodies.

The patient with a tracheostomy has to breathe through this opening, and can no longer speak. Some patients learn to speak by using air swallowed first into the stomach, but this is not always possible. The risk of infections of the lower respiratory tract is high in patients with a tracheostomy because the defense mechanisms of the entire upper respiratory tract have been removed.

Ten percent of those who have been "cured" of laryngeal cancer develop lung cancer at a later stage in their life. This second cancer is almost never curable.

Information box 3.3c-IX

Cancer of the larynx: comments from a Chinese medicine perspective

In Chinese medicine, the symptoms of cancer of the larynx would reflect Phlegm and Blood Stagnation in the Lungs. The long-standing depletion that underlies this has resulted in most cases at least in part from the Toxic Heat and Stagnation that result from cigarette smoking.

The red flags of upper respiratory disease

Some patients with upper respiratory diseases will benefit from referral to a conventional doctor for assessment or treatment. Red flags are those symptoms and signs that indicate that referral should be considered. The red flags of upper respiratory disease are described in Table 3.3c-I. A summary of the red flags in a format designed for quick reference in clinical practice can be found in Appendix III. This gives advice on the degree of urgency of referral for each of the red flag conditions listed.

Table 3.3c-I A16: Red flags of upper respiratory disease

Red flag	Description	Reasoning
A16.1	Features of progressive upper respiratory infection in susceptible people (e.g. frail elderly people, those who are immunocompromised and those with pre-existing lower respiratory disease): cough and fever or new production of yellow-green phlegm, each persisting for >3 days	In healthy people an upper respiratory infection (i.e. affecting any part of the respiratory tract above and including the bronchi) may be protracted but is not necessarily a serious condition. In most cases, as long as there is no breathlessness, or the patient is not a smoker, it is safe to treat conservatively and there is no need for antibiotics In healthy people consider referral if there is no response to treatment within 1–2 weeks However, in elderly people and those who are immunocompromised (including those with chronic diseases such as cancer, kidney failure and AIDS), severe infections can be masked by relatively minor symptoms, and it is advisable to refer any respiratory condition that persists for >3 days People with pre-existing lung disease (e.g. asthma, chronic bronchitis, emphysema, lung cancer, cystic fibrosis) are at increased risk of progressive infection, and similarly merit early referral Smokers commonly do not recover as quickly from upper respiratory infections and early antibiotic treatment may be merited in this case also
A16.2	Features of progression of infection to the lower respiratory tract: moderate to severe breathlessness* with malaise suggests the involvement of the bronchi or lower air passages. Usually accompanied by cough and fever, but may be the only symptom of an infection in elderly people or those who are immunocompromised	Even in healthy people, an infection that descends to below the bronchi is a more serious condition, as the ability of the lungs to exchange carbon dioxide and oxygen will be compromised by the narrowing of the thin airways of the bronchioles and inflammation of the alveoli (air sacs) Breathlessness is a feature of lower respiratory tract narrowing or infection and should be taken seriously, especially in elderly people, those who are immunocompromised, those with pre-existing lung disease (e.g. asthma, chronic bronchitis, emphysema, lung cancer, cystic fibrosis) and smokers All patients with breathlessness resulting from lung infection should be referred for a high priority assessment by a medical doctor A respiratory rate of >30 breaths/minute is a marker of significant breathlessness
A16.3	A single, grossly enlarged tonsil: if the patient is unwell and feverish and has foul-smelling breath, this suggests quinsy	Quinsy is the development of an abscess in the tonsil. It carries a serious risk of obstruction of the airways and requires a same-day surgical opinion Refer urgently if the patient is experiencing any restriction of breathing (stridor may be heard; see A16.5)
A16.4	A single, grossly enlarged tonsil: if the patient appears well, lymphoma is a possible diagnosis	If the patient appears well, consider that a single enlarged tonsil in a young person may, very rarely, result from a lymphoma and should be referred for exclusion of this diagnosis. However, grossly enlarged tonsils are not an uncommon finding in someone who has suffered from recurrent tonsillitis. In this case the tonsils are usually bilaterally enlarged
A16.5	Stridor (harsh, noisy breathing heard on both the in-breath and the out-breath)	Stridor is a noise that suggests upper airways obstruction. It is a serious red flag if it develops suddenly. It suggests possible swelling of the air passages due to laryngotracheitis, quinsy or epiglottitis If restriction to breathing is significant, the patient with stridor will be sitting very still It is important not to ask to see the tongue, as this can affect the position of the epiglottis, and may worsen the obstruction

A16.6	Any new onset of difficulty in breathing in a small child (<8 years), including unexplained blockage of nostril	Always take a new onset of difficulty in breathing in a child seriously, and refer for medical assessment to exclude serious disease. Possible common causes include lower respiratory infections, asthma, allergic reactions, inhalation of foreign bodies and congenital heart disease
A16.7	An unexplained persistent blockage of the nostril on one side in an adult (for >3 weeks)	One-sided blockage of a nostril is unusual in benign conditions (e.g. nasal polyposis). It may be the presenting sign of a carcinoma of the nasopharynx. A one-sided bloody discharge is a warning sign of this

* *Categorization of respiratory rate in adults*: Normal respiratory rate in an adult: 10–20 breaths per minute (one breath is one inhalation and exhalation); Moderate breathlessness in an adult: >30 breaths per minute; Severe breathlessness in an adult: >60 breaths per minute. *Categorization of respiratory rate in children*: The normal range for respiratory rate in children varies according to age. The following rates indicate moderate to severe breathlessness: Newborn (0–3 months): >60 breaths per minute; Infant (3 months to 2 years): >50 breaths per minute; Young child (2–8 years): >40 breaths per minute; Older child to adult: >30 breaths per minute.

3.3d Diseases of the bronchi and bronchioles

This section looks at the diseases that affect the airways of the lower respiratory tract, the bronchi and the bronchioles. The conditions studied are:

- Infections of the airways of the lower respiratory tract:
  - acute bronchitis
  - bronchiolitis
- Asthma
- Chronic obstructive pulmonary disease (COPD) (chronic bronchitis)
- Bronchiectasis
- Cystic fibrosis (CF)
- Cancer of the bronchus (lung cancer).

Infections of the airways of the lower respiratory tract

Acute bronchitis
Acute bronchitis is not dissimilar to many of the infections of the upper respiratory tract described in Section 3.3c. It is frequently the result of a virus infection, and has symptoms of dry cough, and a sensation of tightness or even pain felt beneath the sternum. However, because the bronchi are relatively narrow tubes, the swelling of their lining from inflammation can cause a marked reduction in the amount of air that can freely travel through them. This can lead to wheezing and shortness of breath, although in uncomplicated viral bronchitis these symptoms should not be severe.

Viral bronchitis can very easily become complicated by bacterial infection. In this case infection tends to be due to

one of the bacteria that in health reside harmlessly in the respiratory tract. Bacterial infection is particularly likely to occur in smokers or, ironically, in people who have just stopped smoking – in the latter because the production of thick mucus is temporarily increased.

In bacterial bronchitis the cough becomes productive, and sometimes profuse yellow-green phlegm is coughed up. Despite the relatively deep situation of the infection, most people do not feel extremely unwell, and fever may only be slight. Most recover from this infection as they would from infections higher up the respiratory tract.

 Information box 3.3d-I

Acute bronchitis: comments from a Chinese medicine perspective
In Chinese medicine, the fever, breathlessness and productive cough of acute bronchitis suggest that an invasion of Pathogens such as Wind Cold or Wind Heat has been succeeded by the penetration of Heat to the Qi Level (according to the Six Levels categorization). The Qi Level syndrome that would fit with bronchitis is Lung Heat.

The more pronounced symptoms of bacterial infection suggest that Heat and Phlegm are more marked than in viral infection. This development is more likely in those with a degree of pre-existing Lung Yin Deficiency, which can result from smoking. In a smoker some of the full Heat and Phlegm may also be of internal origin.

As bacterial infection occurs against a background of Lung Deficiency, antibiotics treat only the manifestation of the imbalance, and so the treatment is suppressive in nature. Ideally the patient should receive additional supportive treatment and make appropriate lifestyle changes to achieve full recovery.

Some doctors may prescribe antibiotics such as amoxicillin, tetracycline or erythromycin, although these may not be necessary for recovery in healthy people, and should really be reserved for intractable symptoms lasting for more than five days.

Bronchiolitis

Bronchiolitis is a viral infection of childhood that tends to affect the small air passages of the lungs, although it often begins with one to two days of upper respiratory tract symptoms. The respiratory syncytial virus (RSV) is the most common causative agent. The affected child will suffer from restricted breathing due to the narrowing of the air passages, and will have a rapid and labored breathing rate. Wheezy noises may be heard through a stethoscope, but the most typical finding is widespread inspiratory crackles that are an indication of infection of the bronchioles. In a proportion of cases the lung tissue also becomes infected, and this, as a form of pneumonia, is a much more severe condition. Treatment of bronchiolitis is initially supportive. Steam inhalation is no longer recommended. There are no known medical treatments that can modify the course of infection, and the majority of babies recover within one to two weeks. Occasionally a very unwell child will need to be admitted to hospital for monitoring and consideration of ventilatory support. Red flag signs include cyanosis, poor feeding and a rapid respiratory rate (>50 breaths/minute).

 Information box 3.3d-II

Bronchiolitis: comments from a Chinese medicine perspective

In Chinese medicine wheezy rapid breathing, called Xiao-Chuan, a term that comes from the words meaning wheezing and breathlessness, is seen as the result of Phlegm in the Lungs or Heat in the Lungs. The origin of the Pathogenic Factor is, in part, external, in the form of Wind Heat or Wind Cold, but the deep nature of the condition suggests an underlying internal Pathogenic Factor. As this is a condition almost exclusively affecting children in the first six months of their life, it is possible the illness could be a process by which Heat Toxins[61] absorbed from the womb environment are eliminated.

Asthma

Asthma is a condition that affects 5–8 percent of the population of the UK. In asthma, breathing is impaired due to a narrowing of the airways of the lower respiratory tract.

This narrowing is typically reversible, which means that the difficulty in breathing comes in bouts. The underlying problem in asthma is that the lining of the airways is much too sensitive to a wide range of factors, which, when they occur, lead to a rapid development of inflammation and the production of mucus. This inflammation causes swelling and narrowing of the airways, and the mucus can actually plug up some of the smaller air passages of the bronchioles.

It is possible that repeated episodes of inflammation in asthma may lead to remodeling of the lungs and entrenchment of the disease process. For this reason there is great emphasis on active early medical management of the symptoms of asthma.[62]

Factors related to the triggering of an asthma attack include:

- animal dandruff
- house dust mite and cockroach feces
- pollen and molds
- substances in the diet, such as egg, milk, wheat and fish
- some drugs (especially aspirin, and other non-steroidal anti-inflammatory drugs (NSAIDs) such as ibuprofen)
- industrial fumes, cigarette smoke and other atmospheric pollution
- cold air and exercise
- respiratory infections
- extremes of emotion.

External factors such as animal dandruff and house dust are known as allergens because they can provoke an allergic response. The allergens that affect an individual will be specific to that individual. For example, some people will be sensitive to only one or two of the allergens on this list, such as pollen in the summer. In others the sensitivity is so broad that it may often be unclear why an attack of asthma has developed.

It is known that asthmatics have excessive numbers of a certain sort of leukocyte called a mast cell in their lung tissue. The mast cell is very sensitive to noxious substances, and when it comes into contact with them it releases powerful chemicals such as histamine that stimulate inflammation in the bronchial airways. This is meant to be a protective response to enable the lung to clear irritating material, but is excessive in asthma. It is an example of a condition in which the immune system is overactive.

Many people with asthma also have other conditions that result from an overactive immune system, such as eczema and hay fever. The tendency to be allergic in this way to a wide range of substances is known as atopy, and seems to run quite strongly in families. In these people the diagnosis of atopy can be confirmed by skin-prick tests, in which a minute amount of a number of different common allergens is inserted into the skin by a shallow injection. Atopic people may show a small area of reddening and swelling around the site of the prick over the next couple of days. This is a confirmation of sensitivity to that allergen. Skin-prick tests can be useful for people with atopy as they can identify which of the common allergens should be avoided.

Atopic people with asthma often have characteristic symptoms of allergy from early childhood. However, some people only develop asthma in later life, and these people seem to be less sensitive to the common allergens. In practice, the treatment of both types of asthma is similar, although adult onset asthma tends to be less fully reversible and, because of this, shows some degree of overlap with the syndrome of chronic obstructive pulmonary disease (COPD; see Section 3.3e).

Asthma does seem to be more common in Western cultures, and its reported incidence, particularly in children, is on the increase. The reasons for this are unclear, although some conventional theories attribute the rise to increases in urban living, and exposure to household damp, cigarette smoke and other atmospheric pollutants in industrial countries. This fits with the observation that asthma is a very common finding in some industries in which the workforce is more exposed to certain chemicals in the atmosphere. The hygiene hypothesis is currently popular, which suggests that early exposure to environmental germs from the land and animals is protective against asthma. For example, studies show that children who have grown up on farms or who have been exposed to dogs are less likely to get asthma.[63]

The symptoms of an asthma attack result from the narrowing and blocking of the airways by inflammation and mucus. The attack may develop within seconds to minutes after exposure to an allergen, to cold or extreme emotion, or may be delayed by a few hours. The person will feel increasing difficulty in breathing. Many people find it hard to say whether it is breathing in or out that is most difficult, but lung function tests will often demonstrate a much prolonged expiration time. This is an objective measure of difficulty breathing out.

During an asthma attack, the act of breathing becomes hard work, and because not so much oxygen is reaching the lungs, the breathing rate increases to make up for this. The sensation of not being able to get air into the chest can induce panic in many people, which can further affect the breathing pattern, as well as worsen the asthma attack itself. A common symptom is the production of a wheezy noise, particularly on breathing out, which results from the air whistling through the narrowed airways. However, dry cough may be the only symptom in mild cases, which may confuse the diagnosis, particularly in children.

In mild cases the attack can settle down in minutes to hours, but often the breathing is affected for a few days afterwards, during which time the lungs are particularly sensitive to further attacks.

In severe cases the breathing never fully settles down to normal as the lungs gradually "remodel" in response to recurrent inflammation. The person with severe asthma can be always wheezy and breathless, and may suffer frequent bouts of worsening breathlessness on top of this.

In all cases the symptoms get worse at night. Waking at night with cough or difficulty breathing is an indication that the asthma is quite severe. It is well known that asthma attacks can be at their worst in the early hours of the morning.

In some cases an attack can lead to such an extreme reduction in the width of the airways that the patient is simply unable to inhale sufficient oxygen for their requirements. As the attack worsens, the respiratory rate increases to a severe level (30 breaths/minute or more). A patient in this state will need to hold themselves still and upright and will be reluctant or unable to talk freely. The heart rate becomes rapid (100–130 beats/minute) as a result of the body's response to the stress of not having enough oxygen (adrenaline is released). This extreme condition is unlikely to settle of its own accord and is termed status asthmaticus. All the features described here are red flags of severe disease.

The development of status asthmaticus can be so rapid and extreme that without urgent treatment the person can die. It requires treatment with oxygen and drugs to reverse the narrowing of the airways. This dangerous form of asthma is most likely to occur in those who have suffered from severe asthma for some time. Occasionally, it can develop out of the blue in someone who has previously had only minor symptoms or even no symptoms at all.

Asthma is diagnosed on the basis of the symptoms and by means of lung function tests. These tests indicate that the force and length of expiration is abnormal when the patient encounters one or more of the factors that trigger the attacks. A distinguishing feature of asthma is that this abnormality usually improves when the triggers are removed or when appropriate treatments are given. A chest X-ray image is usually normal in asthma.

The simplest measure of expiration is the peak expiratory flow rate, which is measured using a hand-held peak flow meter. This gives an objective measure of the force with which the person can blow out. The figure obtained has to be adjusted for the patient's size and sex. The patient has to be carefully instructed in how to blow into the meter, or the readings obtained will not be helpful.

The peak flow meter can demonstrate the hour-to-hour variability in peak flow rate that is characteristic of asthma. It is used in general practice and by patients at home to monitor their current state and response to treatment.

Ideally, the peak flow should be in the normal range for the person's size and sex, and should show very little variability at different times of the day.

Figure 3.3d-I shows a graph of the peak flow readings taken three times a day by a person with asthma over the course of two weeks. It can be seen that in the first few days the peak flow measurements show great variation, with the lowest readings occurring in the early morning. In this patient, treatment with corticosteroid medication affects this pattern, leading to a general improvement in peak flow rate and a marked reduction in the variability of the peak flow.

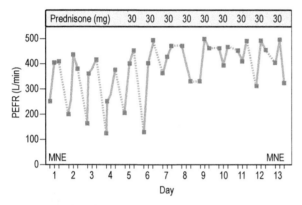

Figure 3.3d-I The day-to-day variability in peak flow rate in a patient with asthma and the response to corticosteroid medication (started on day 5)
MNE: morning, noon and evening

A good measure of successful treatment of asthma is that the hour-to-hour variability of the peak flow measurements is reduced. This is an important point to be appreciated when using peak flow readings to monitor the effects of acupuncture treatment. For useful monitoring it is necessary to look at measurements taken at different times of the day, over the course of a few days, and this, of course, requires the patient's help in taking measurements at home.

The treatment of asthma depends on the severity of the condition. Because it is such an important condition, the British Thoracic Society and Scottish Intercollegiate Guidelines Network have produced guidelines for the management of asthma, which are now highly respected amongst doctors in the UK.[64] These are comparable to the guidelines produced by the National Institute of Health and Care Excellence (NICE) for the management of hypertension, in that they grade the asthma according to certain features, and then recommend treatment and lifestyle advice for each grade of asthma.[65]

The guidelines advise on a stepwise management of asthma, which is summarized in detail in Section 3.1 of the *British National Formulary* (BNF).[66] The general points about

the management of asthma that can be distilled from these guidelines are that there are three broad types of treatment:

- avoidance of triggers (including allergens, smoking and family stress)

- use of drugs called bronchodilators to reduce the narrowing of the airways (by inhaler or tablets)

- use of anti-inflammatory drugs, in particular corticosteroids, to reduce the development of inflammation in the airways (by inhaler or tablets).

All patients with even very mild symptoms may be offered a bronchodilator. This type of drug, usually administered by an inhaler, rapidly reverses the narrowing of the airways in asthma. The drug most commonly prescribed is salbutamol. This is taken whenever breathing becomes limited, although this should not be necessary more than once or twice a day in mild asthma. Salbutamol mimics the effect of adrenaline (the other name for this group of drugs is beta stimulant – the action is directly opposite to that of beta blockers), and can therefore have the side effects of increased heart rate and a sensation of anxiety and sleeplessness, although these would be unusual at a dose of one or two inhaled puffs a day.

In all but the mildest forms of asthma (when salbutamol is required more than three times a week, or more than once at night) the guidance is to add in a regular dose of an anti-inflammatory drug to be used in addition to the bronchodilator. This means that most people with asthma will be prescribed two inhalers, one to be taken when they feel wheezy (the bronchodilator), and one to be taken twice a day (the anti-inflammatory). In adults the most commonly prescribed anti-inflammatory drug is a corticosteroid (e.g. beclomethasone and fluticasone). In children, a drug called sodium cromoglicate may be used first, although many children will eventually be prescribed a steroid inhaler because it seems to work better for them.

Both bronchodilators and anti-inflammatory drugs are taken in mild to moderate cases of asthma by inhaler, because this is known to concentrate the drug in the lungs and thus general side effects to the rest of the body are minimized.

It is important to recognize that to give a steroid inhaler to people with mild asthma is considered good practice in conventional medicine. This is because use of the steroid in all but the mildest cases has been shown to reduce the severity and frequency of severe attacks. Studies indicate that regular inhaled steroids reduce the numbers of cases of status asthmaticus and deaths from asthma.

Important side effects from the steroid inhalers include hoarseness of voice due to an effect on the vocal cords, thrush in the mouth and slight growth retardation in children. All these appear to be significant only when very high doses are given.

In more severe cases of asthma the dose and frequency of bronchodilators and anti-inflammatory drugs is increased. The next recommended step is that a long-acting form of beta agonist (such as salmeterol) is prescribed. Another medication that is currently recommended as an adjunct in asthma that has not responded fully to inhaled beta agonists and steroids alone is one of the leukotriene receptor antagonists such as montelukast. Oral theophyllines are also recommended as an additional type of bronchodilator. If the asthma still fails to settle, regular dosing with corticosteroid tablets may have to be initiated, and for some patients, long-term corticosteroid therapy is a necessity in order to prevent life-threatening exacerbations of the condition.

In an acute bout of asthma, the guidelines suggest that the patient is advised to step up the dose of steroids rapidly in order to control the symptoms, and only to reduce back to the usual dose once the bout has settled down again. In a very severe attack steroids may be given by tablet or even intravenously, and bronchodilators may be given in very high doses via a mask and a machine called a nebulizer. Some patients with severe asthma may have both a nebulizer and access to oxygen at home to deal with sudden severe attacks.

A patient in status asthmaticus is usually treated in hospital with oxygen and intravenous steroids and bronchodilators, and medical care may be offered in the setting of an intensive care unit.

 Information box 3.3d-III

Asthma: comments from a Chinese medicine perspective

In Chinese medicine, the breathing difficulties of asthma have various descriptors including the term Xiao-Chuan, which describes the combination of wheezing and breathlessness that occurs in asthma. However, the differentiation of asthma is complex and depends on the symptoms of the individual.

In most cases, the commonly recognized symptoms point to an underlying Deficiency of the Qi of both the Lungs and the Kidney. Kidney Qi Deficiency appears to be particularly prominent in atopic individuals. In Chinese medicine, Lung Qi is important for the action of expiration and Kidney Qi for inspiration (the Kidneys are said to grasp Lung Qi in inspiration).

Combined Lung and Kidney Qi Deficiency predisposes to Invasion of Wind Cold or Wind Heat, which can in itself lead to an acute bout of asthma. The rapidity with which some attacks follow exposure to certain allergens is characteristic of Wind Invasion. In many cases, mucus and phlegm is a prominent feature, and this would be a manifestation of Accumulation of Phlegm, or Retention of Phlegm Heat. Anger and frustration leading to an asthma attack would be diagnosed as Liver Qi insulting the Lungs.

Bronchodilators allow the relaxation of the tight smooth muscle of the airways and do this by mimicking adrenaline, a hormone released by the adrenal glands. The function of adrenaline is Yang and Moving in nature. Bronchodilators therefore Boost Kidney Yang and also Move Stagnant Qi. Their action is suppressive in nature because they do not deal with the root cause of the problem, which returns when they wear off. It is possible that frequent use of bronchodilators is Depleting to the Kidneys, Lungs and the Heart because they produce excessive stimulation of the functions of these Organs.

Anti-inflammatory drugs appear to Subdue Heat and Phlegm, which could be interpreted as the result of the inflammation and mucus in asthma. They would also appear to Boost Lung and Kidney Qi, as their use prevents further attacks of asthma. Again, these drugs are suppressive because they do not cure the root problem, which will recur, although sometimes at a much later date, when the drugs are withdrawn. This would imply that the removal of the asthma symptoms is at the cost of Accumulation of Heat and Phlegm at deeper levels. Long-term Depletion of the Kidneys and Lungs may result, so that a dependence on the drugs may be induced.

Chronic obstructive pulmonary disease (COPD): chronic bronchitis

Chronic obstructive pulmonary disease (COPD) (a term that embraces the conditions formerly described as chronic bronchitis and emphysema) is a very common degenerative and inflammatory condition of the lungs. It is the result of a combination of recurrent infections and smoking (or other damaging factors including atmospheric pollutants) causing long-term (chronic) changes in the lining of the bronchi and bronchioles. COPD is defined in terms of a restriction in airflow in the lungs, which, unlike asthma, is fixed and not reversible.

One significant change in COPD is that the mucus cells of the respiratory epithelium tend to produce thick, sticky mucus in excess. Because of smoking or pollutants, the cilia are not functioning well, and the mucus cannot be cleared efficiently. These changes in themselves encourage the development of further infections and inflammation of the lining of the air passages. The chronic inflammation leads to swelling of the air passages and thus a reduction in their internal diameter. This restricts easy breathing, and breathing can become labored or wheezy. These changes are what were formerly described as chronic bronchitis, which is actually a very apt descriptive term for the underlying disease processes.

At the same time the delicate structure of the alveoli can also become affected by the chronic inflammatory processes of COPD. The alveolar walls break down, leading to larger air spaces in the depth of the lungs that are less efficient at the task of transfer of gases. This is the process described as emphysema, described in more detail in Section 3.3e.

COPD affects most smokers and is estimated to be grossly under-diagnosed, with one estimate suggesting that 85 percent of people with COPD, almost all of whom will be smokers, have not received a formal diagnosis.[67]

The initial changes in the bronchi and bronchioles are reversible, and the damage to alveoli preventable if the patient can stop smoking. However, in long-standing cases the airways become permanently scarred as a result of the inflammation, and remain narrowed and irregular, and the airspaces in the chest may become permanently inflated and less able to perform their role.

 Information box 3.3d-IV

COPD (Chronic bronchitis): comments from a Chinese medicine perspective

In Chinese medicine, depending on the precise symptoms, the symptoms of COPD could fit with either one of Damp Phlegm or Phlegm Heat Obstructing the Lungs. Both of these are chronic conditions in which the Pathogens are primarily internally generated.

Stopping smoking will both enable the recovery of damaged Lung Yin and remove a potent source of Phlegm and Heat. This is, if course, an energetically appropriate treatment. Antibiotics tend to be suppressive, but may be necessary to prevent progressive damage to the lungs in a persistent case of bacterial infection. Vaccinations do indeed protect against damaging infections, but may introduce additional problems in the forms of Heat Toxins in those who are vulnerable.

Once COPD is established, the patient is more prone to further bouts of acute bronchitis (infections), which then worsen the ongoing inflammation. A vicious cycle of progressive damage is established, particularly if the patient is unable to give up smoking. The damage often goes hand in hand with smoking-related damage deeper in the lung.

The treatment of chronic bronchitis is to offer smoking cessation advice and support, and to avoid pollutants and infections (including offering flu and pneumococcal pneumonia vaccines). Conventional advice is to treat any bacterial infections promptly with antibiotics to minimize further damage to the lining of the air passages.

The more systematic management of COPD as a chronic disease is described in Section 3.3e.

Bronchiectasis

Bronchiectasis is the term used to describe a condition in which the airways have become permanently distorted and dilated, usually as the result of a severe infection. The damaged air passages are unable to be fully cleared of mucus because the cilia on the respiratory epithelium are no longer functional, and this means that chronic infection is commonly present in these parts of the airways.

A person with bronchiectasis will always produce phlegm, sometimes in large quantities, and is more prone to bouts of acute bronchitis, which may, of course, worsen the underlying condition. The phlegm predisposes to further infections, but is also the cause of ongoing inflammation and scarring of the airways. Rarely, the affected area can bleed, and the patient will cough up blood. In some cases this bleeding can be so profuse as to be life-threatening.

The most common cause of bronchiectasis used to be whooping cough (pertussis) in childhood, but this has become much less common as the health of Western populations has improved, and since the introduction of the pertussis vaccination. Now, the most common cause of this condition is the congenital disease cystic fibrosis, discussed in more detail below.

It is very important for the patient with bronchiectasis to clear the excessive mucus that accumulates in the damaged airways. In severe cases, a physiotherapist can help the patient to cough up the phlegm while the patient is in a tipped position (postural drainage).

It is believed that any infections should be treated rapidly with antibiotics so that further damage to the structure of the airways is prevented.

In very severe progressive cases, the only option for the patient is to have a heart-lung transplant. The heart is removed at the same time as the lungs in this condition because it, too, is damaged as a result of the long-term strain of pumping blood through scarred lungs (see Section 3.2f, where it is described how chronic lung disease is one of the causes of chronic heart failure). As with a heart transplant, a heart-lung transplant is a risky procedure for the patient, and requires long-term immunosuppressive medication after recovery from the operation. Only 70 percent of patients who have this operation will still be alive three years after the operation.

Information box 3.3d-V

Bronchiectasis: comments from a Chinese medicine perspective

In Chinese medicine, the signs and symptoms of bronchiectasis would correspond to the chronic conditions of Accumulation of Phlegm or Phlegm Heat Obstructing the Lungs. Although the initial damage may have been triggered by an infection and a Pathogen of external origin, the severity of the condition indicates that the Phlegm and Heat is largely of internal origin.

The tendency to Heat and the destruction of the structure of the lungs implies that the underlying deficiency was originally of Lung Yin. Profuse bleeding and profuse discolored phlegm are both indications of Full Heat.

Postural drainage is an energetically appropriate therapy, as it enables the clearance of Phlegm/Heat, which is, of course, the natural tendency of the body.

Although antibiotics are known to slow the progression of the condition, they deal only with the manifestation of the problem, and are therefore suppressive in nature. Their energetic nature is Cold and Damp, which can predispose to the formation of more Phlegm by injuring the action of Spleen. However, it is difficult to argue against their use in bronchiectasis, as there is good evidence for benefit in terms of prolonged life expectancy. Ideally the patient using them should make appropriate lifestyle changes in terms of diet and emotions, and receive supportive treatment focused on nourishing Spleen and Lung energy.

Cystic fibrosis (CF)

Cystic fibrosis (CF) is a relatively common inherited condition, which usually occurs when a baby inherits a CF gene from each parent. This occurs in just under one in 2000 births. The carriage of one form of this gene is common, with one in 22 Caucasians possessing it. However, most carriers are totally unaware of the fact that they are carriers because the condition is, in genetic terms, a recessive condition. This means that it only manifests if the person carries two CF genes, one from each parent. Because of the nature of the recessive inheritance of the condition, most babies born with CF used not to be diagnosed for some months to years after birth. Some genes lead to more serious disease than others, and so the presentation of the disease in different individuals is wide-ranging in terms of severity.

The main problem in CF is that the mucus produced by the body is excessively thick and sticky. This is of particular significance in the lower respiratory tract, where the healthy production of mucus is an important barrier to disease. This means that a baby with CF will have frequent infections of the lower respiratory tract, including bouts of pneumonia. As the child gets older, phlegmy conditions of the nose and throat, such as sinusitis, also become frequent. The inability to clear the thickened secretions in infection means that the permanent and progressive condition of bronchiectasis may develop early in life, particularly if the condition is not diagnosed until relatively late.

The other major physical problem of CF is related to the digestive tract. Thickened secretions in the pancreas can lead to a failure to produce sufficient pancreatic enzymes. This leads to a form of malabsorption, as described in Section 3.1e. The management of this complication of CF is by means of artificial pancreatic enzymes, which can be taken by mouth with meals.

CF also causes male infertility, as the underlying problem of CF affects the development of sperm. Although women with CF are technically fertile, the ill health caused by the condition leads to failure of ovulation in many women.

CF can also predispose to liver failure and diabetes as a result of the progressive damage to the bile ducts and pancreas.

Diagnosis of CF can now be informed by means of a neonatal test, which, since 2007, has been offered to all babies in the UK as part of the Guthrie blood spot analysis test. If this test is positive, a more specific genetic test for the CF mutations is performed. The definitive diagnosis is made by means of sweat analysis, which reveals abnormally high sodium and chloride levels. This means that most babies are now diagnosed shortly after birth, and this has dramatically improved the prognosis.

Treatment of CF involves promoting physical activity, meticulous attention to clearing of phlegm by postural drainage and rapid treatment of infections with antibiotics. Vaccination against influenza and pneumococcal pneumonia is performed. High antibiotic use leads to problems of antibiotic resistance in many patients with CF, who, by adulthood, will be carrying bacteria that are no longer affected by the common antibiotics. This has become so problematic that patients with CF may be advised not to mix with other patients with CF or another chronic lung disease in order to prevent transmission of these resistant "super-bugs." This has obvious effects in terms of social isolation, particularly when the patient with CF has to be hospitalized. Drugs that break down mucus (dornase alpha) may be administered by means of a nebulizer with some benefit.

Recently, in-depth knowledge of how the gene defect in CF causes faulty mucus production has led to research into the development of some powerful designer drug therapies. CF is one of the few genetic diseases in which the use of a normal gene, cloned into virus vectors from healthy human cells, has been used to produce some benefit to patients. These treatments are still in the experimental stages, and are not yet widely available.

Even in recent decades, people with CF were not expected to live past their mid-teens, but now most people with the disease live well into adulthood. Children born today with CF are expected to live to the age of 40–50, a 10–20 year increase on the median life expectancy of 30 in 1990. This improvement is attributed to early recognition of the disease and skilled attention to the excessive phlegmy secretions and frequent infections. Nevertheless, progressive lung damage due to bronchiectasis or uncontrollable infection or liver failure will eventually lead to an early death in most people with CF. Heart-lung or liver transplant may be available to those whose life expectancy is less than 18 months, but two-thirds of patients in the UK waiting for this procedure will die before a suitable donor organ becomes available.[68]

The genetic test that can reveal carriage of a mutated CF gene is currently only available, for cost reasons, to couples planning to have children who have someone with CF in their immediate family.

Information box 3.3d-VI

Cystic fibrosis: comments from a Chinese medicine perspective

In Chinese medicine, the presentation of CF would carry a similar range of diagnoses to bronchiectasis with Accumulation of Phlegm and Phlegm Heat manifesting on a background of Spleen, Lung and Kidney Deficiency. The severity of the condition in later years would indicate that Stagnant Heat has led to Depletion of Yin and also Blood Stagnation. The inherited nature of the condition and its effect on fertility suggests that Jing Deficiency is the predisposing cause. Malabsorption due to pancreatic failure might be seen as a manifestation of Spleen Qi Deficiency leading to Blood Deficiency.

Cancer of the bronchus (lung cancer)

Lung cancer accounts for 19 percent of cancer diagnoses in the UK, and 27 percent of cancer deaths. In most cases of lung cancer the site of the tumor is in the bronchi or bronchioles. Only 2 percent of all lung cancers actually originate in an alveolus. This is because the main trigger for lung cancer is of external origin, most commonly (in 90 percent of cases) being the carcinogens in cigarette smoke. Other important lung carcinogens include asbestos, iron oxides and environmental radon. Because of the protective nature of the lining of the airways of the lower respiratory tract, toxins such as those contained in cigarette smoke are deposited on the walls of the airways before they have a chance to reach the alveoli.

Lung cancer is the third most common cause of death in the UK after heart disease and pneumonia. It used to be a disease that affected men much more than women, but is now known to be increasing in women. This is attributed to the rapid increase in smoking in women, which began in the middle of the 20th century and is continuing, particularly in younger women.

Lung cancer develops from one of the lining cells of the respiratory epithelium. As it grows to obstruct the airway it can cause symptoms such as a cough, with or without phlegm, or heavy chest pain. Occasionally, a first symptom is coughing up of small amounts of blood, a symptom referred to as hemoptysis. Less common first symptoms result from quite advanced disease, and include breathlessness, loss of weight, hoarseness and enlarged lymph nodes in the neck. Hoarseness can occur because the nerve that supplies the larynx passes deep within the chest and so can be damaged by a spreading lung cancer.

Advanced lung cancer can compress the other structures in the chest cavity to cause difficulty in swallowing and swelling of the face and neck. In an advanced case breathlessness might become very severe, because the growing cancer is secreting fluid that accumulates in the pleural space and compresses the lung (pleural effusion). The presence of the obstructing tumor increases the risk of infection, and pneumonia can develop in advanced disease.

The cancer tends to spread first to the lymph nodes deep within the chest and then most commonly to the bones, leading to deep bone pain and risk of fracture. Spread to the liver and the brain is also fairly common.

A chest X-ray image will reveal the presence of a shadow on the lung field of many people who have symptoms due to lung cancer, although in up to 10 percent of cases a chest X-ray may actually appear normal. The diagnosis is confirmed by examination of the sputum for cancer cells and by means of a bronchoscopy, when a biopsy may be taken for accurate diagnosis of the type of cancer. A computed tomography (CT) scan is usually performed to look for evidence of spread to the lymph nodes or the liver. This is important for staging of the cancer.

Fifteen percent of cases are the rarer and chemotherapy-sensitive small cell cancer, but the remaining 85 percent consist of different forms of lung cancer that are known not to respond well to chemotherapy, and not dramatically well to radiotherapy. Moreover, most of these tumors are too advanced at diagnosis to be removed by surgery. Of the small percentage of patients with cancers that can be removed by surgery, only one-fifth will be still alive after five years. If surgery is not possible, high-dose radiotherapy may slow the progression of the disease, but still has a low overall cure rate. The few cancers that are known to respond to chemotherapy (small cell tumors) do so rapidly and dramatically, but in most cases they tend to recur after a few months. Rarely, chemotherapy can give a few years of remission from the tumor.

Most lung cancers, unless diagnosed very early in their development, are very resistant to modern cancer treatment. Only 5.5 percent of all people treated for lung cancer will be alive ten years after diagnosis, and this figure represents an improvement compared to previous decades. In most people who receive such therapies, the most that can be expected is a few more months of life, with, hopefully, a reduction in distressing symptoms for this period.

Palliative care includes radiotherapy for painful bone tumors and rapidly enlarging tumors in the chest. Corticosteroids and strong morphine-based painkillers can improve mood, appetite and the sensation of breathlessness.

 Information box 3.3d-VII

Lung cancer: comments from a Chinese medicine perspective

In Chinese medicine, lung cancer, like most cancers, may be seen as Phlegm and Blood Stagnation on a background of long-standing Deficiency of Yin and/or Yang. It can be differentiated into various presentations that include Lung Heat and Yin Deficiency, Phlegm Damp Stasis in the Lung, and Blood Stasis with Pathogenic heat, and these may overlap with each other. In lung cancer, which is almost always associated with long-term smoking, the background deficiency is likely to be of Lung Yin. This fits with the recognition that modern treatments, which tend to be Heating and therefore Depleting of Yin, are not very successful in lung cancer. Also, the pattern of Qi or Blood Stagnation from emotional repression is likely to be apparent, and will contribute to the Pathology of Stasis seen in all forms of cancer. All these treatment approaches are, of course, suppressive in nature.

Breathlessness

In contrast to the diseases of the upper respiratory tract, one key feature of diseases of the bronchi and bronchioles is breathlessness. Usually any inflammation above the voice box will not be sufficiently severe as to compromise intake of air to the lungs. Coughs and colds and laryngitis may be uncomfortable, but will not affect the amount of

oxygen reaching the lungs. The exception to this rule is the extreme upper respiratory obstruction that might occur in epiglottitis and inhalation of a foreign body (leading to the harsh inspiratory and expiratory noise of stridor).

Inflammation or constriction of the smaller airways will often lead to reduced exchange of oxygen and carbon dioxide because of the restriction to airflow posed by the narrowed air passages. The brainstem responds to the increased carbon dioxide and reduced oxygen levels in the bloodstream that result from poor gas exchange, and stimulates deeper and more rapid breathing. The patient will experience this as breathlessness.

The normal respiratory rate for a healthy adult is 10–20 breaths/minute. In breathlessness, this rate is increased and, particularly if of recent onset, the patient has a sensation of difficulty in breathing. For the purposes of this section, a respiratory rate of more than 30 breaths/minute is classified as moderate breathlessness, and a rate of 60 breaths/minute is classified as severe breathlessness (see Table 3.3d-I). The corresponding rates for children are higher (see Table 3.3d-II).

Table 3.3d-I Categorization of the respiratory rate in adults

Category	Rate
Normal respiratory rate in an adult	10–20 breaths per minute (one breath is one inhalation and exhalation)
Moderate breathlessness in an adult	>30 breaths per minute
Severe breathlessness in an adult	>60 breaths per minute

Table 3.3d-II Categorization of the respiratory rate in children

Category	Rate
The normal range for respiratory rate in children varies according to age	
The following rates indicate moderate to severe breathlessness:	
Newborn (0–3 months)	>60 breaths per minute
Infant (3 months to 2 years)	>50 breaths per minute
Young child (2–8 years)	>40 breaths per minute
Older child to adult	>30 breaths per minute

Moderate or severe breathlessness of recent onset, which is also associated with a fever, suggests infection of the lungs themselves (pneumonia) rather than the bronchi (bronchitis). This serious condition is now described in Section 3.3e.

3.3e Diseases of the alveoli and pleura

This concluding section on the respiratory system looks at those diseases that primarily affect the deepest parts of the lung tissue – the tiny air spaces called the alveoli. For completeness, the diseases that can affect the pleural linings are also discussed. The conditions studied here are as follows.

- Deep infections of the lower respiratory tract:
  - pneumonia
  - pleurisy
  - tuberculosis (TB)
- Emphysema and chronic obstructive pulmonary disease (COPD)
- Fibrosis of the lung and occupational lung disease
- Pulmonary embolism and infarction
- Common causes of collapse of the lung.

Deep infections of the lower respiratory tract

Pneumonia

Pneumonia is the term used to describe a deep inflammation of the lung tissue that involves the airspaces or alveoli, and is most commonly a result of infection.

Pneumonia is the second most common cause of death in the UK according to the information obtained from death certificates. This is a slightly misleading statistic, however, because very commonly an episode of bronchopneumonia is the final event that causes death in elderly people who have become frail for a variety of other underlying reasons, such as Alzheimer's disease, cancer or chronic heart failure. For this reason, pneumonia has somewhat cynically been termed "the old man's friend" because it can lead to a relatively rapid and pain-free death in people who are reaching the end of their natural lives.

However, pneumonia can also be a devastating and depleting illness in people of all ages, and used to be a dreaded cause of many premature deaths as recently as the earlier decades of the 20th century. In recent years, the improvement in the general health of the population, together with the use of antibiotics, has changed this situation. Nowadays, deaths from acute pneumonia are relatively rare except in those who have some form of immunodeficiency resulting from conditions such as cancer or acquired immune deficiency syndrome (AIDS).

Pneumonia can be caused by a wide range of infectious agents, including viruses, bacteria and fungi. However, in contrast to the other infections of the respiratory tract, which tend to be viral in origin, an episode of pneumonia is more likely to be caused by bacteria, which tend to produce much more severe inflammation and more pus (coughed up as colored phlegm) than viruses. This is an indication that pneumonia is a condition that tends to affect those who are already energetically depleted in some way. In healthy people, the defense mechanisms of the respiratory tract are able to prevent the penetration of external infectious agents to the deep parts of the lung. The most common forms of bacterial pneumonia are caused by bacteria that can reside harmlessly in the respiratory tract of healthy people (most importantly, *Streptococcus pneumoniae* and *Haemophilus influenzae*).

In pneumonia, the inflammation leads to damage to the delicate alveolar lining and accumulation of fluid and cell debris within the air spaces. This causes irritation and a marked reduction in the amount of oxygen that can enter the blood from each in-breath. In the most common form of bacterial infection, the inflammation is confined to a single lobe of one lung. This is termed lobar pneumonia. In other forms of pneumonia, the inflammation can be more widespread, with the smaller bronchioles also becoming inflamed. This is called bronchopneumonia.

The primary symptoms of pneumonia are cough (which may be dry or productive of colored phlegm) and moderate to severe breathlessness. The patient will feel unwell and feverish, although the severity of these symptoms depends on the nature of the infection and the strength of the individual. In some cases the breathlessness can be so severe as to require emergency treatment. The features of severe breathlessness are similar to those of severe asthma. A rapid respiratory rate of 30 breaths per minute or more, needing to sit up and sit still to breathe, and difficulty in talking are serious signs. A blue discoloration of the tongue and lips, known as cyanosis, is a very severe sign indicating that there is insufficient oxygen reaching the blood.

At this stage in a severe infection, the patient may be so ill that they do not have the energy to maintain rapid respirations. Breathing may become shallower and the patient may drift in and out of consciousness. This state, when the level of oxygen in the blood cannot be maintained, is called respiratory failure, and the patient requires emergency treatment to prevent death.

In hospitals the severity of pneumonia is graded according to four parameters (the CRB-65 scoring system). The factors that are recognized to predict a more serious outcome include confusion, rapid respiratory rate (>30 breaths/minute) and low systolic blood pressure, and age greater than 65. A low CRB-65 score helps a doctor to decide that the episode can be safely managed at home.

In all types of pneumonia the investigations and treatment are similar. X-ray images and sputum samples are taken to assess the extent of infection and to diagnose the type of infection. Blood tests can be used to provide evidence either of infectious agents or of a recent immune response, and this can help diagnose the type of infection.

According to the type of infection, appropriate antibiotics are prescribed, initially to be taken by mouth. If breathlessness is severe, the patient is given emergency support in hospital. This may include the administration of oxygen, with antibiotics given intravenously. Oxygen may be administered under a degree of pressure by a close-fitting mask to assist in gaseous exchange (this is known as continuous positive airway pressure (CPAP) or bi-level positive airway pressure (BIPAP)). Occasionally, the patient may have to receive assisted breathing on a mechanical ventilator in an intensive care unit (known as ventilation).

LOBAR PNEUMONIA

Approximately half of all cases of pneumonia are lobar pneumonia, in which the infectious agent is a bacterium called *Streptococcus pneumoniae*. In lobar pneumonia the infection is often confined to a single lobe of one lung and the overlying pleural linings of that lobe. This infection tends to affect people who are depleted in some way or have pre-existing lung damage. It may also follow on from a viral infection of other parts of the respiratory tract.

In this streptococcal pneumonia there is a rapid onset of very high fever, breathlessness and cough. Pain may be felt on inspiration on one side of the chest. A common sign is the development of a cold sore, which is a well-known response to high fever.

Most cases should respond to the antibiotics benzylpenicillin, amoxicillin or erythromycin, although the full period of recovery from the infection is usually long. After treatment has been completed, the patient is frequently left in a state of exhaustion, which can last for some weeks. Chest X-ray images are used to ensure that the infection has cleared from the chest and that there are no other underlying problems in the lung, such as cancer, which may have led to the infection in the first place. Full recovery is less likely in the very frail.

Another severe bacterial pneumonia is caused by the organism *Staphylococcus aureus*, which can reside harmlessly on the skin and in the nose. This organism tends to infect already damaged lungs, and it most commonly occurs when frail individuals develop viral infections such as measles or influenza. Staphylococcal and streptococcal pneumonia account for many of the deaths that occur in epidemics of influenza.

OTHER PNEUMONIAS

Most other common forms of pneumonia are usually less severe than lobar pneumonia. About one-third of community-acquired pneumonias are caused by "atypical" microorganisms, and most commonly *Mycoplasma*. This infection tends to affect younger people, and leads to vague drawn-out symptoms such as headache, mild fever, tiredness and occasional cough. Because of the vague symptoms, diagnosis may be delayed, but usually the infection responds to antibiotics. Occasionally, a protracted state of exhaustion may also result from this infection.

LEGIONNAIRES' DISEASE

Legionnaires' disease is another less common but severe form of pneumonia resulting from an atypical bacterium called *Legionella pneumophila*. This microorganism spreads in water storage systems and gets dispersed in droplets of water emerging from taps and showers. It is contracted by inhalation and leads to a severe systemic disease that can also cause widespread organ failure in severe cases, and especially in older patients. Both Legionnaires' disease and *Mycoplasma* pneumonia respond to antibiotics such as clarithromycin.

OPPORTUNISTIC PNEUMONIAS

Opportunistic diseases are those that affect individuals with immunodeficiency. Opportunistic pneumonias are a significant cause of ill health and death in those who are immunocompromised. Diagnosis may be delayed because these conditions do not often lead to such marked symptoms as other types of pneumonia.

One of the most common types of opportunistic pneumonia in AIDS patients is *Pneumocystis* pneumonia (PCP), caused by a fungus, the spores of which are inhaled from the air. The symptoms may appear gradually over the period of a few weeks, with cough and slight fevers. Without early treatment, the infection can cause severe lung damage, and the patient may eventually require ventilation. This pneumonia responds to antibiotics including cotrimoxazole (Septrin) and pentamidine, although these are most effective if given early in the course of the disease. Patients will then be advised to continue taking low doses of these antibiotics in the long term to prevent relapse of the infection. Dapsone and atovaquone are alternative medications that may be administered in certain cases.

BRONCHOPNEUMONIA

Bronchopneumonia is a form of pneumonia that affects a much-depleted patient and can be caused by a range of the infectious agents already described. In this condition the inflammation spreads to involve a diffuse area of the lungs and bronchioles, and often occurs because the patient is unable to cough up the thickened lung secretions that result from inflammation. This is the form of pneumonia that is commonly the actual cause of death in frail patients who are close to the end of their natural lives.

Pleurisy

Pleurisy is the term used to describe the pain that develops when the pleural lining of the lung is inflamed. The most common cause of pleurisy is infection, although it can also result from lung cancer and also from the lung infarction caused by a pulmonary embolus (see later).

Lobar pneumonia frequently leads to pleurisy because it usually causes inflammation that extends to the outer margins of the lung tissue. Another less serious cause of pleurisy is a virus infection, which can affect the pleural lining without infecting the lung itself.

In pleurisy the patient experiences a localized, sharp and sometimes severe pain that is worse on deep breathing and twisting movements of the chest. The pain is provoked when the two inflamed pleural linings rub against each other. Sometimes this rubbing can be heard as a scratchy noise through a stethoscope.

The treatment of pleurisy is by treating the underlying cause and giving painkillers for relief of symptoms. This is of particular importance in pneumonia as the pain of pleurisy can be so severe as to inhibit deep breathing and coughing, which are important for the healing of the infection. Viral pleurisy, although very painful, will get better spontaneously within a few days.

 Information box 3.3e-I

Pneumonia and pleurisy: comments from a Chinese medicine perspective

In Chinese medicine, an uncomplicated case of pneumonia would correspond to Lung Heat or Lung Phlegm Heat at the Qi Level, according to the Four Levels categorization. The cough and breathlessness are due to Heat or Phlegm Heat obstructing the descent of Lung Qi.

The rapidity of development of some pneumonias, including lobar pneumonia, is an indication that Invasion of Wind Heat can be an initiating cause. The cold sore that commonly occurs in pneumonia is a manifestation of Wind Damp Heat.

As pneumonia frequently occurs on a background of deficiency, this suggests that there is a pre-existing Deficiency of the Lung, probably of Lung Yin, and that the Pathogenic Factors are, at least in part, internally generated as a consequence of the deficiency.

The intense pain of pleurisy would normally be associated with Stagnation of Blood and Qi in the chest. In pneumonia this probably is a result of Heat, and in viral infection may be ascribed to Wind Invasion.

Tuberculosis (TB)

Tuberculosis (TB) is an infection caused by a bacteria-like organism called *Mycobacterium tuberculosis*. This causes a particular form of deep lung infection that is unlike the other forms of pneumonia already discussed.

TB of the lung develops after inhalation of infected droplets, after which the organism settles most often in the upper part of one lung. In most healthy individuals the immune system deals with this primary infection and the person develops immunity without experiencing any symptoms. The organism can also enter the digestive tract through infected milk, but this does not now occur in the UK because of the two practices of screening of cattle for infection and pasteurization of milk.

In depleted individuals in particular, the immune response to the primary infection may lead to a prolonged inflammatory reaction at the site of the infection, after which the infection is not necessarily fully cleared. Instead, a firm nodule is left at the site of this infection, which can be seen on a chest X-ray image, together with enlarged lymph nodes at the center of the chest. In these individuals there might be a vague illness, with fluctuating fever and cough over the course of a few weeks. In some of these cases the inflammation may eventually settle down, but in other cases it can progress over the course of weeks to months to involve more of the lung tissue. This can result in pneumonia and bronchiectasis.

Occasionally, the nodule can break down to release thousands of TB organisms into the rest of the lung and sometimes the bloodstream, which then go on to lead to widespread inflammation in diverse parts of the body, including the bones and the brain. This is known as miliary TB, and is a life-threatening complication of the primary disease.

In the cases in which the inflammation in the nodule of infected tissue has settled down, the problem may recur after many years, when the infection latent in the nodule for all that time becomes active again. This is known as post-primary TB. This usually occurs because the immune system of the person has become deficient in some way. It can occur in old age, or when the person has become ill for another reason, such as cancer or diabetes. For this reason it is often a much more severe infection than the primary infection.

The person with post-primary TB may become gradually more unwell over a period of weeks, with weight loss, exhaustion and night sweats. A persistent productive cough is a very common symptom, and is very significant because the sputum often contains highly infectious TB organisms. At this infectious stage, the diagnosis may not be made for weeks, so the infection may have been spread to many other people before the patient can be treated with antibiotics. Often the symptom that provokes the person to seek medical help is the appearance of blood in the sputum, a common occurrence in established post-primary TB.

Occasionally, the reactivated TB occurs in a different site of the body than the lungs, such as the bowel or the bone, but this is uncommon in the UK.

Diagnosis can be made on the basis of characteristic changes seen on the chest X-ray image, and by examination of the sputum for TB organisms. Sometimes a bronchoscopy is necessary to obtain infected tissue for diagnosis and choice of appropriate antibiotics.

Without treatment some patients with severe primary TB and many patients with post-primary TB would die from progressive damage to the lungs and bodily exhaustion. Severe TB used to be known as consumption because of the way people with TB could waste away whilst the disease took hold in their bodies. Common terminal events used to include profuse bleeding from the lungs or pneumonia.

The incidence and seriousness of the disease has markedly declined in the UK since the beginning of the 20th century. This is largely due to improvements in the general health of the population. In addition, the advent of antibiotics has enabled established cases to be controlled rapidly. Vaccination against TB, introduced in the 1950s, has reduced the risk of contracting the infection in many individuals. However, it has been estimated that one-third of the world's population has latent TB. Because of the prevalence of untreated AIDS cases, TB remains a primary cause of death in sub-Saharan Africa.

Conventional treatment of TB involves a cocktail of antibiotics (including initially all four of rifampicin, isoniazid, pyrazinamide and ethambutol) that has to be taken consistently for six to twelve months to be fully effective. Often the treatment produces relief of symptoms and infectivity in a very short time, and some patients stop taking the medication prematurely. This is more likely to occur in countries in which antibiotics are costly or in short supply, a major problem in the treatment of TB. It is known that if the drugs are not taken continuously, the infection may recur, and antibiotic-resistant types of organism are encouraged to develop. In some developing countries, antibiotic-resistant strains are leading to epidemics of untreatable TB, such as were seen in this country many decades ago. It is estimated that about 4 percent of cases of TB worldwide are resistant to the antibiotics that are normally used for treatment.

The vaccine for TB is known as the BCG, which stands for the French name of the strain of bacterium contained in the vaccine, Bacille Calmette-Guérin. It consists of a strain of organism that is alive but far less virulent than TB. It induces immunity in recipients, leading to a 70 percent reduced risk of developing TB. BCG is only given to those people who can be shown by a skin-prick test (the Heaf test) to have not already built up their own immunity

to the disease. However, because the incidence of TB is falling generally in the UK to very low levels, the practice of vaccinating teenagers routinely with the BCG has been stopped. Vaccination is still offered shortly after birth only to those infants who may be at high risk of coming into contact with the disease early in life.

In order to minimize the spread of disease in the UK, any case of TB that does occur is treated with seriousness. The patient is urged to continue with regular medication for the full recommended time period, and all close contacts during the possible time period of infectivity are traced and tested for active TB by X-ray imaging and skin-prick tests.

In the UK, most new cases of TB occur either in immigrant people who have come from countries in which TB is endemic, often as cases of reactivated post-primary TB, or in elderly people who contracted the primary infection in childhood. There is a worrying increase of TB in homeless people, a problem that is difficult to control because of difficulties in ensuring adequate completion of antibiotic treatment, thorough contact tracing and treatment of infected contacts.

Patients with AIDS are the other population in whom TB is of increasing concern. Because of the immunodeficiency that develops in AIDS, TB can take rapid hold and may be difficult to clear with antibiotics. The patient requires an even longer period on antibiotic treatment, during which time there is a risk of the development of antibiotic resistance. In developing countries in which TB is endemic, the combination of TB and AIDS is a deadly one, leading to many premature deaths.

 Information box 3.3e-II

Tuberculosis: comments from a Chinese medicine perspective

In Chinese medicine, the swelling and inflammation associated with TB could be seen as Phlegm Heat Obstructing the Lungs. The fever and wasting that arise in post-primary infection would be taken as evidence of Depletion of Lung Yin, and when the disease is in an advanced stage, Yang Deficiency becomes apparent. In light of this interpretation, TB may be seen to be energetically comparable to cancer.

TB is essentially a condition that affects people who are already depleted in some way. Because antibiotic therapy does not treat the root cause of the condition, it is suppressive in nature. Nevertheless, there is no doubt that antibiotic therapy is a powerful method of halting the disease.

Emphysema and chronic obstructive pulmonary disease (COPD)

Emphysema is, together with the changes of chronic bronchitis higher up the respiratory tree, a characteristic disease process of COPD. The term refers to a condition in which the delicate structure of the alveoli and the smallest bronchioles has permanently broken down as a result of inflammation in the deep part of the lungs. In some forms of emphysema the tiny walls that separate the alveoli are destroyed, while in others the terminal bronchioles dilate, and in both the air spaces within become enlarged. The dilatation that can occur in these deep parts of the lung in two types of emphysema is illustrated in Figure 3.3e-I.

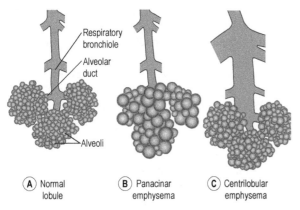

Figure 3.3e-I Diagram showing the dilatation of the air spaces in two forms of emphysema
(a) Normal alveoli. (b) Dilated alveolar spaces in panacinar emphysema. (c) Dilated bronchioles in centrilobular emphysema.

Emphysema can severely impair the exchange of gases that should take place between the walls of the alveoli and the blood in the capillaries, which, in health, form a close network around the alveoli. The response of the body to the resulting impaired uptake of oxygen and accumulation of carbon dioxide is to increase the respiratory rate, so that the patient with emphysema is breathless, particularly on exertion.

In some patients, due to narrowing of the smaller airways by inflammation, air becomes trapped in the dilated alveolar air spaces, which then expand, sometimes to form large air-filled spaces called bullae (singular bulla). The chest of a patient with this problem looks permanently overinflated. Occasionally, a bulla can rupture to release air into the surrounding pleural space. This condition of air in the chest cavity external to the lung is called pneumothorax, and leads to collapse of one of the lungs.

The most common cause of emphysema is smoking. However, the tendency to emphysema does run in families. In susceptible individuals with an inherited tendency, and in particular that which comes from a recessively inherited genetic disorder, alpha-1-antitrypsin deficiency, the effect of smoking is much more marked. This susceptibility is not that rare, as it is estimated that one in ten people carry a defective alpha-1-antitrypsin gene. The inflammation that results from long-standing asthma can also lead to emphysema.

The changes of emphysema commonly coexist with those of chronic bronchitis, described in Section 3.3d. As described in this section, together these conditions contribute to the aforementioned syndrome of COPD. The patient with COPD will therefore have symptoms of cough with phlegm, wheezing and breathlessness that never fully remits. It is not uncommon for patients with COPD to also develop symptoms of asthma, with bouts of increased breathlessness. These can be only partly relieved by bronchodilator and corticosteroid treatments, a characteristic of the reversibility of asthma.

COPD is diagnosed on the basis of impaired results from lung function tests, which involve the patient blowing into a spirometer. This assesses the rate of expiration and the capacity of the lungs to expel air, both of which may be reduced in COPD. Similarly, in COPD there will be a reduced peak flow rate, but usually little of the day-to-day reversibility seen in asthma.

Emphysema and COPD are progressive conditions that will continue to deteriorate if the patient continues to smoke, and so smoking cessation support is a central part of the treatment approach. Patients are also advised to engage in physical exercise and ensure that they maintain a healthy weight. Depending on severity of airways obstruction, patients will be prescribed two types of inhaled bronchodilator – a beta agonist such as salbutamol, and a muscarinic antagonist such as tiotropium. They may also receive inhaled steroids, so the treatment is similar to the stepwise approach in asthma.

Patients with COPD are prone to bouts of acute bronchitis and pneumonia. Each infection is likely to leave the lungs in a worse condition, so that a vicious circle of infection and damage is set up. For this reason, antibiotics are prescribed readily to patients with COPD. Patients who are vulnerable to infective exacerbations may be prescribed "rescue medication" comprising a course of antibiotics and also of oral steroids to use in case.

In very severe disease, the heart comes under strain as it has to pump blood through damaged lungs, and so right-sided heart failure with edema may develop (a condition known as cor pulmonale).

In the end stages of the condition the person with severe COPD may require long-term oxygen therapy (LTOT) to remove the disabling symptom of breathlessness. The patient will need to have oxygen cylinders at home to enable adequate treatment. In many patients, oxygen therapy can prolong life because it helps to relieve some of the pressure on the failing heart muscle. Patients with features of asthma will be prescribed high doses of inhaled bronchodilators and corticosteroids. The usual cause of death in severe COPD is bronchopneumonia.

 Information box 3.3e-III

Chronic obstructive pulmonary disease: comments from a Chinese medicine perspective

In Chinese medicine, the symptoms of COPD would correspond to Accumulation of Phlegm, with Phlegm Heat or Damp Phlegm Obstructing the Lungs. The destruction of the lung tissue that occurs in emphysema represents a background of Deficiency of Lung Qi and Yin. As the condition progresses and leads to respiratory and cardiac failure, an end-stage patient might be diagnosed as Deficient in both Yin and Yang. Severe Deficiency of Heart, Spleen and Kidneys is also likely to feature in the diagnostic picture.

Fibrosis of the lung and occupational lung disease

Fibrosis is the medical term used to describe scarring. In lung fibrosis the scarring affects the alveoli and the smallest bronchioles, and leads to narrowing of the airways and loss of elasticity of the lungs. This can severely impair the action of breathing.

Fibrosis is often the end result of a long-standing process of inflammation, which can result from irritation caused by inhaled substances in the form of tiny particles. Many of these substances are found within industrial settings. For example, coal dust, silica from stone and asbestos can lead to impairment in the function of the lungs in people who have jobs such as mining, stonemasonry and ship-building. Allergy to a mold that grows on stored hay can produce a similar sort of scarring reaction in farm workers, in a condition known as farmer's lung.

Rarely, the fibrosis can be a result of certain prescribed drugs, and can occasionally develop with no obvious cause (when it is known as idiopathic pulmonary fibrosis (IPF) or usual interstitial pneumonia (UIP)). This is a serious progressive disease and carries a poor prognosis. Less than 20 percent of patients diagnosed with IPF will be alive after five years.[69]

The main symptom of fibrosis is progressive breathlessness. In farmer's lung the initial symptoms include fever and increased breathlessness after working with hay. In severe cases the patient will have the blue discoloration of the lips and tongue known as cyanosis. In these severe cases the heart is put under strain because

it has to pump blood through scarred lung tissue, and this can lead to heart failure with edema.

Asbestos is a particularly harmful dust because, in addition to causing inflammation and scarring, it is highly carcinogenic. People who have been exposed to asbestos dust have an increased risk of bronchial cancer, and a very high risk of an otherwise rare cancer of the pleural lining of the lung called mesothelioma. Both these types of cancer are resistant to modern treatments.

Apart from eliminating the cause of fibrosis, the treatment is largely supportive only, as the condition is irreversible. New drugs including pirfenidone may be trialed in advanced cases as these seem to slow the speed of fibrosis, but their use is limited by side effects.

In selected patients lung transplantation may be considered, although this also carries a low survival rate, with only up to 50 percent of patients surviving beyond five years after a lung transplant for this reason.

Patients with IPF have an increased risk of suffering from lung cancer and also right-sided heart failure.

The patient with severe fibrosis will eventually require oxygen therapy to relieve breathlessness and reduce the strain on the heart. Patients in the UK whose fibrosis has resulted from industrial exposure to dusts may be eligible for financial compensation from the government.

 Information box 3.3e-IV

Lung fibrosis: comments from a Chinese medicine perspective

In Chinese medicine, the impaired elasticity and narrowing of the airways of the lungs in fibrosis would correspond to Depletion of Lung Qi (Yang) and Yin. The edema that results from heart failure in chronic lung disease is a form of Kidney and Lung Yang Deficiency. The cyanosis that develops in the end stages of all severe lung disease is a sign of severe Stagnation of Blood due to Yang Deficiency.

Pulmonary embolism and infarction

Pulmonary embolism was introduced in Section 2.2d, in which the disorders of excessive blood clotting were explored, and is described there as a possible serious consequence of deep vein thrombosis (DVT).

Pulmonary embolism is the end result of unwanted material (emboli), usually in the form of blood clots, entering the blood vessels that lead from the right side of the heart to the lungs. This material lodges in the progressively narrowing blood vessels of the lung, and leads to infarction of the part of lung supplied by those vessels. The wider the vessel that is blocked by pulmonary emboli, the greater the amount of lung that is infarcted.

The small clots that can break off from a DVT are probably the most common cause of pulmonary embolism. However, other causes of excessive clotting in the blood, such as serious chronic disease (including cancer), the contraceptive pill and occasionally pregnancy, can also cause the condition without a prior DVT.

A small pulmonary embolism may affect only a tiny part of the lung close to the pleural lining. This will result in death of that part of the lung and a small area of inflammation. The inflammation may cause a temporary bout of pleurisy, but is likely to heal.

If this event occurs a number of times, it can lead to progressive irreversible damage to the lung. After areas of the lung have been infarcted, air can enter the lung, but as the circulation to the lung has been gradually reduced, the exchange of gases is impaired. The patient might become increasingly breathless over the course of a few weeks. The heart comes under strain as the free circulation of blood is impaired, and angina or chronic heart failure might develop.

A medium to large pulmonary embolus suddenly cuts off the blood supply to a much larger portion of the lung. This can be so severe as to lead to acute heart failure and sudden death. If less severe, intense chest pain and breathlessness is experienced, and the patient has to be treated as a medical emergency.

Pulmonary embolism is diagnosed definitively by means of computed tomography angiography of the pulmonary arteries (CTPA). If this is not available, a scintigram scan may be performed. This exposes poorly perfused areas of the lung following an injection of a radioactive tracer chemical. The D-dimer blood test can be used to check to see if thrombosis has occurred (D-dimers are fragments of the clotting protein fibrin, the levels of which are raised shortly after an episode of thrombosis).

In all cases, the aim of treatment is to maximize oxygen transfer, so 100 percent oxygen is administered by means of a mask. Then, in order to reduce the tendency of the blood to clot, a low molecular weight heparin, a rapidly acting anticoagulant medication, is given by injection. If the patient is gravely unwell as a result of a massive embolism, a clot-busting drug such as streptokinase or alteplase may be given to unblock the artery in the lung that contains the clot. These drugs work in the same way as when given for a heart attack.

Once the acute symptoms have been controlled, either warfarin or a novel oral anticoagulant (NOAC) such as rivaroxaban will be prescribed to inhibit the blood clotting in the long term, and will be continued for between six weeks and six months. Patients considered to be at high risk of recurrence of this life-threatening condition may be advised to continue with warfarin therapy for life.

 Information box 3.3e-V

Pulmonary embolism: comments from a Chinese medicine perspective

In Chinese medicine, the symptoms of pulmonary embolism correspond to acute Heart Blood Stagnation, and like a heart attack, may lead to Heart Yang Collapse.

Heparin and warfarin reduce the tendency of the blood to clot, and may be described as Heating.

Collapse of the lung

There are a number of conditions in which the tissue of the inflated lung loses its shape and the open air spaces within it collapse. As described in Section 3.3a, the natural tendency of the elastic tissue of the lung is to collapse down, and this is prevented in health by the integrity of the lining membrane of the pleura, which are normally firmly attached to the walls of the chest cavity.

The most important condition causing lung collapse, of which acupuncturists in particular should be aware, is pneumothorax. In pneumothorax, air comes between the pleural linings and allows the lung to collapse. The rupture of bullae in emphysema is one cause of pneumothorax. However, the most common cause of pneumothorax is when the normal lung is punctured as a result of injury. A broken rib resulting from a traumatic accident can easily puncture the underlying lung, and the air that escapes leads to a pneumothorax.

Pneumothorax is a known, but rare, adverse event arising from acupuncture treatment to the shoulder and chest. The lungs lie only a few millimeters under the skin in some thin people, and so they can easily be reached by even a shallow needle insertion. Usually, a thin needle puncture of lung tissue will not cause a collapse to the lung. However, a rough or repeated insertion may have this unfortunate consequence, particularly in a person affected by a chronic lung disease such as emphysema.

Occasionally, a pneumothorax can occur spontaneously in an otherwise fit young person. This is usually attributed to the presence of a previously undiagnosed bulla that has ruptured because it is much weaker than normal lung tissue. A few bullae can be present from birth in some people, and these localized areas of deficiency could be compared to the occasional weak area of thin rubber that might be found on the surface of a balloon.

Other causes of collapse of the lung include the accumulation of a large amount of fluid in the space between the pleural membranes. Fluid collecting in this space is called pleural effusion, a term first introduced in this text when pleural effusion was described as a possible complication of lung cancer. In this case, the fluid has been secreted by cancer cells. Other sources of fluid include bleeding from an internal chest injury or inflammatory fluid developing as a result of pneumonia, particularly lobar pneumonia.

Figure 3.3e-II is a diagrammatic representation of a collapsed lung surrounded by a pleural space containing air, blood or the fluid that results from inflammation (inflammatory exudate). It illustrates how the lung can contract down to a fraction of its normal size if compressed by fluid or air in the pleural space. As the diagram indicates, the common term for this sort of collapse of the lung is pressure collapse.

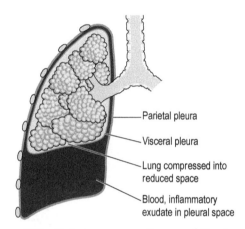

Figure 3.3e-II A pressure collapse of the lung

The other cause of collapse, absorption collapse, is illustrated in Figure 3.3e-III. In this case the whole lung, or just part of it, has collapsed because some or all of the airways have become totally blocked due to an infection or tumor. The lung behind (distal to) this obstruction collapses because the air within it gradually becomes absorbed into the blood, and cannot be replaced. The pleural space then fills with tissue fluid (colored in pale gray in the diagram).

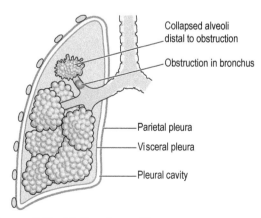

Figure 3.3e-III An absorption collapse of the lung

In pressure collapse, such as pneumothorax, the onset of symptoms is usually sudden. The patient experiences a sudden onset of breathlessness, and often the pain of pleurisy. Usually the patient is not in severe distress, but this depends on the degree of collapse. Occasionally, as can occur with tension pneumothorax, the situation becomes a medical emergency, as the exchange of gases is severely impaired and the patient goes into respiratory failure.

The treatment of lung collapse depends on the cause. Pneumothorax, if mild, can resolve spontaneously over the course of a few days, as the puncture in the lung heals. If air continues to leak out of the lung, the excess air can be drained away by means of a tube inserted into the pleural space through a small incision between the ribs. This allows the lung to re-inflate, and usually the puncture or rupture can then heal naturally. Occasionally, a surgical operation is necessary to repair the damaged lung.

In a similar fashion, fluid in the pleural space can resolve spontaneously, but may also need to be drained away, particularly if it contains blood. In cancer, the fluid may continue to accumulate, and the pleural effusion may need to be drained repeatedly to keep the patient relatively comfortable.

If the collapse has occurred due to obstruction, again, resolution may be possible if the obstruction can be removed. This is not always possible, in which case the lung remains permanently damaged and reduced in capacity.

The sharp pain of pleurisy that commonly accompanies pneumothorax suggests Blood and/or Qi Stagnation. This may purely be the result of an injury, but may develop from internal deficiency (e.g. the rupture of a weak part of the lungs).

 Information box 3.3e-VI

Lung collapse: comments from a Chinese medicine perspective

In Chinese medicine, the breathlessness that results from collapse of the lung might correspond to Deficiency of either one or both of Lung Yin and Qi (Yang), because the underlying problem is of the integrity of the structure of the lung itself.

The red flags of lower respiratory disease

Some patients with diseases of the lower respiratory tract will benefit from referral to a conventional doctor for assessment or treatment. Red flags are those symptoms and signs that indicate that referral should be considered. The red flags of lower respiratory disease are described in Table 3.3e-I. A summary of the red flags in a format designed for quick reference in clinical practice can be found in Appendix III. This gives advice on the degree of urgency of referral for each of the red flag conditions listed.

Table 3.3e-I A17: Red flags of lower respiratory disease

Red flag	Description	Reasoning
A17.1	Features of progressive upper respiratory infection in susceptible people (e.g. frail elderly people, those who are immunocompromised and those with pre-existing disease of the bronchi and bronchioles): cough and fever or new production of yellow-green phlegm, each persisting for >3 days	In healthy people an upper respiratory infection (i.e. affecting any part of the respiratory tract above and including the bronchi) may be protracted, but is not necessarily a serious condition. In most cases, as long as there is no breathlessness, it is safe to treat conservatively, and there is no need for antibiotics In healthy people consider referral if there is no response to treatment within 1–2 weeks However, in elderly people and those who are immunocompromised (including those with chronic diseases such as cancer, kidney failure and AIDS), severe infections can be masked by relatively minor symptoms, and it is advisable to refer any respiratory condition that persists for >3 days People with pre-existing lung disease (e.g. asthma, chronic bronchitis, emphysema, lung cancer, cystic fibrosis) are at increased risk of progressive infection, and similarly merit early referral Smokers commonly do not recover as quickly from upper respiratory infections and early antibiotic treatment may also be merited in this case
A17.2	Any new onset of difficulty in breathing in a young child (<8 years)	Always take a new onset of difficulty in breathing in a child seriously, and refer for medical assessment to exclude serious disease. Common causes include lower respiratory infections, asthma, allergic reactions, inhalation of foreign bodies and congenital heart disease
A17.3	Features of severe asthma, at least two of the following: • rapidly worsening breathlessness • >30 respirations/minute (or more if a child)* • heart rate >110 beats/minute • reluctance to talk because of breathlessness • need to sit upright and still to assist breathing Central cyanosis (see A17.12) is a very serious sign	Severe asthma is a potentially life-threatening condition and may develop in someone who has no previous history of severe attacks. Urgent referral is required so that medical management of the attack can be instigated. Keep the patient as calm as possible while waiting for help to arrive It may be very difficult to differentiate an asthma attack from the more benign situation of panic attack (characterized by a felt experience of intense fear, racing heart, increased depth of breathing, numbness and tingling of the extremities, and mild muscle spasms), and it is possible for the two to coincide, as an experience of breathlessness can trigger a panic reaction. In this situation, the key feature is respiratory rate, and if this does not respond to calming measures within a few minutes, and rebreathing exhaled carbon dioxide (by breathing into a paper bag) within a minute or two, referral needs to be considered. Central cyanosis would never be apparent in a panic attack, so if present, this is an absolute indicator for urgent referral
A17.4	Hemoptysis: any episode of coughing up of more than a teaspoon of blood	Blood-streaked sputum is a common and benign occurrence in upper respiratory tract infections, and is not a reason for referral if the amount of blood is small and infection is self-limiting (i.e. episode limited to the few days when cough from the infection is present) A larger amount of fresh blood may herald more serious bleeding in those with bronchiectasis. It may also be the first symptom of lung cancer or tuberculosis (TB). Blood in the sputum also occurs in the case of pulmonary embolism

A17.5	New onset of chronic cough or deep, persistent chest pain in a smoker	The most common first symptom of lung cancer is a chronic, irritating cough, which may feel different to the clearing of phlegm that characterizes the smoker's cough
		Rarely, lung cancer can cause deep, persistent chest pain, but this is a less usual first symptom
A17.6	Unexplained hoarseness lasting for >3 weeks: may be the first symptom of laryngeal or lung cancer (particularly in smokers >50 years)	Prolonged hoarseness is usually benign in origin and may be diagnosed as chronic laryngitis. This painless syndrome is commonly the result of misuse or overuse of the vocal cords
		However, the possibility of laryngeal cancer in smokers >50 years needs to be considered
		Lung cancer can also be a cause of hoarseness, as the recurrent laryngeal nerve that passes deep in the chest can be damaged by an infiltrating tumor. Again smokers >50 years are a high-risk group
		Referral is advised to exclude these less likely possible causes of chronic hoarseness
A17.7	Features of infection of the alveoli (pneumonia) include: • cough • fever • malaise • >30 respirations/minute (or more if a child)* • heart rate >110 beats/minute • reluctance to talk because of breathlessness • need to sit upright and still to assist breathing Cyanosis (see A17.12) is a very serious sign	Pneumonia means that inflammation (usually as a result of infection) has descended to the level of the air sacs (alveoli) in the lungs. As these sacs are involved in the exchange of gases, breathlessness is always part of the picture of pneumonia. As the infection is so deep, the patient can become extremely unwell and may need hospital treatment
		Use the severity of the symptoms to guide the urgency of the referral
		Severe breathlessness merits urgent referral
A17.8	Features of pleurisy: localized chest pain that is associated with inspiration and expiration. Refer if associated with fever and breathlessness, as this is an indication of associated pneumonia	Pleurisy is the syndrome resulting from inflammation of a region of the pleural lining of the lungs. Inflammation of the pleural lining leads to a localized region of chest wall pain, which worsens with coughing and breathing in
		Pleurisy commonly results from a viral infection, and in this case may be a benign syndrome associated with no other lung damage
		However, pleurisy may be a complication of the spread of pneumonia to the periphery of a lung, in which case, it would be associated with malaise and breathlessness
		Pleurisy can also result from non-infectious causes, such as pulmonary embolism, in which case there will be breathlessness and sometimes expectoration of bloody sputum (see A17.10)
		If clearly associated with an upper respiratory infection and if there is no breathlessness, there is no need for immediate referral. However, a patient with pleurisy will need to be referred if the symptom is not settling within 1–2 days

A17.9	Features of TB infection: chronic productive cough, weight loss, night sweats, blood in sputum for >2 weeks	TB is more common in people who have lived in countries where it is endemic, and in those who live in situations of poverty and in overcrowded damp conditions. It can also develop in people who have close contact with those at high risk
		Referral is for isolation, diagnosis and initiation of a prolonged program of antibiotic therapy. Contacts will be traced and tested for infection if the diagnosis is confirmed
		TB is a notifiable disease**
A17.10	Features of pulmonary embolism: sudden onset of pleurisy (see A17.8) with breathlessness, cyanosis (see A17.12), collapse	Pulmonary embolism is the result of a lodging of a blood clot or multiple blood clots (emboli) in the arterial circulation supplying the lungs (pulmonary circulation). If the blood clot is large there can be a sudden reduction in the oxygenation power of the lung, and this can result in collapse and sudden death. In less severe cases, the infarction of the lung tissue manifests as pleurisy with breathlessness, and blood may be coughed up in the sputum
		This syndrome merits urgent referral for anticoagulation (thinning of the blood)
A17.11	Features of sudden lung collapse (pneumothorax): onset of severe breathlessness; there may be some pleurisy (see A17.8) and collapse if very severe	Pneumothorax can occur spontaneously, or may be provoked by a puncture of the lungs. It is notorious amongst acupuncturists as a possible complication of needling vulnerable points in the thorax, and practitioners should be vigilant that in extremely rare cases the symptoms can develop gradually up to 24 hours after a needle puncture
A17.12	Central cyanosis (as a new finding)	Cyanosis describes the blue coloring that appears when the blood is poorly oxygenated. The oxygen saturation of the blood needs to be less than 85% for cyanosis to become apparent (normal saturation level of the blood is >98%)
		Cyanosis of the extremities is a common finding in extreme cold and is not necessarily a serious sign. It is the result of sluggish circulation in the peripheral tissues, but does not necessarily indicate a generally depleted level of oxygen in the blood
		Central cyanosis from poor oxygenation can be seen on the tongue and in the complexion. Central cyanosis is a very serious sign that the body is failing to maintain adequate blood oxygen levels
		It can be the result of respiratory disease or cardiac disease, in which case there will be associated breathlessness. It can also result from respiratory suppression (e.g. with drugs or neurological disease), in which case the respiratory rate may be lower than normal
		Some people with chronic lung or heart disease may demonstrate central cyanosis yet be in a stable state
		However, if cyanosis is found in an acutely ill patient, this merits urgent referral

* *Categorization of respiratory rate in adults:* Normal respiratory rate in an adult: 10–20 breaths per minute (one breath is one inhalation and exhalation); Moderate breathlessness in an adult: >30 breaths per minute; Severe breathlessness in an adult: >60 breaths per minute.

Categorization of respiratory rate in children: The normal range for respiratory rate in children varies according to age; The following rates indicate moderate to severe breathlessness: Newborn (0–3 months): >60 breaths per minute; Infant (3 months to 2 years): >50 breaths per minute; Young child (2–8 years): >40 breaths per minute; Older child to adult: >30 breaths per minute.

** Notifiable diseases: notification of a number of specified infectious diseases is required of doctors in the UK as a statutory duty under the Public Health (Infectious Diseases) 1988 Act and the Public Health (Control of Diseases) 1988 Act, and more recently, the Health Protection (Notification) Regulations 2010. The UK Health Protection Agency (HPA) Centre for Infections collates details of each case of each disease that has been notified. This allows analyses of local and national trends. This is one example of a situation in which there is a legal requirement for a doctor to breach patient confidentiality.

Diseases that are notifiable include: acute encephalitis, acute infectious hepatitis, acute poliomyelitis, anthrax, cholera, diphtheria, enteric fevers (typhoid and paratyphoid), food poisoning, infectious bloody diarrhea, leprosy, malaria, measles, meningitis (bacterial and viral forms), meningococcal septicemia (without meningitis), mumps, plague, rabies, rubella, scarlet fever, severe acute respiratory syndrome (SARS), smallpox, tetanus, tuberculosis, typhus, viral hemorrhagic fever, whooping cough, yellow fever.

The Blood

3.4

3.4a The physiology of the blood

In this last section of Stage 3, the physiology and pathology of the blood and its associated diseases are explored, although some of the different aspects of the function of the blood have already been described when discussing inflammation, clotting, the immune system and the cardiovascular system.

The composition of the blood[70]

In Section 2.1c it was explained that the blood is composed of fluid called plasma and three types of blood cells: red blood cells (erythrocytes), white blood cells (leukocytes) and platelets (thrombocytes).

The plasma

The plasma forms just over half (55 percent) of the volume of the blood. Plasma consists of water in which a number of substances are dissolved. It is a thick (viscous) fluid, a property resulting from the proteins dissolved in it. One important function of these proteins is to help keep the watery part of the blood within the blood vessels. As the proteins are too large to move out of the blood vessels by diffusion, they maintain a level of concentration in the blood that contributes to its osmotic pressure (see Section 1.1c).

The most abundant of the plasma proteins is albumin, which is similar in structure to the protein of egg white. Albumin is made by the liver, and its main role is to contribute to osmotic pressure. All the plasma proteins, for example, the clotting factors and antibodies, have important functions. The transport proteins are important

in that they help carry some salts and hormones that would otherwise be relatively insoluble in plasma.

Plasma is also the vehicle by which the nutrients and oxygen, which are essential for the life of the cells, actually reach the tissues. Although oxygen tends to be concentrated in the red blood cells, it also has to move freely through the plasma so that it can pass from the alveoli to the red blood cells and thence to the tissues.

As the vehicle for the transport of hormones, plasma is also important for communication between one part of the body and another. For example, thyroid hormone is secreted by the thyroid gland into the bloodstream and carried to all the tissues of the body, and so in this way the plasma is essential for the role of the endocrine system (see Chapter 5.1).

The blood cells

All three types of blood cell originate from the bone marrow. The bone marrow contains a number of immature cells called stem cells, and it is these that are the starting material for all the different subtypes of blood cells, including all the leukocytes, such as macrophages and mast cells, which leave the blood to perform immune functions in the tissues. Figure 3.4a-I gives a diagrammatic representation of how the stem cell is the "great grandparent" of the red blood cell (the erythrocyte), the platelet and the six different categories of white blood cell (the granulocytes and agranulocytes). It is important to appreciate this process before approaching the study of the condition of leukemia.

RED BLOOD CELLS (ERYTHROCYTES)

The primary function of red blood cells is to carry oxygen from the lungs to the tissues. To do this, red blood cells contain an iron-containing protein called hemoglobin, which has a strong affinity for oxygen molecules. Because of its hemoglobin a red blood cell can carry much more oxygen than could be dissolved in an equivalent volume of plasma, and this is essential to enable the blood to carry sufficient oxygen for the body's requirements.

When hemoglobin attracts and holds on to oxygen molecules, it turns bright red, giving the blood its characteristic color. When it releases oxygen, the color of the hemoglobin, and therefore the blood, becomes a more purple shade of red. This is why arterial blood in the body circulation is bright red and venous blood is darker.

Hemoglobin is manufactured within the maturing red blood cell in the bone marrow. Iron, obtained from the diet, is an essential ingredient in this process. The vitamins folic acid and vitamin B12, also obtained from the diet, are important factors that enable the production of healthy red blood cells.

The production of red blood cells is stimulated by the hormone erythropoietin, which is released by the kidneys. The hormone is released when the blood fails to perform its role of oxygenation of tissues in the conditions of anemia and acute blood loss (see Sections 3.4c and 3.4d).

Before the maturing red blood cell leaves the bone marrow to enter the blood, the nucleus breaks down. The red blood cell then takes on a disc-like shape, which enables it to be flexible enough to move in large numbers through the finest capillaries. Once in the circulation, the life of the red blood cell is about 120 days, after which it is broken down in the spleen, the liver and parts of the bone marrow by phagocytic white blood cells. In this process, the iron is removed from the hemoglobin and recycled for further use in the body. The by-product of this process is bilirubin, which is a digested form of hemoglobin, and this is taken up by the liver and excreted into the bile (see Section 3.1a).

The surface of the red blood cells expresses characteristic forms of polysaccharide molecules, and these are the basis for categorizing a person into one of the four blood groups, A, B, AB or O, and also whether they are rhesus (Rh) positive or negative. This terminology reflects the two important ways in which blood groups are classified: the ABO system and the rhesus system.

The ABO system categorizes blood type according to the presence or absence of two genetically determined polysaccharides (antigens) known simply as A and B that are present on the surface of the red blood cell. Group A means that substance A is carried on all the red cells, whereas the red cells of group B carry substance B. The red cells of blood group AB carry both A and B, whereas those of blood group O carry neither.

The rhesus system, at its most simple, categorizes blood into whether or not it carries a particular substance called rhesus D. Rhesus-positive people carry rhesus D on their red cells. The rhesus system is independent of the ABO system.

If blood of different blood groups is mixed, there is a tendency for the red blood cells to clump together and break down. This is called incompatibility, and results from antibodies to foreign blood groups present in the serum of the blood samples. Some combinations of blood groups are much more likely to have this reaction than others. For this reason, before being used in a blood transfusion, donated blood is "typed" to ensure that the ABO and rhesus D factors are exactly the same as those of the intended recipient.

PLATELETS (THROMBOCYTES)

The platelets, like the red blood cells, are cells without nuclei that originate from the bone marrow. Their function is to work together with the clotting factor proteins in the plasma to enable an efficient and controlled clotting reaction (see Section 2.1c).

WHITE BLOOD CELLS (LEUKOCYTES)

The diverse functions of the white blood cells were introduced in the description of wound healing, inflammation and the immune system in Chapters 2.1 and 2.2.

There are two broad groups of white blood cell, which are categorized according to whether or not the cytoplasm contains granules. These are the granulocytes and agranulocytes (see Figure 3.4a-I).

Granulocytes contain granules that consist of chemicals (enzymes) that are important for the destruction of unwanted foreign matter and in the generation of inflammation. Some of the granulocytes are able to phagocytose (see Section 1.1c) small particles such as damaged bacteria. All the granulocytes can move, like an amoeba, out of the blood vessels and into the tissues when their presence is required.

The agranulocytes, which include the lymphocytes and monocytes, do not contain granules. Lymphocytes are the cells that provide the foundation of the immune response. They secrete antibodies in response to antigens and carry specific antibodies on their surface. Monocytes are cells that are able to phagocytose foreign material and debris from damaged and aging cells. Macrophages are a type of monocyte that are plentiful in connective tissue for this purpose.

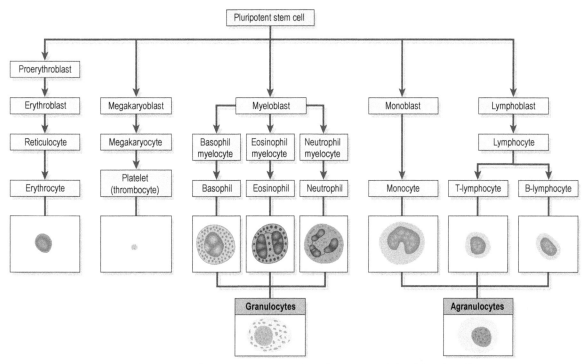

Figure 3.4a-I The stages in the development of the blood cells

The role of the blood

The blood is part of the body that is in constant movement and which by means of the blood vessels reaches all body parts. Its primary role is to transport essential substances from one part of the body to another and to remove waste products.

It is because of the healthy flow of blood that all the cells of the body can have a constant environment.

This environment provides water, nutrients, oxygen, protection, warm temperature, and the perfect balance of acidity and salts, and is also always cleansed of wastes. In short, blood is a cornerstone of the state of balance called homeostasis, and the fact that it is crucial for maintaining balance is, of course, likely to be of interest to those who hold to a holistic approach to medicine.

 Information box 3.4a-I

The functions of the blood: comments from a Chinese medicine perspective

To consider the role of the blood in Chinese medicine, it is useful to list the functions of the substances Blood and Qi as they are generally understood.

The functions of Blood are to:

- nourish
- moisturize
- house the Shen.

The functions of Qi are to:

- transform
- transport
- hold
- raise
- protect
- warm.

The conventional understanding of the function of blood clearly embraces some of the functions of both Blood and Qi in Chinese medicine. The nourishing and moisturizing function of the physical blood is attributed in Chinese medicine to Blood, whereas the transporting, protecting and warming functions are attributed to Qi. Of course, the close relationship between Blood and Qi is recognized in Chinese medicine in the sayings "Blood is the mother of Qi" and "Qi is the commander of Blood."

As always with these comparisons, there are marked differences. The physical blood has no relationship with the mental, emotional or spiritual aspects corresponding to the Shen, the spiritual aspect of the Blood in Chinese medicine.

Information box 3.4a-II

The manufacture of blood: comments from a Chinese medicine perspective

In the physiology of Chinese medicine, Blood is made from Gu (food) Qi, which originates from the Spleen. Gu Qi requires the motive force of Lung Qi to reach the Heart, where it is transformed into Blood. This process is aided by Original (Yuan) Qi and Jing (Essence), which produces marrow.[71]

In this ancient interpretation of how Blood is made there are some clear correspondences with the conventional understanding of the manufacture of blood. The basic materials for the physical blood come from the diet. This includes water, basic nutrients, iron and the vitamins, folic acid and vitamin B12. These can be compared to the Gu Qi made by the Spleen.

The stem cells in the bone marrow are the templates for all the blood cells, and are present in marrow from before birth. These may be comparable to Yuan Qi and Jing. The kidneys also play an important role in the production of blood, in that they secrete the hormone erythropoietin. This could be seen as a physical aspect of Yuan Qi.

The lungs and the heart are important in the circulation of the blood, as they sit at the central point of the circulation. The heart provides the motive force for the blood, and this prevents clotting. The lungs ensure oxygenation of the blood, so that the blood is able to give life to the cells. These organs are essential for maintaining the nature of living blood.

The other Organ that is considered in Chinese medicine to have an important relationship with blood is the Liver. The Liver is considered to be a storehouse for the Blood, particularly when a person is at rest. When the Blood is in the Liver it can be nourished. This is one of the reasons why in Chinese medicine adequate rest is considered to be important for healthy Blood.

In conventional medicine the liver can also be said to store blood, as it holds a large proportion of the circulating blood at any one time. The liver manufactures the plasma proteins and enables an even release of the most basic nutrient, glucose, into the blood. This picture is consistent with the Storing and Nourishing functions of the Liver Organ.

Despite all these correspondences it is important to be clear when talking to patients that the physical blood and the Chinese medicine energetic concept of Blood are not the same thing. The physical blood is a reflection of some of the aspects of Blood, the Vital Substance, but also carries some of the characteristics of Qi.

3.4b The investigation of the blood

Mild forms of the most common non-cancerous diseases of the blood, the anemias, may be investigated and managed solely by a family physician (general practitioner (GP)), who is able to examine the patient and take blood samples to be sent to a laboratory for interpretation.

The investigation of more severe diseases of the blood is carried out by a hospital specialist called a hematologist. A doctor who specializes in hematology has been trained not only in the clinical skills required to examine and treat patients with blood diseases, but also in the examination of samples of blood and bone marrow under the microscope.

The investigation of the diseases of the blood involves:

- a thorough physical examination

- specialized blood tests and examination of a blood film

- examination of a sample of bone marrow

- biopsy and other tests to visualize the lymph nodes.

Physical examination

The physical examination of a patient with a suspected disease of the blood involves the stages listed in Table 3.4b-I.

Table 3.4b-I The stages of physical examination of the blood

General examination for signs of anemia: including pale nails, pale creases in the palms of the hands, general pallor of the skin, sore tongue without coating, and cracked lips in severe cases
Examination of the lymph nodes: to look for the enlargement that can occur in cancers that affect the blood cells
Examination of the heart and lungs: to exclude the rapid heart rate and pulmonary edema that can result from severe anemia
Examination of the spleen and liver: these can become enlarged in various diseases of the blood

Blood tests

A great deal of information can be obtained about the blood from tests that involve the patient in relatively little discomfort. All the tests described below are used in the investigation of a wide range of diseases affecting all the body systems. Because these tests are performed so frequently, they are described in some detail.

Full blood count

The full blood count (FBC) is one of the most commonly performed blood tests. The FBC can give information about all three types of blood cell (red blood cells, white blood cells or leukocytes and platelets).

To perform an FBC, about 5 milliliters of venous blood is taken by syringe, usually from a vein at the elbow (in the approximate area of acupoint Chi Ze, LU-5). This blood is mixed in a tube with an anticoagulant to prevent clotting, and sent to a laboratory where it is examined by means of a cell counter machine. This is able to recognize the various blood cells in the sample by their size, and gives a figure for the numbers of the different sorts of blood cell within the sample. The relative numbers of the different sorts of leukocytes, the concentration of hemoglobin in the sample and the sizes of the red blood cells can also be measured.

These figures are then compared to the normal range of values found in an average population. The FBC can show if there are too many or too few of any one type of blood cell, if the hemoglobin is too low, and if the red cells are abnormal in shape or size.

Blood film

In this examination of the blood, a drop of the blood sample taken for the FBC is placed on a microscope slide and examined by a hematologist. This examination can give more precise information about abnormalities in the shape and structure of the various blood cells.

Erythrocyte sedimentation rate (ESR)

The erythrocyte sedimentation rate (ESR) and the level of C-reactive protein (CRP) are both measures of an active inflammatory response taking place in the body. The ESR is simply a measure of how rapidly the red blood cells settle out of a shaken sample of blood, like particles of mud might settle out of a sample of river water. The rate at which the cells settle is dependent on the proteins such as antibodies in the plasma. The ESR is raised if the body is dealing with an ongoing infection, inflammation, cancer or trauma. The ESR is not very specific, but if raised, is a sign that there is an ongoing state of physical imbalance in the body.

C-reactive protein (CRP)

CRP is one of the plasma proteins, the levels of which rise during inflammation. If the CRP level is raised, the body is dealing with acute inflammation or trauma. This test is therefore a bit more specific than the ESR, but is more expensive to perform.

Serum samples

Serum can be obtained from the blood by allowing venous blood to clot in a test tube. The fluid that separates from the clot is plasma without the clotting factor fibrinogen. This fluid is called serum. A wide range of assays can be performed on the serum sample to investigate diseases that affect the body systems. For example, substances as diverse as vitamin C, insulin, calcium and cannabis are all detected from serum samples, although a separate blood sample is required for each assay.

Contrary to what many patients might expect, a single blood test cannot reveal information about all these diseases and substances. A single sample of about 7 milliliters of blood can only be used for one or two assays. Alcohol, for example, will only be detected if the alcohol assay has been requested. Even if present, alcohol will not be detected if the doctor has requested that the blood is tested only for thyroid hormone.

In the investigation of the diseases of the blood, some of the most commonly performed serum tests are for iron, vitamin B12 and folic acid (also called folate in some texts), all of which are important in the investigation of anemia.

Examination of the bone marrow

In all severe conditions of the blood, including anemia, examination of the bone marrow can reveal whether there are abnormalities in the development of the blood. The blood-forming marrow is a dense blood-like fluid that can be drawn up into a syringe. The removal of the sample of bone marrow involves the insertion of a large needle into the bone of the iliac crest after the area has been numbed with a local anesthetic. Despite the anesthetic this is a much more painful procedure than the simple blood test.

The sample obtained is examined in the same way as the blood film. The bone marrow sample will reveal the shape and structure of the stem cells and the immature forms of the three different types of blood cell.

Biopsy and other tests to visualize the lymph nodes

The two most common forms of cancer that affect the cells of the blood are leukemia and lymphoma. These diseases are the focus of Section 3.4e. In both these conditions the lymph nodes may become engorged with increased numbers of cancerous white blood cells.

In lymphoma, the lymph node is the primary site of the tumor. Surgical removal and examination (biopsy) of an affected superficial node can give valuable information about the tumor. Computed tomography (CT) scans can give more information about the state of lymph nodes deeper in the body. Both these tests can be important for the accurate staging of lymphomas.

3.4c Anemia

Anemia is a term derived from the Greek meaning no blood, and is used to describe the range of conditions that lead to an impairment in the ability of the red blood cells to transport oxygen to the tissues. In a person with anemia, the concentration of hemoglobin in the blood is less than that in healthy people.

In Section 3.4d the ways in which a sudden loss of a large quantity of blood might affect the body are explored. Although this condition also reduces the ability of the blood to transport oxygen to the tissues, this is not the same as anemia. In acute blood loss, the red cells and concentration of hemoglobin are normal, but the volume of the circulating blood is reduced.

It is important at this stage to clarify that the term anemia does not say anything about the underlying disease process. It simply describes the end result. If doctors are to treat anemia effectively, the underlying cause of the problem must first be diagnosed.

Despite the variety of causes of the condition, there are some features that all patients with anemia have in common.

The clinical features of anemia

Symptoms of tiredness, breathlessness and feeling faint, together with the sign of pallor, are characteristic of anemia. In addition, palpitations, chest pain and edema may also be experienced by the patient with severe anemia. There is also a range of other symptoms that are specific to particular types of anemia.

 Information box 3.4c-I

Anemia: comments from a Chinese medicine perspective

The symptoms of anemia and the syndrome of Blood Deficiency in Chinese medicine have some close similarities but are not directly equivalent.

According to Chinese medicine, the general features of Blood Deficiency include the symptoms of dizziness, poor memory, numbness, floaters in the visual field and blurred vision, difficulty in sleeping, depression, anxiety and lack of initiative and the signs of pallor of the face, pale lips and tongue, and dry tongue.

The features that are specific to Heart Blood Deficiency include facial pallor, poor memory, poor sleep and anxiety, and the features that are specific to Liver Blood Deficiency include floaters and blurring of vision, numbness and lack of initiative.

If Blood Deficiency becomes severe it leads to Yin Deficiency. Additional features of Heart Yin Deficiency include palpitations, restlessness, tendency to be easily startled, and dry tongue. Additional features of Liver Yin Deficiency include dry eyes and withered nails.

It is clear from this summary that there are some correspondences between the features of anemia and the features of Blood Deficiency. Nevertheless, anemia and Blood Deficiency are not the same thing. The physical blood embodies some characteristics of the energetic Blood, but equally some of Qi. Therefore, symptoms of Qi Deficiency as well as of Blood Deficiency might well be expected in someone with anemia.

The condition of Blood and Yin Deficiency can exist even when all blood tests show that the level of hemoglobin and the structure and number of the red blood cells are normal. However, it is safe to assume that, if anemia has been diagnosed, Blood Deficiency, as well as some Yin Deficiency and some Qi Deficiency, will be present.

It may be helpful to think of anemia as one possible manifestation of Blood and Yin Deficiency. In anemia, the energetic imbalance of Blood Deficiency has become manifest in a measurable physical change in the hemoglobin levels and red blood cells.

The symptoms of tiredness, breathlessness and depression are a consequence of the cells of the body not receiving the nourishment in the form of oxygen that they require. Oxygen is an essential ingredient in the process of cell respiration, and thus it is understandable how an insufficient supply of oxygen to the tissues of the body can lead to these general symptoms of anemia.

The sign of pallor is due to the reduction in levels of the bright red colored hemoglobin in the blood.

Palpitations and chest pain occur in severe anemia because the heart responds to the reduced level of oxygen in the blood by pumping faster. This has the initially beneficial effect of increasing the amount of oxygen that reaches the tissues at any one time, but can place strain on the heart muscle itself. The symptoms of angina may result in someone who has a degree of atherosclerosis, and occasionally edema may develop as a result of heart failure.

The causes of anemia

The causes of anemia are conventionally categorized into two groups:

- anemia due to impaired production of red blood cells

- anemia due to increased destruction of red blood cells.

Impaired production of red blood cells

Impaired production of red blood cells most commonly results from a deficiency of the three essential factors required for the healthy development of red blood cells: iron, vitamin B12 and folic acid. This leads to an anemia in which the red blood cells produced in the bone marrow are unable to carry the amount of oxygen that could be carried by normal red blood cells.

Another important cause of reduced production of red blood cells is bone marrow failure. The most common cause of bone marrow failure is cancer. Secondary cancer and blood cancers can form in the marrow spaces in the bones and prevent the healthy growth of bone marrow.

Red blood cells are also under-produced in severe chronic disease such as kidney failure (chronic renal failure) or rheumatoid arthritis. In kidney failure the anemia results from insufficient production of erythropoietin, which is normally made by the healthy kidneys. In other chronic diseases, the cause for the anemia is less clearly understood. Anemia of chronic disease (AOCD) may be a mild anemia, but can still be sufficiently severe to lead to symptoms.

Increased destruction of red blood cells

Red blood cells can become prematurely destroyed either because they have become damaged in some way, or because there is excessive enlargement of the spleen, the main organ responsible for the natural breakdown of the red cells. Again, in these types of anemia the number of red blood cells in the blood is reduced.

The inherited conditions of sickle cell anemia and thalassemia are both conditions in which the red cells are abnormal in shape and are more prone to destruction. Both these conditions are examples of anemia due to the premature destruction of red cells.

Anemias resulting from impaired production of red blood cells

Iron-deficiency anemia

Iron-deficiency anemia is the most common cause of anemia in Western countries. Moreover, it is one of the most important causes of ill health worldwide. In developing countries, deficiency of iron in the diet contributes to poor growth and development, and impairs the ability to fight infections. Iron-deficiency anemia is the underlying cause of millions of premature deaths, especially of women in childbirth, babies and children. Iron deficiency can be compounded in people in tropical countries by the anemia that can result from malaria and other parasitic infections.

Iron-deficiency anemia can result either from inadequate amounts of iron-containing foods in the diet, or from excessive loss of the iron contained in the blood. A combination of the two is commonly present.

Iron is initially obtained in infancy from breast milk, although the amount of iron in breast milk is considered to be insufficient as a sole source of iron in children over the age of one. For this reason, many milk formulas produced for bottle feeding are supplemented with iron. After weaning, iron is obtained from foods such as meat and fish, eggs, whole grains and dark leafy vegetables. In the West many processed cereal products are fortified with iron.

In the West, despite an abundance of food, many people are at risk of iron deficiency because of an inadequate diet. People who are particularly at risk are small children, people on long-term slimming diets, vegetarians and vegans, and older people.

Another group of people who are at risk of iron deficiency are those who cannot absorb iron from the diet because of malabsorption (see Section 3.1e).

In health, the body holds a lot of iron in reserve. The bulk of this is held within the hemoglobin of the red cells, and is recycled for further use when the old red cells are broken down by the spleen. The remainder of the body's iron stores is found in the liver and the muscles. The body can withstand a period of weeks of a relatively low intake of dietary iron. However, unless the diet can provide sufficient iron, the store will eventually run out, as iron is gradually lost through sweat and urine as well as through bleeding.

Iron stores run out much more quickly if excessive blood is lost on a recurrent basis. As many blood donors might wish to testify, the body can withstand a significant loss of blood as long as sufficient time is allowed for the iron stores to recover before the next episode of blood loss. However, in some situations a steady loss of iron from long-term bleeding may be too great to be recovered from the diet alone. This most commonly results from heavy menstrual bleeding, or in people who are unknowingly losing just a few milliliters of blood a day into their bowel from gastrointestinal conditions such as a stomach ulcer. In these cases, the iron stores gradually run down until the manufacture of red cells is affected, and then anemia develops.

Pregnancy and the months following childbirth are recognized as times during which the iron stores can become depleted. The pregnant woman loses iron as it passes through the placenta to the developing fetus, and then a large amount of blood can be lost at delivery. The iron stores will be depleted further as the mother breastfeeds.

It is recognized that it is very common for iron stores to be depleted, although not by enough to affect the production of red blood cells and to cause anemia. This is called latent iron deficiency, and is obviously a state in which the body is not in a good state of balance. Latent iron deficiency is not conventionally recognized to be associated with specific symptoms.

When the iron stores are very low, the red cells produced in the bone marrow are small and pale because of the reduced amount of hemoglobin. They are also reduced in number. This pattern is characteristic of iron deficiency, and so a simple FBC can often be all that is needed to confirm the diagnosis. Serum samples will show reduced levels of iron in the blood.

A patient with iron-deficiency anemia will experience all the general symptoms of anemia, their severity depending on how much the level of hemoglobin has been reduced. Additional symptoms that are recognized to occur in iron-deficiency anemia are believed to be a result of deficiency of iron in certain other tissues of the body such as the skin, the mucous membranes and the nails. In severe iron deficiency a patient might have dry skin and a tendency to bruising, concave (spoon-shaped) nails and a sore tongue and cracked lips. The tongue loses its coat and can appear bright red (likened to a beefsteak). In very severe cases, the retina at the back of the eye can show areas of swelling and bleeding, and this carries a risk of blindness.

In all cases of iron-deficiency anemia, the diagnosis alone is not a sufficient basis on which to start treatment. In all cases, the possibility of malabsorption or excessive blood loss should also be excluded, and this may involve the patient in a referral to a gastroenterologist to exclude chronic bowel disease or bleeding from the bowel. A referral to a gynecologist may be made for the treatment of heavy menstrual bleeding (see Section 5.2c).

Dietary causes of anemia can be rapidly addressed by giving the patient iron supplements in tablet form. Ferrous sulfate and ferrous fumarate are two common preparations. Many iron supplements cause gastrointestinal side effects such as nausea, acid indigestion and constipation, although more naturally derived preparations are available (not on prescription) that are claimed to have fewer of these side effects.

Iron supplements are given in pregnancy very often in mild cases of anemia, to counter the anticipated further iron losses that might occur during childbirth and breastfeeding. Unfortunately, the side effects of nausea, indigestion and constipation can be particularly problematic in pregnancy. This is considered important as anemia at the time of labor is associated with poorer outcomes and excess maternal bleeding.

It is only in very extreme cases of anemia, or in cases in which the bowel cannot absorb iron, that iron is given by other means. In these cases iron may be given by intravenous injection, although this carries risks of more severe side effects.

In anemia due to malabsorption or blood loss, the cause of the anemia should be treated in addition to supplementing the iron stores of the body with iron preparations.

 Information box 3.4c-II

Iron-deficiency anemia: comments from a Chinese medicine perspective

In Chinese medicine, the symptoms of iron-deficiency anemia closely correspond to the syndromes of Heart and Liver Blood (and Yin) Deficiency with Qi Deficiency.

Iron-containing foods include meat and fish, eggs, whole grains and dark leafy vegetables. All these foods would be considered in Chinese medicine to Tone (nourish) the Blood.[72]

Latent iron deficiency is not conventionally recognized to lead to any symptoms. However, it is possible that those non-anemic people who experience the symptoms of Blood Deficiency might have latent iron deficiency. This might explain why it is recognized in Chinese medicine that a diet rich in Blood Toning foods can be of benefit to all people with Blood Deficiency, even if they are not anemic. The Blood Toning diet will build up the iron stores of people with latent iron deficiency, and so will help these people regain a more balanced energetic state.

Medicinal iron preparations nourish the Blood but are also Heating in nature and can deplete Stomach Yin. They may also Stagnate Liver Qi.

Vitamin B12 deficiency and pernicious anemia

Vitamin B12 can be obtained from the diet in foods such as meat, fish and eggs, but not from plants. The liver contains a large store of vitamin B12, which will run out only after two years of lack of the dietary vitamin. For this reason dietary causes of vitamin B12 deficiency are rare, except in people on a strict vegan diet.

A healthy stomach is required for the uptake of vitamin B12, because the parietal cells of the stomach lining are the source of a chemical called intrinsic factor, which is necessary for the absorption of the vitamin. People who have had their stomach removed by surgery are prone to vitamin B12 deficiency for this reason. However, the most common condition to affect the stomach and prevent healthy absorption of vitamin B12 is pernicious anemia. In pernicious anemia the parietal cells of the stomach lining are gradually damaged by an autoimmune process. This condition is most common in middle-aged and older women. It tends to run in families, and this suggests an inherited susceptibility to autoimmune disease.

Lack of vitamin B12 leads to impaired development of the red blood cells. The affected cells are larger than normal, but do not contain sufficient hemoglobin for adequate oxygen transport. The general symptoms and signs of anemia are present, although the pallor may have a slight yellowy tinge. Lack of vitamin B12 affects other tissues, and this leads to additional symptoms. As in iron-deficiency anemia, a sore mouth and tongue can develop. However, the most serious symptoms relate to the nervous system.

In advanced pernicious anemia the patient develops numbness and weakness of the limbs, impaired vision, and eventually dementia, as the nerves are deprived of this essential vitamin. Before injectable vitamin B12 supplements were available, the damage to the nervous system led to permanent disability and sometimes death. This explains why this form of anemia was described as pernicious.

The FBC shows the enlarged blood cells suggestive of vitamin B12 deficiency, but the diagnosis is usually confirmed by means of serum tests for vitamin B12. In over 90 percent of patients with pernicious anemia antibodies are found to parietal cells and intrinsic factor, and this is usually sufficient to confirm diagnosis without performing more invasive tests.

If the cause is dietary, vitamin B12 supplements in tablet form can be given. However, in pernicious anemia these cannot be absorbed by the bowel because of the lack of intrinsic factor. Nevertheless, the symptoms of pernicious anemia can be totally reversed by regular injections of vitamin B12. These injections are usually given at three-month intervals for the rest of the patient's life.

Although in pernicious anemia the patient does not usually suffer from any gastric symptoms, the autoimmune process affecting the lining cells of the stomach is a form of inflammation. Because of this, in some patients, it can eventually lead to cancer.

 Information box 3.4c-III

Pernicious anemia: comments from a Chinese medicine perspective

In Chinese medicine, vitamin B12 deficiency may correspond with Heart and Liver Blood and Yin Deficiency. The symptoms of numbness and visual impairment particularly suggest a Deficiency of Liver Blood. The eventual development of dementia suggests that there has been a progression to severe Depletion of Kidney Yin.

The underlying destruction of the lining cells of the stomach could correspond to a deficiency of Spleen and/or Stomach Yin. The yellowish tinge to the pallor also suggests Spleen Deficiency. This fits with the Chinese medicine understanding that a healthy Spleen is necessary for the formation of Blood.

Vitamin B12 supplements nourish the Blood and Yin, and the Liver in particular. They do not address the underlying cause of the pernicious anemia. Although this is technically a suppressive treatment, there is no doubt that it is life-saving.

Deficiency of folic acid

Like vitamin B12, folic acid (folate) is also important for the healthy development of red blood cells in the bone marrow. Folic acid is found in the diet in meat and in dark green, leafy vegetables. The body does not have very rich reserves of folic acid, so dietary lack can lead to anemia within a few months. Elderly people and those who are dependent on alcohol are particularly vulnerable to folic acid deficiency.

The body uses folic acid when there is rapid repair or growth of cells, as it is used up during mitosis. Pregnancy is a time when folic acid stores can become depleted, as the developing fetus uses up the vitamin. Deficiency can also develop when the body is recovering from major trauma, or in a chronic disease, especially in the case of a rapidly growing cancer.

The red blood cells in folic acid deficiency are large, but have too little hemoglobin. These changes are similar to those caused by vitamin B12 deficiency.

Folic acid deficiency leads to the general symptoms of anemia. A sore tongue may also occur, but there are no other additional symptoms. The most serious consequence of folic acid deficiency is on the developing fetus. If the diet in very early pregnancy is inadequate, insufficient folic acid can lead to defective development of the spinal cord in the first few weeks of the life of the fetus, and the neural tube (spinal) defects including spina bifida can result. This is why all pregnant women are urged to take folic acid supplements for the first 20 weeks of pregnancy.

Studies have shown that folic acid supplementation in pregnancy can reduce the frequency of cases of spina bifida.

Diagnosis of folate-deficiency anemia is confirmed by an FBC and a serum test for folic acid (folate).

Symptoms can be reversed by treatment of any underlying cause, and by folic acid supplementation.

Information box 3.4c-IV

Folate-deficiency anemia: comments from a Chinese medicine perspective

In Chinese medicine, anemia due to folic acid deficiency seems to correspond to Deficiency of Heart and Liver Blood and/or Yin. In addition, folic acid seems to play an important role in nourishing the Jing of the fetus, as its deficiency leads to symptoms that Chinese medicine would ascribe to Jing Deficiency.

Bone marrow failure and aplastic anemia

Bone marrow failure occurs when the normal bone marrow is prevented from developing. This can be the result of cancer in the bones taking over the marrow spaces. Another cause is when the marrow is damaged by certain drugs and radiation. Unfortunately, the treatments that are given for cancer can also cause bone marrow failure, although this is usually temporary. Occasionally, infections, including tuberculosis and certain viruses, can damage the bone marrow sufficiently to cause failure. In many cases the cause is unknown, but may be attributed to an autoimmune process akin to autoimmune idiopathic thrombocytopenic purpura (AITP) (see Section 2.1c).

All three types of blood cell can be depleted in bone marrow failure. This leads to three major problems: thrombocytopenia from insufficient platelets, immune deficiency from insufficient white blood cells, and anemia from insufficient red blood cells. Occasionally, only one type of developing cell is affected. If only the red blood cell is affected, the condition is termed aplastic anemia.

A patient with bone marrow failure will suffer from bleeding, opportunistic infections and the severe general symptoms of anemia. All three of these problems can be life-threatening, and the patient will require nursing in a specialized environment. Blood and platelet transfusions and intravenous antibiotics may be necessary. In some cases of unknown cause, the patient might respond to treatment with corticosteroid drugs. If the cause is irreversible, the patient will eventually die, usually from uncontrollable bleeding or from infection. The one treatment available for severe irreversible cases is bone marrow transplantation. This risky procedure is explained in more detail in Section 3.4e.

Information box 3.4c-V

Bone marrow failure: comments from a Chinese medicine perspective

In Chinese medicine, the symptoms of anemia resulting from bone marrow failure point to severe Deficiency of Blood and Yin. The damage to the marrow represents damage to Kidney Yin and Jing.

Anemia of chronic disease

In a wide range of chronic diseases the patient may develop a form of anemia that cannot be helped by supplementing iron, vitamin B12 or folic acid. This form of anemia is poorly understood, but is possibly mediated by inflammatory proteins generated as part of the underlying condition. Usually, anemia of chronic disease is not severe, but will contribute to the general feeling of malaise that accompanies chronic diseases.[73]

In chronic renal failure the anemia has a more understood cause. The damaged kidney is no longer able to produce the hormone erythropoietin, which stimulates the production of red blood cells. In this case the anemia can become very severe, as a result of greatly reduced numbers of red blood cells. This problem can be treated by injections of synthetic erythropoietin. Before this genetically engineered treatment was available, the only alternative for patients was to receive repeated blood transfusions.

Anemias resulting from increased destruction of red blood cells

Inherited anemias

Some people are born with a problem that affects the shape of the red blood cells. The misshapen cells are more fragile than healthy red blood cells. In some of these conditions the underlying problem lies in the structure of the hemoglobin, resulting from a mutation in the genetic code for hemoglobin.

In health, one function of the spleen is to recognize the aging red blood cells, which become fragile and misshapen, and to remove them from circulation. In these inherited disorders the spleen removes and destroys the misshapen cells prematurely, and this is the main cause of the anemia. Sickle cell anemia and thalassemia are two of the most common inherited anemias worldwide.

Sickle cell anemia

Sickle cell anemia is a condition that is particularly common in black Africans. Up to 25 percent of black Africans carry a mutation in the hemoglobin gene that has been inherited from at least one parent. The condition is only very severe if the child has inherited two mutations, one from each parent. If only one gene has been inherited, this is called sickle cell trait, and rarely causes serious problems.

In sickle cell anemia, the hemoglobin has an abnormal shape like a sickle, which becomes most pronounced when there is very little oxygen in the blood. The sickle-shaped cells are very fragile and can be destroyed as they pass through the tiny capillaries of the circulation, and are also removed and destroyed by the spleen. This will occur more often under conditions where the oxygen level in the blood is reduced, such as when the body is using up more oxygen during infection or following trauma, or when the external oxygen levels are low, such as during an airplane flight.

If many red cells are destroyed at once, this can lead to a very severe situation called a sickle crisis. The broken irregular cells can block up the capillaries and lead to multiple small areas of infarction. This can affect all body parts, including the bones, the lungs, the brain, the kidney and the skin.

Severe complications of infarction of these body parts include intense bone pain and chronic infections of areas of dead bone, lung infarction with pleurisy, strokes, kidney failure and skin ulcers.[74]

The patient in a sickle crisis needs intensive hospital treatment. Intravenous fluids and oxygen are given to nourish the tissues and to reverse the sickling of the cells, and strong opiate painkillers are required. A blood transfusion may be necessary. Recurrent sickling crises may lead to progressive disability and premature death.

 Information box 3.4c-VI

Sickle cell anemia: comments from a Chinese medicine perspective

In Chinese medicine, the symptoms of sickle cell anemia would equate to Blood Deficiency and Blood Stagnation, which are worsened under conditions that reduce the availability of oxygen to the tissues. This suggests that the Deficient Lung Qi may be part of the root of this condition. Because sickle cell anemia is inherited, the principal root of the Blood Deficiency would appear to lie in Kidney Jing.

The sickling crisis is an extreme form of Blood Stagnation, which is a consequence of the Blood Deficiency. Oxygen and fluids nourish the Blood, and so help to move Stagnation.

In between sickle crises, the red cells are broken down more rapidly than should occur in health, particularly by the spleen, but the patient is generally well. A blood test will show reduced numbers of red blood cells and the occasional sickle-shaped cell.

A test for sickle cell anemia is now given in the UK to all newborn babies of African descent as part of the heel-prick test. A drop of blood is all that is required to test for the condition. An early diagnosis will give a child the best possible start in life, as the parents can be made aware about how to act to prevent the development of sickling crises.

THALASSEMIA

The term thalassemia comes from the Greek meaning blood like sea water. It refers to a number of similar types of an inherited disorder of hemoglobin. Thalassemia is common in people from the shores of the Mediterranean, from the Middle East, India and Indonesia, and is particularly common in the Greek Cypriot community.

Depending on the nature of the inherited genes, the condition ranges from a mild anemia to one that causes death in childhood. In severe cases, the abnormal hemoglobin leads to fragility of the red cells and premature destruction of these by the spleen from very early infancy. This leads to a much more severe anemia than is found in most people with sickle cell disease.

In the baby with severe thalassemia, the anemia stimulates the release of erythropoietin from the kidneys, which in turn stimulates the increased production of red blood cells in the marrow. However, this has negative consequences in that the bone marrow expands in the soft developing bones and leads to enlargement and thickening of those bones, and particularly the bones of the skull. Despite this response, the red cells produced are not effective in transporting oxygen, and the child needs repeated blood transfusions. Often the spleen is removed in an older child to reduce the rate at which the red blood cells are destroyed.

Although such intensive treatment may allow the child to reach adulthood, repeated blood transfusions cause long-term problems because the iron contained within them cannot be removed rapidly enough from the body. The excess iron is toxic, and can cause severe damage to the heart, liver and endocrine glands. Many people with severe thalassemia will suffer from extreme ill health. Premature death is usual.

In some cases, bone marrow transplantation using marrow taken from a sibling can provide the child with a source of healthy blood cells. This procedure carries great risks, but can reduce disability in early childhood in those children in whom the procedure is successful (see Section 3.4e).

Information box 3.4c-VII

Thalassemia: comments from a Chinese medicine perspective

In Chinese medicine, thalassemia could be equated to severe Blood Deficiency. The effect of erythropoietin on the bone marrow suggests an inherited imbalance in the Kidney Qi. The root of the problem would therefore be a Deficiency of Kidney Jing.

Blood transfusion initially nourishes the Blood and Yin, but the toxicity of the excess iron eventually depletes the Yin and Yang of the deep organs.

Other causes of premature destruction of red blood cells

Red blood cells can be prematurely destroyed for reasons other than inherited defects of the red cell. However, all conditions involving premature destruction of cells will lead to a condition known as hemolytic anemia. If very severe, the accumulation and clumping of damaged red blood cells in the circulation can lead to infarction of tissues.

Another problem results from the excess hemoglobin that is released from damaged red blood cells. This is broken down by the liver and spleen into the yellowish substance called bilirubin. Bilirubin is usually taken up by the liver and excreted as bile. However, the liver cannot cope with this excessive amount of bilirubin, and so it builds up in the bloodstream, leading to jaundice (see Sections 3.1a and 3.1d).

Occasionally, infections and drugs can damage the red cells, leading to premature hemolysis. Malaria is the most common infection worldwide that has this serious consequence. In a case of severe malaria, the rapid destruction of those red blood cells that have been infected by the malarial parasite can lead to strokes and profound anemia with jaundice. The excess bilirubin spills over into the urine and makes it dark in color. This is why another name for severe malaria is blackwater fever.

The other common cause of premature hemolytic damage to red cells is attack by antibodies. This is the fundamental cause of incompatibility of blood in transfusion. A mismatched blood transfusion will lead to damage to the patient's red cells caused by antibodies contained in the transfused blood. In severe cases this can lead to a sudden reduction in the number of red blood cells, fever because of the inflammatory response, and infarctions of diverse body tissues.

Hemolytic disease of the fetus and newborn

Another example of when antibodies can damage red blood cells and lead to hemolysis is when the blood group of a pregnant woman is different to that of her unborn child.

This problem is usually only clinically important when the mother is rhesus negative and the child is rhesus positive. Maternal antibodies to the rhesus factor can cross the placenta and damage the rhesus factor-containing fetal red cells. This can cause severe anemia, jaundice and sometimes death of the unborn baby.

It is recognized that these antibodies develop particularly in women who have already had a rhesus-positive baby, and seem to form just after the first baby is born. Usually, the blood of the mother and fetus do not mix, but it is believed that a little fetal blood enters the mother's circulation during childbirth, and also during miscarriage. This can be sufficient to stimulate the mother's immune system to produce anti-rhesus antibodies, which are then forever present and can cause problems in subsequent pregnancies.

For this reason, the blood group of all women is tested in early pregnancy. An additional test in rhesus-negative women looks for the presence of antibodies to the rhesus factor, and this test is repeated during the pregnancy.

The development of rhesus antibodies to fetal rhesus-positive blood cells can be prevented. After childbirth or miscarriage, all rhesus-negative women are given an immunization of an antibody that can destroy any rhesus-positive cells that may have entered their circulation. This allows the removal of the foreign blood cells before the mother can develop an immune memory to the rhesus factor. This immunization has dramatically reduced the death and disability that can result from rhesus incompatibility in the newborn.

However, not all cases can be prevented. If rhesus incompatibility is suspected in pregnancy, the mother is referred to a specialist in the condition. Advanced techniques can be used to test for anemia in the fetus and to actually transfuse blood while it is in the womb. The baby may require intensive care after birth and treatment for the jaundice that can result from the damage to its red blood cells (see Chapter 5.4).[75]

Information box 3.4c-VIII

Hemolytic disease of the newborn: comments from a Chinese medicine perspective

In Chinese medicine, the symptoms associated with rhesus incompatibility might represent Blood Deficiency and Blood Stagnation. Jaundice is usually ascribed to Damp Heat in the Liver and Gallbladder, and may result from the Blood Stagnation.

The underlying root of the problem is an attack of an essentially normal fetus by antibodies present in the mother's blood. This attack will inevitably damage Jing, as it occurs at such a vulnerable time in fetal development.

Information box 3.4c-IX

The treatment of patients with anemia: advice for complementary health practitioners

A clinical diagnosis of anemia suggests that there is a significant imbalance of Vital Substances (in Chinese medicine this would be framed as Deficiency of Blood and Qi), and so nutritional supplementation and herbal treatments would be appropriate in addition to solely energetically focused treatments such as acupuncture and homeopathy.

In cases of anemia due to poor diet, medicinal supplements of iron, vitamin B12 or folic acid (depending on the underlying cause of the anemia) may be energetically appropriate remedies. All these are available in naturally produced preparations, and are relatively inexpensive compared to herbs.

To recommend supplements it is essential to be sure of the underlying cause of the anemia. Therefore,

it is wise to refer a patient for a conventional diagnosis so that any underlying problem such as blood loss or malabsorption can be excluded, and so that the appropriate supplements can be recommended. This advice is of particular importance in pernicious anemia. If folic acid supplements are mistakenly taken in pernicious anemia, these can lead to worsening of the damage that vitamin B12 deficiency can cause to the nervous system.

The other advantage of a conventional diagnosis is that a full blood count (FBC) can provide a numerical and objective measure of the degree of anemia. This can be a useful benchmark against which to assess the benefits of future treatment.

The red flags of anemia

Some patients with anemia will benefit from referral to a conventional doctor for assessment or treatment. Red flags are those symptoms and signs that indicate that referral should be considered. The red flags of anemia are described in Table 3.4c-I. A summary of the red flags in a format designed for quick reference in clinical practice can be found in Appendix III. This gives advice on the degree of urgency of referral for each of the red flag conditions listed.

Table 3.4c-I A18: Red flags of anemia

Red flag	Description	Reasoning
A18.1	Features of long-standing anemia: any of the general symptoms of anemia should be considered as a reason for referral so that serious treatable causes can be excluded. These include: • pallor • tiredness • palpitations • breathlessness on exertion • feeling of faintness • depression • sore mouth and tongue	Anemia refers to a reduced hemoglobin level in the blood. Hemoglobin is the iron-containing pigment that enables red blood cells to carry high concentrations of oxygen to the tissues. When hemoglobin levels are low, the tissues experience relative oxygen lack Reduced concentration of the pigment in the blood can be seen in the skin as pallor The cardiovascular system responds by increasing the heart rate and the respiratory rate increases, so leading to palpitations and breathlessness Iron stores in the body become low as iron is utilized to the maximum, and the tissue cells suffer, meaning that the person suffers tiredness, depression and sore mouth and tongue, and dry skin and hair Referral is important to establish the cause of the anemia Causes include: • increased blood loss (particularly from menstruation and bleeding from stomach or bowel, and prolonged use of aspirin or non-steroidal anti-inflammatory drugs (NSAIDs)) • reduced production of blood in the marrow (due to poor diet, malabsorption of iron, vitamin B12 or folic acid from the diet, and bone marrow disease) • chronic illness Mild anemia is common and benign in pregnancy

A18.2	Features of severe anemia: the following additional symptoms and signs suggest that anemia is very severe: • extreme tiredness • severe breathlessness on exertion • excessive bruising • severe visual disturbances • chest pain on exertion • tachycardia • edema	See A18.1. Severe anemia puts extra strain on the heart as it attempts to increase oxygen delivery to the tissues by increasing cardiac output. This can lead to cardiac failure and angina
A18.3	Features of pernicious anemia: • tiredness • lemon-yellow pallor • gradual onset of neurological symptoms (numbness, weakness)	Pernicious anemia is a form of anemia that results from an impaired ability to absorb vitamin B12 from the digestive tract. The underlying cause is an autoimmune disease that affects the production of a protein (intrinsic factor) from the stomach. Intrinsic factor needs to bind to vitamin B12 before the vitamin can be absorbed As vitamin B12 is also vital to the health of the nervous system, neurological symptoms can develop if deficiency is prolonged. Treatment involves regular and lifelong injections of vitamin B12

3.4d Acute blood loss, transfusion and disorders of the spleen

This section begins by summarizing the ways in which the sudden loss of a large volume of blood can affect the body. Hemorrhage (meaning flow of blood) is the medical term used to describe blood loss. Severe hemorrhage can lead to a condition conventionally termed shock.

Shock is the result of any condition in which the ability of the blood to transport oxygen and nutrients to the tissues is suddenly reduced. Although blood loss is one major cause, there are a number of other causes that are also discussed in this section.

One important emergency treatment for hemorrhage is transfusion of blood to replace the plasma and blood cells that have been lost. Transfusion can also be used in other conditions, such as in the treatment of two types of anemia already described, thalassemia and rhesus disease of the newborn. The common conditions in which transfusion of blood, or one of its component parts, is performed are explored in this section.

The conditions that can result from diseases of the spleen are described at the end. Strictly speaking, the spleen is part of the lymphatic system, but it is included here because it plays such an important role in the physiology of the blood.

Acute blood loss

The sudden loss of a large volume of blood is a major trauma to the body. It most commonly occurs as a result of physical injury. Road traffic accidents and bleeding during surgery are the most significant causes of sudden blood loss in the UK.

There are also some common internal causes of hemorrhage. These include bleeding from gastrointestinal disease, such as peptic ulcer, and esophageal varicose veins in liver disease. Occasionally, bleeding from a tumor in the bowel or the lung can be very severe. Another site from which a lot of blood can be lost is the uterus, following childbirth or miscarriage.

The body can usually withstand the sudden loss of less than 500 milliliters of blood. This corresponds to about one-eighth of the circulating volume. This is the amount of blood that is withdrawn from the vein of a blood donor in a single donation session. Nevertheless, it is not uncommon for blood donors to feel dizzy or faint immediately after giving blood. This symptom arises because the body has not had time to adjust to the sudden reduction in volume of the blood.

When the blood volume is suddenly reduced as a result of hemorrhage, there is an immediate drop in blood pressure. This can be compared to suddenly releasing air from a bicycle tire so that the tire pressure drops. A sudden drop in blood pressure causes an immediate drop in the amount of oxygen and nutrients that can reach the tissues. The brain responds most rapidly to this change, as it requires an adequate level of oxygen and glucose to function well. The lack of oxygen and glucose in the brain is the cause of dizziness and fainting, and if the drop is very severe the person may lose consciousness.

There are sensors in the circulation that can detect a sudden drop in blood pressure. The most important of these are situated in the aorta and the carotid vessels of the neck. These are part of a negative feedback loop (see Section 1.1c), which ensures that the blood pressure is kept at a steady level. As soon as the blood pressure drops, the sensors trigger a series of bodily changes to ensure that the tissues regain a supply of oxygen and nutrients. It is not necessary to go into too much detail about the mechanism of the negative feedback loop. However, it is helpful to understand that one of the results of a drop in blood pressure is that a range of hormones, including adrenaline, renin and the body's natural steroid, cortisol, is released into the bloodstream. All these hormones have effects on the body that tend to increase blood pressure. They also tend to increase the availability to the tissues of nutrients stored in the body. Adrenaline, renin and cortisol are all released from the region of the body in which the kidneys are located. Adrenaline and cortisol are made in the adrenal glands, and renin in the kidneys themselves.

These responses include an increase in heart rate, constriction of the blood vessels, particularly in the superficial parts of the body (leading to coldness of the hands and feet), conservation of water by the kidneys, release of sugar into the blood from the liver, and the emotional response of panic or fear.

To summarize, after an initial drop in blood volume from hemorrhage, there are a number of bodily responses that have the effect of increasing the supply of blood and nutrients to the tissues, and in particular to the deep organs. From a patient's point of view, the experience of acute blood loss will bring about symptoms of dizziness and feeling faint. There will also be profound symptoms resulting from the bodily reaction to this blood loss. The patient will have a racing heart, and clammy and cold hands and feet. They will pass very little urine. The dizziness and faint feeling might be overcome by a sense of urgency, panic or fear.

If blood loss continues, these bodily reactions are not sufficient to protect the tissues from lack of oxygen and sugar. The patient will feel increasingly cold at their core. The heart rate might slow down again. Faintness and confusion may increase, and gradually the patient will lose consciousness. Without urgent medical treatment, the patient in this state is very close to death.

Shock

Shock is the medical term used to describe the syndrome of these bodily responses to a sudden reduction in the supply of oxygen and nutrients to the tissues. However, sudden hemorrhage is only one cause of shock.

Shock can result from three other medically significant causes: acute heart failure, acute allergic reaction and severe infection.

Shock resulting from acute heart failure

In acute heart failure, the pumping action of the heart suddenly deteriorates. This may be due to cardiac arrest or another arrhythmia, weakening of the heart muscle following a heart attack, or compression of the heart through injury.

Shock resulting from acute allergic reaction (anaphylaxis)

Anaphylactic shock is the most severe form of allergic reaction. In cases of severe allergy there is a dramatic release of a number of chemicals of inflammation into the bloodstream. The function of these in health is to cause dilatation of the blood vessels and leakage of fluid into the tissues. However, in excessive quantities they cause a life-threatening reaction involving widespread swelling of the tissues, spasm of the bronchi and bronchioles (asthma), and a sudden drop in blood pressure.

Shock resulting from severe infection and sepsis

In very severe infection, toxins released by the infectious organism can cause a similar reaction of dilatation of all the blood vessels in the body. This is a life-threatening condition formerly called endotoxic shock, and now described as septicemic shock. The condition that predisposes to shock is called sepsis, some of the markers of which are fever, drop in blood pressure, lethargy, cold extremities and confusion. Patients with sepsis need urgent management in intensive care units as it is a life-threatening condition that can result in multi-organ failure. Sepsis is a condition that may present insidiously and often too late. All patients unwell after having an infectious disease and any with unexplained acute serious illness need to be considered as possibly having sepsis. Septic shock leads to death in 40 percent of cases.[76]

Fainting

Profound emotion can also lead to a sudden drop in blood pressure, so much so as to cause fainting (see Section 3.2a). This reaction will rarely lead to a prolonged condition of shock in the medical sense of the term, because it is so readily reversed by the bodily reactions triggered by the sudden drop in blood pressure. However, technically speaking, for the brief period leading up to the faint, the body is in the state of shock. Although there are no life-threatening consequences, there is no doubt that the body in such a situation has had to respond in a sudden and profound way, and will need some time to recover and regain a state of balance. This temporary but unbalanced state is what is being described when we hear on the news that people involved in traumatic situations have been treated for shock.

The treatment of shock

Treatment of shock should always involve treating the cause with measures including stemming blood loss, treating heart failure and treating any infections with antibiotics.

Treatment of the temporary shock that results from emotional trauma involves allowing the person to rest, giving sweet warm drinks and providing emotional support. However, when the state of shock is very profound and always if sepsis is suspected, this has to be treated as an urgent priority. Patients in severe shock are ideally managed in an intensive care unit, with close monitoring of the important body functions.

In situations in which fluid has been lost from the circulation, it can be replaced by rapid infusions of saline and blood. When it is the cardiovascular system and not the volume of blood that is the problem, a wide range of drugs, including adrenaline, are given to encourage the heart to beat faster and the blood vessels to constrict. The insertion of an intravenous cannula (tube), fed via the superficial veins of the neck deep into the right side of the heart (a central line), may be necessary so that fluid pressures can be assessed accurately.

Information box 3.4d-I

Shock: comments from a Chinese medicine perspective

In Chinese medicine, an emotional or physical shock is believed to Deplete the Kidneys, and in particular, the Jing, which is a deep reserve of condensed Qi. In conventional medicine terms, the body responds to the state of shock by the release of powerful hormones, many of which either originate from or affect the kidneys. This response draws on stored nutrients in the body. Here the possible correspondence with the Chinese medicine view is clear.

In the case of hemorrhage, treatment with blood and fluids is an appropriate energetic remedy because it replaces the lost Blood and Yin. Treatment of other forms of shock with drugs that stimulate the kidneys and cardiovascular system, such as adrenaline, boost Kidney and Heart Yang. In doing so, they draw on the body's deep reserves of Yin and Yang. They are therefore ultimately depleting. Although life-saving in the short term, these treatments are ultimately suppressive in nature, and the patient can ideally take time and treatment to recover from the energetic repercussions of both being so unwell and also receiving such powerful treatments.

Blood transfusion

In many situations the transfusion of whole blood or components of the blood is a life-saving treatment when the body requires replacement of these substances.

Ideally, blood donors are healthy individuals. In the UK volunteer donors are asked a series of screening questions in order to exclude potential donors who may have come into contact with any of the infectious diseases that affect the blood, such as human immunodeficiency virus (HIV) and hepatitis. In addition, a simple blood test is used to exclude people who are anemic.

All donated blood is screened for infectious diseases, such as HIV, hepatitis and syphilis, and is treated to kill infectious agents. The blood is then typed according to the ABO and rhesus blood groups.

In very severe acute blood loss, whole blood is occasionally used as the replacement treatment. However, in most cases the patient only requires one part of the blood. For these cases, the blood is separated into its component parts of plasma, white cells, platelets and red cells. The plasma proteins can be separated from the plasma so that people who are in need of clotting factors or antibodies might be given these factors only.

The risks of blood transfusion

Blood transfusion carries risks, and for this reason should not be performed unless considered absolutely necessary. These risks include the transmission of infection and the problems that can result from incompatibility with the blood of the recipient.

Despite screening and treatment for infections, there is always a risk that donated blood carries infectious agents. Recent history provides tragic examples of the problems caused by the transmission of infections such as HIV and hepatitis C and D via donated blood products. These were infections that, at the time of the transfusions, were not fully recognized. It has been estimated that before hepatitis C testing was introduced in 1991, up to 1 percent of all transfusions led to this form of hepatitis in the recipient. It is very possible that there are still some infections, not yet isolated, which might in the future be found in donated blood.

Although the risks of infection from transfusion of blood products are considered to be very low, they are, of course, increased in those people who require repeated transfusions. This is the reason why so many patients with hemophilia, who need regular transfusions of clotting factors, have developed hepatitis C and HIV in recent years (see Section 2.1c).

The other risk of transfusion comes from incompatibility. Ideally, before each transfusion, the blood of the donor and the recipient is cross-matched. This involves a laboratory test to rule out the possibility of an immune reaction that could lead to damage of either the donated or the recipient's blood cells. The test involves checking that antibodies to the red blood cells are not present. Again, although cross-matching very much reduces the risk of major immune reactions, it is not a fail-safe.

Incompatibility reactions are more common in patients who receive repeated blood transfusions because they gradually build up immunity to all the foreign blood cells that their body encounters. This can become very problematic in conditions such as thalassemia, in which repeated transfusions are necessary.

A mild reaction may simply involve a fever or rash, which settles down over a few hours. This is thought to result from immune reactions between the plasma proteins or white cells of the recipient and donor. Mild reactions are common. However, in rare cases, this reaction is very severe, leading to high fever and a form of anaphylactic shock. In this life-threatening situation the patient may need to be given intravenous adrenaline, antihistamines and corticosteroids to reverse the reaction.

Incompatibility of red cells is a very serious situation. The damaged red cells can clump to cause infarction and will release a lot of hemoglobin into the circulation. This can damage the kidneys, and the bilirubin that is formed leads to a severe form of jaundice.

The clinical uses of transfusion of blood products

Blood is most commonly used in the UK to replace losses that have occurred through hemorrhage from injury, disease or surgery. Unless blood loss is very severe, red cells are transfused, rather than whole blood, as this minimizes the risks of incompatibility from the other parts of the blood. Fluid losses are replaced by intravenous saline solution.

As described in Section 3.4c, red cells are also used in certain types of anemia, such as aplastic anemia and thalassemia, to increase the numbers of red cells in the circulating blood. These transfusions have to be repeated at regular intervals because the life of red cells in transfused blood is no more than one to two months.

Platelets may be used in severe cases of thrombocytopenia and bone marrow failure, to increase the clotting function of the blood.

Plasma is used to provide clotting factors in situations such as severe infection and trauma, when the body's own supply of clotting factors has been used up.

Antibodies can be obtained from the pooled plasma of many donors. These are most commonly used in the practice of vaccination to generate passive immunity. This is only a temporary immunity because the antibodies have a life of about three months. Preparations of human antibodies are called immunoglobulins, and are most useful in vulnerable people who have had recent exposure to a dangerous disease such as rabies, when there is no time for the patient to develop their own immune response.

The various blood products can be irradiated to reduce transfusion reactions or chemically treated to minimize risk of infections.[77]

 Information box 3.4d-II

Transfusion: comments from a Chinese medicine perspective

In Chinese medicine, the transfusion of blood products would appear to be a form of Nourishing Blood and Yin. However, transfused blood can never perfectly match the requirements of the patient. The presence of foreign antigens and antibodies, as well as infectious agents in blood products, is a potential form of Xie Qi, which can have damaging effects on the body by leading to the Invasion of Pathogenic Factors and Depletion of Vital Substances.

Conversely, the donation of blood will Deplete the Blood, Yin and Qi of the donor. Although the lives of many people depend on blood donation, blood donors should be made aware of the way in which it can cause depletion. In fit individuals, the losses can be made up through attention to rest and diet. Blood donation may not be advisable in those who are already deficient in Blood and/or Qi.

Disorders of the spleen

In this concluding section the ways in which the spleen is affected by disease are explored.

The spleen is composed of two different sorts of connective tissue, described as the white pulp and the red pulp. The role of the white pulp is as part of the immune system. This part of the spleen can be compared to a very large lymph node through which all blood flows. The spleen houses many lymphocytes, some of which mature as they rest within it. The spleen is important in the development of immunity to disease and the production of antibodies.

The primary role of the red pulp in health is to ensure the removal of aging and misshapen red blood cells and platelets. This leads to the release of iron and bilirubin into the circulation. This role of the red pulp is also shared by the liver and bone marrow. The red pulp also has the capability of housing bone marrow tissue. This means that, in times of stress, extra blood cells can be made within the spleen. This property is also shared by the liver.

 Information box 3.4d-III

The spleen: comments from a Chinese medicine perspective

The roles of the spleen recognized by conventional medicine cannot be easily directly attributed to the Spleen Organ as described in Chinese medicine. In turn, the digestive function of the Spleen Organ is more properly attributed to the various functions of the conventional gastrointestinal system, to which the spleen, interestingly, is embryologically related. However, the main role of the red pulp of the spleen can be seen to overlap with this digestive function, in that it breaks down the aging blood cells and enables the nutrients contained therein to be recycled for further use in the body.

Another function of the red pulp is that it literally "holds blood." Up to one-third of the platelets available to the circulation are stored within the spleen, from where they can be released when necessary. Here is a remarkable correspondence with the ancient Chinese view that one function of the healthy Spleen is to hold blood and so to prevent bleeding.

The role of the white pulp of the spleen in the immune system much more closely fits with the combined roles of Wei Qi and its foundation Kidney Jing. As discussed in Section 2.1d, these are the Substances that are seen in Chinese medicine to be important in protecting the body from invasion by Pathogenic Factors of external origin.

Rupture of the spleen

Rupture is probably the most common condition to affect the spleen and is a consequence of modern life. This is because the trauma that is associated with a serious road traffic accident very commonly involves the spleen. It is an unfortunate characteristic of seat belts that they can forcefully compress the abdomen in an accident that has occurred at high speed, and in this way the spleen can be damaged. However, the damage that can result from not wearing a seat belt is potentially far more severe than rupture of the spleen.

The spleen has a delicate lining and is very vulnerable to trauma. Once damaged, bleeding from the red pulp of the spleen can be profuse. It is a surgical emergency, often requiring a large transfusion of blood. Occasionally, the damage is so severe that repair is impossible, and the spleen is removed to stop the bleeding.

Loss of the spleen (asplenism)

The spleen is most commonly removed because of damage in traumatic accidents as described above. However, there are certain conditions in which the spleen is removed for medical reasons in a surgical operation known as a splenectomy. These include those conditions in which there is a need to preserve red blood cells or platelets, as these are usually removed by the spleen. Splenectomy may be performed for these reasons in conditions such as thalassemia and thrombocytopenia.

Sometimes the spleen has to be removed because it has become too large. This can be a problem because a large spleen will cause excessive destruction of blood cells and can then lead to anemia and thrombocytopenia.

In the short term, the loss of the spleen leads to a buildup of platelets because these can no longer be removed from the blood as rapidly, and this may lead to problems with excessive blood clotting. However, in a few weeks this problem settles down as the liver and bone marrow begin to take over this role of the red pulp of the spleen.

The major long-term problem with a splenectomy is that there is a risk of the patient developing overwhelming infections. For a reason that is unclear, patients are particularly at risk of infections caused by the very common respiratory bacterium *Streptococcus pneumoniae*. For this reason, all patients are given a vaccination to protect against streptococcal infections. Some patients may be prescribed regular penicillin to reduce further the risk of infections.

Information box 3.4d-IV

Loss of the spleen: comments from a Chinese medicine perspective

In Chinese medicine, loss of the spleen does not directly correspond with Spleen Deficiency, as digestive symptoms are not prominent. Much of the role of the red pulp is not lost, but it is taken over by the liver and bone marrow. The main problem that results from a splenectomy is impaired immunity, and in particular, to an infection that normally leads to Wind Heat progressing to Lung Heat. This suggests that loss of the spleen must in some ways be regarded as equivalent to a form of Depletion of Wei Qi and possibly also of Kidney Jing.

Enlarged spleen (hypersplenism)

In health, the spleen is about the size of a large fist and sits at the back of the abdominal cavity, resting against the tenth to twelfth ribs on the left. It cannot normally be felt on examination of the abdomen.

In certain conditions the spleen can enlarge to an enormous size. Sometimes the spleen can be felt extending below the umbilicus in the front of the abdomen. This can occasionally result from infections, and tropical infections in particular. Infectious mononucleosis (glandular fever) is the most common cause of temporary enlargement of the spleen in the UK, and this leads to its common symptom of pain under the ribs on the left-hand side. Occasionally, the enlargement of the spleen in infectious mononucleosis can be so rapid as to lead to rupture, although this complication is very rare.

Another cause of a much enlarged spleen is cancer of the blood cells (leukemia and lymphoma), described in the next section. In these cancers the spleen enlarges as it fills up with excessive cancerous white blood cells.

The main problem of an enlarged spleen is that it can cause excessive destruction of the red cells and platelets. If this becomes a severe problem, the spleen can be surgically removed.

Information box 3.4d-V

Enlargement of the spleen: comments from a Chinese medicine perspective

The condition of an enlarged spleen can lead to anemia and bleeding due to excessive destruction of the red cells and platelets. This would be consistent with the symptoms associated with Deficiency of Blood and Yin, with Spleen Qi not holding Blood.

The red flags of hemorrhage and shock

Red flags are those symptoms and signs that indicate that referral to a conventional doctor should be considered. The red flags of the conditions discussed in this section are described in Table 3.4d-I. A summary of the red flags in a format designed for quick reference in clinical practice can be found in Appendix III. This gives advice on the degree of urgency of referral for each of the red flag conditions listed.

Table 3.4d-I A19: Red flags of hemorrhage and shock

Red flag	Description	Reasoning
A19.1	Continuing blood loss: any situation in which significant bleeding is continuing for more than a few minutes without any signs of abating (except in the context of menstruation)	An adequate volume of blood in the circulation is essential to maintain the blood pressure required to enable adequate perfusion of the organs and tissues of the body. If blood pressure drops too low, the syndrome of shock develops (see A19.3)
		Shock is defined as a situation in which there is a failure of the circulatory system to maintain adequate perfusion of vital organs
		If bleeding is continuing unabated, the patient needs to be referred for fluid replacement and medical or surgical intervention to prevent further blood loss. This is of particular concern if the bleeding is from an internal location
		Administer basic first aid to accessible bleeding sites while waiting for help to arrive

A19.2	Features of severe blood loss leading to shock: refer if blood has been lost and the following symptoms and signs have been present for more than a few minutes or are worsening: • dizziness, fainting and confusion • rapid pulse of >100 beats/minute • blood pressure <90/50mmHg • cold and clammy extremities	If the symptoms of shock (see A19.3) are developing, this is an emergency situation. Administer basic first aid to bleeding sites. Ensure the patient is lying down and is kept warm while waiting for help to arrive
A19.3	General symptoms of shock or sepsis: • dizziness, fainting and confusion • rapid pulse of >100 beats/minute • blood pressure <90/50mmHg • cold and clammy extremities Refer if these symptoms are worsening or sustained (more than a few seconds)	Shock can result from: • blood loss and extreme dehydration (hypovolemic shock) • an allergic reaction (anaphylactic shock) • overwhelming infection (septic shock) • failure of the heart to maintain an adequate circulation (cardiogenic shock resulting from damage to heart muscle, heart valves or from an arrhythmia) Sustained shock is always a situation in which treatment is required as an emergency, as the vulnerable organs of the brain, kidneys and heart are at risk of damage from inadequate levels of oxygen and nutrients A faint can produce a syndrome that is akin to shock, but the drop in blood pressure is always short-lived and the person should start to recover within seconds. In the case of a faint, the drop in blood pressure follows a sudden slowing of the heart rate. For this reason, a weak and slow pulse would be expected in the few seconds following a faint, and this should return to a normal rate within 1–2 minutes. There is no need to refer in this situation
A19.4	Additional symptoms of anaphylactic shock: • widespread inflammatory response with warm extremities, puffy skin and face, difficulty breathing	In anaphylactic shock the drop in blood pressure is a result of an extreme allergic reaction. In this case, the collapse may be preceded by a patchy swelling of the skin (hives) and worsening asthma. This is an emergency situation, as the symptoms can worsen rapidly to a state of respiratory and circulatory collapse

3.4e Cancer of the blood cells

This section is concerned with the three main types of cancer of the white blood cells: leukemia, lymphoma and myeloma. These are the focus of a single section because, as blood is a fluid tissue, cancer of the blood has characteristics that are different to the solid cancers described in Chapter 2.3.

The cancers of the blood are relatively rare. Leukemia and lymphoma are particularly well known because, although rare, they are two of the most common forms of cancer that affect children and young adults. These are also unusual forms of cancer in that often they can be cured by medical treatment, particularly in young people.

This section focuses on the clinical features and treatment of these three most common forms of cancer.

Leukemia

Leukemia is a term derived from the Greek meaning white blood. This description refers to the fact that the numbers of white blood cells in the circulating blood can be greatly increased in some forms of leukemia. Leukemia results from a cancerous mutation in a single immature white blood cell within the bone marrow. The cancerous change means that this single cell multiplies at an uncontrolled rate, just as occurs in solid cancers.

The cause of leukemia

In children it is now believed that the initial genetic defect that leads to susceptibility to leukemia is present by the time of birth. Then subsequent infections such as influenza or exposure to carcinogens such as X-rays may be the trigger to lead to cancerous change in a white blood stem cell. In most individual cases no definite cause can be found for the cancerous change. However, it is recognized that certain environmental factors increase the risk of leukemia. For example, there is clear evidence of a link between childhood leukemia and maternal exposure to X-rays, and adult leukemia and exposure to radioactive fallout after an atomic explosion, such as occurred in the communities living close to Hiroshima. Certain chemicals, including benzene, and drugs, including some used in cancer chemotherapy, are also known to increase the risk of leukemia.

The tendency to leukemia runs slightly in families, suggesting a genetic susceptibility. It is also more common in people with Down syndrome.

The types of leukemia

There are many different types of leukemia and these can be categorized according to the exact type of white blood cell that has mutated, the surface chemistry of the cancer cells and the form of their chromosomes. Each type of leukemia can also be broadly categorized as either acute leukemia or chronic leukemia. This categorization is made on the basis of the speed of development of the leukemia. Acute leukemia is the type that most commonly affects children and young adults.

Acute leukemia

In acute leukemia the cancerous white blood cells multiply extremely rapidly and cause symptoms because they take over the bone marrow space. This leads to the life-threatening syndrome of bone marrow failure, described in Section 3.4c.

Acute leukemia can be diagnosed on the basis of a full blood count (FBC) and blood film, and a bone marrow investigation, in which the excessive numbers of white blood cells can be clearly measured and seen.

Without urgent treatment, the patient will inevitably succumb to severe infection or hemorrhage within days or weeks of diagnosis. Bone pain may be a prominent symptom.

The treatment of acute leukemia should take place in a specialized environment in which the patient is kept at low risk of infection. Any infections that develop are treated with high-dose intravenous antibiotics. Anemia and thrombocytopenia may require transfusions of red cells and platelets, respectively.

The cancer is treated with cycles of intensive chemotherapy (including drugs such as vincristine, prednisolone, asparaginase and doxorubicin) over the course of six to twelve months. In cases in which it is assessed that there is a high risk of spread of cancer cells to the nervous system, chemotherapy is given into the spinal fluid as well as intravenously. The treatment itself damages the already depleted cells of the bone marrow,

and so the patient has to be intensively nursed during this period. Patients may be given drugs to stimulate the regrowth of healthy white blood cells (colony stimulating factor) during this time. In some types of acute leukemia the cancer cells are rapidly destroyed by the treatment. If the patient can survive the risky period of treatment, they may be left with no measurable evidence of leukemia. However, although there is no evidence of leukemia, it is still possible that a few cancer cells remain in the body. This state is called remission.

In the most common form of childhood leukemia, up to 90 percent of children enter complete remission. However, in adults, and in other forms of acute leukemia, the success rate is not so high. Without more intensive consolidation treatment, after months to a few years the leukemia reappears, this time in a form that is more resistant to treatment. Therefore, to prevent these relapses, further maintenance chemotherapy may be given, or a bone marrow transplant may be performed.[78]

Bone marrow transplant involves replacing the potentially cancer-containing bone marrow of the patient with a sample of healthy bone marrow. This can involve use of the patient's own bone marrow, which is withdrawn by a needle just after remission has been induced by chemotherapy. It can only be hoped that this sample does not contain lingering cancer cells. Alternatively, transplant involves the use of marrow from a donor, who is ideally a close relative of the patient.

The principle of bone marrow transplant is first to totally kill all remaining bone marrow after remission has been induced by high-dose chemotherapy (cyclophosphamide) and irradiation. This is a most risky time for the patient, as all the blood-forming stem cells have been removed and the patient becomes totally dependent for a time on transfused blood products. The healthy bone marrow sample is then injected into one of the patient's veins. The stem cells within the sample find their way into the patient's marrow spaces and start to multiply. If successful, the transplant will "take" and new blood cells will start to be produced.

There is a risk that marrow from a donor will not survive in the patient host because the white cells within it start to damage the patient's tissues, which they recognize as foreign (so-called graft-versus-host disease). This is more likely to occur if a non-relative's marrow is used. To prevent this, the patient has to stay on immunosuppressive medication for life, and so this means accepting all the side effects and risks that this powerful treatment brings (see Section 2.2c).

Up to one-third of patients who receive donated marrow die during the treatment. The risks are lower with the use of the patient's own marrow, but the risks of cancer recurrence are greater. In those who survive the treatment, bone marrow transplant can bring about cure of the leukemia, but in every case a very careful risk-benefit analysis has to be made. For this reason, bone marrow transplants are generally performed in the forms of leukemia that are less likely to respond to chemotherapy alone.

The long-term effects of cancer chemotherapy on children cannot be estimated fully because this form of treatment has only been used widely with success over the past four or five decades. There is no doubt that the physical depletion that results from the toxic drugs and corticosteroids given at such a vulnerable time

in development is great, and problems in lung function, thyroid function, fertility and growth may become apparent. It is increasingly being recognized that the psychological impact of having a life-threatening disease for a period of two years or more in childhood is also very significant. In addition, the time scale and severity of treatment cause shock waves that affect all the close relatives of the sick child.

 Information box 3.4e-I

Acute leukemia: comments from a Chinese medicine perspective

The stem cells in the bone marrow, viewed from the perspective of Chinese medicine, could be seen as one of the physical roots of Blood and Yin, as these are the source of the healthy blood cells. In this way they could be seen as corresponding to Kidney Jing. The stem cells are crowded out in acute leukemia. Therefore, in Chinese medicine acute leukemia could be interpreted as severe Deficiency of Jing, Blood and Yin. The immune deficiency and bleeding suggest that there is additional Deficiency of Spleen and Lung Qi.

The cause of these deficiencies is the rapidly dividing cancerous white cells. External factors such as irradiation and acute infections can trigger leukemia. A possible interpretation is that Toxic Xie Qi has damaged Blood and Fluids and has led to the congealing of Phlegm in addition to profound Depletion of Jing, Blood and Yin. This is an interpretation that accords with the appearance of

the swollen lymph tissue that develops in some forms of leukemia.

Chemotherapy would be seen as Clearing of Phlegm but Depleting of Jing, Blood and Yin because it too destroys bone marrow tissue. This has to be suppressive in nature, because the root cause is not treated. Many individuals, and especially children, can survive this depletion, probably because they have deep reserves of Vital Substances, which can be built up once the Phlegm has been cleared.

Bone marrow transplant literally replaces the lost Vital Substances of Jing, Blood and Yin. However, as with blood transfusion, there is a very high risk of the introduction of Pathogenic Xie Qi with the treatment. Immunosuppressive treatment that is often needed after bone marrow transplant tends to be Heating and Stagnating and Depleting of Blood and Yin.

CHRONIC LEUKEMIA

Chronic leukemia is a disease of older people, and also, occasionally, teenagers. In chronic leukemia, the onset of the disease is much slower than in acute leukemia. The underlying cause is the same, a multiplication of a cancerous white blood cell. Chronic leukemia is also classified on the basis of cell type, and also the chromosomal status of the cells. The different manifestations include chronic myelocytic leukemia (CML), chronic lymphocytic leukemia (CLL), and a cluster of conditions of abnormal cellular development of the bone marrow called myelodysplastic syndromes.

Because of the slow onset, less acute symptoms such as enlarged lymph nodes or recurrent low fevers may be the first symptoms. Sometimes the diagnosis is made by chance because an FBC blood test is taken for another unrelated reason.

As the condition progresses, the multiplication of cancer cells tends to become more active and a transformation to acute leukemia can develop. Treatment with chemotherapy (including chlorambucil, corticosteroids, alpha-interferon and imatinib) can slow the disease, but is not expected

to be curative. However, a few patients can be cured with a combination of chemotherapy and a bone marrow transplant. Even if cure is not achieved, symptoms can be held at bay by intermittent drug treatment, and in some cases they may not necessarily lead to premature death.

 Information box 3.4e-II

Chronic leukemia: comments from a Chinese medicine perspective

The Chinese medicine interpretation of chronic leukemia is similar to that of acute leukemia. The chances of long-term survival are lower, possibly because the reserves of Vital Substances are much lower in elderly people.

Lymphoma

Lymphoma is a tumor of the white blood cells that originates not in the bone marrow but in lymph tissue. The most common site for a lymphoma to develop is in a lymph node, but it can also occasionally emerge from within the lymphoid cells that line the respiratory tract or the gastrointestinal tract.

One type of lymphoma, called Hodgkin's disease, is particularly common in young adults. This tumor predominantly affects the lymph nodes of the neck and is potentially curable. Certain forms of Hodgkin's lymphoma seem to be associated with previous infectious mononucleosis (glandular fever) infection.

As well as an abnormal swelling of a lymph node, Hodgkin's disease can lead to symptoms such as fevers, itching and loss of appetite. Often the disease can be diagnosed early in its development because the swollen lymph nodes in the neck are very noticeable.

Other forms of lymphoma may have similar symptoms, although these can also affect deep lymph nodes or other sites such as the bowel, and so diagnosis may be delayed. In advanced lymphoma, a number of lymph nodes as well as the spleen and liver may be found to be enlarged by cancerous white blood cells. If untreated, lymphoma causes death for reasons similar to other solid tumors.

Early Hodgkin's disease is unusual in that it can be cured by radiotherapy to the affected nodes alone. Although this carries risks of long-term damage to the healthy tissues that have been irradiated, this treatment has a very high cure rate of over 95 percent.

Advanced Hodgkin's disease may also be cured by a combination of chemotherapy (usually the ABVD regimen of adriamycin, bleomycin, vinblastine and dacarbazine) and radiotherapy, although the success rate is lower. If Hodgkin's disease recurs after treatment, it is almost never curable.

Some of the other lymphomas can be cured by radiotherapy alone or by a combination of chemotherapy (including chlorambucil, alpha-interferon, rituximab, and the CHOP regimen of cyclophosphamide, hydroxydaunorubicin, vincristine (Oncovin) and prednisolone and radiotherapy. Most non-Hodgkin's lymphoma is less responsive to treatment, and the tumor eventually reappears in a form that cannot be cured.[79]

Information box 3.4e-III

Lymphoma: comments from a Chinese medicine perspective

In Chinese medicine, lymphoma, like most solid tumors, could be seen as a manifestation of Phlegm with Blood Stagnation against a background of Depletion of Yin and/or Yang.

Myeloma

Myeloma is a rare cancer of those white cells that produce antibodies. It predominantly affects elderly people. The cancerous cells cause three main problems that are characteristic of myeloma.

First, the myeloma cells multiply within bone tissue, and this causes weak areas of bone that are prone to fracture and that are a source of intense pain. Second, the myeloma cells release excessive amounts of protein into the bloodstream. This protein is similar in form to the antibody protein, immunoglobulin, but has no value in protection against infection. In high concentrations it tends to cause damage to the kidneys and can lead to kidney failure. Finally, in advanced disease, the cancerous cells take over the bone marrow and cause bone marrow failure.

The progression of myeloma can be slowed down by chemotherapy. In older patients the chemotherapy used (usually melphalan or cyclophosphamide with prednisolone and thalidomide) has a much lower risk of bone marrow failure than that used in leukemia. In younger people stem cell transplant may be considered after induction with a combination of bortezomib and the potent steroid dexamethasone. Bortezomib is a novel anticancer agent that prolongs the life of anticancer proteins produced by the body.

Eventually, the cancerous cells in myeloma progress to a form of acute leukemia. Patients usually die either from bone marrow failure or from kidney failure. Even with treatment death occurs on average at three to four years after diagnosis, but some live for as long as eight years.[80]

Information box 3.4e-IV

Myeloma: comments from a Chinese medicine perspective

In Chinese medicine, the interpretation of myeloma could be similar to that of leukemia, because the symptoms are comparable. The presence of bone pain suggests that Blood Stagnation contributes to the symptoms.

The red flags of leukemia and lymphoma

Red flags are those symptoms and signs that indicate that referral to a conventional doctor should be considered. The red flags of the conditions discussed in this section are described in Table 3.4e-I. A summary of the red flags in a format designed for quick reference in clinical practice can be found in Appendix III. This gives advice on the degree of urgency of referral for each of the red flag conditions listed.

Table 3.4e-I A20: Red flags of leukemia and lymphoma

Red flag	Description	Reasoning
A20.1	• Features of bone marrow failure: symptoms of progressive anemia (see A18.1) • recurrent progressive infections • progressive easy bruising, purpura (see A1.4) and bleeding	The bone marrow contains the stem cells for the three major cellular components of the blood (red blood cells, platelets and white blood cells) Bone marrow can fail to produce healthy blood cells if infiltrated by cancer, damaged by medication (including cancer chemotherapy) or radiation, and sometimes as a result of an autoimmune disease Bone marrow failure is a life-threatening situation
A20.2	Multiple enlarged lymph nodes (>1cm in diameter), but painless, with no other obvious cause (e.g. known glandular fever infection) for more than 2 weeks	Groups of lymph nodes can be found in the cervical region, in the armpits (axillary nodes) and in the inguinal creases (groin). In health, the lymph nodes are usually impalpable masses of soft tissue, but they can enlarge and become more palpable when active in fighting an infection or if infiltrated by tumor cells. If a number of nodes are enlarged (>1cm in diameter), this may signify a generalized infectious disease such as glandular fever The other important cause of widespread lymph node enlargement (lymphadenopathy) is cancer, and in particular, the cancers of the white blood cells (leukemia and lymphoma) If multiple enlarged lymph nodes are found, it is best to refer for a diagnosis, and as a high priority if the patient is unwell
A20.3	A single markedly enlarged lymph node (>2cm in diameter) with no other obvious cause	Even in the situation of infection it is unusual for a lymph node to become grossly enlarged. Cancerous infiltration can lead to a firm, enlarged lymph node, which may be painless. This is particularly typical of lymphoma Unexplained fever, weight loss and itching are other symptoms which, together with lymph node enlargement, are suggestive of lymphoma

Notes

1   Waugh, A. and Grant, A. (2014) *Ross and Wilson: Anatomy and Physiology in Health and Illness.* Twelfth Edition. Edinburgh: Elsevier, Chapter 12.

2   NHS Choices (2016) 'The Eatwell Guide.' Available at www.nhs.uk/Livewell/Goodfood/Pages/the-eatwell-guide.aspx, accessed on 6 June 2016.

3   National Institutes of Health (2005) 'Omega-3 Fatty Acids and Health.' Factsheet for Health Professionals. Available at https://ods.od.nih.gov/factsheets/Omega3FattyAcidsandHealth-HealthProfessional, accessed on 6 June 2016.

4   US FDA (Food and Drug Administration) (2016) 'Talking about trans fats: What you need to know.' Available at www.fda.gov/Food/ResourcesForYou/Consumers/ucm079609.htm, accessed on 6 June 2016.

5   Dharmananda, S. (1997) 'The use of aromatic agents for regulating Qi, vitalising blood and relieving pain.' Available at www.itmonline.org/arts/aromatic.htm, accessed on 10 June 2016.

6   NHS Choices (2016) 'The Eatwell Guide.' Available at www.nhs.uk/Livewell/Goodfood/Pages/the-eatwell-guide.aspx, accessed on 6 June 2016.

7   Flaws, B. and Wolfe, H. (1983) *Prince Wen Hui's Cook: Chinese Dietary Therapy.* Brookline, MA: Paradigm Publications.

8   Blyth, D. and Lampert, G. (2015) *Chinese Dietary Wisdom: Eating for Health and Wellbeing.* Hartford, CT: Nutshell Press.

9   Deadman, P., Al-Khafaki, M. and Baker, K. (1998) *A Manual of Acupuncture.* Hove, England: Journal of Chinese Medicine Publications.

10 Deadman, P., Al-Khafaki, M. and Baker, K. (1998) *A Manual of Acupuncture.* Hove, England: Journal of Chinese Medicine Publications.

11 Keown, D. (2014) *The Spark in the Machine.* London: Singing Dragon, Chapter 25.

12 Maciocia, G. (1989) *The Foundations of Chinese Medicine.* Edinburgh: Churchill Livingstone, Chapter 13, p.111.

13 Keown, D. (2014) The *Spark in the Machine.* London: Singing Dragon, Chapter 26, p.188.

14 Keown, D. (2014) *The Spark in the Machine.* London: Singing Dragon, Chapter 26, p.186.

15 Keown, D. (2014) *The Spark in the Machine.* London: Singing Dragon, Chapter 27, p.221.

16 Johns Hopkins Medicine (2016) 'Diagnostic digestive procedures.' Available at www.hopkinsmedicine.org/healthlibrary/conditions/digestive_disorders/digestive_diagnostic_procedures_85,P00364, accessed on 10 June 2016.

17 Henderson, R. (2016) 'Gastro-oesophageal reflux disease.' Available at http://patient.info/doctor/gastro-oesophageal-reflux-disease, accessed on 10 June 2016.

18 Henderson, R. (2016) 'Oesophageal cancer.' Available at http://patient.info/doctor/oesophageal-cancer-pro, accessed on 10 June 2016.

19 Knott, L. (2014) 'Gastroenteritis in adults and children.' Available at http://patient.info/doctor/gastroenteritis-in-adults-and-older-children, accessed on 10 June 2016.

20 NICE (National Institute for Health and Care Excellence) (2004) *Dyspepsia: Management of Dyspepsia in Adults in Primary Care.* Clinical Guideline CG17. Available at www.nice.org.uk/guidance/cg17?unlid=715267601201621282322, accessed on 24 November 2016.

21 Knott, L. (2016) 'Acute pancreatitis.' Available at http://patient.info/doctor/acute-pancreatitis-pro, accessed on 10 June 2016.

22 Lowth, M. (2014) 'Primary biliary cirrhosis.' Available at http://patient.info/doctor/primary-biliary-cirrhosis-pro, accessed on 14 June 2016.

23 Tidy, C. (2013) 'Gallstones and cholecystitis.' Available at http://patient.info/doctor/gallstones-and-cholecystitis, accessed on 14 June 2016.

24 Willaby, H. (2012) 'Crohn's disease.' Available at http://patient.info/doctor/crohns-disease-pro, accessed on 14 June 2016.

25 Keown, D. (2014) *The Spark in the Machine.* London: Singing Dragon, Chapter 3, p.11.

26 Waugh, A. and Grant, A. (2014) *Ross and Wilson: Anatomy and Physiology in Health and Illness.* Twelfth Edition. Edinburgh: Elsevier, Chapter 5.

27 Maciocia, G. (1989) *The Foundations of Chinese Medicine.* Edinburgh: Churchill Livingstone, Chapter 6, p.72, Chapter 7, p.84.

28 Greenwood, M. (2005) *Needle Shock: Adverse Effect or Transformational Signal.* Paradox Publishing. Available at https://paradoxpublishing.com/assets/files/publications/articles/aama/vol-16-1-needle-shock.pdf, accessed on 28 June 2016.

29 BHS (British Hypertension Society) (2016) 'BP monitors.' Available at http://bhsoc.org/bp-monitors/bp-monitors, accessed on 28 June 2016.

30 NICE (National Institute for Health and Care Excellence) (2011) *Hypertension in Adults: Diagnosis and Management.* Available at www.nice.org.uk/guidance/cg127/chapter/1-Guidance, accessed on 28 June 2016.

31 Maciocia, G. (1989) *The Foundations of Chinese Medicine.* Edinburgh: Churchill Livingstone, Chapter 6.

32 Deadman, P., Al-Kafaji, M. and Baker, K. (1998) *A Manual of Acupuncture.* Hove, England: Journal of Chinese Medicine Publications, p.207.

33 Maciocia, G. (1989) *The Foundations of Chinese Medicine.* Edinburgh: Churchill Livingstone, Chapter 11.

34 Larre, C., Shatz, J. and Rochat de Vallee, E. (1986) *Survey of Traditional Chinese Medicine.* Paris: l'Institut Ricci.

35 Maciocia, G. (1989) *The Foundations of Chinese Medicine.* Edinburgh: Churchill Livingstone, Chapter 11.

36 Keown, D. (2014) *The Spark in the Machine.* London: Singing Dragon, Chapter 24.

37 Flaws, B. and Sionneau, P. (2001) *The Treatment of Western Diseases with Chinese Medicine.* Boulder, CO: Blue Poppy Press, Chapter 21, 'Coronary Artery Disease'.

38 Flaws, B. and Sionneau, P. (2001) *The Treatment of Western Diseases with Chinese Medicine.* Boulder, CO: Blue Poppy Press, Chapter 61, 'Raynaud's Phenomenon'.

39 Ruli, G. (2013) 'Hypertension.' Available at http://patient.info/doctor/hypertension, accessed on 3 July 2016.

40 NICE (National Institute for Health and Care Excellence) (2011) *Hypertension in Adults: Diagnosis and Management*. Available at www.nice.org.uk/guidance/cg127/chapter/1-Guidance, accessed on 28 June 2016.

41 NICE (National Institute for Health and Care Excellence) (2011) *Hypertension in Adults: Diagnosis and Management*. Available at www.nice.org.uk/guidance/cg127/chapter/1-Guidance, accessed on 28 June 2016.

42 Qrisk.org (2016) 'QRISK®2.' Available at www.qrisk.org, accessed on 3 July 2016.

43 CVriskcalculator.com (2016) 'Heart risk calculator.' Available at www.cvriskcalculator.com, accessed on 3 July 2016.

44 NICE (National Institute for Health and Care Excellence) (2011) *Hypertension in Adults: Diagnosis and Management*. Available at www.nice.org.uk/guidance/cg127/chapter/1-Guidance, accessed on 28 June 2016.

45 National Center for Health Statistics (2016) *Health, United States, 2015: With Special Feature on Racial and Ethnic Health Disparities*. Table 55. Hyattsville, MD. Available at www.cdc.gov/nchs/data/hus/hus15.pdf#055, accessed on 10 December 2016.

46 Siriwardhana, N. (2012) 'Flavonoids may lower the risk of fatal cardiovascular disease.' *Nutrition Remarks*, 11 April. Available at www.nutritionremarks.com/2012/04/11/flavonoids-may-lower-the-risk-of-fatal-cardiovascular-disease, accessed on 3 July 2016.

47 Sambrook, J. (2016) 'Mediterranean diet.' Available at http://patient.info/health/mediterranean-diet, accessed on 3 July 2016.

48 NICE (National Institute for Health and Care Excellence) (2010) *Chest Pain of Recent Onset: Assessment and Diagnosis*. Available at https://www.nice.org.uk/guidance/cg95, accessed on 3 July 2016.

49 NICE (National Institute for Health and Care Excellence) (2008) *Prophylaxis Against Infective Endocarditis: Antimicrobial Prophylaxis Against Infective Endocarditis in Adults and Children Undergoing Interventional Procedures*. Available at www.nice.org.uk/guidance/cg64, accessed on 10 December 2016.

50 Perloff, J. and Warnes, C.A. (2001) 'Challenges posed by adults with repaired congenital heart disease.' *Circulation*. Available at http://circ.ahajournals.org/content/103/21/2637, accessed on 11 July 2016.

51 Waugh, A. and Grant, A. (2014) *Ross and Wilson: Anatomy and Physiology in Health and Illness*. Twelfth Edition. Edinburgh: Elsevier, Chapter 10.

52 Maciocia, G. (1989) *The Foundations of Chinese Medicine*. Edinburgh: Churchill Livingstone, Chapter 8.

53 Keown, D. (2014) *The Spark in the Machine*. London: Singing Dragon, Chapter 26.

54 NICE (National Institute for Health and Care Excellence) (2009) *Amantadine, Oseltamivir and Zanamivir for the Treatment of Influenza*. NICE Technology Appraisal Guidance TA168. Available at www.nice.org.uk/guidance/ta168, accessed on 11 July 2016.

55 Maciocia, G. (1994) *The Practice of Chinese Medicine*. Edinburgh: Churchill Livingstone, Appendices II and III.

56 Flaws, B. and Sionneau, P. (2001) *The Treatment of Modern Western Medical Diseases with Chinese Medicine*. Boulder, CO: Blue Poppy Press, Chapter 20.

57 NICE (National Institute for Health and Care Excellence) (2008) *Respiratory Tract Infections (Self-limiting): Prescribing Antibiotics*. Clinical Guideline CG69. Available at www.nice.org.uk/guidance/cg69/chapter/1-guidance, accessed on 11 July 2016.

58 Balfour, H.H. Jr, Sifakis, F., Sliman, J.A., Knight, J.A., Schmeling, D.O. and Thomas, W. (2013) 'Age-specific prevalence of Epstein-Barr virus infection among individuals aged 6–19 years in the United States and factors affecting its acquisition.' *Journal of Infectious Diseases 208*(8), 1286–1293. Available at www.ncbi.nlm.nih.gov/pubmed/23868878, accessed on 11 July 2016.

59 Gallagher, J. (2014) 'Tamiflu: Millions wasted on flu drug claims major report.' *BBC News*. Available at www.bbc.co.uk/news/health-26954482, accessed on 11 July 2016.

60 Flaws, B. and Sionneau, P. (2001) *The Treatment of Modern Western Medical Diseases with Chinese Medicine*. Boulder, CO: Blue Poppy Press, Chapter 2.

61 Scott, J. and Barlow, T. (1999) *Acupuncture in the Treatment of Children*. Seattle, WA: Eastland Press, p.17.

62 Tidy, C. (2014) 'Asthma.' Available at http://patient.info/doctor/bronchial-asthma, accessed on 12 July 2016.

63 Fall, T., *et al.* (2015) 'Early exposure to dogs and farm animals and the risk of childhood asthma.' *Journal of the American Medical Association Pediatrics 169*(11), e153219. Available at www.ncbi.nlm.nih.gov/pubmed/26523822, accessed on 11 July 2016.

64 British Thoracic Society and Scottish Intercollegiate Guidelines Network (2014) *British Guideline on the Management of Asthma: A National Clinical Guideline*. Available at www.brit-thoracic.org.uk/document-library/clinical-information/asthma/btssign-asthma-guideline-2014, accessed on 11 July 2016.

65 NICE (National Institute for Health and Care Excellence) (2011) *Hypertension in Adults: diagnosis and management*. Available at https://www.nice.org.uk/guidance/cg127/chapter/1-Guidance, accessed on 7 March 2017.

66 NICE (National Institute for Health and Care Excellence) (2015) *Adult and Child over 5 Years*. Available at www.evidence.nhs.uk/formulary/bnf/current/3-respiratory-system/31-bronchodilators/management-of-chronic-asthma/adult-and-child-over-5-years, accessed on 12 July 2016.

67 Tidy, C. (2014) 'Chronic obstructive pulmonary disease.' Available at http://patient.info/doctor/chronic-obstructive-pulmonary-disease-pro, accessed on 12 July 2016.

68 Knott, L. (2015) 'Cystic fibrosis.' Available at http://patient.info/doctor/cystic-fibrosis-pro, accessed on 12 July 2016.

69 Tidy, C. (2015) 'Pulmonary fibrosis.' Available at http://patient.info/doctor/pulmonary-fibrosis, accessed on 12 July 2016.

70 Waugh, A. and Grant, A. (2014) *Ross and Wilson: Anatomy and Physiology in Health and Illness*. Twelfth Edition. Edinburgh: Elsevier, Chapter 4.

71 Maciocia, G. (1989) *The Foundations of Chinese Medicine*. Edinburgh: Churchill Livingstone, p.48.

72 Flaws, B. and Wolfe, H. (1983) *Prince Wen Hui's Cook: Categorization of Foods*. Brookline, MA: Paradigm Publications, pp.143–190.

73 Tidy, C. (2013) 'Anaemia of chronic disease.' Available at http://patient.info/doctor/anaemia-of-chronic-disease, accessed on 13 July 2016.

74 Tidy, C. (2015) 'Sickle cell disease and sickle cell anaemia.' Available at http://patient.info/doctor/sickle-cell-disease-and-sickle-cell-anaemia-pro, accessed on 12 July 2016.

75 Gandhi, A. (2016) 'Haemolytic disease of the fetus and newborn.' Available at http://patient.info/doctor/haemolytic-disease-of-the-fetus-and-newborn, accessed on 12 July 2016.

76 Tidy, C. (2016) 'Sepsis (septicaemia).' Available at http://patient.info/doctor/sepsis-septicaemia-pro, accessed on 12 July 2016.

77 Joint United Kingdom (UK) Blood Transfusion and Tissue Transplantation Services Professional Advisory Committee (2014) *Transfusion Handbook: Blood Products*. Available at www.transfusionguidelines.org.uk/transfusion-handbook/3-providing-safe-blood/3-3-blood-products, accessed on 12 July 2016.

78 Tidy, C. (2013) 'Childhood leukaemias.' Available at http://patient.info/doctor/childhood-leukaemias, accessed on 12 July 2016.

79 Tidy, C. (2014) 'Hodgkin's lymphoma.' Available at http://patient.info/doctor/hodgkins-lymphoma-pro, accessed on 12 July 2016.

80 Tidy, C. (2014) 'Myeloma.' Available at http://patient.info/doctor/myeloma-pro, accessed on 12 July 2016.

THE NERVOUS, MUSCULOSKELETAL AND URINARY SYSTEMS

4.1

The Nervous System

4.1a The physiology of the nervous system

This section focuses on the physiology of the nervous system. Together with the endocrine system, the nervous system is one of the topics explored in this text that arguably has great relevance to the understanding of the physical basis of holistic approaches to healing. Together with the endocrine system, the nervous system is involved in the process of communication of one body part with another. Together, these systems form, from a medical perspective, part of the physical foundation of what makes the body an integrated whole.

It is important to point out here that a prevailing and convincing holistic understanding on interconnectedness (exemplified by Myers (2001)[1] and Keown (2014)[2]) is that the myofascial system (comprising the muscles and the body-wide interconnected web of fascial connective tissue that links them with the periosteum of the bones) is another integrated body system that provides the medium for the communication of energy/Qi between disparate body parts. Whilst there is good embryological and anatomical evidence that this fascial basis for energy flow is consistent with acupuncture meridian theory, the medical establishment still doesn't generally recognize the potentially profound role that fascia and its unique electric properties might have to play in linking the function of diverse body parts. From a medical perspective this role is all down to nervous and endocrine systems.

The complexity of the nervous system is so great that it is very likely that it can never be fully understood by human minds. The number of brain cells alone approximates 10 billion, while the total number of connections made between these cells runs into the trillions. These connections are unique to each individual, not only as a consequence of a particular genetic makeup, but also because these connections continually form and reform in response to the personal experiences of that individual.

In the light of this complexity, even with increasingly complex computer modeling, it makes sense that only the most basic features in this mysterious neural landscape have been understood and described by scientists. The subtleties that form the foundations for many aspects of human experience, such as the diverse emotions and spiritual experiences, have simply not yet been mapped. It is very possible that these experiences, and also some aspects of the subtle phenomena that holistic therapists attribute to the movement of energy described as Qi or Prana, could be explained scientifically if this unmapped part of the nervous system were explored using reductionist experimental methods. However, it may be that such knowledge will always be out of reach of the scientific experiment, being protected within the unique complexity of the structure of each individual's brain.

For this reason it may well be that the mechanism of the more subtle energetic approaches to healing will never be fully explained by science. For example, there is strong scientific evidence to support the role of acupuncture in the modulation of pain, but little or no evidence to explain the more subtle effects on the body's function, emotions, and even the destiny of an individual, as described in Chinese medicine theory. However, this does not mean that a physical mechanism for these subtle effects does not exist, but possibly that it is far too delicate, complex and unique to an individual healing encounter for current scientific experiment (and possibly for the human mind) to explain in physical terms.

This section explores only the most basic of the principles of the physiology of the nervous system. Nevertheless, it might be helpful to consider that the structures described here are those parts of the body that regulate those aspects that many complementary therapists might recognize as essential foundations to health, such as the control of homeostasis, thoughts, emotional feelings and even the spirit.

As there is a great deal of material to study, the section is divided into two parts. If you are following this text as part of a study course, you are recommended to work through this section in two separate study sessions. Part I describes the nervous tissue, which is the basic building material for the nervous system. The three parts of the nervous system, the central nervous system, the peripheral nervous system and the autonomic nervous system, are then introduced. Finally, the central nervous system is explored in more detail. In Part II the peripheral nervous system and the autonomic nervous system are described in more detail.

Part I: The physiology of the nervous system[3]

THE NERVOUS TISSUE
The nerve cells (neurons)

The foundation of the nervous system is the nerve cell, which is scientifically termed the neuron. Nerve cells have the ability to relay messages between each other, and are specialized to perform this role.

The way in which this communication occurs can be compared to an old-fashioned telephone exchange that allows communication to take place between any two households that are connected to that exchange. In a telephone exchange the physical basis of the communication is an electrical current that is conducted from households through telephone wires to the exchange. The telephone acts as the receiver of information, as well as relaying the message from the household at the other end of the line. At the exchange the telephone message from one household can be specifically processed and directed to another household by means of a telephone operating system. The presence of the exchange dramatically reduces the need to have wires linking every home with all the others in the system. Each home needs to be connected only to the exchange, and similarly, each body part needs to be connected only to the central nervous system in order to have a nerve-mediated influence on another body part.

In the nervous system some of the specialized nerve cells are able to receive information from the environment and translate it into an electrical message (akin to the telephone receiver). Nerve cells that receive external information and relay it to the nervous system are known as sensory nerve cells (or effector nerve cells). This term reflects the fact that these nerve cells sense the environment.

Other cells are adapted to act like the telephone wires to the exchange, and relay the message via the spinal cord to other nerve cells or to the brain. The spinal cord and the brain can be seen as the telephone exchange, from which messages originating in the body are redirected to other parts of the nervous system. The nerve cells that link up different parts of the nervous system in this way are sometimes called connector nerve cells.

Within the body's "telephone exchange" the message is processed and leads to one or more response messages, which are relayed back out to the body. The nerve cells that relay messages back out to the body to bring about a change in the body's function are called effector nerve cells or motor nerve cells. In this text the term motor nerve cell is used to describe these nerve cells. It may help to remember this term by reflecting that a motor in mechanical terms is a structure that converts energy into action. It is the same for motor nerve cells, because they allow the transformation of the energy of the electrical message that they are carrying into the action of a contraction of a single muscle cell fiber.

A simple example to illustrate this system is the bodily response to an unexpected pin-prick. The message of pain is sensed and relayed by sensory nerve cells to the spinal cord. Messages returning via motor nerve cells from the spinal cord in response to this pain lead to action in the form of a rapid withdrawal of the body from the offending pin. This example describes the most basic form of reflex, which will be explained in more detail presently.

THE PHYSIOLOGY OF THE NERVE CELL

The membrane that surrounds each nerve cell is very sensitive to changes in its environment. External changes to which a nerve cell is sensitive are termed stimuli (singular stimulus). Sensory nerves, depending on their specific role, can respond to a diverse range of external stimuli, such as pressure, light, heat, cold and irritants. All other nerve cells respond to the stimulus of chemicals called neurotransmitters, which are released from the nerve cells that are near to them.

A stimulus will cause the membrane of a nerve cell to change so that an electrical impulse is transmitted to all parts of the cell membrane. The ability to convert an external stimulus to an electrical charge is called irritability. The transmission of the electrical impulse to all parts of the cell is called conductivity. It is these properties of irritability and conductivity that allow a stimulus at one part of the cell to be transmitted, in an electrical form, to all other parts of the cell.

All nerve cells are closely linked to other nerve cells by means of fine-branching extensions of the cell membrane called dendrites (from the Greek meaning little trees).

Figure 4.1a-I illustrates a generalized nerve cell, and shows the long extension of the axon and the smaller tree-like extensions called dendrites. The branching dendrite-like structures at the bottom of the axons have endings called boutons, which are adapted to release tiny quantities of neurotransmitter chemicals from secretory vesicles inside the cell. The axon is an extension that can be very long, and for this reason it can also be termed a nerve fiber. For example, the nerve cells that relay information from the feet have axons or nerve fibers that run from the spinal cord right down to the toes.

When a nerve cell receives a stimulus, the electrical impulse is conducted to the tips of all the dendrites and also down the length of the axon. Some axons are coated in a white substance called myelin. Although this myelin sheath is simply represented in Figure 4.1a-I, the structure of myelin is actually very complex as it consists of a fine layer of fatty substance secreted between layers of a glial cell membrane wrapped many times around the nerve fiber. The glial cell that forms myelin in this way is called the Schwann cell. Myelin enables these cells to transmit an impulse more quickly than those cells that do not have this coating.

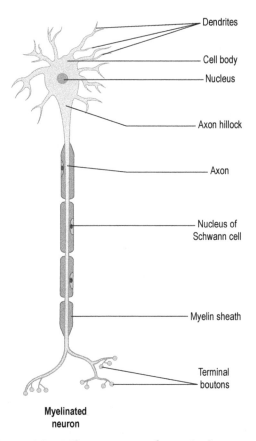

Figure 4.1a-I The structure of a typical neuron

The tips of the dendrites make contact with other nerve cells. In the case of motor nerves, the tips of some of the axons make contact with muscles. The way in which dendrites or axons make contact with other nerve cells is shown in Figure 4.1a-II. This illustrates that the branching ends of the axons come very close to the dendrites of

another nerve cell. However, they do not actually touch, but instead leave a tiny gap called a synapse or synaptic cleft.

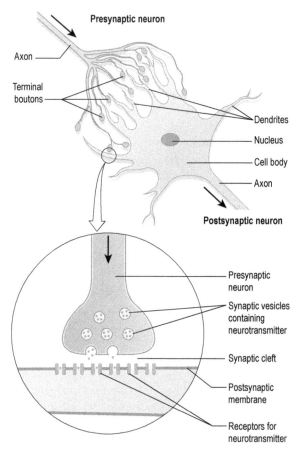

Figure 4.1a-II A synapse

When an electrical charge reaches the branching end of the axon it causes an internal change in the cell, which leads to a release of neurotransmitter from the branching tips of the axon at the terminal boutons. This chemical can diffuse across the synapse, and may act as the stimulus for the nerve cell on the other side of the gap. In some cases the neurotransmitter has the opposite effect and reduces the irritability of the nerve cell on the other side of the synapse. In this case, instead of acting as a stimulus, the neurotransmitter inhibits further stimuli for a brief period. This complex process involving both an electrical charge and a release of chemicals is the basis for communication between nerve cells, and also between a nerve cell and a muscle.

As stated earlier, the number of synapses in the body runs into trillions. Whenever a single cell is stimulated, impulses are transmitted via its axons to a number of other cells. Some of these impulses will lead to the stimulation of a series of cells in connection with the first cell. Of course, all these cells have their own connections with many other cells, and this can lead to a chain reaction of impulses, which can spread through the nervous system.

However, there will also be inhibition of other cells, which may in turn lead to another chain reaction of inhibition of other cells in the nervous system.

This series of chain reactions from a single stimulus is how an experience such as a single pin-prick not only causes a withdrawal from the source of pain, but also leads to the felt experience of pain, an emotional response to the pain, an expressed cry of indignation, and the laying down of memory about the incident, among many other possible responses.

Nerve cells are highly active because they constantly manufacture neurotransmitter chemicals. The manufacture of substances within the cell requires basic nutrients and energy in the form of energy-charged adenosine triphosphate (ATP), and takes place within the endoplasmic reticulum and the Golgi body (see Section 1.1b). The neurotransmitters are exported to the outside environment by the process of exocytosis of vesicles, which is one of the methods of active transport described in Section 1.1b. This process also requires energy in the form of ATP.

Because of its intensive energy requirements, the nerve cell is absolutely reliant on a high level of oxygen and glucose to perform this function. A nerve cell that is even temporarily starved of these nutrients cannot function well, and is more likely to die than some other types of cell. Once a nerve cell has died it cannot be replaced, because nerve cells are one of the few types of cells in the body that do not divide. However, although nerve cells cannot be replaced, new connections between remaining cells can be made, as dendrites from nerve cells can grow out and make new contacts with other cells.

Sometimes the loss of nerve cells can be overcome by this mechanism of new growth, although full recovery may take some time. In other cases, the loss of nerve cells leaves a permanent deficit, as occurs in the case of many strokes.

Glial cells (neuroglia)

Glial cells (also known as neuroglia) are the connective tissue cells of the nervous system. They form about one-third of all nervous tissue. These cells act as the scaffolding that holds the nerve cells in place. Unlike nerve cells, glial cells can replicate. For this reason almost all cancers of the nervous system are derived from the glial cells rather than from nerve cells.

One type of glial cell called the astrocyte protects nervous tissue from toxins in the blood by forming a layer around the blood vessels that enter the nervous system. This is called the blood-brain barrier. Some drugs cannot penetrate the blood-brain barrier, a property that has been utilized by drug manufacturers. For example, the newer types of beta blocker drugs are less likely to cause emotional and sleep disturbance because they have been designed not to be able to cross the blood-brain barrier.

However, many other drugs, such as alcohol and nicotine, cross this barrier very easily.

Another type of glial cell, called the oligodendrocyte, is responsible for the manufacture of the myelin that enables rapid conduction of electrical impulses down the nerve cell axons.

The last category of glial cell, called the microglia, is derived from the leukocyte. This is similar to the macrophage in ordinary connective tissue, and can phagocytose (see Section 1.1c) unwanted cellular material.

The composition of nervous tissue

The nerve cells and the supporting glial cells are the main components of all parts of the nervous system, from the brain and spinal cord, right down to the thread-like branching nerves that penetrate all the body tissues. The structure and consistency of the different types of nervous tissue depend on the relative proportion of cell bodies and axons (nerve fibers).

The tissue that makes up the brain contains many cell bodies and is very soft in consistency, rather akin to a thick blancmange. This explains why it can be so easily damaged by violent shaking or a blow to the head, and why it requires the rigid casing of the skull for protection. The cell bodies are concentrated in particular areas within different parts of the brain and, when very closely packed, have a grayish color. This is the origin of the term gray matter, which in common usage refers to the part of the brain that does the thinking. The nerve fibers or axons running from these cell bodies to different parts of the brain, or down to the spinal cord, tend to run together rather like all the telephone wires running from one group of houses to the exchange. These pathways of thousands of nerve fibers are called tracts. They have a white appearance because of the white myelin, and are described as the white matter.

In the spinal cord, the tracts of nerve fibers are very prominent. Thousands of nerve fibers run up and down the length of the spinal cord, allowing communication between different parts of the body and the brain. These also appear as white matter when the spinal cord is dissected. However, in the core of the spinal cord are dense clusters of the nerve cell bodies of connector and motor neurons. On dissection these are seen as a central H-shaped area of gray matter. Figure 4.1a-III shows a cross-section of the spinal cord, illustrating the appearance of the white and gray matter. Like the brain, the spinal cord is of a very soft consistency and is also vulnerable to injury.

Figure 4.1a-III also shows the two roots of the nerve fibers that leave this part of the spinal cord. These meet to leave the vertebral column as a single spinal nerve containing thousands of nerve fibers. With the exception of the nerves that supply the head and neck, all the bodily nerves originate from spinal nerves. In this case, the word nerve means thousands of nerve fibers bundled together, rather than a single cell (correctly called nerve cell, nerve fiber or neuron).

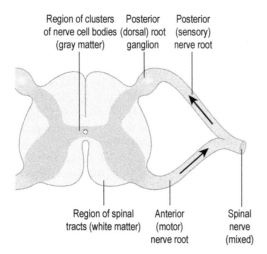

Figure 4.1a-III A section of the spinal cord showing the nerve roots on one side

All the nerves that run outside the spinal cord consist entirely of sensory and motor nerve fibers, and have originated from the anterior (containing motor fibers) and posterior (containing sensory fibers) spinal nerve roots (see Figure 4.1a-III). The cell bodies of the motor nerve fibers sit within the gray matter of the spinal cord. However, the cell bodies of the sensory nerve sit outside the spinal cord, mostly within the spinal root ganglion on the sensory nerve root. This is seen as a swelling in Figure 4.1a-III. The spinal root ganglion is, therefore, a little mass of gray matter. (The sensory nerves of the autonomic nervous system have their cell bodies in ganglia situated further away from the spinal cord, as described later.)

THE PARTS OF THE NERVOUS SYSTEM

The nervous system is conventionally described as being composed of three interrelated parts: the central nervous system (CNS), the peripheral nervous system (PNS) and the autonomic nervous system (ANS).

The CNS consists of the brain and spinal cord. It is protected by a thick fibrous coat and sits within the brain and the vertebral column. The brain is further divided on an anatomical basis into the upper brain (cerebral hemispheres), hindbrain (cerebellum) and brainstem (the midbrain, the pons and medulla oblongata).

The largest part of the PNS consists of 31 pairs of spinal nerves, which emerge from the spinal cord to pass through the spaces between each vertebra and through the holes in the sacrum bone known as the sacral foramina. These nerves contain sensory and motor nerve fibers, and divide to penetrate most of the body tissues. The motor nerve fibers of this part of the PNS are primarily concerned with the voluntary control of muscle action.

The PNS also embraces 12 pairs of cranial nerves, which originate not from the spinal cord but from the lower portions of the brain itself. These also contain sensory and motor nerve fibers. Although some of the motor nerve fibers in the cranial nerves are concerned with the voluntary control of muscular action (e.g. the nerve that supplies the masseter muscle, the muscle of chewing), many carry nerve impulses to control involuntary muscle action (e.g. the vagus nerve, which supplies the cardiac muscle).

Those nerves in the PNS that are involved in the involuntary control of body activity are conventionally considered as a separate system, the ANS. Strictly speaking, the ANS is a subdivision of the PNS.

The central nervous system (CNS)

The CNS consists of the brain and the spinal cord, and sits protected within spaces formed within the bony architecture of the brain and the vertebral column. Figure 4.1a-IV illustrates the structure of the main parts of the CNS. Note that this diagram is not drawn to scale; the spinal cord is, in reality, much longer than indicated in this drawing.

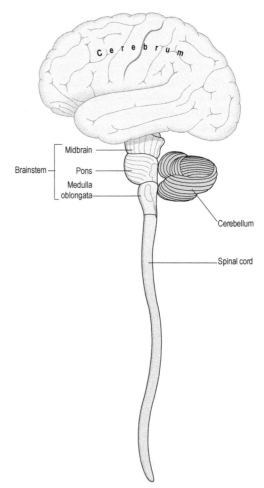

Figure 4.1a-IV The parts of the central nervous system

This delicate nervous tissue of brain and spinal cord is protected within the bony housing of the skull and vertebral canal by three layers of tissue, the dura mater, arachnoid mater and the pia mater, which collectively are called the meninges.

THE MENINGES

The meninges (see Figure 4.1a-V) consist largely of fibrous tissue. The outermost layer, known as the dura mater (dura), is composed of dense white fibrous tissue, the outer layer of which is adherent to the skull, where it forms the periosteum (see Section 4.2a) and the bony margins of the vertebral canal (central canal) right down to the coccyx. In certain regions in the skull the dura splits into two layers, and venous blood courses in the spaces between them in canals called sinuses. An epidural anesthetic is one that is injected carefully in the lumbar region of the spinal cord so that the anesthetic drug collects outside the dura and acts to numb the lower thoracic and lumbar spinal nerve roots as they course down to supply the abdomen and legs.

Figure 4.1a-V The meninges covering the brain and spinal cord

Beneath the layers of the dura is the subdural space. This contains fluid that separates the dura from the next layer, the arachnoid mater, which is also composed of fibrous tissue. The arachnoid mater loosely follows the internal contours of the dura mater. Veins also pass through the subdural space. These can become vulnerable to damage in old age as the substance of the brain shrinks, and there is

more possibility of traction on these vessels if the skull is suddenly moved, as can occur in a fall. This is the cause of subdural hemorrhage (see Section 4.1d).

Beneath the arachnoid mater is the subarachnoid space, which separates the arachnoid mater from the deepest meningeal layer, the pia mater. The delicate pia courses along the surface of the brain and the spinal cord, and in some areas there is quite a pronounced space between it and the arachnoid mater. This space is filled with a fluid known as cerebrospinal fluid (CSF). This space is in connection with the CSF, which bathes internal portions of the brain within the chambers known as ventricles. It is in the subarachnoid space that the major arteries that course along the surface of the brain are located, and it is into this space that blood can leak should one of these arteries become damaged. This is the situation of subarachnoid hemorrhage (see Section 4.1d). A lumbar puncture is an investigation that involves inserting a needle into the region of the subarachnoid space as it widens out in the lower lumbar area below the termination of the spinal cord (see Figure 4.1a-V) so that a sample of CSF can be obtained.

Craniosacral therapists work with what they perceive to be the pulsations of the CSF within the meningeal membranes, transmitted throughout the whole body via the myofascial system. Cranial therapy works to influence deep structures by allowing the release of the myofascial system, through very gentle manipulation techniques, and through such manipulation effect healing at physical, emotional and spiritual levels.

THE CEREBRUM

The cerebrum is the upper part of the brain (see Figure 4.1a-IV), and is divided into two cerebral hemispheres. These have a convoluted surface, giving this part of the brain a cauliflower-like appearance. Despite this visual comparison, the cerebrum is the most complex part of the brain, and is the part that is most enlarged in human beings compared to other animals.

The cerebrum deals with the most complicated aspects of nervous activity. To use once again the example of the pin-prick, although the reflex withdrawal from the pain need not involve the brain at all, the emotional experience of pain, the cry of indignation and the laying down of memory about the event all involve the nerve cells in the cerebral hemispheres. In keeping with this complexity, the cerebrum contains a lot of gray matter (nerve cell bodies) concentrated on its convoluted surface. This part of the cerebrum is called the cerebral cortex. The functions of particular parts of the cerebral cortex have now been extensively mapped. For instance, the voluntary control of movement of all the body parts can be located onto precise segments of a single ridge of cortex, called the motor area, situated on the side of each cerebral hemisphere. The complexity of such representation is illustrated in Figure 4.1a-VI. The mapping of the motor area and other surface regions of the brain has influenced the location of points used in the modern Chinese development of scalp acupuncture.[4]

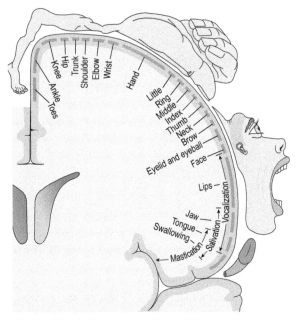

Figure 4.1a-VI The mapping of the motor cortex to bodily function

This diagram illustrates how different strips of the motor cortex have been mapped to regions of muscle function in the body. The distorted humanoid figure is called a homunculus and is drawn to illustrate that some parts of the body (the hand, face and tongue) have disproportionate representation on the motor cortex, in keeping with the complexity of their muscle action.

In order to comprehend the complicated effects of cerebral diseases it helps to understand that, if parts of the cerebrum are lost through injury or disease, the precise function of those parts is also lost. For example, a person who has a small stroke (see Section 4.1d) that damages part of the motor area of the cortex only will suffer an inability to move the corresponding part of their body. In this situation, other functions such as sensation and speech will be unaffected. In contrast, a person who has a stroke that affects the visual cortex only will suffer from visual problems, while movement will be unimpaired.

Tracts of white matter (nerve fibers) descend through the brain from the cerebral cortices (plural of cortex). These connect with other parts of the brain, and also with the spinal cord. The two halves of the upper brain are intimately connected with each other by a wide tract of nerve fibers called the corpus callosum. The tracts of fibers that link the cortices with the rest of the body tend to cross over (decussate) within the brainstem, so that the left side of the brain controls the right side of the body, and vice versa. For this reason the left side of the brain is the dominant hemisphere in a right-handed person.

Deep within the cerebral hemispheres are islands of gray matter called nuclei. These have essential control functions. The largest of these nuclei are the basal ganglia (important for the control of movement), the thalamus (important for the control of sensation) and the hypothalamus (important for the control of the hormones of the pituitary gland and for other aspects of homeostasis such as temperature control).

The main areas and functions of the cerebral cortex are illustrated in Figure 4.1a-VII. The cortices are each anatomically divided into four lobes named after the skull bone that overlies them. Functions can therefore be associated anatomically with lobes; for instance, vision is a function of the occipital lobe. The areas associated with speech production (frontal lobe) and processing of language (temporal lobe) are concentrated on the so-called dominant hemisphere only, which is usually on the left-hand side in right-handed people and the right-hand side in left-handed people. In contrast, the areas responsible for spatial awareness (parietal lobe) tend to be more developed on the non-dominant side of the cerebrum.

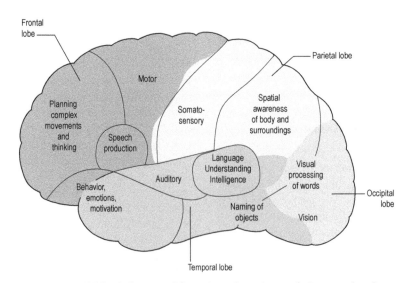

Figure 4.1a-VII The lobes and functional regions of the cerebral cortex

THE BRAINSTEM

The brainstem consists of the midbrain, the pons variolii (the pons) and the medulla oblongata (the medulla) (see Figure 4.1a-IV). These three sections of the brain contain large tracts of white matter that carry nerve fibers between the cerebrum and the spinal cord.

All three of these areas of the brain contain nuclei of nerve cell bodies that have the function of the control of the most basic aspects of maintaining life in a complicated organism. For this reason, the structure of these areas is not too dissimilar to the equivalent parts of the brain in other animals. For example, the control of breathing, heart rate and blood pressure is coordinated by specialized centers of nerve cells in the medulla. Because these functions are all essential for life, these specialized areas of the brainstem are called vital centers. Other centers in this part of the brain control the reflex actions of coughing, vomiting and sneezing.

A specialized area in the brainstem called the reticular activating system (RAS) is responsible for the control of how much sensory information gets through to the cerebral cortex. It is the RAS that controls our level of awareness of the environment, and which allows us to focus on one thing to the exclusion of all others in certain circumstances. It is believed that sleep, a time in which our conscious awareness is very much inhibited, is controlled in part by the RAS.

THE CEREBELLUM

The cerebellum, or hindbrain, sits at the back of the brainstem. A hand placed over the upper part of the back of the neck and supporting the base of the skull (while covering the area that includes acupoints Feng Fu DU-16 and Feng Chi GB-20) will have the palm overlying the cerebellum.

The cerebellum is another control center of the brain. It is responsible for the smooth coordination of movement and balance. To perform this function it receives information from the muscles, ears and eyes about the position of the body.

It is believed that the cerebellum also holds memory about repeated actions, so that with practice these can be performed smoothly and without conscious effort. For example, it is the cerebellum that allows a person who is driving to perform a complex task such as changing gear and signaling when decelerating towards a junction, even while focusing consciously on a conversation on the radio.

In a disease that damages the cerebellum only, the conscious mind and the vital centers are left intact. A person with such a condition will have no problem with thinking and the physical body will be in generally good health. However, balance will be poor, speech will be clumsy and the simplest tasks will have to be performed slowly and deliberately, with many errors of movement occurring as the task is undertaken.

THE SPINAL CORD

The spinal cord is the long extension of nervous tissue that leaves the brain at the base of the brainstem. It projects through the large hole at the base of the skull called the foramen magnum, and extends down as far as the first or second lumbar vertebrae. The spinal cord is protected as it runs in the vertebral canal (also known as the spinal canal), formed by the ring-shaped vertebrae that sit one on top of the other. The solid vertebral bodies lie in front of the spinal cord, and the spinous and transverse processes project out to the back and the side of the vertebral rings that embrace the cord along its length. A section of the thoracic spinal cord is illustrated in Figure 4.1a-VIII.

Figure 4.1a-VIII Horizontal section through the vertebral column and spinal cord at the level of the thorax

As shown in Figure 4.1a-IX, the 31 pairs of spinal nerves leave the cord at regular intervals. These spinal nerves project out of the meningeal membranes, which protect the cord and leave the vertebral column through spaces between the vertebrae. Figure 4.1a-X illustrates the base of the spinal cord as it looks on a vertical section of the vertebral column. This diagram shows how the cord only goes down as far as the first lumbar vertebra. The labels T1, T7, T12, L1, S1 and S3 point to the solid bodies of three thoracic vertebrae, one lumbar vertebra and two of the sacral vertebrae that are fused to form the sacrum bone. This diagram also shows the spinous processes projecting back from the vertebral canal. These processes are linked by a tough fibrous ligament, not shown in this diagram, which runs from the base of the skull to the sacrum. It is this ligament that is penetrated when a lumbar puncture is performed.

Figure 4.1a-IX shows the paired spinal nerves. In this diagram the nerves are cut off just at the point where they exit the vertebral canal between the vertebrae. This shows how the lower thoracic, lumbar and sacral nerves descend by increasing lengths through the vertebral canal before they actually leave the space between the vertebrae.

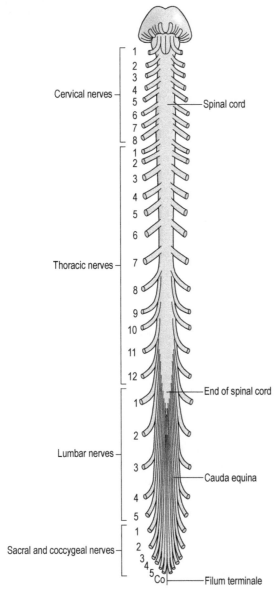

Figure 4.1a-IX The spinal cord and spinal nerves

The first to seventh cervical nerves leave above the corresponding cervical vertebra. However, the eighth cervical nerve leaves below the seventh cervical vertebra. The 12 thoracic and five lumbar spinal nerves all exit below the corresponding thoracic and lumbar vertebrae. The sacral and coccygeal nerves all leave through gaps in the fused sacrum and bones of the coccyx.

With this information it is possible to work out which spinal nerve emerges at a particular spinal level. For example, the level L2/L3, the level at which the acupoints Ming Men DU-4 or Shen Shu BL-23 are situated, is also the level of the emergence of the second lumbar spinal nerve from the vertebral column.

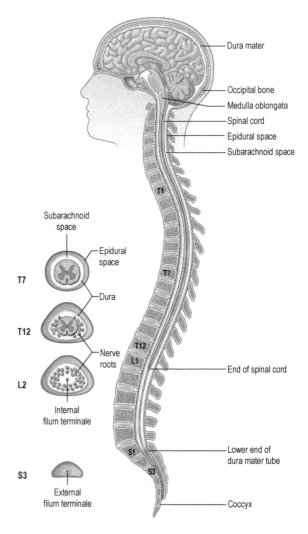

Figure 4.1a-X Section of the distal end of the vertebral canal
This diagram also shows horizontal sections of the spinal column at four levels. These illustrate how the spinal cord terminates at the level of L1/L2 and distal to this only nerve roots travel in the spinal canal.

The spinal cord consists of tracts of white matter containing vertically ascending and descending nerve fibers, and a core of gray matter containing cell bodies. This core is approximately H-shaped when seen in horizontal section (see Figure 4.1a-VIII). Some of the nerve fibers in the white matter of the spinal cord travel to and from the brain, whereas others simply link different levels in the spinal cord.

The spinal cord receives sensory information from most parts of the body below the head and the neck through sensory nerve cells that enter the cord through the sensory root of the spinal nerves. The muscle action within the body is controlled by information carried by motor nerve cells that leave the spinal cord at the motor root of the spinal nerves (see Figures 4.1a-III and 4.1a-VIII).

The gray matter in the spinal cord can be considered as having a similar function to the nuclei of the brain. Some basic aspects of muscle movement are controlled by the clusters of nerve cells in the spinal cord alone. The protective reflex arc and spinal tone are two such aspects that function adequately without any input from the nerve fibers of the brain.

THE PROTECTIVE REFLEX ARC

The protective reflex of withdrawal from pain is one example of a movement that is controlled by the spinal cord alone. Once again the example of the response to a pin-prick of the finger is a useful illustration. In this case, the pain of a pin-prick leads to impulses in the sensory nerves that supply the finger. These travel up the arm to where the nerves enter the spinal cord at the thoracic level of T6/T7. Here the sensory nerve cells make connections with a number of motor nerve cells in the spinal cord by means of connector nerve cells. These motor nerve cells send impulses down to various muscles in the arm and shoulder to cause a withdrawal of the arm from the pain. In such a reflex, the brain is not involved. A diagrammatic representation of a simple reflex arc is given in Figure 4.1a-XI. In this case the diagram illustrates the "knee jerk" reflex that is an involuntary response to the stretch of the patellar tendon.

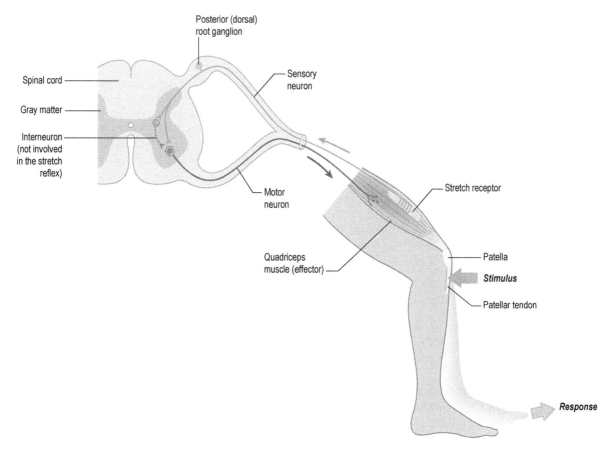

Figure 4.1a-XI A simple reflex arc

SPINAL TONE

The spinal cord is responsible for maintaining a constant level of contraction, or tone, in the body muscles. This is essential as a background on which upright posture and smooth body movements can occur. The existence of this tone is clear in the situation when all connection between the limbs and the brain is lost, as can occur in an injury of the spinal cord. In this situation, the muscles do not just go limp and useless. Instead, they manifest a sometimes intense level of this sustained contraction, a result of impulses from motor nerves originating in the spinal cord. This tone tends to cause the lower limbs to extend out straight, and the upper limbs to flex so that a bend is held at the elbow. This limb position is characteristic of patients who have suffered a spinal injury at a high level such as at the neck. In such patients the involuntary muscular contraction is often over-forceful, and over time the muscles become tight and contracted.

The reason why this excessive level of tone is not experienced in a healthy person is that nerve impulses originating from the brain are transmitted down the spinal cord to partially inhibit the spinal motor nerves, and to reduce the muscle tone to a level that enables upright posture and smooth movements.

Motor nerve cells that originate in the spinal cord are called lower motor neurons. Motor nerve cells that originate in the brain and descend to control the function of lower motor nerves are called upper motor neurons. This distinction is important to make, as it will help in understanding the underlying problems in the severe diseases that cause impaired muscular movement, such as multiple sclerosis, motor neuron disease and stroke.

In a simple reflex arc and the production of tone after a spinal injury it is the lower motor nerves only that are responsible for the muscle contraction. However, in most other movements the action of the lower motor nerve cells has been stimulated or inhibited by the impulses from upper motor nerves originating from the brain.

Part II: The physiology of the nervous system continued

The peripheral nervous system (PNS)

The peripheral nervous system (PNS) consists of all the parts of the nervous system that exist outside the protective skeletal casing of the skull and the vertebral column. It comprises the 31 pairs of spinal nerves and the 12 pairs of cranial nerves. The autonomic nervous system (ANS) is the part of the PNS that is concerned with the involuntary control of the deep organs, blood vessels and glands, and thus it is essential for the maintenance of homeostasis.

THE SPINAL NERVES

The structure of the spinal cord was described at the end of Part I. The 31 pairs of spinal nerves, which each leave the cord at regular intervals (see Figure 4.1a-IX), divide to form the largest part of the PNS.

All the spinal nerves are mixed nerves in that they carry both motor and sensory nerve fibers to all the parts of the body that they supply. In the spinal nerves, the motor nerve fibers are largely responsible for the voluntary movement of the skeletal muscles (this includes reflex actions such as the withdrawal of parts of the body from painful stimuli). However, some of the motor fibers divide away from the spinal nerves close to their exit from the vertebral column to control the contraction of the smooth and cardiac muscle of the blood vessels, deep organs and glands. These functions are mainly not under the control of the will. These involuntary motor nerves are considered to be part of the ANS.

The first pair of spinal nerves (the first cervical nerves) passes out of the vertebral column between the skull and the first cervical vertebra. All the other cervical nerves, the thoracic nerves and the first four lumbar nerves pass out

between the vertebrae that make up the vertebral column. The fifth lumbar nerve exits between the fifth lumbar vertebra and the sacrum. The sacral nerves leave via holes (foramina) within the sacrum, and the coccygeal nerves leave at the level of the fusion of the bones of the sacrum and the coccyx. The names of the spinal nerves are usually abbreviated according to the associated spinal level. For example, the third cervical nerve is called C3, and the fifth lumbar nerve is called L5.

After its exit from the vertebral column, each spinal nerve divides many times to form all the nerves that together carry motor and sensory nerve fibers to most parts of the body below the head and the neck.

THE CRANIAL NERVES

In addition to the spinal nerves, 12 pairs of nerves (the cranial nerves) leave the base of the brain to supply the tissues of the head and the neck. In addition, the tenth cranial nerves (the vagus nerves) each divide to form nerve branches, which extend deep into the thorax and abdomen to supply the deep organs within. The optic nerves, which supply the eye, and the auditory nerves, which supply the ear, are two other examples of cranial nerves.

The cranial nerves are named either by a name derived from a Latin root or by a number (abbreviated as the Roman numeral). For example, the optic nerve is also known as the second cranial nerve (II), and the vagus nerve is also known as the tenth cranial nerve (X).

Unlike the spinal nerves, not all the cranial nerves are mixed nerves. Three of the pairs of cranial nerves carry only sensory fibers (e.g. the optic nerve, which leads from the retina of the eye to the brain). Five pairs carry only motor nerve fibers (e.g. the oculomotor nerves, which supply some of the muscles that move the eye). The remaining four pairs of cranial nerves are mixed nerves. Like the spinal nerves, these four pairs of mixed cranial nerves also carry motor nerves, which are responsible for involuntary action of the muscles that control the functions of the deep organs and glands.

The cranial nerves pass out from the bony skull through holes in or between the cranial bones (e.g. through the hole at the back of the orbit, the cavity that cradles the eyeball).

In this section on the PNS, only those aspects of the cranial nerves that are responsible for sensation and the voluntary control of the skeletal muscles are considered. Those nerve fibers that are responsible for the involuntary control of smooth muscle and cardiac muscle in the blood vessels, deep organs and glands are generally considered as forming a distinct system, the ANS. This system is discussed at the end of this section.

THE DIVISION OF THE SPINAL AND CRANIAL NERVES

Each spinal and cranial nerve branches in a tree-like fashion to supply a particular portion of the body. In the cervical, lumbar and sacral regions, the adjacent spinal nerves intermingle with each other close to the spinal cord before they separate out again into a number of nerve branches that then supply the tissues of the neck, arm, leg and genital areas. This intermingling produces a net-like web of nerves called a plexus. Figure 4.1a-XII illustrates the location of the major nerve plexuses.

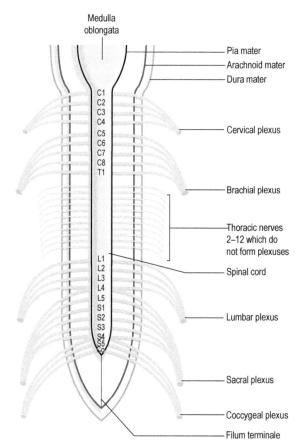

Figure 4.1a-XII Diagrammatic representation of the level of the five major nerve plexuses

The major nerve branches that emerge from the plexuses are given descriptive names derived from Latin. For example, the radial nerve is the nerve in the arm that runs close to the radius bone, and the peroneal nerve describes the nerve in the leg that runs close to the peroneal muscles.

The intermingling of fibers in the plexuses is important to understand because the nerve branches that emerge from each plexus contain nerve fibers that originate from more than one spinal nerve. For example, the sciatic nerve, which emerges from the buttock to descend down the leg, carries fibers that originate from five spinal nerves (L4, L5, S1, S2 and S3). This may seem to be a rather esoteric point, but is very relevant to an understanding of the physical effect of acupuncture and other manipulative therapies.

DERMATOMES

The parts of the body that are supplied by each spinal and cranial nerve are clearly understood. The areas of skin and tissue supplied by the sensory nerves of each spinal nerve have been mapped, and are much the same for each person. These areas are called dermatomes, and are illustrated in Figure 4.1a-XIII. Dermatomes represent those strips of skin and areas of the body that are supplied by the individual spinal and cranial nerves. Although the diagram suggests that there is a clear demarcation between dermatomes, in reality this is not the case, with there being considerable overlap of the regions supplied by adjacent spinal nerves. Nevertheless, these diagrams can be very useful for health practitioners because they indicate which spinal nerve supplies the nerves to whatever body part is a source of symptoms or a focus for treatment. Some dermatomal diagrams also indicate which nerve branch (e.g. the radial nerve or the sciatic nerve) supplies a particular area. Figures 4.1a-XIV and 4.1a-XV show examples of such diagrams for the arm and the leg, respectively.

Figure 4.1a-XIII Dermatomes of the spinal roots and the three divisions of the fifth (V) cranial nerve on the face (the trigeminal nerve)

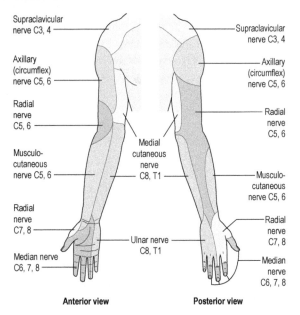

Supraclavicular nerve C3, 4

Axillary (circumflex) nerve C5, 6

Radial nerve C5, 6

Musculo-cutaneous nerve C5, 6

Radial nerve C7, 8

Median nerve C6, 7, 8

Medial cutaneous nerve C8, T1

Ulnar nerve C8, T1

Supraclavicular nerve C3, 4

Axillary (circumflex) nerve C5, 6

Radial nerve C5, 6

Musculo-cutaneous nerve C5, 6

Radial nerve C7, 8

Median nerve C6, 7, 8

Anterior view   **Posterior view**

Figure 4.1a-XIV Dermatomes of the nerves that supply the arms

Although the aim of dermatomal diagrams is to illustrate the distribution of the sensory nerves, they can also give approximate information about the motor nerves that supply the muscles in a particular region. For example, the muscles that control plantar flexion of the wrist and gripping of the fingers are largely supplied by motor nerves that originate from the C6, C7, C8, T1 spinal nerves. Just as they direct the sensory nerve fibers from these spinal nerves away from the area, the ulnar and median nerves and their branches direct these motor nerve fibers to this part of the lower arm.

Ilioinguinal nerve L1

Posterior rami S1, 2, 3

Subcostal nerve T12

Genitofemoral nerve L1, 2

Lateral cutaneous nerve of thigh L2, 3

Obturator L2, 3, 4

Medial and intermediate cutaneous nerves L2, 3

Lateral cutaneous nerve of calf of leg L5, S1, 2

Superficial peroneal (musculocutaneous) nerve L4, 5, S1

Sural nerve S1, 2

Deep peroneal nerve L4, 5

Saphenous nerve L3, 4

Subcostal nerve T12

Iliohypogastric nerve L1

Posterior rami L1, 2, 3

Lateral cutaneous nerve of thigh L2, 3

Posterior cutaneous nerve S1, 2, 3

Obturator nerve L2, 3, 4

Medial cutaneous nerve of thigh L2, 3

Lateral cutaneous nerve of calf L4, 5, S1 of leg

Sural nerve L5, S1, 2

Tibial nerve S1, 2

Anterior view   **Posterior view**

Figure 4.1a-XV Dermatomes of the nerves that supply the legs

Information box 4.1a-I

The dermatomes: comments from a Chinese medicine perspective

The discussion about referred pain illustrates recognition in conventional medicine terms that distant parts of the body are linked because they are associated with the same spinal levels. For example, there is a link in the nervous system between the heart and the front of the arm and the neck. In this example, the spinal levels of C3 through to T6 are linked, probably by connector nerve cells in the spinal cord.

In the examples of referred pain, the site of the pain from these deep organs can relate to the position of channels and points that have a close connection with the treatment of these conditions from the Chinese medicine viewpoint.

The referred pain in a heart attack is felt not only in the center of the chest, but down the arm in the area of the Pericardium and Heart Channels, and up the neck, through which the deep pathway of the Heart Channel runs. The referred pain of cholecystitis is felt at the shoulder, over which the Gallbladder Channel passes. The referred pain of the ovary is felt on the front and inner aspect of the thigh, over which pass the Stomach, Spleen and Liver Channels. In all three conditions, points can be chosen from these Channels to relieve the symptoms.

It is now scientifically accepted that acupuncture has a measurable analgesic effect mediated by impulses traveling up to the spinal cord by sensory nerves. Acupuncture stimulation appears to modulate nervous activity in the spinal cord at the level of the stimulated spinal nerve, which then results in inhibition of pain-carrying nerve fibers associated with the same spinal level. Impulses also travel up from the affected spinal cord level to the regions of the midbrain that deal in the general modulation of pain. This supports the observation that acupuncture can have both a local and general effect on the experience of pain. The neurotransmitters B endorphin and metenkephalin are recognized as two chemical mediators that are instrumental in these acupuncture effects.

The non-analgesic effects of acupuncture are less well explained scientifically. These include improvements in wound healing, nausea reduction, treatment of addiction, improved organ function, stimulation of the immune system and enhancement of mood. However, given the complex interconnections of the nervous and endocrine systems, it is feasible that acupuncture-mediated stimulation of nerves at a particular spinal level may have diverse ramifications both at a neural and the endocrine level.

Keown (2014),[5] however, persuasively argues that acupuncture meridians seem to follow anatomical pathways formed between planes between the connective tissue that divides the various anatomically and embryologically distinct body parts. Fascia is made up from collagen that is a protein with unique piezoelectric qualities. This means that electrical charge is created when its structure is deformed. It is possible that the acupuncture needle stimulates not only the nervous system but also this anatomically hidden system of fascial pathways, and so leads to energetic change in diverse ways.

REFERRED PAIN

Referred pain is the term used to describe the situation in which pain originating in one part of the body is experienced elsewhere. In general, referred pain is felt either as a cutaneous or muscular sensation, when in fact the pathology is in a deeper part of the body. In sciatica, the problem usually lies either in the structure of the lumbar and sacral bones at the base of the back, where there can be bony or muscular impingement on the L5–S3 nerve roots, or in the proximal region of the sciatic nerve itself as it emerges from the sacral plexus and enters the buttock muscles. However, sciatic pain is experienced at the back of the leg and the foot. The pain is experienced in the leg and the foot because the brain misinterprets the origin of the irritation as coming from the distal ends of the spinal nerve branches that terminate in the dermatome, rather than the correct site, which is far more proximally located.

Another cause of referred pain is the pain that originates from the deep organs. Compared to the skin and the skeletal muscles, the deeper body parts do not have a very full sensory nerve supply. For example, there is not a general awareness of how the spleen feels, or of the opening of our heart valves. If a deep organ is in distress, the pain from the organ and its surrounding tissues results in sensory messages that travel to the spinal cord through the spinal nerves that supply nerve fibers to that organ. However, the brain interprets these messages as coming from the nerves that supply its particular dermatome. The organs are connected by nerves often to a number of spinal levels, which means that deep organ pain is often vague and difficult for the patient to localize. In some cases, the dermatome overlies the position of the organ, but in others the pain is felt in a distant site. For example, gallbladder pain may be referred to the shoulder tip, the region of the C4 dermatome, because fibers from the C4 spinal nerve supply the diaphragmatic region as well as the shoulder.

The autonomic nervous system (ANS)

As mentioned earlier in this section, the motor nerve fibers of the spinal nerves and the mixed cranial nerves are involved in the involuntary control of the deep organs, blood vessels and glands. It is this aspect of the function of the nervous system that is called the autonomic nervous system (ANS). The term autonomic refers to the fact that the function of the ANS is largely outside the control of the conscious will.

The ANS controls the automatic functions of the body such as breathing, the pumping of the heart, the maintenance of blood pressure, sweating, salivation and the function of the digestive system. It not only keeps these functions going, but also enables them to be modified so that the total function of the body is responsive to its precise requirements at any one time. For example, the ability of the cardiovascular system to modify the pulse rate and blood pressure according to the needs of the body is mediated by the ANS.

In a healthy person, the ANS is always working to return the body to a state of homeostasis. Often it has to undo the imbalance in homeostasis that has been induced by the actions commanded by the conscious mind. For example, when a person decides to start running for a "not-to-be-missed" bus, the ANS brings about a series of changes in the body to ensure that the cells receive a steady supply of oxygen and nutrients, and that the body does not get overheated. In this sort of situation, it is the ANS that temporarily shuts down unnecessary functions, such as the production of urine and digestion, and speeds up the heart and respiratory rate, increases blood pressure and promotes sweating. The ANS even alters aspects of the mind, so that a state of daydreaming is replaced by one of focus and determination. After the bus has been caught and the pressure is off, the ANS continues to act to ensure that the body gradually returns to a balanced resting state.

The ANS is made up of two parts, which work in an opposing manner. The sympathetic nervous system (SNS) tends to predominate in stressful situations, such as the previously mentioned situation of running for a bus. The parasympathetic nervous system (PSNS) predominates during rest, such as in the recovery period after running for the bus.

THE SYMPATHETIC NERVOUS SYSTEM (SNS)

It might be said that the SNS acts to promote the more Yang aspects of the maintenance of homeostasis. It is most active when the mind has been alerted, or when the body has been injured, and prepares the body for quick responses, including meeting a challenge head on or the decision to escape (fight or flight).

The nerve cells of the SNS originate in the brainstem, and descend to connect with nerves in the spinal cord between T1 and L3. From these levels, fibers leave the spinal cord through the spinal nerves and intermingle with each other in a chain of nervous tissue that runs on either side of the spinal column at the back of the abdominal and thoracic cavities. There are a number of cell bodies, known as the sympathetic ganglia, within this chain of nervous tissue, and thus it can be compared to the gray matter of the brain and the spinal cord (the term ganglion, from the Greek meaning lump, is used in this case to refer to a cluster of nerve cell bodies). Figure 4.1a-XVI illustrates how nerve fibers leave the sympathetic ganglia to travel to all body parts, and indicates the wide range of tissues and organs that are influenced by the sympathetic nerves.

As mentioned above, the sympathetic part of the ANS is sometimes described as the part of the nervous system that prepares the body for fight or flight. It causes physical changes that allow the body to expend energy in a focused way, such as was described in the example of running for the bus. The various actions of the SNS are listed in Figure 4.1a-XVI, and it might become clear that all these changes, such as dilatation of the pupil, inhibition of mucus secretion, increased heart rate and reduced peristalsis, are appropriate ones for a body that is about to go into action.

The SNS also directly stimulates one endocrine gland, the adrenal medulla (the central part of the adrenal gland), which is situated just above the kidneys. This causes the release of the hormones adrenaline and noradrenaline into the bloodstream. These hormones help the body to deal with impending stress, and complement the function of the sympathetic nerves, as they have effects such as stimulation of the heart rate, increase of blood pressure, widening of the bronchioles and increased mental alertness.

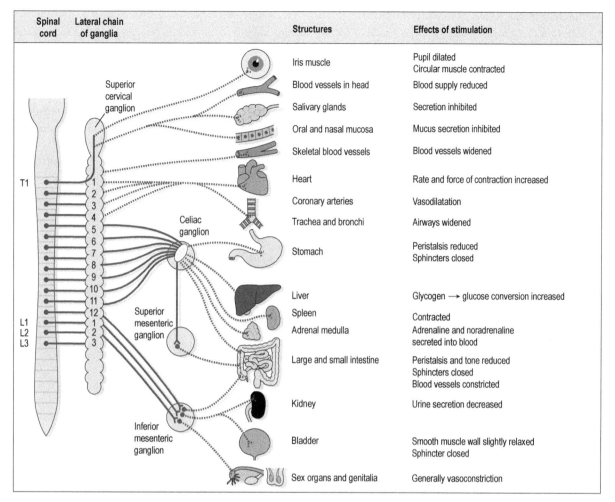

Spinal cord	Lateral chain of ganglia	Structures	Effects of stimulation
	Superior cervical ganglion	Iris muscle	Pupil dilated Circular muscle contracted
		Blood vessels in head	Blood supply reduced
		Salivary glands	Secretion inhibited
		Oral and nasal mucosa	Mucus secretion inhibited
		Skeletal blood vessels	Blood vessels widened
T1		Heart	Rate and force of contraction increased
		Coronary arteries	Vasodilatation
	Celiac ganglion	Trachea and bronchi	Airways widened
		Stomach	Peristalsis reduced Sphincters closed
		Liver	Glycogen → glucose conversion increased
		Spleen	Contracted
	Superior mesenteric ganglion	Adrenal medulla	Adrenaline and noradrenaline secreted into blood
L1 L2 L3		Large and small intestine	Peristalsis and tone reduced Sphincters closed Blood vessels constricted
		Kidney	Urine secretion decreased
	Inferior mesenteric ganglion	Bladder	Smooth muscle wall slightly relaxed Sphincter closed
		Sex organs and genitalia	Generally vasoconstriction

Figure 4.1a-XVI The structure and influence of the sympathetic nervous system

 Information box 4.1a-II

The sympathetic nervous system: comments from a Chinese medicine perspective

The sympathetic chain of ganglions is situated in the part of the back that runs from T1 to L3. This is the part that curves outwards between the natural inward curves formed by the neck and the small of the back. Although all of the back is considered as Yang in Chinese medicine, this section of the back is its most Yang aspect.

A noteworthy point is that the inner line of the Bladder Channel, which is considered in Chinese medicine to have a profound influence on the function of the deep organs, runs on the surface of the skin overlying the position of the sympathetic ganglia. It is possible that needling points along this section of the bladder line may exert a profound influence on the organs by affecting the nerve impulses within the sympathetic ganglia. This nervous tissue is particularly concentrated in three main ganglia: one at the level of T12, one at the level of L1 and one at the level of L3. These would correspond in level to the position of the major points on the back affecting the Spleen, the Stomach and the Kidney (acupoints Pi Shu BL-20, Wei Shu BL-21 and Shen Shu BL-23), respectively.

THE PARASYMPATHETIC NERVOUS SYSTEM (PSNS)

In contrast to the sympathetic system, the PSNS might be described as promoting the maintenance of homeostasis. It is most active when the mind and body are at rest.

The parasympathetic nerves originate in the brainstem and the sacral part of the spinal cord. In particular, the vital centers in the brainstem, which deal with essential functions such as respiration and the heart rate, contain many parasympathetic nerve cells. These nerve cells have fibers that leave the cord either through the four pairs of mixed cranial nerves (the oculomotor, facial, glossopharyngeal and vagus nerves) or within the S2, S3 and S4 spinal nerves. The mixed cranial nerves have parasympathetic branches that extend to supply the deep organs and glands of the head, neck and abdomen down to the upper part of the large intestine. The parasympathetic fibers in the sacral spinal nerves supply the lower part of the large intestine, the bladder and the genital organs. Figure 4.1a-XVII illustrates the structure of the PSNS.

Figure 4.1a-XVII The structure and influence of the parasympathetic nervous system

The PSNS promotes those aspects of bodily function that work to nourish and build up the body's reserves. It enables the body to make use of the resting periods to perform functions such as the digestion of nutrients and the clearance of wastes from the kidneys and the bowel. It is noteworthy that it is when the PSNS is active that sexual function is promoted. This suggests that sex is an activity that ideally takes place when the person is at rest, and has the purpose of nourishing and building up the individual as well as the creation of a new life. It is clear that excessive sympathetic nervous activity, such as would occur in a stressful period or even a situation of excitement, tends to counteract this parasympathetic action, and can lead to impotence.

Figure 4.1a-XVII shows how the various organs and glands are supplied by nerves that originate from the brainstem and the sacral spinal cord. The parasympathetic nerves increase secretions from the eye, the mouth and the digestive tract. Although not indicated in this diagram, the production of mucus of the respiratory tract is also increased. These secretions are all protective and nourishing to the organs that produce them. The heart and respiratory rate slows with parasympathetic stimulation, and digestion, defecation and urination are also promoted.

Information box 4.1a-III

The parasympathetic nervous system: comments from a Chinese medicine perspective

In contrast to the SNS, the outflow of the parasympathetic nerves (PSNS) emerges from the regions of the spinal column in which there is an inward curve (the neck and the small of the back). These could be described as the more structurally Yin regions of the spine because of their inward curvature. The activity of the PSNS aids assimilation and storage of nutrients. It also increases bodily secretions, which are protective and nourishing to the organs that produce them. Such activities would be interpreted as Yin in Chinese medicine terms.

It is interesting to consider that much of the lifestyle advice of Chinese medicine focuses on activities that promote the action of the PSNS. Regular relaxed meals, regular times of sleep, gentle exercise and meditation will all have this effect. The hands-on therapies such as massage, shiatsu and reflexology will tend to stimulate the PSNS. The calming and enabling approach of craniosacral therapy, in particular, focuses on the two regions of the spine from which the parasympathetic nerves emerge.

THE BALANCE BETWEEN THE SYMPATHETIC AND PARASYMPATHETIC SYSTEMS

The PSNS can be seen as the aspect of the ANS that always tends to increase in function when the mind and body is at rest. When the mind and body are at rest, the centers of nerve cells in the brainstem and in the spinal cord automatically cause the PSNS to stimulate all the organs and glands of the body. When the mind is alerted or when the body has been injured, messages are relayed to inhibit the action of the parasympathetic centers in the brainstem, and the sympathetic nerve centers in the brainstem come into action instead.

It would make sense that the periods of stress that lead to sympathetic stimulation should be short-lived, so that a time of parasympathetic stimulation can allow the body to recover from the stress. Dealing with stress is a natural aspect of human life, not least because the creative and competitive aspects of human nature often lead us to instigate situations of stress. This is not necessarily a bad thing, as long as there are adequate periods of recuperation between these stressful episodes.

It is not easy to assess what the ideal balance of parasympathetic and sympathetic stimulation should be, and this ideal may vary from individual to individual, depending on personality amongst other things. However, what seems to be clear is that many people in modern society do not have sufficient periods of parasympathetic activity to make up for the times during which their SNS is overactive.

Information box 4.1a-IV

The autonomic nervous system: comments from a Chinese medicine perspective

The healthy function of the ANS, with an ideal balance between the opposing aspects of the SNS and PSNS, is a fundamental requirement for the maintenance of health, both from a conventional and a Chinese medical viewpoint. It would make sense that the practice of Chinese medicine, which focuses heavily on allowing the body to regain balance, will have profound effects at the level of the ANS. In Chinese medicine, treatments that tonify Yin or treatments that are sedating of excess would seem to promote parasympathetic aspects of function, while treatments that tonify Yang would appear to promote sympathetic aspects of function.

One could argue that, if the more profound aspects of the mechanism of acupuncture are to be communicated to a conventionally trained practitioner, they might best be explained in terms of the function of the ANS. For example, it might be suggested that the acupuncture needle, by stimulating sensory nerves, leads to impulses that arrive at the corresponding spinal level of the spinal cord. It can then be explained that this is scientifically recognized to be one part of the mechanism by which acupuncture leads to the reduction of pain. However, it can also be suggested that these impulses in the spinal cord may also modulate the nervous activity of the ANS, particularly of those autonomic nerves that emerge from the spinal level of the dermatome that is needled. In this way the parasympathetic and sympathetic aspects of the functions of the blood vessels, deep organs and glands may be affected.

One could add that, in most treatments, it would seem that acupuncture, and the lifestyle advice that goes with it, enhances in particular the function of the parasympathetic aspect of the ANS. To support this suggestion, scientific studies of the action of electro-acupuncture have demonstrated that electrostimulation leads to predictable modification of organ function normally controlled by the ANS.[6]

Persistent stress, be it social, spiritual or physical, leads to excessive stimulation of the fight-or-flight response of the sympathetic nerves. Blood pressure and heart rate become persistently high, digestion worsens, blood sugar levels rise, muscle tension is increased and the mind is unable to relax. This, of course, becomes a vicious circle, as a tense body and alerted mind further stimulate the sympathetic nerves. In such a situation, if the body and mind could be allowed to rest, the activation of the PSNS would help the organs to begin the self-healing process of the body. This is why rest is so important, as it allows the heart and blood vessels to relax, nutrients to be well absorbed, wastes to be fully cleared, and muscles and joints to be free of tension.

4.1b The investigation of the nervous system

The investigation of the nervous system is managed within the hospital specialty of neurology. Because most of these investigations are highly technical, most neurological tests are arranged for a patient only after referral to a hospital specialist called a neurologist. An investigation of the nervous system might involve:

- a thorough physical examination

- investigations to examine the structure of the nervous system (magnetic resonance imaging (MRI), computed tomography (CT) scan and angiography)

- examination of the cerebrospinal fluid (CSF) and biopsy

- investigation to examine the function of the brain and spinal cord (electroencephalography (EEG))

- investigations to examine the function of the peripheral nerves (electromyography (EMG) and nerve conduction studies).

These investigations are considered briefly in turn below.

Physical examination

The physical examination of the nervous system involves the stages listed in Table 4.1b-I. Most aspects of the nervous system cannot be examined directly. Instead, much of the examination of the nervous system involves looking for the physical signs that can result from damage to specific parts of the nervous system.

Table 4.1b-I The stages of physical examination of the nervous system

Examination of the general appearance: this can reveal the characteristic features of neurological disease that affect the facial appearance, movements and posture, such as Parkinson's disease and stroke

Examination of the retina: by means of an ophthalmoscope

Examination of the cranial nerves: a systematic examination that tests functions of the body that are controlled by the cranial nerves. These include:

- the sense of smell and taste
- the acuity of vision and the extent of the visual fields
- the eye movements and the reactions of the pupil to light
- the sense of hearing
- the sensation of the dermatomes of the face
- the strength of the facial muscles and the muscles of the palate and the tongue
- the strength of the muscles of the neck and shoulders

Examination of the spinal nerves: a systematic examination that involves testing of the following functions of the spinal nerves:

- the sensation of the skin across the various dermatomes
- the strength of the muscle groups in the limbs
- the stretch reflexes of the important muscle groups such as the triceps, quadriceps and gastrocnemius

Examination of the cerebellum: testing the balance and coordination of skilled movements

Examination of the cerebral cortex: this can include a wide range of specialized tests designed to expose specific defects in functions such as speech, memory and the ability to recognize objects by their shape

Examination of the general appearance

This can reveal the characteristic features of neurological disease that affect the facial appearance, movements and posture, such as Parkinson's disease and stroke.

Examination of the retina by means of ophthalmoscope

This is the one aspect of physical examination that involves direct visualization of an aspect of the nervous system. The retina at the back of the eye consists of layers of specialized sensory nerve cells called rods and cones. All the nerve fibers of these converge at a place called the optic disc, which is located just off the center of the retina. From here they run down the optic nerve to the brain (the diseases that affect the eye are discussed in more detail in Section 6.1d). The appearance of this layer of nervous tissue and the root of the optic nerve can be seen using an ophthalmoscope. In addition to the conditions that affect the eye itself, this examination can reveal changes that occur as a result of increased pressure within the brain.

Examination of the cranial nerves

This is a systematic examination that tests the functions of the body that are controlled by the cranial nerves. These include:

- sense of smell and taste
- acuity of vision and the extent of the visual fields
- eye movements and the reactions of the pupil to light
- sense of hearing
- sensation of the dermatomes of the face
- strength of the facial muscles and the muscles of the palate and the tongue
- strength of the muscles of the neck and shoulders.

Examination of the spinal nerves

This is a systematic examination that involves testing of the following functions of the spinal nerves:

- The sensation of the skin across the various dermatomes: by testing for the ability to sense a pin-prick, heavy pressure and light touch from cotton wool.
- The strength of the muscle groups in the limbs: motor nerves are tested by systematically checking the strength of the various muscle groups of the body.
- The stretch reflexes of the important muscle groups such as the triceps, quadriceps and gastrocnemius: a light hammer is used to test the stretch reflexes of some of the major muscle groups, for example, the knee-jerk reflex. In the knee-jerk test, the hammer is used to apply a sudden stretch to the patellar tendon, which attaches the quadriceps group of muscles, through the patella, to the upper part of the tibia. In healthy people there is a spinal reflex that causes the suddenly stretched muscle to contract. In the knee-jerk reflex the stretch of the patellar tendon causes the lower leg to kick upwards involuntarily as the knee joint is extended

(see Figure 4.1a-XI). In conditions in which the upper motor neurons that descend from the brain to the spinal cord are affected by disease, these reflexes will be excessive as a result of reduced inhibition of spinal tone. The reflexes will therefore be increased in conditions such as stroke or multiple sclerosis. In conditions in which the lower motor neurons that leave the spinal cord to supply the muscles are diseased, the stretch reflexes will be absent. Motor neuron disease is an example of such a condition. Also, any condition that impairs the sensory nerves that supply the tendons will also cause the stretch reflexes to be absent. This can occur in severe diabetes, for example.

Examination of the cerebellum

This involves testing the balance and coordination of skilled movements.

Examination of the cerebellar cortex

The examination of the cerebral cortex can include a wide range of specialized tests designed to expose specific defects in functions such as speech, memory and the ability to recognize objects by their shape.

Magnetic resonance imaging (MRI) and computed tomography (CT) scan

The structure of the brain and the spinal cord can be examined in detail by means of an MRI. The patient lies on a bed that is moved into a cylindrical scanner. A very strong magnetic field is used to produce detailed images of slices of the body. The MRI produces high-resolution images of nervous tissue, and in this respect for many neurological diseases it is a superior investigation to CT scanning (see Figures 4.1b-I and 4.1b-II).

MRI is not believed to carry the long-term risk that results from exposure to the X-radiation of CT scans. However, many patients find this painless procedure an ordeal because it involves spending about 30 minutes keeping very still within the noisy enclosed space of the MRI scanner. Very small children and some adults cannot tolerate this, and may have to be given a general anesthetic to undergo an MRI scan. The patient undergoing a CT scan has a very similar experience, as the external structure of the CT scanner is similar to that of the MRI scanner.

Before the development of CT and MRI scanners, plain X-ray images of the skull and spinal cord were often used, although the information that these tests could give was never very specific.

Figure 4.1b-I CT scan of the brain showing an area of hemorrhage in the cerebellum (arrow)
A horizontal slice taken at the level of the eyes. The eyeballs and optic nerves can be seen anteriorly, and the sphenoid bone of the skull is in the middle of the image.

Figure 4.1b-II MRI scan of the brain showing two areas of subdural hemorrhage (arrows)
A vertical slice showing cervical vertebrae inferiorly. Note the very distinct contrast between the gray and white matter of the brain, a characteristic of a high-definition MRI image.

Angiography

Angiography is described in detail in Section 3.2b on the cardiovascular system. The same technique is used in the investigation of diseases of the brain and spinal cord to produce images of the main blood vessels that lead to and supply the brain, although advances in MRI have led to this procedure being far less frequently performed.

Angiography can reveal the narrowing of the carotid and vertebral vessels in the neck. This narrowing can lead to emboli, and so is a risk for recurrent strokes. Angiography can also show up areas of the blood vessels that are dilated by aneurysms.

Despite being used as part of the prevention and treatment of stroke, an angiography of these delicate vessels in itself carries a risk of stroke. Doppler (ultrasound) imaging is a useful non-invasive alternative investigation for the carotid and vertebral arteries of the neck.

Positron emission tomography (PET) scanning

Positron emission tomography (PET) is a specialized form of CT scanning in which the scan picks up radioactivity from a short acting tracer given to the patient in advance. The tracer is chosen to highlight bodily activity in the area of interest. This test is currently largely used in neuroscience research rather than in day-to-day clinical practice.

Examination of the cerebrospinal fluid (CSF)

A sample of CSF can be obtained by means of the technique known as lumbar puncture. A conscious patient is either seated or lying on their side in the fetal position. A needle is inserted into the L2/3 or L3/4 intervertebral space as far as the subarachnoid space, so that a few milliliters of CSF can be withdrawn.

Lumbar puncture is used most frequently to diagnose the infective organism in meningitis. It can also show characteristic changes in more rare conditions such as multiple sclerosis. The technique can also be used to treat certain diseases of the brain, as drugs can be injected directly into the CSF (e.g. for administering chemotherapy in the treatment of leukemia).

The most common problem that occurs with lumbar puncture is that the patient can suffer from recurrent headaches as a result of the drop in the volume of the lubricating CSF. This complication affects up to one-third of patients. The patient is requested to keep lying down for 24 hours after the procedure in order to prevent this occurring.

The spinal cord terminates above the L2 level, and so there should be no risk of damage to the spinal cord from this test. Nevertheless, the needle can irritate or damage one of the lumbar spinal nerves that descend through the space, so leading to referred pain in the affected dermatomes, and possible numbness and weakness of associated muscles. This is a very rare complication.

It is in the diagnosis of meningitis that lumbar puncture carries the most risk. In severe meningitis, the inflammation of the brain can cause the CSF to be under great pressure. The sudden release of pressure that follows withdrawal of CSF can result in the brainstem being forced downwards against the base of the skull. This can be a fatal complication. Because of this real risk, if possible, all patients with meningitis should have a CT scan to look for signs of brain swelling before the lumbar puncture is performed.

Biopsy

In cases of suspected infection or cancer, a sample of tissue can be removed from the brain or other parts of the nervous system by means of a small probe. The biopsy is guided with the help of CT and MRI scans.

Electroencephalography (EEG)

The technique of EEG can be compared to electrocardiography (ECG) in that it detects electrical changes originating from a deep organ via electrodes placed on the skin. Both techniques are completely non-invasive. EEG exposes the electrical changes that are a reflection of the electrical activity of the brain, commonly called the brainwaves.

The activity of the nerves in the brain leads to characteristic patterns of brainwaves, which vary according to the state of consciousness. The EEG of a person who is actively thinking is different to that of a person who is asleep. The brainwaves in sleep go through phases according to the depth of sleep, so that deep sleep can be differentiated from the dreaming state, in which there are spontaneous bodily movements and rapid eye movements (REM). Interestingly, the brainwaves that occur in a state of deep meditation (alpha waves) are very similar to those that occur in a stage of the healthy sleep cycle. It is known that the alpha brain rhythm is associated with a predominance of the parasympathetic part of the autonomic nervous system (ANS).

In certain diseases, in particular during an epileptic seizure, the brainwaves look abnormal. The EEG is used most commonly to diagnose epilepsy. An EEG study may be combined with a video recording of the patient's behavior, so that in the case of epilepsy a seizure can be captured on video and compared with the brainwaves that were occurring at the same time.

Electromyography (EMG)

This technique measures the electrical activity within a muscle. It involves the insertion of a very fine needle into a muscle. EMG can detect disorders of both the muscle and the motor nerves that supply the muscles.

Nerve conduction studies

This is another type of study that detects electrical changes, this time in the peripheral nerves. In nerve conduction studies one part of the nerve is stimulated with a small electrical impulse. The time for the impulse to be recorded further down the nerve is measured. This test can detect problems that affect the structure of the peripheral nerves (e.g. the damage caused by compression of the median nerve in carpal tunnel syndrome). A particular form of nerve conduction study assesses, by means of a surface electrode, the brain response to the stimulation of the eye or the ear. These cerebral-evoked potentials give information on the health of the neural pathways that link the sense organs with the cerebral cortex.

4.1c Disorders of the central nervous system: impairment of consciousness

Consciousness can be defined as a state of wakefulness in which there is awareness of self and surroundings. It results from the healthy functioning of certain parts of the brain. If these parts are damaged by disease, consciousness can be impaired. This can manifest as sleepiness or confusion, and can progress to stupor, when it is very difficult to rouse the patient to respond to external stimuli. A coma is a state of unarousable unconsciousness. If extreme, there are no responses at all, even to the most painful stimuli.

The cerebral cortices are responsible for the complex higher functions of the brain, including thinking, memory, conscience and will. If a small area of a cerebral cortex is damaged, a clearly defined disability may result. However, if the whole of the cerebral cortex is poorly functioning, such as might occur in advanced dementia or meningitis, confusion followed by a lack of consciousness will develop.

The reticular activating system (RAS) in the brainstem is responsible for wakefulness. It is responsible for switching off the consciousness in sleep, but can also be damaged in certain disease states. In particular, metabolic disturbances, such as hyperglycemia in acute diabetes, uremia in kidney failure or drug intoxication, can affect the functioning of the brainstem and lead to loss of consciousness. Similarly, raised pressure within the skull can cause compression of the brainstem against the base of the skull and lead to loss of consciousness.

Unconsciousness resulting from disease of the cerebral cortex

The cells of the brain, and the cerebral cortex in particular, are very sensitive to anything that disturbs the homeostasis of their immediate environment. Reduction in the levels of oxygen and glucose, or the presence of toxins or certain drugs, can impair the function of brain cells much more rapidly than the cells of many other tissues of the body. Fever is another cause of impaired brain function, particularly if very high or if it rises rapidly. Physical trauma can also lead to a disturbance in the function of the cortex, which may only be temporary. Nevertheless, even if the damage is not long-lasting, a profound change in consciousness can occur for the period leading up to recovery.

This sensitivity to lack of oxygen and glucose, toxins, fever and trauma is very marked in young children and elderly people, which means that a state of confusion or drowsiness can result from what might appear to be a fairly minor bodily disturbance. For example, small children and elderly people can easily become poorly responsive or confused as a result of an infection or a high fever.

The effect of an oxygen or glucose imbalance

In general, even in severe disease, the bodily responses to a disturbance in homeostasis will ensure that an adequate supply of oxygen and glucose to the brain is maintained. The action of the sympathetic aspect of the autonomic nervous system (ANS) is very important in this respect. A simple faint can lead to loss of consciousness, but the sympathetic nervous system (SNS) immediately responds to reverse the impaired blood flow to the brain, so that consciousness returns within a matter of seconds. The sympathetic nerves initiate an increase in the heart and respiratory rate, an increase in blood pressure, and a constriction of peripheral blood vessels so that more oxygenated blood is redirected to the brain and other essential organs. Glucose stores are released from the liver in response to sympathetic nervous activation.

Inadequate oxygen reaching the brain can result from insufficient atmospheric oxygen, such as might occur at high altitude. However, the most common cause is cardiac or respiratory failure, in which the heart and the lungs fail to ensure that sufficient oxygenated blood feeds the brain. For example, confusion and coma can be the result of very severe heart failure or chronic obstructive pulmonary disease (COPD). If these conditions cannot be treated, death will follow.

Insufficient blood glucose can result from the drug treatment of diabetes. This can lead to the progression of confusion, coma and death if not reversed.

The effect of drugs and toxins

The brain cells are also very sensitive to the buildup of certain drugs and toxins. If these are present in excess, consciousness will be impaired, but the dysfunction is very often reversible. In fact, this sensitivity to drugs is utilized in conventional medicine when general anesthetics are administered. Alcohol and sleeping tablets are other examples of widely used drugs that can also easily cause a reversible loss of consciousness.

In certain diseases an accumulation of toxins develops. Kidney and liver failure are both conditions that can lead to confusion and coma for this reason. In both these conditions, without medical intervention the toxins will rapidly lead to death.

Other diseases alter the delicate balance of the chemical reactions that go on within all the cells of the body. These are known collectively as metabolic diseases (metabolic imbalance is classed in Section 2.2a as one of the seven fundamental processes of disease). In some metabolic diseases the balance of acidity and salts in the blood becomes progressively disturbed. These disturbances can affect the function of the brain cells. Often, it is a disease of an endocrine organ that is the cause of this metabolic imbalance. It is for this reason that conditions such as pituitary disease, hypothyroidism and diabetes, if untreated, can lead to coma and death.

The effect of physical trauma

The brain is very vulnerable to physical trauma. A sudden blow to the head or a physical shaking can lead to a degree of swelling of the damaged brain tissue. This leads to an increase of pressure within the enclosed space of the skull. If this swelling is minor it may settle down within hours or days. In such cases the pressure causes a temporary dysfunction of the cortical brain cells and may even lead to a loss of consciousness. As the swelling settles down the patient may recover within a short time and regain normal function, although the patient will often have a period of memory loss relating to the time just before the injury and leading up to the period of recovery. This state is described as concussion.

In a more severe head injury the cells of the cortex and other parts of the brain may sustain permanent injury. If a patient with this sort of injury recovers from the coma, they will be left with a permanent loss of cortical function. If the damage is confined to one area of the cortex, the patient will suffer from a permanent deficit in the function that is controlled by that area of the brain. This is akin to the consequences of a stroke. These focal problems of cortical function are described in Section 4.1d.

More commonly, however, a severe traumatic injury leads to loss of nerve cells throughout the cortex and other parts of the brain, so that the loss of function is much harder to define. In such cases there may be a change in aspects of the personality, memory loss and difficulties with perception and movement. This is the underlying problem that affects boxers who have become "punch drunk." In this case, it is repeated knockouts that have led to a cumulative and permanent loss of brain cells, a condition known as dementia pugilistica.

If the cortical damage is very severe, consciousness may never be recovered. This leads to the condition known as persistent vegetative state (PVS). In PVS the vital functions such as breathing and respiration, and the basic reflexes such as coughing, remain intact, but the patient is unable to perceive anything about the environment and has lost awareness of self.

Unconsciousness resulting from damage to the brainstem

The other major consequence of head injury is that the pressure within the enclosed space of the cranium can increase to such an extent that the deeper parts of the brain such as the brainstem are also compressed. This can result purely from swelling of the brain, but may be compounded by internal bleeding.

The brainstem contains the RAS. If this part of the brain is damaged the patient will lose the state of wakefulness, and if the damage is severe the patient will become unarousable. The most common causes of damage to the brainstem are stroke and raised intracranial pressure.

Brainstem stroke

The brainstem can be damaged by a stroke (see Section 4.1d), which causes a sudden reduction in oxygen supply to this vital part of the brain. Often these strokes are fatal because the vital centers of respiration and heart rate are damaged. Sometimes it is consciousness only that is lost, and this can result in a permanent comatose state.

Sudden raised intracranial pressure

A sudden increase in pressure in the intracranial space (the space within the enclosed skull) can cause severe damage to the brainstem. This is because the brainstem can be rapidly forced down against the opening of the foramen magnum, and thus receives the brunt of the pressure. This situation carries a high risk of death, because the vital centers of the brainstem can be damaged.

A very common cause of this situation is head injury resulting from high-speed road traffic accidents. A combination of brain swelling and bleeding into the brain leads to a rapid rise in pressure within the cranium. In such cases there is a rapid loss of consciousness. A severe warning sign of brainstem damage is that the pupils become tightly constricted. Such a scenario is a neurosurgical emergency. The patient requires surgery immediately to drain any blood and fluid from the brain to relieve the pressure.

Another well-known cause of this sudden increase in pressure is severe bacterial meningitis (see Section 4.1e), in which an infection of the meninges leads to swelling and inflammation. As mentioned in Section 4.1b, in such a case the risk of damage can be increased by the procedure of lumbar puncture.

Information box 4.1c-I

Loss of consciousness: comments from a Chinese medicine perspective

In Chinese medicine, the state of consciousness reflects a healthy Shen. The Shen is the aspect of vital energy that is housed by the Heart Organ. When consciousness is impaired, the Shen is described as Obstructed in Chinese medicine. Obstruction of the Shen is said to occur following Obstruction to the Orifices of the Heart. The Pathogenic Factors associated with this syndrome are Wind, with Fire, Phlegm and Heat or Phlegm and Damp. The underlying mechanism of some of the causes of impaired consciousness described in the text can be attributed directly, from a Chinese medicine viewpoint, to Phlegm or Heat, and the "stirring up" of these by Wind.

The obstruction to blood flow from atheroma, the underlying mechanism of many strokes, might be interpreted as a manifestation of Phlegm in the blood vessels. It is described in Section 5.1c how hypothyroidism is a condition that leads to Accumulation of Phlegm, and in its extreme form can manifest as impaired consciousness. Any form of swelling of the brain will place pressure on the brainstem, and this will affect consciousness. This can result from metabolic diseases, head injury or from a tumor. Swelling of tissues might be understood as a manifestation of Damp or Phlegm.

High fever or infections such as meningitis represent Fire or Heat. Heat and Damp predominate in uncontrolled diabetes. Severe bleeding (reckless hemorrhage) is also seen as a manifestation of Heat. If this occurs into the brain, consciousness will be depressed, and the interpretation might include Wind and Heat obstructing the Orifices.[7]

The role of the brainstem in death

Even if very severe damage is sustained to the cerebral cortex, such as in the case of PVS, life is maintained because the vital centers of the brainstem are intact. Although the causes of death are diverse, the final event that leads to death is always loss of function of the brainstem. It is this relatively small area of the brain which, figuratively speaking, holds the key to life and death.

However, in most deaths, the sequence of events is that the whole brain is affected either by lack of oxygen and glucose in the blood supply, or by an accumulation of toxins. This would be the case in death caused by heart attack, bronchopneumonia or liver failure, for example. This means that the cells of the cerebral cortex as well as those in the brainstem start to dysfunction. The person will drift or fall rapidly into unconsciousness, depending on the speed of events. Once the vital centers of the brainstem stop functioning, death will ensue within seconds to minutes, as the whole of the brain loses its already impaired blood supply.

Raised intracranial pressure

It has just been described how a sudden rise in intracranial pressure can cause severe damage to the brainstem and result in a loss of consciousness. In contrast, there are a number of causes of a gradual rise in intracranial pressure that give rise to less dramatic symptoms.

There are three main reasons for a rise in intracranial pressure: swelling of the brain tissue, accumulation of cerebrospinal fluid (CSF) within the ventricles of the brain, and the development of a swelling or tumor within the brain. The term space-occupying lesion is used to describe the latter cause (the word lesion in medical usage refers to any area of damage to the body that results from a disease process).

In swelling of the brain tissue, the main symptom of raised intracranial pressure is impaired or lost consciousness, because the swelling develops rapidly, usually as a result of inflammation. In contrast, the pressure that develops from accumulation of CSF and most space-occupying lesions (with the exception of the swelling that results from a hemorrhage) is gradual in onset, and impaired consciousness is not a prominent symptom until very late in the progression of the underlying condition.

Swelling of the brain from inflammation

As described earlier, inflammation can result from infections such as meningitis or encephalitis, or can be a response of the brain cells to toxins or drugs. In these sorts of cases the swelling of the brain tissue causes rapid changes in consciousness because it is primarily the cells of the cortex that are affected.

The inflammation of the brain that occurs following trauma can be much more severe, and can lead to compression of the brainstem. Again, in this case there is a rapid loss of consciousness.

Accumulation of cerebrospinal fluid (CSF)

If the CSF cannot drain freely from the ventricles of the brain, the pressure of fluid within the ventricles will build up. The ventricles expand under this pressure and the surrounding brain tissue becomes compressed. This is called hydrocephalus (from the Greek meaning water in the head). Hydrocephalus can result from a congenital malformation of the structure of part of the brain, although the symptoms of this may not become apparent until adult life. In severe cases, the baby is born with an enlarged head, because the increased pressure has caused expansion between the not yet fused bones of the cranium.

Hydrocephalus can also develop in adult life. In most cases this is due to an obstruction in the flow of CSF by a brain tumor or from the scarring that follows an episode of meningitis or a brain hemorrhage. Hydrocephalus is occasionally found through the investigation of an older person with dementia. In these poorly understood cases, the pressure of the CSF is normal and the condition is called normal pressure hydrocephalus.

Space-occupying lesions

A space-occupying lesion refers to any product of a disease process that takes up the limited space within the skull. This may be a brain tumor, an abscess or a collection of blood that has formed following a hemorrhage. All these conditions are described in more detail in the following sections. If the development of the space-occupying lesion is gradual, there will be a gradual increase in pressure within the skull.

The symptoms of a gradual rise in intracranial pressure

The three main symptoms of a gradual rise in intracranial pressure are headaches, vomiting and blurred vision. All these symptoms are progressive over a period of weeks to months. These symptoms should always be regarded as red flags of severe disease.

The headaches are characteristically worse in the morning because the pressure in the skull is increased after a night of lying down. The headache tends to wear off as the day goes on.

The vomiting is also worse in the morning, and need not be accompanied by nausea. This symptom is sometimes described as effortless vomiting. The vomiting is probably a result of pressure on the vomiting center in the brainstem, and so does not have the same prodrome of nausea as might vomiting of gastric origin.

Blurred vision occurs at a later stage, and is a result of pressure on the nerves that leave the brain to supply the retina of the eye. This produces a characteristic swollen appearance of the optic disc when the eye is examined using an ophthalmoscope.

The treatment of raised intracranial pressure

In all cases, whether the onset is rapid or gradual, treatment should be focused on reversal of the cause of raised pressure in the skull. This is undertaken as a matter of urgency.

In hydrocephalus, the CSF can be enabled to drain freely by means of the surgical insertion of a fine tube known as a shunt, which leads from the ventricles of the brain either into a large blood vessel or into the peritoneal cavity. This tube is passed from the brain through the deep tissues of the body and is left in place. It contains a tiny pump, which can be massaged through the skin to prevent it from becoming blocked. There is a risk of infection of this foreign body, so frequent courses of antibiotics may be necessary.

A space-occupying lesion has to be removed or drained by means of surgery. In the case of a brain tumor, after surgery, radiotherapy and steroids may be given to further reduce the size of the mass for as long as possible (see Section 4.1d).

The red flags of raised intracranial pressure

Any patients with undiagnosed features of raised intra-cranial pressure will benefit from referral to a conventional doctor for assessment and/or treatment. Red flags are those symptoms and signs that will indicate that referral should be considered. The red flags of raised intracranial pressure are described in Table 4.1c-I. A summary of the red flags in a format designed for quick reference in clinical practice can be found in Appendix III. This gives advice on the degree of urgency of referral for each of the red flag conditions listed.

Table 4.1c-I A21: Red flags of raised intracranial pressure

Red flag	Description	Reasoning
A21.1	Features of a rapid increase in intracranial pressure: a rapid deterioration of consciousness leading to coma. Irregular breathing patterns and pinpoint pupils are a very serious sign	An increase in pressure within the skull seriously threatens the integrity of the structure of the brain. If the pressure increases rapidly (usually as a result of a sudden intracranial hemorrhage or bleeding from a fractured skull) there can follow downwards pressure via the soft tissue of the brain onto the brainstem
		The brainstem is the seat of the basic vital functions such as breathing and maintenance of consciousness
		As the brainstem is compressed, the patient can lose consciousness, and eventually will stop breathing
		Constriction of the pupils is a result of compression of the nerve that leaves the brain at the level of the brainstem to supply the internal muscles of the eye. This is a grave warning sign of impending serious brain damage
		Ensure that the patient is in a safe and warm place and, ideally, in the recovery position (unless neck trauma suspected) while waiting for help to arrive
A21.2	Features of a slow increase in intracranial pressure: progressive headaches and vomiting over the timescale of a few weeks to months. The headaches are worse in the morning and the vomiting may be effortless. Blurring of vision may be an additional symptom	Intracranial pressure will slowly increase if there is a gradual development of a space-occupying lesion, such as a brain tumor, abscess in the brain or accumulation of poorly draining cerebrospinal fluid. The pressure will be worse when the patient has been lying down, and so the symptoms are characteristically worse in the morning. These include blurring of vision, effortless vomiting (i.e. not much preceding nausea) and headache

4.1d Disorders of the central nervous system: hemorrhage, stroke and brain tumors

This section describes some serious conditions that can affect the function of the brain. It begins with an exploration of the ways in which bleeding within the enclosed space of the skull (intracranial hemorrhage) can affect the brain. It then examines the causes of stroke (one of these being brain hemorrhage) and the physical basis for the many different symptoms of stroke. Finally, the symptoms and treatment of brain tumors are described.

Intracranial hemorrhage

Hemorrhage within the skull has different consequences according to the site of bleeding. Conventionally, bleeding from within the skull is categorized according to its origin in relation to the three meningeal membranes. Extradural hemorrhage refers to bleeding that occurs between the skull bones and the outer dural membrane of the skull. Subdural hemorrhage describes bleeding that occurs between the dural membrane and the arachnoid mater. Subarachnoid hemorrhage refers to bleeding that occurs in the space between the arachnoid and the pia mater; this is the space through which the CSF circulates. Intracerebral hemorrhage refers to bleeding that occurs within the brain tissue itself.

Extradural hemorrhage

This occurs most commonly as a complication of a head injury in which the skull is fractured. The bleeding comes from the damaged blood vessels that normally run up the inside of the skull. Initially, the person who has had the injury may be conscious, but as the blood begins to accumulate along one side of the brain, the brain and brainstem gradually become compressed. Within a matter of minutes to hours the person will develop weakness of one side of the body, confusion and, eventually, coma. Without emergency surgery to drain the blood, the pupils will become constricted and death will follow due to compression of the vital centers of the brainstem.

Emergency surgery involves drilling a hole through the skull bones to drain the blood and surgical attention to any major bleeding blood vessels. In some cases this essential treatment can permit full recovery.

Subdural hemorrhage

A subdural hemorrhage occurs more commonly in elderly people. It is the result of bleeding from the veins that run between the dural and arachnoid membranes. In elderly people the supportive tissues around these veins become weak, so that the veins are liable to break more easily. This can occur as a result of a fairly minor fall or knock to the head. Subdural hemorrhage is more likely if the person is a heavy drinker.

In contrast to extradural hemorrhage, the bleeding is usually much slower. A mass of clotted blood, called a hematoma, develops over the course of days to weeks. This gradually increases the intracranial pressure. The symptoms are of gradually developing drowsiness, confusion and headaches. Because the symptoms are often vague, the condition may not be diagnosed for some time.

The treatment is surgical drainage of the clotted blood, but it may be too late to reverse some of the damage to the brain that has occurred as a result of the bleed.

Subarachnoid hemorrhage

In subarachnoid hemorrhage the bleeding is from the arteries that pass through the subarachnoid space to enter the base of the brain. The bleeding is rapid, and thus symptoms develop quickly. In 80 percent of cases there is an underlying problem in the structure of these arteries, which has commonly been there from birth. The most common form of structural problem is the berry aneurysm (see Section 3.2c), which is a small rounded dilatation of the artery.

The leaking blood mixes with the CSF in the subarachnoid space, and can therefore circulate around the brain and spinal cord. The blood increases the pressure within this space and also stimulates an inflammatory response. The sudden increase in pressure causes an intense headache, which can be described as feeling like a hit to the back of the head. For this reason this type of headache is termed thunderclap headache. The patient is in intense pain and needs to lie still. Vomiting is common. If the bleed is very large, the patient can rapidly become unconscious. In this case the patient will die if this serious bleed is not treated urgently.

The inflammation of the membranes is technically called meningitis, even though there is no infectious cause. This will disturb the function of the brain cells so that, following less severe bleeds, the patient may become drowsy or comatose over the period of a few days after the bleed.

All patients with a sudden onset of a very severe headache that appears out of the blue and that does not abate within a couple of hours should be assessed medically as a matter of urgency. The possibility of a bleed will be assessed by means of a computed tomography (CT) scan, which can confirm the presence of bleeding. If the scan is inconclusive, a lumbar puncture may be performed to look for evidence of blood in the CSF. If bleeding is confirmed, then magnetic resonance imaging (MRI) guided angiography may be used to locate the source of the bleeding. In up to 50 percent of cases of thunderclap headache these tests show no abnormalities, the patient recovers and the diagnosis remains uncertain.

The development of a subarachnoid hemorrhage is a very severe condition. Over half of all patients die before reaching hospital. Up to one-fifth of the remainder will die in hospital because the bleeding cannot be prevented or because the damage to the brain is already very severe. The immediate treatment is bed rest and management of any hypertension. Intravenous steroids and the calcium channel blocker (CCB) nimodipine may be prescribed to reduce brain swelling and prevent spasm of the cerebral blood vessels. Surgical treatments attempt to stop the bleeding from the artery by means of application of a metal clip. Increasingly, angiographic treatments are employed, including the insertion of platinum coils into the damaged blood vessels.

Of the 50 percent of patients who survive a subarachnoid hemorrhage, some will be left with a permanent disability resulting from brain damage, and some will develop hydrocephalus because of the scarring that has resulted from the inflammation. However, others will make a full physical recovery from this life-threatening condition. It is very important that after recovery strict attention to the control of risk factors such as high cholesterol and smoking needs to be maintained.

Information box 4.1d-I

Intracranial hemorrhage: comments from a Chinese medicine perspective

The rapid bleeding and loss of consciousness associated with extradural and subarachnoid hemorrhage suggest that the Chinese medicine diagnosis could be Wind and Extreme Heat causing Obstruction of the Orifices of the Heart. The intense pain that can accompany these conditions reflects Stagnation of Qi and Blood.

In subdural and intracerebral hemorrhage, pain can be a less prominent feature, and the bleeding is more contained. In subdural hemorrhage, the blood congeals to form a mass of clot. In intracranial hemorrhage the underlying cause is usually atheroma in the cerebral arteries. This suggests that Phlegm might be an additional Pathogenic Factor in both these conditions.

Intracerebral hemorrhage

In intracerebral hemorrhage the bleeding occurs deep in the substance of the brain from one of the intracerebral arteries. This is usually a result of weakening of the arteries by atheroma, and may be precipitated by a rise in blood pressure, which puts a strain on the already weakened arteries.

The blood spreads into the surrounding brain tissue and causes damage to the brain cells. It also has effects on more distant parts of the brain due to increased pressure. The result is that a specific aspect of the function of the brain is immediately lost, and very often this is accompanied by a severe headache. Intracerebral hemorrhage is one of the important and life-threatening causes of the condition called stroke, discussed below.

Stroke

Stroke is the term used to describe a condition in which there is a sudden loss of function of part of the brain. The other commonly used medical term to describe a stroke is cerebrovascular accident (CVA).

There are a number of causes of stroke, but cardiac emboli, hypertension and atheroma are the most important underlying conditions. The symptoms of the stroke depend on exactly which part of the brain has been damaged.

Stroke most frequently results from infarction of part of the brain (cerebral infarction). Common causes of a cerebral infarction are the formation of a blood clot that blocks an artery within the brain, and blockage by an embolus (usually a blood clot originating either in the chambers of the heart or from a distorted carotid artery) that has lodged within the artery in the brain. About one-third of strokes result from an intracranial hemorrhage. Although these are usually a result of atheroma in the blood vessels and hypertension, hemorrhage can also occur as a result of trauma.

Rarely, infarction occurs because of inflammation of the arteries of the brain (arteritis). Syphilis used to be one of the most common causes of arteritis of the arteries of the brain, but nowadays most cases are the result of autoimmune disease (most commonly systemic lupus erythematosus (SLE) and temporal arteritis).

A rapidly growing tumor can also mimic a stroke, as it can lead to a sudden loss in brain function. Tumors are another cause of intracerebral hemorrhage, and so can also cause stroke in this way.

The conditions that lead to increased clotting (such as pregnancy) and problems with heart valves and heart rhythm (especially atrial fibrillation (AF)) are important causes of thrombosis and embolism.

Transient ischemic attack (TIA)

A transient ischemic attack (TIA) is the consequence of a small embolus lodging only temporarily within a branch of an artery in the brain. As the embolus usually consists of a tiny blood clot, this can simply break up with time. The temporary blockage of the circulation to the part of the brain causes a loss of function of that part, but only for a period of seconds to a few hours. Because the blockage is temporary, the brain cells can recover, and the person regains completely normal function after the event. If the blockage stays in place for longer than a few hours, the risk of permanent damage to the brain cells increases and full recovery from the event becomes less likely.

Blood clot emboli can arise for a number of reasons. The most common cause is from atheroma in the blood vessels of the neck that lead up to the brain. The carotid arteries (in the region of acupoint Ren Ying, ST-9) are a common site for atheroma. Twisting and compression of the atheromatous vessels of the neck during neck movements may promote the development of emboli relatively easily.

The heart can also be a source of emboli (see Sections 3.2f and 3.2g). The conditions of AF, damaged or replaced heart valves and endocarditis can all lead to the formation of emboli that can travel through the circulation to the brain.

Occasionally, emboli will develop in circumstances in which the blood is more prone to clot. For example, rarely TIAs can occur in women who are pregnant, or those on the combined oral contraceptive pill. They are also more likely in smokers or those with a serious underlying disease such as cancer.

The symptoms of a TIA are indistinguishable from those of a small stroke, the only difference being that they are temporary. Symptoms such as blindness, inability to speak clearly, memory loss and one-sided limb weakness may develop only to recover again within minutes to hours.

A TIA is a serious occurrence because it is a warning of an impending stroke. Statistics show that within five years nearly half of all people who have suffered a TIA will have had a stroke, and a quarter will have died either from heart disease or stroke.

The patient with a TIA is investigated by means of an echocardiogram for underlying causes such as atrial fibrillation and damaged heart valves. A Doppler/ultrasound scan of the vessels of the neck can reveal the presence of atheroma and assess its extent. Angiography can be used to complement this investigation of the arteries of the neck. A CT scan or MRI may be performed to check that there has been no permanent brain damage.

The symptoms of transient ischemic attack (TIA) and stroke

The symptoms of stroke depend on which area of the brain has been damaged and how much damage has been caused. In a TIA or a small stroke, the symptoms generally reflect the fact that the damage is limited to a fairly small part of the brain. On the other hand, a stroke that results from a large hemorrhage or infarction of a major artery may lead to profound disability, coma or instantaneous death.

Nevertheless, there are some relatively small parts of the brain that have important functions, and if these are damaged by a stroke, the patient may be left severely disabled. Problems such as loss of speech, blindness, one-sided weakness of a limb, loss of memory and loss of balance may all result from damage to a relatively small area of the brain. In a TIA these problems are temporary, but in an established stroke these symptoms will persist to a greater or lesser extent.

In contrast, sometimes an established stroke may result in very few persisting symptoms. For example, sometimes a CT or MRI scan performed for another reason may reveal the signs of a past stroke, even though the patient has no history of any symptoms.

A large stroke can cause the loss of a number of functions of the brain. One common form of large stroke is one that affects a deep portion of one part of the cerebrum. This is called a cerebral stroke. A cerebral stroke may result in loss of sensation and movement on the whole of one side of the body. If there is total paralysis of one side of the body this is called hemiplegia, while if there is some muscle strength remaining, the term hemiparesis is used. In hemiplegia and hemiparesis the weakness of the muscles results from damage to the upper motor neurons, which run down the spinal cord. The lower motor neurons, which lead from the spinal cord to the muscles themselves, are left intact. This means that the spinal reflexes that work to provide tone to these muscles are not impaired. Therefore, in hemiplegia and hemiparesis the limbs are not floppy, and instead there is increased muscle tone. The leg tends to assume an extended posture, and the arm becomes flexed at the shoulder and the elbow. The tendon reflexes, if tested using a tendon hammer, are increased. The sensitivity of this reflex is so great that the whole limb can go into an involuntary twitching movement called spasm at unpredictable times. This can be both painful and embarrassing for the patient.

In addition, comprehension and speech may be lost. Loss of speech is termed aphasia, whereas partial impairment of speech is called dysphasia. When the ability to articulate speech has been lost, difficulty in swallowing may also be present. This is a severe symptom as it can cause choking on food and drink.

A stroke to the posterior part of the cerebrum will damage the visual higher centers, so that difficulty in comprehending visual images or total blindness may result.

Strokes that affect the anterior part of the cerebrum may have less clearly defined physical effects, but can bring about a change in personality. Apathy, inappropriate social behavior and impairment of intellectual function are features of anterior cerebral strokes.

A stroke that damages the cerebellum will lead to clumsy movements, awkward speech and inability to maintain a steady balance.

A stroke that damages the brainstem may give rise to extremely severe symptoms because it can damage the vital centers in the brainstem. A brainstem stroke often leads rapidly to coma and death. A smaller brainstem stroke may leave the vital centers intact, but may damage the reticular activating system (RAS) or other centers that deal with bodily reflexes and balance. Therefore, various symptoms such as drowsiness, vomiting, hiccupping and dizziness can result from a less severe brainstem stroke.

One rare form of brainstem stroke causes serious damage to the fibers that link the brain through the spinal cord to the outside world. This stroke will leave the patient conscious, and with intact sight and hearing, but bodily sensation and the ability to move the body is lost. The patient is left totally paralyzed but aware. The only possible form of communication is through blinking of the eyes. The medical term for this condition is locked-in syndrome.

In some people, particularly those with hypertension, a number of small strokes may occur in succession. These lead to a cumulative loss of function of the brain, which may superficially appear to result in a gradual decline in the intellectual and physical ability of the patient. In fact the decline occurs in a number of small steps. Over the course of time, memory and intellect deteriorate, and the patient becomes clumsy. The pattern is very like Alzheimer's disease, but can be distinguished by means of a CT scan or MRI. This condition is called multi-infarct dementia, and is the second most common cause of dementia after Alzheimer's disease. It is also recognized that a stroke may trigger an Alzheimer's-like dementia process.

The treatment of transient ischemic attack (TIA) and stroke

The treatment of TIA is to deal with the underlying cause and thus prevent the occurrence of a stroke in the future. In all cases patients should be prescribed an antiplatelet medicine (see Section 2.2d) to reduce the risk of the formation of emboli. Aspirin is the first choice, but clopidogrel and dipyridamole are two platelet-inhibiting medications that might be used as alternatives. If AF or emboli originating from the heart are confirmed, evidence suggests that warfarin or a novel anticoagulant medication (NOAC) is the most effective anticoagulant to prevent stroke, but otherwise, low-dose aspirin is the drug of choice because of its low risk of side effects. These relatively simple therapies have been shown to be life-saving. AF and endocarditis are treated medically. Statins are usually also recommended. Smokers are urged to give up, and the oral contraceptive pill and hormone replacement therapy should be stopped.

Some patients will respond very well to a surgical operation to remove the atheroma from the vessels of the neck. This operation carries a significant risk (3 percent) of death, and so is only undertaken in those cases in which the potential benefit appears to be high on the basis of general health and angiographic assessment.

There is sadly very little that can be done to reverse the damage to the brain cells that has occurred as a result of a stroke. For this reason, many patients with TIAs or a mild stroke might not even be sent into hospital, although all should be referred to a specialist within the week for confirmation of diagnosis to rule out underlying preventable causes.

Patients who have suffered from a stroke will undergo an MRI or CT scan to determine whether or not the cause is infarction (by thrombosis, embolism, arteritis or compression) or hemorrhage. Tests are performed for underlying conditions, such as atheroma of the neck vessels, hyperlipidemia, hypertension, AF or autoimmune disease, which then can be treated. In the case of infarction, the patient will be prescribed a regular dose of aspirin, dipyridamole, clopidogrel or warfarin to prevent further clotting of the blood. This would not, of course, be appropriate treatment in the case of intracerebral hemorrhage. If the patient can be seen in a specialist unit within three hours of onset of the stroke, clot-busting treatment may be considered for cerebral infarction. The drug tPA (tissue plasminogen activator) may be prescribed under close medical supervision.

Recovery from a stroke is known to be maximized if the patient is referred to a specialist stroke unit. Unfortunately, in the UK there are not enough stroke units to admit every patient who has suffered a stroke. In general, young patients who have suffered a severe stroke are the most likely to receive the specialized care offered by a stroke unit.

The aim of the treatment of stroke is rehabilitation, a process that enables the patient to regain as many of the activities of daily living (such as washing, dressing, self-feeding) as possible. Rehabilitation is not the same as recovery. It involves accepting that a disability is present, and then finding new ways to deal with life's challenges while living with that disability.

One of the principles of rehabilitation is to enable the patient to relearn certain activities so that different parts of the brain can be encouraged to take up the role of those parts that have been permanently lost. In this process, new connections will form between the remaining brain cells, and remarkable recovery can be achieved for up to a year after a stroke, and even after this time the patient may continue to make physical improvements.

Skilled physiotherapy is a fundamental aspect of stroke rehabilitation. The patient is encouraged to start using their muscles as soon as possible after the stroke and to relearn basic activities such as how to balance and walk. The physiotherapist will teach the patient with a hemiparesis how to prevent the limb muscles from becoming tight and contracted.

Speech therapy may be required in cases of aphasia and dysphasia. Speech therapists are also skilled in dealing with difficulties in swallowing.

Occupational therapists work with the patient to help them relearn the more complex activities that are important for a dignified and independent life, such as dressing and washing, making a cup of tea and using the telephone. An occupational therapist might recommend that specialized physical aids such as stairlifts, raised toilet seats and modified kitchen appliances are installed in the patient's home.

A hospital social worker may counsel the patient about the possibility of returning to work and eligibility for various state benefits.

Stroke care is one of the many examples in the care of complicated physical illness in which a multidisciplinary approach is ideal. Hospital doctors, general practitioners (GPs), the therapists described above, and social workers may communicate with each other to coordinate the aspects of care for an individual patient.

The long-term outcome in stroke

The majority of patients who die directly as a result of a stroke will do so within the month following the stroke. Hemorrhagic and large brainstem strokes tend to have the worst outcome. Patients with a large cerebral infarction, particularly one that affects swallowing, also do not generally do very well. This is because the problem of choking on food and drink, combined with impaired free body movement, carries a high risk of the patient developing bronchopneumonia.

Many people who have had a stroke will go on to have a second or third stroke. In the majority of cases, because atheroma is an underlying problem, there is also a high risk of death from a heart attack.

Overall, of those who survive a stroke, about one-third will regain independent activities, and about one-third will require long-term institutionalized care.

Information box 4.1d-II

Stroke: comments from a Chinese medicine perspective

In Chinese medicine, the syndrome that corresponds to most forms of acute stroke is described as Wind Stroke. This term reflects the rapid onset of changing symptoms that occurs in a stroke.

Wind Stroke is seen to occur due to a combination of factors. Wind causes the sudden onset of profound symptoms, and is understood to arise from underlying Liver Yin Deficiency. Symptoms of mental confusion, numbness and slurred speech are described in terms of Phlegm or Phlegm Fire, and stiffness and pain in the limbs in terms of Blood Stagnation. Deficiency of Qi and Blood in the Channels predispose to the invasion of Wind and Phlegm and the development of Blood Stasis in the limbs and face.

In many cases, Depletion of the Kidneys is an important underlying factor. Kidney Yin Deficiency can lead to Liver Yin Deficiency, and then to Liver Yang Rising and Liver Wind. Deficiency of Jing will deplete the Marrow, and this will fail to nourish the Blood. Blood Deficiency and Stasis is the result.

These Chinese medicine interpretations correspond to the modern medical understanding of stroke. In cerebral infarction stroke occurs because of insufficient blood supply to a part of the brain. The Chinese medicine interpretation of this would be Blood Deficiency and Blood Stasis. Very often, atheroma is an underlying problem. Atheroma may be understood in terms of a combination of Phlegm and Stagnation, as it is a substantial obstruction that impedes smooth flow of blood.

The bleeding from an intracerebral hemorrhage is very often associated with atheroma and hypertension. As profuse bleeding represents Heat, the Chinese medicine interpretation of this could be a combination of Wind and Phlegm Fire.

Symptoms such as mental confusion, loss of memory, intellect and personality change are all features of Obstruction of the Orifices of the Heart.

After a stroke the substance of the brain itself is permanently damaged. This might be interpreted as Jing (Essence) Deficiency.

Brain tumors

Tumors within the tissue of the brain are common. Approximately 10 percent of all forms of primary cancer arise from the brain. Secondary brain tumors arising from cancers elsewhere in the body, in particular, from the lung, the breast, the stomach, melanoma and the prostate, are also common, constituting 30 percent of all brain tumors.

Primary brain tumors almost always arise from the neuroglial cells, which form the connective tissue of the nervous system. These tumors tend not to metastasize outside the nervous system, and instead cause damage by spreading within the tissue of the brain.

The symptoms of a brain tumor develop for two main reasons. The first is that the growth causes local damage to the surrounding tissue of the brain. According to the position of the tumor, the symptoms will be similar to those of a stroke affecting the corresponding part of the brain. The main difference is that with a tumor the symptoms are usually progressive rather than sudden in onset.

For example, a brain tumor in one cerebral hemisphere may lead to a gradually worsening numbness and weakness of the opposite side of the body, a hemiparesis. Eventually, total paralysis, a hemiplegia, may develop. All this might occur over the course of days to weeks. In contrast, a stroke in the same part of the brain will lead to a sudden development of a hemiplegia. Sometimes the damage caused by a tumor is a trigger for an epileptic seizure. For this reason any person who has suffered with an epileptic seizure for the first time in their life should be investigated by means of a CT scan or MRI to exclude a brain tumor.

The second problem that can result from a tumor is a gradual rise in intracranial pressure, as discussed in the previous section.

The different types of brain tumors

Approximately 70 percent of primary brain tumors are malignant, the most common being astrocytomas and oligodendrogliomas. These strange names refer to the glial cell of origin of the tumor. Despite being malignant, some of these tumors are slow growing and develop gradually over the course of many years. Others are highly malignant and will cause death within months.

The remaining one-third of brain tumors are relatively benign. These can often be removed surgically, but may have caused irreparable damage to a part of the brain before they are diagnosed. The meningioma arises from the arachnoid membrane and can grow slowly to a large size. This growth will gradually damage a part of the cortex of the cerebral hemispheres by direct pressure. Also, if not diagnosed early, the tumor can lead to a rise in intracranial pressure.

The neurofibroma is a tumor that can arise anywhere in the body from a peripheral nerve. It can develop within the skull from the root of a cranial nerve. The most common significant form of this tumor arises from the auditory nerve (VIII), which arises close to the cerebellum and passes through a hole in the side of the skull to the ear. This tumor is also known as an acoustic neuroma. The symptoms include one-sided deafness and dizziness (vertigo). Eventually, pressure on the cerebellum can cause unsteadiness and clumsy gait (ataxia).

Pituitary tumors

Strictly speaking, pituitary tumors do not arise from nervous tissue, as they originate from the endocrine cells of the pituitary gland. They develop at the site of the pituitary gland, which lies at the base of the brain within the skull, at the level of the eyes.

A growing pituitary tumor can exert pressure on the optic nerves that lead from the eyes to the back of the brain, and so it can cause visual disturbances. It can also lead to symptoms of a gradual rise in intracranial pressure.

Other important symptoms of these tumors result from damage to the pituitary gland or from the production of excessive quantities of a single hormone, or both these problems. These aspects of pituitary tumors are discussed in more detail in Section 5.1e.

The treatment of brain tumors

Many patients with brain tumors and features of pressure effects will initially be given a high dose of a corticosteroid medication called dexamethasone. This has the effect of reducing swelling of the brain tissue and can cause a dramatic reduction in symptoms, irrespective of whether the tumor is malignant or benign.

If possible, the tumor is removed either completely or in part by surgery. This will be curative in operable benign tumors but, as mentioned previously, the patient may be left with a permanent disability due to localized brain damage.

Many patients will require long-term anti-epileptic medication to prevent the seizures that can result from the damage caused by the tumor.

In the case of malignant tumors, chemotherapy and radiotherapy to the brain may also be prescribed. These therapies can slow the progression of the tumor, but are rarely curative. In most patients with malignant tumors the growth will gradually spread again. Only half of patients with a malignant primary brain tumor will still be alive five years after the date of diagnosis.

 Information box 4.1d-III

Brain tumors: comments from a Chinese medicine perspective

As with all forms of cancer, in Chinese medicine the substantial nature of a brain tumor might be interpreted in terms of Phlegm and Blood Stagnation. The fact that the site of the tumor is in the brain suggests that Kidney or Essence Deficiency is the most significant underlying problem that has preceded the development of the Pathogenic Factors.

The signs and symptom of brain tumors are unique to the patient and the diagnosis would be comparable to stroke.

The red flags of brain hemorrhage, stroke and brain tumor

Any patients with undiagnosed features of brain hemorrhage, stroke or brain tumor will benefit from referral to a conventional doctor for assessment and/or treatment. Red flags are those symptoms and signs that indicate that referral should be considered. The red flags of these conditions are described in Table 4.1d-I. A summary of the red flags in a format designed for quick reference in clinical practice can be found in Appendix III. This gives advice on the degree of urgency of referral for each of the red flag conditions listed.

Table 4.1d-I A22: Red flags of brain hemorrhage, stroke and brain tumor

Red flag	Description	Reasoning
A22.1	Progressive decline in mental and social functioning: increasing difficulty in intellectual function, memory, concentration and use of language	Gradual loss of mental function can result from a range of slowly developing brain disorders, including dementia, recurrent small strokes, extradural hemorrhage and a slow-growing brain tumor In elderly people in particular, depression can manifest in this way, and the symptoms may resolve with antidepressant medication
A22.2	A temporary loss of neurological function (usually <2 hours), such as: • loss of consciousness • loss of vision • unsteadiness • confusion • loss of memory • loss of sensation • limb weakness	A temporary loss of neurological function is most commonly seen as part of the syndrome of migraine, in which case it is usually part of a pattern with which the patient is familiar. In migraine, the blood flow to a portion of the brain is temporarily reduced as a result of spasm of an artery. A simple migraine does not merit referral The most common cause of loss of consciousness is a simple faint. This benign syndrome does not merit referral. It is characterized by a low blood pressure and slow but regular pulse, and is triggered by prolonged standing, stuffy conditions and/or emotional arousal. A person who has fainted should start to recover almost immediately after the collapse If these sorts of symptoms occur for the first time, and are not obviously due to a faint or migraine, it is important to exclude the more serious syndrome of transient ischemic attack (TIA), in which a branch of a cerebral artery has been blocked by the temporary lodging of a small blood clot. A TIA is a warning sign of the more permanent damage that results from stroke, and the patient needs referral as a high priority for diagnosis and treatment If the loss of neurological function has occurred within the past 24 hours and is proving to persist for more than 2 hours (a possible stroke), referral should be urgent (see A22.3)
A22.3	A persisting loss of neurological function such as: • loss of consciousness • loss of vision • unsteadiness • confusion • loss of memory • loss of sensation • muscle weakness	Any development of symptoms that suggest a persisting loss in neurological function merits referral to exclude stroke or a rapidly growing brain tumor Some of these symptoms can also result from disease of the spinal cord (e.g. multiple sclerosis) or of a peripheral nerve (e.g. Bell's palsy). Refer urgently if the loss of neurological function has occurred within the past few hours
A22.4	A loss of neurological function that is progressive over the course of days to weeks: this is more suggestive of a brain tumor than a stroke	See A22.3. Progressive symptoms of loss of neurological function are more suggestive of brain tumor or degenerative disease (e.g. motor neuron disease) than stroke. However, multiple small strokes can present in this way

A22.5	Features of a slow increase in intracranial pressure: progressive headaches and vomiting over the timescale of a few weeks to months. The headaches are worse in the morning and the vomiting may be effortless. Blurring of vision may be an additional symptom	Intracranial pressure will slowly increase if there is a gradual development of a space-occupying lesion, such as a brain tumor, abscess in the brain, extradural hemorrhage or accumulation of poorly draining cerebrospinal fluid (CSF) The pressure will be worse when the patient has been lying down, and so the symptoms are characteristically worse in the morning. These include blurring of vision, effortless vomiting (i.e. not much preceding nausea) and headache
A22.6	Features of a rapid increase in intracranial pressure: a rapid deterioration of consciousness leading to coma. Irregular breathing patterns and pinpoint pupils are a very serious sign	An increase in the pressure within the skull seriously threatens the integrity of the structure of the brain If the pressure increases rapidly (usually as a result of a sudden intracranial hemorrhage or bleeding from a fractured skull) there can follow downwards pressure via the soft tissue of the brain onto the brainstem. The brainstem is the seat of the basic vital functions, such as breathing and maintenance of consciousness. As the brainstem is compressed, the patient can lose consciousness, and will eventually stop breathing. Constriction of the pupils is a result of compression of the nerve that leaves the brain at the level of the brainstem to supply the internal muscles of the eye. This is a grave warning sign of serious brain damage

4.1e Disorders of the central nervous system: headache and infections

This section focuses on those conditions that cause the symptom of headache. Headache is very common, familiar to most people. In most cases, headaches have no underlying measurable physical basis. These headaches are usually ascribed a diagnosis of either tension headache or migraine. However, some are much more sinister, for example, the early morning headaches of raised intracranial pressure and the thunderclap headaches of a subarachnoid hemorrhage introduced in Sections 4.1c and 4.1d.

Because recurrent headache is a problem very commonly presented to complementary therapists, the important distinction between benign symptoms and those that should be referred for further investigation is emphasized in this section.

The section concludes with an overview of the different ways in which infection can affect the brain. Three of the most common forms of brain infection are meningitis, encephalitis and brain abscess. All of these have headache as a primary symptom, so it makes sense to include them here.

The mechanism of headache

Contrary to popular understanding, the pain of a headache does not arise from the brain tissue itself. The brain is supplied by hardly any pain nerve fibers. Headache, in fact, results either from sensations that originate from tissues outside the skull (e.g. the blood vessels and muscles of the neck and scalp) or from the tissues that surround the brain within the skull (e.g. the meninges and the blood vessels that supply the inner aspect of the skull bones).

The exact source of the pain in most benign headaches is poorly understood, although tenderness in the muscles of the scalp and neck frequently accompany benign headaches. It is conventionally recognized that the tenderness can be localized by the patient to very precise areas, and these are recognized as muscle trigger points by body therapists and as the equivalent of Ah Shi points in Chinese medicine. It is also well recognized that treatment of trigger points either by massage, manipulation or needling can relieve headache.

Benign headaches

In benign headaches there is no measurable physical basis for the symptoms. Because of this, the symptoms that result from a benign headache, even if very severe and debilitating, are not a source of serious concern to conventional practitioners.

Conditions involving symptoms that have no measurable physical basis are called functional syndromes. Benign headache, such as migraine, is an example of a functional syndrome. It is important to recognize that, although the physical basis is not measurable, it does not mean that there is no physical basis. Instead, the term functional implies that, whatever the mechanism of the underlying cause, it is too subtle to be assessed by currently available medical investigations, and is unlikely to progress to a serious condition.

Tension headaches

Tension or stress headaches are the most common form of benign headache. The most common symptoms of tension headache include a feeling of tightness around the head, a pressure behind one or both eyes, and throbbing or bursting sensations. Usually these symptoms come on gradually, at any time of the day, and will ease off gradually. Sometimes a tension headache can last for days on end.

Many people recognize that certain situations will trigger their symptoms. Very often emotional stress is an underlying factor. In other people more physical causes such as muscle tension around the neck and shoulders, eye strain, sinusitis and toothache precede the development of the headache. Some people can attribute their headaches to certain foods or drinks, such as chocolate, coffee, oranges or alcohol. Headaches of a similar nature are a common symptom accompanying an infection such as a common cold or influenza. Tension headaches are also common premenstrually, in pregnancy and after childbirth.

In the absence of more worrying features, the most common practice is to reassure the patient, who may be concerned about a more serious underlying cause, and to recommend a painkiller. Aspirin and paracetamol are most frequently recommended, although increasingly many people use more potent preparations, including non-steroidal anti-inflammatory drugs (NSAIDs), such as ibuprofen, or morphine-related drugs, such as codeine. It is not uncommon for some people with recurrent tension headaches to self-medicate with the maximum dose of these drugs for days on end.

Many people find that regular massage of areas of chronic tension (trigger points) in the muscles of the neck and the upper shoulders, or corrective chiropractic or osteopathic treatment of the neck, skull and jaw, can prevent tension headaches from developing.

The reassuring feature of a tension headache is that the symptoms are not progressive over the course of a period of weeks to months. In most cases the headaches have a familiar pattern of symptoms, and although they may get worse and more frequent during times of stress, they will settle down again when the pressure is off.

Information box 4.1e-I

Tension headache: comments from a Chinese medicine perspective

The functional syndrome of tension headache can be attributed to a range of Chinese medical syndromes according to the precise nature and location of the symptoms. External Full conditions that can cause headache include Invasion of Wind Cold, Wind Heat and Wind Damp. Internal Full conditions include Liver Qi Stagnation, Liver Yang Rising, Liver Fire Blazing, Stomach Fire and Blood Stagnation. Internal Empty conditions include Blood, Qi and Kidney Deficiency. In all these conditions the underlying pattern leads to a Stagnation of Qi and Blood in the scalp or the neck, and this is the manifestation that leads to the pain.

All painkillers act by moving Qi and Blood. With the possible exception of aspirin in a case of Wind Cold Invasion, none of them addresses the root cause of the imbalance. Aspirin may release the exterior in an Invasion of Wind Cold and so may be an appropriate energetic remedy. All the other preparations seem to be suppressive in nature.

In some types of headache, in addition to the effects of suppressed symptoms, the drug-induced disease caused by the medication may also worsen the root imbalance. For example, aspirin can cause Stomach Heat, and so may worsen the underlying problem in a Stomach Heat headache, even though it can temporarily improve the symptoms. Paracetamol and morphine-related drugs are toxic to the liver, and so may worsen the underlying imbalance in headaches caused by Liver Qi Stagnation and Liver Yang Rising.

Migraine

In contrast to the possible muscular origin of tension headache, the pain of migraine is believed to originate from the blood vessels that supply the brain within the skull. The vessels are thought to constrict and then expand during a migraine attack, and this leads to the symptom of a throbbing headache. The one-sided nature of the syndrome is attributed to the fact that this problem only affects the vessels on one side of the brain.

Migraine is distinguished from tension headache on the basis of some characteristic features. In contrast to tension headache, many people report that a migraine attack might come on at a time when stress has been relieved, such as the weekend after a busy working week. Very often a dietary trigger can be found. Chocolate, coffee, cheese, monosodium glutamate and red wine are among the most common dietary triggers for migraine. The experience of migraine often changes at puberty, during pregnancy or during the menopause. Some people get better and some people get worse after these times of major hormonal change.[8]

The classic syndrome of migraine involves a period of a few minutes to hours of some warning symptoms called an aura, although most patients with migraine (90 percent) do not experience an aura. It is believed that the aura results from constriction of the blood vessels that supply a defined part of the brain. For this reason, the symptoms of an aura can be very like a stroke or TIA.

The most common form of aura that migraine patients experience involves visual disturbances, often including flashing lights or some loss of vision. Some experience a characteristic mood change, dizziness or a strange smell, and others experience a temporary weakness of one half of the body (hemiparesis) or inability to speak (aphasia). About half the patients with migraine and aura in one recent study were shown to have the congenital heart defect patent foramen ovale, and one theory for the mechanism of this link between heart and head is that turbulent blood flow in the heart leads to activated and more sticky platelets arriving at the brain where they might have an increased tendency to clump.[9]

The migraine headache itself is characteristically one-sided, often located behind or above one eye. In a severe case the patient may feel nauseous and may have diarrhea or vomiting. Many people need to lie down in a darkened room. The headache usually lasts for a few hours. When it wears off some people report that they experience a period of a day or so of exhaustion, and some describe a lightened mood, sometimes described as euphoria.

Some migraines are not so severe, and so in many cases it is difficult to distinguish them from tension headaches.

The treatment of migraine involves treatment to relieve the acute attack and treatment aimed at prevention of future attacks. Migraine will settle down without any treatment, but many people find that the pain and nausea is so debilitating that they seek medication. If migraine is relatively infrequent, painkillers are generally prescribed, although commonly much stronger preparations are required to have any effect on the pain of a bad migraine. Tablets that contain a combination of paracetamol and a morphine-related drug such as codeine (co-codamol) are commonly prescribed. Recently high-dose aspirin (900mg) has been found to be particularly effective for the treatment of migraine. Anti-nausea medication such as prochlorperazine or metoclopramide may also be prescribed for an acute migraine attack. Painkillers and anti-emetics may be prescribed in formulations designed for rectal administration if vomiting is a significant problem.

The triptan drugs such as rizatriptan or sumatriptan are prescribed to treat very severe symptoms. These are available in a tablet and injection form, and it is advised that they are taken as early as possible to abort a migraine attack. These drugs give marked relief in over one-third of patients, and so are commonly prescribed. The triptans reverse the dilatation of the blood vessels in the brain, but can have side effects resulting from constriction of other blood vessels in the body. For example, angina is a known side effect. For this reason, triptans should not be given to people with heart disease or uncontrolled hypertension.

To prevent further attacks it is helpful if the patient can determine whether there are any avoidable triggers for the migraine. Keeping a headache diary can be useful in clarifying a link with dietary or other lifestyle factors. The offending trigger can then be avoided if possible.

All women with focal (classic) migraine should use alternative forms of contraception to the oral contraceptive pill, as the risk of stroke is increased in women with migraine who take hormone-containing preparations.

In cases of severe intractable migraine, botulinum toxin (Botox) injections into areas of tension in the neck or scalp may be considered. This treatment may need repeating every few months to maintain its effectiveness.

There is a range of drugs that can be taken regularly to avoid migraine (i.e. for prophylaxis). These tend to be considered if attacks occur more than twice a month. Beta blockers (e.g. propranolol) are currently the medication of choice to reduce the frequency of migraine. Antidepressants such as amitriptyline can also help reduce frequency of attacks.

 Information box 4.1e-II

Migraine: comments from a Chinese medicine perspective

In Chinese medicine, the intensity and one-sided frontal position of the typical migraine suggests that the pain is a manifestation of a Mixed or Full condition. Liver Yang Rising, Liver Fire Blazing and Stomach Heat might all give rise to the symptoms of migraine. A dislike of bright light suggests an imbalance of the Liver. Nausea, vomiting and diarrhea can be attributed to Stagnant Liver Qi invading the Stomach and Spleen.

The fact that migraine is recurrent suggests that there is a long-standing tendency to imbalance of the Liver Organ. Pent-up emotions are likely to be a common underlying cause of Stagnation of Liver Qi. The underlying pathology of dilatation of blood vessels suggests that Heat is present, either as a result or as a cause of the Stagnation.

The simple painkillers tend to move Blood and Qi. The triptans cause constriction of blood vessels, and so could be described in terms of Clearing Heat, but at the expense of causing more Stagnation (constriction of blood vessels) of Blood and Qi. These preparations are all suppressive in nature.

The drugs used to prevent migraine all have in common the tendency to promote Damp or Phlegm or Yang Deficiency, a fact evidenced by the side effects of treatment such as weight gain, coldness, drowsiness and sluggishness. These treatments are all suppressive in nature.

Pizotifen is now a less commonly prescribed preparation. This has the side effect of drowsiness and weight gain, but will often reduce the frequency of attacks. If all these approaches fail, sometimes the anti-epileptic medications valproate, gabapentin or topiramate may be effective for prophylaxis.

The Cochrane Collaboration has confirmed that acupuncture seems to be at least as beneficial as prophylactic medication for the treatment of recurrent migraine.[10]

Cluster headache

Cluster headache is a debilitating form of headache characterized by recurring bouts of intense pain centered over one eye. The bout of pain lasts for up to several hours and can be so severe as to cause vomiting. The affected eye may become bloodshot and the eyelid may droop. The attacks often occur at night, and can recur over a period of about four to eight weeks. Sometimes there can be a long remission of months to years before the next series of attacks.

The frequency of attacks peaks between the ages of 20 and 55, after which they generally become less severe and less frequent. They are more common in men.

The headaches do not appear to be related to migraine. Inhalation of 100 percent oxygen may be prescribed during an acute attack, and drugs as diverse as calcium channel blockers (CCBs), lithium and steroids have been prescribed in attempts at prophylaxis.

Information box 4.1e-III

Cluster headache: comments from a Chinese medicine perspective

In Chinese medicine, the intense pain of a cluster headache represents severe Blood Stagnation in the region of the Gallbladder Channel. In light of the intensity of the attacks, the underlying syndrome would appear to be either Liver Yang Rising or Liver Fire Blazing.

Less benign causes of headache

Conditions such as intracranial hemorrhage and the causes of raised intracranial pressure have been described in earlier sections as very serious causes of headache. The two remaining important serious causes are temporal arteritis, an inflammatory condition that affects elderly people, and the various infections that can affect the brain and the meninges.

Temporal (giant cell or cranial) arteritis

Temporal arteritis is an inflammatory condition of possible autoimmune origin, which almost always affects people over 50. Men are affected more commonly than women. The underlying problem is an inflammation of the blood vessels (vasculitis) of the brain and scalp. In about a quarter of cases the patient also suffers from the condition of polymyalgia rheumatica.

Inflammation of the blood vessels that supply the temples (temporal arteries) is a common feature of the condition. This leads to a severe one-sided headache (in the region of acupoint Tai Yang, M-HN-9), and exquisite tenderness in this region across which the inflamed artery runs. Commonly, tenderness may radiate back over the scalp to the base of the skull on the same side. The artery can be thickened and distorted in shape. There can also be pain in the face, jaw and mouth, particularly on chewing.

The headache and facial pain of temporal arteritis are red flags of a very serious complication of the condition. This is a result of inflammation of the retinal artery, which can lead to sudden and irreversible blindness in one eye.

Temporal arteritis should be referred as a matter of urgency. A blood test generally shows a very high erythrocyte sedimentation rate (ESR) and C-reactive protein (CRP) (see Section 3.4b), which is highly suggestive of the diagnosis. Treatment is urgent administration of high-dose corticosteroids (60mg/day). In most cases this will lead to the reversal of the symptoms, and markedly reduces the risk of developing permanent visual impairment. Rapid withdrawal of this medication may result in recurrence of the symptoms, and the patient may have to remain on very gradually reducing doses of steroids for a period of months to years, while activity of the condition is assessed by means of serial ESR tests.

The diagnosis of arteritis is usually confirmed by means of a biopsy of the temporal artery, although this test is often only performed after treatment has been established.

Information box 4.1e-IV

Temporal arteritis: comments from a Chinese medicine perspective

In Chinese medicine, the pain of temporal arteritis corresponds to Blood Stagnation in the region of the Gallbladder and Stomach Channels. The late age of onset and underlying inflammation suggest that Yin Deficiency (in particular, of Liver Yin) and Heat are underlying factors. As with other autoimmune diseases, Damp and Phlegm are likely to be present. The evidence for this is in the thickened and distorted blood vessels.

The sudden onset of blindness is very similar to that which might occur in a small stroke, and therefore might represent a stirring up of Phlegm by Wind. This Obstructs the Orifices of the Heart (as the Heart, together with the Liver, is the Organ responsible for clear vision), and may lead to a sudden loss of vision.

Infections of the brain

The brain is affected by infectious agents in three ways: meningitis (inflammation of the meninges), encephalitis (inflammation of the substance of the brain) and brain abscess (a localized collection of pus within the brain). Headache is a symptom that is common to all of these serious types of infection.

Meningitis

Meningitis literally means inflammation of the meninges, and can have a variety of causes. Upper respiratory tract organisms are the most common cause of meningitis.

Most often the condition of meningitis gives rise to severe symptoms that develop over the course of a few hours. This is known as acute meningitis, and is most commonly the result of bacterial or viral infection. A more slowly developing form of meningitis is also recognized. This is termed chronic meningitis.

The bacterial causes of acute meningitis can lead to the most severe infections because they tend to cause more pus formation and therefore more damage to the lining of the brain. One of the most common bacterial causes is meningococcus (*Neisseria meningitidis*). This organism leads to an infection called meningococcal meningitis. Two of the other important bacterial causes of meningitis are pneumococcus (*Streptococcus pneumoniae*) and *Haemophilus influenzae*.

Common viral causes of acute inflammation of the meninges include mumps and measles. In general, viral meningitis is less severe than bacterial infection, and is commonly followed by full recovery. In rare cases, infection with the human immunodeficiency virus (HIV) can cause a form of meningitis.

Chronic meningitis is a condition that results from a slowly developing infection. This can be a result of tuberculous infection, or can occur as a form of opportunistic infection in conditions that lead to impairment of the immune system. In acquired immunodeficiency syndrome (AIDS), for example, fungal and tuberculous infection can lead to vague symptoms that develop over the course of a few weeks.

Acute meningitis is characterized by a cluster of symptoms which, if found together, should always be taken seriously. These are severe headache, neck stiffness, confusion and fever. Nausea and vomiting are also commonly present. The headache is characteristically intense. The patient prefers to lie still in a darkened room, sometimes lying with the neck arched backwards. This extended head position is particularly noticeable in young children.

Neck stiffness refers to the resistance that is felt by an examiner trying to move the patient's head freely at the neck. In meningitis there is muscle spasm in the upper back and neck, and free movement is involuntarily resisted.

Fever is usually, but not always, high. In uncomplicated meningitis the patient remains fully conscious, but confusion is a serious sign. In practice, if any patient has a severe headache, nausea and fever, it is wise to refer them to their general practitioner (GP) or medical emergency department for an urgent medical opinion.

Another very ominous sign, which is unique to meningococcal meningitis, is the development of a bruising rash. This rash, which may be confined to only one part of the body, is a result of inflammation of the blood vessels following infection of the blood (septicemia). The blood vessels leak blood into the tissue, so that the marks of the rash look deep red or purplish in color and (unlike most rashes) they do not fade (blanch) when pressure is applied to them. If a person with the symptoms of meningitis develops this rash, they should be referred to hospital as a matter of urgency. Other features of meningococcal sepsis that may precede the rash include cold hands and feet, pain in the legs and mottled skin in a very unwell patient. All these non-specific signs if present with headache should be taken as possible indicators of serious disease.

Without treatment the infection of acute bacterial meningitis can lead to fatal septic shock or may spread into the brain tissue, and the resulting tissue swelling can cause severe pressure on the brain. This will cause the patient to fall into a coma. Death may follow as the vital centers of the brain become irreversibly damaged.

In contrast, an episode of viral meningitis will generally settle down over the course of a few days, although the patient may experience persistent headaches for a prolonged period following the infection.

The treatment for acute bacterial meningitis is primarily by means of intravenous antibiotics. In an urgent case benzylpenicillin or an equivalent antibiotic will be given before any tests are performed because the condition can deteriorate very rapidly. If in hospital, the patient might also be given intravenous steroids to reduce swelling of the brain tissue, and broad spectrum antibiotics are also administered intravenously.

In a less unwell patient, tests to confirm the diagnosis should first be performed before antibiotic treatment is given. These tests include blood samples to culture for bacteria. Many patients are then given a CT scan, which may show the accumulation of pus within the subarachnoid space. If there is no warning sign of increased intracranial pressure from the CT scan, a lumbar puncture (see Section 4.1b) is performed to obtain a sample of cerebrospinal fluid (CSF). The fluid obtained will show increased leukocytes and many bacteria in a bacterial infection. It is very helpful to confirm the type of bacteria so that appropriate antibiotic treatment can be chosen.

Even with rapid and appropriate treatment, 15 percent of patients with bacterial meningitis will die. A proportion of those who recover will have some persisting damage, most commonly deafness due to damage to the nerve that leads from the base of the brain to the ear. Some patients will suffer the long-term effects of inflammation of peripheral blood vessels with loss of fingers and toes or limbs. Many more will suffer from a prolonged syndrome of weakness and recurrent headaches.

In a case of meningococcal meningitis, the close contacts of the patient will also be offered a short course of antibiotic treatment, as it is known that close contacts are more likely than the average person to be carrying the meningococcus as part of the healthy bacteria that reside in their respiratory tract. However, studies of healthy people show that many people (up to 25 percent in some groups of young people) carry this bacterium harmlessly. It remains a mystery why only a tiny proportion of those who carry the meningococcus will actually develop meningitis.

Vaccines are now available to prevent various strains of bacterial meningitis. The *Haemophilus influenzae B* (HiB), pneumococcal and meningitis B and C vaccines are offered to all babies as part of the UK routine immunization schedule at two, three and four months of age. The quadrivalent meningitis vaccine for the four strains ACWY is offered to teenagers in the UK to protect them for the additional risk of contracting meningitis when entering college. These new vaccinations have significantly reduced the impact of bacterial meningitis over the past two decades.[11]

The symptoms of chronic meningitis are much slower to develop. Vague recurrent headaches, low fevers, exhaustion and nausea are typical symptoms, which can be present for weeks before a diagnosis is made. Treatment of chronic meningitis is by means of appropriate antibiotic therapy.

 Information box 4.1e-V

Acute meningitis: comments from a Chinese medicine perspective

In Chinese medicine, the symptoms of acute meningitis would closely approximate to an extreme Wind Heat Invasion. The headache is due to Stagnation of Blood and Qi in the head as a result of Wind. The high fever is a manifestation of extreme Heat. In bacterial meningitis, the development of pus could be seen as an indication that Phlegm and Heat are manifest. Wind, Heat and Phlegm can combine to obstruct the Orifices of the Heart and this can manifest as impaired consciousness.

In conventional medicine terms, antibiotic treatment acts by clearing the pathogens, and this could be described symptomatically in Chinese medicine as Clearing of Wind Heat and Phlegm.

Antibiotics used in meningitis are powerful and broad spectrum, and are recognized to carry the risk of side effects, including anaphylaxis, rashes and digestive disturbances. The drawn-out period of recovery in some people with meningitis could be attributed to Residual Pathogenic Factor, new disturbances introduced by treatment and also Depletion of Blood and Qi as a result of the illness.

Bacterial meningitis is often caused by a bacterium commonly found in the respiratory tract but only affects a tiny minority of individuals. This suggests that an underlying susceptibility, possibly in the form of Wei Qi or Yin Deficiency, might play a part in the development of meningitis.

Encephalitis

Encephalitis is a condition in which the substance of the brain is inflamed. This is a deeper condition than meningitis. In most cases, encephalitis is caused by viruses, although bacteria and fungi are common causes in people who are immunocompromised (e.g. those with AIDS).

Some brain infections lead not to inflammation but degeneration, and result in a syndrome of dementia similar to Alzheimer's disease. Prion disease, such as Creutzfeldt-Jakob disease (CJD) and new-variant CJD (attributed to bovine spongiform encephalitis (BSE) infection), are two examples. Degeneration of the brain is also a late manifestation of syphilis and HIV infection.

In the UK, the most common viruses to cause encephalitis include mumps, measles and herpes simplex, the virus that causes cold sores. Sometimes the infection, such as viral meningitis, is relatively mild. The patient develops headache and fever, but will recover within a few days.

In more severe infections, headaches and fever are followed by drowsiness, confusion and mood changes. Herpes simplex is the most common cause of severe encephalitis in the UK. If untreated, features of localized brain damage, including epileptic fits (see Section 4.1f) and loss of consciousness, might develop. Permanent brain damage, short-term memory loss or death can be the result of severe infections.

Rabies is a well-known form of encephalitis that is transmitted through the bite of an infected animal. Without urgent treatment the encephalitis caused by rabies is always fatal.

Encephalitis is diagnosed by means of CT scans, and MRI and electroencephalogram (EEG) recordings. Herpes simplex infection can be treated with an intravenous antiviral drug called aciclovir, although the impact of this drug on the infection and on long-term recovery is not as marked as is the effect of antibiotics on bacterial meningitis.

The mumps and measles vaccines will protect against encephalitis caused by these viruses, although encephalitis is a very rare complication of these previously common infections. These vaccines are offered to all children in the UK as part of the measles, mumps, rubella (MMR) vaccine. Rabies vaccine is available to protect travelers to areas in which rabies is endemic.

Information box 4.1e-VI

Encephalitis: comments from a Chinese medicine perspective

In Chinese medicine, the symptoms of encephalitis, like meningitis, suggest an Invasion of Wind Heat. Drowsiness and loss of consciousness are a result of Obstruction of the Orifices of the Heart.

Encephalitis is a rare infection, but is caused by common viruses. This suggests that, as with meningitis, there is a pre-existing susceptibility in the patient. Deficiencies of Wei Qi or of Yin are likely to be present in someone who develops viral encephalitis.

Chronic fatigue syndrome (CFS) (formerly known as myalgic encephalitis, ME)

Chronic fatigue syndrome (CFS) is one of the many terms used for an increasingly described syndrome of chronic tiredness and aching muscles. Although CFS can affect all groups of people, it has been reported to be common in young people, especially women, from high-achieving backgrounds, and students who have a tendency to overwork. A history of trauma such as whiplash may also be present. The prevalence is estimated to be 2–4/1000 people in both the UK and the US.

The symptoms that can be experienced in CFS include fatigue (by definition affecting more than 50 percent of the day and lasting over six months), poor concentration and memory, swollen and tender lymph nodes, mood changes, unrefreshing sleep and muscle and joint aches. The nature of the fatigue is characteristic in that muscles become progressively more fatigued with recurrent use. The condition can be extremely debilitating, but is not life-threatening.

CFS is considered by the medical profession to be a functional syndrome. This means that there are no easily measurable physical changes consistently found in patients who complain of the symptoms characteristic of the syndrome.

Scientific studies have shown that the blood supply to parts of the brain is reduced in patients who have the symptoms of CFS, and also that the autonomic nervous system (ANS) reacts differently (i.e. blood pressure reflexes

are not so reactive), which does indicate that there is some physical basis to the condition. It is not clear if these physical changes are simply secondary to the condition and its longevity rather than central to its causation. There is also evidence that there is abnormal mitochondrial function in some patients, which points to problems in the cellular production of energy in the form of adenosine triphosphate (ATP). This is supported by research evidence that treatment with the drug NADP (nicotinamide adenine dinucleotide phosphate), a precursor of ATP, showed some promising results in symptom reduction in CFS. This treatment is not recognized by the medical establishment because of paucity of convincing evidence to support it.

Because of the lack of simple tests to diagnose the condition, CFS is often diagnosed after a long period of excluding other conditions. Although some cases follow a viral infection, such as influenza or glandular fever, this is not a consistent finding, which means that an infective cause is generally not medically recognized. In some cases, the symptoms develop slowly over the course of a few months. In these cases it is often impossible to pinpoint a particular infection that might have been the trigger for the symptoms.

In the UK, most patients who seek help from an NHS doctor will, at best, be offered psychological therapies, including counseling and antidepressant medication, together with graded exercise programs.

Information box 4.1e-VII

Chronic fatigue syndrome: comments from a Chinese medicine perspective

In Chinese medicine the symptoms of CFS correspond to one or more of Residual Pathogenic Factor, Latent Heat or the Lesser Yang pattern according to the Six Stages theory. Damp and Heat and Qi Stagnation are the predominant Pathogenic Factors/Patterns in these conditions. There is often an underlying Deficiency syndrome, such as Qi Deficiency, or Deficiency of Kidney Yin and Yang.

Brain abscess

A brain abscess results from a localized area of pus-producing infection within the brain. The area of pus expands to produce a mass, which compresses adjacent parts of the brain, and so the symptoms of a gradual rise in intracranial pressure can develop (see Section 4.1c).

The source of infection is usually an area of the body that is close to the brain, commonly the middle ear and the sinuses. However, an abscess can develop through spread of infectious organisms in the blood from a more distant source, such as from pneumonia or endocarditis. Although tuberculosis is a rare cause of a brain abscess in the UK, tuberculous brain abscess is relatively common worldwide.

The symptoms of a brain abscess can be very similar to those of a brain tumor (see Section 4.1d), and similarly there can be a long delay before the correct diagnosis is made. The symptoms may persist in a vague form for weeks before the patient becomes very unwell. Common symptoms include vague headache, low fevers and the progressive signs of brain damage, such as hemiparesis or epileptic fits.

The brain abscess is diagnosed and clearly localized by means of a CT scan or MRI. Some abscesses will respond to antibiotic treatment alone, but in many cases a surgical operation is required to drain the pus. However, despite treatment, up to one-quarter of people with a brain abscess will die from the damage caused by the infection.

The red flags of headache

Some patients with headache will benefit from referral to a conventional doctor for assessment and/or treatment. Red flags are those symptoms and signs that will indicate that referral should be considered. The red flags of headache are described in Table 4.1e-I. A summary of the red flags in a format designed for quick reference in clinical practice can be found in Appendix III. This gives advice on the degree of urgency of referral for each of the red flag conditions listed.

Table 4.1e-I A23: Red flags of headache

Red flag	Description	Reasoning
A23.1	Features of a slow increase in intracranial pressure: progressive headaches and vomiting over the timescale of a few weeks to months. The headaches are worse in the morning and the vomiting may be effortless. Blurring of vision may be an additional symptom	Intracranial pressure will slowly increase if there is a gradual development of a space-occupying lesion, such as a brain tumor, abscess in the brain, extradural hemorrhage or accumulation of poorly draining cerebrospinal fluid (CSF). The pressure will be worse when the patient has been lying down, and so the symptoms are characteristically worse in the morning. These include blurring of vision (especially after coughing or leaning forward), effortless vomiting (i.e. not much preceding nausea) and headache
A23.2	A sudden, very severe headache that comes on out of the blue: the patient needs to lie down and may vomit. There may be neck stiffness (reluctance to move the head) and dislike of bright light	The sudden, very severe headache (like a hit to the back of the head) is a cardinal symptom of the potentially devastating subarachnoid hemorrhage. This is a bleed from an area of weakness in one of the arterial branches that course around the base of the brain (the circle of Willis). Subarachnoid hemorrhage may result from an inherited malformation, and so may develop out of the blue in a seemingly fit person
A23.3	A severe headache that develops over the course of a few hours to days with fever, together with either vomiting or neck stiffness. The patient may become drowsy, confused or unconscious. Suggests acute meningitis or encephalitis	Meningitis and encephalitis are infections (of the meninges and brain tissue, respectively) that can be caused by a wide range of infectious organisms Although headache and fever are common co-symptoms in benign infections such as tonsillitis, the triad of headache, vomiting and fever is more suggestive of brain infections, and needs to be treated with caution Additional symptoms, such as reluctance to move the head, arching back of the neck, and dislike of bright lights, may also be present, and if so, are sinister signs. There may be a purpuric rash (see A23.4), but the absence of a rash does not rule out the diagnosis
A23.4	A severe headache that develops over the course of a few hours to days, with fever and with a bruising and non-blanching rash. The patient may become drowsy, confused or unconscious. Suggests meningococcal meningitis	See A23.3. In the form of meningitis caused by *Meningococcus* there can be a serious form of pus-producing infection of the meninges. This carries a risk of septicemia (multiplying bacteria in the bloodstream) and septic shock (see A19.3) Also characteristic of meningococcal septicemia is the development of an irregularly distributed purpuric rash (like a scattering of pinpoint and larger bruises). The spots in this sort of rash do not blanche (go pale) when pressed, unlike the spots in inflammatory rashes such as the rash of measles. This is an emergency situation

A23.5	A severe, one-sided headache over the temple occurring for the first time in an older person	One-sided headaches are common and usually benign, but an unusual, severe, persistent one-sided headache in an elderly person should be taken seriously, as this could reflect the inflammatory condition of temporal arteritis. Temporal arteritis is a form of vasculitis
		In this condition inflammation of the arteries supplying the head can become inflamed and thickened, and this carries the risk of obstruction by blood clot
		There is a significant risk of thrombosis of a cerebral (brain) artery or retinal artery in temporal arteritis and this is minimized by treatment with corticosteroid medication. Temporal arteritis is more likely to develop in people who have also been diagnosed with polymyalgia rheumatica (see A28.3)
A23.6	A long history of worsening (progressive) headaches, with generalized symptoms such as fever, loss of appetite and exhaustion	Recurrent headaches are common and are usually benign. They are often categorized by doctors as either migraine or tension headaches
		Consider referral if there is a progression in severity of the headaches, or if there are other symptoms not usually associated with benign headache, such as fever, loss of appetite, weight loss or other neurological symptoms. Benign headaches should respond significantly to treatment, so also consider referral of recurrent headaches if there is no improvement within 1–2 months

4.1f Disorders of the central nervous system: dementia, epilepsy and other disorders

This section completes the overview of disorders that affect the functioning of the brain. The information covered will fill all the important remaining gaps concerning the conditions that affect the central nervous system (CNS), and for this reason this section introduces a range of very diverse conditions.

The conditions to be explored in this section are:

- Dementia:
  - Alzheimer's disease
  - multi-infarct dementia
  - infectious causes of dementia
- Epilepsy
- Disorders of movement:
  - Parkinson's disease
  - Huntingdon's disease
  - benign (essential) tremor
  - tics and spasms
- Multiple sclerosis (MS)
- Motor neuron disease (MND)
- Cerebral palsy.

Dementia

Dementia is a general term applied to the range of conditions that lead to a widespread and permanent impairment of the function of the cortex of the brain, as well as certain subcortical areas. In most cases this impairment is progressive, so that the patient will suffer a gradual loss of the higher functions for which the cortex of the brain is responsible. This means that memory, thinking, comprehension, calculation, orientation, language and judgment are all gradually impaired.

Despite these losses, consciousness remains relatively intact, so that the person with dementia can remain fully alert until very advanced stages of the condition. Psychiatric problems are well recognized in patients with dementia, particularly in the early stages of a progressive dementia. Depression, paranoia, agitation and aggression are particularly common.

As the damage to the cortex progresses, the person with dementia gradually becomes less able to perform basic activities of daily life, such as washing and dressing. Incontinence can develop and movements become clumsier. Life expectancy is shortened, as in this state the person becomes more immobile and prone to infections. Bronchopneumonia is a common terminal event in patients with advanced dementia.

Dementia can be categorized into pre-senile and senile in onset. This arbitrary classification is used to describe dementia that occurs before and after the age of 70, respectively. There is no clinical distinction between these two classes of dementia.

As the condition of dementia progresses, the impact on the caregiver, often an elderly spouse, becomes very great. The incidence of depression in the carers of people with dementia is known to be high. This is now recognized to be an important problem, so that the ideal approach to the care of a person with dementia should also embrace the needs of the carer of that person. In many cases, as with a severe stroke, a multidisciplinary team of health professionals coordinates the care of a person with dementia.

Information box 4.1f-I

Dementia: comments from a Chinese medicine perspective

In Chinese medicine, dementia corresponds in part to Jing Deficiency, reflected by the fact that the substance of the brain is lost in the progression of the condition. Phlegm and other obstructing Pathogenic Factors (Damp and Heat) would also appear to be prominent in the condition. The difficulties in functions such as thinking, concentration and memory, which in health are the manifestation of a balanced Shen, are often associated with Phlegm Obstructing the Orifices of the Heart.

Alzheimer's disease

Alzheimer's disease is the most common form of progressive dementia. It becomes more common in older age groups, but can develop in people as young as 40. The tendency to develop Alzheimer's disease can run in families, and there is very commonly a strong family history of the condition if the disease develops at a very early age. Alzheimer's disease is also particularly common in people who have Down syndrome, in whom features of this dementia can also appear at an early age.

In Alzheimer's disease there is a characteristic degeneration of the cells of the cortex. Plaques of a thick substance called amyloid develop in the tissue of the brain. There is also a reduction in the quantities of a range of neurotransmitters, including acetylcholine, a fact that has been focused on in the development of drug treatments for the disease.

Ideally, a patient with suspected Alzheimer's disease needs to be investigated carefully in order to exclude treatable causes of cognitive impairment such as hypothyroidism, pernicious anemia and subdural hematoma. This would involve tests of mental ability, blood tests and a CT scan or MRI.

There is now good evidence that the cholinesterase inhibitors such as donepezil, rivastigmine and galantamine cause moderate improvement of memory and motivation at all stages of the disease process, and the drug memantine seems to be of benefit in more advanced stages. It is also always worth treating hypertension in people with Alzheimer's disease, as high blood pressure is linked with worsening disease. Statins are also recommended if the cholesterol levels are raised. Gingko biloba, fish oils and vitamin E are recommended by some therapists as improving brain function, but clinical evidence is not yet conclusive for the benefit of any of these treatments.

Even with drug treatment, the condition is always slowly progressive. Most patients will have died within ten years of the first diagnosis.

Multi-infarct dementia

This second most common form of dementia was explained in Section 4.1d as one of the syndromes that can result from recurrent strokes. The underlying physical problem in multi-infarct dementia is usually atheroma or hypertension, or a combination of both. The manifestation is similar to that of Alzheimer's disease.

Infectious causes of dementia

Various infections can cause a gradual degeneration of the brain tissue and thus lead to a dementia.

The prion diseases Creutzfeldt-Jakob disease (CJD) and new variant CJD are both recognized to lead to a form of rapidly developing dementia due to a characteristic degeneration of the brain tissue. This degeneration has been likened to a sponge, in that multiple tiny areas of brain tissue are lost throughout the brain. The degeneration is not wholly confined to the brain cortex, which means that disorders of movement are also prominent in these conditions.

Although CJD can develop out of the blue for no understood reason, it is also known to have been contracted if a patient is exposed to the nervous tissue of an infected person. Until fairly recently, the surgical use of corneal grafts and injections of hormones, such as growth hormone derived from human brain tissue, were two mechanisms whereby CJD was transmitted from one person to another, symptoms appearing often after a delay of about five years. New variant CJD is believed, but not proven, to originate from the ingestion of nervous tissue in the meat from cattle infected with the BSE (bovine spongiform encephalitis) prion.

The venereal disease syphilis can lead to a form of inflammation and degeneration of the nervous system, which can then progress to the symptoms of a dementia. This is increasingly a very rare condition, because syphilis can be completely cured in its early stages by means of early antibiotic treatment. Before such treatment was available, the syphilis organism could lie dormant for many years after an initial infection, and then reappear in a form that could cause damage to the nerves, spinal cord and brain.

This form of syphilis was termed general paralysis of the insane, because the dementia was combined with impairment of movement and sensation.

HIV is also well known to cause a form of dementia in advanced stages of infection. The development of this dementia is rapid, and is very often the cause of death in people with AIDS.

 Information box 4.1f-II

Alzheimer's disease, multi-infarct dementia and prion disease: comments from a Chinese medicine perspective

In Chinese medicine, the development of amyloid plaques could be interpreted as Accumulation of Phlegm. The general degeneration of the cortex could also reflect Jing Deficiency.

The underlying energetic problem of multi-infarct dementia is likely to be a combination of Phlegm and Blood Stagnation, as these are the Pathogenic Factors that correspond to the development of atheroma. The infarcts that result lead eventually to loss of brain tissue, and this corresponds to Jing Deficiency.

In prion disease, the irreversible change of brain proteins into masses of prion proteins might be suggestive of the Accumulation of Phlegm. The rapid development of symptoms and the irregular writhing and twitching movements that can occur in these disorders suggest that Liver Wind is an additional important Pathogenic Factor.

Epilepsy

Epilepsy is a term used to describe a range of conditions in which the common event is that a large number of nerve cells in the brain discharge simultaneously. A single episode of simultaneous discharge of nerve cells leads to what is termed an epileptic fit or seizure. Epilepsy is only diagnosed if there is tendency to experience recurrent seizures. This affects about one person in 200 of the general population.

An epileptic seizure occurs when the discharge of one set of nerve cells in the brain is not limited adequately. This means that a chain reaction takes place, in which all the adjacent nerve cells discharge and then cause the discharge of their neighboring cells. This chain reaction is sometimes so great that a wave of electrical discharge spreads across the surface of the brain. In other cases the area of discharge is limited to one part of the brain.

This loss of limitation of the nerve cell impulses can occur in any person under certain conditions. For example, extreme lack of oxygen, low blood sugar, very high temperatures or certain chemicals can induce fits in many people. However, in some people fits occur much more readily. It is known that this tendency to epilepsy runs in families.

Alcohol abuse is a well-known cause of fits. These particularly occur either during a drinking binge or on withdrawal of alcohol. Usually the fits will cease if the person ceases drinking alcohol.

Fits are more likely to occur if there is an area of brain damage, even if this area is so small that it does not cause any other problems for the patient. For this reason, epilepsy is a well-known complication of birth trauma (causing brain damage to the baby), brain tumors and abscesses, brain surgery, strokes and head injury. However, in most cases, the reason for the development of epilepsy is unknown, in that there is no identifiable area of brain damage.

The characteristics of an epileptic seizure depend on the site of origin of the discharging brain cells and on how far this discharge spreads across the brain. In current medical practice, epilepsy is classified according to the type of seizure. If a seizure represents a widespread discharge of nerves across the brain, it is known as a generalized seizure, whereas if it is confined to a defined area of the brain it is called a partial seizure. In a generalized seizure consciousness is always impaired or lost.

In established epilepsy, some people will experience a prodrome of a couple of days leading up to a fit, in which there is a subtle change of personality, mood or energy levels. Also, many patients often recognize a warning sensation in the few seconds to minutes prior to seizure, similar to the warning sensation experienced by some migraine sufferers. This warning is also called an aura. In epilepsy, the common types of aura include a characteristic mood, a recurrent memory or a strange smell.

Some sufferers of epilepsy recognize that there are particular triggers for attacks. These include tiredness, emotional upset, high fevers or exposure to rapidly flashing lights.

Generalized seizures: grand mal (tonic-clonic) seizures

In a grand mal seizure the discharge of the brain cells affects the motor cortex so that the muscles of the body are stimulated to contract simultaneously. This causes the body to go rigid, and the patient often lets out a cry before falling to the ground. This state of muscular contraction, which lasts for 10–30 seconds, is called the tonic phase. The muscles then go into repeated and rhythmic cycles of contraction and relaxation, so that the patient lies in an unconscious state while the body undergoes coarse shaking movements. At this stage the patient may froth at the mouth, and can go blue in the face as breathing is impaired. This is called the clonic phase, and usually lasts for a few seconds to a few minutes. During this phase the bladder or the bowel may empty involuntarily.

After the grand mal (or tonic-clonic) seizure the patient can remain in an unconscious or drowsy state for up to several hours. In severe cases, the clonic state does not settle down. This is called status epilepticus, and is a medical emergency if it lasts for more than a few minutes. This is because in status epilepticus there is an increasing risk with time that the brain becomes starved of oxygen and permanently damaged.

The onset of grand mal epilepsy most commonly occurs either between three and seven years of age or in the teenage years. In these cases there is usually no obvious underlying cause. If this form of epilepsy occurs after the age of 25, a distinct area of brain damage, such as a brain tumor or brain abscess, is more likely to be the underlying cause.

Generalized seizures: petit mal (absence) seizures

In petit mal epilepsy the seizure is not associated with any disorder of movement. Instead, the patient suffers a brief (few seconds) loss of awareness known as an absence. To an onlooker, the person suddenly becomes vacant, may even stop in mid-speech or activity, and can go pale. When the seizure is over the person may carry on the activity they were performing as if nothing has happened.

Petit mal epilepsy is most common in young children, who may grow out of it as they enter their teens. Rarely, some children with absence attacks may go on to develop grand mal epilepsy. The condition is sometimes confused with dreaminess, and so may not be diagnosed for some time. This can become a real problem in the education of the child. It is now known that a child with petit mal epilepsy misses out on a lot more learning than would be represented by the time of the absence attacks alone, and can experience learning difficulties without appropriate teaching support.

Partial seizures

In partial seizures only a small portion of the brain is affected by the discharge of brain cells. The resulting seizure can be compared in some ways to a transient ischemic attack (TIA), in which there is also a temporary loss of function of a small area of the brain. In some cases there is also impairment of consciousness.

A motor partial seizure involves the motor cortex on one side of the brain, so that the patient will experience a rhythmic jerking of all or part of one half of the body. In many cases, the development of this type of epilepsy signifies a progressive but localized condition of the brain such as a tumor.

A temporal partial seizure involves the cortex of the temporal lobe of one side of the brain. This can have very diverse symptoms, including the experience of a strange mood or smell, a period of loss of memory, a changed personality state and visual hallucinations. For this reason, temporal lobe epilepsy can easily be misdiagnosed as a psychiatric or personality disorder. These temporal lobe seizures are also known as complex partial seizures.

Diagnosis of epilepsy

The first aspect of diagnosis is to confirm that a fit has actually occurred. This is not always as straightforward as might be expected, as a number of other conditions, including fainting, TIAs and psychiatric disorders, can mimic epileptic fits.

The electroencephalogram (EEG) is used to assess the brainwaves (electrical activity) of the brain. An EEG recording taken during a fit is almost always abnormal. Therefore, the ideal is to obtain an EEG reading when a fit actually occurs. This is not always possible if fits are infrequent.

In some people, the EEG is abnormal in between fits. This is highly suggestive of epilepsy, although this is not always the case. For this reason, a patient with possible epilepsy may be exposed to certain triggers, such as rapidly flashing lights, during the EEG recording, to see if any abnormalities of brain activity are induced.

A CT scan or MRI is always performed to look for any structural abnormalities of the brain. This is of particular importance in adult-onset epilepsy, in which an underlying disease such as cancer or stroke might explain the development of the seizures.

The treatment of epilepsy

An isolated fit is never diagnosed as epilepsy, and so medication would not be offered unless the seizures became recurrent. Nevertheless, an isolated seizure does have considerable impact on the life of an adult patient. In the UK, for example, according to the Driver and Vehicle Licensing Agency (DVLA) legislation, anyone who has had an epileptic fit or unexplained loss of consciousness is not allowed to drive for the following 12 months. Heavy goods vehicle (HGV) drivers who have suffered a seizure will lose their HGV license for the next ten years.

Patients who are prone to recurrent seizures are advised to avoid activities that may put their own lives or those of other people at risk should they happen to have a seizure. For example, activities such as climbing, swimming alone and the use of heavy machinery are discouraged. Driving is permitted in people with controlled epilepsy, as long as there have been no seizures in the daytime for at least one year. Fits that occur during sleep are much more common and are not considered to be a reason to avoid driving, as long as they have occurred only in sleep for over three years.

The treatment of status epilepticus includes first aid measures to ensure that the patient can breathe freely.

The patient should be encouraged to lie on their side in the recovery position and restrictive clothing should be loosened. If the seizure has been ongoing for more than 3 minutes, the medical treatment is a tranquillizer such as lorazepam or diazepam, which is inserted by means of a rectal tablet (suppository) or by intravenous injection. In the very unusual case of this having no effect, the patient will need urgent life support treatment. The patient in resistant status epilepticus may require ventilation in an intensive care unit.

Prevention of recurrent seizures involves prescription of one or more drugs. Different types of seizures tend to respond to different groups of drugs. All these drugs are given the general name of anticonvulsants or anti-epileptics (see *British National Formulary* (BNF), Section 4.8). Anticonvulsant medication acts by preventing the spread of electrical discharge in the brain, which seems to encourage the inhibitory aspect of the nervous system (see Section 4.1a).

All the anticonvulsant drugs have significant side effects. The ideal treatment involves only one of these preparations because it is recognized that side effects are more troublesome and the likelihood of toxicity increases if they are used in combination. It sometimes takes a number of years to establish which medication is the most suitable for a particular patient in terms of effectiveness and minimization of side effects. This is a particularly difficult process in adults who drive, because driving is not permitted in a patient with epilepsy for a year after any change in medication, because of the risk of recurrence of fits.

The drugs most commonly used in generalized epilepsy include carbamazepine, lamotrigine, sodium valproate, topiramate and vigabatrin. Phenytoin used to be widely prescribed, but is less used now as newer agents with better side effect profiles and a lower risk of toxicity have been introduced.

All these medications are introduced initially as the sole drug at a low dose, and gradually increased in dose until the frequency of seizures is brought under control. Sometimes perfect control can never be achieved. Some preparations require the patient to have regular blood tests to ensure that the levels of the drug in the blood are within a safe threshold.

All anti-epileptic drugs in excessive doses lead to a condition of drowsiness, confusion, stumbling speech and staggering gait. Even in safe doses, most patients experience a degree of drowsiness or clumsiness when on medication.

In addition, each drug has characteristic side effects that can have a significant impact on the quality of life. These include rashes, weight gain, swollen gums, dizziness, blurred vision and excessive body hair (depending on the particular drug). The three commonly prescribed preparations, carbamazepine, sodium valproate and

phenytoin, are all potentially harmful to the developing fetus, so pregnancy should be avoided.

Information box 4.1f-III

Epilepsy: comments from a Chinese medicine perspective

In Chinese medicine, the sudden loss of consciousness and spasm of muscles of a grand mal seizure may be described as a manifestation of Liver Wind stirring upwards and causing Phlegm to Obstruct the Orifices of the Heart. A petit mal seizure, although less dramatic, has similar characteristics in terms of sudden onset and loss of awareness. These also imply that Wind and Phlegm are important Pathogenic Factors.

In partial motor seizures, the most prominent feature is the sudden onset of twitching muscles. This is indicative of Wind in Chinese medicine. In partial temporal lobe epilepsy, the various rather vague perceptual symptoms would also appear to result from Phlegm impeding the functions of the Shen. Sudden onsets of conditions are themselves often indicative of Wind.

The underlying syndromes in a person with epilepsy are likely to be those that predispose to the development of Liver Wind and Phlegm. These include Deficiency of Liver and Kidney Yin and Spleen and Stomach Deficiency. In the many cases in which the onset is in childhood, this is highly suggestive that Jing Deficiency is an additional factor.

All anticonvulsant medication is suppressive in nature, as evidenced by the fact that seizures often return with greater severity on withdrawal of medication. The side effects of drowsiness and clumsiness, with dizziness, confusion and loss of balance, if drugs are taken in excessive dose, all suggest that these drugs are Phlegm Forming. The drugs appear to act by damping down the Stirring up of the Wind (their physical action is to increase the action of the inhibitory nerves of the brain), but do not seem to address the main root cause of the problem, which is, of course, the Accumulation of Phlegm.

The various additional side effects are due to drug-induced disease. Swollen gums indicate Heat and Phlegm in the Stomach, and rashes indicate Heat in the Blood. Most of the drugs are toxic to some degree to the liver, and side effects that indicate Stagnation of Liver Qi are also common, including depression and increased risk of suicide.

Withdrawal from anticonvulsant medication should be very slow and controlled because of the high risk of recurrence of seizures. For this reason, drug withdrawal should never be undertaken outside of medical supervision. All patients who withdraw from medication are obliged to abstain from driving for the period of the withdrawal and for six months afterwards.

All patients with epilepsy in the UK should be under the supervision of a hospital neurologist. Some may also have access to a specialist epilepsy nurse, who will be experienced in carefully guiding and supporting patients through the complex medical and social issues that arise from having epilepsy.

Disorders of movement

There are a number of disorders of movement that result from disease of the brain. The most important movement disorder by far, in terms of the number of people affected and its severity, is Parkinson's disease. This was formerly known as paralysis agitans, a Latin term that succinctly describes the distressing nature of the disability that develops in this condition.

Parkinson's disease

Parkinson's disease is a progressive disorder affecting one in 200 of the UK population over the age of 65. It is the result of degeneration of the part of the brain called the basal ganglia. These clusters (nuclei) of nerve cells, situated deep within the cerebral hemispheres, play a role in the smooth control of muscle action.

In most cases the cause of the condition is unknown, although in some there is a family history. Occasionally, Parkinson's disease can develop following a head injury – it is a well-known complication of the frequent knockouts experienced by boxers. In Parkinson's disease, degeneration of a specific part of the basal ganglia, and loss of dopamine-producing cells, leads to a characteristic syndrome of stiffness of muscles, difficulty initiating movements and tremor.

Prescription of some of the major tranquillizer drugs used to treat serious mental illness such as schizophrenia and bipolar disorder is an important cause of a syndrome called Parkinsonism, which is very like Parkinson's disease. This syndrome develops because these drugs lower the levels of a neurotransmitter in the brain called dopamine. The levels of dopamine are known to be disturbed in major mental illnesses. However, dopamine is also important for the normal function of the basal ganglia. Within a few days of the onset of treatment a person on high doses of this sort of medication is very likely to develop the symptoms of Parkinson's disease, including tremor, stiffness of movement and paucity of facial expressions. This syndrome is a significant cause of discomfort and also stigmatization. Parkinsonism is largely reversible on withdrawal of treatment.

The first symptom frequently is of gradual onset of stiffness of muscles initially affecting the limbs, but later involving facial and body muscles. Often the onset of this stiffness is asymmetrical, so that one side of the body is more severely affected than the other.

In addition to this stiffness, a difficulty in initiating movement develops. Actions such as standing from sitting or getting out of bed become difficult. The rapid responsiveness of the facial muscles is lost so that a person with Parkinson's disease can look permanently blank and emotionless. This can, of course, affect social interactions.

A coarse tremor (with a rate of 4–6 beats/second) develops in the hands and limbs, and progresses over a period of years to affect the whole body. This tremor is improved during the performance of an action such as picking something up, and is worse at rest. Strong emotion can also cause worsening of the tremor.

Gradually, the posture is affected, so that the person develops a stoop, and has a characteristic shuffling gait. Balance is impaired, and falls are common. These can have serious consequences in elderly people. Sleep may be impaired, and bowel and bladder function problematic. Depression is a common and serious problem. In late stages of the disease speech becomes difficult to comprehend, and difficulty swallowing and dribbling of saliva are common.

Usually the disease progresses slowly over the course of 10–15 years. Death usually occurs from bronchopneumonia, a result of immobility and the inability to clear secretions from the throat.

The UK National Institute for Health and Care Excellence (NICE)[12] recommends that anyone with suspected Parkinson's disease should be referred at the point of diagnosis to a specialist team comprising a neurologist, physiotherapist and specialist nurse, because of the complex mix of medical and social needs affecting anyone with this diagnosis.

Exercises to maintain mobility and balance are recommended from the outset. For example, tai chi is recognized to help strengthen the postural muscles and prevent falls and may be recommended. Medication is deferred until symptoms are very significant, as it does not prevent progression, and the beneficial effects of the drugs wear off with time.

Parkinson's disease is most commonly treated with two main types of drug. The so-called dopaminergic drugs mimic the action of dopamine. Increasingly, newer agents such as ropinirole and cabergoline may be introduced as the first treatment, but the most established dopaminergics are forms of L-dopa, a chemical precursor of dopamine. The common preparations of this drug are called co-careldopa and co-beneldopa.

The effects of each dose of the dopaminergic type drugs are to reverse the symptoms of Parkinson's disease, but this effect wears off with increasing rapidity as time progresses. This means that eventually the patient may have to take a number of doses throughout the day.

L-dopa preparations can have severe long-term effects on the nervous system (after about five years), which is the reason why treatment is delayed for as long as possible. Immediate side effects include nausea, confusion and hallucinations. Long-term effects include uncontrollable muscle movements. Another problem with long-term treatment is that the periods of relief from symptoms can be interspersed with periods of 2–4 hours of a greatly reduced ability to move (on-off syndrome), which are very unpleasant for the patient. One extra drug, entacapone, which slows the breakdown of the dopa-related drugs by the body, may be prescribed together with dopa-related drugs to prevent on-off syndrome.

Another type of drug, selegiline, may be introduced at an earlier stage in the disease. This drug increases the action of the dopamine that is produced in the brain. It may also be used together with L-dopa preparations, because it seems to overcome, at least for a few years, the rapid end-of-dose deterioration of these drugs. The short-term side effects of selegiline are similar to those of the L-dopa drugs, in that they include nausea and psychiatric disturbances.

Experimental studies involving the insertion of cells removed from the brains of aborted human fetuses into the brains of people with Parkinson's disease have received a lot of media attention in recent years. There have been mixed reports about the benefits of such an approach, which still remains within the realm of research rather than clinical practice.

 Information box 4.1f-IV

Parkinson's disease: comments from a Chinese medicine perspective

In Chinese medicine, a root cause of tremor is considered to be insufficient Blood and fluids to nourish the channels and sinews. This can result from long-standing Qi and Blood Deficiency. The channels and sinews are then vulnerable to Wind. Liver Wind is the most likely description in Chinese medicine for the manifestation of tremor in Parkinson's disease.

Liver Wind may develop as a consequence of Liver and Kidney Yin Deficiency, as it does in the development of Wind Stroke. Liver Yang Rising can also lead to the generation of Liver Wind, so that long-term suppressed emotion may also be causative in Parkinson's disease. Phlegm Heat or Phlegm Fire can be important in some cases, because Phlegm Heat obstructs and dries the channels and sinews.

The drug treatments for Parkinson's disease therefore act by Subduing Wind and Clearing Phlegm. They do not attend to the root cause of the problem, and so are suppressive in nature. Nausea and psychiatric disturbances suggest that these drugs may themselves be Phlegm Forming. The development of chronic disorders of movement after prolonged drug treatment suggests the reappearance of Wind in a different manifestation.

Drugs used in major mental illness that are also a cause of the syndrome of Parkinsonism have a number of features that suggest that they are both Heating and Phlegm Forming. Other side effects of these drugs indicate that they lead to the generation of Wind (the complex energetics of these powerful drugs is discussed in more detail in Chapter 6.2).

Huntingdon's disease

Huntingdon's disease is another degenerative disorder of the deep nuclei in the brain known as the basal ganglia (see Section 4.1a). In this condition, different parts of the basal ganglia are affected than in Parkinson's disease, and the result is a progressive disorder of movement called chorea (from the Greek word meaning dance). Chorea consists of jerky and fidgety extra movements of the limbs and the body, which can progress from one body part to another. Other parts of the brain also degenerate in this condition, leading to a form of dementia.

Huntingdon's disease tends to affect people in middle life. It is almost always inherited from one parent, who passes the gene for the disease to the children. There is a 50 percent chance of a child developing the condition if one parent carries that gene (it is an autosomal-dominant condition; see Section 5.4c).

Because the disease usually develops after childbearing years, it is not usually known that there is a risk of the children having the disease until a few years after they are born, when one parent develops the condition. A genetic test is available that can offer the children of a person with Huntingdon's disease the opportunity of knowing whether or not they too carry the gene.

The progression of Huntingdon's disease is such that death occurs within 10–20 years of diagnosis. There is no satisfactory treatment for the condition. Tetrabenazine may help mitigate the chorea in some patients, but this drug can cause depression, which limits its usefulness.

Information box 4.1f-V

Huntingdon's disease: comments from a Chinese medicine perspective

In Chinese medicine, the dementia of Huntingdon's disease most clearly corresponds to Jing Deficiency. The chorea is the result of Liver Wind, which in this case can possibly be attributed to Kidney and Liver Yin Deficiency.

Benign (essential) tremor

Benign (essential) tremor is a condition in which there is a fine tremor of the limbs, often including the head and the body. This tremor is similar in quality to the tremor that may be experienced by most people in an extreme state of anxiety. The difference with benign tremor is that, although it is worsened by a nervous mood, it is present all the time. The tremor is not as coarse as the tremor of Parkinson's disease, and so the two conditions are easily distinguished by an experienced physician. In some cases the tremor has been present since youth, and in these cases it is often an inherited condition (also autosomal dominant). In other cases the tremor develops as a consequence of aging. Although the tremor may be progressive, it rarely hinders daily activities in a significant way.

Occasionally, beta blockers (propranolol) are given to ease the tremor. This is because they block the action of adrenaline, one of the natural contributors to a benign tremor. Interestingly, alcohol in small doses can also reduce the shaking movements of this condition in some patients.

 Information box 4.1f-VI

Benign (essential) tremor: comments from a Chinese medicine perspective

In Chinese medicine, a benign tremor would normally be diagnosed as a manifestation of Liver Wind. Qi and Blood Deficiency or Kidney and Liver Yin Deficiency may be underlying conditions.

From a conventional medical perspective, the release of adrenaline leads to this physical manifestation of fear. In Chinese medicine, the tremor that results from adrenaline could be described in terms of Empty Heat and Wind, which can result from Kidney Yin that is deficient in relation to Kidney Yang. By blocking the action of adrenaline, beta blockers, which also have side effects of slowed heart rate and feelings of cold and depression, might be seen as Subduing Kidney Yang.

Tics and spasms

There are a few diverse conditions in which repetitive unwanted movements (tics) occur. The most common form of tic is benign and appears in early childhood. The child can pass through a phase of performing habitual movements such as blinking or screwing up the face. These often settle down as the child grows up. More pronounced tics can last throughout life or can develop in adult life. Other conditions can involve unpredictable limb movements, in which the muscles can go into painful spasms (also known as dystonias).

 Information box 4.1f-VII

Tics and spasms: comments from a Chinese medicine perspective

Unpredictable and brisk muscular movements are seen in Chinese medicine to correspond to Liver Wind. If spasm of muscles (interpreted as tendons and sinews in Chinese medicine) is also prominent, this suggests an additional imbalance within the Liver, such as Liver Qi Stagnation or Liver Blood Deficiency.

Multiple sclerosis (MS)

Multiple sclerosis (MS) is a common autoimmune degenerative disease of unknown cause that affects the nerve cells of both the brain and the spinal cord, but not the peripheral nerves. The condition can first appear at any time in teenage and adult life. MS is more common in people who have spent their childhood in countries a long way from the equator (such as northern Europe, Canada and the northern USA). This suggests that there is some sort of environmental trigger that affects a growing child in a cold climate, but no definite trigger has yet been isolated. Some studies of large populations suggest that a diet high in animal fats might be contributory in increasing the risk of MS, but this link has not been proven.

The underlying problem in MS is that small patches, called plaques, develop within the central nervous system (CNS) in which the myelin coating of the nerve fibers has degenerated. It is now recognized that an abnormal immune response is responsible for this damage to the myelin, and axon death follows the loss of the myelin. This means that the ability of the nerves to transmit messages through the affected areas is lost. The plaques can develop in a wide range of sites, and thus can cause a wide range of neurological problems, hence the other name for MS, disseminated sclerosis.

The pattern of the condition is that it commonly starts with a period in which there is a sudden and rapid deterioration of the function of an aspect of the nervous system, sometimes triggered by stress, heat or exercise. Frequent first symptoms include the sudden onset of blurred vision, or numbness and weakness of one or both limbs, or slurred speech. This sudden deterioration is termed a relapse.

In the majority of cases, a relapse is followed after a few weeks by a period in which the symptoms may get partially and sometimes completely better. This improvement is called a remission. However, in most people with MS the period of remission is followed by a further relapse, this time leaving the nervous system in a more damaged state than before. Thus, with a cycle of relapses and remissions, most people with MS become progressively more disabled over the course of 10–30 years. In approximately 30 percent of cases, the remissions are less prominent, and the pattern is instead one of a progressive decline. In a very few cases, the decline between relapses is not so rapidly progressive, and permanent severe disability never develops.

The disabilities that can affect a person with advanced MS depend on the site of the CNS in which the plaques are most prominent. Common problems include temporary visual disturbance, double vision, and weakness and numbness of the limbs due to damage to the nerves that travel down the spinal cord to supply the limbs. Upper motor neurons are affected (see the section "Spinal tone" at the end of Part I, Section 4.1a), leading to increased tone of the affected limbs, and the limbs can easily go into painful spasms. This condition can progress so that the patient becomes wheelchair bound.

Damage to the sensory nerves of the bladder and the bowel can result in incontinence. Damage to the cerebellum can cause difficulty in balance and clumsiness. Speech becomes difficult to understand. Damage in the cortex of the brain can affect personality and intellect. This means that a form of dementia may complicate long-term MS. Even in the early stages of the disease, mood can be affected. In particular, a state of euphoria is well known in people with MS. However, violent mood swings, depression and irritability are also common.

MS may be diagnosed by means of an MRI, which reveals the plaques as small patches throughout the CNS. A lumbar puncture may be performed and characteristic antibodies may be found in the cerebrospinal fluid (CSF).

A person who is suffering from an acute relapse is usually offered treatment of high doses of intravenous corticosteroids (methylprednisolone). Although this treatment seems to reduce the initial extent of the disability experienced during the relapse, there is no evidence that it affects the long-term outcome of the condition. The side effects of these treatments, in particular, weight gain and muscle weakness, can in some cases hinder the person's ability to recover from the damage caused by the relapse.

There is an increasing range of new drugs available that seem to have a modest effect on the relapse rate in primary progressive MS. Interferon-beta, glatiramer and the immunosuppressant azathioprine all seem to reduce the relapse rate, but have a less marked effect on reducing long-term disability. The interferons have side effects including flu-like symptoms and depression, which may make them very difficult for some people to tolerate as long-term treatments.

Natalizumab is a very new drug that carries significant risks of side effects, but seems to lead to an impressive reduction in relapse rate (reduced by two-thirds). It is currently reserved for use only in those patients whose relapses are continuing despite treatment with interferon-beta.

Patients may find that linoleic acid supplements and regular vitamin B12 injections help with chronic tiredness.

The main aspect of treatment in advanced MS is multidisciplinary support of the patient and their family. In this way it is comparable to the treatment of the disability caused by stroke. Physiotherapy is essential to prevent tightening of the muscles of the limbs. Drugs may be prescribed to help mitigate discomfort from spasms and nerve pain. These include the anti-epileptic drugs carbamazepine and gabapentin, and the antidepressant amitriptyline.

 Information box 4.1f-VIII

Multiple sclerosis: comments from a Chinese medicine perspective

In Chinese medicine, MS is a type of atrophy syndrome (Wei Syndrome).[13] It is considered to be a manifestation of a combination of Damp Obstructing the Channels (causing heaviness, numbness and tingling) and Deficiency of Kidney and Liver Yin (causing dizziness, problems with vision, difficulty in urination and weakness of the muscles). Muscle spasms are due to the generation of Liver Wind. A sudden shock leading to Depletion of Spleen and Heart Qi is also considered to be an additional factor in some cases. The observations that MS is more prevalent in a cold climate and in populations that have a diet high in animal fats are consistent with the Chinese medicine interpretation that Damp is an important factor in the development of MS. The sudden onset of symptoms in MS is in keeping with the rapid movement of Wind.

The action of steroid medication might be described in terms of clearing Damp from the Channels. However, its side effects demonstrate that it is in the long-term Damp/Phlegm Forming and Depleting of Yin. It therefore seems to be having a suppressive action in the treatment of MS.

Occupational therapists can advise on methods by which the progressive disabilities can be overcome with the use of physical aids. Advice from a social worker may be needed to discuss plans for future employment and to help acquire appropriate state benefits. The MS Society is a valued source of support for people in the UK with MS.[14]

Motor neuron disease (MND)

Motor neuron disease (MND), as its name implies, is a degenerative condition that affects the motor neurons within the brain and spinal cord. It may help to now turn back to the section entitled "Spinal tone" at the end of Part I, Section 4.1a, to remind yourself of the distinction between upper and lower motor neurons.

MND is much rarer than MS. It tends to affect men in middle life more often than women, and is of unknown cause. The loss of the motor neurons in MND is progressive, and leads to death usually within three years of diagnosis. Rarely, some patients survive for as long as ten years.

There are two main forms of MND. The first, amyotrophic lateral sclerosis (ALS) (also known as Lou Gehrig's disease), includes a subcategory called progressive bulbar palsy (PBP). ALS results from degeneration of motor nerve cells in the motor cortex and the spinal cord, and manifests as progressive weakness, first of the limbs and then of the muscles of speech, mastication and swallowing. In PBP only the upper and lower motor neurons that govern swallowing, speech and chewing are affected. The progression of this form of MND is usually rapid over the course of about three years, and death tends to result from pneumonia resulting from poor swallowing mechanisms and aspiration of fluid into the lungs. PBP tends to run an even shorter course. In about one-third of patients a form of dementia also becomes apparent.

The other form of MND is called progressive muscular atrophy (PMA). This form tends to affect lower motor neurons in the spinal cord. The patient will present with progressive weakness. PMA tends to run a longer course than ALS and is not associated with dementia.

The first symptom to appear depends on which motor nerves are affected first. In the most common form of MND the lower motor neurons that lead to the muscles of the limbs are affected first. This leads to weakness and wasting of the muscles. Eventually, the limbs become flaccid and lifeless. As the nerve cells supplying the muscles die, this causes a fine twitch to be seen on the surface of the muscles, which appears like a constant rippling motion under the surface of the skin. There is no pain or loss of sensation in MND.

In less common forms of MND the upper motor neurons are affected first. If this occurs within the spinal cord, the result is a gradual paralysis of the muscles of the limbs and body, but without the wasting. The tone of the paralyzed muscles is increased, as commonly occurs in multiple sclerosis. Spasm and tightening of the muscles occurs, and this can be very painful.

If the upper motor neurons of the brainstem are affected, this affects the action of the cranial nerves. The patient loses the ability to speak freely, and swallowing becomes difficult. This is the most serious aspect of MND, because impaired swallowing will eventually lead to choking on excess saliva, development of bronchopneumonia and death.

The only drug that is licensed for the treatment of MND is riluzole, which is reported to increase life expectancy in ALS by only three months. Riluzole counteracts the action of the excitatory neurotransmitter glutamate, which is believed to have a causative role in MND, although for reasons which are as yet unclear. Riluzole is only licensed in the UK for use in ALS, and not for PMA.

Information box 4.1f-IX

Motor neuron disease: comments from a Chinese medicine perspective

In Chinese medicine, MND is another atrophy syndrome. The underlying causes could include Invasion of Damp in the Channels, on top of a range of possible conditions of depletion, including Stomach and Spleen Qi Deficiency, Heart and Spleen Qi Deficiency, and Kidney and Liver Yin Deficiency. The rippling of the muscles that follows lower motor nerve degeneration in MND reflects Wind in the Channels.

Cerebral palsy

Cerebral palsy is a broad term used to describe a non-progressive defect within the CNS that occurs either before birth or in early childhood.

The most usual cause of cerebral palsy is that the baby in the womb is starved of oxygen for a short time. This can occur either before or during labor. Another well-known cause is the rupture of blood vessels in the brain of the baby during a traumatic labor. Immature clotting mechanisms mean that even a small injury might lead to a significant bleed and damage to the brain. After birth, the fits that can occur in high fever, or other causes of coma, can leave the baby with an area of permanent brain damage.

Cerebral palsy is much less common than it used to be. Some of this decline can be attributed to improved antenatal care and the specialist care of high-risk pregnancies. Also, two oral doses of vitamin K, a vitamin essential in the production of four of the 12 clotting factors in the liver, are now offered to all newborn babies in the UK to improve immature clotting mechanisms and help prevent intracranial bleeding.

In many cases, cerebral palsy is not diagnosed for some months to years after birth. This is because some of the disabilities that result from the area of brain damage are not apparent in the immature nervous system of an infant. The most common situation is that the baby is found not to be attaining the usual milestones of development (child development is explored in more detail in Chapter 5.4), and is then referred for a neurological examination.

In some cases, the disability is confined to the physical realm. In these cases there may be problems such as a hemiplegia (see "Stroke" in Section 4.1d), paralysis of both legs (diplegia), muscle spasms or difficulties with production of clear speech. Because of the increased tone of the affected limb muscles and problems with spasms, the (now outdated) term spastic used to be applied to children with these sorts of disabilities.

However, many children with cerebral palsy have, in addition to physical problems, learning difficulties, which can vary from being mild to very severe. Epilepsy is also very common in children with cerebral palsy.

It is recognized that early diagnosis is important so that the child can receive appropriate treatment, such as physiotherapy, and the family can be offered support in caring for the child.

> **ⓘ Information box 4.1f-X**
>
> ### Cerebral palsy: comments from a Chinese medicine perspective
>
> In Chinese medicine, the loss of the functioning of an aspect of the brain will nearly always correspond to Jing (Essence) Deficiency. Other syndromes depend on the exact nature of the disability. Phlegm is an important additional factor, particularly in cases in which there is epilepsy or in which intellect has been impaired.

The red flags of dementia, epilepsy and the other disorders of the central nervous system

Some patients with dementia, epilepsy and the other disorders of the CNS will benefit from referral to a conventional doctor for assessment and/or treatment. Red flags are those symptoms and signs that will indicate that referral should be considered. The red flags of these conditions are described in Table 4.1f-I. A summary of the red flags in a format designed for quick reference in clinical practice can be found in Appendix III. This gives advice on the degree of urgency of referral for each of the red flag conditions listed.

Table 4.1f-I A24: Red flags of dementia, epilepsy and other disorders of the central nervous system

Red flag	Description	Reasoning
A24.1	Progressive decline in mental and social functioning: increasing difficulty in intellectual function, memory, concentration and use of language	Gradual loss of mental function could result from a range of slowly developing brain disorders, including dementia, recurrent small strokes, extradural hemorrhage and a slow-growing brain tumor In elderly people in particular, depression can manifest in this way, and the symptoms may resolve with antidepressant medication
A24.2	Recent onset of confusion (i.e. evidence of an acute organic mental health disorder): features may include confusion, agitation, visual hallucinations, loss of ability to care for self	Organic mental health disorders are, by definition, those that have a medically recognized physical cause, such as drug intoxication, brain damage or dementia Organic disorders are characterized by confusion or clouding of consciousness, and loss of insight. Visual hallucinations may be apparent, as in the case of delirium tremens (alcohol withdrawal) Referral has to be considered if it is recognized that the patient or other people are at serious risk of harm if their condition is not disclosed. As it may be very difficult to fully assess this risk, it is advised that, unless there is absolute confidence that the patient is safe, they should be referred to professionals who are experienced in the treatment of mental health disorders Referral in such a situation may result in the serious outcome of the patient being detained against their will in hospital under a section of the Mental Health Act. As this may be a situation in which patient confidentiality may need to be breached, it is advisable, if there is the time to do so, to seek guidance from your professional body about how to proceed

A24.3	A temporary loss of neurological function (usually <2 hours): features may include loss of consciousness, loss of vision, unsteadiness, confusion, loss of memory, loss of sensation, limb weakness	A temporary loss of neurological function is most commonly seen as part of the syndrome of migraine, in which case it is usually part of a pattern with which the patient is familiar. In migraine, the blood flow to a portion of the brain is temporarily reduced as a result of spasm of an artery. A simple migraine does not merit referral
		The most common cause of loss of consciousness is a simple faint. This benign syndrome does not merit referral. It is characterized by a low blood pressure and a slow but regular pulse, and is triggered by prolonged standing, stuffy conditions and/or emotional arousal. A person who has fainted should start to recover almost immediately after the collapse
		If these symptoms occur for the first time, it is important to exclude the more serious syndrome of transient ischemic attack (TIA), in which a branch of a cerebral artery has been blocked by the temporary lodging of a small blood clot. A TIA is a warning sign of the more permanent damage that results from stroke, and the patient needs to be referred as a high priority for diagnosis and treatment
A24.4	A persisting loss of neurological function (lasting >2 hours): features may include loss of vision, unsteadiness, confusion, loss of memory, loss of sensation, muscle weakness	Any development of symptoms that suggest a persisting loss in neurological function merits referral to exclude stroke or a rapidly growing brain tumor
		Some of these symptoms can also result from disease of the spinal cord (e.g. multiple sclerosis) or of a peripheral nerve (e.g. Bell's palsy)
A24.5	A first-ever epileptic seizure:

Generalized tonic-clonic seizure: convulsions, loss of consciousness, bitten tongue, emptying of bladder and/or bowels. This is an emergency if the fit does not settle down within 2 minutes

Generalized absence or complex partial seizures: defined periods of vagueness or loss of awareness, or mood or personality changes

Focal simple seizures: episodes of coarse twitching of one part of the body | Epilepsy most commonly first presents in childhood, and is more common in children who have experienced febrile convulsions. Early diagnosis is important so that early management can help prevent deleterious effects on education and social development. However, it can present at any stage in life, and anyone who may have experienced a first epileptic seizure needs to be referred for diagnosis and advice about driving and personal safety |
		If the seizure occurs during sleep, the only symptom a patient might experience might be a sensation of grogginess in the morning and possibly a wet bed if the bladder has been voided. In such a case, the patient will have no memory of the episode of urination
		Absence and complex partial seizures may also be difficult to recognize, but are important to refer if suspected, as there is real risk of harm if an episode occurs when performing a risky activity such as climbing or driving
		A first epileptic seizure may, rarely, result from a brain tumor
		If a tonic-clonic seizure is ongoing, and particularly if it has lasted for >1 minute, it could develop into an emergency situation, and help needs to be summoned with urgency. It is important to ensure the fitting patient is in the recovery position whilst help arrives
		The patient who has experienced a possible seizure must be urged strongly not to drive until they have received medical advice
A24.6	Progressive coarse tremor appearing in middle to late life	A fine, symmetrical tremor that is worse with anxiety and over-arousal is common and benign, particularly in elderly people
		In contrast, Parkinson's disease presents with a progressive tremor that is far coarser and characteristically causes the movement of repeated opposition of thumb and fingers (the so-called "pill-rolling tremor"). Combined with this there will be increased stiffness of the muscles (the arms will be felt to resist passive movement). Parkinson's disease commonly affects one side more than another in its early stages
		Commonly, treatment is delayed for as long as is reasonable in Parkinson's disease, so there is no need for high-priority referral

4.1g Disorders of the spinal cord and peripheral nerves

This final section is concerned with the neurological disorders that have their origin outside the brain, either within the spinal cord or the peripheral nerves. The conditions to be explored in this section are:

- Disorders of the spinal cord:
  - spinal cord compression
  - spina bifida
  - poliomyelitis (polio)
- Disorders of the spinal nerve roots:
  - lumbar spondylosis and sciatica
  - cervical spondylosis
- Disorders of the nerve plexuses:
  - cervical rib
  - malignant infiltration
- Disorders of the peripheral nerves:
  - Guillain-Barré syndrome (post-infective polyneuropathy)
  - polyneuropathy
  - mononeuropathy from nerve entrapment (carpal tunnel syndrome and meralgia paraesthetica)
  - Bell's palsy and facial weakness
  - trigeminal neuralgia (TGN)
  - multiple mononeuropathies
  - leprosy
  - herpes zoster (shingles)
- Disorders of the neuromuscular junction:
  - myasthenia gravis.

Disorders of the spinal cord

It might be helpful to turn back to Section 4.1a to revise the structure of the spinal cord and how the peripheral nerves arise from it. (This information can be found from the section entitled "The spinal cord" up to the end of Part I, and information on the spinal nerves from the beginning of Part II up to the end of the section entitled "Referred pain.")

Spinal cord compression

The nervous tissue of the spinal cord is very delicate and is vulnerable to permanent damage by compression. Sudden spinal cord compression can result from traumatic injury to the spine in which a fracture or dislocation of one or more vertebrae can cause narrowing of the spinal canal. A more gradual onset of compression can result from a tumor or an abscess developing within the spinal canal. Occasionally, an intervertebral disc can prolapse (slip) and compress the posterior aspect of part of the cord. This rare form of prolapse most commonly affects the sacral levels of the cord. Arthritic changes of the vertebrae can also lead to a deformity of the spinal cord that is so great as to cause compression. This most commonly affects the lower cervical and sacral cord.

The various symptoms of cord compression are the result of the combined damage to the sensitive meninges that surround the cord, damage to the spinal nerves emerging from the cord at the level of the compression, and damage to the nerve cells and nerve fibers situated in the spinal cord at that level. The way in which these symptoms manifest depends, of course, on the level of the compression. For example, a sudden compression at the level of T5 from a fracture dislocation between the T5 and T6 vertebrae will lead to pain in the region of the compression (from damage to the bones and meninges) and pain in the dermatome of skin supplied by the T5 spinal nerves. In this case the area of skin is a band that encircles the chest approximately at the level of the nipple. The pain will be worse on coughing or straining because these actions further increase the pressure within the spinal canal.

The most significant symptoms of compression result from the damage done within the cord itself. This can result in damage to the nerve fibers that travel through the cord at that level. The function of these fibers is to connect all parts of the body supplied by spinal nerves originating at positions lower than that level with the brain.

If the compression is very severe or the cord is actually severed, all connection between those parts of the body supplied by the more distal spinal nerves and the brain is lost. The result is total paralysis of all voluntary muscles in these parts of the body, and total numbness of these parts of the body. For example, in the case of a serious compression at the level of T5, the patient will become paralyzed from the lower chest down and will be numb from the chest down. Voluntary control of the bladder and bowels is lost. Total paralysis of the lower limbs is termed paraplegia (if partial, it is termed paraparesis). However, the spinal reflexes responsible for the maintenance of tone in the lower limbs and for the involuntary control of the bladder and bowel are not affected. The tone of the muscles in the legs can be excessive, because the control that is normally exerted on these reflexes by the brain is lost. This means that muscle spasms can occur. This is the reason for the term spastic paraplegia.

In the case of an injury at the level of the cervical vertebrae (colloquially termed a broken neck), the connection is lost between the brain and the spinal nerves that supply the arms. This means that all four limbs become paralyzed, a condition termed tetraplegia (also known as quadriplegia).

In cervical cord compression the muscles that supply the chest wall are also paralyzed, and this severely impairs the action of inspiration. An injury above the level of C3–4 has the added serious consequence of causing paralysis to the diaphragm, so that unassisted breathing is not possible at all.

In the acute compression of the cord that occurs from traumatic injury, the condition is a surgical emergency. Without very prompt attention, permanent damage to the cord will occur. Even with very careful support, it is rare for a person who has suddenly developed these sorts of symptoms to recover fully from the injury.

A more slowly developing case of compression will, of course, cause a more gradual progression of these sorts of symptoms. For example, the typical scenario that follows from the growth of a tumor within the spinal cord is that pain develops in the dermatome supplied by the spinal root, and there is a gradual and patchy onset of numbness and weakness in the parts of the body supplied by spinal nerves distal to the tumor.

Patients with suspected acute or gradual cord compression are diagnosed by means of an MRI. In many cases of progressive cord damage, urgent removal of the cause of the problem (known as spinal decompression) can arrest the symptoms and may be followed by recovery of some of the lost function. Intravenous steroids may be given in the acute situation to reduce swelling of the cord, and anticoagulants to prevent blood clotting from reduced muscle movement. Tumors may be treated by one or more of surgery, chemotherapy and radiotherapy.

However, following a traumatic compression to the spinal cord, many patients will have to learn to live with a serious and permanent disability. Any patient who develops paraplegia or tetraplegia requires skilled and prolonged nursing care. The ideal is for the patient to be nursed within a specialized spinal unit that puts an emphasis on rehabilitation. The aim of rehabilitation is to enable the patient to return to an active role in society.

Special attention has to be given to the function of the bladder and bowel. In the initial stages after injury the bladder may not void at all. A urethral catheter is intermittently inserted to enable complete drainage of the bladder. This has the potential complication of increasing the risk of infections of the bladder. These bladder infections have a tendency to spread to involve the kidneys in a patient who is immobile. If they occur, they are treated promptly with antibiotics. Some people manage to start to learn to void without use of a catheter at all as the bladder is under reflex spinal control. Others, even without this reflex, can learn to self-catheterize. Elderly people are more likely to have to depend on an indwelling catheter.

Similarly, initially the patient will be fecally incontinent. However, with time the bowel starts to empty regularly and a form of continence can be achieved, although a pattern may take some weeks to establish following the injury.

The problem of permanently contracted muscles has to be avoided. This means that the patient requires intensive physiotherapy to the limbs to enable the muscles to be stretched regularly. Drugs such as baclofen and dantrolene that inhibit spasms are given frequently to prevent contractures. These can have side effects such as severe nausea, confusion and other mental disturbances, which can markedly affect the patient's quality of life. The paralyzed patient has to be turned regularly in bed, or moved in position within a wheelchair, to prevent pressure sores developing. A chronic pressure sore is a serious problem in paraplegia, as once established it is very difficult to heal. The chronic infection from a pressure sore can have a very debilitating effect.

With time, many patients regain mobility with the help of specially adapted lightweight wheelchairs. Although all will continue to require regular support from a multidisciplinary team of carers, many will be able to return to an active life in their own homes.

The patient with a spinal cord injury remains at risk of recurrent infections of the chest and the kidneys. These complications can lead to an early death, either from respiratory failure or from chronic kidney failure.

Other causes of damage to the spinal cord

Some other rare conditions can cause localized damage to the cord, leading to a condition similar to cord compression. For example, vitamin B12 deficiency (pernicious anemia) involves spinal cord damage as well as a form of dementia. Also, occasionally the damage caused by the plaques of multiple sclerosis (MS) can be localized to one part of the cord, and might produce similar symptoms, although in both these conditions the pain is not so prominent. Inflammation of the cord can occur as a result of radiotherapy or some rare infections. This, too, will produce similar symptoms.

 Information box 4.1g-I

Spinal cord injury: comments from a Chinese medicine perspective

In Chinese medicine, the symptoms that arise from severe damage in spinal cord injury correspond to Deficiency of Jing. This is another example of an atrophy syndrome (see Section 4.1f). Numbness and weakness correspond to Damp Obstructing the Channels together with Deficiency of Yin (Kidney and Liver). Spasticity is a manifestation of Liver Wind in the muscles. Lack of control of the urethra and the anus would also fit with severe Kidney Deficiency.

Spina bifida

Spinal bifida is a congenital structural abnormality of the spinal cord in the lumbosacral region. In severe cases, the posterior part of the cord is undeveloped, and the residual part of the cord opens out onto the skin, where it is covered by a membrane-bound sac called a meningocele. This requires immediate surgery at birth to protect the cord from rupture of the sac and subsequent infection. Surgery cannot amend the damage caused by the lack of the nerves in this part of the cord. In severe spina bifida, the child might have a spastic paraplegia, numbness of the lower limbs, and incontinence of the bladder and bowel. In some cases, these problems can be associated with other abnormalities such as hydrocephalus.

In less severe cases the abnormality is not apparent at birth, and only becomes apparent as the child fails to reach the expected milestones of development, such as sitting, crawling and walking. This situation of undiagnosed spina bifida is becoming increasingly rare because the condition can be detected from the prenatal ultrasound scan that most pregnant women in the UK undergo. This means that appropriate care for the child can be offered at a very early stage.

It is now known that adequate dietary levels of certain vitamins early in pregnancy are important in the prevention of spina bifida. In particular, there is very strong evidence that a regular dose of folic acid, taken in the first weeks of pregnancy (ideally from preconception to at least 20 weeks), reduces the risk of this abnormality. It is also for this reason that foods such as bread and breakfast cereals are often fortified with this vitamin.

 Information box 4.1g-II

Spina bifida: comments from a Chinese medicine perspective

In Chinese medicine spina bifida might be described as Deficiency of Jing and Yin together with accumulation of Damp in the Channels. In this case the cause of the Jing Deficiency is congenital rather than severe trauma, but otherwise the energetic interpretation of the syndrome is comparable to that of a spinal cord injury.

The strong link that exists between spina bifida and deficiency of folic acid in pregnancy suggests that folic acid plays a role in Nourishing the Jing of the fetus.

Poliomyelitis (polio)

Poliomyelitis (polio) is a viral infection that has a propensity for the nervous system. The virus is excreted in the feces, and so is passed on through contact with feces. In most cases of polio infection (95 percent) there are very few symptoms. The remaining 5 percent of people who contract the infection suffer from a flu-like illness with muscle aches. However, less than one in five of these will go on to develop the severe condition of paralytic poliomyelitis. In these cases the virus has invaded some of the lower motor nerve cells in the spinal cord that lead to all the voluntary muscles. The result is a paralysis of the affected muscle groups. The paralysis leads to a flaccid limb, without tone, and in this way is different to the paralysis caused by spinal cord compression. There is no loss of sensation in polio.

In paralytic polio the patient experiences a flare up of symptoms about four to five days following recovery from the flu-like illness, a headache (due to a form of meningitis) and the development of weakness of some of the muscles. The muscle weakness is not necessarily symmetrical.

Polio tends to affect children less severely than adults. Whereas a child characteristically might develop weakness in one or both lower limbs, an adult might develop a tetraplegia or difficulty swallowing due to damage to the lower motor nerve cells originating in the cervical cord and the brainstem.

The incidence of polio worldwide has dropped markedly since the introduction of vaccination. It is the aim of the World Health Organization (WHO) to coordinate the vaccination campaign so that polio, like smallpox, becomes totally eradicated. The initial aim of the program was total eradication by the year 2000. This looked tantalizingly close, as in 1994 the Americas were declared polio free, and in 2000 the Western Pacific followed. In 2002 Europe was declared polio free, but in six countries, including Afghanistan, India and Nigeria, the disease remained endemic. Since that time there has been a resurgence of cases in many countries in Africa, not helped by political unrest in many of these countries and the disruption that such unrest causes to the success of health programs.

In the UK almost all of the very few new cases of polio were diagnosed either in people who had contracted the condition overseas or who had developed polio as a result of a very rare complication of the live vaccine (now totally replaced by inactivated vaccine). Nevertheless, in some developing countries polio is still an endemic disease. In these countries, people who have the lifelong disabilities that have resulted from a childhood polio infection (usually a single wasted and useless limb) are a common sight.

Disorders of the spinal nerve roots

The spinal nerves (nerve roots) that emerge from the spinal cord can be selectively damaged in some conditions. These conditions will lead to a characteristic syndrome of one-sided pain, sensory loss and weakness, depending on the site of the damage.

Lumbar spondylosis and sciatica

Sciatica is the term used to describe a pain that has its origin in the lumbar and sacral spinal nerves. This pain is referred down one or both legs, along the distribution of the sciatic nerve. The symptoms include pain and/or tingling that radiates down the buttock and the back of one leg to the foot. There may be patchy numbness of the skin in the region affected by the pain, and weakness of some of the muscles of the lower leg. The pain is typically provoked by movements that affect the lower back, particularly bending forward. Sciatica is often, but not always, associated with low back pain.

Sciatica results from damage to one or more of the lumbar or sacral spinal nerves that emerge from the very base of the spinal cord. The spinal cord actually terminates at the level of L1/L2 vertebrae. The lower lumbar and sacral spinal nerves leave the base of the cord at this level, and then travel downwards within the spinal canal to their points of exit at the sacral and lumbar intervertebral spaces.

The lumbar and sacral spinal nerves can be damaged by anything that compresses them, either as they descend through the spinal canal, or as they emerge through the intervertebral spaces in the lower lumbar or sacral regions of the back. The most common cause of compression of the spinal nerves is the protrusion (prolapse) of an intervertebral disc, either between the L5/S1 vertebrae or between the S1/S2 vertebrae (for more details about intervertebral disc prolapse, see Section 4.2e). Prolapsed discs will tend to compress the L5 and S1 nerve roots.

Figure 4.1g-I illustrates how a prolapsed disc can compress the spinal nerve roots. This diagram shows how the bulging of the posterior part of an intervertebral disc can affect either the spinal nerves (b) or the cord itself (a), depending on the site of the bulge. Bulging that is slightly to one side (b) is by far the more common situation.

Figure 4.1g-I Central (a) and lateral (b) disc protrusion

Diagram showing possible locations of compression of cord and nerve roots as a result of prolapse of a portion of an invertebral disc.

The other common cause of compression of the spinal nerves is osteoarthritis of the vertebrae (see Section 4.2f). The arthritic changes to the vertebral bones can lead to narrowing of the intervertebral spaces as well as of the spinal canal itself.

The term spondylosis is used to describe the degenerative processes that lead to both disc prolapse and arthritic deformity of the vertebrae. Therefore, lumbar spondylosis is the medical term applied to these degenerative causes of sciatica and low back pain.

Sciatica may also occur simply as a result of tension in the muscles and ligaments that support the vertebrae. Tension causes the vertebrae to be squeezed close together and cramps the spaces through which the spinal nerves should exit. This form of sciatica is typically less severe and tends to appear and disappear according to factors such as overwork, tiredness, mood and the weather.

Rarely, a tumor of the spinal canal, or one that is situated close to the lumbosacral spinal column, may cause sciatica. In this case, the sciatica is slowly progressive. Progressive sciatic pain should, therefore, be taken as a red flag of serious disease.

The arthritic changes of lumbar spondylosis may be seen on an X-ray image of the spine, although there is a poor correlation between the changes seen on the X-ray image and the severity of symptoms. The most informative investigation is an MRI, which will usually show the site of the compression of the spinal nerve, and whether or not a disc prolapse is present.

The treatment of sciatica and low back pain is described in more detail in Section 4.2e.

 Information box 4.1g-III

Sciatica: comments from a Chinese medicine perspective

In Chinese medicine, the pain and numbness of sciatica is ascribed to Damp Cold (or, more rarely, Damp Heat) in the Gallbladder and Bladder Channels. An underlying Deficiency of the Kidneys is very often the reason why sciatica has developed.

Cervical spondylosis

The same process of degeneration of the intervertebral discs and the vertebral bones also commonly occurs in the cervical spine. In this case the C7 spinal nerves are most frequently affected. This leads to pain and tingling that radiates down one arm to the hand, numbness of the skin of the arm and weakness of the muscles of the forearm and the hand.

The treatment of cervical spondylosis is discussed in Section 4.2e.

Information box 4.1g-IV

Cervical spondylosis: comments from a Chinese medicine perspective

In Chinese medicine, the symptoms of cervical spondylosis would also be ascribed to Damp Cold or Damp Heat leading to Qi and Blood Stagnation, this time in the channels of the arm. Again, because the degeneration of the spine is the underlying cause, a Kidney Deficiency is likely to be present. Contributory neck and shoulder muscular tension would correspond to Qi Stagnation.

Disorders of the nerve plexuses

The nerve plexuses are the networks of nerves formed by the intermingling of the spinal nerves that supply the arms and the legs. If the nerve plexuses are affected by disease, because a number of peripheral nerves will be damaged, a complex pattern of symptoms can develop.

The two brachial plexuses involve the C5 to T1 spinal nerves, and are situated deep in the upper chest at the level of the clavicle. The nerves that supply the shoulder, the arm and the upper chest emerge from the brachial plexus.

The two lumbosacral plexuses involve the L4 to the coccygeal nerves and are situated deep in the lower abdomen and pelvis close to the lumbar spine and sacrum. The nerves that supply the buttocks, leg and genitals emerge from this plexus.

Cervical rib

The brachial plexus can be affected by a rare condition in which there is an additional rudimentary rib attached to the C7 vertebra, the so-called cervical rib. This can stretch the lower nerve roots of the brachial plexus and cause pain and numbness on the underside of the arm and the ulnar border of the forearm and hand. This extra rib can also compress the major artery that supplies blood to the arm and hand. If one-sided, this can lead to a very weak pulse on that side. Usually, a cervical rib causes no symptoms, but if symptoms do occur, the condition can be treated surgically.

Information box 4.1g-V

Cervical rib: comments from a Chinese medicine perspective

In Chinese medicine, the symptoms of a cervical rib correspond to Stagnation of Qi and Blood in the Heart and Small Intestine Channels of the affected arm. Although the pulse may be very abnormal on the affected side, this perhaps should be taken as a feature of the condition rather than as a reflection of the whole energetic balance of the body.

Malignant infiltration

The more serious condition that can affect the nerve plexuses is infiltration by a tumor. A common cancer-related plexus problem is when enlarging lung cancer invades the brachial plexus having spread from the upper portion of a lung. This causes pain down the arm of the same side and wasting of the muscles of that arm. The pain of cancerous infiltration of the nerves can be very severe.

Information box 4.1g-VI

Malignant infiltration: comments from a Chinese medicine perspective

In Chinese medicine, the pain of malignant infiltration corresponds to Blood Stagnation in the affected channels, and is a manifestation of the underlying cancerous process.

Disorders of the peripheral nerves

The peripheral nerves comprise the cranial nerves and the spinal nerves, and include all the nerves that emerge from the nerve plexuses. These nerves branch to supply all the muscles of the body with motor or autonomic nerve endings. They also carry sensory nerve fibers from all superficial parts of the body. Therefore, a condition that damages a peripheral nerve will have two effects: it will cause weakness and wasting of the muscles supplied by that nerve, and will also cause a loss of sensation of the part of the body supplied by that nerve. Sometimes the affected nerve gives rise to pain or tingling rather than numbness. The pain from a damaged nerve is called neuralgia, and is characteristically severe.

A condition that affects a number of peripheral nerves is called a polyneuropathy, and one that affects a single nerve is called a mononeuropathy. A polyneuropathy typically affects long nerves most severely. This means that the nerves that supply the hands, the legs and the feet are most damaged. The patient with this form of polyneuropathy develops what is called glove and stocking numbness, because of the area of skin affected, and weakness of the muscles of the hands and the legs. Balance can be impaired, because the sensation of the bones of the feet and ankles is also lost.

In both types of neuropathy, if prolonged, the numbness can result in recurrent injury to the affected area, because the protective mechanism of pain has been lost.

Information box 4.1g-VII

Neuropathy: comments from a Chinese medicine perspective

In Chinese medicine, the numbness of neuropathy would usually correspond to Damp and/or Blood Deficiency, and the weakness to Deficiency of Liver and Kidney Yin. This is another form of atrophy syndrome. Injuries that result from the numbness reflect Stagnation of Blood and Qi.

Guillain-Barré syndrome (post-infective polyneuropathy)

This syndrome tends to develop one to three weeks after an infectious illness. It is thought to be the result of autoimmune damage to the peripheral nerves that has been triggered by the infectious process. The patient initially develops a glove-and-stocking numbness, and weakness of the hands and legs. In many patients there is a slow but sure recovery of the nerves over the following few weeks. However, in some cases (about 20 percent) the polyneuropathy is rapidly progressive so that shorter nerves become affected. This includes the respiratory and facial muscles. This deterioration can occur rapidly, over the course of a few days, and can lead to a medical emergency as the patient may require assisted ventilation to support the failing respiratory muscles.

A preparation of antibodies, called gamma-globulin, appears to slow the progress and severity of the condition. This is given to patients with severe Guillain-Barré syndrome.

In severe cases recovery may require several months, during which time the patient is almost totally paralyzed. In these cases recovery is often not complete, so that some residual numbness and weakness of muscles remains. The mortality associated with the severe form of this condition is 10 percent.

Information box 4.1g-VIII

Guillain-Barré syndrome: comments from a Chinese medicine perspective

In Chinese medicine, the peripheral numbness and weakness of Guillain-Barré syndrome, like all forms of polyneuropathy, correspond to Damp in the Channels, with Liver and Kidney Yin Deficiency. In this case the origin of the Damp is possibly a Residual Pathogenic Factor following an infectious disease. Full Heat from an infection may have contributed to weakening of the Yin.

Polyneuropathy in chronic illness

There are a number of chronic conditions in which polyneuropathy can develop. The most common of these is diabetes mellitus, in which, because wound healing is poor, numbness can be a source of serious medical complications. Small wounds to the numb skin of the feet, in particular, can easily develop into chronic ulcers, and eventually the foot may require amputation.

Numbness of the hands and feet can also develop in severe kidney disease and advanced cancer.

Certain vitamin deficiencies, if prolonged, can lead to a polyneuropathy because the vitamins are essential for the maintenance of healthy nerves. In particular, deficiencies of thiamine (vitamin B1), pyridoxine (vitamin B6) and vitamin B12 may lead to nerve damage.

Polyneuropathy caused by toxins

A number of drugs and toxins can damage the peripheral nerves. Alcohol is the most important of these in the UK in terms of number of people affected. With high alcohol intake over a length of time, loss of sensation of the feet and legs and muscle weakness can develop, and lead to a vulnerability to injury and an impairment of balance. Alcohol-related damage to the cerebellum can also impair balance and coordination, and so these harmful effects will be additive. The nerve damage and impairment of coordination may persist even after abstention from alcohol.

Some of the drugs that cause polyneuropathy include phenytoin (an anti-epileptic drug), gold (an antirheumatoid medication), and vincristine and cisplatin (chemotherapeutic drugs).

Mononeuropathy from nerve entrapment

A single peripheral nerve can be damaged by excessive pressure as it passes through the tissues. Some nerves are more vulnerable to this problem than others because they travel through areas that are more vulnerable to damage, or because they pass through a very tight anatomical space.

The loss of function that results from damage to a single nerve is sometimes termed palsy. For example, median nerve palsy is the cause of carpal tunnel syndrome.

Carpal tunnel syndrome is an entrapment neuropathy that results from the compression of the median nerve as it passes over the wrist bones (in the region of acupoint Da Ling, PC-7) to supply the muscles of the thumb and skin of the radial side of the hand. The cause is usually an accumulation of fluid within the limited space of the soft tissue of the wrist (known as the carpal tunnel) through which the nerve passes. Carpal tunnel syndrome can occur out of the blue, but it is often associated with more generalized conditions, in particular pregnancy, hypothyroidism and obesity.

The symptoms include numbness and tingling of the radial side of the hand and weakness of grip. There may be pain and aching in the hand and forearm, which is particularly severe at night, and is helped by dropping the arm out of bed.

Treatment includes taking the pressure off the nerve by splinting the wrist in an extended position. Corticosteroid injections may be given. If the pain and weakness is persistent, a surgical operation is performed on the wrist to reduce the pressure in the carpal tunnel.

Meralgia paraesthetica is an entrapment neuropathy of the lateral cutaneous nerve of the thigh. This is a sensory nerve that supplies the outer aspect of the skin of the thigh. The entrapment occurs as the nerve passes through the femoral canal (in the region of acupoint Qi Chong, ST-30). This causes numbness, tingling and pain on the outer aspect of the thigh.

Meralgia paraesthetica is fairly common in pregnancy and can also be a problem in obesity. This is because in both these conditions there is additional pressure on the femoral canal. If the condition develops during pregnancy it usually settles after delivery.

 Information box 4.1g-IX

Carpal tunnel syndrome and meralgia paraesthetica: comments from a Chinese medicine perspective

In Chinese medicine, the numbness and weakness of carpal tunnel syndrome corresponds to Damp and/or Blood Deficiency, and pain will correspond to Qi or Blood Stagnation. The Pericardium and Lung Channels are particularly affected.

The numbness of meralgia paraesthetica corresponds to Damp and/or Blood Deficiency, and pain will correspond to Qi or Blood Stagnation. The Stomach Channel is affected.

Bell's palsy and facial weakness

Bell's palsy is the result of inflammation of the facial nerve (the seventh cranial nerve), which supplies the muscles of the face. The facial nerve carries very few sensory fibers, which means that numbness is not a typical symptom. It is believed that the inflammation is due to a viral infection of the facial nerve, which causes swelling of the nerve as it passes through the bone of the skull close to the ear.

The symptoms are of a sudden onset of weakness of one side of the face, sometimes following a brief episode of earache on the affected side. The corner of the mouth droops and the eyelid may be unable to close completely. In serious cases this problem, if prolonged, can lead to ulceration of the eye and damage to the cornea. The patient may also notice an altered taste on one side of the tongue.

In most people improvement begins spontaneously after two weeks and complete recovery can be expected, although recovery can be slow and incomplete in a minority of cases. Corticosteroids are often given by mouth for a week or so early in the course of the condition to reduce the swelling and damage to the nerve. This treatment is known to improve chances of recovery. Antiviral medication may also be given, although there is more uncertainty about the benefit of this additional treatment. A minor operation may have to be performed to encourage the eyelid to close and thus prevent ulceration of the cornea of the eye.[15]

A more serious cause of damage to the facial nerve is pressure on the nerve from a brain tumor. For this reason, if a person with Bell's palsy does not start to recover at all within two weeks they may be referred for further neurological investigations including an MRI.

 Information box 4.1g-X

Bell's palsy and facial weakness: comments from a Chinese medicine perspective

In Chinese medicine, the symptom of facial weakness is considered to be caused by Wind Cold Invasion of the Channels of the face. Bell's palsy is attributed to External Wind, whereas facial weakness occurring in a stroke or other severe chronic condition (e.g. cancer or diabetes) may be due to internally generated Wind. A pre-existing Zheng Qi Deficiency and vacuity of channels and collaterals predisposes to this condition.[16]

Weakness of the facial muscles can occur in other conditions. The most common cause is a one-sided stroke, although this will usually be accompanied by symptoms of weakness in other parts of the body. In a stroke, the eyelids and the forehead muscles are not affected.

Myasthenia gravis is a condition that causes a more symmetrical facial weakness; it is described in more detail at the end of this section.

Trigeminal neuralgia (TGN)

Trigeminal neuralgia (TGN) is a condition in which the nerve that carries the sensory nerve fibers that supply the skin and soft tissues of the face becomes excessively sensitive. This nerve is the fifth cranial nerve, also known as the trigeminal nerve. The pain of TGN is experienced as a severe stabbing or electric shock-like sensation that radiates down the face from the area in front of the ear. The condition predominantly affects elderly people.

Light touch, shaving, washing and exposure to a cool breeze can trigger an attack of this pain, which then can occur repeatedly over the course of a period of hours. There may be gaps of weeks to months between attacks.

Although the majority of cases have no precipitating cause, in a significant minority (14 percent) the nerve has been irritated by a structural change such as a tumor or aneurysm. For this reason many cases will be investigated by means of an MRI.

The most effective painkillers for the intense pain of TGN are the anti-epileptic medications carbamazepine, phenytoin, lamotrigine and gabapentin, all of which have an inhibitory effect on the nervous system. In very severe recurrent cases, the nerve may be deadened by injection with alcohol. This will leave the patient with a permanently numb face. Alternatively, in some cases, the blood supply of the nerve root can be decompressed by delicate microsurgery, with good results.

Information box 4.1g-XI

Trigeminal neuralgia: comments from a Chinese medicine perspective

In Chinese medicine, the symptoms of TGN also correspond to Wind or Wind Cold Invasion or other causes of obstruction of the Yang Channels and collaterals of the face. The intense pain indicates Blood Stagnation, which results from the obstruction. The fact that this is predominantly a disease of elderly people suggests that an underlying Deficiency of Yin or Qi is also likely to be present. In some cases, suppressed anger can lead to a stirring of Liver Fire and, in susceptible individuals, lodging of Phlegm Fire in the channels of the face, via the Shaoyang system.[17]

Multiple mononeuropathies

Multiple mononeuropathies is a condition in which a number of peripheral nerves are damaged, but not usually in the symmetrical way in which a polyneuropathy first presents. In the UK, it is most commonly a result of the damage to the circulation to the nerves that occurs in diabetes. The patient with this condition will have repeated episodes in which the function of single nerves is lost. This occurs suddenly as the arterioles that supply the nerves undergo thrombosis.

For example, a sudden onset of numbness and weakness affecting the ulnar side of the hand (ulnar nerve palsy) might be followed by an inability to raise the foot and numbness on the border of the shin (common peroneal nerve palsy), and so on.

Other causes of multiple mononeuropathies include advanced cancer, and HIV infection. Leprosy, described below, is the most important cause worldwide.

Information box 4.1g-XII

Multiple mononeuropathies: comments from a Chinese medicine perspective

As with the other mononeuropathies, the localized numbness and weakness correspond to Damp Phlegm or Wind Obstructing the Channels and collaterals and will be predisposed to by localized Blood Deficiency. The progressive nature of the problem indicates an underlying Deficiency of Yin.

Leprosy

Leprosy is an infection that occurs in tropical and warm temperate regions. It primarily affects the peripheral nervous system, but can spread via the nerves to affect the soft tissues. The infectious agent, *Mycobacterium leprae*, is from the same family as the organism that causes tuberculosis. It is uncertain exactly how the organism is transmitted from one person to another. It is possible that organisms are transmitted by nasal secretions, as it is known that millions of organisms may be expelled from the nose each day by an infected individual. Whether these then infect skin or the respiratory tract of a contact is, as yet, unknown. After the initial infection there can be a delay of a few months to a few years before symptoms appear.

The manifestation of the leprosy infection depends very much on the state of the immune system of the individual. In those with good immunity, the infection is localized to one part of the body and is not contagious. This is known as paucibacillary leprosy or tuberculoid leprosy. In this form of leprosy, a single peripheral nerve becomes damaged and thickened. The skin supplied by this nerve becomes numb and loses some of its pigment. The pale patch that results can have slightly thickened edges. As with other mononeuropathies, the muscles supplied by the nerve become weak and wasted.

In people with poor immunity, the number of nerves affected increases, and the damage done by the organism to the skin supplied by those nerves is greater. This is called lepromatous leprosy or multibacillary leprosy. In severe cases there is a multiple mononeuropathy, with weakness or paralysis of a number of muscle groups, numerous numb patches of skin, and gross thickening of areas of the skin, particularly on the face. In severe lepromatous leprosy, the face can become very deformed by the thickened skin. The inflammation also affects deeper tissues. The cartilage of the nose erodes and the testes atrophy. The prolonged numbness of the limbs leads to loss of fingers and toes as a result of chronic injury not prevented by the usual withdrawal response to pain.

It is no wonder that leprosy used to be such a dreaded disease and that in many countries lepers were exiled from their own communities. Despite this fear, the condition is not very contagious, with only one in 100 of people who have been in close contact with a person with advanced leprosy going on to develop the disease.

Lepromatous leprosy can be treated by long-term antibiotic therapy. Because the bacterium is slow growing, and able to hide within the nervous system, a daily dose of the antibiotic dapsone and low-dose clofazimine is recommended to be taken for a minimum of two years. In addition, additional antibiotics (rifampicin and high-dose clofazimine) are given once a month. This regimen is a difficult one to stick to for anyone, and more so for people who live in poverty in rural areas. Ideally, treatment is administered from a specialist center. In tuberculoid leprosy, six months of treatment is the maximum that would be prescribed to eradicate the infection.

In established leprosy, the damage already done to the nerves, soft tissues and the skin cannot be reversed by drug treatment. Physiotherapy and surgery are also important aspects of the treatment of the deformities caused by this infection.

 Information box 4.1g-XIII

Leprosy: comments from a Chinese medicine perspective

In leprosy, in addition to Damp (numbness) and Blood Deficiency (pale skin patches), the thickening of the skin suggests that Phlegm is an important additional Pathogenic Factor. The fact that an impaired immunity predisposes people to severe leprosy suggests that there is an underlying severe deficiency syndrome. Kidney Yin Deficiency is the most likely. The etiology of leprosy has been associated with invasion of Wind Cold and also the development of Internal Phlegm, Damp and Heat.[18]

Varicella zoster (shingles)

Varicella zoster is the name given to the chickenpox virus. The condition of shingles is a late consequence of a chickenpox infection, and usually occurs decades after an initial childhood infection. It is common, affecting up to 20 percent of people in the UK in their lifetime.

It seems that following some cases of chickenpox the virus is not fully cleared from the body, but instead hides within the sensory nerve cell bodies that sit next to the spinal nerves close to the spinal cord. It is believed that during the episode of chickenpox the virus travels up to this site via the sensory nerve fibers that supply the areas of infected skin. In this way an episode of shingles involves the recurrence of a skin infection by the virus, but this time localized to the dermatome supplied by a single spinal nerve.

The virus spreads from its hiding place close to the spinal cord via the nerve ending of the spinal nerve so that the skin of the dermatome first becomes painful for a day or so, and only then develops crusting and weeping spots akin to the original chickenpox. Shingles is contagious at this stage, although the condition that would be transmitted would be chickenpox rather than shingles. The appearance is of a strip of red crusting skin localized to one half of the body only.

Shingles develops at a time when the natural immunity is low, either as a result of aging, or because of stress or another ongoing illness. In frail people, the skin infection can be very severe and painful. In particular, shingles that affects one of the facial dermatomes can be very debilitating, particularly if it is close to the eye. A shingles infection that affects the nerve that supplies the cornea of the eye (the ophthalmic division of the fifth (trigeminal) cranial nerve) can be so severe as to threaten the sight.

Recovery of the crusting rash occurs over a matter of days. However, in up to one in ten people the area of skin that was affected is left in a very sensitive and painful state. This pain can be intense, prolonged and draining, and does not respond to conventional painkillers. It can last for a period of months to years. In some people, treatment with anti-epileptic or antidepressant medication (e.g. carbamazepine, gabapentin, lamotrigine or amitriptyline) can be of help.

The acute infection of shingles can be treated with the antiviral drug aciclovir given in tablet form. Some studies demonstrate that if this drug is given to people with shingles in its very early stages, the prolonged pain that follows the infection can be reduced in severity.

Information box 4.1g-XIV

Shingles: comments from a Chinese medicine perspective

In Chinese medicine, the rash of shingles may correspond to an Invasion of the Channels by Wind Damp and/or Wind Heat. The obstructing Pathogens may also be internally generated. Damp Heat may be the result of weak Spleen and poor diet, or suppressed emotions may lead to generation of depressive Liver Fire. If very painful, this is suggestive of Heat with Blood Stagnation. Long-term pain and numbness would signify local Deficiency with Blood Stagnation and Phlegm Damp Obstructing the Channels.[19]

Disorders of the neuromuscular junction

The neuromuscular junction is the term given to the specialized synapse at which the branches (dendrites) at the very end of a motor nerve make contact with a muscle fiber. The dendrites of the stimulated nerve release a neurotransmitter into the space of the synapse. Receptors on the muscle fiber respond to these molecules by causing a muscle contraction. The most important disorder of the neuromuscular junction is myasthenia gravis.

Myasthenia gravis

Myasthenia gravis is a term that literally means severe weakness of muscles. It is an organ-specific autoimmune disease of unknown cause, but tends to affect women twice as often as men. Commonly, young adults are affected.

In myasthenia gravis antibodies that target the receptors for the acetylcholine neurotransmitter in the neuromuscular junction are generated. This means that the message of the stimulated motor nerve cannot get through effectively to the muscle to bring about a contraction. In addition, in 70 percent of young patients the thymus gland, a small lump of lymphoid tissue deep in the chest, is found to be enlarged. In a small proportion of these people a tumor, called a thymoma, is found within the thymus.

The characteristic symptom of myasthenia is that muscles are weak, and that the weakness increases after repeated action of a particular muscle. This is known as fatigability. The facial muscles and the muscles that cause flex of the shoulders and hips are most affected. This means that double vision, drooping eyelids, difficulty swallowing and chewing, and difficulty standing from sitting may all occur. In severe cases, the action of breathing may be impaired. However, there is one form of myasthenia in which the eye and eyelid muscles only are affected.

Because the first symptoms are often vague, the patient who complains of periods of weakness and fatigue may not be correctly diagnosed for some time. In most cases there is a gradual, but slow, progression of symptoms. In severe cases respiratory failure may develop.

Diagnosis may be confirmed by testing for antibodies to the acetylcholine receptor. A CT scan should be performed to exclude tumor of the thymus in the chest.

Myasthenia gravis is treated with drugs that prevent the normal removal of the neurotransmitter at the neuromuscular junction. Pyridostigmine is the most widely used drug. The side effects of diarrhea, abdominal pain and excessive salivation are partly a result of the effect this drug has on parts of the body that are not affected by the myasthenia. These drugs do not alter the course of the disease.

In severe cases corticosteroids and other immunosuppressants, such as azathioprine or methotrexate, can also reduce the symptoms by inhibiting the immune damage to the neuromuscular junction.

In people with a large thymus gland or a thymoma, a surgical operation is performed to remove the gland. This operation can also lead to some relief from symptoms in up to half of patients.

The red flags of diseases of the spinal cord and peripheral nerves

Some patients with diseases of the spinal cord and peripheral nerves will benefit from referral to a conventional doctor for assessment and/or treatment. Red flags are those symptoms and signs that will indicate that referral should be considered. The red flags of these conditions are described in Table 4.1g-I. A summary of the red flags in a format designed for quick reference in clinical practice can be found in Appendix III. This gives advice on the degree of urgency of referral for each of the red flag conditions listed.

Table 4.1g-I A25: Red flags of diseases of the spinal cord and peripheral nerves

Red flag	Description	Reasoning
A25.1	Any sudden or gradual onset of objectively quantifiable muscle weakness (e.g. weak grip or difficulty in standing from sitting) For Bell's palsy (facial muscle weakness), see A25.2	It is important to distinguish true muscle weakness from a perception of muscle weakness (a common complaint, particularly in people who are chronically tired or depressed). In true muscle weakness there will be real limitation in performing simple day-to-day activities such as brushing teeth or walking Asking the patient to move muscles against resistance is a simple way of gauging the muscle strength, and is particularly effective in demonstrating if the weakness is asymmetrical (e.g. a one-sided weakness of grip would be very clearly felt on resisted moves of the hands and arms) Muscle weakness may result from conditions of the brain, spinal cord, peripheral nerves and neuromuscular junction, as well as the muscles themselves. As so many of these conditions are potentially serious, it is wise to refer all patients with muscle weakness for a medical diagnosis The rare condition of Guillain-Barré syndrome can lead to a rapidly progressive weakness of the limbs. This would be accompanied by numbness of the hands and feet (it is a peripheral neuropathy). If the patient with these symptoms becomes unable to walk, refer urgently, as the condition, rarely, can progress to affect the respiratory muscles
A25.2	Bell's palsy (facial weakness)	Bell's palsy is thought to be the result of a viral infection affecting the facial nerve. In rare cases it may be the result of a more serious underlying condition, such as tumor, multiple sclerosis or Lyme disease The onset can be dramatic, with one-sided facial paralysis developing over the course of 1–2 days The patient may be unable to move their mouth, lift their eyebrows and, importantly, not be able to close the eye on the affected side Bell's palsy requires high-priority referral, as early treatment with antiviral and corticosteroid medication may improve the chances of full resolution of symptoms. Also, the health of the cornea of the eye needs to be assessed regularly in the early stages (it can become damaged if the eyelid is not able to be closed fully)
A25.3	Features of polymyalgia rheumatica: prolonged pain and stiffness and weakness of the muscles of the hips and shoulders associated with malaise and depression Refer urgently if there is a sudden onset of a severe, one-sided temporal headache or visual disturbances	Polymyalgia rheumatica is an inflammatory condition of the muscles of the shoulders and hips, which predominantly afflicts people >50 years. Because it is inflammatory in nature, there may be associated malaise, but the main symptoms are pain and weakness of the shoulder and hip muscles. Difficulty in standing from a sitting position is a classic sign of hip weakness In polymyalgia rheumatica there is an increased risk of the serious condition of temporal arteritis. Referral is needed for treatment with corticosteroids (see A23.5)

A25.4	Any sudden or gradual onset of unexplained, measurable numbness or pins and needles (either generalized or localized), unless symptoms suggest benign nerve root impingement	Numbness can arise from problems in the brain, spinal cord and the peripheral nerves. All these have potentially serious underlying causes, so if the cause is unclear the patient should be referred for a medical diagnosis
		Vague numbness is a subjective complaint that is commonly described, but when tested the person can actually distinguish between different types of touch on the numb area. Measurable numbness here refers to the finding that there is the inability to distinguish between the pain of a pin-prick and the touch of a piece of cotton wool
		The most common cause of measurable numbness, however, is compression of nerve roots, in either the neck or sacral region, as a result of osteoarthritis of the spine and sacrum or increased muscle spasm
		These are benign causes of numbness, and are distinguished by having a one-sided distribution on either the side of an arm and hand or down the back of the leg (sciatica)
		In this case, if the diagnosis of nerve root impingement is correct, physical treatment (e.g. with acupuncture and massage and specific muscle-stretching exercises) should relieve the numbness as the muscle tension resolves. Refer if there is no improvement in one week and urgently if there are any features of cauda equina syndrome (see A25.5)
A25.5	Cauda equina syndrome: • numbness of the buttocks and perineum (saddle anesthesia) • bilateral numbness or sciatica in the legs • difficulty in urination or defecation • impaired sexual function	The cauda equina (horse's tail) is the bunch of nerves that descends from the bottom of the spinal cord from the level of L1–L2 downwards. These nerve roots supply sensation and motor impulses to the perineum, buttocks, groin and legs
		Cauda equina syndrome suggests the compression of a number of these roots (usually from a central prolapsed disc, but possibly from tumor or other spinal growth). This is a serious situation, as prolonged compression of the perineal nerve supply can lead to permanent problems with urination, defecation and sexual function
		Refer as a high priority
A25.6	The features of early shingles: intense, one-sided pain, with an overlying rash of crops of fluid-filled reddened and crusting blisters. The pain and rash correspond in location to a neurological dermatome. The pain may precede the rash by 1–2 days	Shingles is an outbreak of the chickenpox virus (varicella zoster) that has lain dormant within a spinal nerve root since an earlier episode of chickenpox. It tends to reactivate when the person is run down and exposed to intense sunlight, and is more common in elderly people
		Warn the patient that the condition is contagious, and advise that immediate treatment (within 48 hours of onset of the rash) with the antiviral drug aciclovir has been proven to reduce the severity of prolonged pain after recovery of the rash. For this reason it is necessary to refer as a high priority to a doctor for advice on medical management
A25.7	Trigeminal neuralgia (TGN) (and other forms of one-sided facial pain): lancinating pain on one side of the face, which radiates out from a focal point in response to defined triggers. May be associated with twitching (tic douloureux)	TGN is excruciating facial pain, often triggered by light touch or wind, which radiates from a defined point in a predictable distribution on one side of the face
		The common (and benign) form may be the result of pressure on the trigeminal nerve within the skull by a blood vessel, but is rarely the result of something more serious, such as a brain tumor or multiple sclerosis
		For this reason, a person with unexplained facial pain should be referred for full investigation
		Microsurgical treatments have recently been found to have success in intractable cases

The Musculoskeletal System

4.2

4.2a The physiology of the musculoskeletal system

The musculoskeletal system consists of the bony skeleton, the joints and the muscles. Its functions are to support the soft tissues of the body, to protect the deep organs and to enable the movements of the body. In addition, as described in Stage 3, the bones contain the marrow spaces in which most of the maturation of the blood cells takes place.

This section considers in turn the physiology of the bony skeleton, the joints and the muscles. It is assumed that the reader has a basic knowledge of the shape, position and names of the bones, joints and muscles.

The physiology of the bony skeleton[20]

All bone consists of a combination of a hard, non-living substance containing salts of calcium and phosphorus together with a vast number of living bone cells. The non-living part of bone is structured upon a scaffolding of numerous connective tissue fibers. It is this complex material that persists after death when the rest of the body has decayed. Nevertheless, in life, this seemingly fixed aspect of bone is constantly in a state of change, as the bone cells are always active in reshaping this hard material according to the needs of the body.

There are two main types of bone tissue. Compact bone is a dense but very strong material present in all bones at their margins. Cancellous bone is more spongy and filled with red marrow, and is particularly rich in the shafts of the long bones and the ribs, the center of the vertebral bodies and the core of the pelvic bones. In both types of

bone a rich network of vessels supplies the bone cells, the osteocytes, with blood and lymph fluid.

The bony skeleton is made up of four different types of bone, categorized according to their shape: the long bones (e.g. the femur and the humerus), the irregular bones (e.g. the vertebrae and the carpal bones), the flat bones (e.g. the sternum and the skull) and the sesamoid bones (e.g. the patella and the pisiform bone). In terms of physiology, the important distinction to be made is between the long bones and the three other types of bone (irregular, flat and sesamoid).

Long bones

The long bones (see Figure 4.2a-I) in the body are the radius, ulna and humerus of the arm and the femur, tibia and fibula of the leg. They are characterized by a shaft and two widened ends known as epiphyses. The shaft is composed of dense, strong compact bone, with a central hollow that is filled with fatty yellow bone marrow. The epiphyses are the site of bone growth in the child, and are largely composed of soft, spongy cancellous bone containing bloody red marrow, all bounded by a rim of strong compact bone. The epiphyses are covered with hyaline cartilage in the regions where they make joints with other bones; elsewhere the long bones are bounded by a fibrous coat called the periosteum. Underneath the periosteum lie clusters of osteoblasts and osteoclasts, the bone-forming cells responsible for bone remodeling and production. These cells are stimulated to form and reshape new bone when the periosteum or underlying bone becomes damaged. The design of the long bones confers strength, which is necessary for their main functions of locomotion, posture and manipulation.

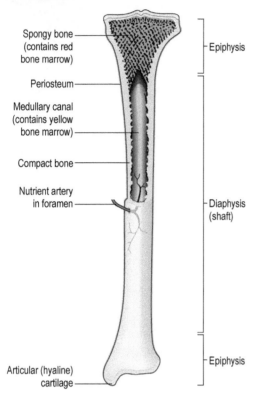

Figure 4.2a-I The structure of a long bone (partially sectioned)

Short, irregular, flat and sesamoid bones

The short bones are less strong than the long bones because they are composed largely of spongy, cancellous, red, marrow-containing bone, and are bounded by a relatively thin protective rim of compact bone. This structure (see Figure 4.2a-II) supports their functions of intricate movements (in the back, hands and feet), protection (skull bones, pelvis and ribs) and bone marrow production.

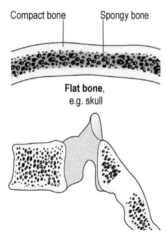

Figure 4.2a-II The structure of flat and irregular bones (sectioned)

The blood-forming marrow

It is the red marrow that is the site of the development of the blood cells. This marrow is abundant in the vertebrae and the flat bones of the skull, ribs, sternum and pelvis.

The growth of bone in childhood and adolescence

An understanding of how bones grow is relevant to the pathology of a number of the diseases of bone. In the fetus there is initially no hard bony material. Instead, at the future site of the long and irregular bones, soft cartilage, a form of connective tissue, appears. At the site of the flat bones a soft tissue membrane develops. Gradually, as birth approaches, osteoblast cells within these areas of soft tissue secrete the hard substance that will form the non-living part of bone. This process of transformation of soft tissue into hard bone is called ossification. When bone has ossified, some of the osteoblasts mature into the bone cells situated deep within bone, where they are known as osteocytes.

This means that in the newborn only a small part of each of the bones is mature hard bone. For example, at the time of birth, only the centers of the skull bones have ossified. The edges of these flat bones are still thick membrane, which allows for some flexibility of movement between the skull bones (very important during childbirth). This soft membrane is most prominent in the diamond-shaped soft spot (the fontanel) that can be felt on the top of the head of most babies under one year of age.

The bones do not fully ossify until early adulthood. Until then, there are still some areas of cartilage or membrane that are actively forming new bone and allowing for growth. Because of this, the approximate age of a child can be estimated from an X-ray image of the bones, which shows the state of progression of ossification of the bones. Puberty is a time during which the surge of sex hormones causes an initial spurt of growth of long bones followed by ossification of the growth centers in the long bones (see Section 5.2a). This is why growth slows considerably once puberty has been reached.

The continued growth of bones

After early adulthood the bones do not change significantly in size. Nevertheless, the osteoblasts remain active in secreting new bone. This laying down of new bone is counterbalanced by the activity of another type of bone cell called the osteoclast. The osteoclasts act continually to digest old bone and to return the calcium, phosphorus and other nutrients within the bone back to the circulation for reuse. This process, known as remodeling, allows bones to become stronger in areas in which there is perpetual physical stress (e.g. the upper part of the femur in someone who is physically active) and allows for the repair of bones in the case of fracture.

The rate of remodeling of bone is influenced by various hormones of the endocrine system. The thyroid hormones, growth hormone from the pituitary gland and insulin from the pancreas stimulate the correct development and ossification of the bones. In puberty, testosterone and estrogen stimulate the growth spurt, and also the changes that differentiate the male and female adult skeletons. Estrogen also helps to maintain the calcium content of bones in premenopausal women. In addition, two hormones secreted from the region of the thyroid gland, calcitonin and parathyroid hormone, are essential in the control of the balance of the activity of the osteoblasts and the osteoclasts.

Vitamin D is an essential factor in the maintenance of the non-living (calcified) part of bone. In vitamin D deficiency the bones become softened. This leads to bowing of the bones during childhood (rickets) and pain and weakness in adulthood (osteomalacia). These conditions are discussed in more detail in Section 4.2d.

The structure of the skeleton

The skeleton can be considered as consisting of two parts: the axial skeleton and the appendicular skeleton. The axial skeleton (shaded bones in Figure 4.2a-III) forms the central bony core of the body, and consists of the skull, vertebral bones, sacrum, coccyx, ribs and sternum. All these bones are either flat or irregular, and so each is composed of a core of red marrow-containing cancellous bone surrounded by a thin rim of compact bone. The skull and the vertebral column support and protect the fragile structure of the brain and spinal cord. The ribs and sternum likewise support and protect the lungs and the heart in the thorax, and the organs of the upper abdomen, including the liver, kidneys, pancreas and the spleen.

The appendicular skeleton (unshaded bones in Figure 4.2a-III) is so called because it consists of the appendages to the axial skeleton. These are the shoulder girdle (clavicles and shoulder blades), the upper limbs, the pelvic girdle (the hip bones) and the lower limbs. The bones of the shoulder girdle and the pelvic girdle are flat bones. The bones of the limbs are either long bones or irregular bones.

The healing of bones

Healthy bones are strong and slightly flexible. In health, bones will only break if exposed to significant trauma. Fractures of healthy bone can be classified as simple, compound or greenstick. If a fracture occurs because the bone is weakened in some way by an underlying disease process, it is described as a pathological fracture.

A simple fracture describes when the ends of the bone do not protrude through the skin, whereas a compound fracture involves a break to the skin by the sharp end of the fractured bone. A greenstick fracture occurs in the flexible bones of young children. In this fracture, the break is incomplete, as the bone is far less brittle than the fully ossified adult bone. This means that the bone bends like a green stick, rather than snapping into two.

The healing of broken bones can be compared to the healing of wounds in that it is the formation of a blood clot in the space between the broken ends that initiates the healing process. Figure 4.2a-IV illustrates the stages in the healing of the broken shaft of a long bone. The blood clot stimulates the inward movement of phagocytes and osteoblasts. The phagocytes remove unwanted debris, while the osteoblasts lay down an initially chaotic mass of new bone called callus. The callus is gradually remodeled by osteoclasts into new, ordered compact bone. In adults this process takes weeks to months, but it is significantly quicker in children.

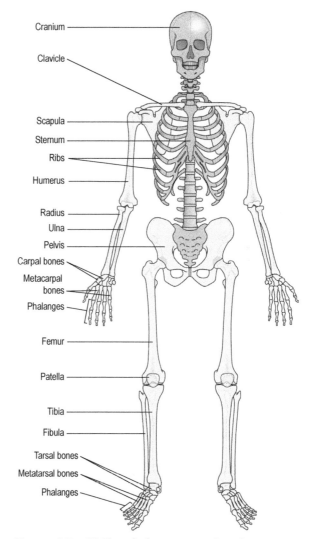

Figure 4.2a-III The skeleton: anterior view (the bones of the axial skeleton are shaded)

Inflamed area

1 — Hematoma and bone fragments

2 — Phagocytosis of clot and debris. Growth of granulation tissue begins

3 — Osteoblasts begin to form new bone (callus)

4 — Gradual spread and mineralization of callus to bridge the gap

5 — Bone almost healed. Osteoclasts reshape and canalize new bone

Figure 4.2a-IV The stages in bone healing

 Information box 4.2a-I

The bones: comments from a Chinese medicine perspective

In Chinese medicine, the bones and bone marrow have a relationship with two of the extraordinary Yang organs: the Bones and the Marrow.

The Marrow corresponds to the substance that nourishes and forms nervous tissue and the bone marrow, and which is produced by Kidney Essence. Therefore, if the Kidneys are Deficient, the bone marrow will be weak.

The Bones correspond directly to the physiological bones. They are nourished by Kidney Essence and Marrow, and will also become weak if the Kidneys are Deficient.

The physiology of the joints

The joints are the sites in the body at which two or more bones come together. They are essential for allowing free, but controlled, movement of the body.

There are three categories of joint in the body: the fixed or fibrous joints (e.g. the sutures of the skull), the slightly movable or cartilaginous joints (e.g. symphysis pubis and intervertebral joints) and the movable or synovial joints (e.g. the elbow, knee and ankle).

Fibrous joints involve two edges of bone that are linked by tough strands of fibrous connective tissue. The suture lines of the skull are an example of fibrous joints (see Figure 4.2a-V). The movement at a fibrous joint is limited.

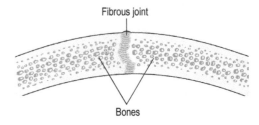

Fibrous joint

Bones

Figure 4.2a-V An example of a fibrous joint: a suture line of the skull

Cartilaginous joints offer the potential for more movement because the bones in these joints are linked by a pad of fibrocartilage, which has more spring and bulk than the fibrous strands of a fibrous joint. In the pubis symphysis and in between the vertebral bodies this fibrocartilage pad has a shock-absorbing function (see Figure 4.2a-VI).

Figure 4.2a-VI An example of a cartilaginous joint: the intervertebral joint

Synovial joints offer the most movement and have the most complex structure (see Figure 4.2a-VII).

Figure 4.2a-VII An example of a synovial joint: section of the knee joint viewed from the side

The internal surface of the bones in synovial joints is lined with glassy smooth hyaline articular cartilage, and the rest of the joint space is bound by a fibrous joint capsule (the capsular ligament). The internal surface of the joint is lined with a fluid-secreting synovial membrane. The term synovial has its root in the Greek word *ovum* meaning egg. This is because the lubricating fluid contained within these joints has been likened in consistency to the white of an egg. The whole joint is given stability by means of fibrous bands (the ligaments) that link the bones and also by the muscle insertions (the tendons) that cross the joint to insert close to its margins.

Some of the synovial joints have unique additional features; for example, the knee joint illustrated in Figure 4.2a-VII contains thickened C-shaped cartilage pads, which sit on the tibial plateau, and two cruciate (crossing) ligaments, which run through the joint space to provide anterior to posterior stability.

Close to the large joints such as the knee, hip and shoulder are fluid-filled sacs lined with synovial membrane called bursae (singular bursa). The purpose of a bursa is

to prevent friction between the layers of tissue overlying the joint.

There is a wide range of structures of synovial joints, although all have the same basic features listed above. Diverse examples include the ball-and-socket joint of the hip, the hinge mechanism of the elbow, the pivot provided by the atlantoaxial joint (between the C1 and C2 vertebrae) and the complementary saddle shapes of many of the small bones of the hands and feet.

Information box 4.2a-II

The joints: comments from a Chinese medicine perspective

The physiological joints are made up of bone, ligaments and synovial fluid, further supported by muscles. In this way their health is dependent on Kidney Essence, Liver Qi and Blood, and Gallbladder Qi, all of which are said to have direct correspondences with these aspects.

The fluid that lubricates the joints in Chinese medicine is called Ye, and is under the control of the Spleen and the Kidneys.

The physiology of the skeletal muscles

The muscles responsible for the movement of the bony joints are all largely composed of skeletal muscle fibers (cells). The muscle fibers run parallel to one another within each muscle, and are bound together by fibrous connective tissue. The muscle fibers converge at two or more fibrous structures, called tendons, at the extremities of the muscle. Tendons usually insert into part of the bony skeleton, but in some muscles they attach to the connective tissue of the skin (e.g. in the muscles of facial expression). The fibrous tissue of muscles (including the tendons) is glistening white and contains blood vessels and fat cells. This is the tissue that gives a raw steak its streaky appearance.

The muscle fibers contract in unison in response to motor nerve impulses (see Section 4.1a). Each muscle fiber receives electrical impulses from a nerve fiber via a specialized synapse called the motor end plate. At this synapse, the electrical impulse traveling down the nerve fiber leads to the release of a neurotransmitter chemical. This chemical stimulates the changes within the muscle fiber that culminate in a temporary contraction. The contraction is sustained only for as long as the nerve continues to stimulate the motor end plate.

Muscles act because they are attached to at least two separate parts of the body, and because they can contract.

When a muscle contracts, it draws the two or more parts of the body to which it is attached closer together, and this leads to movement.

Most skeletal muscles never attain a state of full relaxation. There is always a low level of nervous stimulation to the muscles, which gives them a firmness known as tone. This background level of tone is essential for correct posture. It is generated as a result of reflex nervous activity at the level of the spinal cord, and is modified further by nervous impulses originating from higher control centers in the brain (see Section 4.1a). If the nerve supply to a muscle is cut off, the muscle becomes completely flaccid, and loses the springy quality that is the normal state in good health.

Muscles act in a variety of ways, of which the biceps brachii, the buccinator and the pelvic floor muscles are good examples. These three muscles have the diverse effects of limb movement, facial expression and support of soft tissues respectively. The biceps (brachii) muscle of the upper arm is an example of a muscle that acts over a synovial joint (the elbow). The biceps has two tendon insertions on the scapula at its proximal end and a single distal insertion into the radius. The flat buccinator muscle of the cheek is an example of a muscle that inserts only into the connective tissue of skin to allow for the movements of the mouth. The muscles of the pelvic floor insert into bone (they are slung between the ischium of the pelvis and the sacrum and coccyx), but do not cause movement at a joint. Instead, by contracting they give support to the tissues of the pelvic floor and are important for maintaining continence of feces and urine.

Information box 4.2a-III

The muscles: comments from a Chinese medicine perspective

The muscles are made up of flesh, tendons and sinews. Their health is dependent on healthy Spleen, Liver and Gallbladder Qi.

Spleen Qi is more responsible for the springy fleshy quality resulting from healthy muscle tone, whereas Liver and Gallbladder Qi are responsible for the power of contraction and the movement that results.

The knots and excessive tone often felt in overtense muscles are usually a reflection of Liver Qi (and Blood) Stagnation. This, in turn, is more likely to occur in muscles that are weak as a result of Spleen Qi Deficiency.[21]

Information box 4.2a-IV

The musculoskeletal system: comments from a Chinese medicine perspective

A healthy musculoskeletal system is dependent on the health of the Kidney, Liver, Gallbladder and Spleen Organs. Kidney Essence is of particular importance to the bones. Healthy Blood and Yin are important for lubricating and nourishing the muscles and joints, as well as for preventing Stagnation of Qi. Hence, muscle and joint pains, stiffness or inflamed tendons can result if Blood and Yin, in particular, of the Liver, are deficient.

4.2b The investigation of the musculoskeletal system

Diseases of the bones, joints and muscles are investigated within two distinct conventional specialties. Diseases that are likely to require medical treatment with drugs are referred to a physician known as a rheumatologist, while those conditions that are likely to require surgery are referred to an orthopedic surgeon.

An investigation of the musculoskeletal system might involve:

- a thorough physical examination

- investigations to examine the structure of the bones, muscles and joints (X-ray imaging, ultrasound imaging, magnetic resonance imaging (MRI) and bone scans)

- examination of the blood to look for disturbances in the hormones and chemicals that reflect bone disorders and autoimmune diseases

- examination of the synovial fluid of a joint

- arthroscopy, the endoscopic examination of the interior of a joint.

These investigations are considered briefly in turn below.

Physical examination

The physical examination is a very important aspect of the examination of the musculoskeletal system. A skilled examiner can identify the site and nature of a wide range of musculoskeletal problems without the need for further investigations. For each joint and muscle group there is a range of specific physical tests that can be performed to examine for particular disorders. For example, the FABER (flexion, abduction and external rotation) test is used to examine for a painful disorder of the hip joint.

The physical examination of the musculoskeletal system involves the stages listed in Table 4.2b-I.

Table 4.2b-I The stages in physical examination of the musculoskeletal system

Examination of the gait, posture and general appearance: this can reveal the characteristic features of musculoskeletal disease, such as a characteristic limp, areas of one-sided muscle wasting or postural deformity due to arthritis

Examination of the muscle groups: looking specifically for areas of wasting or fine twitching, feeling for knots or swellings, and assessing the strength of the muscle groups

Examination of the bones: looking specifically for areas of deformity or shortening, feeling for deformity, swellings or areas of tenderness, and percussion of the bones to examine for deep tenderness

Examination of the joints: looking specifically for redness, swelling and deformity, feeling for heat and tenderness, and passively moving a joint to assess range of movement and the strength of the muscles that cause movement of the joint (active movement). In the case of a localized joint problem, the joint is examined using a range of specific tests

---

X-ray imaging

X-ray imaging is the most common investigation performed for musculoskeletal disease. This is because it is relatively cheap, quick to perform, and often produces an excellent picture of the bony structure of the body. The disadvantage of X-ray imaging is that it exposes the patient to radiation, although this is considered to be of minimal risk if X-ray imaging is only required on rare occasions during the lifetime of a patient.

However, X-ray images cannot reveal much information about muscle problems, and will only reveal changes of arthritis at a late stage in the condition, when the bony surfaces of the joint have become eroded. For this reason, the general medical view is that X-ray images are not helpful in the diagnosis of most cases of low back pain, which are usually the result of muscle strain, prolapsed disc or early arthritis, none of which are revealed on an X-ray image.

Ultrasound scan

This can be a useful and non-invasive test for the examination of a joint and the soft tissues that surround it. It is of particular value in the examination of the shoulder.

Magnetic resonance imaging (MRI)

MRI provides very high-quality information about joints and muscles, and reveals the structure of the low back in detail. However, it is expensive and can be uncomfortable for the patient to experience.

Bone scans

Bone scans involve the injection of a radioactive substance into the bloodstream. This substance is concentrated in areas of bone in which there is active growth, which are then revealed by scanning the body for radioactivity. This is useful for revealing areas where there may be a fracture or the site of bone cancer.

A DEXA (dual energy X-ray absorptiometry) scan is a specialized form of X-ray imaging used to investigate the condition of osteoporosis. This form of bone scan does not necessitate injection of a radioactive substance. Instead, it uses a low dose of X-rays to assess the degree of osteoporosis. The DEXA scan is most usually performed in menopausal women and other people at risk of osteoporosis to assess need for medical treatment for this condition.

Blood tests

There are numerous blood tests that can give some information about diseases of the musculoskeletal system. For example, a serum sample can give information about the levels of the mineral salts of calcium and phosphorus in the blood, as well as whether or not levels of hormones such as parathyroid hormone and calcitonin are within the normal range.

The erythrocyte sedimentation rate (ESR) and C reactive protein (CRP) tests can indicate whether an inflammatory process is going on. There is a range of autoantibodies that can be assayed from a serum sample if an autoimmune disease is suspected. In the case of a chronic autoimmune disease, such as rheumatoid arthritis, a full blood count (FBC) may reveal anemia of chronic disease.

Examination of the synovial fluid of a joint

Synovial fluid may be withdrawn from a joint by means of a needle and syringe for examination in the case of arthritis. If the joint is very swollen with fluid, this simple procedure may also give the patient relief from discomfort. In some cases, after withdrawal of the fluid, a corticosteroid drug may be injected directly into the joint through the same needle.

The fluid may reveal the microorganisms and pus characteristic of infection, and so can be a guide for appropriate antibiotic treatment. In the case of arthritis due to simple inflammation (e.g. autoimmune disease or osteoarthritis) the fluid will be clear. In gout the fluid will contain the microscopic crystals that are the cause of the pain.

There is a small risk of introducing infection into the joint with this procedure.

Arthroscopy

Arthroscopy is a procedure that enables the examination of the interior of a joint, usually the knee. It involves the insertion of a fine endoscope into the joint space via a small incision in the skin overlying the joint. A general anesthetic is usually given. In this way, the integrity of the joint cartilage and any other structures, such as ligaments within the joint, can be examined. In some cases, surgery to the damaged structures within the joint (e.g. a tear in the cartilage within the knee) may be carried out at the same time.

Even if no surgery is carried out, many people report that chronic knee pain is relieved (usually temporarily) following arthroscopy.

4.2c The treatment of musculoskeletal pain

This section explores the way in which conventional medicine manages the problem of pain resulting from musculoskeletal disease. The approach to musculoskeletal pain can be broadly categorized into disease modification and symptom relief.

Disease modification involves the use of medication that actually alters the progression of the underlying disease. Because the disease has been slowed or halted, symptoms abate. The disease-modifying treatments are described in the next three sections on diseases of the musculoskeletal system because they vary according to the disease being treated.

Symptom relief involves the use of medication or other therapies to block the sensation of pain. It does not attempt to alter the underlying disease process. Almost by definition, symptom relief is suppressive in nature. The most common form of symptom relief in musculoskeletal pain is the use of painkillers. The medical term for a painkiller medication is an analgesic.

Analgesics in musculoskeletal disease

Musculoskeletal disease is the most common reason for the prescription of analgesics. Analgesics are also used for a wide range of other conditions, including headache, menstrual pain and the pain of cancer. The analgesics used can be broadly categorized into simple analgesics, non-steroidal anti-inflammatory drugs (NSAIDs) and opioid (morphine-like) analgesics. These might be prescribed on their own or in combination with each other. There are, in fact, many analgesic preparations that contain a combination of two drugs that are believed to complement each other in their mode of action (e.g. co-codamol and co-dydramol, which combine paracetamol with codeine and dihydrocodeine, respectively). Other compound analgesics incorporate non-analgesic drugs such as caffeine or decongestant medication.[22]

A vast range of analgesics is available for direct sale to the public. Many of these are compound preparations.

Simple analgesics

The simple analgesics are aspirin and paracetamol. Aspirin is anti-inflammatory in action, which means that it inhibits the chemical communication between the leukocytes that maintain the process of inflammation. Therefore, aspirin acts to reduce the heat (fever), redness, pain and swelling that are characteristic of inflammation. Paracetamol has a poorly understood mechanism of action. It is believed not to be anti-inflammatory. However, its effect is similar to that of aspirin in that it can reduce pain and fever.

Aspirin also reduces the tendency of platelets to stick together. This is why it is of value in the prevention of thrombosis and embolism. For this effect, a very low dose (75mg) is required daily. The analgesic dose is much higher (up to 600mg four times a day).

Aspirin tends to irritate the lining of the digestive tract, although in most cases this effect is mild and painless. However, in some people this can result in severe inflammation, with bleeding into the stomach (gastritis). Other side effects include asthma and rashes. In children under the age of 12 there is a very small risk of a severe form of inflammation of the liver called Reyes syndrome.

Paracetamol has few side effects in low doses, but in overdose it is highly toxic to the liver.

Simple analgesics are recommended for mild pain. Aspirin should not be given to children, and ideally should not be taken at analgesic doses for a long-standing (chronic) condition because of the risk of stomach irritation.

Information box 4.2c-I

Simple analgesics: comments from a Chinese medicine perspective

In Chinese medicine, the reduction in pain from the simple analgesics corresponds to Movement of Stagnation and Clearance of Heat. In pain relief the action is suppressive in nature, as it clears the symptom locally without necessarily addressing the underlying cause.

Aspirin is believed to be generally Warming and Dispersing in nature. In some cases it may enable the Clearing of Wind Cold by causing sweating and the Release of the Exterior. The Warm nature is evidenced by the side effect of Heat in the Stomach. Asthma and rashes suggest that, in some people, aspirin may also depress Lung Qi and permit Wind Heat Invasion.

In high doses, the liver toxicity described in conventional medicine strongly suggests that paracetamol stagnates and damages the Liver Qi from a Chinese medicine viewpoint.

Non-steroidal anti-inflammatory drugs (NSAIDs)

NSAIDs are a family of drugs that have an anti-inflammatory effect similar to that of aspirin. Like aspirin they can reduce pain, fever, redness and swelling, and they also have side effects that include gastric irritation, asthma and rashes. Rarely they can promote cardiovascular thrombotic adverse events.

Commonly prescribed NSAIDs include ibuprofen and diclofenac. Diclofenac is considered to carry more risk of thrombotic events than ibuprofen.

NSAIDs generally have a more powerful effect than aspirin, and are particularly useful in any pain that has inflammation as its root cause. Therefore they are useful in the inflammatory conditions of the musculoskeletal system such as arthritis, tendon and ligament injuries, and most bony pain, including fractures. NSAIDs at maximum dose can be safely used in combination with paracetamol or with opioid analgesics to increase the effect of pain relief.

The side effect of gastric irritation is less marked than for aspirin. Nevertheless, it is recommended that NSAIDs are taken with food. However, NSAIDs can also be toxic to the kidneys in susceptible people, particularly if taken at a high dose for a prolonged period. For this reason they should be used with caution in elderly people or in combination with other medication that may affect the kidney function.

The cyclooxygenase-2 (COX-2) NSAIDs (etoricoxib and celecoxib), which are selective inhibitors, were developed to minimize the risk of upper gastrointestinal bleeding, and short-term data suggest that they do indeed carry a low risk of bleeding events in clinical practice. However, there does seem to be an association between these COX-2 inhibitors and adverse thrombotic cardiac events, and so their use is reserved only for those situations when older-generation NSAIDs cannot be used and risk of cardiovascular disease is low.

For reasons that are unclear, the response in terms of pain relief of an individual to different NSAIDs is unpredictable. For this reason a number of these drugs may be tried in succession before the best effect is found.

Information box 4.2c-II

Non-steroidal anti-inflammatory drugs: comments from a Chinese medicine perspective

In Chinese medicine, the energetic action of NSAIDs is similar to that of aspirin in terms of having a property of Moving Stagnation and Clearing Heat. The side effects suggest that these medications introduce Toxic Heat (rash and gastritis) and can also lead to Stagnation of Blood and Qi (thrombotic events in susceptible people). In the long term, the warming nature of these drugs may deplete Blood and Yin, primarily of the Liver and Kidney (evidenced by long-term damage to both liver and kidney function). They also can adversely affect Lung Qi in some individuals as asthma can be induced by NSAIDs.

Opioid analgesics

Opioid painkillers are so called because their action is similar to that of the naturally occurring drug opium. They all appear to mimic the effect of the body's natural painkillers, the endorphins, and act within the spinal cord and the brain to reduce the sensation of pain.

Opioid analgesics provide strong pain relief, although they do not reduce inflammation directly. They are generally only used in musculoskeletal conditions when pain is very severe (e.g. after acute trauma such as a fracture). They may safely be used in combination with aspirin, paracetamol or NSAIDs. Opioid analgesics include codeine, morphine, buprenorphine, diamorphine (heroin), dihydrocodeine, pethidine and tramadol.

Opioids are highly addictive, and also induce bodily tolerance to the effects of the drug. With recurrent use increasing doses may be required to maintain a steady level of pain relief. They may induce a sense of euphoria or well-being.

The most common adverse side effect is nausea and vomiting. Therefore, anti-sickness medication may have to be prescribed at the same time. Constipation is also a common side effect. With very high doses the depth of breathing may be inhibited, and the patient may fall into a stupor. In overdose, death may result from respiratory failure.

Information box 4.2c-III

Opioids: comments from a Chinese medicine perspective

In Chinese medicine, the pain-relieving effect of opioids would correspond to the Movement of Stagnation. This effect is suppressive in nature, and the side effects indicate profound energetic disturbance. The side effects of euphoria and stupor may reflect the obstructing effect of Heat (at the Blood Level) on the Heart Organ. Constipation may also be a result of Heat, in this case in the Small and Large Intestine. Itch and rashes also are suggestive of Wind and Heat. Suppression of respiration may reflect a Depression of Lung and Kidney Qi. Nausea and vomiting might be seen as a manifestation of Stagnation of Liver Qi and consequent rebellion of Stomach Qi.

In the long term opiates are addictive and promote dependency. The profound effects of Heat on the Heart will lead to Heart Yin Deficiency and also Stagnation of Liver Qi. The person will therefore feel they need more of the drug in a need to deal with the discomfort of these states of imbalance. In the long term the patient on opiates will show signs of Heart/Kidney Yin Deficiency, with Liver and Spleen Disharmony.[23]

Other drugs used for symptom relief in musculoskeletal disease

The two other classes of drugs that are used for symptom relief in musculoskeletal disease are muscle relaxants and corticosteroids.

Muscle relaxants

An important class of drug used to relax tense muscles in musculoskeletal conditions is the benzodiazepine class that includes diazepam and lorazepam. These drugs are most commonly prescribed for their effects in calming anxiety in minor mental illness (see Chapter 6.2).

In certain painful conditions of the joints and muscles, in particular, low back pain, reflex muscle spasm can worsen the underlying pain and may slow healing by making the whole area surrounding the injury rigid. In cases such as these, drugs such as diazepam may be prescribed for a short period (ideally a few days at the most) to relieve the pain and tension caused by the muscle spasm.

The side effects of diazepam include drowsiness and unsteadiness of gait, but these are not usually problematic in short-term use for an acute musculoskeletal problem. Diazepam is also highly addictive, but again, this should not be a problem when used in the short term.

Information box 4.2c-IV

Diazepam: comments from a Chinese medicine perspective

From a Chinese medicine perspective, the calming and slowing effect of benzodiazepines could correlate with a depression of Yang, in particular, of the Liver and Heart. Like alcohol, these medications are considered to be powerfully heating in nature, even though the initial effect is one of sedation. Long-term use will rapidly lead to Liver and Heart Yin Deficiency and so side effects of agitation and heat become manifest, and explain the addictive properties of these medications.[24] Side effects of drowsiness and unsteadiness indicate that in excess it might also be seen as Phlegm Forming.

Corticosteroids

Corticosteroids may be used for their disease-modifying properties in the forms of arthritis that result from autoimmune disease (e.g. rheumatoid arthritis). In this case, they are given regularly by mouth to calm the underlying inflammatory process.

Corticosteroids may also be administered by injection to reduce local inflammation in a wide range of musculoskeletal conditions. The injection can be directed into a joint in cases of arthritis, or around a tendon in cases of tendonitis (e.g. tennis elbow). The injection may bring about rapid relief in the symptoms of inflammation, and can be relatively long acting (days to weeks).

The side effects are mostly a consequence of the locally high concentration of steroids in the tissues. They include wasting of the tissues below the skin (fat atrophy) and, in rare cases, weakening of the connective tissue of the tendons themselves. Occasionally, tendons may rupture as a result. The anti-inflammatory properties of steroids may promote the development of infection (unchecked by the immune system), which can have disastrous effects within a joint.

Information box 4.2c-V

Corticosteroid injections: comments from a Chinese medicine perspective

The effects of corticosteroid injections might be interpreted as Clearing of Heat by Moving of Stagnation. These effects are suppressive. Other side effects (e.g. irritation of the stomach lining and mental agitation) suggest that corticosteroids are actually profoundly Heating in nature, and eventually lead to Qi and Yin Deficiency and accumulation of Phlegm Damp. Fat atrophy and wasting of tendons could be a manifestation of Depletion of Yin and Qi of the tissues.

Non-drug methods of pain relief in musculoskeletal disease

Many patients with chronic musculoskeletal disease are referred to an orthopedic physiotherapist who may use one or more of the following approaches to relieve pain. Unfortunately, because of the time-consuming nature of many of these therapies, they are not always available free of charge within the UK National Health Service (NHS).

Advice and training on posture and physical exercises

This is commonly offered, as it is considered a therapy that can help patients to help themselves. Usually, a few appointments are offered to teach the patient some basic exercises to help strengthen muscles or stretch out tense areas. It is probably true that if all patients could stick to an allotted exercise regimen, much discomfort from muscular and arthritic problems would be relieved. Unfortunately, many people are not able to generate the commitment required for a regular exercise and posture routine, particularly if little long-term follow-up of their progress is arranged.

Manipulation and massage

Some physiotherapists are skilled in the manipulation of joints and massage of tense muscles. Specialized approaches such as osteopathy and chiropractic are rarely available within a state-funded healthcare system, even though there can be much overlap between the therapies offered within these disciplines and physiotherapy. All these therapies can realign displaced skeletal structure, relieve muscle spasm and allow for stretching of tense muscles. They may need to be repeated to be of long-term benefit. Heat and ice packs may also be used to relieve pain and swelling.

 Information box 4.2c-VI

Exercises, massage and manipulation: comments from a Chinese medicine perspective

The Chinese medicine interpretation of appropriate exercise and correction of posture is that it helps to move Stagnant Liver Qi and benefits the Kidneys. This is an energetically appropriate treatment, as long as it is not too strenuous. Tai chi and yoga are examples of exercise programs that offer postures and movements to benefit particular organ systems, in addition to the overall benefit of Moving of Liver Qi and Nourishing Kidney Qi.

Massage and manipulation will enable the Moving of Stagnant Qi and Blood. However, if an underlying imbalance is not attended to, this form of therapy can be suppressive in nature, by dissipating a symptom without addressing the underlying cause.

Ultrasound, TENS and local acupuncture

Physiotherapists use ultrasound, TENS (transcutaneous electrical nerve stimulation) and local acupuncture to relieve the pain in localized musculoskeletal problems. Ultrasound therapy involves focusing ultrasound waves so that they are concentrated at the site of the injury. TENS involves the passage of a low-voltage electrical current across the affected area of the body via electrode pads fixed to the skin. The acupuncture offered by physiotherapists often involves the use of local and tender (Ah shi) points to give pain relief and reduction in spasm.

The mechanism of all three approaches is not clearly understood in conventional terms, although there is a belief that all have a similar action in stimulating suppressive neurotransmitters (including endorphins) within the spinal cord and the brain.

 Information box 4.2c-VII

Ultrasound, TENS and local acupuncture: comments from a Chinese medicine perspective

In Chinese medicine, all three of these treatments will move Blood and Qi Stagnation and may enable the Clearance of Pathogenic Factors. However, if the underlying imbalance is not attended to, all three may be suppressive in action.

Anesthetic and surgical approaches to pain relief

In some cases of severe intractable pain, specialized procedures can be performed to reduce the sensation of pain. These involve the deadening or destroying of nerves or nerve roots within the peripheral nervous system. Anesthetists or surgeons carry out these procedures.

4.2d Diseases of the bones

This section is concerned with the important diseases that affect the bones. The diseases of the bone marrow have already been summarized in Section 3.4e. The conditions studied here are:

- Generalized disorders of the formation of bone:
  - osteoporosis
  - Paget's disease
  - Rickets and osteomalacia (vitamin D deficiency)
- Inherited or childhood bone disorders:
  - achondroplasia (dwarfism)
  - brittle bone disease (osteogenesis imperfecta)
- Infections of the bone:
  - osteomyelitis
- Tumors of the bone:
  - benign tumors
  - malignant osteosarcoma
- Metastatic disease of the bone.

Generalized disorders of the formation of bone

Osteoporosis

Osteoporosis is a term used to describe a condition in which the actual amount of bony material within the bones is decreased, meaning that there are more spaces within the bone tissue. This has the effect of weakening the bones, and the bones look pale on an X-ray image. In lay terms, the bones in osteoporosis are thin. In conventional medical terminology, the term low bone density means the same thing.

The solidity or density of bone normally increases rapidly as a response to the hormone surge of puberty. At this time the bones in a healthy adolescent become more heavy and resistant to fracture. From the age of about 40 onwards there is a progressive natural decline in this density of bone. This decline is called bone loss. In men bone loss

continues gradually into old age. In some women the rate of bone loss increases very rapidly at the menopause, when the natural levels of estrogen suddenly drop, and bone density can suddenly become significantly reduced over a relatively short period of a few years.

Certain factors reduce the rate of bone loss. These include a healthy vitamin- and calcium-rich diet and a moderate level of physical activity from childhood. Weight-bearing physical activity (e.g. walking and running rather than swimming) is known to be particularly important in the maintenance of good bone density.

Factors that increase the rate of bone loss include a poor diet, physical inactivity, reduced levels of estrogen in women (including early menopause), smoking and chronic diseases. The amenorrhea that affects some women athletes and women with anorexia will lead to thinned bones if prolonged. It follows that excessive physical activity may not necessarily be so beneficial to the bones in women. Numerous pregnancies and prolonged periods of breastfeeding will also deplete calcium reserves in the bone. It is now known that it is very significant if any of these factors are present in adolescence, as the bones will then never achieve the optimum starting point of bone density after the growth spurt. This is of concern in Westernized countries today in which adolescents tend to live an increasingly sedentary existence and eat a highly processed diet. In addition, particularly in girls, eating disorders are increasingly prevalent in younger age groups.

Osteoporosis is of enormous health concern in developed countries, in which there is an increasing proportion of the population who are elderly. Osteoporotic hip fractures will affect 15 percent of all women and 5 percent of men from the age of 60. A hip fracture can have disastrous consequences in an older person. A high percentage of people who suffer from these fractures either die as a direct result of the injury or complications of the fracture, or suffer from long-term disability.

The symptoms of osteoporosis can be broadly categorized according to the age and sex of the patient, although there is much overlap between the categories.

In some postmenopausal women a very rapid decline in cancellous bone mass causes the vertebrae in the cervical and thoracic spine to thin very quickly. These spongy bones are then at risk of collapsing under the weight of the head and upper body. This form of crush fracture can be very painful and will lead to progressive bowing forward of the upper back. In extreme cases, the so-called dowager's hump develops. In addition, there is particular thinning of the distal end of the radius, which means that a fall onto the outstretched hand may lead to a fracture of the wrist (Colles fracture).

In more elderly people (over the age of 70) the strength of the compact bone of the long bones is more gradually reduced, and it is at this stage that hip fracture becomes more common. The vertebrae of the spine also soften and compress down, but because the bone loss is less abrupt, sudden painful crush fractures are less common.

The ideal approach to the management of osteoporosis is prevention. Ideally, this begins in adolescence with a calcium-rich diet and regular, moderate weight-bearing exercise. Women in particular are encouraged to keep up a calcium-rich diet, particularly when breastfeeding. Ideally, all people should keep up a steady level of activity throughout adult life in order to minimize the rate of bone loss.

Osteoporosis can be graded in severity by means of a DEXA scan, in which bone density of the lumbar spine and hip are assessed. The results are expressed in the form of a T score, in which a negative value suggests lower than predicted bone density for a young healthy adult. A T score below −1 would lead a doctor to consider preventive medical treatment.

Hormone replacement therapy (HRT) used to be a widely prescribed preventive treatment for osteoporosis in perimenopausal and postmenopausal women. However, recent clinical research following large groups of women on HRT has prompted the UK Committee on Safety of Medicines (CSM) to advise that HRT is no longer recommended as a principal (first-line) treatment for osteoporosis. This guidance has come in the light of the link between HRT and an increased risk of venous thromboembolism, breast cancer, ovarian cancer and endometrial cancer. The clinical studies also demonstrated that HRT has a less protective effect against the development of coronary heart disease than was previously believed, and may even have a deleterious effect if used in older women ten years or more after the menopause.[25]

The bisphosphonates form a class of drugs that is increasingly used in established early osteoporosis. These drugs prevent the action of the osteoclasts in breaking down bone, and do seem to slow bone loss and reduce the fracture rate. Alendronate sodium (alendronic acid) and risedronate sodium are two types of bisphosphonate in common use. Nausea and esophagitis are unwelcome common side effects. A serious dental side effect is osteonecrosis of the jaw, and results from long-term bisphosphonate use, usually in people who have established dental disease. In osteonecrosis there is failure of damaged jaw bone to heal, and this can progress to a state of chronic inflammation in which breaks in the gum lining expose regions of unhealthy bone.

 Information box 4.2d-I

Osteoporosis: comments from a Chinese medicine perspective

In Chinese medicine, the thinning of bones in osteoporosis corresponds to Deficiency of Kidney Essence. The gradual decline in bone density corresponds to the idea in Chinese medicine that Essence gradually declines from its maximum flourishing state in early adulthood. Attention to a healthy diet and moderate exercise will allow for a measured and natural decline of Kidney Yin and Jing, whereas under- or over-exercising and poor diet will Deplete Kidney Yin and Jing. Pregnancy and breastfeeding are draining of Blood and Yin.

The hormone estrogen enables the expression of healthy Spleen Qi and Yin, as evidenced by its beneficial effect on fleshiness and fertility. HRT likewise Boosts Yin, but this may be at the expense of drawing on reserves of Kidney Yin and Jing. The common side effects of HRT include headaches, fluid retention and weight gain. There is also an increased risk of breast, ovarian and womb cancer and venous thromboembolism and stroke. This suggests that HRT might promote Stagnation of Liver Qi and Blood and Accumulation of Phlegm and Damp. These symptoms are a manifestation of drug-induced disease, as HRT is not identical to natural estrogen, nor, if used postmenopausally, is it taken at the time of life when estrogen is produced naturally. As HRT actually suppresses the natural progression to the menopause, these symptoms may even be a form of expression of suppressed imbalance.

By slowing bone loss, bisphosphonates appear to directly Boost the Kidneys and Jing, but are Depleting to Spleen Qi and Stomach Yin, as evidenced by the very common side effects of nausea and esophageal ulceration. This tells us they are suppressive in nature and also powerfully Heating. Osteonecrosis of the jaw is an indication of poor bone health and also localized Heat/Phlegm and Blood Stagnation.

Vitamin D and calcium nourish the bones, and are therefore nourishing to the Kidneys and Jing. In normal dietary quantities this treatment is curative in nature, but the possible adverse cardiovascular effects suggest that excess medicinal calcium may also introduce drug-induced disease (by promoting atheroma development).

Calcium and vitamin D in a low-dose chalky tablet or effervescent preparation are widely prescribed together as a preventive treatment in elderly people, often together with bisphosphonates. This treatment, which is less well supported by evidence of benefit than the bisphosphonates, should be unnecessary if dietary intake is adequate, but a poor diet and poor absorption may work together in old age to reduce intake of calcium.[26] More recently, concerns have been expressed about possible adverse effects on the cardiovascular system from calcium supplementation,[27] but current practice is still to recommend twice daily use in those at risk of osteoporosis.

A late preventive measure is to prevent the occurrence of falls in elderly people. Exercise programs can improve muscle strength and improve balance, and therefore may prevent falls. Regular tai chi classes are one of the active measures that have been shown in experimental studies to reduce the incidence of falls in elderly people.[28]

Paget's disease

Paget's disease is a disease of the aging bones that affects up to 10 percent of adults by the age of 90. In this condition the process of bone remodeling is imbalanced, with both excessive absorption of old bone (by osteoclasts) and excessive formation of new bone (by osteoblasts) taking place.

The affected areas of bone may become enlarged and irregular, but the bones are actually structurally weak and more prone to fracture. An increased blood supply causes the affected bone to feel warmer than other parts of the body. Most patients with Paget's disease have no symptoms, although some bony deformities may be apparent such as bowed shin bones (see Figure 4.2d-I) or an enlarged and irregular skull. The most common symptom, which affects only a minority of patients, is aching in the affected bone. In some people a joint may become arthritic if the bony deformity affects the internal architecture of the joint. Fractures and bone cancer are very rare complications of Paget's disease.

Bisphosphonates (usually alendronate) may be given to treat the symptoms of Paget's disease, because of their effect on the osteoclasts. Surgery is occasionally necessary to correct a severe deformity.

Figure 4.2d-I Bowing of the legs in Paget's disease

Rickets and osteomalacia (vitamin D deficiency)

The main source of active vitamin D for humans is through manufacture of the pro-vitamin in skin that is exposed to sunlight. In most people the diet is only a secondary source of vitamin D. This fat-soluble vitamin is found in animal fats, eggs and fish oils.

However sourced, vitamin D depends on healthy kidneys to be converted to an active form in the body. When converted by the kidneys to the active form, vitamin D enables the hardening of new bone by promoting the absorption of calcium from the blood. In its absence, any new bone formed is too soft.

Rickets is the result of vitamin D deficiency in infancy and childhood, whereas osteomalacia is the result of vitamin D deficiency in adulthood. In Westernized countries, these conditions are particularly common in Asian immigrant girls and women and elderly people. A combination of lack of exposure to sunlight (including constant use of sunblock) and a vegetarian or vegan diet can lead to vitamin D deficiency. Chronic kidney disease is the other important cause of osteomalacia, because the diseased kidneys can no longer activate the vitamin D to a form that is useful to the body.

Rickets is rare in developed countries. When established, there is a characteristic widening of the wrist

---

 Information box 4.2d-II

Paget's disease: comments from a Chinese medicine perspective

In Chinese medicine, the irregular enlargement of the bones and increased blood supply might be seen as corresponding to an Accumulation of Phlegm with Heat. The weakening of the affected bones suggests an underlying Deficiency of Kidney Yin and Essence. The increased risk of cancer is consistent with the development of Phlegm against a background of Yin Deficiency.

As discussed earlier, bisphosphonates Nourish Kidney Yin and Essence, but this action is suppressive. They also have side effects in keeping with a Heating nature.

joints, grooving of the ribs at the level of the diaphragm, and a bowing outwards of the shin bones. The muscles are weak because these, too, depend on vitamin D for an adequate supply of calcium.

In adulthood, osteomalacia causes vague aches in the bones and muscle weakness, which may lead to a waddling gait in advanced cases. Small areas of bone fracture can develop.

Simple attention to diet and safe exposure to sunlight can reverse cases of osteomalacia and prevent rickets. Low-dose vitamin D supplementation is now recommended as a precautionary measure in the UK for pregnancy and also for infants.

With the recent development of easy and accurate blood testing for vitamin D levels, low blood levels of this vitamin have been found to be very common, and particularly so in winter. In one study over 30 percent of adults and children in the UK were found to have low vitamin D levels in the winter.[29] It is currently not clear to what extent low vitamin D levels in the blood correlate with disease, but recommendations are that patients who are found to be vitamin D deficient (and there are indeed many of them) should take vitamin D supplementation.

 Information box 4.2d-III

Rickets and osteomalacia: comments from a Chinese medicine perspective

In Chinese medicine, the symptoms of both rickets and osteomalacia correspond to Jing and Qi Deficiency (weak bones, tiredness and aching). Vitamin D nourishes the Kidney Qi and Jing.

Inherited or childhood bone disorders

Achondroplasia (dwarfism)

Achondroplasia (dwarfism) is an autosomal-dominant inherited genetic condition in which there is defective formation of bone and cartilage. This causes the long bones to fail to lengthen fully during childhood. An adult with achondroplasia has a trunk of normal length, but very short and broad legs and arms. The skull is enlarged in size and the face appears small, with a depressed nasal ridge. Because of the way this condition is inherited, there is a 50 percent chance of the children of a person with achondroplasia also developing the disorder.

 Information box 4.2d-IV

Achondroplasia: comments from a Chinese medicine perspective

In Chinese medicine, the underlying problem of maturation of bone in achondroplasia suggests Jing Deficiency. Problems resulting from distorted bony architecture, enlarged tonsils, recurrent ear infections, excessive weight gain and obstructive sleep apnea suggest that this is a condition in which there is a tendency for Phlegm/Damp to Accumulate.

Brittle bone disease (osteogenesis imperfecta)

The term brittle bone disease is used to describe a group of inherited conditions in which there is a defect in the structure of collagen, the connective tissue that supports bone. This means that the bones are unusually brittle.

In very severe types of this condition, the newborn baby develops multiple fractures and bony deformities. Early death is almost inevitable. In less severe forms, the child may be more prone to recurrent fractures, but may grow up to lead a relatively normal adult life as the bones strengthen in puberty. In one of the most common forms of brittle bone disease (osteogenesis imperfecta tarda) a cluster of other features is also often present, including deafness (otosclerosis), heart valve disorders, weak teeth and a blue discoloration to the whites of the eyes. This form of brittle bone disease is autosomal-dominantly inherited, which means that the gene defect will be passed down to 50 percent of the children of someone with the condition.

 Information box 4.2d-V

Brittle bone disease: comments from a Chinese medicine perspective

In Chinese medicine, brittle bone disease corresponds to Kidney Essence Deficiency. The recurrent fractures, deafness and bluish tinge to the sclera all point to a Kidney imbalance.

Infections of the bone

Osteomyelitis

Osteomyelitis is the term used to describe an infection that has developed within bone tissue. It can develop as a result of direct contamination of bone, as might occur following a compound fracture, or from a traumatic penetration of the flesh, such as a gunshot wound. Alternatively, bacteria from an infected site (such as a boil) elsewhere in the body can lodge in the bone from the bloodstream.

People who have a depleted immune system from malnutrition or another chronic illness are more prone to osteomyelitis. Also, those with sickle cell anemia may be particularly prone to developing infection in the areas of infarcted bone that can result from the condition.

Another cause of osteomyelitis is tuberculosis (TB). The bones are a favored site for infection in which the TB bacterium can thrive. A common location for tuberculous osteomyelitis is in the vertebrae. In this case, it can lead to collapse of the vertebrae.

Osteomyelitis is very difficult to treat because the bone tissue is relatively poorly supplied with blood and immune cells. It is common for an acute infection to become chronic. In some cases an abscess containing pus develops within the bone. This may start discharging through a sinus out onto the skin or towards other body parts (see Section 2.2b).

Treatment might involve a long course of high-dose antibiotics, in some cases initially given intravenously to maximize the concentration of drug in the bloodstream. In persistent cases the area of infected bone may need to be surgically excised. Some cases of chronic osteomyelitis will never heal fully.

 Information box 4.2d-VI

Osteomyelitis: comments from a Chinese medicine perspective

In Chinese medicine, the infection of osteomyelitis might be seen as corresponding to Heat or Damp Heat against a background of Kidney or Jing Deficiency.

Tumors of the bone

Benign tumors

Occasionally, a smooth, rounded, hard lump of dense bone and cartilage tissue grows from the surface of a bone. This benign bony lump, known as an osteochondroma, is particularly common in the facial bones. In addition, chondromas, benign bony lumps derived from cartilage, can develop usually from the ends of the bones of the fingers and toes. Both these forms of benign growth are often painless, and once developed may change either very slowly or not at all. They are usually only removed for cosmetic reasons.

Occasionally, an area of dense bone develops deep within the bone tissue. This benign condition, known as osteoid osteoma, can lead to a sensation of deep throbbing pain because of the increased pressure within the bone. It is a recognized cause of intense bone pain in young adults. In this case, a surgical operation might be performed to remove the internal growth of dense bone tissue.

 Information box 4.2d-VII

Benign bone tumors: comments from a Chinese medicine perspective

The dense tissue of benign tumors of the bone is likely to be described as a manifestation of Phlegm. Pain would suggest additional Blood Stagnation.

Malignant osteosarcoma

Osteosarcoma is a rare primary cancer of bone tissue. It most commonly affects children and young adults, with boys being more commonly affected than girls. However, it can also affect elderly people, and sometimes occurs as a very rare complication of Paget's disease.

This malignant tumor commonly develops close to the end of a long bone, especially the femur, in young people. The symptoms include deep pain, a limp and fever.

A plain X-ray image is often sufficient to confirm a diagnosis of malignancy, but a biopsy of the bone is performed to grade the tumor.

Treatment is by means of immediate amputation, as the tumor is very aggressive and needs to be removed to avoid rapid progression. This treatment, together with intensive chemotherapy (doxorubicin and cisplatin), has improved a previously very poor average length of survival, and total cure is now achieved in approximately 50 percent of cases.

 Information box 4.2d-VIII

Osteosarcoma: comments from a Chinese medicine perspective

The fact that osteosarcoma is usually a young person's disease suggests that there is an underlying inherited weakness, possibly of Jing. The tumor itself is often regarded, like most tumors, as a manifestation of Phlegm and Blood Stagnation.

Metastatic disease of the bone

Secondary bone cancer is by far the most common form of bone cancer. Cancers that are particularly likely to metastasize to bone include cancers of the lung, breast, prostate, thyroid and kidney.

The most common symptom of secondary bone cancer is pain, which can be very intense and boring in quality. The bone may be particularly tender to percussion (tapping with the fingertip), which is a feature of deep bone pathology. In some cases the first symptom is an unexpected (pathological) fracture. The fracture is the result of the underlying weakness of the cancerous bone. As secondary cancer indicates that the condition is in an advanced stage, the patient may also experience symptoms of exhaustion, fevers, weight loss and appetite loss.

In addition to the solid cancers, myeloma is a cancer of the white blood cells that particularly affects the bone (see Section 3.4e). Myeloma tends to cause multiple small erosions in the bone. When myeloma is in an advanced stage, the weakening caused by these erosions can be similar in effect to that of severe osteoporosis. The patient becomes prone to fractures, particularly of the marrow-containing ribs and vertebrae, and also the potentially dangerous syndrome of hypercalcemia as calcium is released from bone into the bloodstream.

Treatment of secondary bone cancer is almost never curative, because the disease is at such an advanced stage. Nevertheless, chemotherapy may be given to slow the progression of the disease and reduce its severe symptoms. Pain can be reduced by means of analgesics; NSAIDs can be particularly effective in bone pain. Localized radiotherapy to an affected bone might also temporarily reduce pain significantly. Bisphosphonates can be given in intravenous infusion to treat hypercalcemia.

 Information box 4.2d-IX

Secondary bone cancer: comments from a Chinese medicine perspective

In Chinese medicine, the pain of secondary bone cancer indicates Blood Stagnation against a background of severe Kidney Deficiency. Hypercalcemia manifests with tiredness and thirst and dehydration. It could be described in terms of extreme Yin Deficiency.

The red flags of diseases of the bones

Some patients with bone diseases will benefit from referral to a conventional doctor for assessment and/or treatment. Red flags are those symptoms and signs that will indicate that referral should be considered. The red flags of the diseases of the bones are described in Table 4.2d-I. A summary of the red flags in a format designed for quick reference in clinical practice can be found in Appendix III. This gives advice on the degree of urgency of referral for each of the red flag conditions listed.

Table 4.2d-I A26: Red flags of diseases of the bones

Red flag	Description	Reasoning
A26.1	Bone pain: pain originating from bone is characteristically fixed and deep. It may have either an aching or a boring quality. Tenderness on palpation and on percussion (weighty tapping, with the fingertip, of the skin overlying the bone) indicates a structural abnormality such as a fracture Boring central back pain at night suggests that the origin is the bones rather than muscles. This symptom might suggest bone cancer	It is worth referring any severe or persistent pain that you believe to be originating from bone, as this may originate from an infective, cancerous or degenerative condition of the bone Possible causes of bone pain include traumatic bruising or fracture, osteomyelitis (bone infection), tumor, Paget's disease, osteoporosis and osteomalacia The collapse of vertebrae in osteoporosis can lead to a sudden onset of vertebral pain and pain radiating around to the front of the body along the line of the affected spinal nerve. Although not usually serious in itself, an osteoporotic collapse needs to be referred for consideration of medical management of the osteoporosis and exclusion of weakening of the bones due to cancer deposits, as this can mimic osteoporosis

4.2e Localized diseases of the joints, ligaments and muscles

In this and the following section the diseases of the joints, ligaments and muscles are studied together, because symptoms arising from these three different structures often overlap, and under certain conditions may co-exist. This section focuses on conditions that are localized to a single part of the body only, while the following section explores those diseases that tend to affect a number of muscles and joints in the whole body (generalized or systemic diseases).

The conditions considered here are:

Localized disease processes affecting the joints, ligaments and muscles

- Localized joint disorders:
  - arthritis
  - damage to internal structures of the joints
  - joint cysts and ganglions
- Bursal disorders:
  - bursitis
- Ligament disorders:
  - sprains
  - hypermobility
- Muscle disorders:
  - myofascial nodules (trigger points)
  - muscle cramp
  - torn muscle and muscle hematoma
- Tendon disorders:
  - tendon strains and rupture
  - tendonitis and tenosynovitis
  - enthesopathy
  - repetitive strain injury (RSI)
  - tendon swellings (trigger finger)
- Fascial disorders:
  - fasciitis
  - Dupuytren's contracture
  - carpal tunnel syndrome.

The following specific disorders of the musculoskeletal system are all manifestations of one or more of the disease processes listed above. These disease processes are described in detail in this section. Table 4.2e-I clarifies which disease processes are relevant for each of these specific disorders, so the underlying pathology of each can be more clearly understood.

Specific disorders of the various anatomical regions

- The neck:
  - muscle pain
  - spondylosis
  - whiplash
- The shoulders:
  - frozen shoulder
  - subacromial bursitis
- The elbow:
  - epicondylitis
  - bursitis
- The hand and wrist:
  - tenosynovitis
  - ganglion
  - Dupuytren's contracture
  - trigger finger
- The lower back:
  - muscular lower back pain
  - spondylolisthesis
  - spondylosis
  - disc prolapse
  - spinal stenosis
- The hip:
  - osteoarthritis
  - bursitis
  - femoral neck fracture
- The knee:
  - medial and lateral ligament strain
  - patellar bursitis
  - chondromalacia patellae
  - meniscal and cruciate ligament tears
  - Baker's cyst
- The lower leg, foot and heel:
  - hallux valgus and bunion
  - plantar fasciitis
  - Achilles tendonitis
  - tear of Achilles tendon
  - calcaneal bursitis
  - shin splints.

Localized joint disorders

Arthritis

The main pathological processes to affect the internal structure of the joints are inflammation and degeneration. The term arthritis, literally meaning inflammation of the joints, is confusingly often used to describe both these processes.

A wide range of different factors can cause arthritis. It may affect a single joint, or may occur as part of a generalized or systemic disease in which a number of joints are affected. In systemic arthritis the joints are often affected in a symmetrical fashion.

In inflammatory arthritis, the affected joints tend to be hot and painful. In synovial joints, the inflammation affects the synovial membrane lining the interior of the joint. The inflammation can then lead to excessive fluid production from the membrane and, if prolonged, damage to the cartilage of the joint. The inflamed joint is therefore swollen, and may become deformed as the internal structure becomes destroyed.

Inflammatory arthritis of a single joint can result from infection within the joint, a condition known as septic arthritis. This infection can originate from another site in the body, or can arise as a result of a penetrating injury into the joint. Joint infection is very serious because, like osteomyelitis, the infectious agents are relatively protected from the immune system and thus the infection can progress rapidly. The production of pus can result in permanent inflammatory damage to the interior of a joint.

In septic arthritis, the patient becomes very unwell with a red, tense and very painful joint and a high fever. However, these symptoms may be less marked in people with chronic illness, such as diabetes or rheumatoid arthritis, or in elderly people. The treatment is urgent hospitalization and administration of antibiotics, ideally by intravenous injection for the first week. Up to 12 weeks of antibiotic treatment may be given to ensure eradication of the bacterium.

Some infectious diseases, for example, gonorrhea, can lead to a generalized form of inflammatory arthritis (see Section 4.2f).

Crystal arthritis is a form of non-infectious inflammatory arthritis that can appear very like septic arthritis. It is caused by the formation of small crystals within the joint fluid that are highly irritating and thus cause inflammation. Gout is the most common form of crystal arthritis (see Section 4.2f).

Bleeding is another cause of inflammation in a joint. This usually occurs as a result of an injury, but may occur spontaneously in a person who suffers from a clotting disorder such as hemophilia. The technical term for blood in a joint space is hemarthrosis. The blood cells within the joint break down and are highly irritating to the synovial membrane. They then induce severe inflammation.

Like infection, a hemarthrosis can also result in permanent damage to the structure of the joint. This is one mechanism for the severe disability that can develop in people with hemophilia.

Other non-infectious systemic conditions can affect the joints, leading to a generalized inflammatory arthritis. The underlying cause of inflammation may be a deposition of autoantibodies within the joint, as occurs in rheumatoid arthritis and systemic lupus erythematosus (SLE). In other conditions the direct cause may be unclear (e.g. in ankylosing spondylitis and inflammatory bowel disease). If the inflammation occurring in these conditions is prolonged, the joints may become permanently deformed (for more details on generalized arthritis, see Section 4.2f).

The joints can also become damaged as a result of a process that is largely degenerative, and which leads to thinning or destruction of the protective cartilage that covers the ends of the bones within the joint. This process, known as osteoarthritis, is loosely described as wear and tear by many doctors to their patients. Osteoarthritis is more likely to occur in joints that have become damaged through injury or overuse, or in those that are held slightly out of alignment due to chronic muscle tension. Conversely, wear and tear may occur because of excessive laxity of the ligaments (hypermobility), so that the joint is repeatedly taken through a much wider range of movements than those for which it is designed. A rather confusing lay term for hypermobility is double-jointedness.

Generalized osteoarthritis usually occurs as part of the aging process and tends to affect the joints in a symmetrical fashion (see also Section 4.2f).

Damage to internal structures of the joints

As described in Section 4.2a, some of the synovial joints contain additional structures. The joint between the femur and the tibia at the knee is a good example of such a joint. First, it contains two C-shaped pads of cartilage (the menisci), which act as cushions for the condyles of the femur on the table of the tibia. Second, two thick ligaments (cruciate ligaments) cross within the joint to prevent the joint from dislocating in an anterior or posterior direction. An injury to the knee, particularly if the joint is twisted, can cause a tear in the cartilage or a rupture of one of the two ligaments. The pain and disability resulting from damage to these structures might be intensified by the swelling caused by bleeding into the joint, known as a traumatic hemarthrosis.

A torn cartilage (meniscus) may prevent full mobility of the joint. A sign of this is that the joint may lock in a flexed position. Particles of broken cartilage can also impair the mobility of the joint and be a cause of pain and inflammation. A torn cruciate ligament will reduce the support to the knee joint and cause it to be prone to further injury. In both situations, if not well healed, the risk of future osteoarthritis of the knee is increased. Injuries of the internal structure of the knee can be clearly visualized by means of an MRI (magnetic resonance imaging). Injuries to either the cartilage or the cruciate ligaments usually require surgical repair if severe. This may be performed by means of the arthroscope.

Information box 4.2e-I

Arthritis and damage to internal structures of the joints: comments from a Chinese medicine perspective

In Chinese medicine, the pain of arthritis is usually described as a form of Painful Obstruction Syndrome and is a manifestation of Blood and Qi Stagnation. In most cases there is also evidence of a Pathogenic Factor (Bi Syndrome). Inflammatory arthritis always involves Heat, but Wind and Damp may also be present. Degenerative arthritis may simply reflect underlying Deficiency, particularly of the Kidneys, but very often Damp or Cold has also lodged in the affected joints to give symptoms of stiffness and deep pain.

The pain from an injury to the internal structures of the joint may well reflect Blood and Qi Stagnation. If adequate healing fails to occur, chronic Qi and Blood Deficiency of the joint can develop, and Pathogenic Factors such as Damp and Cold may invade.

A deformed joint, which is very commonly the long-term outcome of arthritis, is a manifestation of Phlegm (Bony Bi).

Joint cysts and ganglions

These are fluid-filled cysts that appear close to the margin of a synovial joint. The cyst is an out-pouching of the synovial membrane, and is filled with synovial fluid. Cysts generally appear as part of a degenerative process. The most common site for a joint cyst is at the edge of the wrist joint, where it appears as a smooth, firm, slightly compressible lump (ganglion). Joint cysts at the back of the knee (Baker's cysts) may also be degenerative, but can develop as part of a generalized inflammatory disorder such as rheumatoid arthritis. Joint cysts are usually painless, but may ache or lead to restriction of movement of the affected joint.

Occasionally, the cyst can burst and release fluid into the surrounding tissues. This may lead to resolution of the problem, although commonly the cyst will reform. Rupture of a large cyst such as a Baker's cyst can cause marked inflammation. In the case of a Baker's cyst the inflammation can mimic that of a deep vein thrombosis (DVT) because the released fluid tracks down the muscles of the calf to cause a tender and swollen calf muscle.

The most effective form of treatment of these cysts is surgical removal. Fluid can be drawn out of the cysts by syringe for relief of discomfort, but fluid tends to re-accumulate in a short space of time.

Information box 4.2e-II

Joint cysts and ganglions: comments from a Chinese medicine perspective

In Chinese medicine, the development of a painless joint cyst would possibly be described as Accumulation of Phlegm caused by Stagnation of Body Fluids.

Bursal disorders

Bursitis

A bursa is a space lined with synovial membrane and filled with fluid. Its function is to reduce friction to the tissues surrounding a joint. A bursa can become inflamed, particularly if the tissues surrounding the joint are under excessive pressure or misuse. This condition is known as bursitis and is characterized by the bursa swelling up with excess fluid, and becoming hot, red and painful. Student's elbow (the olecranon bursa), housemaid's knee (suprapatellar bursa) and clergyman's knee (prepatellar bursa) are three examples of bursitis from pressure and over-use.

Bursitis is usually treated by means of rest of the over-used tissues and NSAIDs. In persistent cases, a corticosteroid injection might be used to reduce the inflammation.

Information box 4.2e-III

Bursitis: comments from a Chinese medicine perspective

In Chinese medicine, an attack of bursitis might be described as local Blood and Qi Stagnation with Heat. Damp may be an additional Pathogenic Factor if localized swelling is prominent. Pain would indicate local Stagnation of Qi and Blood.

Ligament disorders

Sprains

The ligaments are the tough fibrous structures made of fibrocartilage that bind bone to bone around the joints. Some ligaments fuse into the joint capsules (also known as the capsular ligament), while others are external to the joint. In some cases the ligaments are found within the synovial joint cavity (e.g. the cruciate ligaments).

In the case of an injury that puts a stretching tension on a ligament, some or all of the fibers in a ligament may become torn, and bleeding can occur in the ligament tissue. A common example of this is the injury that might occur when someone turns on their ankle, so that the ligament that links the external malleolus of the fibula to the talus of the foot (in the region of acupoint Qiu Xu, GB-40) is suddenly stretched. This sort of injury is called a sprain.

In a mild injury only a few fibers of the ligament are torn. The person may feel momentary discomfort, but the problem then subsides. In a more severe tear there may be marked swelling and bruising from the damaged ligament, and the injury may take weeks to heal. A severe tear, even when healed, may leave the joint vulnerable to a recurrence of the injury, as the repaired ligament is never quite as strong as before. This problem of persistent weakness is due to the fact that ligaments do not heal as efficiently as other tissues such as skin or muscle.

The conventional way of treating an acute ligament strain involves **R**est of the affected area, application of **I**ce to reduce swelling, use of a **C**ompression tubular bandage, and **E**levation of the affected part to reduce swelling (a treatment approach known as RICE). This reduces the amount of bleeding into the ligament, but will slow healing if prolonged. RICE can be maintained for the first 24 hours after the injury. Thereafter, gentle heat applied to the injury will be more beneficial. Some severe ligament tears may require physiotherapy, a plaster splint or surgery to allow optimum healing.

Information box 4.2e-IV

Acute sprain: comments from a Chinese medicine perspective

In Chinese medicine an acute sprain might correspond to acute Blood and Qi Stagnation. Chronic weakness of a previously sprained ligament corresponds to local Qi Deficiency, and the area may become vulnerable to invasion by Pathogenic Factors (especially Damp and Cold).

Hypermobility

Hypermobility is a term used to describe excessive joint laxity. Some people are born with this tendency. In some cases it may be the result of a rare inherited deficiency of connective tissue. Hypermobility may also be acquired through long-term strenuous stretching exercise, such as gymnastics, particularly if performed during childhood. Although the joints of most adults are far too inflexible, a hypermobile joint is not necessarily a good thing. This is because the increased range of movement puts excessive strain on the internal structures of the joint and may lead to the development of osteoarthritis in later life.

Information box 4.2e-V

Hypermobility: comments from a Chinese medicine perspective

In Chinese medicine, the range of movement associated with hypermobility is the result of a deficiency in the correct tensile properties of the ligaments and tendons. This might be interpreted in terms of a Deficiency in Liver Blood and Qi. Joint damage resulting from this might correspond to Stagnation of Blood and Qi and also Invasion of Pathogenic Factors (Heat, Damp and Phlegm), all as a result of the pre-existing Deficiency of Blood and Qi.

Muscle disorders

Myofascial nodules (trigger points)

Myofascial nodules are lumps, commonly called knots, which can be felt within the body of tense muscle. They are often very tender. Myofascial nodules consist of a localized area of tensely contracted muscle fibers. If a nodule has only recently developed, deep massage of the area of the knot may cause it to relax and disappear. More long-standing nodules may become fixed as structural changes take place in the tensed area of muscle tissue.

These nodules are commonly found in the muscles of the back of the neck, upper back and shoulders, lower back and overlying the sacrum. In particular, the trapezius muscle is commonly affected. The nodules can develop in any skeletal muscle as a result of excessive tension held in the muscle body. They are often the underlying cause of musculoskeletal pain when there is no other structural damage to be found. Muscle tension may have a postural or an emotional root, and is very commonly a combination of the two. It can also develop as a result of a local painful musculoskeletal condition. For example, pain from disease of the intervertebral joints in the lower back can lead to tension (spasm) of the lumbar muscles. This initially protective reflex can result in the development of painful myofascial nodules in the lumbar muscles and, if the joint problem persists, may become chronic in nature.

The pain from myofascial nodules can cause tension to spread to other local muscle groups, so that a whole anatomical region, in particular, the shoulder and back of the neck, can become stiff and knotted. Often, pain is referred to other parts of the body. For example, headache is a very common consequence of muscle tension in the shoulders and upper neck. The patient will tend to want to rub or hold the affected area, and the pain can be greatly helped by a prolonged stretch of the affected muscle, application of warmth or massage. Acupuncture is medically recognized to be an effective treatment for tender myofascial nodules (also known as trigger point acupuncture).[30]

Information box 4.2e-VI

Myofascial nodules: comments from a Chinese medicine perspective

In Chinese medicine, myofascial nodules correspond to areas of Qi and Blood Stagnation. Sometimes they are at the site of known acupuncture points, and can be viewed as a form of Ah shi point. This has implications for how the nodules are treated. They point to disharmony in the Organ that dominates the area in which the nodule has developed. Very commonly, this disharmony is within one of the Yang Officials, in particular the Gallbladder, Small Intestine, Triple Burner or Bladder. Referred pain is commonly felt along the pathway of the associated channel.

Treatment directed at the trigger points alone, such as massage, cupping and acupuncture, can be very helpful in relieving symptoms, but may not deal with the deep root of the problem (usually a form of deficiency or repetitive damage due to poor use). If this is the case, the patient will need to return again and again for treatment, and the practitioner needs to consider additional methods of treatment to focus directly on the root problem.

Muscle cramp

Cramp is a sudden painful contraction of a large muscle group. The mechanism of cramp is poorly understood, but is commonly explained as a result of buildup of waste products in a muscle. This theory fits with the observation that cramp commonly occurs in over-exercised muscle in which the requirements of the metabolism of the muscle may exceed the blood supply. Cramp in the legs (particularly in the calf and feet) becomes increasingly common in old age. In this case, it must be distinguished from the cramping pain that can result from arteriosclerosis of the arteries of the legs.

An acute cramp may be relieved by forcibly stretching the muscle. Chronic night-time cramps may be relieved in some people by the medication quinine sulfate taken on a regular basis.

Information box 4.2e-VII

Acute cramp: comments from a Chinese medicine perspective

In Chinese medicine, an acute cramp signifies Deficiency in Liver or Spleen Organs and the intense pain would correspond to Blood and Qi Stagnation. It may be that Stagnation is arising as a result of chronic Blood and Qi or Yin Deficiency, but it may also represent invasion of Cold/Damp into vacuous channels and collaterals.

Torn muscle and muscle hematoma

Just as a ligament can be torn during an acute injury, so can the fibers of a muscle. Muscle fibers can tear when unexpected strain is placed on a muscle group, especially if those muscles are contracted. This injury commonly affects the hamstring muscles (at the back of the upper leg) and the abdominal muscles, both in the context of strenuous exercise. The term strain is used to describe a torn muscle or tendon.

An area of torn muscle will become inflamed as a result of cell damage and bleeding, and if the tear is severe the affected area may become tender and warm. Rarely, a large bleed into the body of the muscle may lead to the formation of a tender, hot lump called a hematoma. This is a common occurrence in people who have a disorder of clotting such as hemophilia.

Usually, muscle tears heal well because muscle fibers have a very good blood supply. Like ligament sprains, the tear is treated medically with RICE (see above) for the first 24 hours. This treatment helps to prevent excessive bleeding into the area. A hematoma may impair healing as the mass of clotted blood can be a continuing trigger for inflammation, and scarring and contracture of the muscle can develop. For this reason, a large muscle hematoma may have to be drained surgically to permit full healing. Muscle contractures are a serious consequence of muscle bleeds in hemophilia.

Information box 4.2e-VIII

Muscle tears: comments from a Chinese medicine perspective

In Chinese medicine, a muscle tear corresponds to Blood and Qi Stagnation. A hematoma reflects Blood Stagnation with Heat. Scarring of a poorly healed muscle reflects local Blood and Qi Deficiency, with persistent Qi Stagnation. Invasion of Cold and Damp into the local channels and collaterals may complicate a chronic muscle tear.

Tendon disorders

Tendon strains and rupture

As the tendon is the site at which the muscle inserts into bone, tendon strains also result from acute trauma or misuse of muscles. The strain can occur at the very point at which the tendon inserts into the bone, or at any position along a tendon up to its insertion into the muscle belly. In very severe cases the tendon can be totally ruptured. One example of this is rupture of the Achilles tendon, which can occur following a forceful landing on the feet when the gastrocnemius muscle is contracted.

Tendons do not heal as well as muscle tissue, as their structure and blood supply is more like that of ligaments. Treatment of a severe tendon strain involves RICE (see above), followed by prolonged immobilization of the area. If there has been a rupture, reparative surgery may be necessary. If the injury is less severe, gentle use of the affected tendon may actually aid healing.

Information box 4.2e-IX

Tendon strains: comments from a Chinese medicine perspective

A tendon strain corresponds to Blood and Qi Stagnation. If healing is poor, this is due to long-term local Depletion of Blood and Qi, with or without Invasion of Cold and Damp.

Although sprains and strains commonly affect young healthy people, they are more likely to occur within the context of an underlying state of Blood and Qi Deficiency or Stagnation. For example, a Liver Blood Deficient person who turns their ankle might be more likely to sustain an injury to the ankle ligaments than someone who is in good health.

Tendonitis and tenosynovitis

Tendonitis is a term used to describe a condition in which tendons become inflamed. Some tendons, for example, the extensor tendons of the hand, travel within fluid-filled sheaths, which protect and lubricate the tendons. If these tendons become inflamed, the term tenosynovitis more correctly describes the condition.

The most common cause of tendonitis is repetitive misuse of the muscles attached to the inflamed tendon. For example, repetitive use of clippers or scissors may lead to tenosynovitis of the extensor tendons of the hand, and repetitive twisting actions of the wrist may lead to tendonitis of the tendon of the extensor carpi radialis as it inserts into the lateral epicondyle of the elbow (known as lateral epicondylitis or tennis elbow).

Tendonitis presents with inflammation of the area affected, and pain on performing the movement that has caused the problem. In tenosynovitis, the tendon sheaths may be swollen with fluid, and crackling sensations (crepitus) may be felt over the affected area if the tendons are moved.

Conventional treatment is with NSAIDs and advice to rest the affected part. Many cases will settle down over two to three days, but in some cases they can become chronic. In such cases, a corticosteroid injection may be offered.

Information box 4.2e-X

Tendonitis and tenosynovitis: comments from a Chinese medicine perspective

In Chinese medicine, tendonitis and tenosynovitis represent severe Blood and Qi Stagnation with Heat. They often occur against a background of local or general Blood and Qi Deficiency (possibly caused by the overuse of the area). Liver Blood Deficiency is a common underlying deficiency.

Enthesopathy

Enthesopathy is the medical term used to describe inflammation of the area at which a tendon or ligament inserts into the bone in the region of a joint. Strictly speaking, tennis elbow is an example of an enthesopathy. Enthesopathy may also occur as a result of a more generalized inflammatory condition such as rheumatoid arthritis or ankylosing spondylitis (see Section 4.2f).

Repetitive strain injury (RSI)

Repetitive strain injury (RSI) is a term used to describe a painful condition that affects the muscle groups that have to perform repetitive movements, often in the context of a stressful work situation. More recently, the terms work-related upper limb injury and chronic upper limb pain syndrome have been introduced to describe the same condition. RSI is a well-recognized problem affecting people engaged in work that demands repetitive movements, for example, typing or the playing of a musical instrument. It is also recognized that there are often underlying emotional or stress-related problems which can predispose a person to developing RSI. The cause of the pain can be one or both of small muscle and tendon strains or chronic tendonitis.

Initial treatment may involve rest, which often means time off work. Ideally, the sources of stress in the working environment should be tackled. Advice about posture and personal stress management might be given. The Alexander technique can be of particular benefit.[31] It is not uncommon for patients to be prescribed counseling, beta blockers or antidepressants to deal with the underlying emotional issues.

Information box 4.2e-XI

Repetitive strain injury: comments from a Chinese medicine perspective

In Chinese medicine, the pain of RSI represents Blood and Qi Stagnation, but in view of the fact that there is an underlying imbalance of muscle and soft tissue, there is likely to be an underlying condition of Deficiency, in particular, of Liver Blood Deficiency and Spleen Qi Deficiency.

Tendon swellings (trigger finger)

Trigger finger is a condition in which a swelling develops on a flexor tendon of a finger just at the point at which it enters the tendon sheath. This is usually a painless condition, but can cause a problem in free movement of the finger. The affected finger tends to lock in a fully flexed position, and will only open with a degree of force, and with a clicking sensation.

De Quervain's syndrome is pain and swelling over the region of the styloid process of the radius (in the region of acupoint Yang Xi, LI-5) because of thickening of the tendons of abductor pollicis longus and extensor pollicis brevis. The pain is felt most strongly when lifting an object in the manner of pouring from a teapot.

A local corticosteroid injection may reduce the swelling on the tendon. Severe cases may be offered surgery.

Fascial disorders

The fascia is the term used to describe the fibrous connective tissue that surrounds the muscles and tendons and holds them in place. In some parts of the body the fibers of the fascia coalesce to form thick sheets of tissue, which have both a protective and structural role. For example, the palmar and plantar fasciae are sheets of connective tissue that lie within the palm of the hand and sole of the foot, respectively. These overlie and protect the flexor tendons of the hands and feet. The fascial layers form the boundaries to compartments within the body, and between these compartments are virtual spaces between fascial layers that can be more easily separated by surgeons cutting across the fascial planes. It has been argued by authors, including Myers (2009)[32] and Keown (2014),[33] that the fascial compartments form an energetic link between distant parts

of the body, and that the spaces between them may provide the physical substrate for the acupuncture meridians.

Fasciitis

Fasciitis is a condition in which there is inflammation of the fascial tissue. The most common site for this to occur is in the sole of the foot (plantar fasciitis). Plantar fasciitis can occur as a result of excessive walking, but may also develop as part of a more generalized inflammatory disorder such as ankylosing spondylitis (see Section 4.2f).

Fasciitis can be very painful. It is treated with rest of the affected area, NSAIDs and, occasionally, corticosteroid injections.

Dupuytren's contracture

Dupuytren's contracture is a disorder in which bands of the palmar fascia become thickened and contracted. If severe, over the course of months to years the contraction can pull the fingers, particularly the fourth and fifth fingers, into a permanent state of flexion. Most commonly, this disorder affects middle-aged men and has no obvious cause. In some cases there may be an associated liver disorder or alcohol problem.

Information box 4.2e-XII

Dupuytren's contracture: comments from a Chinese medicine perspective

In Chinese medicine, as this is an inflammation and thickening of fascial connective tissue, which is a substance that has a role both of Binding (Liver) and Supporting (Spleen), Dupuytren's contracture might represent Liver Blood Deficiency, Spleen Qi Deficiency and Liver Qi Stagnation, leading to Accumulation of Phlegm in the channels and collaterals. Because of the affected area that is invariably the palmar aspect of the 4th and 5th metacarpals, this suggests an underlying imbalance in the Heart or Pericardium Organs.

Carpal tunnel syndrome

The carpal tunnel is a space running through the wrist that is bounded by a band of thick fascia (the flexor retinaculum), which helps to hold the small bones in place. Figure 4.2e-I illustrates the structure and location of the flexor retinaculum. Inflammation of the soft tissue within this space can cause compression of the median nerve. This leads to the symptoms that comprise carpal tunnel syndrome. This condition, an entrapment neuropathy, is described in Section 4.1g.

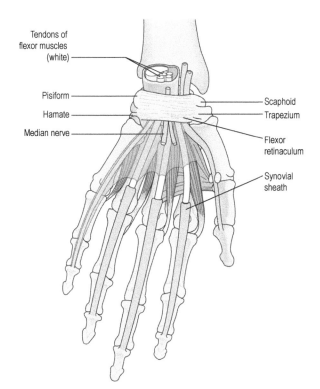

Tendons of flexor muscles (white)

Pisiform
Hamate
Median nerve

Scaphoid
Trapezium
Flexor retinaculum
Synovial sheath

Figure 4.2e-I The carpal tunnel and synovial sheaths in the wrist and hand (palmar aspect)

Specific localized problems according to anatomical region

Specific localized musculoskeletal problems were listed at the beginning of this section. All these conditions result from one or more of the types of muscle and ligament disorder described above. The nature of the pathology of each of these conditions is listed in Table 4.2e-I. It can be seen from this table that the pathology of most of these conditions has already been described, and so by using Table 4.2e-I as a guide, the underlying disease process for each of these conditions can be understood. The underlying pathology of each of these conditions is described in detail in the body of the text.

Table 4.2e-I The pathology of the common localized musculoskeletal disorders

Anatomical region	Name of condition	Underlying pathology
Neck	Muscle pain	Muscle strain and myofascial nodules
	Spondylosis	Degenerative arthritis and nerve compression
	Whiplash	Complex ligament sprains, and muscle and tendon strains
Shoulders	Frozen shoulder	Tendonitis or inflammation of the fibrous ligaments of the joint capsule
	Subacromial bursitis	Bursitis
Elbow	Medial and lateral epicondylitis	Tendonitis
Hand and wrist	Tenosynovitis	Tenosynovitis
	Ganglion	Joint cyst
	Dupuytren's contracture	Fascial contracture
	Trigger finger	Tendon swelling
Lower back	Muscle pain	Muscle strain and myofascial nodules
	Spondylolisthesis and spondylosis	Degenerative arthritis and nerve or spinal cord compression
	Disc prolapse	Degenerative arthritis of a fibrous joint
	Spinal stenosis	Degenerative arthritis and nerve compression
Hip	Osteoarthritis	Degenerative arthritis
	Trochanteric bursitis	Bursitis

Knee	Osteoarthritis	Osteoarthritis
	Medial and lateral ligament strain	Chronic sprain
	Patellar bursitis (housemaid's and clergyman's knee)	Bursitis
	Chondromalacia patellae	Degenerative arthritis
	Meniscal and cruciate tears	Degeneration of the structures inside a joint
	Baker's cyst	Joint cyst
Lower leg, foot and heel	Hallux valgus and bunion	Degenerative arthritis and bursitis
	Plantar fasciitis	Fasciitis
	Calcaneal bursitis	Bursitis
	Achilles tendonitis	Tendonitis
	Achilles tendon tear	Strain
	Shin splints (pain in the front of the calf from overuse, common in joggers)	Fasciitis of the tibialis anterior muscle fascia

The exception to this rule relates to those conditions that are the most common cause of pain in the neck and the lower back. A summary of these conditions now follows.

Chronic neck and back pain

In many cases, chronic neck and back pain begins simply as a result of long-standing tension in the supporting muscles of the neck and back. The muscles in such a case will feel tense and have knotted areas containing myofascial nodules that are particularly tender. It is at this stage that treatments such as massage, osteopathy and acupuncture can be most effective, and may be curative.

Spondylosis

If muscle tension is held for a long time, fibrous changes develop within the muscles, with the result that they lose their ability to fall into a fully relaxed state. Moreover, some of the myofascial nodules can become permanent fibrous structures. The continual tension placed on the fibrous joints of the vertebral column is likely to speed up the degenerative process of osteoarthritis which, as previously discussed, is a natural tendency of aging joints. However, held tension is not the whole story. Some people are more likely to develop osteoarthritis than others simply because of an inherited tendency to the condition.

Osteoarthritis of the fibrous intervertebral joints leads to deformity of the vertebral bodies, and pain and stiffness of the facet joints, which in health permit free movement of one vertebra upon another. The most characteristic deformity is the development of bony outgrowths, called osteophytes, which project horizontally outwards from the bodies of the vertebrae. Together, these bony changes are called spondylosis. Spondylosis develops most prominently in the cervical and lumbar spine, but can appear at any intervertebral joint. Cervical and lumbar spondylosis is described in Section 4.1g.

The osteophytes in spondylosis may place pressure on local tissues, including nerve fibers, and be an additional cause of pain. Therefore, the symptoms of spondylosis might include chronic pain, stiffness and reduction of free movement. There may also be referred pain in the distribution of an affected nerve root (e.g. lumbar and upper sacral spondylosis is one possible cause of the compression on nerve roots leading to sciatica).

It makes sense that spondylosis can be prevented by attention to preventing held muscle tension earlier in life. Regular gentle stretching exercise, a focus on good posture and relaxation will help minimize the tendency to the formation of spondylosis, and will also reduce its symptoms.

Intervertebral disc prolapse

The increased pressure on the fibrous pad (disc) that separates the individual vertebrae may cause a protrusion of its soft core (known as a herniation or prolapse), so that a bulge projects, usually postero-laterally, out of the joint.

Intervertebral disc prolapse may lead to pressure on one of the posterior nerve roots of the spinal cord and, if this is the case, will cause symptoms of pain, numbness and weakness affecting the distribution of the nerves in the nerve root. There may be additional back pain, as the injury may trigger increased muscle spasm in the surrounding area. Sometimes the prolapse can occur gradually as a response to chronic muscle tension, but will often develop suddenly because of an acute increase in pressure within the disc. Common causes of acute herniation of a disc are digging and lifting of heavy weights. In a weak back, a small turn or a cough may be enough to cause an acute prolapse.

Disc prolapse can affect young people, in whom the cause is excessive tension of the muscles of the lower back. In some cases there is also a degree of inherited structural deformity of the vertebrae or their ligaments. In later life, disc prolapse is also associated with the changes of spondylosis, in which case a degree of degeneration of the intervertebral disc may have predisposed to the condition.

In both spondylosis and disc prolapse there are underlying structural changes that are often irreversible. Nevertheless, exercises and lifestyle changes focusing on the reduction of muscle tension may well be of benefit in reducing symptoms, but are unlikely to cure the problem completely.

In conventional medical practice the pain of spondylosis and disc prolapse is notoriously difficult to investigate and treat. The symptoms of both can be indistinguishable from the pain and nerve compression caused by simple muscle tension or muscle strains. The bony changes of spondylosis can be seen on an X-ray image, but are very commonly not associated with pain, so that such images are usually unhelpful. The investigation of choice is an MRI, because this can differentiate between bone, muscle and nerve root, and can often show the precise physical cause of the pain. MRI is uncomfortable for the patient and expensive, so its use is usually reserved for severe intractable cases of low back and neck pain.

Treatment initially involves pain relief, usually with a combination of paracetamol and an NSAID. In an acute situation, opiate analgesics and muscle relaxants may be needed in the short term to relieve pain and reduce spasm of the supporting muscles. In persistent or severe cases, the patient may be offered advice and treatment from a physiotherapist. In some cases, surgery may be required to decompress the soft tissue around compressed nerve roots, remove the bulging part of a prolapsed disc, or to stabilize the intervertebral joints.

Information box 4.2e-XIII

Low back and neck pain: comments from a Chinese medicine perspective

In Chinese medicine, low back and neck pain usually correspond to a combination of Damp and Cold Invasion, Blood and Qi Stagnation and underlying Deficiency, usually of the Kidney/Bladder and Liver/Gallbladder Organs. Treatment will involve using local and distal points from the Channels related to these Organs and also from the Governor (Du) Channel. The Huatuojiaji points that lie just 0.5cun lateral to the Du points overlie the facet joints and the multifidus muscle, and are also valuable in treating pain related to the spine.[34]

The red flags of localized disorders of the diseases of the joints, ligaments and muscles

Some patients with localized disorders of the joints, ligaments and muscles will benefit from referral to a conventional doctor for assessment and/or treatment. Red flags are those symptoms and signs that will indicate that referral should be considered. The red flags of the localized disorders of the joints, ligaments and muscles are described in Table 4.2e-II. A summary of the red flags in a format designed for quick reference in clinical practice can be found in Appendix III. This gives advice on the degree of urgency of referral for each of the red flag conditions listed.

Table 4.2e-II A27: Red flags of localized diseases of the joints, ligaments and muscles

Red flag	Description	Reasoning
A27.1	Features of traumatic injury to a muscle or joint: • sudden onset of pain or swelling in a joint suggesting possible bleeding into the joint (hemarthrosis) • sudden severe pain and swelling around a joint with reluctance to move (sprain or strain, or possible fracture) • sudden onset of tender swelling in a muscle (possible hematoma) • locking of the knee joint (meniscal cartilage tear)	If there are any of these features of traumatic injury to a muscle or joint, it is wise to refer for appropriate immediate assessment (including X-ray imaging) and orthopedic management The Rest/Ice/Compression/Elevation (RICE) formula should be considered if there is significant inflammation (redness and swelling). "Rest" means ensuring that the injured region is immobilized, and this needs to be effected by means of recognized first aid approaches (e.g. splints, bandages, slings)

A27.2	Features of intervertebral disc prolapse and severe nerve root irritation: sudden onset of low back pain so severe that walking is impossible (severe sciatica); difficulty urinating or defecating	In most cases disc prolapse is not an emergency condition, and may do very well with appropriate complementary medical and massage techniques. Even with sciatic pain it might be expected that appropriate use of many physical therapies might bring relief without need for referral
		In most cases the referred pain and weakness indicates compression of one or more of the L3, L4, L5 or S1 nerve roots, and the symptoms are usually one-sided. Expect at least partial relief of these symptoms within a few days of treatment
		However, medical treatment (anti-inflammatory and muscle relaxant medication) can be very useful if the pain is very severe and there is a lot of muscle spasm, which is not responding to physical therapies
		Difficulty in urination or defecation and sacral numbness are rare but serious signs that indicate compression of the delicate lower sacral roots (cauda equine syndrome). If these symptoms are apparent, refer for assessment as a high priority (see A27.3)
A27.3	Cauda equina syndrome: • numbness of the buttocks and perineum (saddle anesthesia) • bilateral numbness or sciatica in the legs • difficulty in urination or defecation • impaired sexual function	The cauda equina (horse's tail) is the bunch of nerves that descends from the bottom of the spinal cord from the level of L1–L2 downwards. These nerve roots supply sensation and motor impulses to the perineum, buttocks, groin and legs
		Cauda equina syndrome suggests the compression of a number of these roots (usually from a central prolapsed disc, but possibly from tumor or other spinal growth). This is a serious situation, as prolonged compression of the perineal nerve supply can lead to permanent problems with urination, defecation and sexual function
		Refer as a high priority
A27.4	Features of septic or crystal arthritis: a single, hot, swollen and very tender joint. Patient is unwell. Not usually associated with injury, but may occasionally be caused by a penetrating injury of the joint space	A hot, swollen joint is a sign of possible joint infection. This presents a grave risk to the health of the joint, and needs to be referred so that infection can be excluded
		However, the most common cause of a single, hot and swollen joint is gout (crystal arthritis), which may respond well to complementary medicine alone. If this is the case, the doctor may wish to prescribe anti-inflammatory medication, but after diagnosis has been confirmed it is worth using simple complementary treatments in the first instance and reserving medication if no improvement is apparent within 3–7 days
A27.5	Unexplained, intense, persistent shoulder pain unrelated to shoulder movement (for >2 weeks)	Shoulder pain that seems to be unrelated to shoulder movement might be referred from a tumor at the apex of the lung (Pancoast tumor). The common (and benign) causes of shoulder pain include frozen shoulder, shoulder impingement syndrome and acromioclavicular joint inflammation; all are characterized by pain or weakness when attempting to use the affected shoulder. Refer any case in which the pain is not improving with treatment or in which the pain is unrelated to movement

4.2f Generalized diseases of the joints, ligaments and muscles

In Section 4.2e those conditions of the joints, ligaments and muscles that are localized to a single part of the body only were explored. This section discusses those generalized (or systemic) diseases that tend to affect a number of muscles and joints in the whole body.

The conditions considered here are:

- Arthritis:
  - osteoarthritis (OA)
  - rheumatoid arthritis (RA)
- Arthritis in other autoimmune diseases:
  - systemic lupus erythematosus (SLE)
  - ankylosing spondylitis
  - psoriatic arthritis
  - gout
  - arthritis due to infection
- Disorders of the muscles and ligaments:
  - Fibromyalgia (fibrositis)
  - polymyalgia rheumatica (PMR) and temporal arteritis
  - muscular dystrophy.

Arthritis

The different types of arthritis are summarized in Section 4.2e. In this section, those generalized conditions that manifest in these diverse forms of arthritis will be described.

Osteoarthritis (OA)

As explained in Section 4.2e, osteoarthritis (OA) is a progressive degenerative disorder of the synovial joints. It is the commonest joint disorder, affecting women three times more than men, and is usually symmetrical.

Figure 4.2f-I illustrates the parts of the body that tend to be affected by OA. It can be seen that the hips, knees, ankles and small joints of the fingers (metacarpophalangeal and interphalangeal joints) are most commonly affected.

The underlying process of disease in OA is focal degeneration of the hyaline cartilage that lines the ends of the bones inside a synovial joint. By a mechanism that is poorly understood, in some cases the bone around the joint also degenerates and becomes deformed in shape. The edges of the bony joint become lipped with spiky protuberances of bones called osteophytes (literally meaning bony leaves). Figure 4.2f-II illustrates the cartilage

thinning and osteophyte formation in early OA of the knee joint.

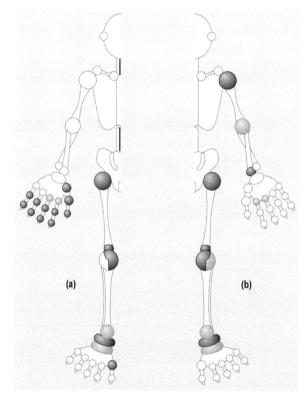

Figure 4.2f-I Typical distribution of the joints affected in generalized osteoarthritis

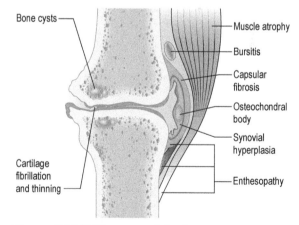

Figure 4.2f-II Diagram of the knee showing early osteoarthritis

The development of OA is so common in old age that it can almost be seen as part of the normal aging process. Most people over 60 will have features of OA on X-ray images, even if they have no symptoms.

The tendency to develop a severe disabling form of OA may be genetically inherited. In addition, any joint that has been subjected to stress or trauma in earlier life is more likely to develop OA with the progression of time. For this reason, being overweight increases the risk of developing OA of the hips and the knees. Strenuous exercise is not good for the joints. It is known that people who are involved in high-impact weight-bearing exercise (running, aerobics, squash, tennis, etc.) are more likely to develop OA of the hip and the knee.[35] Also, joints that are not held in correct alignment due to anatomical deformity, hypermobility of ligaments or chronic muscle tension are more prone to developing OA. Another factor that may make the development of OA worse is a diet low in the natural antioxidants found in a varied range of fruit, vegetables and seeds.

The development of severe symptoms of OA may be prevented by attention to the following:

- avoidance of repetitive stressful use of the joints earlier in life (such as might occur in competitive sports and certain occupations)

- loss of weight (symptoms are much worse in obese people)

- adoption of exercise routines that relax and strengthen the muscles around the joints so that the joints are held in the correct anatomical alignment (gentle swimming, tai chi and gentle yoga can all be very helpful in relieving the chronic pain of OA)

- maintenance of a diet rich in antioxidants.

Joints affected by OA can ache, and tend to feel stiff in the morning, although gentle mobilization will improve this stiffness. Heat often helps the pain. A severely affected large joint may accumulate excess synovial fluid, and can appear puffy.

In many people, particularly women, the first features of OA may be a painless deformity of the small joints of the hand. This commonly starts to occur in late middle age, often around the time of the menopause in women. The distal interphalangeal joints and the first metacarpophalangeal joints are particularly affected. Irregular swellings protrude from the edges of the bone at these joints, so that the ends of the fingers develop a characteristic deformity (known as Heberden's nodes) (see Figure 4.2f-III). In some people this process, known as nodular OA, will cause achy pain and inflammation of the joints of the hand. In most painful cases the pain and the swelling will settle down over the course of a few years, although the deformity of the joints will persist, and may progress.

Less commonly in nodular OA, the minor changes in the hands are accompanied by aching and stiffness of the large joints, which in some cases progresses steadily to a disabling condition. The hips and/or the knees are the most commonly affected joints. Hip pain tends to be felt deep in the low buttock (often in the region of acupoint Huan Tiao GB-30) and radiates into the groin. Weight-bearing exercise is uncomfortable. The knee pain

of OA is felt deep in the joint and may be associated with crunching noises (crepitus) as the joint is moved. In both types of OA the muscles that support the joint may become very thin and wasted. This appears to be a reflex response to the pain in a joint, although it is not helpful for the patient. The weakened muscles cannot support the joint as well, and may contribute to worsening of the symptoms.

Figure 4.2f-III Nodal osteoarthritis
Heberden's nodes of the distal interphalangeal joints, and marked deformity of the middle finger proximal interphalangeal joint.

Degeneration of the joints can also affect the intervertebral joints, in particular, of the cervical spine and the lumbar spine. These changes may or may not co-exist with symptoms of OA elsewhere in the body. These are the changes known as cervical spondylosis and lumbar spondylosis discussed in the previous section.

OA can lead to marked deformity, such as significant bony swelling around the joints of the hands and the knee, but may give rise to very few symptoms. In these cases there is no need for treatment. If symptoms develop, the patient could first be advised about lifestyle changes, such as attention to a healthy diet and weight loss, and be given a simple exercise routine to strengthen the affected joints. Most conventional practitioners would be happy for their patients to seek complementary approaches, such as acupuncture, for the symptoms of early OA, although the UK National Health Service (NHS) does not usually provide these.

Analgesics form the mainstay of the medical treatment approaches for OA. Paracetamol is usually recommended first, before the potentially harmful anti-inflammatory NSAID medication is introduced. Corticosteroids may be injected into affected joints, but it is recognized that this procedure cannot be performed repeatedly as the risks of side effects from this powerful medication are cumulative. Glucosamine is a supplement that is possibly of benefit in mild to moderate OA when prescribed on a once daily basis, although recent analysis of scientific trials has laid doubt on former claims to its effectiveness.[36]

In very severe OA of the large joints, joint replacement surgery can transform the pain and disability caused by the condition. In both hip and knee replacement surgery, the worn-out ends of the bones forming the joint are removed and replaced by plastic or metal replacement parts or prostheses. These do not provoke an immune response because they are not of antigenic material, and many patients recover remarkably quickly from the operation. In about 1 percent of operations a serious complication such as infection or loosening of the joint prosthesis develops. The patient will then require a repeat operation, but the chances of full recovery are diminished. Thrombosis of the leg veins is also a possible complication, although all patients are now protected from this by means of injected anticoagulant medication given during the period of the operation and hospital stay.

A replacement joint will ideally last about ten years before it may need further replacement, but many joints appear to survive longer than this.

 Information box 4.2f-I

Osteoarthritis: comments from a Chinese medicine perspective

In Chinese medicine, the presenting features of OA would be described as Bi Syndrome. The aching and stiffness is characteristic of Cold (Painful) and Damp (Fixed) Bi, whereas the deformities that develop in the late stages of the condition reflect Phlegm (Bony) Bi. There is always an underlying Deficiency of the Kidneys, and particularly so in OA of the knee in which there may also be a Deficiency of the Spleen/Stomach. OA of the hip suggests that there is an additional imbalance of the Gallbladder and Liver Organs.

The analgesics used in OA are suppressive in nature. Joint replacement does not affect the underlying imbalance, but strengthening the integrity and mobility of the joints would appear to be a local form of Nourishing Kidney and Liver Qi and Yin. If it is effective, glucosamine might be described as a Kidney Yin Tonic.

Rheumatoid arthritis (RA)

Rheumatoid arthritis (RA) is a symmetrical inflammatory and deforming arthritis. It is the result of an autoimmune process. The underlying problem in RA is that the body develops autoantibodies that are targeted at the synovial membrane that overlies the cartilage within synovial joints. Other tissues may well be affected by autoimmune damage. This means that RA is an example of a multisystem autoimmune disease.

The synovial lining of the joints in RA becomes very inflamed and thickened. It spreads within the joint space as a boggy tissue called pannus and deprives the cartilage in the joint of nutrients. Pannus also causes thinning and destruction of the bone adjacent to the joint. As the disease progresses, the joint becomes more deformed.

RA is common, affecting 1–3 percent of the population, but is far less common than OA. It generally starts at an earlier age than OA (from age 30 to 50) and affects women more commonly than men, particularly in younger age groups. There is a tendency for it to run in families, but less markedly so than for OA.

Smoking is an important risk factor in RA.

A majority of cases flare up in the winter, and it is more common in damp and cold climates.

RA can affect children. Childhood arthritis has slightly different features to adult RA and is discussed in more detail in Chapter 5.4.

The first symptoms are pain and stiffness of the joints associated with a sense of illness and fever. Stiffness is characteristically worse in the morning and, unlike the stiffness of OA, which improves within a few minutes with movement, may persist for more than an hour after waking. The joints most commonly affected are the small joints of the hands and feet, and the wrists, elbow, knees and ankles. The affected joints are usually warm, tender and slightly swollen. In some people the condition begins with brief episodes of inflammation of a single joint, which may only last for one to two days, and then eventually develops into a more generalized form of arthritis.

Up to 25 percent of cases of RA can be expected to recover completely after the initial flare-up. In some cases the acute condition lasts only a matter of months before it settles down again without leaving any permanent damage, and in other cases, despite a course of a few years, the condition settles down leaving only minimal damage. However, the usual pattern is that the initial condition persists, flaring up from time to time, and over the course of a few years leads to progressive damage to the joints and other parts of the body. In these cases, the initially swollen joints become permanently deformed by the development of pannus within the joint.

In very severe cases the following problems may develop:

- In the hands and feet the fingers and toes tend to point in the ulnar direction, and assume permanent misshapen positions (see Figure 4.2f-IV).

- The muscles around the shoulder may waste and the tendons may rupture, leading to an inability to perform basic activities of daily living such as washing and dressing.

- The knees may become very swollen and deformed, although the hips are only rarely affected.

- RA in the neck can be very serious because parts of the bony vertebrae may become weakened or destroyed. The vertebrae may slip slightly against one another and place excessive pressure on the spinal cord. This may lead to spinal cord compression that requires emergency surgery (see Section 4.1g).

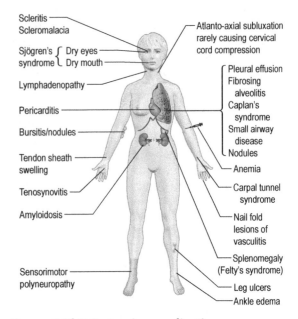

Figure 4.2f-V Systemic complications of rheumatoid arthritis

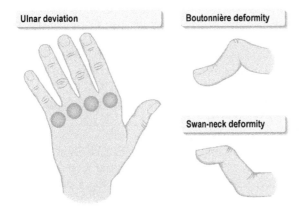

Figure 4.2f-IV Characteristic hand deformities in rheumatoid arthritis

The other parts of the body that can become affected in RA are shown in Figure 4.2f-V. Other aspects of musculoskeletal damage include muscle wasting around affected joints, as also occurs in OA. The tendons can become inflamed (tendonitis), which means that they can become swollen, painful and may rupture. The synovial membrane inside a bursa may also become inflamed, leading to a tense, swollen, hot lump within the soft tissue close to a joint (bursitis). Another cause of lumps in the soft tissue is the formation of nodules. These lumps are unique to RA. They tend to form close to the elbow and other parts of the body exposed to recurrent pressure. Nodules are the result of a focus of autoimmune damage within the soft tissue.

The autoimmune process of RA can also lead to progressive scarring of the lung tissue, damage to single nerves (mononeuropathy) and polyneuropathy (see Section 4.1g), inflammation of the whites of the eye (scleritis), dry eyes, kidney damage and inflammation of the small blood vessels of the skin (vasculitis). In addition to these problems, anemia of chronic disease and depletion of immune cells may also occur.

RA is diagnosed on the basis of the characteristic clinical features, X-ray images of the joints and by means of blood tests. In RA a full blood count (FBC) blood test will often reveal anemia of chronic disease. The erythrocyte sedimentation rate (ESR) and C-reactive protein (CRP) are raised, indicating an inflammatory process (see Section 3.4b). In about 70 percent of cases a particular antibody, called rheumatoid factor, is present in the serum. These so-called seropositive cases of RA are more likely to progress to severe multisystem forms of the disease. It follows that in 30 percent of cases this specific antibody is not detectable, and in these instances a further test for an antibody called anti-cyclic citrullinated peptide (anti-CCP) may be performed.

Treatment involves both symptom control, usually by means of NSAID medication, and a disease-modifying approach. Disease-modifying antirheumatic drugs (DMARDs) are prescribed because they tend to inhibit the destructive inflammatory process, and it is recommended that they are initiated once a diagnosis of RA has been made. Some DMARDs are immunosuppressants used in other conditions such as cancer control. DMARDs include azathioprine, ciclosporin, leflunomide, sulfasalazine, methotrexate, gold (auranofin), penicillamine and hydroxychloroquine. Methotrexate and sulfasalazine are the most commonly prescribed DMARDs. All DMARDs have a number of potentially serious side effects. These include damage to the blood cells, liver damage, kidney damage, visual damage and severe skin rashes, depending on the individual drug, and many patients on DMARDs will need regular monitoring by means of blood tests to ensure that dangerous side effects to medication are not developing.

Because the patient requires monitoring for adverse effects and response to treatment, all patients with RA are best managed by a hospital specialist. Usually only one drug is prescribed at a time, and it is initially given for a few weeks to months to see how well the patient responds. Poor response or the development of side effects will necessitate a change to another DMARD.

Corticosteroids given by tablet are powerful disease-modifying drugs, but are used only in very severe intractable cases of RA because of the problems with long-term side effects (see Section 2.2c). Corticosteroids are also given in RA by injection into inflamed joints or around inflamed tendons. In cases in which there is multisystem involvement, with the threat of damage to major organs such as the kidney, corticosteroids used to be the only option available to prevent disease progression.

A new range of immune system-modifying drugs are now increasingly being prescribed instead of oral steroids in severe cases of RA that are unresponsive to DMARDs. These modulate the action of a mediator of the immune response called cytokines, including tumor necrosis factor (TNF), which is recognized to be overactive in RA. These drugs include infliximab and adalimumab (anti-TNF antibodies) and etanercept (a TNF receptor blocker).[37]

Physiotherapy is an important aspect of the treatment of RA. In acute flare-ups, the damage to the joints can be minimized by splinting the joints in a fixed position. In between flare-ups, graded exercises and hydrotherapy can aid mobility and muscle strength.

Surgery may be performed for a range of reasons in severe RA. The excess pannus in an inflamed joint can be removed surgically to minimize deformity early in the condition. Surgical alteration of the shape of some of the bones close to the joints may relieve pressure points that have developed as a result of joint deformity. With advanced technology, the large joints of the body can now all be replaced with plastic and metal prostheses. In the case of impending cervical cord compression, a surgical approach may be necessary to stabilize the cervical vertebrae.

 Information box 4.2f-II

Rheumatoid arthritis: comments from a Chinese medicine perspective

In Chinese medicine, the initial presentation of RA with hot and stiff joints corresponds to Hot and Damp (Fixed) Bi. In some cases, Cold and Damp Bi may have been the first presentation, but the Cold rapidly turns to Heat. The progression of the condition to the development of permanent deformity is an indication of the Accumulation of Phlegm (Bony Bi). Rheumatoid nodules also correspond to Phlegm. The wasting of muscles and tendons, the weakening of the bones and damage to other systems of the body indicate a severe underlying Deficiency of Spleen Qi, Liver Yin and Kidney Yin and Yang.[38]

NSAIDs are warming and initially Clear Heat by Moving Stagnation. DMARDs and corticosteroids also have Warming properties. The long-term problem with these drugs is that they appear to Deplete Blood and Yin, as evidenced by blood disorders and heat symptoms. All the drugs used to treat RA are suppressive in nature.

Arthritis in other autoimmune diseases

A few of the other multisystem autoimmune diseases involve the musculoskeletal system, and this is the reason for their alternative collective name of rheumatic autoimmune disease. These include systemic lupus erythematosus (SLE), systemic sclerosis and dermatomyositis.

Systemic lupus erythematosus (SLE)

The most common of the multisystem conditions to affect the joints is systemic lupus erythematosus (SLE). SLE is a condition in which autoantibodies also cause damage to the kidneys, skin and hair follicles, the lining of the lungs and the heart, as well as the joints. It tends to affect women significantly more than men. The diagnosis can be confirmed by the presence of antinuclear antibodies (present in 95 percent of cases) and anti-double-stranded DNA antibodies (present in 60 percent of cases). The affected patient suffers from symptoms in episodes known as relapses. These can then subside (remit), leaving disease-free intervals. Important symptoms include tiredness and fever, a facial rash, and muscle and joint aches. A serious relapse can involve symptoms of damage to deep organs, including the heart, lungs, kidneys and brain, and if signs of organ damage are apparent, immunosuppressant drugs including hydroxychloroquine, cyclophosphamide and high-dose corticosteroids may be prescribed. Low-dose steroids or azathioprine may be used as maintenance treatment to prevent relapses occurring in vulnerable patients in remission. More recently, the cytokine modulator drug rituximab, which targets the overactive B-lymphocytes in SLE, has shown some promising benefits.

Ankylosing spondylitis

Ankylosing spondylitis is an inflammatory arthritis that primarily affects the vertebrae and sacroiliac joints. It tends to cluster in families, and its effects are more serious in men than women.

The cause of the inflammation is unknown, although it is known that almost all people who develop ankylosing spondylitis are more likely to have a certain type of genetic makeup (known as HLA B27), which is found in 8 percent of the population. It is believed that this genetic constitution gives susceptibility to developing the condition. There is as yet no evidence of any autoimmune damage in ankylosing spondylitis.

The condition usually first presents in early adulthood, with episodes of pain affecting the sacroiliac joints. This pain can radiate into the buttocks. As with most forms of arthritis, the pain and stiffness are worse in the morning. At an early stage of the disease the patient may also be prone to other inflammatory musculoskeletal conditions, such as inflammation of the joints between the ribs over the front of the chest (costochondritis) or within the soft tissue of the heel (plantar fasciitis). Inflammation of the interior of the eye (uveitis) is also relatively common in people with ankylosing spondylitis. In some people the large joints, in particular, the hip, are affected.

 Information box 4.2f-III

Ankylosing spondylitis: comments from a Chinese medicine perspective

In Chinese medicine, the symptoms of ankylosing spondylitis of stiffness, rigidity and pain in the sacroiliac joints and hips suggests a diagnosis of Qi Stagnation in the Liver and Gallbladder Channels against a background of a Kidney Deficiency. Cold and Damp are likely to be contributory in the chronicity of the problem, and the development of bony deformities is suggestive of Phlegm Formation.

The symptomatic treatments, NSAIDs and sulfasalazine, are both Warming in nature and can Move Stagnation, although in the long run will be Depleting to Yin and Blood. A gentle exercise program is an energetically appropriate approach, as it will enable the Movement of Stagnation and prevent Phlegm Accumulation without being depleting.

In severe cases, the mobility of the sacroiliac joints and the intervertebral joints gradually becomes greatly reduced as bony osteophytes grow out and cause the bones to fuse across the joints (the term ankylosing refers to this phenomenon). In severe cases, the ribs cannot expand freely as their joints are also affected, and breathing becomes labored. The thoracic part of the chest and the neck can become very bowed, so much so that the person may be unable to look straight ahead. Fibrosis of the lungs may also develop and contribute to restricted breathing.

This severe degree of rigidity can be prevented, at least in part, if the condition is diagnosed early and the patient is encouraged to perform regular back exercises. NSAIDs and COX-2 inhibitors may be prescribed for their symptom-relieving properties, as pain relief will enable exercises to be performed more freely. The new anti-TNF drugs adalimumab and etanercept, which are known to be of benefit in advanced RA, are licensed for use in ankylosing spondylitis.

Although the majority of patients with ankylosing spondylitis live normal lives, nearly a fifth become moderately to severely disabled by the condition.

Psoriatic arthritis

Psoriasis is a common inflammatory scaling disorder of the skin (see Section 6.1c). Up to 8 percent of people with psoriasis will develop one of a number of forms of arthritis. In some cases the arthritis appears before the skin disorder. It can be triggered by exposure to damp and cold climates.

The arthritis is typically symmetrical and inflammatory in nature. The most common form involves the finger joints only, and in this case deformities and pitting of the nails are common. In other forms the arthritis can be much more widely distributed and can be very similar to RA. In addition, it is not uncommon for tendonitis and bursitis to occur. It is a characteristic of psoriatic arthritis that, as well as the synovial membrane becoming inflamed, the bone adjacent to the joint can become eroded. In less than 5 percent of cases this bony erosion is so severe that the integrity of joints is seriously compromised (see Figure 4.2f-VI).

Figure 4.2f-VI X-ray image of feet in psoriatic arthritis, showing deformities of the toes
The circled area shows a total loss of bone on the head of the fourth metatarsal, and a hollowing of the proximal end of the fourth proximal phalanx.

In most cases NSAIDs are all that is needed to provide symptom relief. In more serious cases, sulfasalazine or other immunosuppressants may be prescribed to control the progression of the disease.

Information box 4.2f-IV

Psoriatic arthritis: comments from a Chinese medicine perspective

In Chinese medicine, the diagnosis of psoriatic arthritis is similar to that of RA, in that it would correspond to a form of Damp and Hot Bi against a background of Deficiency. In some cases this may be precipitated by an initial invasion of Damp Cold. In psoriasis the scaling, inflamed skin would be attributed to Heat (and sometimes Phlegm/Damp) upon an underlying Deficiency of Blood and Yin.

Gout

Gout is an inflammatory arthritis that results from the formation of crystals of uric acid (also known as urate) within the synovial fluid. Uric acid is a by-product of the normal metabolic processes of the body. It is produced in excess if there is a high amount of cholesterol, beer, offal, fish, shellfish, yeast extract and fructose syrup in the diet, or if there is a high turnover of cells in the body, such as might occur in cancer. Uric acid is usually excreted by the kidneys so that its levels do not rise too high. However, excretion from the kidneys may be impaired in certain situations, including following excessive exercise, in starvation and following excessive alcohol intake. Certain drugs, including thiazide diuretics and aspirin, can also impair the excretion of uric acid. Gout is more common if the patient has high cholesterol or if they are obese.

If the concentration of uric acid in the blood becomes too high, which might occur as a combination of excessive production of uric acid and impaired excretion, crystals of uric acid can come out of solution within the synovial fluid. The crystals are engulfed by leukocytes, but this then causes these cells to rupture and release inflammatory chemicals into the joint. This triggers the process of inflammation.

Commonly, the arthritis of gout is confined to a single joint, often the first metatarsophalangeal joint (at the base of the big toe). However, large joints, such as the knee or ankle, might also be affected. The affected joint becomes acutely inflamed and swollen, and is intensely painful. The attack may be precipitated by a binge of drinking and eating to excess or by a period of dehydration. Not uncommonly, a prescription of diuretics can provoke an attack. Men are affected more often than women, and attacks are more likely in older people. Less commonly, the arthritis can be more generalized, and affects a number of joints. This form of gout is more prevalent in elderly people.

If the uric acid level is very high, the crystals may form not only in the joint but also in the soft tissues. This leads to large inflamed white deposits called tophi. Tophi might appear in various sites, including the tissues surrounding joints and the ear lobes. In these cases there is a possibility that crystals may also be deposited within the delicate tissue of the kidney. This is a serious situation that requires prompt medical treatment.

Gout is diagnosed by examination of joint fluid for crystals (not always performed) and by a serum blood test for uric acid levels, which will show high-normal to high levels.

An acute attack of gout is treated by encouraging a high fluid intake, and prescription of NSAIDs to calm down the inflammation and relieve the intense pain. The medication colchicine or corticosteroids might also be prescribed to help calm down an acute attack.

If attacks are frequent and do not respond to dietary advice and alcohol reduction, allopurinol is prescribed to be taken on a regular basis. This drug reduces the production of uric acid in the body. A severe but very rare side effect is depletion of blood cell production in the marrow. More commonly, skin rashes may occur.

Information box 4.2f-V

Acute gout: comments from a Chinese medicine perspective

In Chinese medicine, the intense pain of acute gout would correspond to Heat and Damp Bi. Tophi would be described as a manifestation of Phlegm/Fire. Foods that precipitate attacks tend to be Damp Heat forming, such as alcohol, shellfish and fructose syrup. The most likely site for an attack is the big toe, and this position might suggest an underlying Liver or Spleen disharmony. An underlying Deficiency of Kidney Yin may also be present.

Arthritis due to infection

A temporary generalized arthritis is a very common occurrence either during or following a number of viral infections. For example, the childhood infection of rubella often causes joint aches, particularly in adults who contract the infection. Chickenpox, glandular fever and mumps are other common causes. In some cases the aching of the joints can persist for a few days to weeks after the infection has settled down.

Some bacterial infections may also affect the joints. The most common of these in the UK is the sexually transmitted disease of gonorrhea. The infection by the *Gonococcus* bacterium spreads from the genital tract, and leads to a fever and a prolonged period of joint aches and swelling. Gonococcal arthritis is most common in women and men who have sex with men. It responds to antibiotic treatment.

Information box 4.2f-VI

Arthritis associated with acute infections: comments from a Chinese medicine perspective

In Chinese medicine, acute arthritis associated with infection might correspond to Wind and Heat Bi following an Invasion of Wind Heat.

In some susceptible patients an inflammatory arthritis (not unlike early RA or ankylosing spondylitis) develops as a delayed reaction to infection by some of the gastrointestinal or sexually transmitted organisms (including *Salmonella*, *Shigella* and *Chlamydia*). In most cases this arthritis will settle down within weeks, but in some a progressive condition develops. In severe cases, attacks of uveitis might occur, and episodes of tendonitis and plantar fasciitis can develop (as can occur in ankylosing spondylitis). This reactive arthritis is treated with NSAIDs. If the arthritis is progressive, DMARDs and corticosteroids, as used in RA or ankylosing spondylitis, may be prescribed. The new anti-TNF drugs adalimumab and etanercept may have a role in severe, unremitting cases.

Information box 4.2f-VII

Reactive arthritis: comments from a Chinese medicine perspective

The Chinese medicine interpretation of reactive arthritis would be similar to that for RA or ankylosing spondylitis. In reactive arthritis, it is likely that the initial infection has led to the accumulation of the Pathogenic Factors of Damp and Heat.

Rheumatic fever is a rare complication of infection with the *Streptococcus* bacterium (most commonly in the form of tonsillitis). It is much more common in the Middle and Far East, Eastern Europe and South America. It mostly tends to affect children and adolescents. In this condition the bacterial infection triggers a delayed autoimmune response, which primarily affects the joints but can also affect the heart, skin and nervous system.

Rheumatic fever follows on from a streptococcal infection with a sudden onset of high fever, joint pains and malaise. The joints are red, swollen and exquisitely tender,

and the pain and swelling flits from one joint to another. In some cases there are irregularities of the heart rhythm and heart murmurs due to inflammation of the pericardium and heart valves. There may also be a pink skin rash, which spreads across the skin. A very severe late complication is Sydenham's chorea (also known as St Vitus' dance), which is a disorder of movement and speech resulting from damage to the nerve centers deep in the brain.

Treatment of rheumatic fever includes bed rest and antibiotics to eradicate the streptococcal infection. The joint pains respond to high-dose aspirin. Corticosteroids may be given to limit damage to the heart.

In most cases the symptoms subside within three weeks, but in some patients symptoms persist for much longer and the arthritis can become long-standing.

About one-tenth of those who experience inflammation of the heart and valves in the acute infection will go on to develop progressive valve damage in late adulthood (see Section 3.2g).

Information box 4.2f-VIII

Rheumatoid arthritis: comments from a Chinese medicine perspective

In Chinese medicine, an attack of RA might be diagnosed as Wind Heat Invasion with Wind (Moving) and Heat Bi. The development of cardiac complications suggests that the Heat in this condition can be very Full and can damage Heart Yin.

Generalized disorders of the muscles and ligaments

Fibromyalgia (fibrositis)

Fibromyalgia is a term used by some conventional practitioners to describe a condition in which the muscles, particularly of the back and shoulders, are tense and very tender. The tenderness is often focused in certain defined areas called trigger points. By definition, several knots or areas of very tense muscle (myofascial trigger points) are found in diverse muscle groups. Fibromyalgia is recognized to be more common in women and to be associated with emotional disharmony of one sort or another.

A patient with the symptoms of fibromyalgia may also suffer from the symptoms of other functional conditions such as irritable bowel syndrome (IBS), chronic fatigue syndrome (CFS), premenstrual syndrome (PMS) or recurrent headaches.

Fibromyalgia is not a well-understood condition in Western medicine. Patients with severe symptoms may be referred to pain management clinics. NSAIDs may be given to relieve the pain, and counseling or antidepressants may be considered to treat the emotional foundation of the condition. It is recognized that the trigger points may be relieved by corticosteroid injections, deep massage or acupuncture.

Information box 4.2f-IX

Fibromyalgia: comments from a Chinese medicine perspective

In Chinese medicine, the pain of fibromyalgia represents Liver Qi and Blood Stagnation. The fact that the muscles and flesh in diverse body regions are tender and painful suggests there may be an underlying Deficiency of Spleen Qi and/or Liver Blood and Kidney Yin, and the chronicity in some cases suggests that Wind Damp Heat is part of the diagnostic picture. Very substantial myofascial nodules can be attributed to Phlegm.[39]

Polymyalgia rheumatica (PMR) and temporal arteritis

Polymyalgia rheumatica (PMR) is an inflammatory condition of the arteries that leads to severe pain and stiffness in the large muscle groups of the shoulders and hips. Like another inflammatory disorder of the arteries, temporal arteritis (see Section 4.1e), it is a condition that primarily affects elderly people, and women are affected more commonly than men.

The patient is often unwell, with fever, exhaustion and depression. Getting up from sitting or lifting arms to head height might be difficult because of muscle weakness in the muscle groups around the hip and shoulder.

There may be an overlap with the symptoms of temporal arteritis. If a one-sided headache develops, it should be treated very seriously as a warning sign of an impending loss of vision or stroke.

In terms of blood test abnormalities, PMR is associated with a raised ESR, mild anemia and a raised alkaline phosphatase level on testing of liver function.

Treatment is initially with a moderate dose of corticosteroids (10–15mg/daily), which always leads to a dramatic reduction in symptoms and an improvement in well-being. Most people need to be on this medication for at least a year, and for about a quarter of these this treatment has to be lifelong in order to keep symptoms at bay.

As long-term steroid treatment can cause osteoporosis, patients being treated for PMR will also often be prescribed bone-protecting drugs such as bisphosphonate, calcium and vitamin D.

Information box 4.2f-X

Polymyalgia rheumatica and temporal arteritis: comments from a Chinese medicine perspective

In Chinese medicine, the symptoms of arteritis might suggest Heat and Stagnation in the blood vessels. As this is a condition of elderly people, there is a possibility that the Heat may have been generated as a result of chronic Deficiency of Kidney Yin. The intense aching and stiffness of polymyalgia is also a reflection of severe Qi Stagnation, and its distribution often relates to the Gallbladder and Bladder Channels.

Corticosteroids are Warming in nature and Clear Stagnation by Moving Qi. In the long term they will further Deplete Kidney Yin and Jing.

Muscular dystrophy

The muscular dystrophies are a group of inherited disorders that result in a progressive degeneration of skeletal muscle. In some forms the cardiac muscle is also affected.

Duchenne muscular dystrophy is the most common form, affecting 1 in 4000 male infants. The genetic defect leads to an absence of a protein essential for the maturation of skeletal muscle. The muscular dystrophy becomes obvious in early childhood, when the child loses the ability to run with ease or to stand up from the floor without support. By the age of ten the muscles of the limbs are very wasted, and the child becomes severely disabled. Death is inevitable between the ages of 15 and 25, and usually results from respiratory infections.

There are less severe forms of muscular dystrophy. Of the two next most common forms, one results in a severe but not life-threatening disability by early adulthood, and the other causes a relative muscle weakness, particularly of the upper body, but life expectancy is normal.

For all forms of muscular dystrophy, the only treatment is supportive, including physiotherapy to prevent muscle contractures. Genetic counseling with respect to future pregnancies may be offered to parents and siblings.

Information box 4.2f-XI

Muscular dystrophy: comments from a Chinese medicine perspective

In Chinese medicine, the symptoms of muscular dystrophy would indicate Jing Deficiency. Weak and wasted muscles are an indication of particular Deficiency of Spleen and Liver Qi.

The red flags of generalized disorders of the joints, ligaments and muscles

Some patients with the generalized disorders of the joints, ligaments and muscles will benefit from referral to a conventional doctor for assessment and/or treatment.

Red flags are those symptoms and signs that indicate that referral should be considered. The red flags of the generalized disorders of the joints, ligaments and muscles are described in Table 4.2f-I. A summary of the red flags in a format designed for quick reference in clinical practice can be found in Appendix III. This gives advice on the degree of urgency of referral for each of the red flag conditions listed.

Table 4.2f-I A28: Red flags of generalized diseases of the joints, ligaments and muscles

Red flag	Description	Reasoning
A28.1	Features of a degenerative arthritis that may benefit from joint replacement: severe disability from long-standing pain and stiffness in the hips, knees or shoulders	Complementary medical treatment such as acupuncture and osteopathy can be very helpful supportive treatment in advanced osteoarthritis of the hip, knee or shoulder. Referral needs to be considered if the condition is deteriorating to a point at which the activities of daily living are becoming compromised. Refer early, as the patient may need to be put on a waiting list, meaning that surgical treatment may only come after a delay of some weeks to months
A28.2	Any features of an inflammatory arthritis: symmetrical pain, stiffness and swelling of the joints, or symmetrical stiffness and pain in the sacroiliac joint. May be associated with a fever or sense of malaise	All episodes of inflammatory arthritis (distinguished from osteoarthritis (OA) by fairly rapid onset, over days to weeks rather than months to years, joint swelling, fever and general malaise) are best investigated by a conventional practitioner so that autoimmune disease or other serious underlying disease can be excluded. Some forms of inflammatory arthritis are erosive, and powerful medical approaches should be considered to prevent progression and permanent joint damage
A28.3	Features of polymyalgia rheumatica (PMR): prolonged pain and stiffness and weakness of the muscles of the hips and shoulders associated with malaise and depression. Refer urgently if there is a sudden onset of a severe, one-sided, temporal headache or visual disturbances	PMR is an inflammatory condition of the muscles of the shoulders and hips that predominantly afflicts people over the age of 50. Because it is inflammatory in nature there may be associated malaise, but the main symptoms are pain and weakness of the shoulder and hip muscles. Difficulty in standing from a sitting position is a classic sign of hip weakness

There is an increased risk of the serious condition of temporal arteritis (see A23.5). Referral is advised so that the patient can be offered the medical treatment of corticosteroids |

The Urinary System

4.3

4.3a The physiology of the urinary system

The urinary system consists of the kidneys, the ureters, the bladder and the urethra. An alternative name is the renal system, although strictly speaking, renal (from the Latin term for kidney) is a term that refers to the kidneys alone. The Greek word for kidney is *nephron*, and hence the study of the kidneys is called nephrology.

The component parts of the urinary system are illustrated in Figure 4.3a-I. It can be seen how the kidneys are situated in the upper part of the back of the abdomen. They rest, protected against the ribs, between the levels of T11 and L3. The influential acupoints on the back of the Kidney Organ (Shen Shu, BL-23) lie directly over the lower parts of the kidneys. The ureters run from the medial aspect of each kidney, down the posterior border of the abdominal cavity, to open into the bladder. The bladder sits protected within the pelvis. Note from the diagram how small the bladder is. Even when uncomfortably full the bladder rarely rises very much higher than the level of the pubic symphysis (the region of acupoint Qu Gu, RN-2). The urethra (a very similar name to that of the more proximal ureter, but a different anatomical structure) is the tube that links the bladder to the external world. It is very short in women, but longer in men because of its passage through the penis.

The major function of the kidneys is to maintain homeostasis of the composition of the blood by excreting wastes and controlling the concentrations of the various mineral salts within the blood. They do this by the formation of urine, which is a solution of wastes and salts. Other important functions of the kidneys include the control of blood pressure, control of the development of red blood

cells by the secretion of the hormone erythropoietin, and production of active vitamin D.

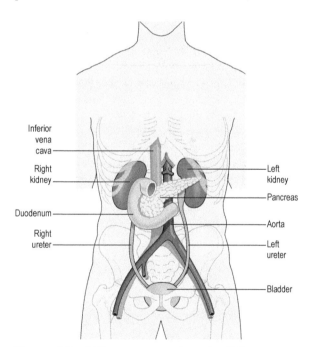

Figure 4.3a-I The component parts of the urinary system (excluding the urethra) and related abdominal structures

The function of the ureters is to allow the free drainage of the urine into the bladder. The bladder is a reservoir that contains this steady flow of urine from the kidneys until there is an appropriate time for its expulsion. This happens through the process of urination (also known as micturition) in which the bladder contracts and the urine passes through the urethra and out of the body.

The physiology of the kidneys[40]

The position and structure of the kidneys

The kidneys sit at the back of the upper abdominal cavity embedded in fat. The adrenal glands sit on the top of each kidney, but do not have a direct link with the role of the urinary system. However, both the adrenal glands and the kidneys have functions that would be understood in Chinese medicine as being related to the Kidney Organ. The kidneys sit very close to a number of other deep organs, including the spleen, pancreas, liver, duodenum and the large intestine.

The tissue of the kidney consists of thousands of tiny tubes called nephrons. Each of these tubes has its origin in the outer parts of the substance of the kidney (the renal cortex). The nephrons converge to open out into wider tubes called collecting tubules, which drain into a space in the core of the kidney called the renal pelvis. The renal pelvis drains downwards into the ureter. The collecting tubules are situated in the deeper tissue of the kidney that is known as the renal medulla. Figures 4.3a-II and 4.3a-III illustrate the external and internal structure of the kidneys in some detail. Figure 4.3a-II shows the position and size of the adrenal glands, and Figure 4.3a-III indicates the location of the renal cortex, medulla, pelvis and ureter.

These diagrams clarify how the kidneys receive their blood supply from a large branch of the aorta called the renal artery. This artery branches within the substance of the kidney to provide each nephron with its own arteriole. The blood supply to the kidney is very rich. About a quarter of all the blood that has left the heart is directed from the aorta through the kidneys. This is very important because it ensures that the blood undergoes a continual and efficient process of being cleansed and returned to a state of balance.

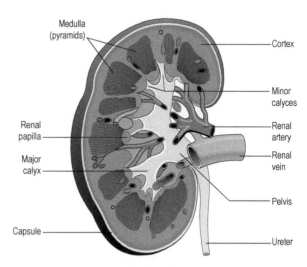

Figure 4.3a-III Longitudinal section of the right kidney

The formation of urine in the kidneys

Figure 4.3a-IV shows how the blood that reaches the nephron first enters a cluster of capillaries called the glomerulus. Here, because of a sudden restriction of easy flow, fluid containing salts, wastes and water is forced out of the glomerulus. From here this fluid passes into the cup-like origin of the nephron. However, substances such as plasma proteins and blood cells are too large to be squeezed out, and so these remain within the blood vessel. This process of draining water and small molecules from the blood into the nephron is called simple filtration.

This fluid then drains down through the tube of the glomerulus towards the collecting tubule. However, it does not yet have the composition of urine. During its passage through the nephron some of the fluid and the salts are reabsorbed back into the bloodstream. The diagram indicates how the arteriole travels on to supply the rest of the nephron with a blood supply for this purpose. Substances can also be secreted from the blood in the arteriole into more distal parts of the nephron.

These two processes of reabsorption and secretion not only make the original fluid that has been drained out of the glomerulus much more concentrated (it is nearly 200 times as concentrated as plasma fluid), but they also allow for a subtle control of its composition according to the body's requirements. For instance, if the person is dehydrated, more water than normal is reabsorbed, and if the person is depleted in salts, more salts are reabsorbed.

The reabsorption and secretion of the fluid in the nephron are under the control of a number of hormones, including parathyroid hormone from the tiny parathyroid glands in the neck (which regulates calcium and phosphate levels), antidiuretic hormone (ADH) from the pituitary gland (which regulates the concentration of the blood) and aldosterone from the adrenal glands (which regulates the amount of sodium and potassium in the blood).

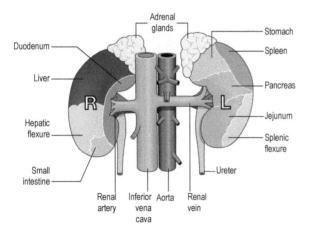

Figure 4.3a-II Anterior view of the kidneys illustrating proximity to overlying abdominal organs

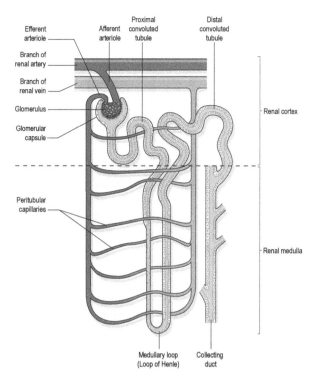

Efferent arteriole

Afferent arteriole

Proximal convoluted tubule

Distal convoluted tubule

Branch of renal artery

Branch of renal vein

Glomerulus

Glomerular capsule

Renal cortex

Peritubular capillaries

Renal medulla

Medullary loop (Loop of Henle)

Collecting duct

Figure 4.3a-IV A nephron and the associated blood vessels

The fluid that leaves the nephron to enter the collecting tubule and thence the renal pelvis has the composition of urine. This yellow-colored fluid consists mostly (96 percent) of water, with a further 2 percent being urea (the waste product of protein metabolism) and the remaining 2 percent comprising a range of other salts including sodium, potassium and uric acid. In a healthy adult, approximately 1–1.5 liters of urine are passed a day, although this can vary from as little as 500 milliliters to as high as 3 liters, depending on the balance of fluid intake and other fluid losses.

Diuretic drugs that act on the kidney tend to inhibit the amount of water that is reabsorbed, and so increase the volume of urine entering the renal pelvis. Some diuretic drugs may also affect the reabsorption of salts. This is why some diuretics can lead to sodium or potassium depletion, and others may cause a buildup of uric acid (predisposing to an attack of gout).

The kidneys and the formation of red blood cells

Erythropoietin (EPO) is a hormone that is made within the kidneys and is released into the bloodstream in response to low levels of oxygen. It is an essential factor in the production of red blood cells from the bone marrow. When blood oxygen levels drop, the secretion of EPO is stimulated, and this in turn increases the production of red blood cells from the bone marrow. These blood cells are then available to carry more oxygen, and thereby to increase the level of oxygen in the blood.

The kidneys and the control of blood pressure

Healthy kidneys are essential for the control of blood pressure, and disease of the kidneys is one of the causes of hypertension. In addition, the kidneys act in a situation of shock (low blood pressure) to conserve fluid, and so to prevent its loss into the urine. There are at least two important hormone systems that cause the kidney to excrete more fluid when the blood pressure is high and to conserve fluid when the blood pressure drops.

The hormones involved in the kidneys' control of blood pressure include aldosterone, renin, angiotensin I and II, and atrial natriuretic factor (ANF). ACE (angiotensin-converting enzyme) inhibitors and angiotensin II receptor blockers are drugs used in the treatment of hypertension and heart failure. They act by blocking the formation of one of these hormones (angiotensin II).

The kidneys and vitamin D metabolism

Although vitamin D is mostly manufactured as a response to the action of sunlight on the skin, it requires conversion within the kidneys to become active in the body. For this reason, kidney disease can be a cause of the disease of weakening of the bones known as osteomalacia.

The physiology of the ureters

The ureters receive a steady flow of urine from the renal pelvis at a rate of 20–100 milliliters/hour. These structures run down the back of the abdominal cavity and enter the bladder where it sits within the pelvis. The flow of urine is aided by waves of muscular contractions that are generated by the smooth muscle fibers within the ureter walls.

The urine that enters the bladder passes through a narrowing, akin to a valve, as it enters the bladder. This important structure prevents the return of urine back into the ureter (known as reflux) from the bladder. The urine enters the bladder in little spurts, which occur every 10 seconds or so.

The physiology of the bladder

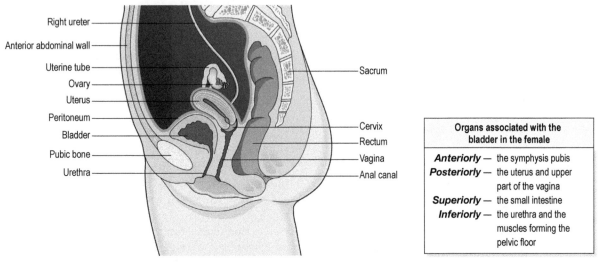

Figure 4.3a-V The pelvic organs associated with the bladder in the female

Organs associated with the bladder in the female
Anteriorly — the symphysis pubis
Posteriorly — the uterus and upper part of the vagina
Superiorly — the small intestine
Inferiorly — the urethra and the muscles forming the pelvic floor

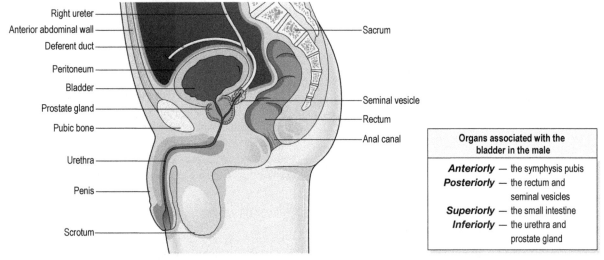

Figure 4.3a-VI The pelvic organs associated with the bladder in the male

Organs associated with the bladder in the male
Anteriorly — the symphysis pubis
Posteriorly — the rectum and seminal vesicles
Superiorly — the small intestine
Inferiorly — the urethra and prostate gland

The bladder is a hollow, pear-shaped organ, the function of which is to act as a reservoir for urine. Figures 4.3a-V and 4.3a-VI above show a vertical section through the pelvis of a woman and a man, respectively. These diagrams illustrate the position of the bladder within the pelvis. Note how in the woman the bladder sits just in front of the cervix and womb. In the man the prostate gland sits at the neck of the bladder, surrounding the first part of the urethra.

The bladder is lined by a form of epithelium called transitional epithelium that has the ability to stretch. Within the wall of the bladder are sheets of smooth muscle, which together are called the detrusor muscle. When the detrusor muscle contracts, it forces urine out through the urethra.

In a healthy adult the desire to urinate arises when the bladder contains more than 300 milliliters of urine. At this stage, the stretch of the bladder muscle stimulates nerve impulses so that the bladder contracts spontaneously (this is a spinal reflex). Indeed, this is what occurs both in the newborn and in someone who has had a spinal injury. However, in the healthy adult, although the sensation of a desire to urinate occurs at this stage, the brain exerts an inhibitory control on this reflex until an appropriate time arises for it to occur. This voluntary control of bladder function is usually learned during the third year of life.

The physiology of the urethra

The urethra is the canal that leaves the neck of the bladder and links it to the exterior. In women, the urethra is about 4cm long, and it opens to the exterior just in front of the vaginal orifice. In men, the urethra first passes through the tissue of the prostate gland and then travels through the length of the penis to the orifice at the tip of the glans penis. Ducts open out into the first part of the male urethra through which the seminal fluid and semen are passed during ejaculation.

In both women and men the urethra passes through the region of the body called the perineum that forms the floor of the pelvis. In doing so, it passes through the pelvic floor muscles, which are slung between the pubic bone and the base of the sacrum and coccyx.

At the origin of the urethra is a smooth muscle ring called the internal urethral sphincter. This is generally maintained in a state of contraction, thus holding the urine within the bladder. In addition to the internal sphincter, the muscles of the pelvic floor provide an additional external urethral sphincter as a result of their generally high level of tone. Together, these factors exert a closing pressure on the urethra, which is released when the person intends to urinate.

 Information box 4.3a-I

The urinary system: comments from a Chinese medicine perspective

According to traditional Chinese medicine, the functions of the Kidneys and Bladder are considered to be as follows.

The Kidneys:

- store Essence (Jing) and control birth, growth, reproduction and development
- produce Marrow, fill up the brain and control bones
- govern water
- control the reception of Qi
- open into the ears
- manifest in the hair
- control the lower two orifices
- house the Will.[41]

The Bladder:

- removes water by the power of Qi transformation.[42]

According to Chinese medicine, it is not only the Kidneys and Bladder that play a part in fluid balance and the excretion of waste. The Lungs, Spleen, Small Intestine and Triple Burner also have specific functions, which are described by Maciocia (1989).[43] These can be summarized as follows.

The Lungs control dispersing and descending. The Lungs have the function of spreading the body fluids around the body in the form of a fine mist. If impaired, fluid may accumulate in the form of edema (often of the face).

The Lungs regulate the water passages. The Lungs also direct fluids down to the Kidneys and Bladder. If this function is impaired there may be urinary retention.

The Spleen governs transformation and transportation. One aspect of this is the transformation, separation and movement of fluids. In Chinese medicine the dirty part of the fluids ingested gets sent to the Small Intestine. If this function is impaired, Phlegm or Damp will Accumulate, sometimes in the form of edema.

The Small Intestine controls receiving and transforming and separates Fluids. The Small Intestine first receives food and drink from the Stomach. The Clean part is sent to the Spleen, and the Dirty part to the Large Intestine (solid) and to the Bladder (fluid). This function of separation is powered by Kidney Yang.

The Lower Burner aspect of the Triple Burner is directly related to the excretion of fluids. This is the aspect that directs the separation of the food essences into a Dirty and Clean part, and which facilitates the excretion of the dirty fluid as urine. In this way the Lower Burner is a summary of the function of the Spleen and Small Intestine.

So here it becomes clear that the Chinese medicine interpretation of the function of the urinary system is not that straightforward. First, most of the functions of the Kidney Organ do not relate directly to functions of the urinary system (e.g. storage of Essence, production of Marrow (with the exception of the effect of EPO on red blood cell production), reception of Qi, opening into the ears, manifesting in the hair and housing Will power). Second, the actual function of the urinary system, which is to permit the continual cleansing of the blood of wastes and the removal of excess fluid into the urine, would seem to be controlled in Chinese medicine by a number of Organs (i.e. Kidney, Bladder, Stomach and Spleen, Small Intestine and the Triple Burner).

It is important to bear this in mind when considering specific diseases of the urinary system, and attempting to draw conclusions about a Chinese medicine interpretation. An imbalance in the urinary system may therefore be described in terms of pathology of one or more of these six Chinese medicine organs.

4.3b The investigation of the urinary system

Diseases of the urinary system are investigated within three distinct conventional specialties. Medical conditions that affect the kidney are treated by a renal physician within the specialty of renal medicine or nephrology. Conditions that affect the ureters, bladder and urethra, and also those conditions of the kidney that may require surgery, are treated by a surgeon called a urologist within the specialty of urology. Conditions that affect the male reproductive organs are also commonly treated by a urologist. However, those conditions that result from sexually transmitted diseases are treated by a genitourinary physician within the specialty of genitourinary medicine or sexual medicine.

The investigation of the urinary system

The investigation of the urinary system involves:

- a thorough physical examination
- urine examination
- blood examination to check for anemia, to assay waste products and salts in the serum, and to look for autoantibodies and other markers of specific diseases
- imaging tests to examine the structure of the urinary system, including ultrasound scan, computed tomography (CT) scan and plain X-ray images
- imaging tests to examine the function of the urinary system, including intravenous urography, cystourethrography and radioactive isotope scans
- examination of the inside of the bladder (cystoscopy)
- biopsy of the kidneys
- urodynamic studies.

These are each considered briefly in turn below.

Physical examination

The physical examination of the urinary system involves the stages listed in Table 4.3b-I.

Table 4.3b-I The stages in the physical examination of the urinary system

Examination of general appearance for the pallor of anemia and the smoky yellow tinge of uremia (this develops in chronic renal failure)

Assessment of blood pressure

Examination of the ankles for evidence of edema

Examination of the abdomen for abnormal enlargement of the kidneys or a distended bladder (the kidneys and bladder are usually not palpable in the abdominal examination, so if they can be felt, this is a sign of distension or enlargement)

Examination of the male genitalia and prostate gland: the prostate gland is examined by means of the insertion of a gloved finger through the anus into the rectum

Examination of the female genitalia: internal vaginal examination can identify uterine prolapse and posterior prolapse of the bladder wall, both causes of urinary incontinence

Urine examination

The most commonly performed urine tests require a midstream sample of urine (MSU). This means that the specimen is taken only after a flow of urine from the urethra has been established. The sample should ideally be free from contamination by the bacteria of the skin, although this is not always possible to ensure, particularly when collecting urine from small children. Any sterile container is suitable for a urine specimen.

Healthy urine is pale yellow and clear. The first urine passed in the morning is usually the most concentrated, and can have a deep amber color. Visual assessment of urine may reveal a pink discoloration suggestive of blood or cloudiness suggestive of infection. Both these findings are abnormal, but commonly result from benign causes. For example, a large amount of beetroot in the recent diet as well as some medications can cause the urine to become pink.

The simplest quantitative test of urine involves dipping the urine with a plastic strip that holds tiny indicator cards. These cards change color according to the concentration of a range of factors within the urine. Use of the plastic dipsticks, commonly termed stix or multistix, can give an instantaneous indication of the amount of sugar, blood, protein and white blood cells in the urine, to name just a few of the variables that can be detected. This test is not as reliable as a laboratory test, but is very commonly used in general practice to check for blood in the urine (hematuria), to give an indication of undiagnosed or poorly controlled diabetes, and to give added weight to a provisional diagnosis of urine infection.

Urine may then be sent to a laboratory for microscopic examination. This may reveal the presence of microorganisms and excessive white blood cells in the case of infection. It will also confirm the presence of red blood cells in the urine. In the diseases (classed as glomerulonephritis) that affect the structure of the tubules of the kidney, unusual tube-shaped casts of protein may be seen in the urine.

The urine can also be analyzed for the substances that are dissolved within it. In addition to the usual body wastes, drugs and hormones can also be found in the urine. Therefore, a urine test can detect the presence of illicit drugs or increased levels of hormones. There is very little protein to be found in healthy urine, but in severe kidney disease it may be present in vast quantities. Both the total protein and the albumin (the most common protein in the plasma) levels may be assessed from a urine sample. A 24-hour collection of urine may be used to quantify accurately the protein loss in kidney disease, and can also be used to assess the rate at which blood is filtered by the kidneys (glomerular filtration rate).

Blood examination

A serum sample of blood can be analyzed to reveal the disturbances in blood chemicals that result from kidney failure. In particular, the by-products of protein metabolism (urea and creatinine) may be increased in quantity. In severe kidney disease there may also be disturbances of the concentration of the basic mineral salts, such as sodium, calcium and potassium, in the blood. The level of creatinine may be inserted into a mathematical formula that incorporates the age, ethnicity and sex of the patient to generate an estimate of the amount of fluid filtered by the kidneys in a fixed amount of time. This is the estimated glomerular filtration rate (eGFR), which is a useful indication of the progression of chronic kidney disease (CKD), a condition that becomes increasingly prevalent with aging.

Other factors that indicate a specific cause of kidney disease may also be assayed (e.g. autoantibodies in systemic lupus erythematosus (SLE)). In disease of the prostate gland, a particular protein called prostate-specific antigen (PSA) is assayed, as this is more likely to be raised if cancer is present.

A full blood count (FBC) may reveal the anemia of chronic disease that can accompany chronic kidney disease.

Imaging tests to examine the structure of the urinary system

Ultrasound, magnetic resonance imaging (MRI) and CT scans are used to visualize the shape of the kidneys, ureters and bladder. The images obtained may be used to examine gross defects, such as the presence of cancer or obstruction to the outflow of urine from the bladder, but cannot reveal the more subtle changes that occur in most diseases of the urinary system. An ultrasound scan obtained by means of a probe passed into the anus may also be used to examine the prostate gland.

A plain X-ray image, although it cannot show any detail about the soft tissues, may be used to reveal the presence of kidney stones, also known as calculi. Figure 4.3b-I shows the X-ray images of the passage over time of a calculus down the left ureter.

Figure 4.3b-I X-ray images of calculi (ureteric stones) at different levels of the left ureter

A catheter (a plastic tube) may be passed into the bladder via the urethra to inject a dye that is opaque to X-rays into the bladder. This test, known as cystography or urography, can show up defects in the structure of the bladder.

Imaging tests to examine the function of the urinary system

Until recently, the most commonly performed of the imaging tests of function would involve the intravenous injection of a solution that contained iodine. This solution, when concentrated, shows up on X-ray images. After injection, serial X-ray images can be taken of the abdomen. The whole procedure, known as an intravenous urogram (IVU) or excretion urogram, reveals the passage of the dye through the urinary system, from when it is first concentrated from the blood by the kidneys and then drained into the bladder. This test can reveal abnormalities in the structure of the kidneys and ureters, as well as in their function of filtering the blood. An excretion urogram is shown in Figure 4.3b-II. An increasingly popular and more accurate form of the IVU is the CT urogram in which the CT scanner is used to locate the obstruction in the urinary system instead of a series of X-ray films.

The function of the bladder may be visualized by requesting the patient to urinate after dye has been inserted into the bladder for cystography. An X-ray image taken during contraction of the bladder will reveal any abnormalities in the way in which it empties. This test is known as micturating cystourethrography (MCU).

A radioactive chemical (containing a radioactive isotope) known as DMSA can be used to assess the filtration function of the kidneys more accurately than the IVU. As in the IVU, DMSA is injected intravenously, and is filtered and concentrated in the kidney. The amount of radioactivity that builds up in the kidneys over the next few hours is then assessed by means of a gamma scanner. The radioactivity dies off very quickly, and so this test is not considered to be harmful to the patient.

Figure 4.3b-II Excretion urogram showing a pale patch of contrast in the calyx of the left kidney
The pale patch represents a large calculus (kidney stone).

Cystoscopy
In cystoscopy, a fiber-optic telescope is inserted into the urethra so that the inside of the bladder can be seen directly. The patient is usually heavily sedated, or has a general anesthetic. Biopsies of the bladder can also be taken by means of the cystoscope.

Renal biopsy
Under guidance from an ultrasound scan, a needle may be directed through the skin into the kidney to remove a small sample of tissue for examination. This procedure carries a small but significant risk of bleeding into or around the kidney.

Urodynamic studies
Urodynamics is the study of the pressure of the urine in the bladder and the flow of the stream of the urine from the urethra. Specialized tests to measure the pressure within the bladder and the flow rate are used mostly to investigate the underlying problem in cases of incontinence or obstructed flow of urine. Urodynamic studies may be used in combination with MCU.

4.3c Diseases of the kidneys

The conditions studied in this section are:

Part I: Disease processes that affect the kidney:

- glomerulonephritis – nephritic syndrome and nephrotic syndrome
- acute and chronic pyelonephritis
- kidney and ureteric stones
- polycystic kidney disease
- interstitial nephritis
- hemolytic uremic syndrome
- hypertension and the kidneys
- diabetes and the kidneys
- cancer of the kidney

Part II: Serious consequences of disease of the kidney:

- acute kidney injury (AKI)
- chronic kidney disease (CKD).

All the common diseases of the kidney described in this section may be so severe as to lead to either sudden (acute) or gradual (chronic) failure of the kidney to perform its necessary functions.

Part I: Disease processes that affect the kidney

Glomerulonephritis
Glomerulonephritis is a term used to describe a broad range of conditions that affect the structure of the cup-like origin of the tubules in the kidney and the cluster of blood vessels within this cup known as the glomerulus. In glomerulonephritis the filtering process is impaired. This has the consequence that red blood cells and protein may leak out of the blood into the urine, and also that excess salts, wastes and water may be retained in the circulation.

In medical textbooks, the condition of glomerulonephritis may be categorized according to the precise pathological changes occurring in the glomerulus, and these categories are assigned descriptive terms such as minimal change, membranous glomerulonephritis and mesangiocapillary glomerulonephritis. This categorization, which is based on the results of kidney biopsy and is important for predicting prognosis, does not relate directly to the condition that may have caused the disease process. For this reason it is not described further in this section.

THE CAUSES OF GLOMERULONEPHRITIS

Glomerulonephritis can result from a variety of underlying disease processes, but also commonly develops without any obvious cause. In many cases the problem results from the deposition of autoantibodies within the glomerulus. Autoantibodies stimulate the immune response, and the inflammation that results leads to glomerular damage. Autoantibodies may develop as a delayed response to infection, as part of an established autoimmune disease such as systemic lupus erythematosus (SLE) or as a reaction to certain drugs. They may also account for many of the cases of glomerulonephritis of unknown cause.

The *Streptococcus* bacterium, which is a common cause of sore throat and tonsillitis, used to be a very common cause of antibody-related glomerulonephritis. Post-streptococcal glomerulonephritis tends to lead to a characteristic cluster of symptoms known as nephritic syndrome or acute nephritis (see below). Bright's disease is an old-fashioned name for nephritic syndrome. This term used to be almost synonymous with post-streptococcal kidney disease.

Other infectious agents that may cause the development of damaging autoantibodies include viruses, such as measles and hepatitis, bacteria, such as *Salmonella*, and parasites, such as malaria.

Glomerulonephritis may also be part of the disease process of a multisystem autoimmune disease. SLE is the most common specific autoimmune disease known to cause glomerulonephritis. In SLE, chronic kidney disease (CKD) resulting from severe persistent cases of glomerulonephritis is the most common cause of death.

Some drugs may also trigger the development of damaging autoantibodies. The drug that most commonly has this effect is penicillamine, which is prescribed as a disease-modifying treatment in rheumatoid arthritis.

THE CONSEQUENCES OF GLOMERULAR DAMAGE

The effects of glomerulonephritis can be broadly divided into four categories, although in practice, for any individual patient, it may be difficult to assign them to a category. The categories are:

- hematuria (blood in the urine)

- proteinuria (protein in the urine)

- nephritic syndrome (blood and protein in the urine, with high blood pressure and edema)

- nephrotic syndrome (excessive protein in the urine leading to severe edema).

HEMATURIA AND PROTEINURIA IN GLOMERULONEPHRITIS

Some forms of glomerulonephritis cause sufficient damage to the glomerulus to bring about a leakage of red blood cells, protein or both. This leakage may not be sufficiently severe to be visible to the patient, and instead may be picked up on routine urine testing. Greater numbers of red blood cells might cause the urine to appear pink or smoky colored, and excess protein might cause the urine to appear frothy. There may be no other symptoms.

Nevertheless, despite the mildness of the symptoms, the finding of even small amounts of blood or protein in the urine in the absence of urinary infection can be a warning sign of a progressive disease of the kidney. CKD can be the long-term consequence of glomerulonephritis that may be signaled by hematuria or proteinuria. For this reason, all patients who are found to have unexplained hematuria or proteinuria above a certain level will be referred to a renal physician for further investigations.

Some forms of glomerulonephritis that cause hematuria or proteinuria may respond to treatment with immunosuppressant drugs, including corticosteroids. Other immunosuppressant medications that may be prescribed at the same time include azathioprine, cyclophosphamide and chlorambucil. All these drugs can have a wide range of toxic effects.

Information box 4.3c-I

Glomerulonephritis: comments from a Chinese medicine perspective

In Chinese medicine, the underlying pathological process of damage to the structure of the kidney in post-streptococcal glomerulonephritis (leading to acute nephritis) suggests that Internal Heat (which may have had External origins if following an infection) is impairing the normal function of Lung/Spleen and Kidneys to transform and move water. Blood in the urine can be a result of transmission of Heart Fire via the Small Intestine or Damp Heat in the Bladder. Protein in the urine may be interpreted as the draining of Essence from the Kidneys.

In other forms of glomerulonephritis Heat Toxins are not part of the picture and instead Wind, Qi Stagnation, Blood Stasis or Damp lead to the impairment of the normal handling of body fluids by the three key organs. Kidney disease is more likely if there is pre-existing Lung, Kidney and Spleen Deficiency. Blood Stasis is more likely in elderly people. Flaws and Sionneau (2010) state that the most common form of chronic glomerulonephritis is said to be "Spleen-Kidney Yin and Yang Vacuity with Blood Stasis."[44]

The predominant energetic effect of immunosuppressant drugs such as azathioprine and cyclophosphamide is that of Heat and they may cause severe damage to Blood and Yin.

NEPHRITIC SYNDROME
(ACUTE NEPHRITIS OR BRIGHT'S DISEASE)

Nephritic syndrome is a term used to describe a glomerulonephritis that causes severe symptoms to appear rapidly. In nephritic syndrome the patient, commonly a child, becomes unwell with fever, vomiting and pain in the back. There may be a history of a streptococcal infection within the past two to four weeks, although streptococcal infection is not always the cause. The face becomes puffy with edema and blood pressure is raised. The urine may be pink or smoky colored by red blood cells. In severe cases the production of urine becomes severely reduced as the filtration function of the kidney is extremely impaired. The patient is then at risk of death from acute kidney failure or malignant hypertension.

A patient with nephritic syndrome requires close medical observation. In most childhood cases there is full recovery from the condition after four to seven days, although a minority of cases take a more chronic course. In contrast to the forms of glomerulonephritis that cause hematuria and proteinuria alone, most of these chronic cases of nephritic syndrome do not respond to immunosuppressant drugs. In post-streptococcal nephritis a course of penicillin is given to ensure eradication of the *Streptococcus*.

Information box 4.3c-II

Nephritic syndrome: comments from a Chinese medicine perspective

In Chinese medicine, some of the symptoms of nephritic syndrome would appear to result from Full Heat. This may originate from a Wind Heat Invasion in the case of post-streptococcal disease. Heat in the Heart is transmitted via the Small Intestine to the Bladder, causing scanty urination and hematuria. Heat obstructing the Orifices of the Heart may lead to the confusion and coma that result from acute renal failure.

Hypertension in nephritic syndrome can lead to convulsions. In Chinese medicine terms these are most likely to result from Heat causing damage to Kidney Yin. Liver Yin is then not nourished, and this leads to Hyperactivity of Liver Yang, which rises and stirs up Liver Wind.

A sudden development of facial edema would be described as Invasion of Wind Water. Proteinuria is a manifestation of Essence draining from the Kidneys.

In acute cases, as the tissue of the kidneys recovers, the toxins and excess salts that have built up in the body are cleared by means of profuse urination. However, in rare cases, the patient may die during the acute illness from acute renal failure and from damage caused to the brain by a rapidly rising blood pressure. Convulsions may develop in these severe cases. This consequence can be prevented with the help of emergency dialysis, which takes over the function of the failing kidney (see later).

In the more chronic cases, and more commonly in adults, there may be persisting damage to the kidneys. This damage can progress to chronic kidney failure over the course of months to years.

NEPHROTIC SYNDROME

Other forms of glomerulonephritis cause the filter of the kidney to leak large amounts of protein. This protein is lost into the urine, which becomes frothy as a result. The main plasma protein to be lost is albumin, but other proteins, including immunoglobulin (the protein that forms the plasma antibodies), are also lost. Nephrotic syndrome describes those cases when excessive amounts of protein are lost into the urine. As albumin is the most abundant plasma protein, this is found in high concentrations in the urine.

Other causes of nephrotic syndrome include the kidney damage that develops in some cases of diabetes, rare drug reactions and allergic reactions.

It is important for the plasma to be maintained at a certain concentration to give it sufficient osmotic pressure to remain in the circulation. The protein albumin plays a vital role in giving the plasma this adequate level of concentration. If albumin is lost, the plasma becomes too dilute, and the plasma fluid tends to move by osmosis into the more concentrated tissue fluid. Excessive fluid collecting in the tissues is called edema. In nephrotic syndrome, the severity of the proteinuria results in severe edema. The patient develops very swollen ankles and legs, and eventually fluid collects in a wide range of body regions, including the abdomen, within the lungs, the facial tissues and the genitalia.

In nephrotic syndrome, changes in the constitution of the plasma mean that clotting becomes a problem, and there is an increased risk of venous thrombosis. Loss of antibodies means that the patient with nephrotic syndrome is more prone to infection. Hyperlipidemia can also develop.

The patient with nephrotic syndrome is treated by means of diuretic medication to encourage loss of the excess tissue fluid, and restriction of salt in the diet. ACE inhibitor medication is prescribed, as this tends to reduce proteinuria, partly by reducing blood pressure. Anticoagulant medication may be given by injection to prevent blood clots. Statins may be prescribed to reduce the hyperlipidemia. Some cases will respond to corticosteroid medication or to other immunosuppressant drugs; this is particularly true in many of the cases that start in childhood.

In children, the underlying glomerulonephritis will very often (in 95 percent of cases) disappear after a few weeks of treatment with corticosteroids. In many of these cases the remission is permanent, and the kidneys return to a healthy state. In most adults, and the remaining childhood cases, a more chronic course develops, in which the proteinuria has to be controlled by ongoing immunosuppressant medication. In some cases the damage to the kidney progresses and CKD results.

Information box 4.3c-III

Nephrotic syndrome: comments from a Chinese medicine perspective

In Chinese medicine, the excessive edema and proteinuria of nephrotic syndrome is associated with a chronic Deficiency of the Lungs, Spleen and Kidneys. The accumulation of edema corresponds to Damp or Damp Heat.

Proteinuria is seen as the draining of Essence from the Kidneys. The Deficiency of Original Qi of the Kidneys that results gives rise to Stagnation of Blood, as Original Qi is necessary to enable smooth movement of Blood in the vessels. This is reflected in the increased risk of thrombosis in nephrotic syndrome.

Acute and chronic pyelonephritis

Pyelonephritis is a term that describes the inflammation that results from infection in the kidney. In most cases this infection has spread from the bladder. Acute and chronic pyelonephritis are two distinct syndromes with different manifestations.

ACUTE PYELONEPHRITIS

Acute pyelonephritis is usually the result of a spread of a bacterial infection in the bladder. It is an uncommon consequence of a bladder infection, and usually indicates underlying chronic disease or depletion in the patient. The exception to this is in pregnancy, when apparently healthy women can develop a kidney infection. This vulnerability in pregnancy to kidney infection is believed to be the result of the effect of the hormone progesterone that causes excessive relaxation of the valve at the site of the insertion of the ureters into the bladder.

The diseases that may predispose to acute pyelonephritis include diabetes and those conditions that result in damage to the structure of the urinary tract. Therefore, the presence of kidney stones and inherited abnormalities of the structure of the kidneys are risk factors for kidney infections. In addition, anything that obstructs the easy flow of urine from the bladder will increase the risk of bladder infections and kidney infections. Prostate disease in men is the most common cause of obstruction to the flow of urine (see Section 4.3d).

The symptoms of acute pyelonephritis include high fever, malaise and loin pain. The urine is often cloudy, and may contain many white and red blood cells and bacteria. In most patients the attack will settle with a course of appropriate antibiotics. However, in rare cases, some areas of the kidney may be scarred and be left with a permanently reduced function. In those who are susceptible, recurrent attacks may cause progressive kidney damage. For this reason, antibiotic treatment is considered to be essential in the treatment of kidney infections.

Information box 4.3c-IV

Acute pyelonephritis: comments from a Chinese medicine perspective

In Chinese medicine the symptoms of acute pyelonephritis correspond to Damp Heat in the Bladder. There is usually an underlying Deficiency of Kidney Yin, which predisposes to the development of Damp Heat. Severe pain would be described in terms of Qi and Blood Stasis as a result of Toxic Heat and Damp.

CHRONIC PYELONEPHRITIS (REFLUX NEPHROPATHY)

Chronic pyelonephritis and reflux nephropathy are synonymous terms used to describe a long-standing condition of the kidneys that results from repeated kidney infections. It is now believed that in many cases the damage to the kidneys actually began in childhood as a result of an anatomical abnormality of the ureters. This abnormality is a weakness of the valve that normally prevents reflux of urine from the bladder into the ureters. The vesico-ureteric reflux (VUR) that results allows the passage of any bacteria in the bladder up the ureters towards the kidneys. In many cases, VUR affects only one of the two ureters.

This problem can begin in infancy, and in particular in baby girls, in whom the passage of bacteria into the bladder is a fairly common event. In a healthy bladder, this transient infection is cleared, usually with few symptoms. However, in the case of a baby with VUR, bacteria may start to colonize in the kidneys. This might be the cause of a feverish illness, but alternatively can lead to a more slowly developing but progressive scarring of the affected kidney. This underlying infection may remain undetected for years. A chronic infection of the kidney can then become the source of repeated bladder infections.

It is now considered good medical practice to refer all children who suffer from recurrent bladder infections for investigation of the urinary tract to exclude VUR. Sadly, in many cases of VUR, many years elapse before the underlying cause is diagnosed, by which time permanent scarring of the kidney may have developed.

If VUR is diagnosed before damage to the kidney has developed, the renal function of the child is closely monitored and urine infections are rapidly treated. It is no longer considered helpful to operate to correct VUR, but in some cases it may be considered appropriate to remove a much damaged kidney if only one side has been affected, as this would otherwise remain as a persistent source of recurrent infections.

The condition that results from long-term scarring of the kidneys due to VUR is termed chronic pyelonephritis or reflux nephropathy. The affected patient may suffer from long-term ill health and recurrent urinary infections. The damage to the kidney, if severe, is progressive and can lead to hypertension and, eventually, CKD in adulthood.

 Information box 4.3c-V

Chronic pyelonephritis: comments from a Chinese medicine perspective

In Chinese medicine, reflux nephropathy represents Kidney Yin Deficiency against a background of Jing Deficiency. These deficiencies predispose to Damp Heat in the Bladder, which can further worsen the underlying Yin Deficiency.

Kidney and ureteric stones (calculi)

KIDNEY STONES

Kidney stones are the result of crystals forming in concentrated urine from substances that usually remain dissolved in the urine. The most common form of stone is made of calcium oxalate, but calcium phosphate and uric acid are also common constituents. Some individuals have a tendency to form these crystals more than others, often for reasons that are unclear. However, there are some known risk factors for the development of kidney stones.

A state of dehydration, which can occur in hot, dry climates or hot working environments, will lead to the production of very concentrated urine. Kidney stones are therefore more common in people living in hot countries, in particular, in the Middle East.

High levels of various substances including calcium salts, oxalic acid and uric acid in the urine can also lead to stone formation. Calcium appears in excess in the urine in people who have too much calcium or vitamin D in their diet. This also occurs in those who have a disorder of the metabolism of their bones that causes too much calcium to be released from the bones into the bloodstream. This can develop in advanced bone cancer, in people who have to undergo prolonged bed rest, and in cases in which the

parathyroid glands are overactive. Oxalate can appear in excess in the urine from an excessive dietary intake of spinach, rhubarb and tea. Excessive uric acid is found in the urine if there is a high dietary intake of cholesterol, beer, offal, fish and shellfish. It also occurs in conditions in which there is a high turnover of cells in the body, such as in cancer. There can also be an inherited tendency to the excessive production of oxalic and uric acid in the urine.

A crystal is more likely to develop in concentrated urine if there is a particle within the urine or an irregularity in the urinary tract around which it can form. Therefore, the sludge that can develop in the urine in urinary infections can encourage stone formation. Recurrent infections can lead to the formation of very large irregular stones.

Kidney stones cause damage in a variety of ways. They can lodge in the form of tiny crystals within the substance of the kidney and there act as a focus for inflammation. The damage that can result from stones can also be a focus for acute pyelonephritis. Alternatively, larger stones can obstruct the outflow of urine from the kidney. This might result in increased pressure and dilatation within a large section of a kidney, and eventually loss of function of that portion of the kidney. A stone that dislodges from the kidney and impacts within a ureter can cause excruciating colicky pain as the ureter contracts in a wave-like pattern around the obstruction.

URETERIC STONES

Very often kidney stones that leave the kidney cause no symptoms and are passed painlessly via the urine out of the urethra. The most common symptom is pain as the stone travels down the ureter towards the bladder. In many people this pain is transient, and the pain subsides once the stone has left the ureter. However, in those in whom the stone impacts in the ureter, the pain can be very intense. The pain of a ureteric stone tends to peak every few minutes and radiates from the loin (kidney area) round to the suprapubic area. In men the pain can radiate into the testicle on the affected side. In some cases the stone can damage the lining of the ureter and can cause a small amount of blood to enter the urine.

A ureteric stone may totally obstruct the flow of urine from the kidney on the affected side. In this case, as well as being very painful, it is a threat to the health of the kidney, as obstructed urine places pressure on the kidney tissue.

A ureteric stone can be diagnosed on the basis of the history alone, but is confirmed by means of a plain X-ray image and, if this is not clear, a CT scan. An ultrasound scan will reveal whether or not the impacted stone is causing any back pressure within the kidney.

If the pain is very intense, the patient is given intramuscular non-steroidal anti-inflammatory drugs (NSAIDs) or opiate pain relief. This may actually allow movement of the stone, as analgesic drugs can cause the ureters to relax, as well as relieving pain. However, stones larger than 1cm in diameter usually require surgical removal.

The development of the endoscope has meant that kidney and ureteric stones are less of a problem to remove than they used to be. Keyhole surgery, which relies on an endoscopic technique, is usually possible for renal stones (percutaneous nephrolithotomy). This means that the patient is only left with a tiny scar. Alternatively, ultrasound shock waves (lithotripsy) can be directed towards the impacted stone, which may then break up so that the fragments pass into the bladder. In intractable cases, an operation is required that leaves the patient with a diagonal scar in the loin (kidney) region.

The best treatment for kidney and ureteric stones is prevention. Those who are at increased risk of developing stones are advised to maintain a high fluid intake. In stone formers, dietary sources of calcium and oxalic and uric acids should be kept to a minimum.

Information box 4.3c-VI

Kidney and ureteric stones: comments from a Chinese medicine perspective

In Chinese medicine, the formation of stones is equated with Phlegm. Excessive Damp Heat on a background of Kidney Yin Deficiency is likely to be a precursor to this. According to Flaws and Sionneau (2010),[45] stone formation in the kidney is very much the outcome of harmful lifestyle and may be engendered by "…damp, hot environment, external contraction of wind, damp, heat evils, over eating acrid, hot, fatty sweet foods, lack of constancy between anger and joy, or excessive bedroom taxation…" They go on to say several patterns may present simultaneously in a single case, explaining, by example, that it is not uncommon to see "liver-spleen disharmonies complicated by yin vacuity, damp heat and blood stasis."

The sometimes intense pain of ureteric stones results from Blood Stagnation. Analgesic drugs move Stagnation in the short term.

Miscellaneous disorders of the kidney

Polycystic kidney disease

Autosomal-dominant polycystic chronic kidney disease (ADPCKD) is a relatively common inherited disorder of the kidneys in which the kidneys develop large fluid-filled cysts during adult life. It affects 1 in 1000 people. The cysts gradually destroy the substance of the kidney leading to CKD in middle to late adult life. The first symptoms are usually hematuria or loin pain (i.e. pain in the kidney area) as a cyst ruptures. Occasionally, severe hypertension or the

development of chronic kidney disease is the first sign of the disease. People with ADPCKD are also more prone to developing kidney infections, liver cysts, mitral valve problems and subarachnoid hemorrhages.

There is no treatment for ADPCKD except for management of the symptoms of pain, hypertension and CKD (see later). Patients may be screened by means of cranial arteriography for the berry aneurysms that can predispose to subarachnoid hemorrhage.

There is a genetic test for ADPCKD so that people from affected families can be screened for the disease, and so that those who are planning a family can receive genetic counseling.

Information box 4.3c-VII

Polycystic kidney disease: comments from a Chinese medicine perspective

In Chinese medicine, the symptoms of polycystic kidney disease are a manifestation of Deficiency of Kidney Jing and Yin. As time goes on, Blood Stagnation and Damp Heat will become more apparent in the form of episodes of painful cyst rupture, recurrent infections, blood in the urine and eventual renal failure.

Interstitial nephritis

Like glomerulonephritis, interstitial nephritis (also termed tubulointerstitial nephritis) is a form of inflammation of the tissue of the kidney. In this case, the inflammation is not of the glomerulus, but of the tissue that surrounds the tubules.

The most common cause of this inflammation is the infection of acute pyelonephritis, but there are important non-infectious causes that are more likely to lead to permanent kidney damage. The most important non-infectious cause in developed countries is the recurrent use of analgesic tablets. The most troublesome drug from this point of view used to be a paracetamol-like drug called phenacetin, although doctors in the UK no longer prescribe this. Paracetamol is far less likely to have this effect on the kidneys. However, the NSAIDs may also, on rare occasions, cause this condition if taken on a repeated basis over the course of three years or more. A prescription of this length is not uncommon in many people with chronic musculoskeletal disease.

Analgesic-related interstitial nephritis can result in a long-term scarring of the kidney tissue, which can develop into CKD. For this reason, anyone who is taking NSAID-related analgesics on a long-term basis should have regular blood tests to check the function of the kidneys.

Progressive interstitial nephritis can also result from some chronic diseases, most importantly diabetes and sickle cell disease.

Information box 4.3c-VIII

Interstitial nephritis: comments from a Chinese medicine perspective

In Chinese medicine, the symptoms of interstitial nephritis suggest a progressive Depletion of Kidney Yin. The damaging effect of analgesic drugs could be attributed to their Heating properties.

HEMOLYTIC UREMIC SYNDROME (HUS)

Hemolytic uremic syndrome (HUS) is a condition in which the primary problem is the formation of fibrin and the breakdown of the red blood cells within the small blood vessels of the circulation (hemolysis). In HUS this serious complication usually follows an infection, particularly of the gastrointestinal or respiratory tracts. A specific strain of the bacterium *Escherichia (E.) coli* (known as O157) has recently been associated with HUS. It is believed that in HUS the infectious agent somehow causes damage to the lining of the blood vessels, which then triggers the clotting cascade and damage to the red blood cells.

This damage affects the renal arterioles in particular, with the result that the glomeruli become damaged. The affected patient, commonly a child, develops hematuria and high blood pressure, and kidney function starts to deteriorate. In some cases this deterioration is so rapid that it leads to acute renal failure. However, in most cases, with adequate medical supervision, there can be full recovery from the condition. An outbreak of *E. coli* O157 food poisoning in Scotland in 1996 was complicated by the development of HUS in a number of patients. The mortality in this outbreak demonstrated that the complications of HUS were more likely to be fatal in older people.

Information box 4.3c-IX

Hemolytic uremic syndrome: comments from a Chinese medicine perspective

In Chinese medicine, the interpretation of HUS would be similar to that of acute nephritic syndrome, in that an invasion of Wind Damp Heat is the initiating factor. Hematuria corresponds to Heat transmitted from the Small Intestine, or to Damp Heat in the Urine. The Full Heat causes damage to Kidney Yin, which, in those who are depleted already, such as elderly people, can have life-threatening consequences.

HYPERTENSION AND THE KIDNEYS

Hypertension can in itself cause damage to the kidneys. One of the effects of hypertension is that it causes narrowing and rigidity of the blood vessels by the process of arteriosclerosis. This results in a reduced blood supply to the kidney and also in structural damage to the glomeruli. The reduced delivery of oxygen to the kidneys triggers a hormonal response that is intended to improve the blood supply to the kidneys in the situation of shock. This response involves hormones called renin and angiotensin, which both act to increase the blood pressure. What would be an appropriate response in the case of shock is actually an inappropriate response in the case of arteriosclerosis, as a vicious cycle of increasing hypertension is set up. The ACE inhibitors and angiotensin II receptor antagonists are classes of antihypertensive medication that act to prevent the action of angiotensin, and so directly break this negative cycle of events.

The damage to the glomeruli also reduces the function of the kidneys, so that in some people with sustained hypertension permanent renal impairment can develop.

Kidney disease can itself be a cause of hypertension, because it, too, can lead to the inappropriate production of renin and angiotensin. Kidney disease also leads to the retention of salt and water in the circulation, which also tends to increase blood pressure. These factors can cause a vicious circle of escalating hypertension, as the hypertension in kidney disease further reduces the blood supply to the already damaged kidneys.

Information box 4.3c-X

Hypertension and the kidneys: comments from a Chinese medicine perspective

In Chinese medicine, the hypertension that results from underlying kidney disease might result from Deficiency of either Kidney Yin or Yang, or both. Kidney Yin Deficiency is seen to predispose to the development of Liver Fire, and Yang Deficiency to the Accumulation of Phlegm Damp. In severe kidney disease, it is likely that a combination of these two syndromes contributes to the development of the hypertension.

For this reason, many patients with diverse forms of kidney disease will develop hypertension. In acute kidney disease, such as the nephritic syndrome and HUS, the rise in blood pressure can be very rapid, whereas in CKD a more gradual rise is usual. Patients with one-sided kidney disease can also develop hypertension in later life. This is an important reason why some people will have a diseased kidney surgically removed (e.g. in one-sided reflux nephropathy).

The treatment of hypertension resulting from kidney disease involves strict attention to a reduction of salt in the diet, and the use of diuretics and ACE inhibitors.

DIABETES AND THE KIDNEYS

The kidneys can be damaged in a variety of ways in diabetes mellitus. Diabetes is a condition in which a persistently raised blood sugar level leads to damage of the small and medium-sized blood vessels. This damage affects the renal arteriole and the glomerulus.

In up to one-third of patients who have been diagnosed with type 1 (juvenile onset) diabetes, serious damage to the kidneys will become apparent in later life. The glomerular damage leads to progressive proteinuria, which if unchecked can lead to nephrotic syndrome. The reduction in the blood flow resulting from the narrowed renal arteriole can cause hypertension, which can, in turn, further worsen the glomerular damage. On top of these two causes of kidney damage, the diabetic patient is also prone to urinary infections because of excessive amounts of glucose in the urine. These infections can lead to acute pyelonephritis in the already damaged kidney. CKD is a common end result of diabetic kidney disease.

The rate of progression of diabetic kidney disease can be prevented by meticulous control of the blood sugar. Patients are advised to undergo regular screening for traces of protein in the urine and blood tests for abnormalities of kidney function such as a decline in the eGFR. It is considered very important that hypertension is controlled to a level of less than 130/80mmHg, ideally by ACE inhibitors, and that any urine infections are treated rapidly by means of appropriate antibiotics.

Cancer of the kidney

The most common tumor of the kidney is renal cell carcinoma. This affects men approximately twice as often as women, and has an average age of onset of 55.

The presenting symptoms are usually hematuria or loin pain, although diagnosis may not occur until after more generalized symptoms of cancer such as fever and weight loss have developed. In localized renal cell carcinoma, the treatment involves removal of the affected kidney. In some patients this surgery can be curative. Surgery may also be performed if the cancer has already spread to lymph nodes and other organs (in particular, the other kidney, liver, bone and lungs). In about one-fifth of patients with metastatic disease, chemotherapy with alpha-interferon and interleukin-2 can give a very good response rate in the short term. However, the long-term outlook is poor for those with metastases, with only 5 percent still alive after five years from diagnosis, compared with 45 percent for those who present without metastases.

The kidney is also the site for one of the most common tumors of infancy known as a nephroblastoma (Wilms' tumor). Common first symptoms of this tumor are hematuria and abdominal swelling. Wilms' tumor has a much better prognosis than renal cell carcinoma, in that most children are cured of this tumor by a combination of surgery, radiotherapy and chemotherapy.

Information box 4.3c-XI

Cancer of the kidney: comments from a Chinese medicine perspective

In Chinese medicine, a tumor of the kidney may represent Phlegm and/or Blood Stagnation. A Deficiency of Kidney Yin and/or Yang with underlying local Stagnation of Qi is likely to be an underlying predisposing factor. In Wilms' tumor and other renal tumors of childhood inborn Jing Deficiency is contributory. Toxic Heat originating from the Womb may also be a contributory Pathogenic Factor.

Part II: Serious consequences of disease of the kidney

The most serious consequence of kidney disease is that the kidney totally fails to perform its functions of filtering the blood and forming concentrated urine. If these functions are lost, fluid, salts and waste products build up in the blood to cause severe illness. If there is an abrupt failure of the kidney function occurring over the course of hours to weeks this is termed acute renal failure. In contrast, the term chronic kidney disease (CKD) is used to describe a gradual loss of kidney function, which can develop over the course of weeks to years. Patients who are developing CKD may experience a sudden rapid deterioration of renal function, in which case the term acute on chronic renal failure may be applied.

Acute kidney injury (AKI)

THE CAUSES OF ACUTE KIDNEY INJURY (AKI)

Acute kidney injury (AKI) can have a variety of causes. A potentially reversible cause is an insufficient blood supply to the kidneys. This means that the kidneys are simply unable to perform their filtration function adequately because they are not receiving sufficient fluid to do so. This can result from sudden blood or fluid loss. Therefore, hemorrhage from serious trauma, fluid loss from burns, and dehydration from severe diarrhea and vomiting can all lead to AKI in this way. The impaired blood supply that can result from a heart attack or heart failure can also cause AKI for the same reason. However, in these cases, as long as the situation of impaired blood supply does not continue for too long, the AKI can be reversed if the blood supply can be restored to normal.

AKI can also result from damage to the tissues of the kidney. Most commonly, this form of AKI is due to a condition known as acute tubular necrosis, in which the cells of the tubules die for a variety of reasons. The most common reason for this to occur is a prolonged reduction of blood supply to the kidneys for the reasons listed above. The cells die simply because of lack of oxygen and basic nutrients. Toxic reactions to drugs are also a recognized cause of this form of AKI. Diuretics, NSAIDs and ACE inhibitors are well known for causing this severe reaction in very rare cases.

The kidney tissue can also be damaged by hemoglobin circulating free in the blood. This reason for AKI most commonly develops following a serious traumatic accident, during which damage to blood vessels and tissues leads to the release of hemoglobin from the blood cells. In this case the damage caused to the kidneys by the hemoglobin is often compounded by a sudden loss of blood supply to the kidneys.

AKI can also develop in pregnancy. The most common cause is the complex cycle of events that develops starting with pre-eclampsia. In this condition of late pregnancy, the initial signs of raised blood pressure and loss of protein in the urine can be overtaken by a serious condition called eclampsia, in which the blood pressure rises to life-threatening levels and the tubular cells of the kidney die from the resulting poor blood supply. Patients with eclampsia can die from a combination of malignant hypertension and AKI. Another cause of AKI during pregnancy is the sudden blood loss that can occur either from a tear of the placenta (abruptio placentae) or from the womb after the delivery of the baby.

The symptoms of acute kidney injury (AKI)

AKI initially presents with the formation of very small quantities of urine. Then the levels of toxins such as urea and creatinine start to rise rapidly in the blood as the kidneys are unable to clear them. This condition, known as acute uremia, will lead to nausea, drowsiness, fits and eventually coma, depending on the rate of accumulation of the toxins. The patient may develop symptoms from overload of fluid in the circulation, including breathlessness due to pulmonary edema. The situation of uremia resulting from AKI is a medical emergency. Ideally, patients with AKI should be nursed in an intensive care setting.

The treatment of acute kidney injury (AKI)

The treatment depends very much on an accurate diagnosis of the underlying cause of the AKI. In the situation in which a temporary impairment of blood supply to the kidney is suspected, the prime aim of treatment is to restore the blood supply to the kidney. This may mean giving a blood transfusion in the case of severe hemorrhage, or a fluid infusion in the case of dehydration. In the case of heart attack or heart failure, drugs may be given to improve the pumping action of the heart. If there has been no damage to the tubular cells of the kidney, these treatment approaches may be sufficient to reverse the AKI.

If the AKI is due to damage to the tubular cells, the cause of the damage needs to be removed. Shock or dehydration needs to be treated, but with great care, as fluid overload is a potential problem with AKI. Toxic drugs are withdrawn in the case of drug-related tubular necrosis. In the case of eclampsia, delivery of the baby by cesarean section can halt the negative cycle of events.

Assuming that the cause of the AKI can be removed, the patient with tubular damage then requires intensive care to support them over the period of the next 7–21 days, which is the time required for the damaged tubular cells to recover. Early specialist care in this situation is vital, as the patient will require very careful monitoring of the circulatory and urinary systems, and may require emergency dialysis (see later) to clear excess fluid, salts and toxins from the blood.

Up to 50 percent of people who suffer from acute tubular necrosis will die from the acute illness. Many who survive will regain normal function of the kidneys. However, a proportion will be left with permanent damage, which may lead to a state of chronic renal failure.

 Information box 4.3c-XII

Acute kidney injury: comments from a Chinese medicine perspective

In Chinese medicine, AKI may correspond to Depletion of Kidney Yin and Yang with sudden Accumulation of Heat and Damp (as evidenced by fluid overload). It might result from Invasion of Toxic Heat (e.g. when induced by drugs) or by severe Stagnation and Depletion (e.g. when induced by trauma and hemorrhage). Fits and coma correspond to the Stirring up of Liver Wind (following severe Kidney Yin Deficiency) and to Heat obstructing the Orifices of the Heart.

Chronic kidney disease (CKD)[46]

The symptoms of chronic kidney disease (CKD)

Chronic kidney disease (CKD) is a term used to describe a state of gradually deteriorating kidney function. It is defined if GFR has been consistently shown to be reduced below an ideal level for more than three months. It has been estimated that approximately 8 percent of the adult population in the UK may suffer from CKD according to its current medical definition (as based on reduction of GFR). Many of these people will be in the very early pre-symptomatic stages of GFR that may never progress to develop into severe disease.

In advancing CKD the ability of the kidneys to filter the blood and concentrate the urine is lost over a period of weeks to years. Over this time the levels of urea and creatinine in the blood raise slowly, eventually causing the patient to feel unwell and the skin to itch, as a result of the toxic urea in the blood (a state described as uremia).

This state of uremia is only life-threatening when the levels of urea and creatinine reach very high levels. Features of fluid retention, with edema, may develop, and the blood pressure tends to rise. Loss of the hormone erythropoietin (EPO) from the failing kidneys leads to a severe form of anemia. Loss of the ability to activate vitamin D contributes to a form of osteomalacia. Impotence is also a known consequence of CKD.

THE CAUSES OF CHRONIC KIDNEY DISEASE (CKD)

CKD can develop as a result of a wide range of disease processes. These include diabetes, hypertension, glomerulonephritis (all forms), infection (in particular, infection leading to reflux nephropathy following VUR), interstitial nephritis, damage by kidney stones and congenital abnormalities (including polycystic kidney disease). In addition, any of the causes of AKI may lead to permanent kidney damage if not successfully treated. Diabetes accounts for half of all cases of symptomatic CKD and hypertension for a further quarter, most of which develop in the eighth decade of life.

One other important cause of CKD is obstruction to the outflow of urine. The underlying causes of this problem are discussed in Section 4.3d, as it primarily relates to the bladder and prostate gland. As urine outflow obstruction is usually gradual in onset, the damage caused by back pressure on the kidneys is also gradual, but can be so severe as to lead to CKD. A sudden obstruction to the ureter from a large ureteric stone can cause a sudden onset of acute renal failure in someone who has only one kidney.

THE TREATMENT OF CHRONIC KIDNEY DISEASE (CKD)

In the early stages of CKD the patient may remain without symptoms and the condition is only apparent through recognition of abnormal blood test results such as a low eGFR or a high creatinine level. In symptomatic cases the symptoms can be controlled by means of salt, potassium, phosphate and protein restriction, and meticulous attention to blood pressure control. A genetically engineered form of EPO is now available so that the severe anemia of chronic disease can be prevented. Activated vitamin D can be given in the form of a drug, although this has to be monitored

with care, as there is a risk of developing excessive levels of calcium in the blood. All this treatment should be provided and monitored by a team of specialist physicians based within a hospital renal unit.

The ideal treatment for CKD is prevention of progression, and so accurate treatment of the cause and meticulous attention to blood pressure and blood sugar levels (in diabetes) is crucial. Once the inevitable progression appears to be apparent, the best treatment is considered to be kidney transplantation at an early stage in the disease, before the health of the body has been too affected by the long-term state of uremia. If a suitable kidney for transplantation is not immediately available, the patient will eventually require regular dialysis to take over the detoxifying and fluid-balancing functions of the failing kidneys.

Dialysis

Dialysis is a general term that is used to describe any method by which the blood is filtered artificially. In hemodialysis, the blood of the patient is redirected through a machine designed to filter the blood of toxins and to remove excess fluids and salts. The flow of blood through the machine must be rapid for the dialysis to work adequately. To enable this to happen, a surgical operation is performed whereby the blood in an artery (usually the brachial artery at the elbow) is directed into a local vein. This operation, known as creating a fistula, leads to the formation of a pulsatile and tense blood vessel that lies close to the surface of the skin. A fistula (see Figure 4.3c-I) permits ready access to a good blood supply for the purposes of hemodialysis.

Figure 4.3c-I An arteriovenous fistula in the right forearm: the arrow points to a surgically enlarged blood vessel that allows for easy access in dialysis

At the time of hemodialysis, a large-bore needle is inserted into the fistula so that blood can be passed through the dialysis machine. This blood is returned to the body through another needle inserted into a distal portion of the fistula. The whole process takes about 4–5 hours and needs to be repeated two or three times a week. If the frequency of dialysis is too low, the patient will develop signs of chronic uremia, including tiredness, itching and poor sleep.

Hemodialysis is an efficient method of dialysis, but carries some problems for the patient. First, it is disruptive to normal life to have to attend the hemodialysis unit on a frequent basis; and second, some people feel quite unwell from the rapid changes in blood composition that result from hemodialysis.

Peritoneal dialysis (chronic ambulatory peritoneal dialysis (CAPD)) is a form of dialysis that does not require the blood to be circulated through a machine. Instead, it relies on the peritoneal space (the space inside the abdomen that surrounds the abdominal organs) to be the site of dialysis. For peritoneal dialysis to take place, a soft plastic tube (catheter) has to be inserted by a surgical procedure so that it rests permanently with its tip in the peritoneal space. The location of the CAPD catheter is shown in Figure 4.3c-II.

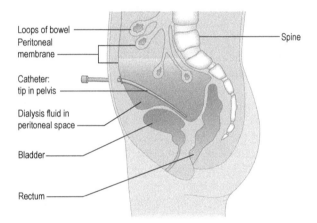

Loops of bowel
Peritoneal membrane
Catheter: tip in pelvis
Dialysis fluid in peritoneal space
Bladder
Rectum
Spine

Figure 4.3c-II The position of the catheter used for chronic ambulatory peritoneal dialysis (CAPD)

Peritoneal dialysis can be performed by the patient at home. In peritoneal dialysis 1.5–3 liters of sterile dialysis fluid are drained into the peritoneal space through the plastic tube and kept within the space for 20–30 minutes. The peritoneal lining acts as the kidney, and toxins and excess salts and fluid can move out of the blood in the abdominal tissues by diffusion into the dialysis fluid. After about half an hour the fluid is drained back out of the abdominal space through the tube by the patient and discarded. This all has to be performed with a strict attention to sterile procedure, as infection in the peritoneal space can lead to severe illness.

Some patients can continue for years being fully reliant on one of the forms of dialysis to perform the function of their failed kidneys. However, the problem remains that the life of a dialysis patient is dominated by the technicalities of the dialysis, and also with dealing with its complications.

Moreover, dialysis can never fully reverse the state of chronic uremia, so that the patient will always be less well than someone with normal kidney functioning. A successful kidney transplant offers much more day-to-day freedom and well-being than dialysis, but unfortunately is not possible for all people with CKD.

Kidney transplantation
The success of transplantation depends on the availability of a donor kidney who is as accurately matched to the tissues of the recipient as possible. The ideal is for a patient to receive a kidney from a twin, in which case there is no risk of rejection of the donated organ by the immune system. Kidneys from any other source will carry antigens on the kidney tissue that are recognized as foreign by the recipient's body.

It is understood that the kidneys from some donors carry more foreign antigens than others. The process of tissue typing involves comparing the antigens on a donor kidney with those of the potential recipient. Only if a fairly close match (it will never be perfect) is achieved will the transplantation operation go ahead. Once the kidney has been transplanted, the recipient will have to remain on lifelong immunosuppressant medication to prevent rejection of the donated organ.

Donor kidneys most often come from young people who have suffered an accidental death. The ideal situation is that the kidney is removed from a patient who has suffered brainstem death, but whose vital functions have been maintained by means of a life-support machine. In this situation the donated kidney is likely to be very healthy.

In the UK, the removal of the organ always requires the consent of the patient's family if the donor is under 16, and usually also requires evidence that the patient wished for their organs to be donated after death. After tissue typing, the pattern of antigens in the donor kidney is compared with those of all the patients on the national waiting list for transplantation. A combination of close match and urgency of need are the criteria by which a suitable recipient is chosen. The transplantation operation is then organized as a matter of urgency. However, because of the low availability of organs, many patients remain on the waiting list for years.

In rare cases, the organ may be removed from a living close relative who wishes to donate one of their kidneys. The donor, whether alive or dead, is always screened thoroughly for evidence of infectious disease and cancer, but the risks of transmitted disease from the donor organ can never be ruled out totally.

The operation itself carries risks, particularly if the patient is in a fairly advanced state of CKD. In particular, the blood supply to the new organ may be lost because of thrombosis. In some patients, the new organ becomes damaged by the inflammation resulting from rejection by the immune system. These rejection episodes are particularly common in the first few months after transplantation. Most are reversible by treating with increased doses of immunosuppressant medication, but some lead to death of the new organ.

A combination of immunosuppressant drugs is used in transplant patients. These most commonly include corticosteroids, and the drugs azathioprine, ciclosporin and tacrolimus. The latter two drugs, like many of the early antibiotics, are derivatives of naturally occurring fungi.

All these drugs can have serious side effects. Azathioprine may cause bone marrow failure, ciclosporin can cause kidney damage, and tacrolimus can damage the kidneys and the nerves. All these drugs will also depress the healthy response to infection, so that the transplant patient is more at risk of developing opportunistic infections.

However, despite the risk of side effects and infections, many patients who have had a successful transplant are able to tolerate these drugs and continue to live a normal life.

 Information box 4.3c-XIII

Chronic kidney disease: comments from a Chinese medicine perspective

In Chinese medicine, the features of CKD correspond to severe Depletion of Kidney Yin and Yang. This is always associated with Depletion of Lung and Spleen Yang, evidenced by accumulation of fluid in the lungs and periphery, exhaustion and yellow coloration. Fluid retention and hypertension might represent accumulation of Phlegm and Damp. Flaws and Sionneau (2010) suggest that in CKD the function of the Triple Burner is compromised so that "clear qi is not able to rise and be upborne, while turbid qi is not able to gain precipitation and be downborne."[47] Damp is not cleared and thus can stagnate and combine with Heat to produce Phlegm and Stasis Heat.

Anemia corresponds to Blood Deficiency, and osteomalacia to Jing Deficiency. The itch, drowsiness and coma that develop in advanced uremia may be consequences of Heat and Phlegm, which eventually obstruct the Orifices of the Heart.

The action of dialysis probably permits some clearance of Accumulated Pathogenic Factors, including Heat and Damp, and acts by supporting the Kidney Yin and Yang.

Transplantation might be considered to Nourish Kidney Yin and Yang, although at the cost of the introduction of Pathogenic Factors in the form of foreign antigens (Wind Heat and Wind Damp most commonly). Immunosuppressant medication is suppressive in nature and may introduce Heat Toxins, but is necessary to prevent the negative effect of these Pathogens.

The red flags of diseases of the kidneys

Some patients with diseases of the kidneys will benefit from referral to a conventional doctor for assessment and/or treatment. Red flags are those symptoms and signs that indicate that referral should be considered. The red flags of the diseases of the kidneys are described in Table 4.3c-I. A summary of the red flags in a format designed for quick reference in clinical practice can be found in Appendix III. This gives advice on the degree of urgency of referral for each of the red flag conditions listed.

Table 4.3c-I A29: Red flags of diseases of the kidneys

Red flag	Description	Reasoning
A29.1	Blood in the urine: • refer all cases in men • refer in women, except in the case of acute urinary infection	The most common and benign cause of blood in the urine in women is bladder infection (cystitis). If the symptoms are suggestive of this diagnosis (burning on urination, low abdominal pain, cloudy or blood-stained urine), there is no need to refer straight away. Treat with complementary medicine, recommend a high fluid intake, and refer only if symptoms are not settling within three days However, blood in the urine is not normal in men, who should be protected from infection by the relatively long male urethra Refer all cases of blood in the urine in men, and in women if there are either no other symptoms (blood may be coming from the kidney or from a tumor) or if the pain is felt also in the loin (suggesting a spread of infection to kidneys)

A29.2	Unexplained edema (excess tissue fluid, manifesting primarily as ankle swelling extending to more than 2cm above the malleoli)	Edema means excess tissue fluid. It tends to manifest in the lower regions of the body, first appearing as ankle swelling. It can also become apparent as abdominal and scrotal swelling
		Mild ankle swelling can develop as a result of inactivity and overheating, but should never extend to more than a couple of centimeters above the malleoli (ankle bones)
		If the edema is severe, it may affect the lower part of the calf and can also accumulate in the scrotum, buttocks and lower abdominal tissue
		If the edema is due to excess tissue fluid it will tend to "pit," meaning that sustained pressure will leave an indentation in the skin
		Edema can have a range of causes, and most of these, including kidney disease and chronic heart failure (see A14.1), are potentially serious. If the patient is accumulating significant edema (more than mild ankle swelling), they should be referred for investigation of the cause
A29.3	Acute loin pain: often comes in waves; patient may vomit and collapse	This is characteristic of an obstructed kidney stone. The pain may radiate round to the suprapubic region, particularly if the stone moves some way down the ureter. Encourage drinking of fluids and refer urgently
A29.4	Persistent loin pain (i.e. pain in the flanks either side of the spine between the levels of T11 and L3)	Persistent achy pain in one or both loins might be an indication of kidney infection or other kidney disease. It would be wise to refer if there is no obvious muscular explanation. Refer as high priority if coexistent with symptoms of cystitis (see A29.1) or generalized infection (e.g. fever and malaise)
A29.5	Features of acute pyelonephritis (kidney infection): fever, malaise, loin pain and cloudy urine suggest an infection of the kidneys	While bladder infections are usually self-limiting, particularly in women, the situation is more serious if there are features indicating that the infection has ascended the ureters to affect the kidney. Acute pyelonephritis carries a risk of permanent scarring of the kidneys, and merits prompt medical attention (treatment with antibiotics)
A29.6	Features of vesico-ureteric reflux (VUR) in a child: any history of recurrent episodes or a current episode of cloudy urine or burning on urination should be taken seriously in a prepubescent child	Urine infections are common in young children, but need to be taken seriously, particularly if there is a history of recurrent infections. The small child is more vulnerable to VUR, which means that when the bladder contracts some urine is flushed back towards the kidneys. In the case of infection of the bladder, VUR can lead to infectious organisms causing damage to the delicate structure of the kidney. Sometimes this damage occurs with very few symptoms, but if cumulative and undetected can lead to serious kidney problems and high blood pressure in later life
		For this reason, it is wise to refer all prepubescent children with a history of symptoms of urinary infections to exclude the possibility of VUR
A29.7	Hypertension of any level with established kidney disease	Always refer for medical management, as blood pressure should be maintained below 130/80mmHg in people with kidney disease. There is a much greater risk of worsening kidney damage in patients with hypertension

4.3d Diseases of the ureters, bladder and the urethra

In this section the diseases of the ureters, bladder and the urethra are considered together. These all share the function of collecting urine as it drains from the kidney.

The conditions studied here are:

- Urinary tract obstruction:
  - hydronephrosis
  - prostatic enlargement
- Infections of the lower urinary tract:
  - cystitis (bladder infections)
  - prostatitis
  - urethritis
- Incontinence:
  - stress incontinence
  - urge incontinence
  - overflow incontinence
  - neurological incontinence
- Tumors of the lower urinary tract:
  - cancer of the bladder
  - prostate cancer.

Urinary tract obstruction

The outflow of urine from the urinary tract can be blocked at any level in its passage from the pelvis of the kidney down to the distal urethra, and this can impact on the function of the kidneys, either suddenly or gradually. For example, kidney stones can lodge in the ureter to cause acute one-sided urinary obstruction. In contrast, the condition of chronic kidney disease (CKD) can develop from gradual obstruction of the outflow of the lower urinary tract (e.g. in prostate disease).

There are numerous possible causes of obstruction to the outflow of urine from one or both kidneys. Internal obstruction to the urine flow in the ureters may result from stones, blood clots or urinary tumors. External compression of the ureters may be the result of intra-abdominal cancer or the enlargement of the womb that occurs in pregnancy.

Obstruction of the ureters is usually one-sided, and will affect the function of the kidney on that side. In most cases of one-sided ureteric obstruction, the filtering function of the kidneys is not jeopardized because the other kidney is able to perform this role alone. However, if the other kidney is diseased or missing, ureteric obstruction will lead to acute renal failure if not adequately treated.

Obstruction of the flow through the bladder and the urethra will always affect both kidneys, as the pressure of the accumulating urine builds up within both ureters. Causes include large bladder tumors, impaired muscle contraction of the bladder (due to a neurological disorder that affects the nerve supply to the bladder) and enlargement of the prostate gland in men. Tightening (stricture) of the urethra can develop as a consequence of infection or damage, and this, too, may be sufficient to cause partial or complete obstruction.

Hydronephrosis

Prolonged urinary obstruction leads to a condition of one or both kidneys called hydronephrosis. In hydronephrosis the affected kidney becomes dilated with the accumulating urine, and the ureter becomes distended down to the point of the obstruction. If the obstruction occurs suddenly, the buildup of pressure in this system is acute and can lead to a rapid loss of function of the affected kidney(s). The more usual case is that the obstruction is partial or gradual, in which case the function of the affected kidney(s) is progressively reduced, but not lost totally.

Hydronephrosis can be seen by means of an abdominal ultrasound scan, but the best test to confirm its presence is the computed tomography (CT) urogram, because this can also reveal loss of function of the affected kidney(s).

Symptoms of urinary obstruction

The symptoms of gradual obstruction may be minimal in the early stages, although, if affecting both kidneys, will lead to the symptoms of CKD if persisting for some time (see Section 4.3c). If one-sided obstruction is gradual, there may actually be no symptoms. This is not necessarily a good thing, because the obstruction may have led to total loss of function of the kidney before the diagnosis is made.

In some cases the distension of the kidneys, particularly if rapid in development, will cause loin pain. The pain is worsened by drinking a large volume of fluid. Sudden obstruction of the ureters by a stone or blood clot will lead to the characteristic pain of ureteric colic.

If an obstruction affects both sides of the urinary system, the patient will notice a sluggishness of urine flow, or no urine flow at all if the obstruction is sudden and total. In sudden obstruction of the urethra, the bladder becomes very distended over the course of a few hours. This condition, known as acute retention of urine, can be extremely uncomfortable. In severe retention, the top of the distended bladder can be felt as high as the level of the umbilicus (it normally never raises above the level of the pubic bone).

Gradual obstruction of the urinary tract leads to stagnation of urine flow, and this can predispose to the development of infection, particularly if the bladder is affected. Cystitis and acute pyelonephritis may therefore also complicate the condition of urinary obstruction.

Prostatic enlargement

In men, the prostate gland sits at the base of the bladder, where it encircles the first section of the urethra. Enlargement of the prostate gland, known as benign hyperplasia, is a very common feature of aging in men, and commonly becomes apparent after the sixth decade of life. In some men this enlargement causes narrowing of the urethral passageway through the prostate so that the free flow of urine is restricted.

A less common cause of prostate enlargement is prostate cancer. Often, in cases of prostate cancer, benign hyperplasia coexists. The diagnosis of prostate cancer should be considered in all men who have symptoms of an enlarged prostate.

A first symptom of prostatic enlargement is that the urine flow becomes less powerful than it used to be. There may be difficulty starting the flow (leading to a need to wait for a few seconds to start to urinate) and also some dribbling at the end of urination. As the condition progresses, these symptoms worsen. The patient might have to get up more than once a night to pass urine, and each time he may need to stand for some minutes while waiting for a small dribble to appear. In severe prostatic obstruction the quality of life can be markedly diminished.

The muscle wall of the bladder is affected by having to deal with the increased pressure of urine within it. In mild cases, the muscle wall thickens so that the bladder can still perform its function of emptying all the urine within it. However, in severe prostatic disease the muscle eventually weakens so that the bladder cannot fully expel all the urine. There is then an increased risk of infection due to stagnation of urine in the bladder. The increased pressure is transmitted to the ureters, which dilate, leading to hydronephrosis.

Patients with symptoms should be investigated to exclude the possibility of prostate cancer and also of damage to other parts of the urinary system. In all but the mildest cases, further tests should be carried out to check that the kidney function and emptying of the bladder is normal. At the least, this would require an ultrasound scan of the bladder while voiding urine, and a serum blood test for kidney function.

Those with distressing symptoms and all those with features of impairment of bladder and/or kidney function will be offered medical treatment. Some patients will respond very well to drugs such as tamsulosin, doxazosin and finasteride, although many people cannot tolerate these drugs because of side effects of dizziness and tiredness (tamsulosin and doxazosin) and impotence (finasteride).

Treatment of severe prostatic enlargement involves surgery. The most common operation performed makes use of an endoscopic tool inserted via the urethra to cut a wider channel through the prostate. Operations of this type, known as transurethral resection of the prostate (TURP), or the less invasive transurethral incision of the prostate (TUIP), carry a risk of hemorrhage into the urethra. To minimize this risk, the patient is left with an indwelling plastic catheter in the urethra for a few days after the operation. This keeps the enlarged channel through the urethra open and compresses any bleeding points. The bladder is continually flushed with saline through this tube for the first couple of days to prevent the accumulation of clots in the bladder or the urethra.

Nevertheless, with TURP blood loss is common, and patients who have had this operation frequently require a blood transfusion, or at least iron tablets, after the operation. In most cases the operation will reduce symptoms and improve quality of life, as well as relieve the pressure on the kidneys. Impotence and infertility (due to ejaculation of semen into the bladder) are common side effects following TURP, but are less problematic after TUIP.

 Information box 4.3d-I

Urinary obstruction: comments from a Chinese medicine perspective

In Chinese medicine, urinary obstruction in general would correspond to Deficiency of Kidney Yang, the motive force of the Kidneys. There may also be Deficiency of Spleen Yang. Ming-Men Deficiency is a specific syndrome of old age and chronic illness, in which weakness of the Ming Men (which then fails to warm the Spleen and Kidney Yang) causes lack of strength when urinating.

Retention of urine is usually thought to correspond with Damp or Damp Heat in the Middle Jiao, against a background of Spleen and Kidney Yang Deficiency.

Kidney failure following on from obstruction is an indication of Kidney Yin Deficiency, which often coexists with Kidney Yang Deficiency. Infections represent Damp in the Bladder. An enlarged prostate may be said to represent the accumulation of Phlegm.

Infections of the lower urinary tract

Cystitis (bladder infections)

The infections of the lower urinary tract originate from bacteria, which most usually have entered the urethra through its external orifice. Very commonly, bacteria from the patient's own healthy bowel bacteria are the cause. The most common organisms recognized to cause bladder infections (cystitis) include *Escherichia (E.) coli*, and *Proteus* and *Enterococcus* species.

Bacteria are more likely to enter the bladder in women, because of the short female urethra, and in young children (especially girls) who wear diapers. Postmenopausal women are even more prone to infections because of the change in the urethral lining that occurs after the menopause. The physical stress on the female urethra from sexual intercourse can precipitate a first attack of cystitis (formerly termed honeymoon cystitis). The insertion of a plastic catheter into the bladder is also a known risk factor for cystitis.

It is also believed that changes to the healthy bacteria of the vagina can increase the risk of cystitis in susceptible women. Tight clothing, over-washing, or the use of perfumed soaps or talcum powders may all have this effect.

Once bacteria have entered the bladder, they have to multiply and cause damage to lead to a case of cystitis. In most people, the flow of urine in a healthy bladder can prevent this, and simply washes the bacteria out of the bladder again. Cystitis is therefore more common in those who have obstruction to the flow of urine and those who drink very little fluid. It is also more common in children with vesico-ureteric reflux (VUR) and people with diabetes.

Cystitis is more common in pregnancy because of combined hormonal and pressure effects on the urinary system. These reduce the smooth, free flow of urine through the ureters and bladder of a pregnant woman.

Cystitis is considered to be usually a mild condition that clears to leave no persisting damage to the urinary system. It is believed only to be of serious consequence to those who already have underlying disease of the urinary system. In these cases the infection may become recurrent and can cause worsening of the underlying condition.

Cystitis can also predispose to the development of kidney stones in those who are susceptible to forming them.

The symptoms of cystitis include painful and difficult urination and low abdominal pain. The urine may be smelly, cloudy or blood stained, but can appear clear, even in established infection. In severe cases the patient can feel very unwell, with fever and malaise. These general symptoms are more usual if the infection spreads up the ureters to involve the kidneys (acute pyelonephritis), in which case loin pain is often experienced. In young children, the symptoms are less specific. A child with cystitis may simply appear unwell with fever and irritability.

In most cases a simple bout of cystitis will clear of its own accord. The symptoms and speed of clearance can be helped by drinking plenty of fluids. Drinking cranberry juice is sometimes recommended by conventional doctors. Most doctors in the UK will readily prescribe an antibiotic because the response to this treatment is very rapid.

Often this treatment is given blind in the form of a broad-spectrum antibiotic that is likely to target the most common organisms. In most cases a short course of one to three days may be sufficient to clear the infection from the urinary system, so side effects are minimized.

A case of cystitis in someone who has an underlying problem of the urinary system, or in someone with diabetes, is treated more intensively. A sample of urine is taken to ensure that it is clear what type of organism has caused the infection. In this case antibiotics are strongly advocated, and the course may last five to seven days. The antibiotics are chosen to target the particular organism identified from the urine culture. In the case of people who suffer from recurrent infections, long-term antibiotic treatment might be recommended in an attempt to clear the urinary system of any bacteria that may be being harbored in an area of damaged tissue.

Some people experience the distressing symptoms of cystitis despite all tests of the urine being returned as normal. In some of these cases the patient may be shown to have a physical cause such as a sexually transmitted infection of the urethra, or inflammation of the urethra following sexual intercourse. In other cases, emotional stress may be a prominent feature, and the symptoms may be classed as a functional disease (irritable bladder) akin to irritable bowel syndrome (IBS).

 Information box 4.3d-II

Cystitis: comments from a Chinese medicine perspective

In Chinese medicine, urinary infections of the bladder often represent Damp Heat or Damp Cold in the Bladder. There is likely to be an underlying Spleen or Kidney Qi or Yang Deficiency. In chronic cases Liver Qi Stagnation may also be a complication and will manifest in the form of intermittent chronic low abdominal pain.

Prostatitis

On rare occasions a bacterial infection can spread from the urethra to affect the prostate gland that then becomes inflamed and swollen. The symptoms of prostatitis include pain in the perineum and the testicles, and occasionally a discharge from the urethra. Prostatitis may be a complication of a sexually transmitted disease, but may simply complicate a urinary infection.

Prostatitis is difficult to treat, as the infection is deep seated. A four- to six-week course of antibiotics may be prescribed.

Information box 4.3d-III

Prostatitis: comments from a Chinese medicine perspective

In Chinese medicine, prostatitis represents Damp Heat in the Lower Jiao often complicated by Qi Stagnation. Emotional frustration is a common etiological factor. Over time the Stagnation and Stasis can lead to more intense perineal pain, a manifestation of local Blood Stasis. In chronic cases there will be Depletion of Kidney Yin and Yang.

Urethritis

Inflammation of the urethra is almost always a complication of a sexually transmitted infection such as gonorrhea or *Chlamydia*, although other bacteria may be implicated. Urethritis is the most common diagnosis made in clinics for sexually transmitted diseases, and diagnosis is suggested by the finding of characteristic white blood cells in the urethra. Most cases will respond to appropriate antibiotic treatment.

Urethritis may be a marker of more serious sexually transmitted infections such as HIV or hepatitis B. In those cases where a diagnosis has been made it is very important to perform a full sexual health screen, to attempt to trace and treat sexual contacts, and to counsel against high-risk sexual behavior.

Incontinence

Incontinence is defined as a condition in which there is an involuntary flow of urine from the bladder through the urethra. A small degree of incontinence is an extremely common, but under-reported, symptom, particularly in women after they have had children. Incontinence is often a cause of great distress, but may be under-diagnosed because of embarrassment.

Stress incontinence

Stress incontinence is an involuntary leakage of urine that occurs when a relatively full bladder is exposed to an additional external pressure. The leakage is due to weakness of the external urethral sphincter, which consists of the muscle of the pelvic floor (the perineal muscles). This muscle group can become weakened by childbirth and also by losing tone through aging. The atrophy of the urethra that follows declining levels of estrogen after the menopause can lead to the worsening of stress incontinence. In some female patients stress incontinence coexists with a degree of prolapse of the womb, another long-term muscular problem associated with childbirth.

In stress incontinence, the patient, who is almost always a woman, will lose an amount of urine upon laughing, coughing or sneezing. In mild cases, the leakage can be contained by a thin sanitary towel, but in more severe cases a much larger volume of urine can be lost.

Urge incontinence

Urge incontinence also affects women much more frequently than men. In this condition, the bladder muscle becomes unstable and may suddenly contract with little or no warning. There may be a sudden and intense urge to urinate, which cannot be suppressed for more than a few seconds, meaning that the patient has to rush to find a toilet. Flooding is an unfortunate consequence of urge incontinence.

Frequently, stress and urge incontinence coexist. Sometimes an increase in pressure within the abdomen can trigger not only a small stress incontinence leakage, but also a full contraction due to bladder instability.

Overflow incontinence

Overflow incontinence is a problem that results from obstruction to the outflow of urine from the bladder. The overflow occurs when the bladder is already quite distended with urine, and the pressure within is high. This form of incontinence is usually in the form of slight dribbling. It is most commonly caused by prostatic enlargement.

Treatment of stress, urge and overflow incontinence

Treatment of these forms of incontinence depends on an accurate diagnosis of the cause. Urodynamic studies are used to assess the changes in pressure within the bladder and the flow rate of urine as it empties. These can help distinguish between urge and stress incontinence in particular.

Mild urge and stress incontinence can both respond very well to simple lifestyle advice. A trained incontinence adviser is invaluable in enabling patients to follow this advice correctly. Stress incontinence may be improved dramatically by means of regular perineal exercises that build up the strength of the pelvic floor muscles. Younger women can use the same exercises after childbirth to prevent the development of stress incontinence. Urge incontinence can be helped by bladder training, which involves following a program of regular and complete emptying of the bladder and avoiding certain dietary triggers which are known to irritate the bladder (e.g. caffeine).

Medication may be prescribed to help prevent incontinence. Drugs such as oxybutynin calm down an overactive bladder muscle and so may be of help in urge incontinence. Duloxetine is an antidepressant that is also licensed for the treatment of stress incontinence.

There is a wide range of incontinence pads and aids available that may help cope with a mild problem. In men a condom (sheath) can be used to drain leaked urine down a plastic tube into a bag discreetly attached to the thigh.

For more severe stress incontinence, surgical repair of the weak supporting muscles of the bladder may be recommended. The repair operation may be performed at the same time as a hysterectomy to correct the problem of a prolapsed womb.

Neurological incontinence

In neurological incontinence the control of the bladder is lost because of damage to the nerves that supply the bladder. This might be the result of disease of the brain or spinal cord (e.g. stroke, multiple sclerosis or spinal injury) or the result of a disorder that causes damage to the peripheral nerves (e.g. diabetes).

In this condition, because the incontinence is often total, the treatment that offers the patient the most freedom in daily life is an indwelling plastic catheter. This plastic tube allows drainage of the urine from the bladder into a plastic bag, which can be emptied at intervals. The main disadvantage of indwelling catheters is that they are frequently the cause of recurrent urinary infections. When possible, patients can be taught to "intermittently self-catheterize," which means that the catheter is used only for voiding the bladder at intervals (usually four times a day) and so does not need to be indwelling.

Information box 4.3d-IV

Incontinence: comments from a Chinese medicine perspective

In Chinese medicine, incontinence corresponds to either Lung Qi Deficiency, a Deficiency of the Kidneys, or both. The Kidney Deficiency can be of Yin or Yang. Kidney Qi not Firm describes a syndrome of nocturnal incontinence. It is an aspect of Kidney Yang Deficiency.

Tumors of the lower urinary tract

The most important tumors to affect the urinary tract are those of the bladder and of the prostate. The rare forms of cancer that affect the ureters and urethra are similar in type to the cancer that more commonly develops in the bladder.

Cancer of the bladder (transitional cell carcinoma)

Malignant tumors of the bladder affect men four times more often than women. They are associated with cigarette smoking and also exposure to certain drugs and environmental toxins. Bladder cancer has been linked to industrial exposure in the rubber and chemical industries. The tropical infection schistosomiasis is an important worldwide cause of bladder cancer. In schistosomiasis, the cancer results from the chronic inflammation of the bladder caused by the disease.

The first symptom of bladder cancer is usually blood in the urine. Alternatively, the first symptoms may mimic a bout of cystitis, including pain on urination and abdominal pain. In the case of cancer these symptoms will not respond fully to antibiotic therapy.

The diagnosis may be suggested by an ultrasound scan, but is confirmed by means of a cystoscopy during which a biopsy of the tumor can be obtained. If the tumor is localized it may be successfully treated by burning (diathermy) with an electrical probe inserted via the cystoscope. The patient will then be instructed to return for a check cystoscopy at regular intervals to look for and treat any recurrences of the tumor. Four out of five patients who have a localized bladder tumor will still be alive five years after the first diagnosis, and a proportion of these will be cured.

A more advanced tumor may be treated with a variety of approaches, including infusion of chemotherapy into the bladder, radiotherapy and surgical removal of the bladder. There is very little chance of cure of bladder cancer if the cancer has spread to other tissues at the time of diagnosis.

Information box 4.3d-V

Cancer of the bladder: comments from a Chinese medicine perspective

In Chinese medicine, bladder cancer corresponds to Phlegm and/or Blood Stagnation. Environmental Heat Toxins may be etiological factors. Blood in the urine suggests Heat. There is always an underlying Deficiency of Kidney Yin and/or Yang.

Prostate cancer

Prostate cancer is a very common development in the aging prostate gland. In many cases the cancer is slow growing and causes few symptoms. It is estimated that 80 percent of men have islands of cancer cells within their prostate gland by the age of 80, but only in a minority of these will the cancer cells be any threat to their health. More malignant prostate tumors grow to a size that causes urinary obstruction. The cancer spreads very commonly to bone, so that bone pain may also be a first symptom.

A malignant prostate may feel hard and irregular on rectal examination, but this is not a reliable sign.

An ultrasound scan of the prostate may reveal a characteristic irregular swelling of the gland, and can give a good estimate of the size of the tumor for the purposes of staging.

A blood test for a chemical called prostate-specific antigen (PSA) is more likely to show a raised PSA level if cancer is present, but the results of this test can be confusing, which has brought its value as a cancer screening test into question. Because of a high incidence of both false-positive and false-negative results, the PSA test is more useful in terms of monitoring response to treatment of established cancer rather than in diagnosis.

Prostate cancer can only be confirmed definitively by means of tissue biopsy. The tissue sample may be obtained by means of a trans rectal ultrasound (TRUS) guided approach or at the time of a TURP for prostatic enlargement. X-ray imaging or a bone scan may be performed to exclude or assess the presence of bony metastases. This is important for the staging of the tumor. Localized prostate cancer is assigned a Gleason Score, which rates the invasiveness of the tumor on a scale from 2 to 10. This score is based on the microscopic appearance of the biopsy. A Gleason Score of 6 or less indicates that the cancer is not likely to spread beyond the prostate gland.

Treatment of symptomatic disease confined to the prostate involves removal of the prostate gland or radiotherapy. Removal of the prostate gland carries the risks of incontinence and impotence (erectile dysfunction). In localized prostate cancer, radiotherapy can take the form of the insertion of radioactive pellets into the prostate gland, which then act over the course of time. This treatment is known as brachytherapy. If the disease has spread outside the prostate gland, radiotherapy can again be beneficial. Radiotherapy carries no risk of incontinence, but does carry a significant risk of erectile dysfunction.

Drugs may be used to hinder the further spread of prostate cancer that has already spread beyond the prostate gland. It is known that the cancer regresses if the effects of testosterone can be eliminated. A radical solution to this used to be removal of the testes, but currently most men prefer to take tablets (cyproterone) or have a regular injection (e.g. goserilin) that acts to suppress the action of testosterone in the body. These approaches carry the side effects of loss of libido and hot flashes.

The prognosis in most cases of metastatic prostate disease is not very good. The majority of patients are not alive five years after diagnosis, although it must be remembered that many patients are elderly at diagnosis, so in some of these cases death may not be a direct result of the prostate cancer.

 Information box 4.3d-VI

Prostate cancer: comments from a Chinese medicine perspective

In Chinese medicine, prostate cancer corresponds to Phlegm and/or Blood Stagnation against a background of severe Deficiency, in particular, of Kidney Yin and Yang. Bone pain is a manifestation of Blood Stagnation.

The red flags of diseases of the ureters, bladder and the urethra

Some patients with diseases of the ureters, bladder and the urethra will benefit from referral to a conventional doctor for assessment and/or treatment. Red flags are those symptoms and signs that indicate that referral should be considered. The red flags of the diseases of the ureters, bladder and the urethra are described in Table 4.3d-I. A summary of the red flags in a format designed for quick reference in clinical practice can be found in Appendix III. This gives advice on the degree of urgency of referral for each of the red flag conditions listed.

Table 4.3d-I A30: Red flags of diseases of the ureters, bladder and the urethra

Red flag	Description	Reasoning
A30.1	Acute loin pain: often comes in waves; patient may vomit and collapse	This is characteristic of an obstructed kidney stone. The pain may radiate around to the suprapubic region, particularly if the stone moves some way down the ureter. Encourage drinking of fluids and refer urgently
A30.2	Blood in the urine (hematuria) or sperm (hemospermia): • refer all cases in men • refer in women except in the case of acute urinary infection	The most common and benign cause of blood in the urine in women is bladder infection (cystitis). If the symptoms are suggestive of this diagnosis (burning on urination, low abdominal pain, cloudy or blood-stained urine), there is no need to refer straight away. Treat with complementary medicine, recommend a high fluid intake, and refer only if symptoms are not settling within 3 days However, blood in the urine is not normal in men, who should be protected from infection by the relatively long male urethra Refer all cases of blood in the urine in men, and in women if there are either no other symptoms (blood may be coming from the kidney or from a tumor) or if the pain is felt also in the loin (suggesting spread of infection to the kidneys) Hemospermia is alarming to the patient but usually benign, as it can result from slight trauma to the genitals. Nevertheless, refer non-urgently to exclude a serious cause
A30.3	Features of recurrent or persistent urinary tract infection: episodes of symptoms including some or all of cloudy urine, burning on urination, abdominal discomfort, blood in urine and fever, especially if occurring in men	Urinary tract infections are generally self-limiting and should clear up within five days. Refer anyone who has persistent symptoms in order to exclude an underlying disorder of the urinary system. Recurrent or persistent infections are particularly uncommon in men, and are more likely to signify an underlying disorder of the urinary tract than when they occur in women
A30.4	Features of a urinary tract infection in a patient in one of the following vulnerable groups: • pre-existing disorder of the urinary system • diabetes • pregnancy • paraplegia	Refer a patient who develops symptoms of a urinary tract infection straight away for treatment if there is an underlying vulnerability such as known disease of the urinary system (e.g. kidney disease, kidney stones, bladder cancer, enlarged prostate gland), diabetes or pregnancy or if the ability to sense and void the bladder is impaired because of paraplegia In both pregnancy and diabetes there is a far higher risk of the infection ascending the ureters and damaging the kidneys In pregnancy urinary tract infections may also increase the risk of early labor or miscarriage
A30.5	Features of moderate prostatic obstruction: enlargement of the prostate gland leads to symptoms such as increasing difficulty urinating and the need to get up at night to urinate (nocturia)	Benign prostatic enlargement is common, and the symptoms may respond to complementary medical treatment such as western herbs or acupuncture. However, the same symptoms can be caused by a prostatic tumor, and so it is wise to refer for further investigations, including physical (rectal) examination, kidney function tests and a blood test for prostate-specific antigen (PSA)
A30.6	Features of acute pyelonephritis (kidney infection): fever, malaise, loin pain and cloudy urine suggest an infection of the kidneys	While bladder infections are usually self-limiting, particularly in women, the situation is more serious if there are features indicating that the infection has ascended the ureters to affect the kidney. Acute pyelonephritis carries a risk of permanent scarring of the kidneys, and merits medical attention (treatment with antibiotics)

A30.7	Features of *vesico-ureteral reflux* (VUR) in a child: any history of recurrent episodes or a current episode of cloudy urine or burning on urination should be taken seriously in a prepubescent child	Urine infections are common in young children, but need to be taken seriously, particularly if there is a history of recurrent infections. The small child is more vulnerable to VUR, which means that when the bladder contracts, some urine is flushed back towards the kidneys. In the case of infection of the bladder, VUR can lead to infectious organisms causing damage to the delicate structure of the kidney. Sometimes this damage occurs with very few symptoms, but if cumulative and undetected, can lead to serious kidney problems and high blood pressure in later life. For this reason, it is wise to refer all prepubescent children with a history of symptoms of urinary infections to exclude the possibility of VUR
A30.8	Bedwetting in a child: if persisting over the age of 5	Consider referral if the child is over 5 years, so that physical causes can be excluded and parents can have access to expert advice
A30.9	Incontinence: if unexplained or causing distress	A mild degree of stress incontinence (leakage of a small amount of urine when coughing or laughing) is common and benign in women, particularly after childbirth and the menopause. However, uncontrollable losses of large volumes of urine are not normal, nor is bedwetting when asleep. In these cases investigations are merited to look for treatable causes (e.g. a prolapsed uterus, prostatic obstruction and nocturnal seizures). Also refer so that the patient can have access to guidance and support from an incontinence specialist nurse

Notes

1   Myers, T.W. (2001) *Anatomy Trains*. Edinburgh: Churchill Livingstone.
2   Keown, D. (2014) *The Spark in the Machine*. London: Singing Dragon, Chapter 17.
3   Waugh, A. and Grant, A. (2014) *Ross and Wilson: Anatomy and Physiology in Health and Illness*. Twelfth Edition. Edinburgh: Elsevier, Chapter 7.
4   Dharmananda, S. and Vickers, E. (2000) 'Synopsis of scalp acupuncture.' Available at www.itmonline.org/arts/newscalp.htm, accessed on 13 July 2016.
5   Keown, D. (2014) *The Spark in the Machine*. London: Singing Dragon, Chapter 17.
6   Mayor, D. (2007) *Electroacupuncture: A Practical Manual and Resource*. Edinburgh: Churchill Livingstone, pp.66–67.
7   Flaws, B. and Sionneau, P. (2001) *The Treatment of Modern Western Medical Diseases with Chinese Medicine*. Boulder, CO: Blue Poppy Press, Chapter 11.
8   Tidy, C. (2014) 'Migraine management.' Available at http://patient.info/doctor/migraine-management, accessed on 18 July 2016.
9   Reismann, M. and Fuller, C.J. (2009) 'Is patent foramen ovale closure indicated for migraine?' *Circulation: Cardiovascular Interventions 2*, 468–474. Available at http://circinterventions.ahajournals.org/content/2/5/468.full, accessed on 18 July 2016.
10 Linde, K., Allais, G., Brinkhaus, B., Manheimer, E., Vickers, A. and White, A.R. (2009) 'Acupuncture for migraine prophylaxis.' *Cochrane Database Systematic Reviews*, 21 January, 1. Available at www.ncbi.nlm.nih.gov/pubmed/19160193?dopt=Abstract, accessed on 18 July 2016.
11 Knott, L. (2014) 'Meningitis.' Available at http://patient.info/doctor/meningitis-pro, accessed on 18 July 2016.
12 NICE (National Institute for Health and Care Excellence) (2006) *Parkinson's Disease in Over 20s: Diagnosis and Management*. Clinical Guideline [CG35]. Available at www.nice.org.uk/guidance/cg35, accessed on 12 December 2016.
13 Maciocia, G. (1994) *The Practice of Chinese Medicine*. Edinburgh: Churchill Livingstone, Chapters 28, 29.
14 Tidy, C. (2015) 'Multiple sclerosis.' Available at http://patient.info/doctor/multiple-sclerosis-pro, accessed on 17 July 2016.
15 Payne, J. (2016) 'Facial nerve palsy.' Available at http://patient.info/doctor/facial-nerve-palsy, accessed on 18 July 2016.
16 Peng, Q.-H. and Frank, C. (2014) *TCM Case Studies; Eye: Ear, Nose and Throat Disorders*. Beijing: People's Medical Publishing House, excerpt on Bell's palsy. Available at http://sixfishes.com/blog/the-treatment-of-bells-palsy-in-tcm, accessed on 18 July 2016.
17 Flaws, B. and Sionneau, P. (2001) *The Treatment of Modern Western Medical Diseases with Chinese Medicine*. Boulder, CO: Blue Poppy Press, Chapter 70.
18 Ashmead, A.S. (1894) 'Traditional treatment of leprosy in Japan and China.' *Journal of the American Medical Association XXII*(17), 605–608. Available at http://jama.jamanetwork.com/article.aspx?articleid=445678, accessed on 18 July 2016.
19 Flaws, B. and Sionneau, P. (2001) *The Treatment of Modern Western Medical Diseases with Chinese Medicine*. Boulder, CO: Blue Poppy Press, Chapter 31.
20 Waugh, A. and Grant, A. (2014) *Ross and Wilson: Anatomy and Physiology in Health and Illness*. Twelfth Edition. Edinburgh: Elsevier, Chapter 16.
21 Legge, D. (1997) *Close to the Bone: The Treatment of Musculoskeletal Disorder with Acupuncture and Other Traditional Chinese Medicine*. 2nd edition. Sydney, NSW: Sydney College Press.
22 NICE (National Institute for Health and Care Excellence) (2016) *British National Formulary: 4.7 Analgesics*. Available at www.evidence.nhs.uk/formulary/bnf/current/4-central-nervous-system/47-analgesics, accessed on 21 July 2016.
23 Buoyancy Foundation of Victoria (2010) *Effects of Drug Use: Traditional Chinese Medicine Perspective*. Available at http://buoyancy.org.au/resources/useful-info, accessed on 21 July 2016.
24 Rosenberg, Z. (2015) 'A Chinese look at Western pharmaceuticals.' Available at www.acupuncture.com/herbs/pharma.htm, accessed on 21 July 2016.
25 Medicines and Healthcare Products Regulatory Agency (2007) *Hormone Replacement Therapy: Updated Advice*. Available at www.gov.uk/drug-safety-update/hormone-replacement-therapy-updated-advice, accessed on 21 July 2016.
26 Sunyecz, J. (2008) 'The use of calcium and vitamin D in the management of osteoporosis.' *Journal of Therapeutics and Clinical Risk Management*, August, 4(4), 827–836. Available at www.ncbi.nlm.nih.gov/pmc/articles/PMC2621390, accessed on 21 July 2016.
27 Paziana, K. and Pazianas, M. (2015) 'Calcium supplements controversy in osteoporosis: A physiological mechanism supporting cardiovascular adverse effects.' *Endocrine*, April, 48(3), 776–778. Available at www.ncbi.nlm.nih.gov/pubmed/25687221, accessed on 21 July 2016.
28 Cochrane Bone Joint and Muscle Trauma Group (2012) *Cochrane Database of Systematic Reviews: Interventions for Preventing Falls in Older People Living in the Community*. Available at http://onlinelibrary.wiley.com/doi/10.1002/14651858.CD007146.pub3/abstract, accessed on 21 July 2016.
29 NICE (National Institute for Health and Care Excellence) (2014) Press release archive: 'Millions of people at risk of low vitamin D need better access to supplements to protect health, says NICE.' Available at www.nice.org.uk/news/press-and-media/millions-of-people-at-risk-of-low-vitamin-d-need-better-access-to-supplements-to-protect-health-says-nice, accessed on 21 July 2016.
30 Unverzagt, C., Berglund, K. and Thomas, J. (2015) 'Dry needling for myofascial trigger point pain: A clinical commentary.' *International Journal of Sports Physical Therapy 10*(3), 402–418. Available at www.ncbi.nlm.nih.gov/pmc/articles/PMC4458928, accessed on 21 July 2016.
31 RepetitiveStrainInjury.org (2010) 'Treating repetitive strain injury.' Available at www.repetitivestraininjury.org.uk/treating-rsi.html, accessed on 21 July 2016.
32 Myers, T. (2009) *Anatomy Trains: Myofascial Meridians for Manual and Movement Therapists*. Edinburgh: Elsevier.
33 Keown, D. (2014) *The Spark in the Machine*. London: Singing Dragon.
34 Legge, D. (1997) *Close to the Bone: The Treatment of Musculoskeletal Disorder with Acupuncture and Other Traditional Chinese Medicine*. 2nd edition. Sydney, NSW: Sydney College Press.

35 Hunter, D. and Eckstein, F. (2009) 'Exercise and osteoarthritis.' *Journal of Anatomy 214*(2), 197–207. Available at www.ncbi.nlm.nih.gov/pmc/articles/PMC2667877, accessed on 21 July 2016.

36 Arthritis Research UK (2010) 'Glucosamine sulphate trials for osteoarthritis.' Available at www.arthritisresearchuk.org/arthritis-information/complementary-and-alternative-medicines/cam-report/complementary-medicines-for-osteoarthritis/glucosamine/glucosamine-sulphate-oa.aspx, accessed on 21 July 2016.

37 Tidy, C. (2015) 'Management of rheumatoid arthritis.' Available at http://patient.info/doctor/management-of-rheumatoid-arthritis, accessed on 22 July 2016.

38 Flaws, B. and Sionneau, P. (2010) *The Treatment of Modern Western Medical Diseases with Chinese Medicine.* Boulder, CO: Blue Poppy Press, Chapter 63.

39 Flaws, B. (2000) *Curing Fibromyalgia Naturally with Chinese Medicine.* Boulder, CO: Blue Poppy Press.

40 Waugh, A. and Grant, A. (2014) *Ross and Wilson: Anatomy and Physiology in Health and Illness.* Twelfth Edition. Edinburgh: Elsevier, Chapter 13.

41 Maciocia, G. (1989) *The Principles of Chinese Medicine.* Edinburgh: Churchill Livingstone, p.96.

42 Maciocia, G. (1989) *The Principles of Chinese Medicine.* Edinburgh: Churchill Livingstone, p.117.

43 Maciocia, G. (1989) *The Principles of Chinese Medicine.* Edinburgh: Churchill Livingstone, Chapters 8, 9, 13.

44 Flaws, B. and Sionneau, P. (2010) *The Treatment of Modern Western Medical Diseases with Chinese Medicine.* Boulder, CO: Blue Poppy Press, p.156.

45 Flaws, B. and Sionneau, P. (2010) *The Treatment of Modern Western Medical Diseases with Chinese Medicine.* Boulder, CO: Blue Poppy Press, pp.526–530.

46 Tidy, C. (2014) 'Chronic kidney disease.' Available at http://patient.info/doctor/chronic-kidney-disease-pro, accessed on 2 August 2016.

47 Flaws, B. and Sionneau, P. (2010) *The Treatment of Modern Western Medical Diseases with Chinese Medicine.* Boulder, CO: Blue Poppy Press, p.171.

THE ENDOCRINE AND REPRODUCTIVE SYSTEMS AND CHILD HEALTH

5.1

The Endocrine System

5.1a The physiology of the endocrine system[1]

It has already been explained in this book that the nervous and endocrine systems together are considered by conventional medicine as the foundation of that which makes the body an integrated whole. This is because they are both concerned with communication between one body part and another.

In the nervous system, the communication between one nerve and another takes place at a junction called the synapse. At the synapse, the release of a tiny amount of a chemical known as a neurotransmitter enables a change that has taken place in one nerve cell to be transmitted to other nerve cells. In the endocrine system, the communication is also based on the release of chemicals. These chemicals, released by specialized endocrine cells, are known as hormones. Endocrine cells may be grouped together in organs known as endocrine glands, but can also be found loosely distributed within many of the organs and tissues of the body.

In contrast to neurotransmitters, hormones stimulate changes in bodily cells only after traveling to local tissues via the tissue fluid, or to distant sites through the bloodstream. However, once hormones reach their target cells, the way in which they lead to internal changes within those cells is remarkably similar to the effect of neurotransmitters on target nerve cells. Both hormones and neurotransmitters connect with protein receptors on the target cell membrane. Through this connection, these chemicals lead to a change in the internal physiology of the cell. As increasing numbers of these chemicals are discovered and their functions described, it is becoming clear that many of those which act as hormones in the body can also be found within the nervous system, where they function as neurotransmitters.

Through communication by means of hormones, the endocrine system encourages the state of homeostasis to be maintained within the body. In order to fulfill this role, the endocrine system has always to be responsive to changes in the internal and external environments of the body.

Cholecystokinin (CCK) (originating from cells in the duodenum), adrenaline (from the adrenal medulla), erythropoietin (EPO) (from the substance of the kidney) and testosterone (from the testes) are examples of hormones that have their impact on the digestive, cardiovascular, blood and reproductive systems, respectively. CCK and EPO are examples of hormones that are not released from specific endocrine organs. CCK is released from endocrine cells scattered within the wall of the duodenum, and EPO is released from endocrine cells within the tissue of the kidney. In contrast, adrenaline and testosterone are examples of hormones that originate from specialized endocrine organs, namely, the adrenal glands and the testes, respectively.

The organs of the endocrine system

This section focuses on the most basic physiology of those endocrine organs that are affected in the important endocrine diseases. These are:

- the pituitary and the hypothalamus

- the thyroid gland

- the adrenal glands

- the endocrine part of the pancreas (pancreatic islets).

The role of the parathyroid glands in calcium homeostasis is described in Sections 4.2a and 4.3a. The function of the ovaries and testes will be explored in Section 5.2a. The pineal gland and thymus gland will not be discussed further in this text.

Figure 5.1a-I illustrates the anatomical location of the organs of the endocrine system.

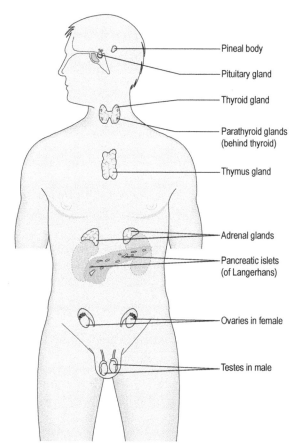

Figure 5.1a-I The anatomical location of the organs of the endocrine system

The negative feedback loop

The negative feedback loop is the basic mechanism that underlies the action of these hormones in maintaining balance. It requires a detector to recognize a move away from balance, a control center that recognizes when the move has been so great that something has to be done about it, and an effector to bring about a change in the body to reverse the imbalance. A thermostat is a mechanical example of the negative feedback loop in action. The detector in this case is a thermometer. The control center is the mechanism that is set to recognize when the temperature falls outside a desired range. The negative feedback loop is based on maximum desired temperature. When the temperature becomes too high, the effector, in this case, the heating element, is switched

off until the time when the temperature drops within the desired range once again.

These rather abstract concepts, which were first introduced in Section 1.1c, can now be placed in more concrete terms. Endocrine cells play the role of both detector and control center, while the release of hormone corresponds to the effector of the negative feedback loop. As a thermostat is designed to keep ambient temperature constant, the endocrine negative feedback loops work to keep bodily variables such as blood sugar or blood calcium at a steady level. This section offers many more examples of this negative feedback loop in action (e.g. see Table 5.1a-I), as each of the important endocrine organs is described in turn.

Table 5.1a-I The release of cholecystokinin (CCK): an example of the negative feedback loop in the regulation of hormones

The endocrine cells of the duodenum are specialized to detect increased levels of fat within the duodenum. They do this by means of specialized proteins on their cell membranes which, when they come into contact with fat, lead to internal changes within the cells. In this case the internal change is the onset of the manufacture of CCK

The control aspect is that it is only when the amount of fat is at a certain level that these cells are stimulated to release CCK into the bloodstream

CCK is the effector that travels within the bloodstream to lead to an appropriate release of bile from the gallbladder, which in turn helps to digest the fats. The release of CCK only ceases when all the fat has been digested and has left the duodenum

CCK also acts at the exocrine pancreas to stimulate the release of fat-digesting enzymes (amongst others) into the duodenum. This is another example of a negative feedback loop in action

The pituitary and the hypothalamus

The pituitary gland is a pea-sized organ that projects downwards from an area at the base of the brain called the hypothalamus. The site of the pituitary is deep within the head, approximately at the level of the bridge of the nose (see Figure 5.1a-II). The extra acupoint Yin Tang, which is considered in Chinese medicine to have a profound influence over mental functions, overlies the region of the pituitary and hypothalamus.

A stalk projects downwards from the hypothalamus through which nerve fibers pass into the pituitary. A delicate network of blood vessels connects the two areas through this stalk. These blood vessels carry hormones from the hypothalamus to the pituitary.

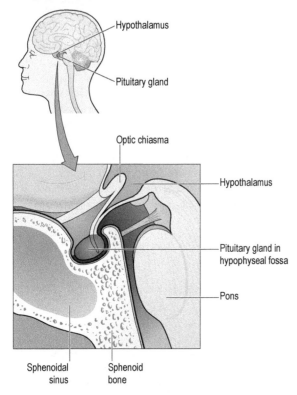

Figure 5.1a-II The position of the pituitary gland and its associated structures

An alternative term for the pituitary gland is the hypophysis. The term adenohypophysis refers to the anterior portion of the pituitary, which contains endocrine cells. The adenohypophysis is the source of six different hormones. The term neurohypophysis refers to the posterior portion of the pituitary gland. This part receives nerve fibers from the hypothalamus, and is the source of two additional hormones that are secreted directly into the bloodstream from the endings of these nerves.

Together, the hypothalamus and the pituitary perform a vital control function in the endocrine system. The hormones secreted by the hypothalamus and the pituitary affect the function of other endocrine organs, including the thyroid gland, the adrenal gland and the sex organs.

The hormones of the hypothalamus are either secreted into the general bloodstream by the nerve endings of the neurohypophysis, or carried within the blood vessels of the pituitary stalk to act on the adenohypophysis. In contrast, all the hormones released by the pituitary gland travel within the bloodstream to have effects on distant endocrine organs as well as other parts of the body.

At least 13 hormones are released by the hypothalamus and the pituitary gland. All of these are commonly described by conventional practitioners by their initials rather than their full medical names, and include growth hormone (GH), thyroid-stimulating hormone (TSH), adrenocorticotrophic hormone (ACTH) from the pituitary,

and growth hormone-releasing hormone (GHRH), corticotropin-releasing hormone (CRH) and gonadotropin-releasing hormone (GnRH) from the hypothalamus.

It is helpful to understand that the hormones of the hypothalamus are the mechanism by which the hormones of the pituitary are controlled. For example, the release of GH from the pituitary gland can be increased and decreased by two different hormones (GHRH and growth hormone-inhibiting hormone, GHIH) from the hypothalamus. This is one example of the close connection between the nervous system (hypothalamus) and the endocrine system (pituitary gland).

The hypothalamus lies deep within the substance of the brain, and so can be influenced by complex internal factors, including the stage of psychological development and the emotions. This might explain why such factors can have profound effects on hormone-controlled events such as childhood growth, timing of puberty and breast milk production.

Table 5.1a-II lists the six hormones that are produced by the adenohypophysis.

Table 5.1a-II The hormones released from the anterior pituitary gland (adenohypophysis) and their functions

Hormone	Function
Growth hormone (GH)	Stimulates growth in many tissues
Thyroid-stimulating hormone (TSH)	Stimulates the production of thyroid hormones
Adrenocorticotrophic hormone (ACTH)	Stimulates the production of cortisol from the adrenal gland
Prolactin (PRL)	Stimulates breast milk production
Follicle-stimulating hormone (FSH)	Stimulates the development of the ovarian follicle (the first half of the menstrual cycle)
Luteinizing hormone (LH)	Stimulates ovulation and the maturation of the ruptured follicle (corpus luteum)

The hormones oxytocin and antidiuretic hormone (ADH) are released from the neurohypophysis, but have their origins within nerve cells within the hypothalamus.

Growth hormone (GH)

GH stimulates the continued growth of the skeleton, muscles and soft tissues, including the major organs. This growth is not only essential during childhood, but is also important for the maintained health and liveliness of these tissues throughout adult life. GH affects the metabolism of the body, meaning that it alters the rate at which the complex chemical processes of the bodily tissues take place. Under the influence of GH, the rate of protein and collagen synthesis increases, and the amount of sugar in the blood tends to rise to meet the body's increased requirements for energy.

Information box 5.1a-I

Growth hormone: comments from a Chinese medicine perspective

A Chinese medicine energetic interpretation of this hormone has to be complex, as GH affects the functioning of diverse tissues at a fundamental level. Its role in continued growth suggests that its control is an aspect of Kidney Essence. Its role in the appropriate use of nutrients to build up the physical substance of the body suggests that it also plays a role in the transformation of Qi. Its control, therefore, can also be seen as an aspect of Original Qi and, in particular, Spleen Qi. Original Qi is, of course, closely related to Kidney Essence.

In excess, GH leads to thickening of soft tissues and broadening of the bones (see Section 5.1e). This might be interpreted as accumulation of Damp and Phlegm. This again suggests that appropriate secretion of GH is an aspect of the healthy function of the Spleen Organ. In deficiency lack of GH manifests as stunted growth, an expression of Jing Deficiency.

Oxytocin

Oxytocin is important for contraction of the uterine muscle during labor and for the expression of breast milk during suckling.

ADH, TSH, ACTH, FSH, LH and PRL

The role of ADH was mentioned in Section 4.3a. This hormone is released in response to an increased concentration of the salts in the blood. It reduces the amount of water that is lost through the urine, and is important in the control of the homeostasis of the concentration of the blood. TSH and ACTH relate to the healthy function of the thyroid and adrenal glands, respectively. PRL, FSH and LH are all important in the physiology of the reproductive system. The function of these five pituitary hormones is described in more detail in Section 5.2a.

The thyroid gland

Figure 5.1a-III illustrates the thyroid gland, which is a bow tie-shaped organ situated just below the level of the laryngeal prominence (Adam's apple) in the neck. The bow tie shape is a result of the gland being formed by two lobes

separated by a narrow bridge of tissue called the isthmus. In health, the thyroid gland can be felt as a small region of vague softness below the voice box. This can be felt to rise and descend during swallowing.

Figure 5.1a-III The thyroid gland and its associated structures

The thyroid gland contains endocrine cells, which secrete two hormones, thyroxine (also known as T4) and tri-iodothyronine (T3). The thyroid gland draws upon iodine from the diet to manufacture sufficient quantities of these hormones. Iodine is found in seawater, and also in plant and animal products that originate from areas close to the sea. For this reason, iodine deficiency may occur in regions of the world that are distant from the sea, especially landlocked countries. However, in many developed countries, such as the UK, table salt contains additional iodine, meaning that iodine deficiency is rarely a problem.

The thyroid hormones T4 and T3 are both released in response to TSH from the pituitary. The release of TSH is primarily controlled by the release of TRH (thyroid-releasing hormone) from the hypothalamus. This is the mechanism whereby the activity of the brain affects thyroid function.

Like GH, the thyroid hormones play an important role in physical growth and the rate at which the cells of the body convert nutrients into energy (the metabolic rate). They are also important in the healthy development of the growing nervous system, the appropriate function of the cardiovascular system and the smooth functioning of the gastrointestinal system. If in excess, the thyroid hormones can cause an increased use of bodily nutrients, leading to the production of heat, weight loss, feelings of nervousness, a rapid heart rate and increased peristalsis in the bowel.

The negative feedback loop of control of the thyroid hormones is affected by factors such as exercise, stress, low blood glucose and malnutrition. All these factors increase the release of TSH from the hypothalamus, and thus increase the release of T4 and T3. Conversely, raised levels of thyroid hormones in the bloodstream will inhibit the release of TRH from the hypothalamus and TSH from the pituitary gland.

Information box 5.1a-II

Thyroid hormones: comments from a Chinese medicine perspective

The Chinese medicine energetic interpretation of the thyroid hormones is complex. The thyroid hormones are important for growth and the appropriate use of nutrients at a cellular level. Both these aspects of their role suggest that their control reflects an aspect of Kidney Essence and Original Qi.

The consequence of an excessive secretion of thyroid hormones is the generation of a state similar to the general pattern described as Yin Deficiency (feelings of heat, anxiety and rapid heart rate). Insufficient secretion of thyroid hormones leads to a state that includes feelings of cold, lassitude, weight gain and slow heart rate (see Section 5.1c), which together can be compared to the pattern of Yang Deficiency. Thus these patterns suggest that the appropriate control of the thyroid hormones reflects an aspect of the fundamental balance of Yin and Yang.

As the seat of Yin and Yang lies within the Kidney Organ, here is another example of how the function of the thyroid gland might be closely related to the Kidney Organ in Chinese medicine. This fits with the fact that the deep pathway of the Kidney Organ passes through the throat and ends at the root of the tongue. Interestingly, the root of the tongue is the origin of the tissue of the developing thyroid gland in the embryo.

Parathyroid hormone (PTH) and calcitonin

Calcitonin is another hormone secreted by the thyroid gland. Together with the parathyroid hormone (PTH), it plays a role in calcium homeostasis. PTH is secreted by the cells of the four tiny parathyroid glands situated deep within the tissue of the thyroid gland.

Information box 5.1a-III

Parathyroid hormone and calcitonin: comments from a Chinese medicine perspective

In Chinese medicine terms, the role of both these additional hormones secreted by the thyroid gland can also be linked to the Kidney Organ, in that they are fundamental to the health of the bony skeleton.

The adrenal glands

The adrenal glands are situated on top of the kidneys, deep in the back of the abdomen, approximately at the level of the lumbar vertebrae L1 and L2. Each gland contains two distinct areas of endocrine tissue. The outer part of each gland is called the cortex, and this is the source of three types of steroid hormones, known as glucocorticoids, mineralocorticoids and androgens. The androgens secreted by the adrenal cortex are male sex hormones, but have a minimal effect in comparison to the effect of those secreted by the sex organs. The inner part of the adrenal gland is called the medulla. The adrenal medulla is the source of two hormones, adrenaline and noradrenaline, which play an important role in the sympathetic nervous system (SNS).

Glucocorticoids

The glucocorticoids include cortisol and corticosterone, and are essential for life. Their release is stimulated via the pituitary (by ACTH). Glucocorticoids are released in times of stress, and their levels also peak early in the morning in preparation for the time of waking up. They affect the way in which glucose is handled in the body, and increase the retention of salt and water in the body.

These hormones have the effect of preparing the body for sustained physical activity such as occurs on waking. They both enable the storage of glucose, and also increase its availability by breaking down other substances such as protein. By retaining salt and water, they increase the blood pressure, which is an appropriate response, if controlled.

Excessive stress will lead to excessive secretion of these hormones, and this can contribute to raised blood sugar (diabetes), muscle wasting and hypertension. Corticosteroids are synthetic forms of these hormones.

Mineralocorticoids

Aldosterone is the main mineralocorticoid hormone. It is secreted in response to a fall in sodium, and enables more sodium and water to be retained by the kidneys. It is also secreted in response to a reduced flow of blood in the kidneys (which stimulates the release of renin).

Aldosterone secretion, by increasing sodium and water retention, has the effect of raising the blood pressure. In the situation of prolonged stress, excessive secretion of this hormone will also contribute to hypertension.

Noradrenaline (norepinephrine) and adrenaline (epinephrine)

Noradrenaline and adrenaline are released in response to activation of the SNS. Noradrenaline leads to increased constriction of blood vessels and so tends to raise the blood pressure. Adrenaline prepares the body in diverse ways to prepare for flight or fight. In a situation of prolonged stress, both these hormones will contribute to the development of hypertension. In addition, adrenaline will lead to a sensation of anxiety, increased breathing rate and, eventually, weight loss.

In summary, the hormones of the adrenal gland function to enable the body to cope appropriately with the demands of physical and emotional stress. However, if stress is prolonged, this response can be harmful, as it can contribute to the development of hypertension, weight loss and diabetes.

Information box 5.1a-IV

The hormones of the adrenal glands: comments from a Chinese medicine perspective

Again, from a Chinese medicine point of view, the energetic interpretation of these hormones is challenging. In health, they all help the body to deal appropriately with physical and emotional demands, by ensuring adequate supplies of glucose to all the tissues and an adequate level of blood pressure. This can be equated to the role of Original Qi and Kidney Yang, which are both aspects of the function of the Kidney Organ.

In conditions of prolonged stress, the hormones are secreted in excess. The problems of excessive blood sugar and hypertension suggest an imbalance of Spleen Qi and hyperactivity of Kidney Yang. Features of Accumulation of Damp and Phlegm may be observed in glucocorticoid and mineralocorticoid excess (see Section 5.1e). A more detailed Chinese medicine interpretation of the diverse effects of excessive synthetic corticosteroids can be found in Section 2.2c.

The pancreas

As explained in Section 3.1a, the pancreas plays an important exocrine role in the production of several digestive enzymes, which are released into the duodenum to break down the nutrients in food leaving the stomach. Studded within the exocrine tissue of the pancreas are little islands (islets) of endocrine cells, which secrete a range of hormones. These hormones are important for controlling the way in which the body utilizes glucose after it has been absorbed into the bloodstream. In a way this can also be seen as an aspect of the digestive function.

Insulin and glucagon are two well-recognized hormones secreted by the islets of the pancreas. These two hormones act in complementary ways to ensure that the cells of the body have access to a continuous supply of glucose, whatever the external conditions may be. This means that, whether the prevailing condition is one of feast or famine, the body tissues can be adequately nourished, at least in the short term.

Insulin

Insulin is secreted in response to a rise in blood sugar, and acts to reduce the blood sugar levels so that they do not exceed a healthy level for the tissues of the body. It does this by:

- stimulating the conversion of excess blood glucose to glycogen, which can then be stored in the liver and muscles

- preventing protein and fat from being converted into sugar (thus counteracting one action of thyroxine)

- enabling the cells to take up glucose from the bloodstream (in the absence of insulin, cells are simply unable to utilize the glucose, however much there may be in the bloodstream, a state compared to "starvation in the midst of plenty").

Glucagon

Glucagon is released in response to decreased levels of glucose in the bloodstream and acts to increase the blood sugar levels. It does this by:

- stimulating the conversion of glycogen stored in the liver into glucose

- stimulating the production of glucose from the breakdown of fats and proteins.

Information box 5.1a-V

Insulin and glucagon: comments from a Chinese medicine perspective

The Chinese medicine interpretation of the endocrine aspect of the pancreas might be that it is also associated with the Spleen Organ. By ensuring an adequate level of glucose in the bloodstream, it continues the role of the digestive tract in providing nutrition for the cells of the body.

This concludes a brief introduction to the organs of the endocrine system. Perhaps more so than for any other system, the delicate nature of the function of this system can only really become apparent after studying what happens when the system becomes out of balance. This will be explored in the following sections of Chapter 5.1.

5.1b The investigation of the endocrine system

The investigation of the endocrine system

The investigation of the endocrine system is usually carried out within the hospital specialty of endocrinology. A patient with a suspected endocrine disease may be referred either to an endocrinologist or to a general physician (GP) with expertise in endocrinology.

The investigation of the endocrine system includes:

- a thorough physical examination

- blood tests to assess the levels of hormones in the blood

- urine tests to assess the levels of hormones excreted in the urine

- more complex blood and urine tests to assess the response of hormones to various stimuli (stimulation and suppression tests)

- imaging tests (in particular, computed tomography (CT) scan and magnetic resonance imaging (MRI)) to visualize the structure of the endocrine organs.

Physical examination

With the exception of the thyroid gland and the testicles, most of the deep-lying endocrine organs cannot be examined directly as part of the physical examination. However, much information can be gained by looking for the effects on the body that can result from endocrine disease.

The physical examination of the endocrine system involves the stages listed in Table 5.1b-I.

Table 5.1b-I The stages in physical examination of the endocrine system

Examination of the general appearance: this can reveal the characteristic features of many of the endocrine diseases, which can lead to marked changes in physical appearance. These include weight loss or weight gain, reduced or excessive body hair, changes to the texture of the skin and loss of muscle bulk. It is often possible for an experienced physician to be fairly sure of a diagnosis from a patient's physical appearance alone

Careful examination of all the other systems of the body: as the endocrine diseases commonly result in changes in diverse body systems, a careful systematic approach to examination can reveal many characteristic changes, such as the increased pulse rate found in hyperthyroidism, or the changes of the retina that can develop in diabetes mellitus

Blood and urine tests

Simple blood tests can be used to assess the levels of the hormones in the blood. In some cases, the results alone may indicate an endocrine disease. For example, in suspected thyroid disease the most common first tests to be performed are serum tests to assess the levels of TSH, T4 and T3. Levels of these hormones that fall outside the normal range would be suggestive of thyroid disease. Such tests are easy for the doctor to perform, and not too inconvenient for the patient.

However, in other cases, because the level of the hormone varies dramatically throughout the day, and also according to individual need at the time, a single blood test cannot offer such conclusive results.

Sometimes a patient might be requested to collect all their urine over the course of 24 hours so that levels of hormone can be assessed from the urine. This has the advantage of overcoming the problem of varying levels throughout the day, but is well known for not being a very accurate method of assessment. Moreover, many patients find this an inconvenient and embarrassing test to perform.

Blood and urine tests may also be used to assess the effects on the body of the hormone in question. The most commonly performed test of this type is the assessment of the glucose (sugar) levels in the blood and the urine in cases of suspected diabetes mellitus. A raised blood glucose level is an indication of a lack of insulin, which is the underlying problem in diabetes mellitus. In both cases, a helpful result can be obtained by applying a drop of blood on a test strip, or by dipping a test stick into the urine.

The most accurate and clinically relevant form of assessing the blood glucose level is to take a specimen when the patient has been fasting for some hours. The least accurate means is to look for glucose in the urine. The latter may be performed to provide a very general overview of the problem, but the gold standard, the fasting blood sugar test, is obviously more inconvenient for the patient.

Stimulation and suppression tests

Stimulation and suppression tests are more complex forms of blood and urine tests. They usually involve assessing the hormonal response that takes place over a few hours following a certain stimulus given to the body. For this reason, the patient may need to spend a day or more in hospital for such tests to be performed. The stimulus is chosen to be something that would normally significantly increase (stimulation test) or decrease (suppression test) the level of the hormone in question.

In general, the stimulation test is used to investigate a disease resulting from insufficient hormone, and a suppression test is used to investigate a disease resulting from excessive secretion of a hormone. For example, suspected diabetes might be confirmed by using the glucose tolerance test. In this test, a patient who has been fasting from the previous evening is given a glucose drink at a set time in the morning. Blood tests are taken at defined time intervals, including one just before the set time of the drink. The blood glucose can then be seen to rise and fall from the fasting period to a few hours after the drink. In health, the blood glucose never exceeds a predictable normal level, but in mild diabetes it may be seen to rise to above a healthy level, even though the level might then drop to within a healthy range after some time. Such an abnormality might not be picked up by a simple blood sugar test. The glucose tolerance test is an indirect form of a stimulation test. The glucose drink should, in health, lead to a release of insulin. The release of insulin in turn should prevent the rise in blood sugar from going too high. The fact that this fails to happen is an indication of insufficient release of insulin.

Another example is the test for a person with suspected disease of the adrenal cortex (Addison's disease). In this case the patient is given an injection of a synthetic form of the pituitary hormone ACTH. In health, this hormone stimulates the release of cortisol and corticosterone from the adrenal cortex. In a patient with Addison's disease, timed blood tests reveal a much lower rise in cortisol in the blood than would be expected. This is another example of a stimulation test that can reveal insufficient production of a hormone.

Stimulation and suppression tests are based on the complexities of endocrine physiology, a clear understanding of which is a challenge even for qualified doctors. From the perspective of a complementary medical practitioner, the important fact to appreciate about the investigation of endocrine disease is that a patient with suspected endocrine disease may be required to spend some time in hospital undergoing such tests.

Imaging tests

Very commonly, endocrine disease results from structural damage to an endocrine gland. In such cases the use of complex soft tissue imaging tests, such as the CT scan and MRI, can be helpful in defining the extent of the damage and whether or not the problem is operable.

For example, the pituitary gland can be clearly revealed by means of an MRI. Figure 5.1b-I shows an MRI image of the pituitary. This image represents the upward growth of a pituitary tumor. Such growth can have marked endocrine consequences (as well as being very likely to impair vision by upwards pressure on the crossing of the optic nerve tracts), and is a cause of chronic headaches.

Figure 5.1b-I MRI scan indicating a large pituitary tumor (extensive growth indicated by arrows)

5.1c Diseases of the thyroid gland

The conditions explored in this section are:

- Enlargement of the thyroid gland: the causes of goiter:
  - simple goiter
  - diffuse goiter
  - multinodular goiter
  - thyroid nodules and thyroid cancer
- Hypothyroidism:
  - autoimmune hypothyroidism
  - iodine deficiency

- congenital hypothyroidism
- damage to the thyroid gland
- pituitary disease
- Hyperthyroidism (thyrotoxicosis):
  - Graves' disease
  - toxic nodular disease and thyroid cancer
  - acute thyroiditis
  - pituitary disease.

Enlargement of the thyroid gland: the causes of goiter

An enlarged thyroid gland is called a goiter. Large goiters are visible as a fullness of the neck, whereas smaller goiters can only be felt on examination. A goiter is considered to be present if it can be felt as a swelling that moves up and down with swallowing. This swelling is more than the vague softness that is usually felt in the region of the thyroid gland. Most goiters are small, and may not be noticed by the patient.

A goiter can become so large as to cause symptoms. The most common symptom is of visible swelling and the cosmetic problems that accompany this. Only in rare cases are there other symptoms. These include discomfort in the neck, difficulty swallowing and restricted breathing.

A goiter does not necessarily mean that there is a problem with the production of the thyroid hormones. The various causes of goiter are described below.

 Information box 5.1c-I

Goiter: comments from a Chinese medicine perspective[2]

In Chinese medicine, the development of a goiter suggests the presence of Phlegm. The position of the goiter corresponds to the pathways of the Stomach and Large Intestine Channels, and so might also suggest imbalance in one or both of these Organs. Spleen Qi Deficiency and Accumulation of Damp are common predisposing factors. If additional symptoms, such as discomfort or difficulty in swallowing, are present, this suggests additional Qi Stagnation or Blood Stagnation.

Simple goiter

A simple goiter is a diffuse enlargement of the thyroid gland of unknown cause. It is not associated with any disturbance of the thyroid hormones. However, a simple goiter is most commonly seen in young women, either during puberty or during pregnancy, which implies that its development may be triggered by hormonal changes.

In most cases the simple goiter is small in size, and can regress if it appears during a time of hormonal change such as pregnancy. However, in some cases, surgery may be performed because of cosmetic unsightliness or, more rarely, because of pressure symptoms. The surgery leaves the patient with a horizontal scar that lies just above the level of the sternal notch (the region of acupoint Tian Tu, RN-22).

Diffuse goiter

A diffuse swelling of the thyroid gland can develop for other reasons. Three fairly common autoimmune processes (atrophic thyroiditis, Hashimoto's thyroiditis and Graves' disease) are well recognized to cause a diffuse enlargement of the thyroid. All three of these conditions may also be associated with the syndromes of hypothyroidism and hyperthyroidism. In all these conditions, antithyroid antibodies lead to immune damage to the gland, which can result in tissue swelling. As with the simple goiter, autoimmune diffuse goiter is more common in women than in men.

More rare causes of a diffusely enlarged goiter in the UK include viral inflammation and iodine deficiency. In some developing countries, iodine deficiency is a common problem, and can lead to the development of a massive goiter (endemic goiter).

Multinodular goiter

A multinodular goiter is, as its name suggests, a thyroid gland that is enlarged due to the development of numerous benign nodules of thyroid tissue. This may, but not always, have the consequence of the production of excessive thyroid hormones, leading to the state of hyperthyroidism. This form of goiter is considered to be the result of a degenerative process of aging.

Multinodular goiter is more common in elderly women, and may also be associated with local symptoms due to pressure effects from the irregularly enlarged gland.

Treatment for multinodular goiter is by means of surgery if there are symptoms due to pressure. Surgical removal of the thyroid is also performed if hyperthyroidism is present.

Thyroid nodules and thyroid cancer

Occasionally, a goiter presents as a result of a single enlarged area within a normal gland, known as a solitary nodule. This is often caused by the same degenerative process that causes a multinodular goiter, but on rare occasions may also be a manifestation of tumor of the thyroid gland, and for this reason it requires careful investigation.

A tumor of the thyroid gland most commonly arises from the cells that produce the thyroid hormones. However, excessive production of these hormones is only a rare consequence of these tumors. This form of thyroid cancer is categorized as either a papillary, follicular or anaplastic carcinoma, according to the findings on examination of a biopsied tissue. Other more rare causes of a tumor within the thyroid gland include cancer of the calcitonin-producing cells (medullary carcinoma) and lymphoma.

Papillary and follicular carcinomas are by far the most common type of thyroid cancer. They are more common in young people and in women. They are often diagnosed before they spread from the thyroid gland, and are treated by total removal of the thyroid gland (thyroidectomy). A radioactive form of iodine is then given. This is concentrated by any remaining thyroid tissue, and is intended to kill off any remaining cancer cells. The majority of people who have this treatment at an early stage will have no recurrence, particularly if the diagnosis is made early in the disease. This treatment does, however, render the patient dependent on lifelong thyroid hormone replacement.

If not treated early in their course, papillary and follicular thyroid carcinomas tend to spread to the lungs and bones. Anaplastic carcinoma is a disease of elderly people, and is a much more aggressive tumor. It spreads rapidly to local tissues and is usually fatal.

Information box 5.1c-II

Thyroid cancer: comments from a Chinese medicine perspective

In Chinese medicine, carcinoma of the thyroid gland is also a manifestation of Phlegm, although pain in a rapidly enlarging nodule would indicate additional Blood Stagnation with Heat. As with all cancers, an underlying severe Deficiency of Yin and Yang is likely to be present.

Hypothyroidism

Hypothyroidism is the term applied to the syndrome that results from inadequate production of the thyroid hormones. Another term that is commonly used to describe hypothyroidism is underactive thyroid gland. Figure 5.1c-I lists some of the most common symptoms and signs that characterize this condition.

Symptoms		Signs
Tiredness		Mental slowness
Loss of appetite		Dementia
Weight gain		Dry thin hair and skin
Cold intolerance		Puffy eyes
Depression		Obesity
Poor libido		Hypertension
Joint and muscle aches		Hypothermia
Constipation		Bradycardia
Heavy periods		Cold peripheries
Psychosis		Edema
Confusion		Deep voice
		Goiter
		Anemia

A history from a relative is often revealing
Symptoms of other autoimmune disease may be present

Figure 5.1c-I The symptoms and signs of hypothyroidism

Many of the features of hypothyroidism result from the slowing down of the energy-producing processes of the cells. In health, these processes are dependent on the stimulus of thyroxine to allow the body to transform nutrition into energy. This is vital for continued activity, growth and maintenance of body temperature.

In early stages of the condition the patient will first experience symptoms of tiredness, sensitivity to cold and depression. It is only as the condition progresses that the more obvious features begin to appear, and dryness of skin and thickening of subcutaneous tissues (myxedema)

becomes apparent. Therefore, the syndrome can be present for months or even years before a diagnosis is made. In elderly people, the diagnosis can be missed until very severe features such as confusion, dementia or hypothermia develop. In its most severe form, hypothyroidism can result in loss of consciousness, a condition termed myxedema coma. This is a medical emergency.

In most cases the diagnosis becomes clear following a blood test for TSH and T4. In established hypothyroidism due to thyroid disease, the T4 level is below the normal range, and the TSH is raised. The raised TSH level is the result of the response of the hypothalamus and the pituitary gland to the persistently low levels of thyroid hormones. In more borderline cases, the T4 levels are normal but the TSH is raised. This suggests that the failing thyroid gland is responding to the increased TSH and is managing to produce sufficient thyroid hormones. Patients with this sort of result may be treated conservatively (watching and waiting) or may be treated with thyroxine tablets if they have symptoms (see below).

Treatment of most cases of hypothyroidism is with synthetic thyroxine (T4) in tablet form. This drug has the same structure as the natural hormone, but of course cannot currently be given in a dose that is tailored to the precise hour-to-hour needs of the body. The severe symptoms of hypothyroidism will abate over the course of a few months of adequate therapy, although swings in energy and mood may persist. Treatment is generally continued for life. The dose of the thyroxine is altered according to the results of regular blood tests for TSH and T4, and also the patient's symptoms.

Hypothyroidism affects approximately 2 percent of women and 0.2 percent of men in the UK, although its subclinical presentation is likely to be much more common than this.[3]

Autoimmune hypothyroidism

The most common cause of hypothyroidism is a progressive autoimmune process that tends to run in families, and that affects women more than men. Specific blood tests will reveal antibodies that are specific for thyroid cells, and that lead to wasting of the thyroid tissue and accumulation of immune cells in the gland. Two pathological processes are described to account for autoimmune hypothyroidism, namely, Hashimoto's thyroiditis and atrophic thyroiditis. However, in practice it is not possible to distinguish between the two conditions without performing a biopsy because the clinical presentations can be identical. Autoimmune thyroiditis may either present with a firm, rubbery goiter or no goiter at all. Treatment with thyroxine tablets will reverse the effects of this autoimmune destruction of the thyroid, but will have no effect on the root cause, for which there is no accepted treatment.

 Information box 5.1c-III

Hypothyroidism: comments from a Chinese medicine perspective

In Chinese medicine, the syndrome of hypothyroidism primarily corresponds to Depletion of Spleen and Kidney Yang. In chronic cases the dry skin indicating Blood Deficiency and thickened tissues indicating Damp and Phlegm Accumulation become apparent, both a consequence of Deficiency of Spleen Yang. Interestingly, a yellow coloring (the cause, in part, of the characteristic peaches and cream complexion) is well known in hypothyroidism. Qi Stagnation and Blood Stasis may also complicate the chronic case, manifesting as aches and pains and depressed mood.

Appropriate thyroxine replacement can be interpreted as being Nourishing to Spleen and Kidney Yang. However, depending on the cause of hypothyroidism, it can be considered as either suppressive or curative. In cases in which there is some residual function of the thyroid gland, the treatment may be considered suppressive in that it does not target the root cause, and has the effect of inhibiting the natural response of the pituitary gland in producing TSH, which in turn stimulates the thyroid gland. However, in cases in which the gland has totally ceased to function, the treatment transforms the energetic imbalance and is undoubtedly curative in nature.

 Information box 5.1c-IV

Autoimmune hypothyroidism: comments from a Chinese medicine perspective

In Chinese medicine, the symptoms of autoimmune hypothyroidism correspond to Kidney and Spleen Yang Deficiency, leading to accumulation of Damp and Phlegm. This is consistent with all forms of hypothyroidism. The inherited tendency to an autoimmune process also suggests an underlying Jing Deficiency.

Iodine deficiency

In areas in which dietary iodine is insufficient, endemic goiter may be common. In endemic goiter, the thyroid gland is basically healthy, but cannot make thyroid hormones because of insufficient iodine. The pituitary responds to low levels of thyroid hormones by producing high levels of TSH. The TSH stimulates the thyroid tissue excessively, and this causes the goiter. The goiter of iodine deficiency can develop into a huge irregular unsightly mass that is commonly seen in middle-aged people who live in landlocked developing countries such as Nepal. In some cases there may be mild hypothyroidism, but in many cases the excess stimulation is sufficient to cause the thyroid to manufacture sufficient thyroxine for the body's needs. Treatment of iodine deficiency is with dietary iodine replacement.

Information box 5.1c-V

Iodine replacement: comments from a Chinese medicine perspective

In Chinese medicine, iodine replacement might be seen as nourishing to Spleen and Kidney Yang.

Congenital hypothyroidism

Congenital hypothyroidism is a condition in which the newborn baby is unable to produce thyroid hormones, most commonly because of an undeveloped thyroid gland. Because thyroid hormones are essential for healthy growth and development of the nervous system, if untreated this condition inevitably leads to poor health, permanent learning difficulties and short stature. The term cretin was previously used to describe children who suffered the long-term effects of untreated hypothyroidism. As the problem affects 1 in 4000 births, cretinism used to be one of the most important causes of mental retardation.

Information box 5.1c-VI

Congenital hypothyroidism: comments from a Chinese medicine perspective

In Chinese medicine, the mental and growth retardation resulting from congenital hypothyroidism would be regarded as a manifestation of Jing Deficiency. By preventing this problem, thyroxine might be seen as nourishing Jing, as well as nourishing Kidney and Spleen Yang. In this context the treatment is curative in nature.

In developed countries, severe problems from this condition have become extremely rare since the introduction of screening for hypothyroidism within the first few days of birth. A drop of blood is obtained from a prick to the baby's heel, and is placed on a card. It is then analyzed for TSH and T4. If hypothyroidism is detected, the child is treated with daily thyroxine for life. This treatment reverses the problem before permanent developmental damage can occur.

Damage to the thyroid gland

Physical damage to the thyroid gland can lead to reduced production of the thyroid hormones. Surgical thyroidectomy and medical (radioactive iodine) treatment of the thyroid gland for cancer or hyperthyroidism are both known to result in hypothyroidism. Lifelong thyroxine replacement may be necessary after such treatments. Other drugs are known to reduce the production of thyroid hormones. One of the most commonly prescribed is lithium, which is prescribed by psychiatrists for bipolar disorder. For this reason, people taking lithium are recommended to undergo regular blood tests for the thyroid hormones.

Pituitary disease

A very rare form of hypothyroidism springs from damage to the pituitary gland rather than the thyroid gland. In this case, the problem is the result of inadequate production of TSH. The most common cause of damage to the pituitary gland is a benign tumor. Pituitary hypothyroidism is also treated by means of synthetic thyroxine given as tablets.

Hyperthyroidism (thyrotoxicosis)

Hyperthyroidism is a syndrome that results from excessive levels of thyroid hormones. It is also known as overactive thyroid or thyrotoxicosis. It is a more common condition than hypothyroidism, and tends to affect younger people. It is more common in women than men. Figure 5.1c-II lists some of the most common symptoms and signs that characterize this condition.

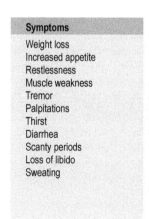

Symptoms	Signs
Weight loss	Tremor
Increased appetite	Restlessness
Restlessness	Sweating
Muscle weakness	Irritability
Tremor	Tachycardia
Palpitations	Warm peripheries
Thirst	Exophthalmos
Diarrhea	Goiter
Scanty periods	
Loss of libido	
Sweating	

Figure 5.1c-II The symptoms and signs of hyperthyroidism

Most of these symptoms result from the effects of the increased thyroid hormones on the chemical processes going on within the cells. Increased amounts of the energy from food are diverted away from storage and tissue growth and into heat-producing metabolism. The patient therefore feels the characteristic restlessness, heat intolerance and raging appetite, despite an increased intake of food. The unmistakable changes that can affect the eyes (see Figure 5.1c-III) only occur in the form of hyperthyroidism called Graves' disease (see below). These result not from excessive thyroid hormones, but from the effect of the autoantibodies that are the cause of Graves' disease.

Figure 5.1c-III Exophthalmos in Graves' disease

 Information box 5.1c-VII

Hyperthyroidism: comments from a Chinese medicine perspective

In Chinese medicine, many of the features of hyperthyroidism correspond to the clinical picture of Yin Deficiency. Kidney Yin Deficiency is likely to be the root deficiency, although the features indicate that Deficiency of Heart and Liver Yin are also part of the picture. Raging appetite, psychosis and bloodshot eyes all suggest Full Heat, as these symptoms correspond to Stomach Fire, Phlegm Fire Obstructing the Orifices of the Heart, and Liver Fire.

Flaws and Sionneau (2010)[4] explain that hyperthyroidism is a consequence of frustrated emotions, which lead first to Stagnation and then to Full Heat (Liver Fire). It is the Liver Fire that then damages the Yin of diverse organs (Stomach Spleen, Heart and Kidney), and which also encourages the accumulation of Damp and Phlegm that may manifest in the form of a goiter, but which can also contribute to mental disturbances.

In early stages of hyperthyroidism the patient may complain only of anxiety or sleeplessness, and it is only in a more progressed stage of the condition that more obvious features such as weight loss and eye changes become apparent. In very severe cases the changes to the cardiovascular system can become life-threatening, as the overstimulated heart fails to cope with the work it has to perform. This can result in the development of atrial fibrillation or heart failure. In some cases the patient can become increasingly restless and irritable, and this can tip over into a full-blown psychosis, with delusions and the development of personality change.

Graves' disease[5]

Graves' disease is by far the most common cause of hyperthyroidism. It is the result of the development of autoantibodies to thyroid cells. However, in contrast to autoimmune hypothyroidism, these antibodies tend to act rather like TSH, and initially stimulate rather than damage the thyroid cells. This has the result of causing excessive production of thyroid hormones.

Other autoantibodies that develop in Graves' disease also cause damage to the soft tissue of the eyes. This can have very severe consequences. Swelling of the soft tissue behind the eyes causes the eyes to bulge forward (see Figure 5.1c-III). This can sometimes be so severe that the eyelids are unable to close properly. Compression of the optic nerve behind the eye can threaten sight.

A diagnosis of advanced Graves' disease is often clinically obvious. However, in all cases a diagnosis of hyperthyroidism is confirmed by a blood test for TSH and T3, wherein the T3 levels are raised and TSH levels are very low. In addition, a blood test for the characteristic antibodies can confirm a diagnosis of Graves' disease.

There are three options for the treatment of Graves' disease. The most often first used treatment are the drugs carbimazole or, if this is not tolerated, propylthiouracil. These antithyroid drugs act within two to three weeks to inhibit the production of the thyroid hormones, but the patient has to continue treatment for some months after this initial response. Beta blockers, such as propranolol, may also be given in the early stages to control symptoms such as anxiety, restlessness and palpitations. In about half of all patients these treatments are effective in restoring the thyroid activity to normal in the long term, but the remaining half of patients given oral medication relapse within two years of treatment. They then have to turn to another treatment option.

Carbimazole has a rare serious side effect in that in 1 in 1000 people it can suppress the activity of the bone marrow and lead to a life-threatening reduction in white blood cells. Other common side effects include nausea, rashes and itching.

An alternative treatment option to drug therapy is surgery to the thyroid gland. In this case some of the thyroid gland is removed (subtotal thyroidectomy) in the hope that this will restore normal function. The operation carries risks of damage to the nerve that supplies the vocal cords (in 1 percent) and also damage to the parathyroid glands, leading to problems in calcium balance (in 1 percent). More importantly, in up to 10 percent of people the operation is followed by hypothyroidism, requiring lifelong thyroxine replacement. In over 3 percent hyperthyroidism recurs after the operation.

An increasingly popular treatment option is the use of radioactive iodine therapy. This relies on a drug containing an iodine isotope which, when taken as a drink, is concentrated by the body in the thyroid tissue. The radioactivity causes progressive damage to the thyroid cells over the course of the next few months and can reverse the hyperthyroidism. Some people experience worsening of their symptoms before they get better with this treatment. Early concerns about increased risk of cancer do not appear to be founded. Because of these concerns, this therapy used to be reserved for elderly people, but is now increasingly being offered to younger people.

The most important complication of radioactive iodine therapy is progressive development of hypothyroidism. Because of this problem, patients are required to have regular blood tests to monitor thyroid hormone levels after both subtotal thyroidectomy and radioiodine treatment.

 Information box 5.1c-VIII

Treatment of hyperthyroidism: comments from a Chinese medicine perspective

In Chinese medicine, carbimazole, by inhibiting the excessive production of the thyroid hormones, seems to calm Liver Fire. Rashes and the very serious side effect of bone marrow suppression may be evidence of suppression of this Heat to different and possibly deeper energetic levels of the body, or simply the manifestation of Toxic Heat introduced by a chemically damaging drug.

Radioactive iodine and surgery act in a different way because they actually lead to loss of thyroid tissue. They must also result in the Clearance of Heat in that they reduce the symptoms of hyperthyroidism. The fact that both these therapies have a high long-term incidence of hypothyroidism implies that they are ultimately Depleting of Qi, and in particular, of Kidney Yang.

Toxic nodular disease and thyroid cancer

A multinodular goiter or a single nodule (see earlier in this section) in the thyroid gland can occasionally produce excessive thyroid hormones, in which case the conditions are termed toxic multinodular goiter and solitary toxic nodule, respectively. The clinical picture is similar to that of Graves' disease, but without the eye changes. These forms of hyperthyroidism rarely respond to carbimazole, and so are treated with either surgery or radioactive iodine.

Acute thyroiditis

Acute inflammation of the thyroid gland may follow a viral infection or, rarely, develop in a mother after delivery of a baby. The thyroid gland becomes slightly swollen and tender. There may be features of hypothyroidism or hyperthyroidism, but these are usually self-limiting.

Pituitary disease

A TSH-secreting tumor of the pituitary gland is an extremely rare cause of hyperthyroidism. Treatment necessitates surgery to the pituitary gland rather than any of the aforementioned approaches to hyperthyroidism of thyroid origin.

The red flags of diseases of the thyroid gland

Some patients with diseases of the thyroid gland will benefit from referral to a conventional doctor for assessment and/or treatment. Red flags are those symptoms and signs that indicate that referral should be considered. The red flags of the diseases of the thyroid gland are described in Table 5.1c-I. A summary of the red flags in a format designed for quick reference in clinical practice can be found in Appendix III. This gives advice on the degree of urgency of referral for each of the red flag conditions listed.

Table 5.1c-I A31: Red flags of diseases of the thyroid gland

Red flag	Description	Reasoning
A31.1	Goiter: refer only if symptoms of hyperthyroidism or hypothyroidism are present (see A31.2 and 31.3), or if the goiter is tender, irregular or noticeably enlarging	A goiter is an enlarged thyroid gland. It can be felt and seen in the lower half of the neck, where it tends to fill the hollow that lies over the trachea and above the manubrium. A small, symmetrical goiter is a not uncommon finding in women, particularly in puberty and pregnancy, and if no symptoms are associated, need not in itself be a cause for referral
A31.2	Features of hypothyroidism (symptoms and signs tend to be progressive over the course of a few months). Symptoms: tiredness, depression, weight gain, heavy periods, constipation, cold intolerance Signs: dry puffy skin, dry and thin hair, slow pulse	The symptoms of hypothyroidism (underactive thyroid gland) overlap with those of depression, but a simple blood test can differentiate between the two syndromes If prolonged, the state of hypothyroidism can have significant deleterious metabolic consequences, and medical replacement therapy is advised if it is not responding to complementary medical treatment
A31.3	Features of hyperthyroidism (these tend to be progressive over the course of a few months). Symptoms: irritability, anxiety, sleeplessness, increased appetite, loose stools, weight loss, scanty periods, heat intolerance Signs: sweaty skin, tremor of the hands, staring eyes, rapid pulse	The symptoms of hyperthyroidism overlap with those of an anxiety disorder, but a simple blood test can differentiate between the two syndromes If prolonged, hyperthyroidism can have a significant impact on the cardiovascular system, and medical treatment is advised if not responding to complementary medical treatment High-priority referral may be indicated if the patient is very agitated, or if cardiac symptoms (chest pain, palpitations or breathlessness) are present

5.1d Diabetes mellitus

Diabetes mellitus is the medical term used to refer to the syndrome that results from excessive levels of glucose (sugar) in the blood. In diabetes mellitus, raised blood glucose, conventionally termed hyperglycemia, is the result of failure of the body either to produce adequate amounts of insulin or to respond to insulin properly (insulin resistance), or both.

The term diabetes mellitus is derived from the Greek meaning excessive flow of urine (diabetes) that is very sweet (mellitus). The term is often shortened to the single word diabetes, although this does not clearly distinguish it from the much more rare condition known as diabetes insipidus. In diabetes insipidus there is excessive flow of very dilute urine (hence the adjective insipidus), which is the result of inadequate production of the pituitary hormone ADH.

The pancreatic hormone insulin plays two very important roles in the control of blood glucose. First, it ensures that the level of blood glucose never rises above a level that is healthy for the body. Second, it enables the cells of the body to take up glucose from the bloodstream. Without insulin, the cells cannot use the glucose circulating in the bloodstream, and will die rapidly unless

the situation is reversed. For this reason, lack of insulin has been compared to the situation of "starvation in the midst of plenty."

The effects of diabetes are threatening to health in two broad ways. First, in acute diabetes an extreme lack of insulin leads to excessively high levels of blood glucose. This leads in a short space of time to the severe problems of dehydration and ketoacidotic coma. Second, in chronic diabetes, uncontrolled raised levels of blood glucose over the course of years have deleterious consequences on the various systems of the body.

The different types of diabetes

The most common forms of diabetes are known as type 1 and type 2 diabetes. These were formerly called juvenile-onset and late-onset diabetes because, in general, type 1 diabetes affects young people and type 2 diabetes affects older people. However, this is by no means always the case, and so these terms have been largely abandoned in medical texts. Nevertheless, they still persist in common language, presumably because they are more descriptive.

Gestational diabetes is diabetes that becomes apparent in pregnancy. This carries a risk for the mother and the child and is increasing in prevalence in the developed world, most likely as a result of increasing prevalence of maternal obesity.

Maturity-onset diabetes of the young (MODY) is a less common inherited form of diabetes in which young people develop hyperglycemia. This form of diabetes is much more sensitive to antidiabetic medication and rarely needs treatment with insulin.

Type 1 diabetes (insulin-dependent diabetes)

Type 1 diabetes develops following total failure of the insulin-producing cells of the pancreas to produce insulin. Once developed, it is irreversible, and without insulin replacement treatment it would lead to death within days. The most common time of onset is between the ages of 10 and 13. For an unknown reason, the incidence has very much increased in recent years, particularly in children.

Type 1 diabetes used to be named insulin-dependent diabetes mellitus (IDDM) because of the patient's absolute need for insulin replacement. Juvenile-onset diabetes was also a previously preferred descriptive term for type 1 diabetes because it primarily develops in children and young adults. However, both these terms are no longer used by doctors as type 2 diabetes is increasingly also treated with insulin and is also becoming apparent in younger people.

It is understood that type 1 diabetes develops because of autoimmune damage to the insulin-producing cells of the pancreas. Islet cell antibodies become apparent in the circulation years before clinical features of type 1 diabetes appear. The tendency for this to happen runs in families, but the actual trigger for the condition is not understood. The rapidly rising incidence suggests an environmental cause. Viral infection in early childhood is conventionally considered to be a possible trigger.

Clinical features of type 1 diabetes

In the early stages of type 1 diabetes there is still some residual production of insulin, so the symptoms appear gradually. However, the severity of the symptoms means that this form of diabetes is usually diagnosed within days to a few weeks of onset. The first features include a general feeling of malaise, weight loss, thirst and increased urination.

All these symptoms are a result of the lack of insulin. Malaise and weight loss are due to the inability of the cells of the body to utilize the glucose they need, and thirst and increased urination are the consequence of increased levels of glucose in the blood. The glucose reaches such a high concentration in the blood that it starts entering the urine from the kidneys. The high level of glucose in the urine then encourages extra water to enter the urine from

the bloodstream by the process of osmosis. The result is that large amounts of sugar-containing urine are produced, and the patient has to drink excessively to make up for this fluid loss.

If the condition is not treated as an emergency, eventually the levels of blood sugar become extremely high, and the patient becomes increasingly dehydrated. More importantly, the cells are deprived of glucose, and the body tries to derive energy by breaking down body fat and protein. Eventually, coma develops, as a combined result of dehydration, the buildup of waste products from the breakdown of fat and protein, and the increased acidity of the blood that follows from this.

In the severe stages of acute diabetes, the patient becomes on the edge of a diabetic coma. In this situation, the patient becomes confused, dehydrated, the breathing is labored and the breath has a characteristic slightly sweet smell. In this state, nausea, vomiting and severe abdominal pain are common.

Treatment of acute type 1 diabetes

Treatment is always a matter of emergency. If a coma has developed, the patient should be nursed in intensive care, as extremely careful control of the body chemistry is required. The main requirements are to replace fluids and to administer insulin, both of which are done in the initial stages by means of an intravenous drip.

If there are no complications, with this treatment the patient may be stable enough within a few days to eat and drink, and to no longer require an intravenous drip. From then on the patient will require regular injections of insulin, in doses tailored to meet individual day-to-day requirements. Most hospitals now have specialist diabetes nurses, whose role is to facilitate the newly diagnosed diabetic person's return to normal life. The initial meetings with this nurse specialist should ideally take place during this first hospital stay.

Treatment in the long term will focus on regular (three- to six-monthly) monitoring of blood sugar and examination to check for signs of diabetes-related damage. Ideally the patient with type 1 diabetes should remain lifelong under expert medical supervision. Long-term management of diabetes is described later in this section.

Type 2 diabetes

Type 2 diabetes (formerly known as non-insulin-dependent diabetes mellitus or NIDDM) develops because of a combination of factors that affect the body's utilization of glucose. The first is that the pancreas starts to fail to produce adequate amounts of insulin. This lack of insulin is not total, and in most cases at least half the insulin-producing cells remain functioning. The second factor is that the body tissues become less sensitive to the insulin that is secreted, a condition termed insulin resistance. This latter factor is much more of a problem if the patient is overweight.

Type 2 diabetes is very common in older people. The age of onset is usually between 50 and 70, although on rare occasions it can develop in young people, particularly if obesity is present. In the UK, over 10 percent of people over the age of 70 have this form of diabetes. It is very much more likely to develop if a close relative has been diagnosed with type 2 diabetes. It is also common in certain ethnic groups, in particular in those with South Asian, African or Caribbean ancestry.

Although the tendency to develop type 2 diabetes is strongly inherited, it is very much a disease of affluent populations. Obesity is present in 80 percent of patients with type 2 diabetes. A poor diet, with a high content of fatty and sugary foods, and low levels of exercise also contribute to the development of type 2 diabetes.

A syndrome similar to type 2 diabetes can also be triggered by certain drugs (most commonly thiazide diuretics and corticosteroid drugs) and in gestational diabetes that is seen during pregnancy. In these cases the clinical features may subside on withdrawal of the drugs or on delivery of the baby. However, in people who develop this form of temporary diabetes, it is known that there may be a tendency to develop type 2 diabetes at a later stage in life.

Clinical features of type 2 diabetes

The onset of type 2 diabetes may be much more insidious than in type 1 diabetes. In some cases the patient may live for years with a raised level of blood glucose and be unaware of the fact. Sometimes, the diagnosis is only made after the patient has suffered a severe complication of prolonged hyperglycemia such as a heart attack.

Most cases are diagnosed because of a combination of vague symptoms such as tiredness, frequent urination and thirst. Because of the vagueness of the symptoms, the patient may often have not felt right for some time before going to ask advice about the problem. This is in contrast to the rapidity of the onset of type 1 diabetes.

The diagnosis of diabetes may also be made following routine urine or blood testing of patients who have visited a hospital doctor or a general practice for an unrelated reason. This is a practice that is very much encouraged, as it is known that early diagnosis may result in lifestyle changes and treatment choices that can prevent severe complications later on in the disease.

Treatment of acute type 2 diabetes

Only rarely do patients with type 2 diabetes require hospital admission to control their diabetes after first diagnosis. However, in some cases, the blood glucose level can rise so high that the patient can become severely dehydrated.

This can become a medical emergency, and particularly in older people.

Usually, the newly diagnosed patient with type 2 diabetes is not acutely unwell. In this case they may first be encouraged to control their diabetes with lifestyle changes alone. In some people, a combination of attention to diet, cutting out alcohol, losing weight and increasing gentle exercise can be sufficient to control the problem entirely.

Long-term management of type 2 diabetes is described later in this section.

Diabetes and the kidneys

In chronic diabetes hyperglycemia causes progressive damage to the blood vessels of the kidneys and to the gradual development of chronic kidney disease (CKD) and specific conditions such as nephrotic syndrome. The increased incidence of urine infections (including cystitis and pyelonephritis) contributes to the kidney damage in diabetes. Kidney damage is the leading cause of premature death in insulin-dependent diabetic people. Moreover, diabetes is the cause of 50 percent of cases of significant CKD.

Diabetes and the eyes

Diabetes can lead to progressive damage to the small blood vessels of the retina. It can increase the risk of blockage of the blood vessels, unhelpful over-proliferation of tiny blood vessels in the eye, or retinal bleeding, all of which will impair the function of the retina in vision. These changes can lead to permanent impairment of sight and, in some cases, blindness.

Diabetes and the nervous system

Damage to the small blood vessels that supply the nervous system can lead to death of the peripheral nerves. This can lead to a progressive loss of sensation and muscle strength in the characteristic glove and stocking distribution of a polyneuropathy. Alternatively, single nerves may suddenly die, leading to the features of a mononeuropathy. In this case the diabetic person might develop symptoms such as weakness of a muscle group in a limb or double vision.

The autonomic nerves can also be affected, leading to problems such as diarrhea, erectile dysfunction, dizziness on standing and difficulty in passing urine.

Diabetes and the skin

The skin becomes vulnerable to damage in diabetes for three reasons. Poor circulation to large and small blood vessels impairs the nourishment of the skin. Infections of the skin are more likely and, for these two reasons, wounds are less likely to heal. This means that small injuries can become enormous problems for a diabetic person. A small wound might develop rapidly into an ulcer if not treated with adequate care. The third reason is that loss of sensation, in particular, to the feet, means that small injuries are more likely, and are not protected because the patient is unable to feel pain.

Long-term management of diabetes

There are two central aims in the long-term management of diabetes:

- prevention of the recurrence of the acute state of hyperglycemia and dehydration

- prevention of the long-term complications of diabetes, which result from chronically raised levels of blood glucose.

The long-term management of diabetes is discussed under the following subheadings:

- lifestyle factors

- medical control of hyperglycemia

- screening for complications.

It is recognized that the adequate control of diabetes requires consistent attention to all three of these areas to achieve the best outcome for the patient. Education of the patient and their family is a necessary prerequisite to achieving the aims of long-term management. Ongoing support and education is, therefore, a core part of the management of diabetes.

Lifestyle factors

In both types of diabetes, careful attention to certain lifestyle factors is fundamental to achieving long-term control of the condition.

Diet is crucial in the management of both type 1 and type 2 diabetes. For both, a diet that minimizes sudden peaks in blood glucose and which is low in unhealthy lipids is strongly advocated. Such a diet would be high in complex carbohydrates, such as sweet potatoes, pasta and brown rice (ideally comprising over one-half of the total diet). Ideally, foods that have a low glycemic index should be chosen over those that lead to a very rapid delivery of sugar to the bloodstream. Refined sugar (cakes, sweets and biscuits) should be kept to as low a level as possible and alcohol should be cut out or kept to a minimum. Plenty of vegetables are advised. Fruit needs to be taken with caution even though the sugars in fruits are less rapidly absorbed than refined sugars, and fruit juices avoided altogether. Fats need to form much less than one-third of the diet, and unhealthy saturated fats and trans fatty acids should be minimized. Protein should come in a low-fat form, such as lean meats, fish, pulses and eggs, and should also comprise no more than one-third of the diet.

Apart from a relative reduction in the amount of fruit, such a diet is no different from a typical healthy eating diet that would be advocated for anyone by a conventional medical practitioner. This means that the diabetic person should not feel set apart by having to attend to this sort of dietary advice. However, in practice, because of cultural values about food, many people find a healthy diabetic diet difficult to follow.

Moderate exercise is also strongly advised, because physical fitness contributes to a smooth control of blood glucose. Moreover, physical exercise is known to improve blood lipid levels.

Smoking is a particular problem in diabetes because it also is very damaging to the circulation. People with diabetes will be counseled about stopping smoking.

Medical control of hyperglycemia[6]

In type 1 diabetes, because the insulin-producing cells of the pancreas have totally and permanently failed, insulin replacement is an essential aspect of the control of hyperglycemia. In people with type 2 diabetes, although lifestyle changes may be sufficient to achieve adequate control, additional medical treatment will be required for most. Oral antidiabetic tablets, glucagon-like peptide-1 (GLP1) injections and insulin are the options for the medical treatment of type 2 diabetes. Hyperglycemia is measured most accurately by means of a blood test which quantifies the percentage of blood cells which have glucose bound to them. This measurement, known as HbA1C, only responds slowly to changes in treatment and is considered a more helpful measurement of diabetic control than the rapidly changing blood glucose measurement. It is known that the higher the HbA1C level, the greater the risk of cardiovascular, renal and visual complications. Ideally people with diabetes should aim to keep the HbA1C less than 6.5 percent (less than 5.5 percent would be considered to be a non-diabetic level).

NON-INSULIN ANTIDIABETIC DRUGS

Oral antidiabetic drugs are medications that act either to increase the release of insulin from the remaining cells in the pancreas, or to increase the body's sensitivity to insulin. There are now many classes of antidiabetic drugs that have been developed over recent years and which commonly are prescribed in combination with each other. These are sulphonylureas (which include glipizide and gliclazide), biguanides (the most commonly prescribed of which is metformin), rapid-acting insulin secretagogues (repaglinide and nateglinide), glitazones (of which pioglitazone is the only one considered safe for prescribing), DPP4 inhibitors (gliptins) and SGLT2 inhibitors. Each of these acts in unique and specific ways to reduce the levels of glucose in the blood. Some act at the liver and some peripherally to influence the use of glucose by the tissues. The SGLT2 inhibitors increase glucose excretion by the kidney.

Metformin is currently considered the first-line treatment for type 2 diabetes. Its advantages are that it carries no risk of hypoglycemia and does not induce weight gain. Disadvantages are that a lot of people develop digestive side effects. Sulphonylureas are the second-line choice, and are generally better tolerated than metformin. However, one unfortunate side effect is that they promote weight gain, and may cause the blood sugar to drop too low (hypoglycemia). DPP4 inhibitors can also be used for single drug treatment in type 2 diabetes.

If a single antidiabetic drug is not sufficient to achieve control of HbA1C after three months in type 2 diabetes, two types of drug may be used in combination. Diabetic doctors tend to follow guidelines that advise how to add in new drugs in a logical way. The SGLT2 inhibitors are the most recently developed antidiabetic medications and tend to be reserved for those cases in which all other medications are not well tolerated.

The injectable GLP1 drugs may then be added to oral medication in some cases. These have a beneficial side effect of suppressing appetite and inducing weight loss, but are very expensive to use and offer only a modest improvement in HbA1C.

If all these medications fail to reduce the blood glucose sufficiently, insulin will be prescribed as a next step.

Glitazones are generally reserved for cases in which metformin, sulphonylureas and insulin fail to suit the patient. They carry a known risk of inducing heart failure, which means the patients for whom they are prescribed need to be monitored carefully.

INSULIN

Insulin is used in all cases of type 1 diabetes, and in cases of type 2 diabetes in which adequate control cannot be achieved by diet and medication alone. Insulin has to be given by injection. The needles used are very fine, so that the pain of injection is far less than that felt with a blood test or immunization. The insulin is usually administered from a cartridge loaded into a pen-shaped device. The patient can then inject varying doses from the pen. Patients are taught to inject themselves into a pinch of the skin over the upper arm, buttock, thigh or the abdomen, and to vary the site of injection to avoid cumulative damage to the skin and soft tissues.

Animal-derived bovine or porcine insulin used to be the only insulin available, but over the past 20 years human insulin has become the most commonly prescribed. This is manufactured by means of a process that involves genetically engineered bacteria. Whereas bovine or porcine insulin is similar to, but slightly different in structure from, human insulin, genetically engineered insulin is identical in structure to natural human insulin. Insulin is produced in three forms: short-, intermediate- and long-acting insulins. As their names suggest, these different preparations act over varying timescales in the body after injection.

As opposed to using fixed doses of insulin a day, whenever possible, patients are taught to vary their doses of insulin according to their diet, level of exercise and the results of blood tests. They do this by using combinations of short- and intermediate-acting insulins given throughout the day. Most people require between two and four separate injections a day.

The ideal aim is to keep the level of blood glucose within a certain range. It is now accepted, at least for type 1 diabetes, that the more that this ideal can be attained, the lower the risk of long-term complications. However, this is a taxing and complex process, and requires consistent attention to daily variations in diet and blood test results. Because of this, some people are much more able than others to control their diet and judge what doses of insulin they require, and so achieve better control of blood glucose. Some people may find the demands of a varying daily dose of insulin too difficult to deal with, and so will be prescribed a regular daily regimen of injections. The disadvantage of this is that blood sugar control is bound to be less than perfect, but this may be the only option for some people.

Some forms of diabetes are much more difficult to control than others, even with meticulous attention to diet and insulin dosage. If severe, these forms of diabetes are termed brittle, and are unfortunately bound to result in higher rates of long-term complications.

HOME MONITORING OF BLOOD GLUCOSE

Although an ideal situation might be that the diabetic person is able to respond to minute-to-minute changes in blood glucose with an appropriate dose of insulin, this is not practical for daily life. Instead, the patient has to respond to as many blood test results as are acceptable. Nowadays, blood glucose levels can be fairly accurately assessed at home by means of a hand-held glucometer test. This involves placing a drop of blood on a test strip, which is then inserted into the glucometer. This can be performed many times a day as required, and can inform what the next dose of insulin should be. Some patients rely on a device that measures blood sugar levels continuously throughout the day via a sensor attached to the skin. This technology is not currently widely available to all patients. Alternatively, a nurse can perform this test if the patient is unable to do it themselves, although this will not, of course, be possible on a frequent basis.

Urine stix tests are easier for the patient to perform, but are less accurate. They are useful in that they can indicate that the blood sugar has been very high over the preceding few hours. They may induce a false sense of good control, even when this is not the case, as the blood glucose has to be very high in some people before glucose appears in the urine.

Screening for complications

Screening for the complications of diabetes is a third essential aspect of treatment. This can be performed largely within general practice, although it is usual for most people with type 1 diabetes to attend a specialist hospital clinic at least annually. At the diabetes check-up appointment, the general practitioner (GP) or hospital specialist should perform a physical examination to look for complications such as raised blood pressure, skin damage and numbness, and damage to the retina. Raised blood pressure is treated very attentively with drugs, as it is recognized that uncontrolled blood pressure can hasten kidney damage as well as increase cardiovascular complications. Any wounds to the skin should be given expert nursing care to promote healing. A urine test will be performed to look for protein and glucose and a blood test to check for HbA1C levels, high cholesterol and adequate kidney function. All patients should attend an eye clinic at least annually so that the retina can be examined for unhealthy changes. Laser treatment can be administered at the same appointment, and this can prevent progression of eye disease.

A multidisciplinary approach to diabetes management

The management of diabetes requires input from a range of medical disciplines. Because of this, ideally, a team of specialists including the GP, diabetologist, community diabetes specialist nurse and eye specialist might liaise to ensure a consistent approach.

Hypoglycemia

Hypoglycemia is a term used to describe a fall in the blood glucose level to below the normal range. Mild hypoglycemia leads to a bodily response that induces feelings of panic or agitation, dizziness and sweating. The pupils are dilated. These features are largely a result of the reflex release of the hormone adrenaline from the adrenal gland. Hypoglycemia, when very severe, leads to glucose starvation of the brain cells, which, in a short space of time, leads to confusion and loss of consciousness. Death will follow if the blood glucose levels are not restored rapidly.

Hypoglycemia and diabetes

Severe hypoglycemia most commonly results from an inappropriately high dose of antidiabetic medication. Both the sulphonylurea class of antidiabetic drugs and insulin can induce a state of hypoglycemia that is so severe as to be life-threatening. A common scenario is that a diabetic

person whose disease is controlled on a regular dose of tablets or insulin either misses a meal or undertakes more exercise than is usual for them. In the initial stages, the person will feel agitation, sweating, a racing heartbeat and dizziness. It is important that people with diabetes become familiar with this pattern of symptoms, which are commonly described as a hypo. If nothing is done to remedy this stage, the person can become so confused that they are no longer able to help themselves. This is a dangerous situation, as the person can then begin to lose consciousness.

Treatment for a hypo in diabetes is to restore the blood glucose level back to normal. In the early stages of the condition, eating some sweet food may be sufficient to bring this about. Most diabetic people on medical treatment will carry biscuits or glucose tablets on their person for dealing with a developing hypo as soon as possible. A glucose drink is also a very rapidly absorbed source of glucose. An alternative treatment is to inject a synthetic form of the hormone glucagon. This has the same effect as eating glucose in that it enables the release of glucose from glycogen stores in the liver. The advantage of glucagon is that it can be given quickly when the person is confused or comatose.

One problem that develops in advanced diabetes is the inability to detect the early warning signs of a hypo. It is very important that friends and family are primed to recognize the confusion, irritability and clumsiness that can result, and are educated about encouraging sweet food intake and on how to administer glucagon.

Once a hypoglycemic coma is established, treatment must be given in hospital as a matter of urgency. Glucose is injected into a vein and glucagon is given at the same time. As long as brain damage has not occurred, the patient should make a rapid recovery back to full consciousness.

Other causes of hypoglycemia

Severe hypoglycemia can result from much more rare medical conditions. The most important of these is a tumor of the endocrine cells of the pancreas called an insulinoma.

The term hypoglycemia is frequently used to describe a state that is experienced by seemingly healthy people, who become pale, weak and sweaty if meals are overdue. This condition, medically described as reactive hypoglycemia, is much more common in young women than in men. A rapid intake of sweet or starchy food will reverse these symptoms. This syndrome is not conventionally recognized to be a dangerous manifestation of hypoglycemia, and studies of people experiencing these symptoms have shown a very poor correlation of symptoms with low blood glucose levels.

The term reactive describes the fact that blood sugar levels can drop rapidly shortly after an intake of very sweet food because the pancreas releases insulin in response to a peak in blood sugar. This rebound effect can take the blood sugar levels to lower than what is normal for that person, and this is believed to give rise to the symptoms.

Medical advice is to avoid refined sugars and eat more complex carbohydrate and fiber-rich food, and also to eat frequent small meals and avoid fasting. Alcohol and cigarette smoking can exacerbate reactive hypoglycemia. Reactive hypoglycemia often improves as the young person reaches middle age, and this could be a result of acquiring appropriate dietary habits with experience.

Secondary diabetes

Diabetes may also develop as a result of other disease processes in the body, in which case it is called secondary diabetes. These causes include other pancreatic diseases (e.g. chronic pancreatitis) and other endocrine diseases that affect the body's utilization of glucose (e.g. Cushing's disease). In these cases the main treatment is of the underlying disease. However, if there has been permanent damage to the pancreas, the patient is treated in the same way as a patient with primary type 1 or type 2 diabetes.

 Information box 5.1d-I

Diabetes: comments from a Chinese medicine perspective

In Chinese medicine, acute diabetes is referred to as the thirsting and wasting disease (Xiao Ke). There are three components to the untreated condition, which are each related to one of the three Jiao. Excessive drinking is related to Upper Jiao Wasting and is attributed to Lung Yin Deficiency with Heat. Excessive eating is related to wasting of the Middle Jiao, and this in turn is attributed to Stomach Yin Deficiency with Dryness and Stomach Heat. Excessive urination is related to Lower Jiao Wasting and this is attributed to exhaustion of Kidney Yin and Kidney Jing. Untreated acute diabetes can, therefore, be summarized in terms of Yin Deficiency with accumulation of Heat or Fire.

Flaws and Sionneau (2010) explain that Spleen Qi Deficiency is always an underlying predisposing imbalance in adult onset diabetes, whereas in children the predisposition is "natural endowment" (Jing) insufficiency.[7]

The diverse complications of long-term hyperglycemia suggest that the energetic interpretation of long-term diabetes is more complicated, and all can be attributed to the long-term effects of Spleen Qi Deficiency with Heat and Damp, and their Stagnating effects, which will eventually manifest as Phlegm and Blood Stagnation. The vascular complications of stroke, heart attack and poor circulation are suggestive of Qi Deficiency with Qi and Blood Stagnation and Accumulation of Damp or Phlegm. Numbness may relate to Blood Deficiency, Damp or Phlegm. Poor healing with a tendency to infections might relate to Blood and Qi Deficiency with Damp or Damp Heat.

In long-term diabetes, therefore, there is a state of overall deficiency together with accumulation of certain Pathogenic Factors. In particular, there are features of Yin, Qi and Blood Deficiency, together with Accumulation of Heat, Stagnation, Damp and Phlegm. Dietary sugar is energetically Damp and Heat forming. It might be concluded from this that hyperglycemia is a condition of Damp Heat.

Treatment with diet and exercise alone serves to nourish deficiency, reduce dietary sources of Damp and Heat, and clear Stagnation. Antidiabetic drugs and insulin, by reducing blood glucose levels and enabling the cells to utilize glucose, might be interpreted as both Clearing Damp Heat and Nourishing Yin. Because antidiabetic medication can never be administered in precisely appropriate doses, it can have side effects of hypoglycemia and weight gain. Weight gain indicates that whilst the action is to clear Damp Heat, nevertheless, the side effect is Accumulation of Phlegm Damp, and is therefore suggestive of suppression of symptoms to another bodily level.

Hypoglycemia is a manifestation of Liver and Spleen disharmony usually with Spleen Qi as the root disturbance. When acute it also manifests with symptoms in keeping with Heart Qi/Blood Deficiency, with anxiety and palpitations and feelings of faintness.

The red flags of diabetes mellitus

Some patients with diabetes will benefit from referral to a conventional doctor for assessment and/or treatment. Red flags are those symptoms and signs that indicate that referral should be considered. The red flags of diabetes mellitus are described in Table 5.1d-I. A summary of the red flags in a format designed for quick reference in clinical practice can be found in Appendix III. This gives advice on the degree of urgency of referral for each of the red flag conditions listed.

Table 5.1d-I A32: Red flags of diabetes mellitus

Red flag	Description	Reasoning
A32.1	Confusion/coma with dehydration (hyperglycemia)	Confusion and coma are serious symptoms of uncontrolled diabetes (when the levels of glucose in the blood become too high) and are urgent red flags in their own right
		If there is any uncertainty whether the cause of the confusion is due to hyperglycemia or hypoglycemia it is wise to administer glucose if the patient is able to take this, or glucagon (by injection) if the patient possesses this treatment. These measures will do no harm if the cause is hyperglycemia, but can be life-saving if the cause is hypoglycemia
		If the patient is losing consciousness, ensure they are kept in a safe place in the recovery position until help arrives
A32.2	Hypoglycemia (due to effects of insulin or antidiabetic medication in excess of bodily requirements): agitation, sweating, dilated pupils, confusion and coma	Confusion/coma can also be the consequence of a hypoglycemic attack (a result of an excessive reaction to insulin or antidiabetic medication). This can be helped by urgent administration of glucose in a readily absorbable form (e.g. a glucose drink) or glucagon (by injection) if the patient possesses this treatment
		If in doubt about the cause of the confusion in a diabetic patient, it is always appropriate to give glucose, as it is safe to do this whatever the cause
		If the patient is losing consciousness, ensure they are kept in a safe place in the recovery position until help arrives
A32.3	Poorly controlled type 1 or type 2 diabetes: short history of thirst, weight loss and excessive urination, which is rapidly progressive in severity	Thirst and excessive urination are due to the osmotic effect of glucose in the urine
		Weight loss occurs because the tissues are unable to utilize the glucose in the situation of a lack of insulin
		The patient is at high risk of coma because of rising levels of lactic acid
		Refer as a high priority, and urgently if there are any signs of clouding of consciousness
A32.4	Untreated type 2 diabetes: general feeling of malaise, with thirst and increased need to urinate large amounts of urine, which develop over the course of weeks to months	In type 2 diabetes the onset is more gradual and the situation is less urgent. Sustained levels of hyperglycemia put the patient at increased risk of heart disease, kidney disease, vascular disease and chronic infections. Referral for medical assessment and advice is recommended
A32.5	Increased tendency to infections such as cystitis, boils and oral thrush (candidiasis)	Increased tendency to purulent, urinary and skin infections may indicate underlying type 2 diabetes
		Any infections in diabetes merit high priority referral for consideration of treatment
A32.6	Poor wound healing, especially in the feet and legs	Increased tendency to poor wound healing may indicate underlying type 2 diabetes
		Any poorly healing wounds in diabetes merit high priority referral for consideration of treatment
A32.7	Hypertension of any level in diabetes	Always refer for medical management. Medical guidelines advise that blood pressure should be maintained below 130/80mmHg in people with diabetes because of the much greater risk of vascular and renal complications that can result from high blood pressure

5.1e Diseases of the adrenal gland and the pituitary gland

In comparison with the diseases of the thyroid gland and diabetes mellitus, the other endocrine diseases are rare. However, they can have long-term debilitating and sometimes life-threatening consequences, and for this reason merit further study.

The diseases studied in this section are:

- Diseases of the adrenal gland:
    - Cushing's syndrome
    - Addison's disease
    - Conn's syndrome
    - pheochromocytoma
- Diseases of the pituitary gland:
    - pituitary tumor and hypopituitarism
    - acromegaly and gigantism
    - short stature
    - Cushing's disease
    - diabetes insipidus
- Other endocrine effects from tumors.

Diseases of the adrenal gland

Cushing's syndrome

Cushing's syndrome is the term used to describe the symptoms and signs that result from a long-term excess of glucocorticoid hormones (such as cortisol and corticosterone) in the body. Cushing's syndrome can also result from long-term prescription of corticosteroid medication. This medication-induced form of Cushing's syndrome is, in fact, by far the most common form.

Disease of the adrenal gland can also be a cause of Cushing's syndrome. In this case, the excess glucocorticoid results from the growth of a benign or malignant tumor of the endocrine cells of the adrenal cortex. Figure 5.1e-I lists some of the most common symptoms and signs that characterize this condition.

If untreated, Cushing's syndrome is a dangerous condition. Uncontrolled hypertension and increased blood glucose levels increase the risk of coronary heart disease. Premature death can occur from heart attack, heart failure or infection.

 Information box 5.1e-I

Cushing's syndrome: comments from a Chinese medicine perspective

In Chinese medicine, Cushing's syndrome would appear to embrace Kidney and Jing Deficiency (weak bones, vulnerability to infection), Spleen Deficiency (a tendency to bruising and stretch marks, weak muscles) and Accumulation of Damp/Phlegm (weight gain, hypertension and extreme mood disturbances). There are also features of Full Heat (acne, raised blood sugar, tendency to gastritis and stomach ulcers). Medical corticosteroids, described by Flaws and Sionneau (2010)[8] as windy, acrid medicinals, are given to suppress inflammation and pain, and do so by out-thrusting Heat and forcefully moving Qi. Both actions are ultimately depleting, leading to Yin Deficiency and damage to Yang Qi, with resulting Accumulation of Heat and Phlegm Damp.

Symptoms		Signs
Abdominal weight gain, depression, scanty periods, thin skin, easy bruising, acne, facial hair, muscular weakness, poor growth in children		Moon face (fat deposition around face), acne, hirsutism, central obesity, thin skin, with stretch marks, bruising, hypertension, osteoporosis, proximal muscle wasting

Figure 5.1e-I The symptoms and signs of Cushing's syndrome

Addison's disease

Addison's disease most commonly results from an autoimmune loss of the endocrine cells of the adrenal cortex. The most significant consequence of this is that the adrenal gland gradually loses the ability to secrete sufficient cortisol and corticosterone. There is also loss of the ability to secrete aldosterone and the adrenal sex steroids. In common with many of the autoimmune diseases, Addison's disease primarily affects women of middle age. However, there are other, more rare causes of adrenal insufficiency. The next most common cause is secondary cancer (metastases) developing in both adrenal glands. In certain cancers there is a marked tendency for secondary cancer to develop in the adrenal glands, and

thus to destroy the healthy endocrine tissue. Figure 5.1e-II lists some of the most common symptoms and signs that characterize Addison's disease.

Symptoms
A short history of:
weight loss, weakness, fever, scanty periods, depression, nausea, vomiting, fainting and abdominal pain

Signs
Pigmentation around new scars and on creases of palm, postural drop in blood pressure, wasting, dehydration, loss of body hair

Figure 5.1e-II The symptoms and signs of Addison's disease

Addison's disease can be fatal within weeks to months if untreated. A severe complication of the undiagnosed condition is the Addisonian crisis. This is a consequence of an exposure to a stressor such as a severe infection or an accident. Because the body is unable to manufacture the steroid hormones that are required to cope with situations of stress, a person with Addison's disease can collapse with abdominal pain, vomiting and shock in such situations. This situation is treated as a medical emergency.

Long-term treatment of Addison's disease is with daily doses of synthetic corticosteroid medication (cortisol or prednisolone) and a synthetic form of a hormone similar to aldosterone (fludrocortisone). This treatment has to be continued for life.

 Information box 5.1e-II

Addison's disease: comments from a Chinese medicine perspective

In Chinese medicine, the features of Addison's disease largely correspond to Kidney and Spleen Yang Deficiency. The dark pigmentation is consistent with a problem affecting the Kidney Organ.

Conn's syndrome

Conn's syndrome is a condition that usually results from an aldosterone-secreting tumor of the adrenal cortex. Aldosterone is responsible for maintaining salt and water balance and blood pressure. Excess secretion of aldosterone initially leads to high blood pressure. If this situation is untreated, the disturbance to the salts in the

blood (low potassium) can become so severe as to be life-threatening. Conn's syndrome is an important cause of unexplained hypertension in young people.

Treatment is by means of surgical removal of the tumor. If this is not possible, a particular form of diuretic (spironolactone) can be used to counteract the effects of the excessive aldosterone.

Pheochromocytoma

A pheochromocytoma is a very rare tumor that secretes the catecholamine hormones adrenaline and noradrenaline in excess. The tumor usually develops from the endocrine cells of the adrenal medulla. However, in 10 percent of cases the tumor develops at another site in the sympathetic nervous system (SNS) (usually alongside the spinal column). A patient with such a tumor may experience symptoms due to excessive release of the catecholamines. These might include panic attacks, palpitations, tremor and hypertension.

On diagnosis, the patient may initially require drug treatment to counteract the effects of the catecholamines (including beta blocker medication). Only once the drugs have been given for long enough for the patient to regain a stable state can an operation be performed to remove the tumor.

Diseases of the pituitary gland

Pituitary tumor and hypopituitarism

Pituitary tumors are the most common cause of pituitary disease. They may cause problems simply as a result of their growth into local tissue. Also, as occurs with some adrenal endocrine tumors, diverse syndromes can result from excessive hormone secretion from a pituitary tumor.

However, tiny tumors of the pituitary, known as microadenomas, are very common incidental findings on an MRI (magnetic resonance imaging) of the brain, and may never develop to lead to any symptoms.

The pituitary gland is cradled in a small cavity in the base of the skull just behind the sinus spaces at the side of the nose. The stalk of the pituitary lies very close to a crossing of the two optic nerves that carry nerve fibers from the back of the eye to the occipital lobe at the back of the brain.

A tumor of the pituitary can cause increased pressure within this bony cavity, and so can only easily expand upwards towards the stalk. This means that, as it grows, a pituitary tumor may readily cause loss of function of some or all of the remaining gland. This leads to a state known as hypopituitarism. In hypopituitarism, there is impaired or absent secretion of the pituitary hormones. GH and LH are commonly affected first, but with progression of the tumor, FSH, ACTH and TSH will also be affected. Paradoxically, PRL may be secreted in excess in such cases.

Symptoms of hypopituitarism include loss of libido, impotence and menstrual disturbances due to loss of the control of such functions by LH and FSH. Excessive prolactin may lead to inappropriate secretion of milk from the nipples (in men and women) and infertility. Lack of GH, ACTH and TSH will all contribute to a condition of tiredness, slowness of thought and action (secondary hypothyroidism), and low blood pressure (secondary Addison's disease).

A pituitary tumor can also spread to damage other structures in the region. Headaches (due to local invasion of the bone and meninges) and impairment of vision (due to damage to the optic nerves) can be the first symptoms indicating local spread of the tumor. Double vision can also develop as a result of damage to the cranial nerves that supply the muscles of the eye.

Some pituitary tumors may also secrete a particular pituitary hormone in excess. The most common hormones that are secreted include PRL, GH and ACTH. PRL-secreting tumors may lead to inappropriate milk production and infertility. The syndromes of excessive GH secretion (acromegaly and gigantism) and ACTH secretion (Cushing's disease) are described below.

An MRI is used to diagnose pituitary tumors. The patient has also to undergo detailed testing for visual defects. These tests can provide an additional indication of the extent of local spread of the tumor. Specific stimulation and suppression blood tests may be performed while the patient is in hospital in order to test for syndromes of hormone insufficiency or excess.

The tumor can be excised surgically, most often by a route that crosses the nasal (sphenoidal) sinus space through the nose. If the tumor is very large it is accessed via the frontal bone in the forehead.

Radiotherapy can be focused on the pituitary area in those cases that are partially or totally inoperable.

Medication (using a drug called bromocriptine or octreotide) can cause tumor shrinkage in some cases (in particular, in those that secrete prolactin). Bromocriptine or cabergoline may also be prescribed simply to reduce the symptoms of hyperprolactinemia.

In the case of hypopituitarism, the impaired secretion of pituitary hormones is treated by means of lifelong replacement with synthetic steroids, thyroxine and sex hormones.

Acromegaly and gigantism

Acromegaly and gigantism are the two possible consequences of excessive secretion of GH. These conditions almost always result from a GH-secreting pituitary tumor.

Acromegaly (literally meaning big extremities) is the syndrome that results when the GH excess develops in adulthood. The high levels of GH will promote bone and soft tissue growth. It will also tend to increase the blood glucose level, and so is a rare cause of secondary diabetes. It can cause enlargement of the heart and a change in the dimensions of the large blood vessels, which together may have the outcome of heart failure and hypertension. It is also recognized that additional cancers are more likely to develop, presumably a consequence of the general growth-promoting properties of the hormone. Figure 5.1e-III lists some of the most common symptoms and signs that characterize acromegaly.

Symptoms		Signs
Change in facial appearance, enlarged hands, feet and hat size, headaches, poor vision, excessive sweating, tiredness, scanty periods, deep voice		Coarse facial features, and thick greasy skin Lower jaw projects further than upper jaw, gaps between teeth, spade-like hands and feet, hypertension, edema, weakness of muscles, glucose in the urine

Figure 5.1e-III The symptoms and signs of acromegaly

In the extremely rare situation of a GH-secreting tumor occurring in childhood, the condition of gigantism will occur. In this situation, because the bony epiphyses have yet to fuse, the excess hormone promotes growth of the long bones as well as the other tissues. This condition was the underlying cause for the tall stature of many of the record-breaking tallest men and women of the world in the 20th century. Sadly, if untreated, gigantism leads to early death, usually from heart failure.

The treatment for acromegaly and gigantism is by means of treatment of the pituitary tumor (see above).

Short stature

A lack of GH is a rare but important cause of poor growth in childhood. The more common causes of poor growth are explored in detail in Chapter 5.4.

Cushing's disease

Cushing's disease is the result of excessive secretion of ACTH by a pituitary tumor. This was the mechanism of the syndrome that was initially reported by Cushing, and so this is why it is described as his disease.

The clinical features of Cushing's disease are very similar to those of the causes of Cushing's syndrome (see above). However, there are three other important features in Cushing's disease:

- pigmentation of the skin (due to the effect of ACTH on the melanin-producing cells of the skin)

- low levels of potassium in the blood (due to the effect of ACTH on the release of aldosterone)

- general features of a pituitary tumor with hypopituitarism may also be present.

Diabetes insipidus

Diabetes insipidus is a condition that develops as a result of lack of ADH (antidiuretic hormone). The consequence of this lack is that there is excessive production of very dilute urine (up to 10–15 liters per day in an adult), together with a compensatory increase in thirst. If very severe, the patient cannot keep up with the fluid requirements, and dehydration can result.

One of the most common causes of diabetes insipidus is surgery for a pituitary tumor, although in most cases this is only a temporary problem. Pituitary tumors themselves only rarely cause diabetes insipidus, because the ADH is actually produced in the hypothalamus, and even if the posterior pituitary is damaged, its production and release is not affected. Other more rare causes of reduced production of ADH include radiotherapy to the pituitary area and head injury.

Inherited diabetes insipidus may be the consequence of a defect in the hypothalamus, or of an abnormal response of the kidney to a normal level of ADH.

The treatment of diabetes insipidus is, ideally, of the underlying cause. Otherwise, a synthetic form of ADH, called DDVAP, can be given by nasal spray or injection once or twice daily.

Other endocrine effects from tumors

Apart from the tumors of endocrine tissue, other tumors can occasionally cause a syndrome resulting from excessive hormone production. This phenomenon is often the consequence of the secretion of hormone-like proteins from certain tumors that have become poorly differentiated (anaplastic).

The most common examples include the secretion of PTH-like protein from lung and breast cancers (particularly after there has been secondary spread), ADH-like protein from lung cancer, and ACTH from lung, thyroid and carcinoid tumors. Because these effects usually occur when the tumor is at quite an advanced stage, the treatment of the syndromes that result from the excessive hormones is usually palliative.

The red flags of the less common endocrine diseases

Some patients with the less common endocrine diseases will benefit from referral to a conventional doctor for assessment and/or treatment. Red flags are those symptoms and signs that indicate that referral should be considered. The red flags of the less common endocrine diseases are described in Table 5.1e-I. A summary of the red flags in a format designed for quick reference in clinical practice can be found in Appendix III. This gives advice on the degree of urgency of referral for each of the red flag conditions listed.

Table 5.1e-I A33: Red flags of the less common endocrine diseases

Red flag	Description	Reasoning
A33.1	Features of Cushing's syndrome: weight gain, hypertension, weakness and wasting of limb muscles, stretch marks and bruises, mood changes, red cheeks and acne	Cushing's syndrome is due to chronically raised levels of corticosteroids, and may result from excessive bodily production or from medical treatment. It carries serious health consequences in terms of increasing the risk of high blood pressure, diabetes and osteoporosis. Refer if the cause is unknown
A33.2	Features of Addison's disease: increased skin pigmentation, weight loss, muscle wasting, tiredness, loss of libido, low blood pressure, diarrhea and vomiting, confusion, collapse with dehydration	Addison's disease is due to a lack of bodily corticosteroid, and the symptoms may develop gradually or may result in a sudden collapse. The syndrome can also result from a sudden withdrawal from high doses of prescribed corticosteroid In both cases the situation is a medical emergency
A33.3	Features of the growth of a pituitary tumor: progressive headaches, visual disturbance and double vision	The pituitary gland is situated at the base of the brain in the region of the crossing of the optic nerves and the passage of the cranial nerve that supplies the eye muscle A tumor of the pituitary gland may cause early visual disturbance and double vision It can also cause the syndrome of hypopituitarism (see A33.4)
A33.4	Features of hypopituitarism: loss of libido, infertility, menstrual disturbances, tiredness, low blood pressure, inappropriate lactation	The pituitary gland is the source of the endocrine hormones, which regulate growth, metabolism and the reproductive system. Damage to the pituitary gland can result in a complicated pattern of endocrine disturbance. If the cause is a pituitary tumor, the tumor bulk can also cause characteristic problems (see A33.3)
A33.5	Features of hyperprolactinemia: inappropriate secretion of milk and infertility	Prolactin may be secreted in excess in all forms of pituitary disease, and so inappropriate secretion of breast milk is a red flag of a pituitary tumor However, in most cases inappropriate secretion of milk has a benign cause, or may be the response to medications such as the contraceptive pill
A33.6	Features of acromegaly (growth hormone excess): change in facial appearance (coarsening of features), increased size of hands and feet, enlarging tongue, deepening voice, joint pains, hypertension, breathlessness	Acromegaly commonly results from a pituitary tumor, and so symptoms of pituitary tumor growth (see A33.3) may also be present

The Reproductive System

5.2

5.2a The physiology of the reproductive system[9]

The function of the reproductive system in both sexes is to ensure the reproduction of the human species. To do this, first, the reproductive system of each sex has to be able to produce healthy sex cells or gametes. These are the ova (singular ovum) from the female, and the spermatozoa (sperm) from the male. A second function of the reproductive system of each sex is to enable the meeting of these gametes to enable fertilization following the act of sexual intercourse.

The gametes originate from specialized cells called germ cells, which are formed within the ovaries in females and the testes in males. The gametes are the result of the particular form of cell division known as meiosis.

It is the role of the female reproductive system to provide a suitable environment for the implantation and nourishment of the fertilized egg, known as the zygote. This role continues for the 40 weeks of pregnancy, as the zygote divides and enlarges through the stages of embryo and fetus in the womb. The female reproductive tract then has to ensure the safe expulsion of the fetus during labor. Finally, it has to undergo all the changes of the postnatal period, which allow the woman to return, as much as possible, to her pre-pregnant state.

This chapter focuses on the male reproductive system and the non-pregnant female reproductive system. The study of the male reproductive system is conventionally termed andrology, and the study of the non-pregnant female reproductive system is termed gynecology (derived from the Greek words for man and woman, respectively). Chapter 5.3 is then dedicated to the conditions of pregnancy, labor and the postnatal period. The study of these conditions is conventionally referred to as obstetrics. This section considers the physiology of the male and female reproductive system in turn, and concludes with a brief discussion about the physiology of sexual intercourse.

The physiology of the male reproductive system

The male reproductive system consists of the testes, epididymis, urethra, penis and associated glands, including the prostate gland. Figure 5.2a-I illustrates the anatomy of this system and Figure 5.2a-II shows the structure of the testis and scrotum in more detail.

The testes are the paired male sex glands, or gonads, and sit suspended from the perineum within the sacs formed by the scrotum. The two main products of the testes are spermatozoa (originating from the germ cells of the seminiferous tubules) and the male sex hormone testosterone (originating from the interstitial cells of Leydig).

The pituitary gland produces follicle-stimulating hormone (FSH) and luteinizing hormone (LH), which play an important role in the function of the testes. FSH stimulates the production of spermatozoa from the germ cells. LH stimulates the production of testosterone from the testes. The levels of both these hormones surge at puberty.

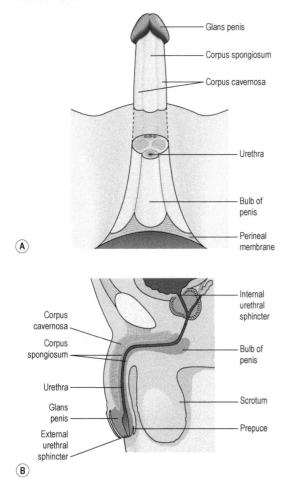

Figure 5.2a-I The anatomy of the male reproductive system

a) Interior of erect penis. b) Lateral view of male genitalia and bladder

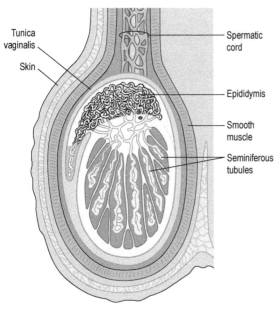

Figure 5.2a-II The anatomy of the testis and the scrotum

A mature sperm cell has a head, a body and a motile tail, which propels the sperm cell forwards by means of a whip-like motion. The formation of sperm is most efficient at about 3°C below body temperature, which is aided by the fact that the testes sit in the scrotum. Spermatozoa are secreted from the germinal cells of the testis into the epididymis. The epididymis is a complex of very fine tubules, which store and direct spermatozoa towards the vas deferens. Testosterone is secreted from the cells of Leydig directly into the bloodstream. Thus the testis is, strictly speaking, both an exocrine and an endocrine gland.

The spermatic cords emerge from a gap in the musculature above the inguinal ligament and provide the testes with a blood and nerve supply. They also contain the vas deferens. The purpose of the vas deferens is to carry the spermatozoa away from the testes and the epididymis, and to lead towards the urethra, from which the spermatozoa can be ejaculated. It is this tube that is severed and tied off in the procedure of vasectomy.

The prostate gland and seminal vesicles are exocrine glands that produce nutrient-rich lubricating fluid to maximize the survival of the spermatozoa and also to promote comfortable sexual intercourse. The seminal vesicles each open out into the distal portion of the two vas deferens, and the prostate gland is situated at the base of the bladder at the point at which the vas deferens ducts enter the urethra. The prostate hugs the most proximal region of the urethra, which is why this portion is described as the prostatic urethra. The fluids produced by these glands mix with the spermatozoa in the urethra during ejaculation to form semen.

The onset of puberty in the boy

The pituitary gland responds to hormonal changes in the maturing hypothalamus to trigger the changes of puberty in both boys and girls. In both, puberty is preceded by a surge of growth hormone (GH) from the pituitary gland, and this becomes manifest as a pre-pubertal growth spurt. Then, in both, the pituitary starts to produce increasing quantities of LH. In boys, this stimulates the interstitial cells of the testes to produce testosterone, and it is testosterone that influences the tissues of the body to change and allows the secondary sexual characteristics to emerge.

These include:

- enlargement of the testicles, penis and scrotum

- pubic hair growth in the groin and axilla

- increased facial and body hair, and thickening of the skin

- enlargement of the vocal cords and breaking of the voice

- increased muscle mass and bone density.

Information box 5.2a-I

The male reproductive system: comments from a Chinese medicine perspective

In Chinese medicine, the male reproductive system is dominated by the Kidney and Liver Organs. Healthy Qi and Kidney Essence (Jing) are key substances essential for male reproductive health.

The Kidney and Liver Channels pass across the anatomical location of the male genitalia. In sexes, sexual maturation and fertility is underpinned by Jing, which is recognized to flow in eight-year cycles in men. Healthy Qi enables a healthy sexual response.

The Kidney Organ is said to control the two lower orifices. This is reflected in the fact that impotence and inappropriate seminal emissions are features of Deficiency of both Kidney Yang (including Kidney Qi not firm) and Kidney Yin. In contrast, the Liver Organ appears to have more bearing on the external genitalia. Damp Heat in the Liver can manifest as soreness or itchiness of the scrotum, whereas Cold in the Liver Channel can give rise to deep pain in the scrotum.

The physiology of the female reproductive system

The female reproductive system lies at a deeper level in the body than in the male (see Figures 5.2a-III and 5.2a-IV). The ovaries sit deep in the basin formed by the pelvis, and lay either side of the womb (uterus). The ovaries are positioned close to the openings of two tubes (the fallopian tubes) that extend sideways from the uterus. The uterus is a pear-sized organ sitting just behind and above the bladder, protected in front by the bridge formed by the pubic bone. The neck of the uterus (the cervix) opens into the bodily space called the vagina. The entrance of the vagina, the vulva, is surrounded by the fleshy lips of the labia minora and labia majora in the perineum.

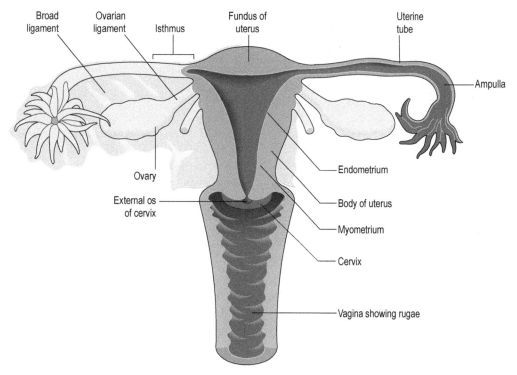

Figure 5.2a-III The uterus and ovaries in the pelvis (anterior view)

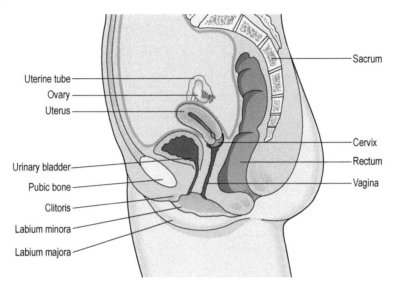

Figure 5.2a-IV The female reproductive system in the pelvis (lateral view)

The system in more detail

THE VAGINA

The vagina is a tube-like space with tough muscular walls. It is approximately 8cm long. The interior of the vagina is kept moist by secretions that originate from tiny glands in the cervix. The lining of the vagina is colonized by healthy bacteria called *Lactobacillus acidophilus*. These secrete an acid called lactic acid, and so keep the interior of the vagina slightly acidic. Lactobacilli are the same type of bacteria that are used to turn milk into live yoghurt. The acidic environment created by the *Lactobacillus* helps keep the growth of less desirable bacteria and yeasts at bay.

In young girls, the opening of the vagina is partially closed by means of a thin sheet of tissue called the hymen. A small opening in the hymen permits the escape of menstrual blood at the onset of puberty. The hymen is always stretched during first intercourse. Tearing of the hymen with a small amount of bleeding can happen at first intercourse, or may occur earlier in an active teenager. The finding of a torn hymen in a prepubescent child is not normal, and is an indicator of possible sexual abuse.

THE UTERUS

The uterus is a hollow organ with three narrow openings formed by the cervix and the two fallopian tubes. The wall of the uterus is composed of a thick layer of smooth muscle called the myometrium. The lining of the uterus is called the endometrium. This is composed of columnar epithelium and contains a large number of mucus-secreting glands. The thickness of this layer varies throughout the monthly menstrual cycle.

The endometrium extends to the lower third of the narrow entrance to the cervix, which is known as the cervical canal. Below this there is a transition to squamous epithelium, which lines the vagina.

THE FALLOPIAN TUBES

The fallopian tubes receive the ovum from the ovary and aid its transport towards the space within the body of the uterus. To do this, the fallopian tubes have frond-like projections at their distal ends. These fronds and also the interior of the fallopian tube are lined with ciliated epithelial cells. When the ovum is released, ciliary movement wafts the ovum into and through the tube. The fallopian tube is the usual location for the fertilization of the ovum and the spermatozoon. The fertilized zygote is then transported into the endometrium in preparation for implantation by means of the ciliary movement of the lining of the fallopian tubes.

THE OVARY

The ovary is the female sex gland or gonad. The ovary originates from exactly the same embryonic tissue as the testis. During development of the male fetus, this embryonic tissue, originally positioned in the abdomen, develops into the testis and migrates into the scrotum under the influence of male sex hormones. In the female fetus, in the absence of these male hormones, the tissue remains where it is and develops into the ovary.

The ovary is the site for the maturation of the ova, and this takes place during the course of the first half of the menstrual cycle, during which usually only a single ovarian follicle enlarges. Ovarian follicles each consist of a single ovum and are lined by ovarian cells. By the time the female baby is born, her ovaries contain all the ova, each within its own ovarian follicle, which will be released during her childbearing years.

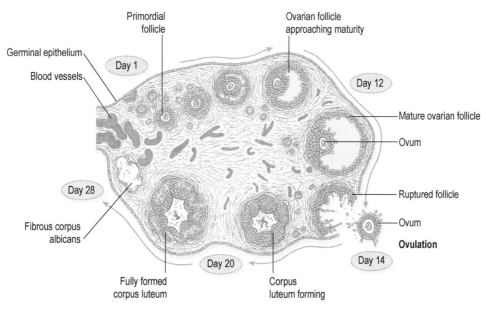

Figure 5.2a-V Section of the ovary showing the development of one follicle over the course of one month

During the first half of the menstrual cycle, a single ovarian follicle begins the process of maturation (see Figure 5.2a-V). This involves the follicle enlarging and developing a fluid-filled cavity over the course of approximately 14 days. This so-called mature Graafian follicle then merges with the outer part of the ovary and ruptures to release the single ovum into the space surrounding the ovary. This process of rupture and release is what is termed ovulation. The whole process is stimulated first by FSH from the pituitary gland, and this explains its name. FSH is the same hormone that in men stimulates the development of spermatozoa from germinal cells.

During the first 14 days of the menstrual cycle, the multiplying follicle cells secrete the female sex hormone estrogen, also under the influence of FSH. The rising estrogen levels have a suppressive (negative feedback) effect on the secretion of FSH. As the FSH levels start to drop, the pituitary then releases a surge of a second hormone, LH. It is this hormone that stimulates ovulation. After ovulation, the remaining follicle develops into a body known as the corpus luteum (the origin of the term luteinizing hormone). Under the influence of LH the corpus luteum no longer produces estrogen, and instead releases the other female sex hormone, progesterone.

The corpus luteum matures and then degenerates over the course of the next 14 days. As the corpus luteum degenerates, it ceases to produce progesterone. However, if fertilization occurs, this degeneration does not happen, and instead the corpus luteum continues to develop. This is a result of the multiplying cells of the zygote that secrete the hormone human chorionic gonadotropin (HCG). This stimulates the corpus luteum and prevents its degeneration.

Thus, in early pregnancy the progesterone levels continue to rise.

To summarize, after puberty, the ovarian follicle is the source of a cyclical release of the female sex hormones. Estrogen is released in the first half of the menstrual cycle, and progesterone in the second half of the menstrual cycle. This cycle is controlled by the cyclical release of the pituitary hormones FSH and LH.

The onset of puberty in the girl

As is the case for boys, in girls the onset of puberty is also stimulated by a rise in the production of FSH and LH. This usually occurs between the ages of 10 and 14.

Two to three years prior to this surge in FSH and LH in both boys and girls there is an increase in the release of GH from the pituitary gland. The release of GH stimulates the growth spurt that occurs in children just before puberty. In girls, the rise in FSH and LH stimulates the production of increasing amounts of estrogen from the follicle cells of the ovaries. Initially, these pituitary hormones are not present in sufficient quantities to stimulate ovulation. However, the estrogen produced affects diverse body tissues to bring about the early changes of puberty, including breast development and the growth of pubic hair. As puberty approaches, the levels of FSH and LH increase until ovulation is stimulated.

At approximately the same time as the onset of ovulation, menstruation begins. The onset of menstruation is termed the menarche. It is recognized that ovulation may occur for a few cycles before the first menstrual bleed. This means that there is a possibility of pregnancy even before menstruation has started.

The onset of puberty in both girls and boys in Westernized cultures is occurring at an increasingly early age. The average age of onset of menstruation is four years earlier now than it was a century ago.[10] This suggests that it is not purely biological programming that stimulates the dramatic increase in the release of FSH and LH that initiates puberty. It is now believed that both nutritional and psychological factors also play a part in this hormonal change. These are believed to influence the physiology of the pituitary via the production of specific hormones from the hypothalamus.

A child who is less well nourished is more likely to experience a delayed onset of puberty. Conversely, a child who achieves a degree of psychological maturity, particularly with regard to understanding or experience of sexual matters, appears to experience an earlier onset of puberty. Both these factors tend to promote the earlier onset of puberty in girls who grow up in modern cultures.

MENSTRUATION

The changes that take place in the ovary after the onset of ovulation have a cycle of approximately 28 days, although any interval between 22 and 35 days is considered conventionally to be within the normal range. These changes are mirrored by cyclical changes in the uterus and vagina as well as many other tissues in the body. They are the result of the rise of estrogen in the first half of the cycle and in progesterone in the second half of the cycle.

Estrogen can be considered as a hormone that stimulates fleshiness. In the first half of the cycle, it continues to promote the healthy development of the breasts and pubic hair. It also stimulates and maintains the changes to the skin, body fat and bony skeleton (in particular, the hips and pelvis) that are characteristic of the female body. In the uterus, it stimulates a thickening of the endometrium, with the development of deep mucus-forming glands and a rich supply of blood vessels. About three days before ovulation thick sticky mucus is secreted from the cervix. This mucus encourages the passage of spermatozoa at the time when the woman is likely to be most fertile. This phase of the menstrual cycle is termed the proliferative phase, a term that refers to the changes taking place in the endometrium at that time.

Estrogen promotes fleshiness of the tissues of the vagina and the labia majora and minor. It also promotes the vaginal secretions that are particularly important for comfortable sexual intercourse.

Progesterone can be considered to be the hormone that prepares the body for pregnancy and promotes the first three months of pregnancy. After ovulation, the rising levels of progesterone stimulate a watery swelling of the endometrium and the production of thick mucus. This mucus is believed to encourage the passage of the spermatozoa into the fallopian tubes, where fertilization

can take place. The changes in the endometrium provide a suitable environment for the zygote. If implantation does not occur, at about 6–8 days after ovulation, the corpus luteum starts to degenerate, and progesterone levels drop. It is this drop that causes the lining of the endometrium to start to break down, culminating in menstruation at 14 days after ovulation. There are thus two distinct phases to this second half of the menstrual cycle, termed the secretory phase and the premenstrual phase (see Figure 5.2a-VI).

Figure 5.2a-VI Diagrammatic summary of one female menstrual cycle

Normal menstruation takes place over the course of three to seven days. As blood, endometrial lining cells and tissue fluid are shed, chemicals are released that stimulate the muscle wall of the uterus to contract, so that bleeding is minimized, and the products are effectively cleared from the uterus. This contraction is the cause of the cramping pain of menstruation. A degree of pain is therefore considered to be normal from a conventional perspective. It is helpful to understand that menstrual blood is not pure blood. A heavy period may not necessarily indicate a large loss of blood cells, as much of the volume of what is lost may be tissue fluid.

While menstruation is occurring, the release of FSH initiates the next cycle, with the stimulation of the maturation of another ovarian follicle. This is why the first day of the menstrual bleed is conventionally considered to be the first day of the whole menstrual cycle.

The menopause

The menopause is the term commonly used to describe the time in life, usually between the ages of 45 and 55, when menstruation ceases. Strictly speaking, the conventional use of the term menopause is to describe the precise time of cessation of menstruation. The term climacteric is used to describe the period of approximately ten years that precedes and follows this event.[11]

The aging ovaries are the cause of the onset of the climacteric. Gradually, the ovaries become less and less responsive to the pituitary hormones. This means that more and more of the menstrual cycles fail to lead to ovulation, and the production of estrogen drops. The rate of drop in estrogen levels varies widely between women, and this might explain why some women experience more profound symptoms than others during the climacteric.

Other features of a lack of estrogen include a reduction in the strength of the pelvic floor muscles, with increased risk of prolapse of the vagina and uterus. Urinary problems, including urinary infections and stress incontinence, can occur because of a combination of reduced pelvic floor tone and changes in the lining of the skin around the opening of the urethra.

The notorious hot flashes are a consequence of a rapid drop in estrogen levels. The symptoms of these include bouts of profuse sweating and heat intolerance, often occurring at night. These can be accompanied by a range of bodily and psychological symptoms, which are not conventionally considered to be necessarily related to a lack of estrogen.

A lack of estrogen also promotes loss of calcium from the bones. This can occur very rapidly during the climacteric and can result in the symptoms of osteoporosis.

As the ovaries become less responsive to the control of the pituitary hormones, menstrual cycles become increasingly irregular. Some women experience increased frequency of menstruation, sometimes with excessive bleeding, for months to years, before the menopause. Usually just before the menopause the periods become lighter and more infrequent.

As the climacteric approaches, women become increasingly infertile as fewer and fewer cycles lead to ovulation. However, onset of the menopause does not necessarily mean that ovulation has ceased. In some women ovulation may still occur for a short time. This explains why it is that, in very rare circumstances, pregnancy can still happen after a woman's periods have ceased. Women who reach the menopause before the age of 50 are counseled to continue to use contraception for two years after the menopause, and those over 50 are advised to continue using contraception for one year.

The breasts

The breasts develop in the female under the influence of progesterone and estrogen during puberty. Each breast contains a lot of fatty tissue in which numerous exocrine glands, called lobules, are embedded. The lobules are responsible for milk production. During lactation milk is secreted from the lobules into ducts called lactiferous ducts. Before these open out into the nipple, each duct widens into a reservoir for milk called a sinus. The health of both the lobules and this fatty tissue is maintained up until the time of the menopause by estrogen released by the maturing ovarian follicles.

The breast is prepared for milk production during pregnancy by the influence of estrogen and progesterone. Milk production is stimulated by two pituitary hormones: prolactin (PRL) stimulates the formation of milk in the lobules, and oxytocin stimulates the contraction of the ducts and sinuses, which leads to the letdown of milk towards the nipple. Suckling is one stimulus for the release of these two hormones.

Information box 5.2a-II

The female reproductive system: comments from a Chinese medicine perspective

From a Chinese medicine perspective, the physiology of the female reproductive system is complex. The extra Yang Organ, the Uterus, is the central organ, but the Spleen, Stomach, Liver, Heart and Kidneys all have important roles. The four Extraordinary Vessels, the Ren Mai, Du Mai, Chong Mai and Dai Mai, are important regulatory Channels. Additional Channels, the Bao Mai and Bao Luo, which link the Uterus with the Heart and the Kidneys, respectively, are also important for the regulation of the female reproductive system.

Blood and Kidney Essence (Jing) are the important substances for a healthy female reproductive system. It is Heart Blood that fills and nourishes the Uterus, and so the Spleen and the Liver Organs are responsible for the manufacture and the smooth movement of this Blood. However, Jing is required in addition to Heart Blood for menstruation to occur, as it is the basis of the menstrual blood. In women, Jing is believed to flow in seven-year cycles. The Spleen and Jing may be the foundation of the action of estrogen, as together they give rise to fleshy characteristics, fertility and strong bones.

The deep origin of all three of the Extraordinary Vessels (Ren Mai, Du Mai and Chong Mai) is the region of the Kidneys. These then all flow through the energetic region described in Chinese medicine as the Uterus before reaching their more superficial pathways.

The Chong Mai, as the Sea of Blood, has a strong influence on menstruation. The Chong Mai is linked to the Stomach Channel via ST-30 (Qi Chong). This explains how nausea can be a problem in conditions such as dysmenorrhea and morning sickness.

The Ren Mai governs the cervix, vagina and the vulva. It also helps to provide the other Yin substances important in female reproductive physiology (Yin, Essence and Fluids), as it is the Sea of the Yin Channels. It is therefore important in the regulation of fertility, puberty, pregnancy and the menopause.

Because of its complex pathway, the Du Mai also influences the vagina and the vulva. The Du Mai together and the Ren Mai together can be seen as two branches of one circuit that interlinks the Uterus with the other Organs. The Dai Mai encircles the waist, and so crosses the leg channels. In this way it influences the smooth flow of Qi in the Liver Channel and harmonizes the Kidneys and the Spleen.

The relative strength of the organs and substances in the four menstrual phases correspond to the physiological phases understood in conventional terms. These are (with conventional terms in parentheses):

- Menstruation: Blood is moving, and is reliant on smooth Liver Qi and Liver Blood.
- Postmenstrual (proliferative phase): Blood and Yin are Empty and Chong Mai and Ren Mai are Empty.
- Mid-cycle (secretory phase): Blood and Yin fill up in Chong Mai and Ren Mai.
- Premenstrual (premenstrual phase): Yang Qi Rises and Liver Qi Moves. This phase does not occur if implantation takes place.

At the climacteric, there is a decline in the Kidney Essence and in the Qi and Blood of the Ren Mai and Chong Mai. There is thus a general drying up of body fluids (Yin Deficiency). This culminates in the cessation of menstruation.

The physiology of sexual intercourse

Sexual intercourse is necessary for natural conception to occur. It enables the meeting of the spermatozoa and the ovum in the fallopian tubes. It is, of course, also a very important aspect of bonding in human relationships.

Despite the overt differences, the physiological processes that take place during sexual intercourse are very similar in men and women. The sexual act, for both men and women, has been described as taking place in five phases, although these phases tend to merge into one another. These phases are:

- Sexual desire: the emotional/mental response to the thought, sight, touch or smell of another person.

- Sexual arousal: following sexual desire, physical changes take place in the sex organs (genitalia). The penis and clitoris become erect and the vagina becomes lubricated. The nipples can become erect. The heart rate can increase. There is a strong desire for sexual intercourse. This phase is mediated by the parasympathetic aspect of the nervous system.
- Plateau: sexual pleasure is intensified and sustained before and after penile penetration has taken place. This phase is also mediated by the parasympathetic nervous system.
- Orgasm: orgasm usually results in ejaculation of semen in men. In penile/vaginal intercourse, the semen is directed deep into the vagina, close to

the entrance of the cervical canal. Ninety percent of women are able to achieve orgasm, although only 25 percent will be able to reach orgasm through penile penetration into the vagina alone. There are rhythmic contractions of the perineal muscles of the women at orgasm. These contractions encourage the upward movement of the semen towards the cervix. The orgasmic phase is mediated by the sympathetic aspect of the nervous system.

- Resolution: after orgasm, both partners are relaxed, and the body gradually returns to a non-aroused state. In this phase the parasympathetic nervous system is dominant. The resolution state encourages rest, and for the woman this is the ideal state for the continued passage of the spermatozoa into the cervical canal and thence into the uterus.

5.2b The investigation of the reproductive system

The investigation of the female reproductive system is usually carried out within the hospital specialty of obstetrics and gynecology. The hospital specialist who deals with the all the disorders of the non-pregnant female reproductive tract is called a gynecologist. However, breast disorders are, in general, managed by a general or a specialist breast surgeon.

Disorders of the male reproductive system are often investigated within the surgical specialty of urology. In some hospitals there may be a dedicated andrology unit.

Sexually transmitted diseases are usually managed within the hospital specialty of genitourinary medicine (GUM). In the UK, in contrast to all other hospital specialties apart from accident and emergency medicine, patients can self-refer to a GUM department. The content of each consultation is kept strictly confidential and is not even revealed to the patient's general practitioner (GP).

The investigation of the female reproductive system

The investigation of the female reproductive system includes:

- a thorough physical examination, including internal examination of the uterus and ovaries

- blood tests and urine tests to assess hormone levels

- examination of samples of vaginal mucus

- cervical cytological examination (Pap smear)

- imaging tests (in particular, pelvic ultrasound, endoscopy of the vagina and the womb, laparoscopy and hysterosalpingography) to visualize the structure of the reproductive organs

- biopsy of the endometrium.

Gynecological physical examination

The main part of the gynecological examination is the internal pelvic examination. For this examination the woman has to lie on her back, with knees bent and feet apart. In the first part of the examination the doctor inserts two gloved fingers of the right hand into the vagina, whilst palpating the suprapubic area of the abdomen with the left. In this bimanual examination the shape of the cervix can be assessed, and structural problems of the uterus and the ovaries may be detected. The doctor then inserts an instrument made of metal or plastic called a speculum into the vagina. The speculum parts the soft tissue of the vaginal walls, and allows the doctor to see the cervix. A speculum is necessary to perform a cervical cytological examination (Pap smear) test.

If the patient can relax, these tests should not be painful. However, many patients find these procedures undignified or embarrassing. They can be very traumatic for those with a past history of sexual difficulties or abuse. The muscle tension that results from resistance to the idea of these tests can make insertion of the examining fingers or the speculum much more difficult, and potentially painful.

Blood and urine tests

Blood tests may be taken to examine the levels of FSH, LH and the sex hormones. As all these hormones vary dramatically throughout the menstrual cycle, it is important to record the time of day and the day of the cycle on which the test is taken.

Urine may also be examined for hormone levels. The most commonly performed urine test is the pregnancy test. This looks for the rising levels of HCG that appear shortly after implantation of the fertilized ovum (zygote).

Examination of vaginal mucus

A sample of vaginal mucus can be obtained by means of a swab inserted during a speculum examination. This test may be performed to investigate possible infectious disease, in which case the swab is sent to a laboratory to look for evidence of microorganisms.

Alternatively, the mucus may be examined as part of natural family planning and also in the investigation of infertility. The patient can be taught to examine her own mucus, and to look for the characteristic changes in consistency that occur at ovulation. When the mucus is at its most profuse and sticky, ovulation is occurring and fertility is at its peak.

The postcoital test is a test of the cervical mucus taken within eight hours of intercourse and is timed to occur in the two days leading up to ovulation. In this test the mucus should contain sperm. The test is to examine whether or not the sperm are able to penetrate the mucus in a normal way. If they cannot, this may suggest a condition in which the mucus contains antibodies that are specific to the antigens on the sperm, and which prevent the sperm from penetrating the cervical opening.

Cervical cytological screening (formerly known as the Pap smear test)

The cervical screening test is designed to examine for early precancerous changes to the cervical cells. The aim is to detect such changes at a time when they can be simply treated by local laser treatment or excision.

In the cervical screening test, the opening to the cervix is visualized by means of a speculum. The cervix is then swept gently with a brush to obtain a sample of the mucus. This process should be painless. The end of the brush is then stirred into a fluid designed to maintain living cervical cells. The sample of cell transport fluid is then sent to a cytology laboratory for microscopic examination. The examination looks for abnormally shaped (dysplastic) cervical cells, which may be an indication of early cancer. It is also possible to test for the very common wart virus (human papilloma virus, HPV) infection as part of the examination. This is now widely performed to offer more prognostic information. The cervical screening test is offered to all women in the UK between the ages of 25 and 65 at regular (three-yearly and then five-yearly) intervals as part of a national screening program.

Cervical screening is not wholly reliable, in that many women who have no physical abnormality will have unclear smear test results and will have to be recalled for re-examination (false-positive results), and some cervical cancers will be missed (false-negative results). Many women are recalled for the more invasive colposcopy treatments on the basis of slight abnormalities that may never have developed into cancer.

There is ongoing debate over whether the cost of the program and its inconvenience to many women is outweighed by the advantages of the early detection of cancer in a few. However, it has been estimated that the UK cervical screening program saves about 3000 lives per annum by preventing the development of advanced cervical cancer. There was a 43 percent reduction in cervical cancer incidence from 1987 to 1997 in the UK that followed the introduction of the screening program.

The introduction of HPV vaccination in teenage girls is likely to impact positively on the incidence of cervical cancer in the long term. It may be possible that the rates of this cancer may drop to such an extent that there will no longer be a need for the screening program.[12]

Imaging tests and biopsy

Because the uterus and ovaries are deep organs, imaging tests are very often necessary to provide more information.

The pelvic ultrasound scan is a non-invasive examination that can provide very useful information. The test usually involves the use of a vaginally inserted probe so that the uterus can be examined from within the bowl of the pelvis. Tumors and cysts of the ovaries and uterus can be visualized by means of an ultrasound examination. The formation of the Graafian follicle can be seen, and so ultrasound can give an indication of healthy ovulation.

Endoscopy of the vagina (colposcopy) is a test that requires the insertion of a vaginal speculum. A colposcope (a form of endoscope) is used to provide detailed images of the surface of the cervix, and permits the removal of cervical biopsies and treatment of the cervix. This investigation is most commonly used to provide more information and treatment after an abnormal cervical cytology test.

Endoscopy of the uterus (hysteroscopy) requires the insertion of a fine endoscope into the uterus via the cervical canal. This is usually performed in an outpatient setting in a conscious patient. The test can be uncomfortable, as the cervix is very sensitive. Hysteroscopy is used in the investigation of menstrual disorders, and is the means by which samples of the endometrium may be obtained for microscopic examination.

Laparoscopy is a procedure in which a fine endoscope is inserted into the peritoneal cavity that surrounds the pelvic organs. The endoscope is inserted via a small incision made adjacent to the umbilicus. Laparoscopy can reveal the details of the external anatomy of the ovaries and the uterus. It can visualize ovarian cysts and the changes that occur in endometriosis. Laparoscopy is also the means by which some important gynecological procedures can be performed. These include sterilization, removal of ovarian cysts and removal of eggs for assisted-fertilization techniques.

Hysterosalpingography (HSG) is a test to examine the interior anatomy of the fallopian tubes. A dye that is opaque to X-rays is injected into the cervical canal, and X-ray images taken of the pelvic area. The dye can reveal the interior shape of the uterus and fallopian tubes, and thereby whether or not the fallopian tubes are blocked.

Endometrial biopsy is performed by means of hysteroscopy. A sample of the lining of the womb is removed from a conscious patient by means of a spoon-shaped instrument called a curette. The patient is likely to experience cramping pain and some bleeding after this procedure.

A less invasive method of obtaining endometrial samples is by means of a fine-ended suction instrument called a Pipelle curette. This samples far less endometrium but still has a greater than 90 percent detection rate for endometrial cancer.

The investigation of breast diseases

The investigation of breast diseases includes:

- physical examination of the breasts and armpits
- withdrawal of fluid from cysts and biopsy
- ultrasound scan
- mammography.

Physical examination of the breasts and armpits

Physical examination of the breasts involves observation for lumps or asymmetry, and systematic palpation for lumps. The examination should extend into the axilla (the armpit), into which the breast tissue extends. The axillary lymph nodes are also examined.

Women should be encouraged to perform this examination on themselves on a regular basis. The techniques of breast self-examination can be learned from a GP or practice nurse.

Fluid drainage and biopsy

Some lumps in the breast are cysts that contain fluid. This fluid can be withdrawn by means of a fine needle and syringe, and then examined under a microscope. A wider needle and syringe may be used to obtain a sample of the cells in a lump. Alternatively, a minor operation might be required to remove a small sample of tissue for a biopsy.

Ultrasound scan

An ultrasound scan is commonly used in the investigation of breast lumps in outpatients. The scan can clearly demonstrate the fluid within breast cysts, and also indicate any irregular areas of growth, which may be suggestive of breast cancer.

Mammography

Mammography is the term given to describe X-ray examination of the breasts. This test is offered to women in the UK aged 50–70 at one- to three-year intervals as part of the National Health Service (NHS) breast screening program.

Mammography is given with the intention of detecting breast cancer in an early (operable) stage. Like the cervical smear test, it is not a wholly reliable test, in that many women who have normal results will have to be recalled for re-examination (false-positives), and some breast cancers will be missed (false-negatives). Also, as for the cervical smear test, there is ongoing debate over whether the cost of the program and its inconvenience to many women are outweighed by the advantages of the early detection of cancer in a few.

The investigation of the male reproductive system

The investigation of the male reproductive system includes:

- a thorough physical examination, including examination of the testes and penis
- blood tests to assess hormone levels and to look for tumor markers
- semen analysis
- visualization of the testes and prostate
- biopsy.

Physical examination of the male reproductive system

The examination of the male reproductive system involves inspection and visualization of the male genitalia and palpation of the scrotum. Palpation will reveal the shape and consistency of the testes, and also the spermatic cords and the epididymis. The inguinal (groin) lymph nodes are also examined. Men should be encouraged to examine their own testes on a regular basis. The techniques of testicular self-examination can be learned from a GP or practice nurse.

The prostate is examined by means of digital rectal examination (i.e. the physician inserts a gloved finger into the anus).

Blood tests

Blood tests can be used to assess levels of FSH, LH and the sex hormones, although these tests are much more commonly performed in women than in men.

Testicular cancer and prostate cancers can secrete characteristic chemicals known as tumor markers, such as prostate-specific antigen (PSA). Blood tests may be taken for tumor markers in the diagnostic stages of cancer, but also during treatment to assess progress.

Semen analysis

A fresh sample of semen that has been obtained by masturbation can be submitted to a range of tests to assess fertility. The volume and consistency of the semen, the number (sperm count) and the shape and movement of the spermatozoa can be analyzed and compared to the normal ranges.

Visualization of the testes and prostate

The structure of the testes and prostate may be examined in more detail by means of an ultrasound scan. The examination of the prostate requires the insertion of an ultrasound probe into the rectum.

Biopsy of the testes and the prostate

In cases of suspected cancer, biopsy of the testes or prostate may be necessary.

The investigation of sexually transmitted diseases

The investigation of sexually transmitted diseases includes:

- physical examination
- examination of discharges
- blood tests.

Physical examination

Many sexually transmitted diseases have characteristic symptoms and signs. Physical examination of the external genitalia in men and women, and the vagina, cervix and uterus in women, may reveal some of the characteristic features of these diseases.

Examination of discharges

Samples of vaginal or penile discharges may be taken by means of a swab to examine for evidence of microorganisms and viruses. In women, often three swabs are taken, two from the cervical opening (os) and one from the vagina. The most common organisms that are isolated include *Candida*, *Gonococcus*, *Chlamydia*, *Trichomonas* and *Gardnerella*.

Blood tests

Blood tests can provide evidence of a sexually transmitted infection. These include the test for human immunodeficiency virus (HIV), in which antibodies to HIV are indicative of infection. Blood tests can also reveal evidence of infection by hepatitis B and C and syphilis.

GU clinics offer the HIV test on a strictly confidential basis. Because of the consequences of being tested as HIV-positive, patients may be offered pre-test and post-test counseling, irrespective of whether the test is positive or negative.

5.2c Disorders of menstruation and the menopause

The conditions explored in this section are:

- Amenorrhea and oligomenorrhea – primary amenorrhea:
  - non-structural causes
  - congenital defects
- Amenorrhea and oligomenorrhea – secondary amenorrhea:
  - non-structural causes
  - primary ovarian failure
  - endocrine causes
  - polycystic ovary syndrome (PCOS)
- Menorrhagia:
  - dysfunctional uterine bleeding
  - uterine fibroids and endometrial polyps
  - pelvic inflammatory disease (PID)
  - hypothyroidism
  - metrorrhagia
- Premenstrual syndrome (PMS)
- Dysmenorrhea
- Problems during the menopause.

Amenorrhea and oligomenorrhea

Amenorrhea is defined as total lack of menstruation. It may be primary or secondary. Primary amenorrhea means that there has never been an onset of menstruation. This diagnosis is made if the menarche has not occurred by the age of 16.

Secondary amenorrhea indicates a cessation of menstruation. This diagnosis is made when menstruation has ceased for more than 70 days. Oligomenorrhea indicates infrequent periods with a cycle length of greater than 35 days. In general, the causes of oligomenorrhea are the same as those of secondary amenorrhea.

Primary amenorrhea
NON-STRUCTURAL CAUSES OF PRIMARY AMENORRHEA

In most cases of primary amenorrhea there is no structural abnormality. There may instead be an inherited tendency to have a late onset of menstruation. There may be other factors, such as chronic illness, an eating disorder or excessive exercise, which have delayed the onset of menstruation. These inhibit the onset of menstruation by causing a reduction in the release of the pituitary hormones LH and FSH.

CONGENITAL CAUSES OF PRIMARY AMENORRHEA

More rare structural causes of primary amenorrhea include congenital defects of the ovaries, uterus, vagina or hymen. In all but the first of these conditions, the other features of puberty will appear normally. Turner's syndrome is a relatively common chromosomal disorder in which the affected woman has underdeveloped ovaries, and often first presents with primary amenorrhea and failure to develop the other secondary sexual characteristics of puberty.

Primary amenorrhea is usually investigated if menarche has not occurred by the age of 16. A physical examination is performed, and blood tests are taken to look for FSH, LH and the sex hormones, including testosterone. Prolactin (PRL) levels and thyroid function are also assessed. If it is found that the ovaries are not responding to the pituitary hormones (suggesting congenital disorders of the ovary such as Turner's syndrome), hormone replacement therapy (HRT) containing estrogen and progestogen is prescribed so that the beneficial effects of estrogen on the bones are maintained.

If the problem lies in factors that lead to underproduction of sufficient pituitary hormones, such as over-exercise or anorexia nervosa, then ideally these factors should first be remedied. In these cases estrogen lack is a real concern, as HRT does not seem to offer the benefit in terms of protection from osteoporosis as might be expected, possibly because of poor nutritional status.

Secondary amenorrhea and oligomenorrhea

The most common cause of secondary amenorrhea is pregnancy. This common cause may actually be a possibility that has been overlooked by the patient, but needs always to be considered in any case of absence of menstrual bleeding.

NON-STRUCTURAL CAUSES OF SECONDARY AMENORRHEA

In most cases of secondary amenorrhea there is no physical abnormality, because most commonly it develops as a response to factors that affect the release of pituitary hormones. Conditions such as chronic illness, eating disorders and over-exercise, already described as causes of primary amenorrhea, can also lead to cessation of periods after a normal menarche. Less seriously, episodes of physical or emotional stress, such as exams or overseas travel, might cause amenorrhea for a short time. Teenage girls are particularly prone to stress-related amenorrhea. For this reason, secondary amenorrhea is usually not investigated until it has persisted for at least six months.

PRIMARY OVARIAN FAILURE

This is a rare and irreversible cause of secondary amenorrhea. In most cases the cause is unknown. In some cases there may be autoimmune damage to the ovaries. In this condition the ovaries simply stop producing follicles, and the woman enters an early menopause (defined as menopause occurring before the age of 40). Women with primary ovarian failure are offered HRT until the age of 50 in order to prevent the development of osteoporosis. Conception may still be possible with assisted conception techniques.

ENDOCRINE CAUSES OF SECONDARY AMENORRHEA

Some cases of amenorrhea are the result of endocrine diseases, for example, hyperthyroidism or excessive prolactin secretion, in which case the treatment is primarily treatment of the underlying cause.

POLYCYSTIC OVARY SYNDROME (PCOS)

In up to one-third of women at some point in their lives the ovarian follicles do not develop properly. The ovary becomes enlarged, with four or more enlarged but intact follicles (cysts). This situation is often associated with irregularity of menstruation, but is not a cause for concern. However, a subgroup of women with polycystic ovaries may be diagnosed with polycystic ovary syndrome (PCOS), when the condition is associated with weight gain, oligomenorrhea or amenorrhea, excessive body hair in a male distribution and infertility. It is believed that insulin resistance and over-secretion of insulin might be the fundamental problem in this form of PCOS.

This hormonal imbalance is believed to affect the LH surge from the pituitary gland (so preventing rupture of the ovarian follicles and causing infertility) as well as leading to excessive formation of male sex hormones (which cause excessive body hair and also acne). PCOS is associated with a greater than average risk of non-insulin-dependent diabetes mellitus, high blood pressure and cardiovascular disease. There is also a small increased risk of cancer of the womb and of the ovaries.

PCOS is very common, affecting between 5 and 15 percent of women. However, only a few will exhibit the more severe manifestations of the syndrome.

In PCOS, ultrasound examination of the ovaries shows unruptured ovarian follicles and a blood test reveals an imbalance in the levels of FSH and LH and in some cases raised levels of testosterone and PRL.

As part of the treatment for PCOS the patient is advised to lose weight, stop smoking and to increase participation in gentle exercise, as these changes can normalize insulin levels. The antidiabetic drug metformin may be prescribed, as it reduces insulin resistance, particularly in anyone who is classified as overweight according to their body mass index (BMI >25).

If amenorrhea is the primary problem, the combined oral contraceptive pill is prescribed to induce regular menstruation and protect the woman from endometrial cancer.

If fertility is the primary concern, the drug clomiphene may be prescribed to induce ovulation in PCOS. If this fails to help with conception, surgical drilling of the ovaries can reduce the production of unnecessary sex steroid hormones and improve fertility rates.

Excessive male-pattern body hair in PCOS can be treated by means of medication. The oral contraceptive may be effective in reducing the hairiness. Alternatively, the drug cyproterone acetate may be prescribed. This has the effect of opposing the action of the male sex hormones.[13]

Amenorrhea: comments from a Chinese medicine perspective

In Chinese medicine, amenorrhea (no periods) may be an Empty or a Full condition. The empty conditions include Jing Deficiency, Blood Deficiency, Spleen and Kidney Deficiency, and Liver and Kidney Deficiency. The Full conditions include Cold in the Uterus, Phlegm or Qi/Blood Stagnation. Oligomenorrhea (late periods) might indicate Blood Deficiency, Cold in the Uterus, Kidney Yang Deficiency or Qi Deficiency.

PCOS with its association with weight gain, acne and hirsutism is likely to involve Phlegm Damp and Liver Qi disharmony.

Menorrhagia

Menorrhagia is defined as menstrual bleeding that is too heavy, and specifically relates to a menstrual loss of more than 80ml/month. However, in practice the degree of menstrual loss is very difficult to assess. Usually loss is expressed in terms of the number of tampons or towels required, and the numbers of episodes of flooding.

The main health consequence of menorrhagia is blood loss. This can, in severe cases, lead to iron-deficiency anemia, as the loss of iron in the menstrual blood is too great to be replaced by the diet alone. Very rarely, the blood loss is so profuse as to require emergency treatment with transfusion.

However, for most people, the main problem with menorrhagia is the inconvenience of having a prolonged and heavy monthly bleed. Although many women feel tired and uncomfortable during a heavy period, they may never lose sufficient blood to become clinically anemic.

Dysfunctional uterine bleeding

The most important and common category of menorrhagia (the cause in 40–60 percent of cases) is functional menorrhagia.[14] This means that there is no structural or readily measurable cause for the bleeding. The term dysfunctional uterine bleeding (DUB) is applied to a range of syndromes, all of which involve heavy bleeding. In DUB the bleeding is usually regular. If the pattern of bleeding is chaotic and with no predictable pattern, the term metrorrhagia is applied.

DUB is most common just after the menarche and in the years leading up to the menopause. Usually, the underlying problem is a defect in the maturation of the ovarian follicle or the formation of the corpus luteum. The reasons for this are usually unclear, although the root lies partly in the control of the whole process by the pituitary gland. This explains, of course, why emotional and mental factors can play an important role in the development of heavy periods.

The defective follicular development may cause the levels of estrogen and progesterone to become subtly unbalanced, and thus cause the heavy bleeding. However, most women with DUB demonstrate no measurable abnormalities in the release of pituitary or sex hormones that might support this theory.

The pattern of problematic bleeding varies according to the precise underlying problem. In some cases the spotting and blood loss occurs for some days before the onset of menstruation. This bleeding may start at the time of ovulation (mid-cycle bleeding). In other cases there is slight bleeding or spotting for some days after the period.

In less common cases the underlying problem is that ovulation does not occur (anovulatory cycles), and the lining of the womb becomes thickened by excessive estrogen production. This form of DUB is common just before the menopause. The time between periods becomes longer (up to six to eight weeks), but when the period comes it is very heavy, and can be associated with flooding.

Another problem that can occur in the few years before the menopause is a result of fluctuating levels of estrogen from the failing ovary. The result is more frequent periods, which may also be heavy, and flooding.

Investigation of persistent DUB is important to eliminate more serious causes (see later). If no physical cause is found, treatment is primarily directed at controlling bleeding. In women who have developed anemia, iron tablets may be prescribed in the short term. Very rarely, a blood transfusion may be necessary to replace blood that has been lost rapidly.

Simple medications that may be used to reduce the volume of heavy bleeds include non-steroidal anti-inflammatory drugs (NSAIDs) such as mefenamic acid. Tranexamic acid is a drug that inhibits the breakdown of blood clots, and this may be used to halt a heavy bleed, but must be avoided if the patient has any risk factors for thrombosis.

DUB can also be treated by means of hormonal drugs. Contraceptive methods can be helpful for many women. The oral contraceptive pill, the progesterone-containing intrauterine device, progesterone implants or injections will all control heavy bleeding. These treatments will, of course, also prevent pregnancy. In some women, withdrawal from these treatments after a few months may result in normalization of the periods.

Norethisterone is a synthetic progesterone (progestogen) that is commonly prescribed in cases of very severe bleeding to control premature breakdown of the womb lining. This is taken daily from day 5 to day 25 of the cycle. In most women this will keep a bleed at bay until the tablets are stopped. Withdrawal of the tablets on day 26 leads to a withdrawal bleed. This treatment is continued for four to six menstrual cycles, and may be sufficient in some women to normalize their periods.

In resistant cases, surgical treatments may be offered. Dilatation and curettage (D&C) is the surgical procedure in which the lining of the womb is scraped away with a curette. It is a low-risk procedure and can bring about a temporary (four to six months) relief from heavy bleeding. This procedure carries risks of perforation and endometrial adhesions and is less commonly used where hysteroscopy (below) is an option.

A more permanent approach is to remove the lining of the uterus by heat or laser via a hysteroscope. This procedure, which requires a one- to two-day stay in hospital, is called endometrial ablation. This procedure causes sterility, but is less invasive than a hysterectomy. In about 80 percent of women who have this procedure there is either total loss of or a relative reduction in periods.

Hysterectomy is now performed less commonly for DUB because the recent developments of drug treatments, and in particular, the progestogen-releasing intrauterine system (Mirena) and endometrial ablation, are effective and are much less risky alternatives.

Uterine fibroids and endometrial polyps

The most common structural cause of menorrhagia is the presence of one or more fibroids. These are benign tumors of the uterine muscle, and are known to develop in up to 20 percent of women over the age of 30, although very often they do not give rise to symptoms. In some women fibroids are associated with menorrhagia and dysmenorrhea. Endometrial polyps are fleshy outgrowths of the endometrial lining, which may also be associated with menorrhagia.

Pelvic inflammatory disease (PID)

Pelvic inflammatory disease (PID) is a chronic inflammatory condition of the lining of the womb, which is a long-term consequence of infection by a sexually transmitted disease. Menorrhagia can be a complication of PID.

Hypothyroidism

Hypothyroidism is an endocrine cause of menorrhagia. It must not be forgotten as a possibility, as it has profound health consequences, but is readily treatable.

Metrorrhagia

Metrorrhagia is the term used to describe bleeding that has no regular pattern. In some cases it may be difficult to differentiate between metrorrhagia and DUB with irregular spotting either side of a regular period.

Metrorrhagia should be investigated seriously as it may indicate a serious structural problem of the endometrium or cervix, and in particular, cancer.

Information box 5.2c-II

Menorrhagia: comments from a Chinese medicine perspective

In Chinese medicine, menorrhagia can be classified according to the pattern of bleeding. These patterns are: heavy periods, flooding and trickling, long periods and bleeding between periods. The causes of these may either be Full or Empty. Empty conditions include Qi Deficiency, Kidney (and Liver) Yin Deficiency with Empty Heat, and Spleen and Kidney Yang Deficiency. Full conditions include Qi and Blood Stagnation, Blood Heat and Damp Heat.

Metrorrhagia can be classified within the pattern of irregular periods. Causes of irregular periods include Liver Qi Stagnation, Kidney Yin Deficiency and Kidney Yang Deficiency. Maciocia (1998) explains that as regularity of menstruation depends upon a "rhythmic ebb and flow of Blood and Essence" then the Kidneys and Liver are always implicated in irregular bleeding.[15]

Premenstrual syndrome (PMS)

Premenstrual syndrome (PMS) is a functional condition that involves low mood and uncomfortable physical symptoms. PMS occurs from any time in the second half of the menstrual cycle (between ovulation and the first few days of menstruation). PMS is more common between the ages of 30 and 40. At the onset of menstruation, or during the period, the symptoms disappear and the woman may even feel euphoric for a few days. The symptoms of low mood and physical discomfort start again after ovulation. It is estimated that up to 8 percent of women experience PMS-related symptoms and that in up to 20 percent of these the mood and physical disturbances of PMS are so severe as to disturb day-to-day living and personal relationships, and to lead them to seek medical help.[16]

The perimenstrual syndrome is a particular pattern of PMS that is described as occurring in the two to three days prior to menstruation.

The emotional and mental symptoms of PMS include irritability, anxiety, depression, tearfulness and confusion. Sweet cravings may be prominent in some people. Physical symptoms include abdominal bloating, breast tenderness, swelling of the ankles, headache, nausea and clumsiness.

In perimenstrual syndrome, the most common symptoms are tiredness and headache in the two days prior to menstruation. Migraine can occur during this time in some women. There may also be bloating and abdominal pain.

The cause of PMS is not clearly understood. Theories that propose a hormonal cause have not been consistently supported by experimental measurement of hormone fluctuations in women with PMS. Recent theories propose that the primary issue is serotonin deficiency, and that this leads to extreme sensitivity to hormone-related changes in the menstrual cycle.

Treatment of PMS ideally should begin with lifestyle advice. Dealing with stress is probably the most important, but in many cases, this is the most difficult lifestyle factor to deal with. In some women, normalization of diet and adoption of whole foods can be very helpful. Regular exercise can also be very beneficial for some people.

Vitamin B6 (pyridoxine) and oil of evening primrose are two relatively natural prescribed medications that can be of help for some people. The drug bromocriptine may also be useful in reducing symptoms of breast tenderness.

For some women the regular cycle induced by the oral contraceptive pill can be helpful, presumably because it provides a regular level of (synthetic) estrogen and progesterone.

Selective serotonin reuptake inhibitor (SSRI) antidepressants taken in the second half of the cycle may also be useful in some women.

Agnus castus fruit extract is a herbal remedy that has good scientific evidence supporting the fact that it can be of help in up to 50 percent of people.[17]

If the problem is very severe, some women are offered surgical treatment. The most invasive approach is to remove the womb and both ovaries and then treat with HRT.

which begin after the onset of menstruation and usually last for less than 24 hours. They may be so severe as to lead to vomiting. Up to three-quarters of young women experience some form of primary dysmenorrhea. The problem usually improves as the woman gets older, and may be markedly better after childbirth.

Secondary dysmenorrhea, by definition, has an underlying physical cause. The most common causes are endometriosis or pelvic inflammatory disease (PID). Fibroids may also be a cause of secondary dysmenorrhea. Secondary dysmenorrhea tends to begin a few days before the onset of menstruation and can continue throughout the period of bleeding. In practice, it may be difficult to distinguish primary from secondary dysmenorrhea on the basis of symptoms alone.

Drug treatment of dysmenorrhea involves two main approaches. Suppression of ovulation by means of an estrogen and progesterone (combined) oral contraceptive may be preferred by many young women who also desire an effective contraceptive method. The progesterone-only pill may also be effective in minimizing menstrual blood loss and pain even without suppressing ovulation. Increasingly the long-acting progesterone-only contraceptives, and in particular, the levonorgestrel-containing intrauterine system (Mirena), are chosen to suppress menstrual bleeding and pain. Alternatively, non-steroidal anti-inflammatory drugs (NSAIDs) may be very effective in reducing the intensity of the pain. Commonly prescribed NSAIDs include mefenamic acid and ibuprofen.

Information box 5.2c-III

Premenstrual syndrome: comments from a Chinese medicine perspective[18]

In Chinese medicine, PMS may be the outward manifestation of Full or Empty patterns. The Full patterns are Liver Qi Stagnation and Phlegm Fire Harassing Upwards. The Empty patterns are Liver and/or Heart Blood Deficiency, Liver and Kidney Yin Deficiency, and Spleen and Kidney Yang Deficiency. Emotional strain, overwork and a Phlegm-forming diet are key etiological factors.

Dysmenorrhea

Dysmenorrhea is painful menstruation. This can be classified into two broad types, which may overlap. The first type, primary dysmenorrhea, classically starts shortly after the menarche and peaks between the ages of 15 and 25. In primary dysmenorrhea there are severe crampy pains,

---

Information box 5.2c-IV

Dysmenorrhea: comments from a Chinese medicine perspective

In Chinese medicine, dysmenorrhea is the result of insufficient menstrual Blood or poor movement of the Blood. According to Maciocia (1998),[19] the Empty patterns that are associated with dysmenorrhea include: Qi and Blood Deficiency, Yang and Blood Deficiency and Kidney and Liver Yin Deficiency. The Full patterns include Stagnation of Qi, Blood Stagnation, Stagnation of Cold, Damp Heat with Blood Heat, and Liver Qi Stagnation turning to Fire (Full patterns). Even the Empty patterns will be complicated by Qi or Blood Stagnation for pain to become apparent. For this reason, emotions that negatively affect the Liver are very much implicated in the pathology of dysmenorrhea. Other factors that predispose to Stagnation in the Uterus are Cold and Damp, and the deficiency that results from overwork, poor diet and childbirth.

Problems during the menopause

The menopause and the climacteric, the period of time within which the menopause occurs, are natural physiological events, and like the menarche represent a time of transition from one stage of reproductive life to another. Although it occurs at a time in life when the body functions associated with fertility are ceasing to be active, a healthy climacteric should not be dominated by negative symptoms. Studies indicate that up to 25 percent of Western women have no symptoms during the menopause. However, 35 percent have mild to moderate symptoms and 40 percent suffer from severe symptoms.[20] This is in contrast to the findings from studies of women across the world. In some cultural groups the menopause marks a transition to a stage in life that offers more freedom and respect. In these cultures the symptoms reported are of far less concern to the women. Hot flashes seem to be in particular a Western woman's concern.[21]

Hot flashes (hot flushes)

Hot flashes are attributed to the response of the body to dropping levels of estrogen. During the flash there is often a feeling of heat centered on the face, which can then spread to other parts of the body. The flash lasts for up to 3 minutes, and may be associated with a rise in temperature. At their worst, hot flashes may lead to sweating at night, with loss of sleep and tiredness in the day. Many other less specific symptoms, including aching joints, headaches, palpitations, dizziness, irritability and depression, may also be experienced.

Hot flashes can begin some years before the menopause, but peak one to two years before the periods stop. They may also persist for years after the menopause.

Vaginal dryness

Vaginal symptoms tend to occur later in the climacteric than hot flashes. The most usual complaint is of dryness or burning. Some women experience painful intercourse, which can have a considerable effect on intimate relationships.

The changes in the epithelium of the vagina also affect the urethra, and this can have the consequence of recurrent urinary tract infections. These changes, together with laxity of the muscles of the pelvic floor, can lead to urinary incontinence (usually stress incontinence).

Ischemic heart disease and osteoporosis

These more long-term problems that can follow the menopause are due to the reduction in the protective effect of estrogen on the arteries and the bones.

Psychological effects of the menopause

Emotional symptoms, including anxiety and depression, are common during the climacteric. The fact that these are more prominent in women from Westernized cultures suggests that there is a culture-based perceived threat of what will happen after the menopause. This may be a result of the emphasis in modern cultures on the importance of youthfulness and vitality, and the decreasing emphasis on the importance of the wisdom that comes with age and experience.

Studies suggest that patterns of sexual desire and drive may not be significantly changed in most women after the menopause, but that in a minority of women they are impaired. According to one North American study, being troubled by low desire was an issue for 10 percent of young women, 12 percent of perimenopausal women and 7 percent of women over 65.[22] These figures suggest that the majority of menopausal women are not troubled by changes in sexual desire. Deterioration in sexual satisfaction is more likely if a woman's satisfaction with her sex life was not so good prior to the menopause. Not all changes in sexual satisfaction in middle life are solely due to the menopause. In the menopause years there may also be a marked change in sexual drive and sexual responsiveness of the male partner, which will, of course, impact on the sex life of perimenopausal women in heterosexual relationships. This is the consequence of a decline in the levels of testosterone, which begins approximately after the age of 50.

Diagnosis of the menopause

As the menopause approaches, the ovary becomes less responsive to the pituitary hormones, and so produces less estrogen. The pituitary response to this is to produce more FSH. As the woman approaches the menopause, the FSH starts to spike, consistent high levels of which are diagnostic of impending ovarian failure.

For this reason, many doctors will choose to test for FSH levels in order to confirm that symptoms such as hot flashes or mood swings are the result of failing ovaries. However, in most women the diagnosis is obvious from the age of the woman and the clinical picture alone. In these cases a blood test is unnecessary. Moreover the FSH does not prove a consistently high level, but instead it will indicate what the FSH level is at the point of the blood test, and so cannot in itself confirm menopause. The FSH test is more useful for excluding possible perimenopause in women younger than the age of 40 who are experiencing menstrual irregularities.

Hormone replacement therapy (HRT)

HRT used to be commonly prescribed to counteract the major menopausal symptoms, which include hot flashes and vaginal dryness, and to prevent the long-term complication of osteoporosis. These symptoms and complications result from the declining levels of estrogen from the failing ovaries, and by providing estrogen HRT counteracts this decline.

However, this pattern of prescribing was affected in 2002–03 by analyses of studies of large numbers of women taking HRT, namely, the Women's Health Initiative and the

Million Women Study. These seemed to suggest that the benefits of HRT in terms of protection from osteoporotic fracture and colorectal cancer were outweighed by an increase in incidence of breast cancer, strokes and cardiovascular disease. For this reason, HRT ceased to be prescribed as a first-line treatment for the prevention of the development of postmenopausal osteoporosis. Since that time the figures from these studies have been examined in more detail, and the current view is that HRT is likely to be of more benefit than risk to women below the age of 60, and it is in older women that the adverse consequences of HRT are concentrated. HRT is still widely recommended and prescribed, but knowledge of the risks has resulted in it being less widely used than before 2002.

HRT is currently considered to offer benefits in terms of stopping hot flashes, improving mood and sleep, reversing vaginal dryness and urinary symptoms, maintaining bone strength, reduction in colorectal cancer, and may possibly even protect against Alzheimer's disease and coronary artery disease when taken before the age of 60.[23]

The significant risks are still recognized to be promotion of breast cancer, strokes, thrombotic events, ovarian cancer, endometrial cancer and gallbladder disease, but these are considered to be outweighed by the benefits.

The therapeutically significant part of HRT consists of a synthetic or naturally derived form of estrogen. As it is not healthy for the uterus to be exposed to estrogen alone (as unopposed estrogen can promote the development of endometrial cancer), most preparations also contain a synthetic progesterone-like compound known as a progestogen. This additional progestogen is only necessary for those women who have an intact uterus. Those who have had a hysterectomy can be prescribed estrogen-only HRT.

HRT comes in the form of tablets, skin patches or implants. In women with an intact uterus who are still menstruating, the treatment may be prescribed so that a period is induced every 28 days. In this case the treatment consists of a regular daily dose of estrogen, and a dose of progestogen to be taken on only up to half of the days of the cycle. The period is, in fact, a withdrawal bleed that follows the start of the time when the progestogen is not taken. In women who have stopped menstruating, a steady combination of estrogen and progestogen is prescribed to minimize the tendency for the endometrium to build up under the influence of estrogen, and so the risk of any bleeding is minimized.

Before prescription of HRT the doctor needs to ensure that the woman is in good health. In particular, HRT is not advisable if there is any evidence of breast or endometrial cancer, liver disease or a history of recent thromboembolism. The blood pressure is checked, because in some women HRT may cause a rise in blood pressure.

HRT is recommended for a maximum of ten years only, although five is now considered an ideal time period for its use. After this time women are encouraged to wean off the medication to prevent a sudden return of menopausal symptoms.

Postmenopausal bleeding

An unexplained episode of bleeding after the menopause (postmenopausal bleeding) is a red flag of cervical or endometrial cancer, and needs to be referred for investigation. If the woman is on cyclical HRT, postmenstrual bleeding would be defined as any bleeding that occurred outside the time of the usual withdrawal bleed. Cervical or endometrial cancers together are the cause of one-fifth of postmenopausal bleeds. Less worrying causes include cervical polyps (fleshy outgrowths) and inflammation of the vaginal lining. Intermenstrual bleeding in premenopausal women is much more likely to have a benign cause, but nevertheless must be referred for investigation if persistent or significant in volume.

 Information box 5.2c-V

The menopause and hormone replacement therapy: comments from a Chinese medicine perspective

According to Chinese medicine, the menopause is the natural consequence of the decline in Jing that occurs in seven-year cycles in women. Hence the natural age of the menopause would be expected to be at 49. Studies of groups of women from diverse cultures all confirm that the median age of the menopause is 50–51, and, unlike the declining age of menarche, this age has not changed over the centuries.

The menopause does not always present with a disease pattern. When it does, the symptoms of the menopausal syndrome are considered in general to be a consequence of the Decline in the Jing, in its Yin and/or Yang aspect, although Kidney Deficiency may also be combined with excess patterns.

The patterns that are associated with menopausal symptoms include Kidney Yin Deficiency, Kidney Yang Deficiency, Kidney and Liver Yin Deficiency with Liver Yang Rising, Kidneys and Heart not harmonized, Accumulation of Phlegm and Stagnation of Qi, and Blood Stagnation. Emotional stress plays a significant role in determining whether menopausal symptoms arise. Other factors that will impact on the experience of menopause are overworking, depletion during pregnancy and childbirth and dietary imbalance.[24]

HRT can benefit symptoms presumably because estrogen is nourishing to the Spleen and to Yin (the Yin aspect of Essence), as evidenced by its beneficial effect on fleshiness and fertility. However, this effect is suppressive, and it may generate its benefits at the expense of drawing on deep reserves of Spleen Qi, Kidney Yin and Jing. The progestogen in HRT is often blamed for the common side effects, which include headaches, fluid retention and weight gain. This suggests that progestogens (together with estrogens) tend to cause Accumulation of Damp and Qi Stagnation. This fits with the physiological effect they have of causing the lining of the womb to become thicker and more edematous. It is only on withdrawal of the progestogen that breakdown of this thick lining occurs and bleeding takes place. There is also an increased risk of blood clots and breast, ovarian and womb cancer with HRT, which suggest that HRT may induce Stagnation and/or Accumulation of Phlegm on a background of Kidney Deficiency.

The red flags of disorders of menstruation and the menopause

Some patients with disorders of menstruation and the menopause will benefit from referral to a conventional doctor for assessment or treatment. Red flags are those symptoms and signs that indicate that referral should be considered. The red flags of disorders of menstruation are described in Table 5.2c-I. A summary of the red flags in a format designed for quick reference in clinical practice can be found in Appendix III. This gives advice on the degree of urgency of referral for each of the red flag conditions listed.

Table 5.2c-I A34: Red flags of disorders of menstruation and the menopause

Red flag	Description	Reasoning
A34.1	Primary amenorrhea: onset of periods delayed until after age 16	Refer any girl for investigation who has not achieved first menstruation by age 16
A34.2	Secondary amenorrhea: for >6 months	Refer if there have been no periods for 6 months
A34.3	Menorrhagia: with features of severe anemia (tiredness, breathlessness, palpitations on exertion)	Menorrhagia (heavy periods) can be the sole cause of significant anemia, and merits prompt referral for investigation and treatment of the cause Menorrhagia may result from fibroids, endometriosis or an ovarian cyst
A34.4	Metrorrhagia: bleeding between periods that has no regular pattern. This includes postcoital bleeding (bleeding after intercourse)	Irregular periods are common, but bleeding that seems to fall outside the normal confines of a 2–5 day menstrual bleed might, rarely, signify a uterine or cervical tumor In younger women, unexpected bleeding is more likely to signify a sexually transmitted disease, most commonly chlamydia Breakthrough bleeding is common in women on the contraceptive pill, but this usually falls into a regular pattern Refer for further investigation if this happens on more than two occasions
A34.5	Postmenopausal bleeding: any unexplained bleeding after the menopause	Predictable bleeding after the menopause is normal with hormone replacement therapy (HRT) Otherwise, any episode of postmenopausal bleeding is a red flag for uterine or cervical tumor. Other causes include uterine polyps
A34.6	Vaginal discharge: after menopause	Vaginal discharge is not normal after the menopause, particularly if offensive or blood-stained. Refer to exclude infection or carcinoma

A34.7	Vaginal discharge: before puberty	Vaginal discharge is not normal before puberty, particularly if offensive or blood-stained. However, the cause is usually benign resulting from over-growth of yeasts or bacteria. Rarely it may be a marker of abuse. Always refer for medical advice (see A40.34)
A34.8	Vaginal discharge: in fertile years	It is normal for there to be a cyclical production of a non-offensive creamy vaginal discharge that peaks in volume around the time of ovulation
		If the discharge becomes offensive or itchy, this may be a sign of bacterial or yeast over-growth and could indicate a sexually transmitted infection
		A patient with unusual discharge can have a confidential consultation at a genitourinary medicine (GUM) clinic, or see the GP for testing (see A35.1)
A34.9	Vaginal itch (if prolonged)	Vaginal itch is a common side effect of thrush (candidiasis) and sensitivity to soaps and bath products, so refer only if prolonged for >1 week and not responding to advice and simple treatment
		Consider the possibility of atrophic vaginitis in postmenopausal women. This can respond to hormone creams
		Also, rarely, itch can develop due to lichen sclerosus and vulval cancer
		Consider the possibility of abuse in children (see A40.34). Always refer children with this symptom for investigation

5.2d Sexual health and sexually transmitted disease

The term sexual health is used conventionally to embrace both the physical and psychological aspects of sexuality. For there to be good sexual health, sexual relationships should be physically and emotionally satisfying for both partners, and they should also carry no risk of unwanted pregnancy or transmission of disease.

Sexual dysfunctions

It is increasingly recognized that sexual satisfaction does not necessarily depend on both partners experiencing all the stages of the sexual experience described in Section 5.2a. However, lack of satisfaction with sexual experience is common. The problem often lies in a combination of unrealistic expectations of what should happen, and a lack of communication between the partners. For example, it may be expected that women should always achieve orgasm during penile intercourse, when in fact this is only possible for 25 percent of women. Other factors that can affect satisfaction in sexual performance include low sex drive, performance anxiety, chronic illness, alcohol or drug abuse, and prescribed medication. Even if these factors are ruled out, sexual dissatisfaction is very often a marker of a problem in the relationship between the sexual partners rather than an isolated sexual problem.

There are a number of specific sexual dysfunctions that may also be the result of one or more of these factors that affect sexual experience. A sex therapist is a psychiatric practitioner who is skilled in the diagnosis of these dysfunctions, and who can offer treatments, which range from simple education and couple counseling to prescription of medication. However, because of embarrassment, most of these dysfunctions are not discussed with health professionals, and so many people do not have access to the support that might benefit them.

Low sex drive (lack of libido) and impotence

Sexual drive varies markedly between individuals. A low sex drive is not necessarily a sign of a dysfunction. Sex drive normally declines with age, and particularly so for men over the age of 50. In general, low libido is believed to affect women more than men. One recent study of students suggests that up to 10 percent of women and 5 percent of men have very low incidence of sexual fantasies or desire for sexual activity.[25] Increasingly low libido, if lifelong, is being recognized as a sexual orientation (termed asexuality) and as such is not a sexual dysfunction.

Sex drive is influenced by psychological factors. A new onset of reduced sex drive can be a manifestation of a deteriorating relationship or depression. Traumatic sexual experiences in the past can have a great impact on sex drive.

Impotence is the inability to achieve orgasm, and often includes the inability to maintain an erection in men (erectile dysfunction). Lack of libido and impotence may go together, but not always. Isolated erectile dysfunction (ED) with no lack of libido is more likely to have an underlying physical cause.

An important physical cause of low sexual drive and ED is chronic illness, particularly if the illness affects a part of the body that is associated with sexuality, such as the prostate, breast or the cervix. Certain chronic diseases, such as diabetes and peripheral vascular disease, can lead to ED because they result in impairment of blood and nervous supply to the genital regions. Endocrine disease such as Addison's disease or hypothyroidism may directly affect libido by affecting the secretion of pituitary hormones. Recreational drugs, including alcohol and heroin, are well known to reduce libido and lead to ED. It may be possible to link a recent onset of loss of sex drive with a prescription of medication. Drugs that are well known to cause low sex drive and/or impotence include diuretics, beta blockers and the newer forms of antidepressants.

For men who experience ED, medical or physical methods may be recommended to aid maintenance of erection. A drug from the phosphodiesterase-5 inhibitor family, such as sildenafil citrate (Viagra) or tadalafil, may be prescribed. A single dose can be taken by mouth about an hour before intercourse to increase penile blood flow. Both these treatments carry the risk of inducing a painful sustained erection, which may require emergency treatment. These treatments are not advisable in those who have coronary heart disease or who are taking nitrate medication.

A simple physical approach to ED is a plastic pump device that encourages erection by means of suction to a vacuum chamber held around the penis. The erection is maintained by means of a ring applied to the base of the penis. Up to 74 percent of patients who use this aid achieve orgasm.

Neither of these methods will directly improve an underlying lack of libido, unless the reduced libido was a result of the emotional response to ED.

Premature ejaculation

In premature ejaculation, the man fails to sustain an erection because ejaculation occurs either before or just after penetration. This problem usually has an emotional cause, often rooted in performance anxiety, and can respond well to sex therapy.

Dyspareunia

Dyspareunia refers to painful intercourse in women and is a relatively common condition that can lead to a complete loss of sexual activity. Dyspareunia may have medical causes. Inflammation of the womb or ovaries in conditions such as pelvic inflammatory disease (PID) or endometriosis will result in pain experienced during deep penile penetration (i.e. during thrusting). This problem, termed deep dyspareunia, is highly suggestive of an underlying physical problem. However, problems in the vagina, such as postmenopausal dryness and vaginal infections, can cause pain very early in penetration. This problem is termed superficial dyspareunia.

Superficial dyspareunia can also result from lack of lubrication and insufficient relaxation of the perineal muscles at the time of attempted penetration. This may be because penetration has been attempted before the woman is aroused. The pain that results can cause a negative cycle of loss of sexual desire and increased tension.

Vaginismus is the term given to a severe form of spasm that affects the perineal muscles at the time of penetration. Vaginismus may totally prevent penetration. Factors such as lack of sexual knowledge, guilt about sexuality and a childhood sexual assault may be underlying issues in a woman who suffers from these functional causes of superficial dyspareunia.

In dyspareunia, any underlying physical cause should be treated first. Sex therapy counseling and the self-insertion of vaginal dilators of graded size can be effective in non-physically (functional) based dyspareunia.

 Information box 5.2d-I

Impotence: comments from a Chinese medicine perspective

In Chinese medicine, impotence is usually attributed to Kidney Deficiency. During erection Blood and Qi Essence from the Kidneys accumulate in the Penis and during intercourse Yang is exchanged for the female partner's Yin. The Liver Organ plays a role in the sexual act in the moving of Qi. The Liver Channel circulates around the genitals to support their function. Deficient Kidneys and Stagnation of Liver Qi will both impair sexual function.

Lack of sexual drive indicates a Deficiency of the Fire of the Gate of Life (Ming Men), which is an expression of Kidney Yang. Excessive sexual activity will Deplete Blood and Kidney Qi in the man and lead to Deficiency of this Ministerial Fire. Other factors that can impair the Ministerial Fire are the emotions of fear or fright, the frustration that Stagnates Liver Qi and worry which impair the function of the Spleen and Heart and which affect the health of the Blood. Damp Heat from diet (including alcohol) can also congeal in the Liver meridian and impair erectile function.[26]

Non-physical dyspareunia has features that suggest Stagnation of Liver Qi and Blood.

Sexually transmitted disease (STD)

Sexually transmitted disease (STD) is the term given to infections acquired through sexual intercourse. Increasingly, the term genitourinary (GU) infection is used in preference to STD, because the term STD may be stigmatizing. Also, not all sexually transmitted diseases are acquired solely by sexual intercourse.

Since the emergence of HIV (human immunodeficiency virus) infection in the 1980s, there has been increasing emphasis on the prevention of STDs by means of safe sex practices. The first message of safe sex is that it is always possible that one or both partners may be carrying infections that can be transmitted during intercourse. Therefore, unless it is within the context of a long-term relationship, patients are always counseled to take precautions if planning to have intercourse. Ideally, promiscuity should be minimized. Condoms are considered to be the best barrier method for protecting both men and women who practice penile, oral and anal sex. The cap, spermicidal creams and the oral contraceptive pill also carry a degree of protection, but should not be relied on solely as effective barriers to disease.

In the UK, the Department of Health coordinates the promotion of the messages of safe sex. These messages are propagated to the general public via family planning clinics, GUM clinics, abortion advice centers, general medical practices, schools and the media.

The infections discussed in this section are:

- Vulvovaginal and penile infections:
  - genital herpes
  - genital warts
  - syphilis
  - infections that cause vaginal discharge
- Infections of the internal genital organs:
  - gonorrhea
  - chlamydia
  - pelvic inflammatory disease (PID)
- General infections due to sexual transfer of body fluids.

Vulvovaginal and penile infections

GENITAL HERPES

Genital herpes is caused by transmission of the herpes simplex virus (HSV). This is the same type of virus that causes cold sores on the mouth and nose. However, in most genital cases, the actual strain of HSV is different from the one that most commonly causes cold sores.

The first (primary) attack of genital herpes is usually the worst. In this primary infection, a crop of itchy and painful sores develop on the vulva and the vagina or the head (glans) of the penis usually about 7–14 days after exposure to the virus. The patient is unwell, with a fever, and there may be tender enlarged lymph glands in the groin. Urination may be difficult. Sometimes these symptoms occur only after a long delay (i.e. years) after the first exposure.

Exposure to the virus is very common. One in ten people carry the genital strain of HSV, but not everyone who is exposed will generate the painful symptoms. The prevalence of HSV carriage suggests that nevertheless it is very transmissible. Many carriers of HSV are oblivious of the fact that they might potentially transmit an STD through sexual contact.

The infection heals over the next seven days with crusting of the spots. Thirty percent of people experience recurrence of the attack (secondary herpes), as the virus is never fully cleared from the body. The attack is usually limited to a smaller area of the genital organs and is often progressively less painful in each recurrence. Less than half of the people who have had primary genital herpes have more than one recurrent attack. Recurrence is more common in the second half of the menstrual cycle, during periods of stress and in hot weather.

The person is only infectious during an attack and its recovery phase. Recurrent herpes is a very serious condition during pregnancy, as it can severely infect a baby during delivery. If a woman goes into labor with active herpes, a cesarean section is advised. In severe cases, antiviral drugs (including aciclovir) may be prescribed on a long-term basis to prevent attacks. However, in most cases these are not prescribed, and the recurrence subsides naturally within a few days.[27]

 Information box 5.2d-II

Genital herpes: comments from a Chinese medicine perspective

In Chinese medicine, the symptoms of genital herpes correspond to Wind Damp Heat. It primarily affects the Liver Channel. Local Deficiency of Blood and Kidney Qi will predispose to recurrent attacks.

GENITAL WARTS

Genital warts are the result of infection by certain strains of the human papilloma virus (HPV). The genital wart strains (most commonly HPV6 and HPV11) are different from those strains of HPV that cause bodily warts (which occur most commonly on the hands and knees). The virus causes a benign growth of epithelial tissue, which develops into cauliflower-shaped bumps on the vulva, vagina, cervix and penis, and also around the anus. The genital wart, like the bodily wart, is painless, and, especially in women, may not be noticed by the patient. Sometimes the patient complains of itching or burning from the area where warts have developed.

HPV infection is very common; up to 30 percent of sexually active adults have evidence of current or past infection. The infection is clinically important because particular strains of HPV (subtypes 16, 18 and 33) are known to induce precancerous changes in mucosal cells of the cervix, penis and oral cavity, even when no warts are apparent. For this reason, HPV testing is performed as part of cervical screening protocols.

HPV carriage is very common after initial infection, but most women develop immunity to the virus and clear the infection completely. In a minority carriage of the virus is prolonged over years, and it is these people who are more vulnerable to cancerous change. There is no known treatment for HPV carriage except for regular screening for precancerous change.

Warts can be treated by repeated weekly application of the drug podophyllin, which burns the wart away. The patient can apply a weaker form of this drug on a daily basis in between clinic visits to maximize the chances of cure. Imiquinod cream is an alternative topical preparation that may be prescribed for self-treatment. Larger warts can be burned by means of a laser or heat probe, or frozen by means of a liquid nitrogen spray. Recurrence of the warts is common after both these treatments.

Information box 5.2d-III

Genital warts: comments from a Chinese medicine perspective

In Chinese medicine, the genital wart is viewed as a manifestation of Toxic Damp and Heat. Chronic Spleen and Kidney Deficiency will predispose to infection. In the long term the Toxic Damp can lead to Stagnation and Blood Stasis and this is the causation of cancerous change. Wang and Prodoehl (2016) explain that "those who smoke, endure excessive stress, overwork, indulge in sexual activity with multiple partners, and use the contraceptive pill long term are the ones who tend to suffer from spleen and kidney deficiency," and so are vulnerable to chronic HPV infection.[28]

HPV vaccination can prevent infection by particular virus subtypes, and is ideally administered before the individual is sexually active. The Gardasil vaccine induces immunity to the strains most likely to induce cancerous change (HPV16 and 18) and also genital warts (HPV6 and 11). In the UK this vaccine is offered currently only to teenage girls as part of the national vaccine program. There is a strong argument for making the vaccine available to boys as well, particularly as it is increasingly recognized that

HPV infection is implicated not only in cervical cancer but also in penile and oral cancer.

SYPHILIS

Syphilis is caused by infection with the bacterium *Treponema pallidum*. Partly because of access to adequate antibiotic therapy, it is now a relatively rare condition in the UK. However, it is still common in developing countries and, worryingly, its incidence is rising sharply in the developed world.

Infection with syphilis occurs in three stages. The primary stage is called a chancre, a thickened lump that forms in the genital area within two to twelve weeks of sexual contact with an infected person. The skin on top of the chancre breaks down, but is often painless. It is this stage that is highly infectious, but like genital warts, it is often unnoticed by the patient.

After healing of the chancre there may be a delay of some weeks before the appearance of secondary syphilis. In most people there is a flu-like illness, with swollen lymph nodes, a characteristic skin rash, and the development of warty genital lumps. In some cases there might be more severe inflammation of a deep organ, such as hepatitis or meningitis.

Secondary syphilis will abate after three to twelve weeks if untreated, but can recur, due to persistence of the organism, in a more severe form as tertiary syphilis. In this stage the infection can cause large ulcerating lumps, called gummas, in a wide range of tissues. The heart and blood vessels can be affected, and a form of dementia (neurosyphilis) may develop. The condition termed general paralysis of the insane, familiar in the setting of Victorian asylums, was a result of the combined features of untreated syphilis.

These later stages of syphilis are now very rare in developed countries because the earlier stages respond well to treatment with a one-month course of penicillin or doxycycline.

Information box 5.2d-IV

Syphilis: comments from a Chinese medicine perspective

In Chinese medicine, the formation of warty lumps in all three stages of syphilis suggests that the underlying pathology is similar to HPV with the generation of Toxic Damp. The recurrence of the condition in a flu-like secondary form suggests that Toxic Heat is also present from the primary infection. The profound disturbances seen in tertiary syphilis indicates that the presence of these persistent pathogens has led to Accumulation of Damp Phlegm, Transformation into Fire and eventual Depletion of Yin and Yang of diverse Organs, and in particular, the Lung, Spleen, Liver and Kidney.

Vaginal discharge

Vaginal discharge is a common complaint, but may be physiological rather than the result of an infection. Physiological discharge is odorless, does not cause itch and varies in quantity throughout the cycle. Nevertheless, it may be profuse and a source of embarrassment or discomfort. Benign changes of the cervix, called cervical erosions, and fleshy cervical polyps may be physical causes of excessive physiological discharge. Both these problems can be treated fairly simply in an outpatient procedure that involves a colposcopy.

A serious cause of vaginal discharge is vaginal, cervical or uterine cancer. In these cases the discharge is more likely to be of recent onset, varying in a way that is not related to the menstrual cycle, and may be smelly or blood stained. A discharge fitting this description should always be taken seriously, but particularly so in postmenopausal women, in whom these cancers are more common.

Candida (yeast) infection (thrush)

Candida is the most common infectious cause of vaginal discharge. As yeasts form about 5 percent of the healthy organisms in the vagina, a candidal yeast infection usually represents an overgrowth of these yeasts rather than a new infection. Candidal infection in women usually arises internally, but can also be sexually transmitted. In contrast, sexual transmission is a common cause of genital candidal infection in men.

Candida develops very readily in some people, who may suffer from recurrent bouts. In susceptible people, an outbreak may be triggered by sexual intercourse, tight clothing, over-washing, use of a different soap or a course of antibiotics. However, serious underlying causes, including immunodeficiency and diabetes mellitus, must be excluded in people who suffer from recurrent episodes.

Genital thrush causes itchy plaques of white discharge that may overlie red inflamed areas of epithelium. The itch can be intensely irritating, particularly in women, and may cause difficulty in urination.

Conventional treatment of *candida* infection is with antifungal medication. In a mild case, application of a cream containing clotrimazole may be sufficient to alleviate the symptoms. In more severe cases, this drug can be administered by means of a course of vaginal tablets (pessaries). Recurrent thrush may be treated with oral antifungal medication. Fluconazole is the most commonly prescribed preparation. Some women rely on recurrent treatments with these antifungal medications to keep their symptoms at bay.

Gardnerella infection (bacterial vaginosis)

Gardnerella infection is another example of an overgrowth of healthy organisms. *Gardnerella vaginalis* is a bacterium that comprises up to 30 percent of the normal population of bacteria in a healthy vagina. In overgrowth, this bacterium causes the discharge to become more watery, and to have a characteristic fishy smell. This condition has been termed bacterial vaginosis (BV). There is usually no discomfort in BV. It is recognized that pregnant women with BV are more likely to go into premature labor, and this has led to debate about whether women with BV should be treated early in labor with antibiotics.

Treatment of BV is with a single high dose of the antibiotic metronidazole (Flagyl) or with a five-day course of lower dose of the same antibiotic if in pregnancy.

Trichomonas infection

Trichomonas vaginalis is a bacterium that comprises up to 7 percent of the healthy bacterial population in the vagina. *Trichomonas* infection is another form of bacterial overgrowth that may also be sexually transmitted. It causes a moderate to profuse discharge, which can cause intense itching in women. If severe, the discharge can have a green and frothy appearance.

Treatment of *trichomonas* infection involves a one-week course of metronidazole. The male partner may be advised also to take this antibiotic to prevent reinfection of his partner.

Information box 5.2d-V

Vaginal discharge: comments from a Chinese medicine perspective

In Chinese medicine, vaginal discharge (leukorrhea) represents Damp in the Lower Jiao. Itching, redness and a colored or smelly discharge all suggest Damp Heat, whereas white, watery discharges are more suggestive of Damp Cold. If a vaginal discharge is bloody and thick and associated with other signs of Full Heat, it may be attributed to the more profound disturbance of Toxic Heat. An underlying Deficiency of Kidney Qi or Spleen Qi (with or without Liver Qi Stagnation) will predispose to thin discharges and the presence of Pathogenic Factors to thicker discharges.[29]

Infections of the internal genital organs

Gonorrhea

Gonorrhea is caused by infection with the bacterium *Neisseria gonorrheae* (gonococcus). In women, the infection initially presents with urinary symptoms and a vaginal discharge. There is a risk of transmitting the infection to a baby during labor, in which case a severe form of conjunctivitis can result.

In men, there may also be urinary symptoms, and a slight pus-like discharge from the urethra. This condition is called urethritis. Urethritis may be caused by a number of organisms in addition to the gonococcus.

In many of these initial infections, particularly in women, symptoms may be so mild that they are ignored. This means that there is high risk of transmission of the infection at this stage. The real problems of gonorrhea come if the infection spreads internally. In women, the next site of infection is the cervical canal, and thence the lining of the uterus. This can lead to the chronic condition known as pelvic inflammatory disease (PID). In men the gonococcus can spread to cause a chronic infection of the prostate, epididymis and the testes. Occasionally, the infection can enter the bloodstream. A feverish illness develops, characterized by painful joints and a widespread rash. This form of gonorrhea is more common in women.

Gonorrhea is treated by means of antibiotics. A single dose of the two antibiotics ceftriaxone and azithromycin is the recommended treatment for uncomplicated cases, but long courses of these antibiotics may be required to treat chronic infections including PID. Gonorrhea often coexists with chlamydia infection, so the antibiotics are chosen to cover for this infection also. Ideally, all sexual contacts should be traced and treated.

Information box 5.2d-VI

Gonorrhea: comments from a Chinese medicine perspective

In Chinese medicine, the symptoms of gonorrhea are attributed to Damp Heat in the Lower Jiao. In severe cases, gonorrhea can manifest as Wind Heat on the Exterior (rashes and fever) and Wind Damp (arthritis). Liver Qi Stagnation and Spleen Deficiency predispose to Damp Heat, and Kidney and Liver Deficiency predisposes to genital vulnerability and to Damp Heat manifesting in the Lower Jiao. Depending on the balance between Deficiency and Pathogenic Factor, all genital tract infections may either be predominantly Empty or predominantly Full; the nature of the symptoms and signs will inform the practitioner which aspect to treat as a priority.

CHLAMYDIA

Chlamydia trachomatis is an infection that commonly coexists with gonorrhea. It is a very common cause of urethritis (also known as non-gonococcal urethritis (NGU)). Like gonorrhea, chlamydia can ascend in the male urethra to cause prostatitis and epididymitis. In women, the infection can be a cause of discharge, but more importantly may spread via the cervical canal to be a cause of PID. If the

baby develops the infection during passage through the birth canal, conjunctivitis and pneumonia can result.

Chlamydia infections are treated with a different class of antibiotics to gonorrhea. Azithromycin or doxycycline are most commonly prescribed to be taken by mouth for between a single day and two weeks. Ideally, sexual contacts should be traced and treated.

Information box 5.2d-VII

Chlamydia: comments from a Chinese medicine perspective

In Chinese medicine, chlamydia infection, like gonorrhea, would also be a manifestation of Damp Heat in the Lower Jiao.

PELVIC INFLAMMATORY DISEASE (PID)

Pelvic inflammatory disease (PID) is the term given to the syndrome that arises as a result of chronic infection of the uterus, fallopian tubes and ovaries (the female internal genital organs). It is believed that over half of these infections are caused by chlamydia and a smaller proportion by gonococcus. However, there are a number of less common organisms that may also cause PID. Commonly PID develops without any preceding symptoms.

The risk of PID is reduced by use of barrier methods of contraception and the contraceptive pill, but the risk is increased in users of the intrauterine device (the coil).

The most common symptoms of an acute infection include severe abdominal tenderness and pain (with deep dyspareunia), and high fever. In an advanced infection, pus may collect in a fallopian tube, leading to a severe illness akin to appendicitis. Infection may also spread to the space surrounding the ovaries.

In its more chronic form, PID may lead to pelvic discomfort, particularly during intercourse, and a long-standing feeling of being unwell. There may be menorrhagia or secondary dysmenorrhea. Internally, the genital organs may become stuck together (with adhesions) and scarred.

A serious long-term consequence of acute and chronic PID is infertility, as the scarring and adhesions may prevent ovulation or implantation of the fertilized ovum. Another important complication of infection is that there is an increased incidence of ectopic pregnancy in women who have had PID. These long-term effects of untreated PID are becoming more common, as unprotected sex, particularly amongst teenagers, is increasingly prevalent.

PID is treated with combined antibiotics such as doxycycline and metronidazole, which may be given intravenously in severe acute infections. Surgery may be necessary in cases in which pus has accumulated. However, as many cases are chronic, the diagnosis may not be made until permanent damage to the internal genital organs has occurred.

Information box 5.2d-VIII

Pelvic inflammatory disease: comments from a Chinese medicine perspective

PID begins with a vaginal infection such as chlamydia or gonorrhea that are described in Chinese medicine in terms of Damp Heat in the Lower Jiao. These infections are predisposed to by Kidney and Spleen and Liver Blood Deficiency and Liver Qi Stagnation. PID is clearly a more profound disturbance, and deep pain is evidence of additional Blood and Qi Stagnation in the uterus.

General infections resulting from sexual transfer of bodily fluids

Although their symptoms do not directly affect the reproductive system, the sexually transmitted infections hepatitis B and C (see Section 3.1d) and HIV are most commonly transmitted through the exchange of bodily fluids during sexual intercourse. These infections are prevented by attention to the practice of safe sex.

HIV INFECTION AND AIDS

HIV is carried in body fluids. Close contact with infected body fluids together with a break in the normal barrier of the skin is necessary for HIV to be transmitted. Sexual contact and childbirth provide these conditions, as does transmission of human fluids by a hypodermic needle.

Infection can be prevented by taking antiretroviral medication immediately after an at-risk procedure or exposure. This is called post-exposure prophylaxis (PEP).

The presence of the virus in the bloodstream leads to an immune response that then causes the flu-like syndrome characteristic of many viral infections. Some people experience glandular fever-type symptoms at this time but only between 20 and 60 percent have a perceptible illness at this time of "seroconversion." Although antibodies are clearly formed at seroconversion, they are most often unable to clear the HIV from the body. This is because the virus is able to penetrate into leukocytes (T lymphocytes) via the CD4 protein receptor, and in this way hide from the immune response. In this intracellular state the HIV remains and multiplies, dividing with the lymphocytes over a period of years, until gradually the function of those cells becomes impaired. The presence of the virus leads to ever reducing numbers of lymphocytes over time as their early death is promoted by the presence of the virus.

After recovery from the initial infection with HIV, the patient may be without symptoms for many years. It is only when the T lymphocyte level has reached a critically low point that the first symptoms appear, most commonly in the form of persistently enlarged lymph nodes and then with unusual presentations of infectious disease.

In the UK HIV infection tends to be diagnosed before the T lymphocytes have reached this level as confidential HIV testing is very accessible and very much promoted in sexual health settings, and is also performed routinely in early pregnancy. Nevertheless it is estimated that 25 percent of people in the UK who have HIV infection are unaware of their infectious status.

Typical infections that are characteristic of HIV infection and that are described as the AIDS-related complex (ARC) include widespread oral *candida* (thrush), severe seborrheic dermatitis (see Section 6.1c), recurrent outbreaks of herpes and shingles together with night sweats, diarrhea and weight loss.

ARC is a prodrome for the stage of severe immunodeficiency that is known as AIDS (acquired immunodeficiency syndrome). In this stage the patient may develop much more serious unusual infections and also cancers. Infections that are seen often in AIDS and that are diagnostic of this stage include pneumocystis pneumonia, recurrent bacterial or viral pneumonia, *candida* of the bronchi and esophagus, tuberculosis (TB), widespread *cytomegalovirus* (CMV) disease with loss of vision and cryptosporidiosis diarrhea. Typical cancers include lymphoma, cervical cancer and a form of skin cancer called Kaposi's sarcoma (see Section 6.1c).

In advanced disease, the nerve cells of the brain may also be damaged by cytokines produced by virus-infected immune cells. This leads to a form of dementia resulting from a process called progressive leukoencephalopathy. As mentioned in Chapter 2.4, HIV is therefore an example of an infection that can cause degeneration as well as both inflammation and also disorder of the immune system. The nervous system complications of AIDS also include toxoplasmosis and lymphoma of the brain.

It is now recommended that antiretroviral treatment (ART) using combinations of two or more antiviral drugs is started as early in the infection as possible. This not only maximizes the chance of preventing onset of advanced disease, but also dramatically reduces infectiousness and transmission of the virus to others. Initial therapy is usually with three antiviral drugs: efavirenz plus tenofovir or abacavir, plus lamivudine or emtricitabine.

HIV infection used to be a dreaded illness that had a life expectancy of ten years after infection, and which was characterized by profound illness and cognitive decline in the latter stages. ART has transformed the outcome of HIV infection into a chronic condition that is compatible with a long lifespan.

Taking ART can be a challenge and may cause difficult side effects. The medications are for life and need to be taken according to a strict schedule to prevent replication of the virus. Common side effects include appetite loss, unusual distribution of body fat (lipodystrophy), diarrhea, fatigue, unhealthy changes in blood cholesterol, depression, nausea and rashes.

All patients with HIV infection are advised to have the pneumonia and flu vaccines.

If levels of the T cells decline to a low level, patients may also be recommended to take other antibiotic medications to ward off some of the common infections that can develop in AIDS.[30]

HIV infection in infancy and childhood is described in Section 5.4d.

 Information box 5.2d-IX

HIV infection and AIDS: comments from a Chinese medicine perspective

The Chinese medicine interpretation of HIV infection, as a modern disease, cannot be drawn from the classic texts, but established AIDS has many of the features of cancer.

The initial infection in adults has the features of an Invasion of Wind Heat Damp. The eventual development of depletion of T lymphocyte function suggests that this Toxic Heat Pathogen has penetrated into the Interior to damage the Blood and Yin. Immune deficiency resulting from the deterioration of the function of the white blood cells (T leukocytes) in the marrow corresponds to severe Kidney Deficiency, which is presumably a result of this initial insult. The lymph node enlargement, infections and tumors that characterize AIDS correspond to a combination of Phlegm, Damp, Heat and Blood Stagnation, all of

which may have accumulated as a consequence of the Kidney Deficiency together with Spleen Deficiency.

Treatment principles in HIV infection would usually include clearance of Heat and Damp Phlegm, movement of Stagnation and support of the Upright Qi and Spleen and Kidney Function.

The antiviral medications must have Cooling properties and appear to Invigorate Blood and Yin and Clear Phlegm. Their action is suppressive in nature; it is well recognized that viral replication will start again even with a short gap in treatment. The diverse side effects are evidence of toxicity and suggest Spleen Deficiency (diarrhea and nausea and loss of appetite), formation of Damp and Phlegm (lipodystrophy) and Stagnation of Liver Qi (depression) and also Toxic Heat (rashes), which may come as a result of Damp and Stagnation.

The red flags of sexually transmitted diseases

Most patients with an STD will benefit from referral to a conventional doctor for assessment or treatment. Red flags are those symptoms and signs that indicate that referral

should be considered. The red flags of STDs are described in Table 5.2d-I. A summary of the red flags in a format designed for quick reference in clinical practice can be found in Appendix III. This gives advice on the degree of urgency of referral for each of the red flag conditions listed.

Table 5.2d-I A35: Red flags of sexually transmitted diseases

Red flag	Description	Reasoning
A35.1	Vaginal discharge: if irregular, blood-stained or unusual odor	A slight, creamy vaginal discharge is usual, and tends to increase and become more elastic around the time of ovulation. An increase in this sort of discharge is normal in pregnancy
		If an irregular pattern of blood staining, volume, itchiness or odor develops, investigation is merited to exclude sexually transmitted disease (STD). This is of particular importance in pregnancy, as some STDs can threaten the health of the fetus
		If an STD is suspected, advise the patient to visit the genitourinary medicine (GUM) department for a confidential consultation in the first instance
		Thrush (candidiasis) does not necessarily merit referral, as it can subside by means of conservative measures and is not usually considered to be contagious. If recurrent and troublesome, consider referral to investigate a possible underlying cause, such as diabetes or immune deficiency
A35.2	Vaginal discharge: after menopause	Vaginal discharge is not normal after the menopause, particularly if offensive or blood-stained. Refer to exclude infection or carcinoma
A35.3	Vaginal discharge: before puberty	Vaginal discharge is not normal before puberty, particularly if offensive or blood-stained. However, the cause is usually benign over growth of yeasts or bacteria
		Consider the possibility of abuse in children (see A40.34). Always refer children with this symptom for investigation
A35.4	Discharge from penis	Always refer, as this may indicate an STD. If an STD is suspected, advise the patient to visit the local GUM department for a free of charge confidential consultation in the first instance
A35.5	Sores, warty lumps or ulcers on the vagina or penis	These are very likely to be manifestations of a sexually transmitted infection such as herpes or genital warts. Rarely, they may be cancer. Refer to the GUM department for a confidential consultation in the first instance for investigation
A35.6	Pelvic inflammatory disease (PID) (chronic form): vaginal discharge, gripy abdominal pain, pain on intercourse, dysmenorrhea, infertility	Chronic PID poses a threat to fertility and may suggest the person has been infected by an STD. If an STD is suspected, advise the patient to visit the GUM department for confidential consultation or to the GP if symptoms are causing a lot of distress and merit prompt treatment
A35.7	Pelvic inflammatory disease (PID) (acute form): low abdominal pain with collapse, fever	Acute PID poses a serious risk to fertility. Refer urgently for antibiotic treatment. Acute PID may present as the acute abdomen (see A6.8)
A35.8	First outbreak of genital herpes: A cluster of painful ulcers on penis, vulva or around the anal margin. Associated with a feeling of malaise. Inguinal nodes (groin) may be enlarged and tender	Refer to the GUM department for same-day treatment as early oral antiviral medication will reduce the length of the painful symptoms and may also reduce the risk of recurrences of the outbreak
A35.9	Outbreak of genital herpes (see A35.8) in the last trimester of pregnancy	Refer to GP or midwife for discussion of birth plan, as there is a risk of transmission of herpes virus to the baby during delivery
A35.10	Offensive, fishy, watery discharge (possible bacterial vaginosis (BV)) in pregnancy	Refer for treatment, as BV leads to an increased risk of early labor and miscarriage

5.2e Contraception

Contraception is conventionally considered to have important health benefits. The first is the reduction in the risk of unwanted pregnancies and their unfortunate consequences, induced abortions. An indirect benefit of this is what has been euphemistically termed "family planning." This is the concept that when pregnancies occur they do so at the time when the woman and her partner are both physiologically and psychologically prepared for them. Moreover, if pregnancy can be delayed until after a woman has reached the age of at least 20, that pregnancy is more likely to be uncomplicated. It is also recognized that if subsequent pregnancies can be spaced by two years or more, the mother has a chance to regain a level of strength that will help both her and her family cope with them. The other major health benefit of certain forms of contraception is that they can be used to prevent the transmission of sexually transmitted diseases (STDs).

However, it can be argued that it is the advent of readily available contraception that has encouraged the rise in sexual activity that has taken place since the 1960s, particularly in young people. And this rise in sexual activity has been accompanied by a rise in unwanted pregnancies and STDs. Nevertheless, there is no doubt about the fact that if contraception is used appropriately, these problems could be avoided. However, whilst contraception mitigates the risks of infection and pregnancy that result from sexual freedom, each method of contraception introduces different risks and also side effects. For this reason, contraception is neither an easy option for many users nor a panacea.

Contraceptive services are provided in the UK under the National Health Service (NHS), and are available free of charge from family planning clinics and general practices. Currently, all contraceptives, including condoms, are available free of charge to NHS patients. In other developed countries, however, it is more usual for individuals to have to fund their own birth control.

The free provision of contraception services in the UK is a reflection of the fact that, since the early part of this century, family planning has been seen as an important mechanism to promote the control of the size of families and the prevention of unwanted pregnancies. The raison d'être of the UK National Birth Control Council, founded in 1930, was that "married people may space or limit their families and thus mitigate the evils of ill health and poverty." Since the 1960s, the use of contraceptives has been increasingly promoted outside the bounds of marriage to encourage safe sex practices. Nevertheless, the UK has a high rate of teenage pregnancy and abortion compared with some other European countries (notably the Netherlands).

Failure rates

Failure rates are a means of expressing the effectiveness of a contraceptive method. No contraceptive method is perfect in preventing pregnancy. Usually the decision about which contraceptive to use is based on a process of weighing up the convenience of the method to the individual (or the couple) and the risks of ill health it might cause against its risk of failure.

Contraceptive failure rates can be expressed in terms of the number of pregnancies that occur in 100 women using the method for one year (pregnancies per 100 woman-years). If no contraceptive protection is used, the pregnancy rate is 85 per 100 woman-years (i.e. 85 percent of sexually active women will fall pregnant within one year of stopping contraception), and failure rates of contraception can be compared to this figure.

For all but the long-acting methods of contraception, failure rates vary dramatically according to the commitment of the user of the method. For example, natural family planning is generally not widely recommended in the NHS because of a measured high failure rate (20–25 pregnancies per 100 woman-years), but if used correctly, it can be an effective and empowering method of birth control. The measured failure rates come from studies involving a broad range of users. In general, most contraceptive methods, if used correctly, are more effective than the failure rates suggest.

Failure rates are all much lower in women who are approaching the menopause, as natural fertility is declining at this time. This means that certain contraceptives (e.g. the diaphragm) may be acceptably safe methods for older women, but less reliable in very fertile women under the age of 30–35.

Methods of contraception

Contraceptive methods are usually grouped into the following categories:

- barrier methods
- intrauterine devices (IUDs or IUCDs)
- hormonal methods
- surgical methods
- natural methods.

Barrier methods

Barrier methods do not prevent the production of the spermatozoa (sperm) or the ovum, but act as a barrier to prevent their meeting. The most commonly used barriers are the condom (or sheath) in men and the cap/diaphragm in women.

THE CONDOM (SHEATH)

The condom is a latex sheath that has to be rolled onto the erect penis, ideally before any genital contact has taken place. The additional use of spermicidal cream is strongly recommended to increase effectiveness.

Failure rate: 12 per 100 woman-years.

Advantages: Simple, cheap and relatively non-invasive. Prevents fertilization. Prevents STDs. The failure rate can be further reduced by concurrent use of spermicidal gel.

Disadvantages: Cannot be used until the arousal stage in sex, and so may be put on too late (i.e. after the release of sperm containing fluids from the penis). There is a risk of the condom splitting if it is not put on correctly. Allergy to creams or latex is increasingly common. Many young people find condoms off-putting, and so do not use them.

THE DIAPHRAGM AND CAP

These are flexible discs or cones of latex that can be inserted into the vagina up to a few hours before intercourse to cover the opening to the cervical canal. The latex barrier should then be left in place for at least six hours. It is only effective if used together with a spermicidal cream. The cap needs to be the correct size, and so a clinic appointment is required for a fitting. This fitting should be repeated annually, and also after pregnancy.

Failure rate: 30 per 100 woman-years.

Advantages: Simple and relatively non-invasive. Prevents fertilization. Prevents STDs. Can be inserted before sexual intercourse has started. Is usually not seen or felt by either partner. Can be cleaned easily and used again and again.

Disadvantages: A high failure rate in young women. Some women find it difficult or impossible to use. Can cause thrush and cystitis in susceptible people. Allergy to creams or latex is increasingly common.

Intrauterine devices (IUDs or IUCDs)

It has been known for centuries that a foreign body in the uterus prevents implantation of a fertilized egg. An IUD, formerly known as "the coil," is a delicate copper-containing nylon device that is inserted via the cervix in an outpatient clinic, and can remain in place for up to ten years. The insertion can be uncomfortable, but does not require a general anesthetic. IUDs have nylon strings that are left to protrude through the cervix for ease of removal. The intrauterine part of the device has fine copper wire wound around its stem.

There is an ethical issue with IUDs in that they do not prevent fertilization. Instead they prevent implantation of the fertilized ovum. From the viewpoint of a number of world religions, this is akin to abortion, and is therefore not an acceptable contraceptive method for some.

Failure rate: 0.22 per 100 woman-years.

Advantages: If no side effects occur, the IUD can be completely forgotten, and remains effective for up to ten years.

Disadvantages: Painful insertion. There is a risk of introduction of infection (with a risk of pelvic inflammatory disease, PID). Risk of perforation of the uterus. Can cause heavy periods and cramping pain. Increased risk of ectopic pregnancy.

Hormonal methods

Hormonal methods use synthetic estrogen and/or progestogens to influence fertility, either by preventing ovulation or by causing changes to the endometrium and cervix that prevent implantation.

INJECTABLE AND IMPLANTABLE PROGESTOGEN

Both these approaches involve the administration to the woman of slow-release synthetic progestogen (similar in function to natural progesterone). The progestogen is given either by injection (lasting for one to three months) or by means of a subcutaneous implant (lasting for up to three years). The implant is inserted under the skin by means of a minor operation, which can be performed by a medical practitioner or nurse. The high dose of progestogen that is released prevents ovulation (via inhibition of the pituitary release of LH and FSH) in the same way that progesterone released by the placenta inhibits ovulation during pregnancy.

Failure rate: 0.3 per 100 woman-years.

Advantages: A very reliable method. Prevents ovulation, and therefore no fertilization should occur. There is no risk of forgetting to use it, or of errors in using it. Progestogens are not considered to have the serious adverse effects on health that estrogens have.

Disadvantages: High doses of progestogens can lead to mood changes and weight gain. Acne is a less common side effect. Usually the periods stop entirely, but some women suffer irregular and heavy bleeding. This is a particular problem in the first few months after the insertion of an implant. Once the injection has been given it cannot be reversed, and so any side effects have to be borne for up to three months. The contraceptive implant insertion and removal procedures may result in surgical damage to nerves or arteries. If side effects occur with implants, the implant can be removed, but this requires a minor operation. A major problem with the injectable progestogen is delayed return of fertility after stopping the contraceptive methods, and so it should not be used in women who are planning a family in the near future. Long-term use of the contraceptive injection may be associated with a reduction in bone density (osteoporosis).

Intrauterine progesterone-only system (IUS)

The intrauterine progesterone-only system (IUS) is a form of IUD designed to release a steady amount of progestogen into the uterine cavity. The IUS has the advantage over the coil in that it can be used in women who tend to suffer from heavy menstrual bleeding. In those women who tolerate this method, periods may become very light or even absent. The risk of ectopic pregnancy is lower with the IUS than with the simple IUCD.

Progestogen-only pill (POP) or mini-pill

The mini-pill contains a low dose of progestogen, and is taken daily at a fixed time of day. Low-dose progestogen inhibits the implantation of a fertilized ovum by altering the quality of the mucus in the cervix and the womb lining. It may also prevent ovulation. The dose is not sufficient to prevent ovulation reliably in most women.

Failure rate: 3 per 100 woman-years.

Advantages: Low dose, so fewer side effects than the injection. Carries none of the serious risks of the combined pill. Can be used by breastfeeding mothers. Can reduce the discomfort of painful, irregular or heavy periods.

Disadvantages: Requires a regulated lifestyle, as the pill must be taken within the same two-hour period every day to remain effective (with the exception of desogestrel, which can be taken within a 12-hour time window). Can have unpredictable effects on periods: some women have no periods at all, some fall into a 28-day cycle with a light period, but many continue to have irregular bleeding. Side effects include weight gain, acne and mood changes.

Combined oral contraceptive pill (COCP) or "the pill"

The COCP ("the pill") contains a combination of estrogen and progestogen, and is usually taken for 21 days of a 28-day cycle. The seven-day gap allows a withdrawal bleed, which is not a true period. Some preparations include seven dummy pills to be taken during this gap to reduce the risks of forgetting to start the next course. Most preparations contain a fixed dose of hormones, but some vary the proportions of hormones throughout the cycle, in an attempt to reflect the natural pattern of hormonal change. These triphasic pills are believed by some doctors to be less likely to give rise to problematic bleeding. There are a number of preparations, and this offers a choice of a range of doses of estrogen, and type of progestogen, each of which has a different side effect profile and risk of failure. It often takes a few attempts to find a preparation that suits an individual woman. The COCP has a dual action, both inhibiting ovulation and also, like the mini-pill, affecting the quality of the cervical mucus.

The major health issue with the COCP is that the high dose of estrogen increases the risk of thrombosis. It also increases the risk of cancer of the breast and cervix, but is considered to be protective against cancer of the ovary and uterus. In most women whose risk of thrombosis is very low, the additional risk from the pill is considered to be extremely low. It is often quoted that the risk of thrombosis associated with pregnancy is much higher than is incurred by taking the pill. Nevertheless, the risk is real, and may be significant in those women who have other risk factors for thrombosis. Women who are obese, who smoke, who have a family or a past history of thrombosis, those with a past history of breast cancer and those with liver disease should be advised to choose an alternative form of contraception. Women with visual migraine are at risk of suffering stroke when taking the COCP, and should be advised to choose another contraceptive method.

As surgery increases the risk of thrombosis, women on the pill who are due to have a major operation will be advised to use an alternative method of contraception for the few weeks either side of the operation date.

An additional problem is that the progestogen in the pill tends to have an adverse effect on the lipids in the blood, and so may accelerate the development of atherosclerosis. Another circulatory side effect, which affects about 2 percent of women who take the pill, is a significant rise in blood pressure. For this reason, all women on the pill are advised to have a medical assessment that includes blood pressure measurement every six months.

The use of the pill is known to decrease the risk of certain cancers, but may increase the risk of breast cancer. The risk of ovarian cancer is decreased by 40 percent and endometrial cancer by 50 percent. However, breast cancer is slightly more common in women taking the pill, although current theories propose that this risk only affects a small subgroup of women who are particularly susceptible to early-onset breast cancer. For this reason, a family history of early-onset breast cancer is a reason to avoid using the pill.

There are many other less serious side effects that can affect certain women who take the pill. For some of these side effects a change to another preparation of the pill may resolve the problem. However, for some women the side effects are so severe that they prevent them continuing with this form of contraception. Common side effects of the pill include acne, mid-cycle spotting or bleeding, dry eyes, gallbladder disease, nausea, mood changes, weight gain, increased vaginal discharge, headaches and migraine. Of all these, migraine has to be taken very seriously, particularly if it is focal in nature. Women who develop visual migraines while on the pill should be changed to another form of contraception because of a possible increased risk of stroke.

Despite all these risks and side effects, many women find the pill improves their quality of life, over and above the sexual freedom it offers. The pill can transform the symptoms of premenstrual syndrome (PMS), dysmenorrhea and menorrhagia. In some women the skin texture improves when on the pill. Others may report an increase in sexual desire and general well-being. Because of its effects on cervical mucus, the pill is also believed to reduce the risk of PID. It is the contraceptive method chosen by over half of all women in the UK under 30.

One form of the pill contains in place of the progesterone a drug called cyproterone that acts by opposing the effects of testosterone. This has the additional effect of improving acne and male-pattern body hair, and may be prescribed for these reasons alone. However, this preparation has a particularly adverse effect on the balance of lipids in the blood, and should ideally not be prescribed for too long because it may accelerate the development of atherosclerosis.

Failure rate: 0.005–0.30 per 100 woman-years (very low).

Advantages: Very reliable if taken correctly. Still reliable if the pill is forgotten for up to 48 hours, so is more suitable than the POP for those with a chaotic lifestyle. Some women find problems such as premenstrual tension and painful periods improve when taking the pill. Sex life often improves, possibly because of freedom from fear of pregnancy. In combination with progestogens, estrogens reduce the risk of ovarian and womb cancer.

Disadvantages: The COCP does require a degree of discipline to be taken correctly, and so is not suitable for some people with an irregular lifestyle. A missed pill at certain times in the cycle can permit ovulation. Many people suffer side effects, including headaches, nausea, low libido, weight gain, acne, mood changes and breakthrough bleeding. Other problems with the COCP include interactions with other medication, with the common result that the effectiveness of the pill is reduced – certain antibiotics can reduce the absorption of the pill. Women should be counseled carefully about this potential problem, and should rely on additional methods, such as condoms, when they are taking certain medications.

EMERGENCY CONTRACEPTION (THE MORNING-AFTER PILL)

Emergency contraception (postcoitus pill, PCP) consists of a single dose of medication that is designed to prevent implantation of an embryo that might have formed as a result of unprotected sex. There are two forms of PCP. First, high-dose progesterone (levonorgestrel) may be given within 72 hours of unprotected sex. It prevents pregnancy in over 95 percent of cases if given within 72 hours (hence the name morning-after pill is a misnomer), and is more likely to be successful the sooner it is given.

High-dose levonorgestrel works primarily by altering the nature of the cervical mucus and the womb lining to prevent implantation, but in some cases it can inhibit ovulation.

The alternative form of PCP is the newer product ulipristal, which is marketed as being active in preventing conception if taken within 120 hours after unprotected sex.

Advantages: Effective.

Disadvantages: A common side effect of both medications is nausea, which can be problematic for absorption of the pills if vomiting occurs. There is a range of other medication-related side effects that might affect a minority of individuals. PCP carries the same ethical problems as the IUD and the mini-pill, because it does not necessarily prevent fertilization.

Information box 5.2e-I

Hormonal contraception: comments from a Chinese medicine perspective

In Chinese medicine, the hormonal methods of contraception would be interpreted as having significant energetic effects, as evidenced by their broad range of side effects.

The progesterone-only methods have side effects that include weight gain, acne, mood changes and amenorrhea. In the long term, the high-dose methods (injection and implants) may lead to osteoporosis by preventing the natural production of estrogen. They mimic natural progesterone that is released in the second half of the menstrual cycle when the Yang Qi is more exuberant. Synthetic progesterone is considered by Rosenberg (2000) as a "Qi raising medicinal" with "Damp and Congestive qualities" which "tends to enter and accumulate in the Liver and Stomach Channels."[31] Its side effects suggest that the negative effects may be manifestations of Accumulation of Damp Heat, Stagnation of Qi and Depletion of Kidney Qi. All three of these factors might explain its effect in reducing fertility.

The combined pill also has side effects that suggest Accumulation of Damp and Stagnation of Qi. These side effects include weight gain, acne, mood changes, headaches and migraine. The additional effects on the circulatory system suggest that the Stagnating effect is more powerful than with the progesterone-only methods, and the adverse effect on blood lipids suggests Accumulation of Phlegm. The increased risk of breast cancer in some women is more evidence of a tendency to cause Blood Stagnation or Accumulation of Phlegm.

Estrogen at physiological levels appears to relate to Spleen Qi, Yin and Blood by promoting fleshiness and moistness of tissues, and it prepares the endometrium for implantation. It makes sense that it, too, has a Stagnating and Damp quality. Estrogen in the premenopausal years is known to lead to thickened endometrium which, when unopposed by natural progesterone, can continue to thicken and even transform into cancerous tissue. In the combined pill the synthetic estrogen is at a much higher dose than physiological levels. This inhibits the pituitary surge that leads to ovulation. In addition to Stagnation and Damp Phlegm Accumulation, Maciocia (1998) observes that the combined pill tends to first cause Blood Deficiency in those who have taken it for some time.[32]

Some women report an improvement in mood, skin and menstrual irregularities when on the pill. This can be explained as symptoms that have been suppressed rather than transformed, as they tend to recur on withdrawal of the pill.

Surgical methods

The surgical methods of contraception are very reliable, although even these have a failure rate. Patients are counseled that both vasectomy and tubal ligation (sterilization by cutting and clipping the fallopian tubes) are to be considered irreversible procedures. It is conventionally believed that these procedures should only be offered to those individuals who have made an informed and considered long-term decision about not having any more children. They should only very rarely be performed in those under 30 or those who have never had children.

Both vasectomy and tubal ligation can be reversed surgically, but a return to fertility cannot be guaranteed. The longer it has been since the initial operation, the lower the chances are of restoring fertility.

Vasectomy

The vasectomy operation can be performed very quickly as an outpatient procedure. A small incision is made in the scrotum, and each vas deferens tube is cut. The two ends of the cut tube are then stitched (tied off). Testosterone is produced as normal, and so, in theory, sex drive should not be affected. Moreover, spermatozoa are also still produced, but these get reabsorbed from the epididymis. A man who has had a vasectomy will still ejaculate, because the production of seminal and prostatic fluids is not affected by the procedure. Recent studies have shown a 10 percent increased risk of prostate cancer in those who have had a vasectomy, although no causal link has yet been proven.[33]

Failure rate: 1 in 2000 over a lifetime (very low).

Advantages: Very reliable. No need to be concerned about contraceptive methods from a few weeks after the operation.

Disadvantages: Not effective straightaway. Semen samples are required at 8 and 12 weeks postoperatively to check that no sperm are present. The procedure should be considered irreversible. There is a small risk of chronic testicular pain and other complications of surgical procedures such as local hemorrhage. There is possibly an increased risk of prostate cancer.

Tubal ligation (sterilization)

In tubal ligation, the fallopian tubes are cut and clipped (tied off) by means of a laparoscopic operation. This is a more invasive procedure than vasectomy, and requires a general anesthetic. There is an increased risk of ectopic pregnancy after tubal ligation.

Failure rate: 1 in 200 over a lifetime.

Advantages: Fairly reliable. There is no longer a requirement for other contraceptive methods.

Disadvantages: The procedure should be considered irreversible. There is a small operative risk from the surgical procedure itself. The risk of ectopic pregnancy is increased.

 Information box 5.2e-II

Sterilization: comments from a Chinese medicine perspective

From a Chinese medicine viewpoint, it is possible that the surgical methods of contraception prevent a free flow of bodily fluids. Although semen is seen as Essence in a material form, and its loss is Depleting to the man, nevertheless, ejaculation may be important for preventing Stagnation of Qi in the pelvic area. The same could be said about the way in which sterilization prevents the release of the ovum. Moreover any intra-abdominal procedure in a woman is likely to lead to adhesions and there is a risk of Qi and Blood Stagnation as a result of the damage caused, and in the man, local Qi and Blood Stagnation in the scrotum as a result of surgical severing of tissues.

The link of vasectomy with an increased incidence of prostatic cancer is consistent with the idea that vasectomy causes Qi and Blood Stagnation.

Natural methods

Natural methods of contraception do not rely on barriers or drugs. Instead, they are dependent on the couple having an awareness of the way in which conception occurs, and how fertility varies throughout the woman's menstrual cycle.

COITUS INTERRUPTUS

The oldest method of contraception, coitus interruptus, is arguably the most natural method, and the method used by nearly 4 percent of women in a marital or consensual sexual union worldwide.[34] In coitus interruptus the man withdraws from the woman just before ejaculation. This is still the favored method for some ethnic groups across the world (it is the preferred method in over 30 percent of those studied in Armenia and Azerbaijan), particularly in those for whom other methods of contraception are considered unethical or inaccessible.[35] The problem with this method is that drops of semen containing thousands of spermatozoa are released from the penis before ejaculation. Therefore, even if carefully practiced, coitus interruptus carries a real, albeit reduced, risk of pregnancy. The failure rate is estimated to be very high, at 30–40 pregnancies per 100 woman-years.

PERIODIC ABSTINENCE (THE RHYTHM METHOD)

Periodic abstinence is another natural method also favored by an estimated 3 percent of couples worldwide. This requires the couple to be aware of the days in the cycle in which the woman is most fertile. Sexual intercourse is then avoided on those days. The fertile period is the time that spans from five days before ovulation to two days after ovulation. Ideally, a couple who plan to use this method should have guidance from an experienced teacher of the natural methods of family planning.

For a woman with a regular cycle, there are some physiological changes that allow her to predict on what day of the cycle ovulation will occur. The most reliable of these are the changes in the consistency of the cervical mucus. At the beginning of the cycle (days 1–7) there is very little mucus. Conception is very unlikely to occur during these dry days. From days 8 to 14 of a 28-day cycle the mucus becomes more profuse. Initially it is cloudy in color and thick in texture, but on the day before ovulation it becomes clear and slippery. At ovulation the mucus is clear and stringy. This change in the mucus is an indication that the woman is at her most fertile day of the cycle. To be able to rely on these changes, the woman has to be able to find her own cervix, and examine her own mucus, ideally first thing in the morning. After a few cycles, she will become aware on what day she tends to ovulate.

An additional indicator of ovulation is that in some women there can be a definite rise in body temperature just before ovulation. The temperature should be taken first thing in the morning and charted throughout the cycle. It is currently taught that temperature changes should only be used in conjunction with assessment of cervical mucus, because if used alone it is known to be quite unreliable.

Some women prefer to use fertility devices such as the Persona ovulation monitor to help them differentiate between fertile and infertile times. These devices rely on regular tests of early morning urine samples. The contraceptive failure rate with reliance on Persona has been estimated at an impressive 6 per 100 woman-years.

For those women who have a regular cycle, and who are prepared to examine their own cervix and mucus or regularly test their urine, these methods can be very reliable. However, for those who have a very irregular cycle, this method cannot be so depended upon. In these women, ovulation can happen unpredictably, occasionally even as early as during the menstrual bleed. Moreover, there are many women who do not wish to be so introspective about their own bodies and who would find the idea of examining mucus distasteful. Furthermore, for some couples, the idea of abstinence from sexual intercourse for seven days is not acceptable. For this reason, some couples may generally rely on this method, but also use a barrier method on the fertile days.

5.2f Infertility

Infertility is defined arbitrarily as the inability of a couple to conceive within 12 months, despite having regular unprotected intercourse. By this definition, infertility affects up to 15 percent of couples, although many of these will conceive naturally at a later date. It is only in a very few cases that the diagnosis of absolute infertility can be made.

For most couples there is a combination of factors that result in reduced fertility, but not a total inability to conceive. This is an important point from the perspective of an acupuncturist, as it implies that for most couples there is scope for treatment to increase the chances of conception. By optimizing the conditions for conception to take place (e.g. by Nourishing Blood and Tonifying the Kidneys), acupuncture may encourage an improved balance of health to enable conception to occur in those with relative infertility.

In some cases of apparent infertility, it may be found that the couple is having sex on an infrequent basis, and not consistently at the woman's most fertile time. If this is the underlying issue, conception may be more likely to occur after the couple have been given advice about how to determine the fertile days in the cycle according to the principles of natural family planning (see Section 5.2e). A couple will not usually be referred for investigation or treatment until after 12–18 months of having regular intercourse during the fertile times of the woman's menstrual cycle.

In about 25 percent of couples who are referred for investigation, no physical abnormality is detected. Despite normal ovulation and healthy semen, conception does not occur. There is no agreed conventional explanation for this problem. Some specialists suggest that this form of infertility is due to a defect in the development of the corpus luteum, which then leads to failure of implantation of a fertilized egg (see later).

In 30 percent of cases a dysfunction in the production of healthy semen is found and in over 65 percent of cases the reproductive system of the woman is found to have an abnormality. In up to 40 percent of cases both partners may each have a condition that contributes to the difficulty in conception.

Investigation of infertility

Investigation of the man
The main test required is semen analysis. Even if the spermatozoa are found to be abnormal, if the couple wishes to use assisted conception techniques (see later), the woman will also be expected to undergo full investigations. This is because combined problems with infertility are not uncommon.

Investigation of the woman
Investigation of the woman involves a general physical and gynecological examination to look for evidence of gross physical abnormalities such as endocrine disease, fibroids or pelvic inflammatory disease (PID). A blood test may be taken in the second half of the cycle to assess the level of progesterone to determine whether or not ovulation is occurring, and to test for hormones including FSH, LH, testosterone, thyroid hormones and prolactin (PRL) in the first half of the cycle to look for evidence of conditions such as polycystic ovary disease, hyperprolactinemia, thyroid disorders or ovarian failure.

Tests to visualize the structure of the internal genital organs include ultrasound scan, laparoscopy and hysterosalpingography. An ultrasound scan will reveal gross defects of the uterus and ovaries, and can also visualize ovulation. A laparoscopy will reveal the changes of endometriosis. The hysterosalpingography can reveal whether or not the fallopian tubes are patent.

Investigation of the couple
If the results of all the tests described above are normal, a postcoital test may be performed. A positive postcoital test indicates whether or not the sperm can easily penetrate the cervical mucus.

The causes of infertility

Defective semen
Although it is commonly assumed that infertility is usually a problem with the woman, in many cases some deficiency in the quantity or quality of the spermatozoa is found. In most of these cases a reduction in normal spermatozoa

(low sperm count) is found. Established causes of a low sperm count include past infection with mumps virus, late descent of the testes and treatment with anticancer drugs. Lifestyle factors such as poor diet, overwork, tight-fitting underwear, smoking and alcohol use are all recognized to impact on semen quality. Over the past few decades the average sperm count has declined markedly. A range of dietary and environmental factors has been suggested to explain this drop, but no single cause has been proven. It is known that an individual's sperm count can vary over time, and may increase if factors such as diet and stress levels can be attended to. Moreover, in cases of reduced sperm count, normal conception may still be possible, as even if the sperm count is less than half the normal number there are still well over a million spermatozoa in an ejaculate of normal volume (2–3 milliliters).

The spermatozoa might be found to be abnormal in structure or movement. In these cases, assisted conception may be necessary. In rare cases, there may be total absence of spermatozoa, in which case use of donor semen is the only option available for the couple who wish to conceive.

In other cases erectile problems are the cause for infertility. If this problem cannot be alleviated but the man can ejaculate through masturbation, then assisted intrauterine insemination (IUI) can be of value.

 Information box 5.2f-I

Defects in sperm count or motility: comments from a Chinese medicine perspective
In Chinese medicine, defective semen is a manifestation of Deficiency of Kidney Essence (in its Yang aspect). Damp Heat may also be considered to be a cause of male infertility in some cases.

Anovulation
Problems with ovulation are the cause of 5–25 percent of cases of infertility. A complete lack of ovulation is termed anovulation. The causes of anovulation are the same as the causes of amenorrhea (see Section 5.2c). Women who suffer from amenorrhea are also very likely to be infertile, although this is not always the case. However, it is also possible for a woman to have a menstrual cycle that appears normal but during which there is no ovulation (an anovulatory cycle).

Anovulatory cycles are common at the extremes of a woman's reproductive years. These may be increased in frequency by factors that affect the release of the pituitary hormones, such as ongoing stress, poor diet or over-exercise. A period of anovulation can follow the withdrawal from a long-term prescription of a hormone-based contraceptive.

In particular, the progesterone injection can have this effect for some months after withdrawal. Other physical causes of anovulation include ovarian damage by drugs or surgery, primary ovarian failure and polycystic ovary syndrome.

Information box 5.2f-II

Ovulatory failure: comments from a Chinese medicine perspective

In Chinese medicine, ovulation depends primarily on Blood and Kidney Essence and healthy Liver Qi. If any of these are impaired, ovulation may fail to occur. Lack of ovulation may be caused by a Full pattern. For example, Damp, Heat and Liver Qi Stagnation are all contributory in the development of the infertility of polycystic ovary syndrome.

Defects in the development of the corpus luteum

As mentioned, some experts attribute cases of unexplained infertility to a failure in the implantation of a fertilized egg. It has been proposed that a defect in the corpus luteum may cause this form of infertility because it leads to a poorly developed endometrium in the second half of the menstrual cycle. It is suggested that a short luteal phase (less than ten days) may be suggestive of a corpus luteum defect.

The problem with this theory is that there is no simple test available that can reliably demonstrate possible defects in corpus luteum development. There are also no clearly defined treatments to reverse this theoretical condition, although progesterone or *human chorionic gonadotropin* (HCG) treatment may be prescribed. However, in common with other functional conditions, this problem is possibly amenable to complementary medical approaches.

Information box 5.2f-III

Corpus luteum defects: comments from a Chinese medicine perspective

In Chinese medicine, the stage of the menstrual cycle in which the endometrium is being prepared for implantation corresponds to the stage in which Blood and Yin are filling the Ren (Directing) and Chong (Penetrating) Vessels. A corpus luteum defect is a physiological description and not a known disease, but its suggested manifestation is failure in implantation in the second half of the cycle. In theory, it might, therefore, correspond to Deficiency of Blood and/or Kidney Essence (in its Yin aspect). As well as nourishing Blood and the Kidneys, treatment should also involve invigorating the Ren and Chong Vessels.

The Pathogenic Factors of Cold, Damp and Blood Stasis may also prevent implantation, and so could be underlying factors in a case of infertility of no measurable physical cause.

Fallopian tube damage

The most common cause of damage to the fallopian tubes is the scarring and adhesions that result from pelvic inflammatory disease (PID). The inflammation and damage that may result from an ectopic pregnancy can also cause permanent damage to one fallopian tube. The structural damage resulting from these conditions may impair the transport of the ovum, and so prevent fertilization.

Information box 5.2f-IV

Fallopian tube obstruction: comments from a Chinese medicine perspective

In Chinese medicine, fallopian tube damage might correspond to one or more of the Full patterns that can cause infertility. Damp Heat, Toxic Heat or Blood Stagnation may be underlying Pathogenic Factors.

Structural problems of the uterus or vagina

A physical disorder of the structure of the uterus or vagina is another cause of infertility. Together, uterine and fallopian tube disorders are important factors in 15–25 percent of cases of infertility.

Endometriosis is a common disorder in which the uterine wall is distorted by the development of cysts lined with endometrial tissue within its muscular walls. Endometriosis is often associated with infertility, although whether the condition is the cause of infertility is still unclear. Fibroids, if very large, are very occasionally found to be the cause of infertility, but in most cases they do not prevent the development of a healthy pregnancy. Rarely, an inherited structural defect of the vagina or uterus is the cause of infertility. In some cases, these defects can be amended surgically.

Information box 5.2f-V

Endometriosis: comments from a Chinese medicine perspective

In Chinese medicine, endometriosis corresponds to Blood Stagnation in the Uterus.

Fibroids also correspond either to Blood Stagnation or Phlegm Damp and can result from a combination of local deficiency, Cold, Damp foods and environment and emotional frustration. Both Blood Stagnation and Phlegm Damp are factors that can impair implantation.

Structural defects of the womb might be regarded as a manifestation of Jing Deficiency.

The treatment of infertility

For some of the causes of infertility the underlying condition can be treated, and this can lead to conception. If the underlying problem cannot be remedied, the assisted methods of conception, which include in vitro fertilization (IVF), can offer a chance of pregnancy that until a few decades ago would not have been thought possible. However, there are some forms of infertility in which it is not possible to obtain the gametes from one or both partners. In these cases, donor gametes (ova or spermatozoa) may enable a pregnancy to be achieved. Each of these approaches to the treatment of infertility is now discussed in turn.

Treatment of the underlying condition

Functional lack of ovulation may be treated by supporting the woman in making appropriate lifestyle changes, such as reducing stress levels, attaining a healthy body weight and reducing excessive exercise.

Endocrine disorders, such as hypothyroidism, and pituitary tumors, can be treated successfully by means of drugs and/or pituitary surgery. Fallopian tube blockage may be treated by means of microsurgery, although the success rate is low (within two years after the operation, only 20–40 percent of women will have conceived). Other structural disorders of the uterus and vagina, including inherited defects and fibroids, may also be treated surgically.

The symptoms of endometriosis are generally treated with a range of hormonal drugs.

In cases of anovulation that do not respond to lifestyle changes, including polycystic ovary syndrome, drug treatment can be used to stimulate the ovary to produce eggs. The most common drug used is clomifene. This drug acts by stimulating a surge in FSH and LH, which in turn promotes ovulation in up to 80 percent of women. It is not uncommon for more than one ovum to be released

with this treatment, and thus there is a risk of multiple pregnancies. More than half of all women who manage to ovulate with this treatment will fall pregnant.

The side effects of clomifene include enlargement of ovarian cysts and the development of endometriosis. Nausea, vomiting, abdominal pain, weight gain and depression are common. There is a health concern about using such drugs for too many cycles, as they are known to increase the risk of ovarian cancer. For this reason, the drugs are generally only prescribed for fewer than six menstrual cycles. If clomifene fails to stimulate ovulation, there is a range of ovary-stimulating hormonal drugs (gonadotropins) that have a similar effect which may be prescribed by a fertility specialist.

Information box 5.2f-VI

Ovarian stimulants: comments from a Chinese medicine perspective

From a Chinese medicine viewpoint, the induction of ovulation at a time when it would not naturally have occurred might be interpreted as Depleting of Blood and/or Kidney Essence, as these are the substances that enable ovulation to occur. The side effects associated with the use of clomifene suggest that it also leads to Liver Qi Stagnation and Accumulation of Damp/Phlegm, and the risk of ovarian cancer suggests that in some cases Blood Stagnation might develop.

New assisted techniques of conception

There are a number of methods currently used in intractable cases of infertility that enable the meeting of the parents' gametes. Apart from assisted insemination with the partner's sperm (see below), all these techniques depend on inducing a state of superovulation in the woman. This means that an ovary-stimulating drug is given to the woman to induce the development of a number of ovarian follicles at the same time.

The ovaries are prepared for this stimulation by first administering a drug by daily injection or nasal spray for two weeks, to prevent the release of FSH and LH from the pituitary. This means that the levels of natural estrogen drop, and a range of side effects, including hot flashes, palpitations and sweating, develop. After 2–3 weeks, a preparation of FSH and LH is given by injection to stimulate superovulation. This causes the ovaries to swell to over twice their normal size. The development of the follicles is monitored by means of regular ultrasound scans.

When the follicles are ready to rupture, the released eggs are harvested by means of a surgical technique that accesses the ovaries via the vaginal wall. The eggs are then taken to a laboratory to be examined and prepared for fertilization. Only the healthy eggs are saved. Some of these eggs may be frozen and stored for future attempts at fertilization or for donation to women who are unable to produce their own.

The emotional consequences to the couple of this aspect of assisted techniques are not to be underestimated. First, the different stages of ovary-stimulating medication have a wide range of physical and psychological side effects. While experiencing the effects of this medication, the woman has to make repeated visits to the fertility clinic for scans whilst the follicles are developing, and ultimately for the harvesting operation. After all this has happened, there is a possibility that the embryos formed from the eggs generated may either be unhealthy or may fail to implant. The couple then has to decide whether or not the whole cycle should be repeated. It is estimated that one-third of women undergoing assisted conception techniques experience anxiety or depression, and one in seven becomes severely distressed.

In some health districts in the UK, limited cycles of assisted conception are funded by the National Health Service (NHS). In others, the couple has to pay a considerable sum for each attempt (cycle) at implantation. The cumulative cost of successive cycles is another factor that can add to the stress of a couple who have decided to opt for assisted conception.

Assisted insemination with husband's sperm (AIH)

AIH involves injection of the partner's sperm directly into the uterus by means of a fine tube inserted into the cervix. This technique is used in cases in which the sperm are unable to penetrate the cervical mucus. It might also be used in cases in which there are psychological or physical problems, such as erectile dysfunction or vaginismus, which may prevent normal intercourse. AIH is the least invasive of the assisted conception techniques, and carries very few risks over and above those of normal sexual intercourse. The risks of surgical penetration of the cervix, although very low when in experienced hands, include introduction of infection into the womb and traumatic damage to the cervix and endometrium.

In vitro fertilization (IVF) and zygote intrafallopian transfer (ZIFT)

In vitro fertilization (IVF) and zygote intrafallopian transfer (ZIFT) involve harvesting of eggs, and subsequent fertilization of these with the partner's sperm in a laboratory. The term in vitro literally means in glass, and

refers to the test tube (in fact, a flat-lidded glass or plastic dish) in which fertilization takes place.

Around the same time as harvesting, the partner or donor is required to produce a sperm sample. The sperm is washed and prepared so that only fast-moving sperm cells are selected. The egg and sperm are then mixed over the next 16–20 hours. Any fertilized eggs are placed in an incubator for the next two to six days, after which the most healthy-looking one or two embryos are selected for transfer. As this process is going on the woman is given further medication to help prepare the womb for implantation.

Up to three fertilized eggs are either returned directly to the woman's uterus, or are allowed to make a few divisions before they are returned as embryos (two to three days) or even blastocysts (five to six days) to the uterus via a thin plastic catheter passed through the cervix.

Successful implantation depends very much on the age and health of the woman. The success rate is nearly 40 percent for women under 35 but drops to 1.2 percent for those aged over 44. The percentage of these pregnancies that survive for the full term is lower. A significant proportion of all pregnancies end in miscarriage within the first few weeks, and this is also true for pregnancies that follow from assisted conception. This means that the stress on the couple is not lifted once a successful implantation has occurred. Because two or three embryos are transferred to the uterus in each cycle, there is also an increased chance of multiple pregnancies with these techniques.

Gamete intrafallopian transfer (GIFT)

Gamete intrafallopian transfer (GIFT) involves the direct transfer of unfertilized eggs and sperm into the fallopian tube to allow the formation of a zygote in a natural environment. This process, which can be performed directly after the eggs have been harvested, is less costly than IVF, but is not always the most suitable technique in some cases of infertility. The implantation rate of GIFT is 30–40 percent per cycle, which is higher than for IVF.

Intracytoplasmic sperm injection (ICSI)

Intracytoplasmic sperm injection (ICSI) involves the in vitro injection of sperm into the cytoplasm of the egg. It enables fertilization in cases in which the sperm have a reduced ability to move or are much reduced in number. ICSI is more costly than IVF, but has a higher success rate per cycle, with implantation occurring in 50 percent of cycles. This high success rate may be a reflection of the fact that ICSI is used in cases in which the problem lies in defective semen, and so in these cases it is more likely that the woman has no physiological barrier to fertility. It is possible to extract sperm from the epididymis or testicle by means of a minor operation, and this means that ICSI may be an option for men who suffer from total erectile failure or who have had a vasectomy.

Use of donor gametes

In some cases of infertility, one or both partners are unable to produce gametes at all. In these cases pregnancy may be possible with the use of donor sperm or donor eggs.

DONOR INSEMINATION (DI) OR ARTIFICIAL INSEMINATION (AI)

In the rare cases of total lack of sperm production, donor sperm may be used to enable conception to occur. This technique, known as donor insemination (DI), has been used successfully for decades. The semen may be donated by a friend or family member, or may be obtained from a sperm bank. The samples of semen held in a sperm bank originate from paid volunteers who have been carefully screened to reduce the risk of transmission of infectious or congenital disease. The couple can select which donated sample is used according to broad characteristics of the donor such as height and skin color. Personal details of the donor are maintained on a Human Fertilization and Embryology Association (HFEA) register. In the UK, all children born after April 2005 have the right to find out the identity of the donor from this register should they wish to at any stage in their life.

The success rate of DI is high, with over 65 percent of women conceiving within a year of using DI on a monthly basis. DI carries a very small risk of the transmission of infectious disease, although this is minimized by screening of donors and also the donated semen.

USE OF DONOR EGGS

As assisted conception techniques are increasingly popular, there is greater availability of donor eggs. These eggs can be fertilized with the male partner's sperm either in vitro or within the female partner's fallopian tube (using GIFT) to enable a pregnancy to occur. As with DI, the donor may be a friend or a family member, but this is not as simple a process for the donor as it is for DI. This is because the donated eggs have to be artificially stimulated and harvested in the same way as they are in the assisted conception techniques.

Surrogacy

Surrogacy is the method whereby the donor of the eggs also carries the pregnancy to full term after donor insemination by the male partner's semen. Commercial surrogacy is illegal in the UK, but couples may travel to countries such as the US where it is available on a private basis, although this inevitably carries significant financial and emotional costs. The couple may experience the pregnancy vicariously by keeping in regular touch with the surrogate mother. There are complicated ethical and legal issues that arise from questions about ownership of the child. This is not an approach that is recommended in conventional clinics.

 Information box 5.2f-VII

Assisted conception techniques: comments from a Chinese medicine perspective

From a Chinese medicine viewpoint, use of assisted fertility techniques raises some important questions about the long-term effects on the health of the woman and also the child. The use of drugs to induce superovulation are likely to be Depleting of Blood and Kidney Essence, as well as being a possible source of the introduction of patterns and Pathogenic Factors such as Toxic Heat and Damp. The damage caused by laparoscopy and cervical instrumentation will also lead to local Blood and Qi Stagnation and possible introduction of Toxic Pathogenic Factors.

In Chinese medicine, the conditions of conception and the early days of embryo development are considered to be fundamental in establishing the Essence of the child to be. Ideally, the parents should be in good health and in a calm emotional state. In contrast, the stress of these techniques may mean that both partners are both physically and psychologically drained at the time of conception. In the case of IVF, the environment for the conception could not be more different than the very Yin space offered by the fallopian tube. These techniques all involve a scientifically observed conception illuminated by the bright lights of a laboratory.

Moreover, the ovum used in such a conception would not have naturally matured at that time, and in the case of ICSI, the sperm would not have naturally been able to penetrate the ovum. This raises questions about the health of the individual gametes, and so will have consequences on the Essence of the child to be. Current studies suggest that the long-term health of babies born as a result of assisted techniques is not as good as those conceived naturally. Birth defects are 30–40 percent more likely to occur. In other words, the risk of an abnormality affecting a child born by assisted reproductive techniques is approximately 1.26 times that of the risk in a naturally conceived pregnancy. Developmental issues are also becoming apparent, particularly in multiple births. It is not possible to discern to what degree either the genetic inheritance of these children (i.e. from often older parents with possible pre-existing health problems) or the IVF process itself have contributed to these findings.[36]

Any complementary medical concerns about the energetic effects of assisted conception are speculative. There is no doubt that these techniques have enabled thousands of couples the opportunity of having a much wanted child. Statistics suggest that over 1 percent of all births in the UK in 2012 were attributed to IVF conception, and this frequency is even higher in some other European countries. The positive aspects of this outcome must not be underestimated. One important role we can have as complementary medical practitioners is to be able to support couples who have chosen to take this route, so that their health and emotional state can be optimized at the time of conception, embryo transfer and during the subsequent duration of pregnancy.

5.2g Structural disorders of the female reproductive system

The conditions studied in this section are those in which the underlying problem is primarily structural. They include:

- Inherited defects of the female reproductive system:
  - imperforate hymen
  - septate uterus and vagina
  - intersex disorders
- Benign structural disorders of the female reproductive organs:
  - cervical and endometrial polyps
  - fibroids
  - endometriosis
  - ovarian cysts
  - benign ovarian tumors
- Cancer of the female reproductive organs:
  - ovarian cancer
  - vulval cancer
  - cervical cancer
  - endometrial cancer
- Prolapse and displacement of the female reproductive organs
- Common surgical treatments:
  - hysterectomy
  - oophorectomy
  - repair operations for prolapse.

Inherited defects of the female reproductive system

Imperforate hymen

The hymen is a thin sheet of tissue that partially closes the entrance to the vagina. Normally it has a small opening through which the menstrual blood can flow at the menarche. In rare cases, the hymen does not have this opening. Ideally, this problem is found during the medical examination of a newborn baby girl, but the condition may be missed. If the problem is not detected before the onset of puberty, at the onset of menstruation the menstrual blood cannot appear. Instead, the blood builds up within the vagina and uterus. This may not necessarily cause symptoms, but can present with abdominal pain and urinary difficulties. The problem may actually not be diagnosed until the periods are noticed to be very late, and the girl is sent for investigations for primary amenorrhea.

The treatment is by means of minor surgery, in which a small incision is made to allow the accumulated fluids to disperse naturally.

Imperforate hymen is the most common inherited defect of the vagina and uterus.

Septate uterus and vagina

Septate uterus and vagina are more rare conditions in which the structure of the vagina, uterus or both is divided into two halves by a wall (septum) of tissue. This problem may not come to light until the woman suffers from recurrent miscarriages, or when the fetus does not lie in the normal head-down position in late pregnancy.

In some cases of septate uterus, surgical removal of the septum can reduce the risk of recurrent miscarriage.

Intersex disorders

Intersex disorders are rare conditions in which incomplete development of the sexual organs has resulted in the formation of genitalia with a structure that is between that of a boy and a girl. They develop as a result of an imbalance in the hormonal environment of the fetus.

In a male fetus both normal development of the external genitalia and also normal descent of the testes are dependent on the secretion of hormones from the developing pituitary and adrenal glands. There are two rare conditions (congenital adrenal hyperplasia and testicular feminization) in which these hormones are not formed properly. In these conditions, the external genitalia are either underdeveloped, or do not develop at all. In testicular feminization the child will look like a girl. The diagnosis may only be made when this female (but genetically male) child fails to menstruate at puberty.

Information box 5.2g-I

Congenital abnormalities of the uterus and ovaries: comments from a Chinese medicine perspective

In Chinese medicine, all these inherited conditions are regarded as manifestations of Jing Deficiency.

Benign structural disorders of the female reproductive organs

Cervical and endometrial polyps

The word polyp refers to a fleshy growth that develops from a thin stalk of tissue. Cervical polyps are common, benign outgrowths of the epithelium of the cervix. They usually produce no symptoms. In some cases they may lead to excessive physiological discharge. Occasionally, they may bleed irregularly, and in this way may mimic the symptoms of endometrial cancer. They can be removed very easily by means of a minor operation.

Endometrial polyps are fleshy outgrowths of the endometrium in the uterus. These, too, can lead to irregular bleeding. They may also be a cause of menorrhagia. They can be removed by means of a curette inserted during hysteroscopy.

Fibroids (uterine myomata)

Fibroids are benign tumors of the uterine muscle and can vary in size from that of a pea to a football. They are known to develop in up to 20 percent of women over the age of 30, and are more common in women who have had either one or no children. It is not unusual for a woman to have a number of fibroids of different sizes within her uterus. The fibroid is dependent on estrogen to grow, and so will very often shrink to a small size after the menopause.

Fibroids do not usually give rise to symptoms, especially if they are small. In some women, they are associated with menorrhagia and dysmenorrhea. Very rarely, large fibroids may be associated with infertility or recurrent miscarriage. A large fibroid may also cause pelvic or back pain, dyspareunia or problems with urination.

In most cases fibroids are not considered to be a cause for concern and as such do not need to be treated. In cases in which mild symptoms develop late in the woman's reproductive years, the best management is often considered to be waiting until the menopause has occurred, after which the symptoms will almost always abate.

A very large symptomatic fibroid can be treated surgically. Sometimes the fibroid alone will be removed (myomectomy), but very often the whole uterus is removed (hysterectomy). A myomectomy may lead to reduced fertility, but 40 percent of women who wish to conceive after this operation will still be able to do so. A hysterectomy is commonly advised for those women who are not concerned about fertility, because fibroids have a tendency to recur. The surgical approach of hysterectomy is discussed at the end of this section.

Uterine artery embolization is a newer surgical technique, in which the aim is to deprive the fibroid of its blood supply. This procedure requires shorter hospital stays and has a shorter recovery time than a hysterectomy, but up to a quarter of women may require further treatments to ensure symptom control.

The drugs goserilin and buserilin are LH analogues. They inhibit the release of FSH and LH, and so lead to a reduction in the natural production of estrogen. These drugs can be useful medical options for the treatment of fibroids in people who do not wish to undergo surgery. Side effects include menopausal symptoms of hot flashes, dry vagina and loss of bone density, a reflection of the fact that the drugs reduce the level of estrogen in the body. It is well recognized that growth of the fibroids can recur after the course of treatment has ended.

Information box 5.2g-II

Uterine polyps and fibroids: comments from a Chinese medicine perspective

In Chinese medicine, a fibroid, as a substantial mass, may be seen as a manifestation of Blood Stagnation and/or Phlegm in the uterus. Cervical polyps and endometrial polyps may be considered to have similar pathology. Any factors that might lead to stagnation and accumulation of Pathogens could be etiological factors, including local deficiency, Cold Damp Invasion, Stagnation of Liver Qi from frustrated emotions, and Damp Phlegm-forming food or environment.

Endometriosis

Endometriosis is a common disorder of unknown cause in which the uterine wall is distorted by the development of cysts of endometrial lining within its muscular walls and in other sites outside the uterus. The current theory for the origin of endometriosis is that small pieces of the endometrium can separate from the uterine wall during menstruation and seed in different locations. Although the uterine muscular wall is the most common location for endometriosis (in which case it may be termed adenomyosis), other sites include the ovary, the bowel and the peritoneal lining that surrounds the bowel and the other pelvic organs.

This displaced endometrium is still responsive to changes in the female hormones, and will build up and break down throughout the menstrual cycle. If the location is deep in some other tissue (e.g. of the ovary or the uterus wall), the menstrual blood cannot escape. This blood instead collects within the tissue to form what are descriptively termed chocolate cysts. The formation of these miniature cysts is a source of pain, which peaks premenstrually and during the period. Endometriotic cysts can be seen during a laparoscopy, when they appear as black spots, likened to the appearance of a burnt match head, on the surface of the uterus, peritoneal wall and ovaries. If the location of the cyst is on the peritoneum, the blood can escape to the peritoneal space and can be highly irritating. Again, this pain is worst during the time of the period.

It is estimated that endometriosis is present in about 5 percent of menstruating women. In many cases of endometriosis, there are no symptoms. However, symptoms can be severe. They include menorrhagia, dysmenorrhea, dyspareunia and infertility. Pain is often the most prominent symptom. In some cases it can persist throughout the menstrual cycle, but it is usually worst around the time of the menstrual bleed.

Adenomyosis and endometriotic cysts of the ovary can be detected by the relatively non-invasive test of intravaginal ultrasound scanning, but the gold standard for diagnosis is laparoscopy. Magnetic resonance imaging (MRI) may also be used to detect peritoneal deposits.

There is a range of drugs that may be used to treat the symptoms of endometriosis. Non-steroidal anti-inflammatory drugs (NSAIDs) such as mefenamic acid may be useful for suppressing pain. All the other treatments are intended to cause regression of the pain-inducing cysts. For this purpose, these drugs need to be taken for three to twelve months, after which time there may be a long-term reduction in symptoms. The drugs act by reducing the influence of estrogen on the cysts, which then shrink in size and become permanently scarred. The choice of drug is largely based on whether or not the symptoms can be tolerated.

In some women, the combined oral contraceptive pill or a high-dose progesterone-only pill (e.g. medroxyprogesterone acetate) may reduce or eliminate symptoms. Long-acting progesterone preparations, such as the depot injection Depo-Provera, and the progesterone-containing intrauterine device (IUD), can also alleviate symptoms very effectively. However, these treatments are not suitable if infertility is the primary concern.

The LH-releasing hormone analogues buserilin and goserilin are also prescribed. These are given by means of nasal spray or a monthly depot injection over the course of three to six months. During this time symptoms will abate, and this effect can be sustained. These drugs reduce the release of FSH and LH, and so the levels of estrogen drop, thus inducing a temporary menopause. Side effects include hot flashes, night sweats and amenorrhea. Bone loss is a potential problem and limits the time for which these medications can be prescribed.

The outcome of drug treatment depends on the initial extent of the endometriosis. In 30 percent of cases the disease regresses totally, in 60 percent there is partial regression, and in the remaining 10 percent there is no significant effect. In about half of those treated successfully, the disease recurs within five years.

Surgery is an alternative treatment for endometriosis. This is most effective if the ovaries are removed at the same time as the cysts are excised or cauterized. In some severe cases, hysterectomy may also be performed. Obviously, this radical approach is not suitable for women who still want to have children. Less radical surgical approaches, such as cautery of individual cysts, have been shown to improve fertility in the year following the intervention.

 Information box 5.2g-III

Endometriosis: comments from a Chinese medicine perspective

In Chinese medicine, endometriosis would appear to correspond to Blood Stagnation in the uterus. The formation of blood-containing cysts may also indicate the presence of Phlegm or Phlegm Heat. Its symptoms are painful periods and infertility and so the range of syndromes that might present with a diagnosis of endometriosis might also include Qi Stagnation, Cold in the Uterus and Damp Heat. Deficiency of Qi, Blood and Yang, particularly when relating to the Liver and Kidney, can predispose to these conditions.

Functional ovarian cysts

A cyst is a fluid-filled swelling. In the ovary, cysts may be part of the normal follicular changes that take place in a menstruating woman, in which case they are known as functional cysts. Cyst formation in the ovary is part of the natural physiology of the development of the ovarian follicle in the first half of the menstrual cycle. As the follicle matures, fluid forms within it, only to be released when the follicle ruptures at the middle of the cycle. Just before rupture, the normal ovarian follicle can reach a size of up to 2cm in diameter.

The most common cause of a symptomatic cyst in the ovary is failure of this process of rupture. Instead of rupturing at mid-cycle, the ovum-containing cyst continues to enlarge as it accumulates fluid. In some cases this does not produce any symptoms, but in others the enlarging cyst continues to produce estrogen, and this can result in menorrhagia and an irregular length of cycle. The causes of this failure are unclear, but are probably rooted in an imbalance in the release of FSH and LH from the pituitary gland.

Alternatively, failure of degeneration of the corpus luteum in the second half of the menstrual cycle can also lead to cyst formation. In this case there may be excessive production of progesterone, giving rise to the symptoms of late periods or amenorrhea.

Polycystic ovary syndrome is the other common condition associated with benign cyst formation.

If followed by serial ultrasound scans it is seen that most functional ovarian cysts will disappear within two to three months. If ovarian cysts persist, the fluid within should be withdrawn by means of a minor operation so that a diagnosis of cancer can be excluded. If symptoms persist, or if the cyst is irregular in shape, the cysts are surgically removed. This operation is not believed to affect the function of the ovary.

Large ovarian cysts may cause symptoms in a number of ways. A very large cyst (more than 10cm in diameter) may cause discomfort as a result of pressure on other structures in the abdomen. Occasionally, a cyst will rupture, with a release of blood-stained fluid. This can be very irritating to the peritoneum, and can present as an acute abdomen (see Section 3.1d), particularly if the blood loss is severe. An enlarged cyst may also cause the ovary to twist around the stalk of tissue that contains the vessels providing its blood supply. This condition, called torsion of the ovary, gives rise to severe pain as the ovary is threatened with infarction. Torsion may settle as the stalk untwists, but otherwise requires an emergency operation. If the torsion settles, an operation to remove the cyst will be performed to prevent recurrence.

Benign ovarian tumors

Tumors of the ovary are common, and may also be cystic in nature. Ninety-five percent of ovarian tumors are benign in nature. One-quarter of these are found to be functional cysts (see above) and just under half of the remainder are growths known as cystadenomas. Like functional cysts, other forms of ovarian tumor may also produce symptoms resulting from rupture, release of fluid and torsion. Some of these tumors (mucinous cystadenomas) can reach an enormous size and can cause abdominal swelling and discomfort. Others give rise to symptoms because they produce excessive sex hormones. Excessive estrogen may give rise to irregular menstrual bleeding, whereas excessive testosterone can lead to masculinization.

Occasionally, the tumor is only diagnosed when a routine ultrasound scan is performed in pregnancy. The mass of the tumor may cause problems in labor, and if it is large, a surgical operation may be performed to remove it, ideally before the 30th week of pregnancy.

Benign tumors arising from the germ cells (immature egg cells) may also develop. These tumors are known as teratomas. Teratomas may contain a range of tissues, including bone, cartilage, hair and brain. As these tumors may be malignant, they are always removed.

If an ovarian cyst or tumor is seen by means of ultrasound scan, the clinical dilemma is whether it is benign and can be safely left alone, or whether it is malignant and needs removal. The shape of the tumor as seen on an ultrasound scan can be helpful, but is not absolutely diagnostic (an ultrasound scan will positively detect 89 percent of ovarian cancers). The risk that an ovarian cyst or tumor is malignant is greater if the levels of a tumor marker called CA-125 are high. Women are therefore assigned a risk score depending on age, ultrasound appearance and the CA-125 level. In younger women with a low risk score, the cyst may simply be monitored by means of regular ultrasound scans or fluid removed for examination by means of laparoscopy. Postmenopausal women with ovarian tumors are generally considered to be at greater risk of ovarian cancer. Those with a low risk score may be managed either by regular ultrasound screening or, if there is any concern, by laparoscopic removal of the ovaries only. Postmenopausal women with a high-risk score are advised to have the tumor removed by means of total hysterectomy together with bilateral oophorectomy (removal of the ovaries).

 Information box 5.2g-IV

Ovarian cysts and tumors: comments from a Chinese medicine perspective

In Chinese medicine, ovarian cysts and tumors might correspond to Blood Stagnation and/or Accumulation of Damp/Phlegm.

Cancer of the female reproductive organs

The most common cancers of the female reproductive organs are cervical cancer, endometrial cancer and ovarian cancer. A less common cancer, vulval cancer, accounts for about 3 percent of all cancers of the reproductive tract. The other cancers, which affect the vagina and the fallopian tubes, are very rare, and are not discussed further here.

Ovarian cancer

Ovarian cancers usually affect postmenopausal women. They have very few early symptoms, and so may not be diagnosed until they are at an advanced stage. First symptoms may include abdominal discomfort and swelling from accumulation of fluid (ascites) in the abdominal cavity. Other symptoms of advanced cancer, such as weight loss and loss of appetite, may also be present.

In rare cases there is a strong family history of postmenopausal ovarian cancer. It is argued that women who have a strong family history of ovarian cancer (i.e. those with two or more close relatives with ovarian cancer) should be offered the choice of surgical removal of the ovaries at the time of the menopause as a preventive treatment, as the lifetime risk of developing ovarian cancer is up to 40 percent in such people.

Treatment of the tumor depends on the exact type of the cancer, which is determined by means of examination of a biopsy. Extensive surgery is recommended for most ovarian cancers, although one rare type is known to respond well to radiotherapy. After surgery, chemotherapy including cisplatin and paclitaxel (Taxol) is given in three-week cycles. Taxol is a drug, derived from the yew tree, which was first introduced by naturopaths. Nevertheless, these treatments in combination are highly toxic to the body, and side effects are very common.

In those cases in which the cancer is confined to the ovary, surgery can be curative. However, in more than 70 percent of cases the cancer has extended beyond the ovary at the time of diagnosis, and in these cases the five-year survival is less than 25 percent, despite the use of surgery and combination chemotherapy.

Vulval cancer

Vulval cancer is usually a cancer of elderly women. Itch is the most common presenting symptom, and may have been tolerated by the woman for some time before a diagnosis is made. Because the diagnosis is often delayed, in many cases metastatic spread to the local lymph nodes is also discovered at the time of diagnosis.

Treatment of vulval cancer discovered at an early stage is excision of the vulva. Radiotherapy is then given to the lymph nodes. If treated at this stage there is a very good chance of cure. If metastatic spread has occurred, much more tissue is removed, and all the lymph nodes in the groin and pelvic area are also excised. This radical operation can be complicated by poor wound healing and persistent leg edema.

Vulval cancer may be preceded by years by a chronic change to the vulval skin known as lichen sclerosus. In this occasionally precancerous condition, white plaques develop on the skin of the vulva. These may be asymptomatic or may cause intense itching over the course of many years. In some people, the atrophic patches of skin can contract to lead to painful fissures and dyspareunia. Lichen sclerosus can also affect the skin of the anus, and the foreskin and glans penis in men. It is treated by means of high-dose steroid creams and regular monitoring for cancerous change.

Vulval intraepithelial neoplasia (VIN) is a more sinister precancerous change of the vulva, which may not necessarily even itch. VIN describes a region of vulval skin that has actually begun to show cancerous change. Like cervical intraepithelial neoplasia (CIN), VIN is associated with previous wart virus infection.

VIN appears as deficient white patches on the vulva, without the thickening characteristic of lichen sclerosus. In general, VIN is treated by means of regular monitoring, as the risk of full cancerous change is about 5 percent. More advanced cases are treated by means of excision, but this carries the risk of sexual dysfunction.

Cervical cancer

Cervical cancer most commonly develops close to the vaginal opening (external os) of the cervical canal. It almost exclusively affects women who have been sexually active. There is increasing evidence that prior infection with certain strains of the wart virus (human papilloma virus, HPV) is associated with the development of cervical cancer. Over 80 percent of women with cervical cancer have evidence of wart virus infection (particularly type 16). It is believed that certain types of wart virus are carcinogenic because they inactivate tumor suppressor genes.

However, the virus can be found in the cervix without there being a history of sexual intercourse, and also, in most cases, infection with the virus will not lead to cancer. One theory is that additional factors are required to allow a cancer to develop. These include smoking, and infection with other sexually transmitted agents, including the herpes virus.

Cervical cancer is one of the few cancers that can be detected by means of a fairly simple test at an early stage. This test is the cervical cytology screen (previously known as the Pap smear). It is believed that in the very early stages of the cancer, the nuclei of the epithelial cells of the cervix undergo a characteristic change in shape. At this stage, the presence of these pre-cancer cells does not necessarily mean that a cancer will develop. In fact, it is now known that, in some women, these abnormal cells will disappear with time, and without the need for treatment. Nevertheless, this stage, known as pre-cancer, is believed to be a strong indicator of the development of an established cancer of the cervix within a timescale of 5–10 years.

The cervical cytology test can distinguish between different stages of progression of the pre-cancer according to the shape of the nuclei in the cells detected. These stages usually correspond to pathological changes in the lining cells of the cervix epithelium known as CIN1, CIN2 and CIN3. These changes can only formally be diagnosed by colposcopy, but the degree of abnormality of cells seen in the cytology testing stage can indicate these pathological states of progression of cervical pre-cancer. Examination of the cytology sample can also indicate the presence of active infection by the wart virus. Whereas wart virus infection alone carries a low risk of progression, CIN1 and CIN2 indicate a progressively high risk of the development of cancer in the future. CIN3 is considered to be highly predictive of the presence of a tiny tumor (carcinoma in situ).

However, up to 15 percent of pre-cancers or cancers will not be detected by a cervical smear (i.e. the test has a 15 percent false-negative rate). This is because it cannot be ensured that all parts of the cervix can be sampled evenly by the brush or spatula, even if the test is performed as carefully as is possible. There is also a false-positive rate in that not all women who have a positive smear test are destined to go on to develop cancer. Nevertheless, a positive test will usually be followed by more invasive investigations or treatment.

The smear test is now offered in the UK to all women above the age of 25 initially at three-year intervals, and is continued until the woman reaches 65. The further investigations and treatment choices offered to the woman depend on the results of the test.

The possible outcomes of a smear test are:

- Normal (negative) test: return for a smear test after three years.

- Inconclusive result: repeat the smear as soon as possible.

- Borderline changes with no HPV DNA demonstrated: treat as normal test.

- Borderline changes with HPV DNA not tested for: repeat in six months.

- Borderline changes with HPV DNA demonstrated: refer for colposcopy test.

- Moderate or severe abnormality of cells (dyskaryosis): refer for colposcopy (a colposcopy is an invasive visual examination of the cervix at which tiny biopsies of the cervix are taken. These can confirm whether or not the CIN changes are present).

- CIN1: this is considered a low risk change. The woman is recalled for repeat cytology examination in a year.

- CIN2 and CIN3: examine the cervix by means of colposcopy, and biopsy the affected area of epithelium to exclude cancer. Destroy the affected area by means of laser, cold probes or heat probes. Large loop excision of the transformation zone (LLETZ) using a hot wire loop is the most commonly performed treatment for small regions of cellular abnormality. If the region of abnormality extends into the os, treatment may involve the removal of a cone-shaped wedge of tissue surrounding the cervical canal (cone biopsy). Repeat smear tests at six-month intervals for one year and at yearly intervals thereafter are required to test for permanent resolution of the CIN changes.

- Biopsy shows carcinoma in situ: treat by means of hysterectomy. The cure rate is very high if the cancer is caught at this stage.

Although colposcopy is uncomfortable, most women who receive this treatment for CIN1–3 will have normal smear test results after five years of follow-up. This means that the progression to cancer is extremely rare, even in those women who are found to have abnormal smear results.

Nevertheless, colposcopy for CIN is uncomfortable and embarrassing for most women. It can be painful and may be followed by a prolonged period of vaginal bleeding as the treated cervix recovers. Moreover, it may have been unnecessary in a proportion of women, as the CIN changes can resolve without the need for treatment. It is estimated that 40–60 percent of CIN1 smears will regress to normal without treatment, but this figure is much lower for CIN2 and CIN3.

An abnormal smear test result is frightening and confusing for many women, who may interpret it as a diagnosis of cancer (which it is not). There is a conventional argument that the burden in terms of inconvenience and worry on the millions of women involved is very significant in terms of well-being. It is argued that, together with the financial cost of the UK national cervical smear program, these negative factors are not outweighed by the benefit of the detection of cancer in a few women.

Although this is a powerful argument, it is difficult for a government to dismantle a cancer screening program once it is in place, particularly if it is successful in detecting most of the early cases of a cancer. It is important to recognize that these are cases that are unlikely to have otherwise come to light until the cancer had reached a much more advanced stage (see below). Published figures suggest that early detection of cervical cancer by means of the cervical smear test prevents premature death, with an estimate of 4500 lives saved each year because of cancers prevented as a result of the UK screening program alone.[37]

ESTABLISHED CERVICAL CANCER

Established cervical cancer is most common in women aged 45–55, although there has been a recent trend for it to appear in increasing numbers of younger women. First symptoms include unexplained vaginal bleeding.

Bleeding after intercourse is particularly suggestive of cervical disease.

If undetected, cervical cancer spreads outside the lining of the cervix, upwards to involve the uterus, and downwards to involve the vagina. Early involvement of lymph nodes is common, which means that cure of many cases of established cervical cancer is unlikely.

Treatment depends on the stage of the cancer. Radical hysterectomy (while preserving the ovaries) is very often a curative treatment for small cancers confined to the cervix (five-year survival for 80–90 percent). In more advanced disease, radiotherapy will also be offered. This involves administering radiation from both an external and a vaginal source. In very advanced cancers, radiotherapy and chemotherapy will be combined, although cure is very unlikely if the cancer has spread beyond the cervix and the upper third of the vagina.

Human papilloma virus (HPV) immunization

In the UK, HPV immunization with quadrivalent vaccine (Gardasil) is part of the routine immunization program for girls aged 12–14, ideally before they have become sexually active (see Section 5.2d). The quadrivalent vaccine is designed to generate immunity to the wart virus types 16 and 18, which are the two subtypes most strongly associated with carcinogenesis.

Endometrial cancer

Endometrial cancer is most common in women aged 55–65. It is believed that the hormone estrogen may be contributory in the causation of endometrial cancer, particularly if its effects on the lining of the womb are unopposed by progesterone. Estrogen causes thickening of the lining of the womb. If progesterone is also produced by the corpus luteum, the womb lining will soften and break down in the second half of the cycle. If the corpus luteum does not develop properly, the endometrium continues to thicken, and this thickening may eventually progress to cancer. Preparations of hormone replacement therapy (HRT) that do not contain progesterone, and polycystic ovary syndrome and obesity (which both lead to an altered balance of sex hormones in the body), are also associated with an increased risk of endometrial cancer for this reason.

The first symptoms of endometrial cancer are usually either a bloody vaginal discharge or frank bleeding. Because of the age range in which this cancer is most common, this symptom often occurs after the menopause, and is soon noticed by the patient as abnormal. This means that 75 percent of endometrial cancer is at a very early stage at the time of diagnosis.

The cancer tends to spread to affect a wide area of the endometrium before penetrating to the deeper levels of the muscle of the womb. The diagnosis is suggested by a thickening of the endometrium seen on an ultrasound scan, and confirmed by means of Pipelle suction curettage or hysteroscopy and biopsy of the lining of the womb.

The treatment of early endometrial cancer is removal of the womb and ovaries (hysterectomy and oophorectomy). In some, but not all, early cases, the pelvic lymph nodes may also be removed. The five-year survival in these cases is 80 percent.

If the tumor is considered to be deeply advanced into the muscle wall of the womb, radiotherapy or hormone treatment is also given. Radiotherapy has the disadvantage of causing scarring of the vagina, which may affect future intercourse.

In advanced cases, hormone treatment is given, involving a high dose of a synthetic progestogen. This inhibits growth of the tumor, but is a palliative, rather than curative, treatment.

> ### Information box 5.2g-V
>
> ### Cancers of the female reproductive system: comments from a Chinese medicine perspective
>
> In Chinese medicine, cancers of the female reproductive organs correspond to Blood Stagnation sometimes with Accumulation of Phlegm, on top of an underlying severe Deficiency of Qi, Blood Yin or Yang. Deficiency in the Chong and Ren Mai, together with Qi Stagnation and/or Invasion of Damp (sometimes via sexually transmitted infections), Cold and the effects of exogenous estrogen, can all predispose to Stagnation and Damp Phlegm Accumulation in the Uterus.

Prolapse and displacement of the female reproductive organs

Prolapse is a term that is used medically to describe the movement of part of the body away from its usual anatomical position. When applied to the female reproductive organs, prolapse refers to a descent of the womb and/or the vagina down towards the vulva. This usually results from the weakening of the surrounding supporting muscles and tissues of the pelvic floor. In contrast, a displacement is a condition in which the position of the womb is abnormal in terms of angulation.

Uterovaginal prolapse

A degree of prolapse of the womb down into the vagina is common as women reach postmenopausal years. Sometimes part of the vaginal wall alone may sag downwards, without any descent of the womb. These conditions are more likely to be severe if there is a history of recurrent or difficult childbirth. Obesity can also exacerbate the problem.

If it is only the vaginal wall that sags downwards, this is called first-degree prolapse. The patient may then feel a lump in the vagina. An additional problem that occurs with prolapse of the anterior vaginal wall is that the bladder can also sag into the vagina (a condition called cystocele). This is thought to increase the risk of bladder infections and incontinence. If it is the posterior vaginal wall that is weak, then either the wall of the rectum or a loop of bowel can drop into the vagina to form the lump (a rectocele), which is felt by the patient. This can cause difficulties in defecation.

A second-degree prolapse is defined as a prolapse of the womb into the vagina so that it may actually project lower than the vulva if the woman strains in some way. The woman may have to push the lump back in place with her fingers if this occurs. In a third-degree prolapse, the womb is permanently prolapsed outside the vulva.

All degrees of uterovaginal prolapse may be a cause of persistent discomfort, particularly on urination or defecation. They may also increase the risk of urinary infections and incontinence.

Mild cases may improve with pelvic floor exercises, which can strengthen the supporting muscles of the pelvic floor. In more severe cases, one non-surgical approach to treatment is to insert a ring pessary into the vagina. In some cases this polythene ring may be all that is required to hold the uterus in place. The ring pessary requires three-monthly removal for cleaning and an annual check-up, but in the interim period should need no other medical attention.

Surgical treatments for prolapse involve either hysterectomy with repair of the prolapsed vaginal wall, or an operation to hitch up the position of the womb.

Displacement of the uterus

Normally, the uterus is situated above the vagina with a slight forward tilt. This means that in most women the cervix is felt on examination to point towards the back. In about 10 percent of women, the uterus tips backwards, and the cervix is felt to point forwards. This may simply be the way the uterus has developed, or can be a result of fixation by the scarring that can develop in endometriosis or pelvic inflammatory disease.

In most cases, the uterus is mobile. A mobile backwards-facing (retroverted) uterus is not believed to be associated with any symptoms or with any problems in either conception or pregnancy.

Symptoms only occur when the uterus is fixed in a backwards position. In these cases, the woman may experience dyspareunia, chronic pelvic pain and backache. These symptoms may sometimes, but not always, be helped by an operation to correct the position of the uterus.

Information box 5.2g-VI

Prolapse of the uterus: comments from a Chinese medicine perspective

In Chinese medicine, prolapse of the uterus corresponds to Deficiency of Spleen and/or Kidney Qi. In particular, there is Sinking of the Spleen and/or Kidney Qi.

A fixed retroverted uterus with associated pain and discomfort might correspond to Qi and Blood Stagnation in the pelvis.

Common surgical treatments

Hysterectomy

Hysterectomy is a procedure whereby the whole uterus is removed surgically. Ideally for the patient, this is performed by means of an incision made in the vaginal walls, as this procedure is less invasive than the alternative. However, if more extensive surgery is required, an abdominal incision may be necessary. Hysterectomy performed by the transvaginal route has a shorter recovery time than surgery by the abdominal route.

Simple hysterectomy was formerly performed for a wide range of gynecological conditions simply because, by removing the offending organ, it was seen to provide the ultimate cure. However, it is increasingly appreciated that the long-term psychological and physical complications make it a less ideal option than it was previously believed to be. Therefore, fewer hysterectomies have been performed in recent years, and other approaches, including drug therapy and endometrial ablation, are increasingly chosen as the first treatment option.

The reasons for performing a hysterectomy include severe dysfunctional bleeding and dysmenorrhea, symptomatic fibroids, endometriosis, prolapse of the uterus and gynecological cancer. In all cases, the potential benefits of the operation have to be weighed against the risks. Although hysterectomy will alleviate the immediate symptoms of the underlying condition, it is a major operation. Therefore, it carries the risks that are associated with all major surgical procedures.

Most women require at least six weeks to return to usual activities, and may not feel right for six months or more. Hysterectomy is irreversible, and so will deny the woman the future option of having children. About 5–10 percent of women suffer from persisting bladder and bowel complications after the operation. There is also a recognized link between hysterectomy and an early menopause (even if the ovaries are conserved).

A range of psychological complications can follow hysterectomy. Conventionally, these are believed to relate, in part, to the way in which the woman was prepared for the operation, but may also result from the loss of an organ that plays an important, albeit subtle, role in sexual and general well-being. These include loss of sexual desire, inability to achieve orgasm, anxiety and depression.

 Information box 5.2g-VII

Hysterectomy: comments from a Chinese medicine perspective

In Chinese medicine the loss of a vital organ will represent loss of Blood and Qi, and the surgical procedure will be a cause for local Blood and Qi Stagnation. There is a particular association between the Uterus and the Heart, as they are linked by the Bao Mai or Uterus Vessel (see Section 5.2a). Therefore, even when hysterectomy is a life-saving treatment, loss of the uterus might be expected to lead to a degree of imbalance in the Blood and Qi of the Heart Organ, as well as the Kidney and Liver. The surgery does not cure the underlying imbalance and, according to Maciocia (1998),[38] this imbalance, usually Stagnation of Blood and Qi, will be retained in the region, and may instead manifest in the form of bladder symptoms.

Oophorectomy

Oophorectomy is the surgical removal of the ovaries. Oophorectomy alone may be performed for benign ovarian disease (usually on one side only). More commonly, oophorectomy is performed together with hysterectomy. The reasons for combined oophorectomy and hysterectomy include gynecological malignancy, and any of the reasons for hysterectomy, particularly if they occur after the menopause. The ovaries are very often removed at the same time as a hysterectomy in postmenopausal women, because it is believed that after the menopause the ovaries are redundant pieces of tissue that have the potential of becoming cancerous.

The risks of the operation are similar to those of hysterectomy alone. In premenopausal women, oophorectomy will result in a premature menopause. In these cases, HRT is started at the same time as the operation, to prevent the dramatic effects of the sudden withdrawal of estrogen, including loss of bone density (osteoporosis) that would otherwise occur.

Repair of vaginal prolapse

The operation that is performed to treat vaginal prolapse is called a vaginal repair. In this operation, a portion of the lax vaginal wall is removed, and the prolapsed bladder wall or bowel is encouraged to return to the correct anatomical position.

These operations have been shown in long-term surgical studies to reduce the serious symptoms of incontinence.

A vaginal repair (colporrhaphy) may be all that is needed to treat cystocele or a rectocele. In this operation the vaginal wall is opened and the fibrous tissue behind strengthened to prevent future prolapse of the bladder or rectum.

Uterine prolapse can be treated by means of hysterectomy and vaginal repair, but this operation is not suitable for those women who wish to have children in the future. There is an alternative type of operation in which the cervix is excised, and the uterus is held in place by means of hitching it to natural ligaments, as well as repairing any additional laxity of the vaginal walls. Although fertility is preserved, the excision of the cervix means that the chances of conception are reduced by this operation. There is also a risk of recurrence of the prolapse. Less drastic surgical techniques involve using a mesh to hitch up the vagina or uterus to fixed structures such as the pelvic ligaments or sacral bone. As with the vaginal repair, symptoms of incontinence and discomfort may improve after these operations.

The red flags of the structural disorders of the female reproductive system

Some women with structural disorders of the reproductive system will benefit from referral to a conventional doctor for assessment or treatment. Red flags are those symptoms and signs that indicate that referral should be considered. The red flags of the structural disorders of the female reproductive system are described in Table 5.2g-I. A summary of the red flags in a format designed for quick reference in clinical practice can be found in Appendix III. This gives advice on the degree of urgency of referral for each of the red flag conditions listed.

Table 5.2g-I A36: Red flags of structural disorders of the female reproductive system

Red flag	Description	Reasoning
A36.1	Primary amenorrhea: after age 16	Refer any woman for investigation who has not achieved first menstruation by age 16
		If secondary sexual characteristics are developing normally, this might suggest an imperforate hymen or, rarely, an intersex disorder
A36.2	Menorrhagia: with features of severe anemia (tiredness, breathlessness, palpitations on exertion)	Menorrhagia (heavy periods) can be the sole cause of significant anemia, and merits prompt referral for investigation and treatment of the cause
		Menorrhagia may result from fibroids, endometriosis or an ovarian cyst
A36.3	Postmenopausal bleeding: any unexplained bleeding after the menopause	Predictable bleeding after the menopause is normal with hormone replacement therapy (HRT)
		Otherwise, it is a red flag of uterine or cervical tumor. Refer for further investigation
A36.4	Metrorrhagia: bleeding between periods that has no regular pattern. This includes postcoital bleeding (bleeding after intercourse)	Irregular periods are common, but bleeding that seems to fall outside the normal confines of a 2–5 day menstrual bleed might, rarely, signify a uterine or cervical tumor
		In younger women with unexpected bleeding it is more likely to signify a sexually transmitted disease, most commonly chlamydia
		Breakthrough bleeding is common in women on the contraceptive pill, but this usually falls into a regular pattern
		Refer for further investigation if this happens on more than two occasions
A36.5	Pelvic pain or deep pain during intercourse	Refer as a high priority if pelvic inflammatory disease is a possibility (see A35.6 and A35.7)
		Otherwise refer routinely so that investigations into the cause can be arranged (may also be the result of endometriosis, fibroids or ovarian cysts)
A36.6	Abdominal swelling: discrete mass in the suprapubic or inguinal region	Always refer for investigations if a mass is felt (possible fibroids, ovarian cyst, tumor, pregnancy)
A36.7	Abdominal swelling: generalized	Refer if the swelling is diffuse and increasing over days to weeks (possible fluid accumulation from a tumor (ascites))
		Other possibilities include multiple fibroids, pregnancy and simple weight gain
A36.8	Vulval itch or vaginal discharge in postmenopausal women	Vaginal itch is a common side effect of thrush (candidiasis) and sensitivity to soaps and bath products, so refer only if prolonged for >1 week and not responding to advice and simple treatment
		Consider the possibility of atrophic vaginitis in postmenopausal women. This can respond to hormone creams
		Also, rarely, itch can develop due to lichen sclerosus and vulval cancer
A36.9	Lump in vulva	This is usually benign (Bartholin's or sebaceous cyst), but refer for advice about excision and to exclude vulval carcinoma or warts
A36.10	Lump in testicle/scrotum	Most scrotal lumps are benign, e.g. varicocele and sebaceous cyst, but rarely can be testicular cancer. Refer for further investigation
A36.11	Acute testicular pain: radiates to groin, scrotum or lower abdomen	Refer any sudden onset of severe testicular pain (radiates to groin, scrotum or lower abdomen). This could signify inflammation of the testicle (orchitis) or a twist of the testicle (torsion). If the pain is very intense (with collapse and vomiting), refer as an emergency

A36.12	Chronic dull testicular pain: radiates to groin, scrotum or lower abdomen	If the testicular pain is more of a long-lived discomfort, this could either be chronic epididymitis or varicocele, and merits a medical examination and further tests
A36.13	Precocious puberty: secondary sexual characteristics before age 8 in girls and 9 in boys	Refer if secondary sexual characteristics begin to appear before age 8 in girls and 9 in boys so that an unusual endocrine cause can be excluded
A36.14	Delayed puberty: secondary sexual characteristics not apparent by age 15 in girls and 16 in boys	Refer if secondary sexual characteristics have not started to appear by age 15 in girls and 16 in boys. Refer if menstruation has not begun by the time of a girl's 16th birthday (primary amenorrhea)

Pregnancy and Childbirth

5.3

5.3a The physiology of pregnancy and childbirth

Chapter 5.2 described the roles of the reproductive system of both the male and female, including the production of gametes, and the provision of an environment in which these gametes can meet to produce a zygote. This section explores what happens following the time of conception, which is when the gametes meet, and follows the stages of development of the embryo and fetus, together with the physiological changes that occur in the mother at this time. The section concludes with a description of the physiology of childbirth and of the puerperium, which is the six-week period that follows childbirth, during which time the mother's body begins to return to its pre-pregnant state.

The formation of the embryo

Conception

Conception is the term used to describe the fusion of one of the millions of spermatozoa in the ejaculated sperm with the ovum, so forming a fertilized egg (zygote). In natural conception this fusion most commonly occurs in one of the fallopian tubes, within a few hours of ovulation. It is estimated that the ovum is viable for no more than 48 hours. This provides the spermatozoa with a relatively short window of opportunity to meet up with the ovum in any one menstrual cycle.

A spermatozoon reaches the fallopian tube from the vagina by means of the waving action of its flagellum (the tail-like process that projects from its cell membrane). The energy required for this feat of long-distance swimming is derived from nutrients contained in the seminal fluid.

The exact timing of the fertile period is unpredictable, as it depends on the timing of ovulation, which is variable even for women with regular menstrual cycles. It is recognized that women with regular cycles can ovulate earlier than day 7 and later than day 21 in a 28-day cycle. This, of course, has implications for the natural family planning methods that can be used either to plan conception or to prevent pregnancy. This is why recognition of the changes in the consistency of cervical mucus is so important for the success of these methods.

Out of the millions of spermatozoa that are ejaculated, only a few hundred reach the fallopian tubes. When these spermatozoa reach the ovum, only one will be permitted to penetrate the cell membrane of the ovum. As soon as penetration has occurred, there is a change in the cell membrane that prevents the remaining spermatozoa from attaching (see Figure 5.3a-I). The nuclei of the male and female gametes contain only 23 single chromosomes, rather than 23 pairs. After fusion of the ovum and sperm, their nuclei fuse to form 23 pairs of chromosomes, giving a combination of genes that is totally unique to that zygote. Within a few hours this new nucleus divides, and the zygote begins to form into the ball of cells known as the embryo.

Figure 5.3a-I A recently fertilized ovum after a single division of the nucleus
Spermatozoa that did not manage to penetrate the egg can be seen outside the cell membrane.

Implantation

The tiny ball of cells of the embryo is propelled down the fallopian tube, and thence into the uterine cavity by means of the wave-like action of the ciliary epithelium of the fallopian tube. As the embryo continues to divide, a fluid-filled cavity forms in its middle. By about seven days after fertilization, the outer layer of the developing embryo has differentiated into cells that can penetrate deeply into the endometrial lining. It is these cells that will form the placenta. These outer cells have proteins on their surface that can recognize and attach to the endometrial lining. This attachment occurs seven to ten days after conception. After attachment, these outermost embryonic cells release a hormone known as human chorionic gonadotropin (HCG) into the bloodstream of the mother. This hormone signals to the corpus luteum in the ovary that pregnancy has occurred, and thus triggers the chain of physiological effects that are indicators to the mother of the start of pregnancy.

It is speculated that the reason for infertility in those couples who are shown by investigations to have no obvious physical abnormality is due to a failure in implantation. In these couples, despite healthy-looking sperm and normal ovulation, pregnancies do not occur. Subtle defects in the formation of the corpus luteum may lead to a poorly developed endometrium in the second half of the menstrual cycle. A poorly developed endometrium may either prevent implantation from occurring at all, or may be the cause of a very early miscarriage. This problem can result from an imbalance in the production of the pituitary hormones, follicle-stimulating hormone (FSH) and luteinizing hormone (LH), which may, in turn, be influenced by variables such as emotional stress, poor diet and tiredness.

Development of the embryo after implantation

After implantation, the identical cells forming this initially tiny hollow ball continue to multiply and differentiate.

Differentiation is the term given to the process whereby cells with an identical set of chromosomes become specialized to form all the different tissues of the body. At implantation, the outer portion of this ball of cells forms into the embryonic part of the placenta. Within the ensuing 14 weeks, tiny blood vessels form within this tissue. This fleshy mass encourages a reciprocal development of the endometrial lining into which it penetrates. A very rich blood supply forms as this tissue develops, in which maternal and embryonic blood vessels run very close to one another. This permits an exchange of oxygen and nutrients from the mother's blood to that of the embryo, but without any mixing of the two blood supplies. As well as oxygen and nutrients, drugs and toxins are able to cross this boundary between the mother and the embryo. It is this combination of maternal and embryonic tissue that is destined to form the placenta. The placenta will be the source of nourishment for the baby until the time of delivery.

Another portion of the hollow ball of embryonic cells is destined to become the embryo itself. This portion develops within the fluid-filled cavity. By two weeks there is a definite lengthening of this mass of cells, so forming the primitive spinal cord. By three weeks a primitive heart has formed, with vessels connecting to those of the placenta. By four weeks a tube has formed from top to bottom, which will later develop into the gastrointestinal system, and by six weeks the first features of the kidneys and sex organs have appeared. By seven weeks all the important organs have appeared. By this time there is a distinct form to the head, with bumps for the nose and ears, and also to the limbs, with tiny buds for the fingers and toes (see Figure 5.3a-II).

Figure 5.3a-II The development of the embryo at (a) six weeks and (b) nine weeks of gestation

The sac of fluid within which the embryo develops is called the amniotic sac, and the fluid within this sac is called amniotic fluid. The embryo is suspended in the fluid by a bridge of tissue known as the umbilical cord. The blood vessels that link the embryo to the placental blood supply pass through the umbilical cord. The amniotic fluid serves as a protective space for the fetus, which, until the very last weeks of pregnancy, can permit unrestricted movement of the developing limbs. This fluid serves to keep the skin moist and nourished, and is also a space into which the first urine is excreted.

The stage of pregnancy (gestation) is dated in a different way to the actual age of the embryo from the time of conception. Gestation is the term used to describe the time elapsed since the date of the last menstrual period. This is, of course, on average two weeks longer than the actual time after conception. For example, in a woman who is eight weeks pregnant, the embryo is in fact only six weeks old.

Many women will be unaware of the possibility of pregnancy for the first eight weeks of gestation, and this is particularly the case for those women who have a light bleed at four weeks, despite the fact that they are pregnant. The embryo is particularly vulnerable to nutritional deficiencies, drugs and toxins in this short time. Therefore, the only way by which a woman can ensure optimum health for her developing baby is to start making lifestyle changes before she falls pregnant. This is the foundation of the practice of giving pre-conceptual advice to couples who are planning to have a baby. The importance of giving pre-conceptual advice is emphasized in both conventional and alternative practice.

Pre-conceptual advice

From a conventional medical perspective, a couple planning to conceive should be aware that all drugs and toxins to which the mother is exposed might also affect the developing embryo. The prospective parents will be advised to stop smoking and to avoid alcohol and other recreational drugs. A healthy diet is advised. Ideally, if possible, all therapeutic drugs should be avoided for a few weeks before conception. Women who have been taking the contraceptive pill might be advised to stop this form of contraception for at least three months before trying to conceive. The only nutritional supplement that is routinely advised are the vitamins folic acid and low-dose vitamin D. Deficiency of dietary folic acid is strongly linked with an increased incidence of spinal cord defects, including spina bifida. The advice is to take a daily supplement of this vitamin from the time of trying to conceive to at least 20 weeks of gestation. Alternative practitioners may advise a wide range of other nutritional supplements, including zinc, manganese and selenium.

Development of the fetus to the time of delivery

From about ten weeks of gestation the embryo is termed a fetus. The fetus has primitive limbs and facial features, and all the rudimentary organs in place. At this time the fetus is about 2.5cm in length.

Nourishment of the fetus

The fetus obtains the nutrients it requires from the mother's circulation. It is generally believed in conventional medicine that, except in cases of extreme starvation, the fetus can obtain all it needs from the mother's bloodstream, and so will not necessarily suffer if the mother is unable to have a good diet, due, for example, to morning sickness. Deficiency of folic acid in the first trimester, and of vitamin D throughout pregnancy, are exceptions to this, as these are routinely recommended as supplements in pregnancy. This is in contrast to the perspective of Chinese medicine, in which the precise content of the diet of the pregnant woman is believed to have a very important bearing on the health of the developing organs of the fetus.

However, the mother may suffer as her nutrients are being diverted to nourish the developing fetus and support the growth of the placenta. Deficiencies of iron and calcium are well recognized to affect women in pregnancy. These can than lead to anemia and weak teeth. It is very likely that many more vitamin and mineral deficiencies can occur, which may partly explain the specific food cravings that many women experience during pregnancy. Although some of the foods craved may be bizarre in nature, the most common cravings are for fruit juice and dairy products, indicating a need to replace vitamins such as vitamin C and minerals such as calcium.

The main source of energy for the fetus is glucose. Glucose is also used to make the fats required by the fetus. Excessive glucose, a problem that occurs in maternal diabetes, will stimulate growth and cause excessive fat formation, and so can lead to an overlarge baby. Maternal amino acids are used to make the proteins required to build the structure of the tissues of the fetus. The wastes that the fetus produces are removed by the placenta into the maternal blood.

The fetal circulation

The circulation of the fetus has some important differences to that of a newborn baby. The blood enters the fetus through the umbilical cord, and first passes through the liver. It is then pumped through the heart, and thence to the rest of the body, before being redirected out through the umbilical cord. One major difference in this circulatory pattern is that relatively little blood is passed through the lungs, which in the fetus are filled with fluid, and are not a source of oxygen. To enable this circulation pattern to occur, the fetal heart retains a hole in its central wall, which permits the exchange of blood between the right and left sides of the heart.

At birth, the lungs are expanded suddenly with the baby's first cry. This expansion diverts a lot of blood into the vessels of the lungs for the first time. This has the remarkable effect of altering the pressure of blood within the rest of the fetal circulation so that the hole in the heart is closed by means of a flap of tissue, and the blood flow in the umbilicus diminishes markedly. Within a matter of seconds the whole pattern of blood flow in the fetus is transformed. Within a few minutes the pulsation of blood in the umbilical cord stops, and the cord can be tied off. What used to be the life source for the fetus now becomes a redundant stump, commonly known as the "belly button."

The fetal digestive system

The gastrointestinal tract is relatively quiet in the fetus. As the fetus matures, it swallows amniotic fluid, which is then absorbed through the intestines and then excreted back into the amniotic fluid cavity by the kidneys. By the end of pregnancy the intestines of the fetus contain a black sticky form of feces called meconium. This is composed largely of epithelial cells that have been shed from the growing intestinal lining.

The fetal lungs

The fluid in the developing fetal lungs is in direct communication with the amniotic fluid through the mouth and nose. A circulation of this fluid is maintained by the breathing movements that occur with increasing regularity in the developing fetus. As the fetus reaches full maturity, the lungs secrete an oily substance, called surfactant, into the alveoli. After birth, surfactant enables the newly expanded air spaces to remain in their patent state. In premature babies, insufficient surfactant can result in a tendency for the alveoli to collapse. Deficiency of surfactant is one of the causes of the severe respiratory problems that can affect premature babies.

The fetal immune system

The immune system of the fetus begins to develop by week 20 of pregnancy. After this time the fetus is able to produce its own antibodies. Nevertheless, this response is not fully mature until some weeks after birth. The fetus gains extra protection from infection in the womb by maternal antibodies, which are able to cross the placenta. These antibodies have a life of a few weeks, and so continue to protect the newborn for a couple of months or so after the birth.

The progression of all the changes that occur in the fetus during its development are summarized in Table 5.3a-I.

Table 5.3a-I The stages in the development of the fetus

Age of gestation	Length of fetus	Stage of development of fetus
14 weeks	6cm	All organs present in rudimentary form
		Limbs, muscles and bones all formed; baby has free movement
		Sex organs developed
		Heartbeat strong and fast
15–22 weeks	16cm	Hair, eyebrows, fingernails and fingerprint all formed; eyelids remain closed
		Baby's movement can be felt by the mother
23–30 weeks	24cm	Movement is vigorous; baby can respond to touch and sound
		Baby can swallow, may get hiccups
		Urine is formed by the kidneys
		Eyelids open from time to time
At 28 weeks the baby has a good chance of survival if born prematurely		
31–40 weeks		Fat is laid down beneath the skin of the baby, making it plump and less wrinkly
At 34 weeks most babies find a head-down position, and movements become more restricted due to lack of space		

The physiological changes of pregnancy

The hormones of pregnancy

The developing embryo secretes the hormone HCG into the endometrium very soon after implantation. This means that at about day 21 after the last menstrual cycle the ovaries receive a signal that implantation has occurred. HCG stimulates the corpus luteum to continue to produce estrogen and progesterone. Without this stimulus, the corpus luteum would degenerate rapidly, and the resulting drop in estrogen and progesterone would lead to menstruation within a few days.

HCG is produced in large amounts during the first third (trimester) of the pregnancy. It is this hormone that can be detected from a sample of the mother's urine and is used as the means of testing for pregnancy. A simple HCG test, which can be purchased at a pharmacy, can indicate pregnancy even earlier than week six of gestation (two weeks after the missed period).

Estrogen is secreted in increasing amounts throughout pregnancy. This is initially produced by the corpus luteum, but is later produced by the placenta. This hormone brings about the increased fleshiness that is characteristic of pregnancy. The cervix becomes swollen and soft, and the breasts and nipples enlarge. Estrogen also stimulates the production of increased vaginal discharge that is a normal feature of pregnancy. It also promotes an increased blood supply to all tissues. The amount of blood pumped through the heart increases, and the blood vessels dilate. In healthy pregnancies this results in a drop in blood pressure. The healthy glow commonly seen in middle to late pregnancy is a result of the effect of estrogen on the blood supply to the skin.

Like estrogen, progesterone is also produced initially by the corpus luteum, and then by the placenta. One important action of progesterone is to cause muscle and ligamentous relaxation. This effect is very marked on the muscular wall of the uterus, but excessive relaxation of the smooth muscle of the esophageal sphincter, the bowel and the ureters may also occur. This effect of progesterone can result in some of the most common minor complications of pregnancy, including heartburn, constipation and tendency to urinary infections. Relaxation of the ligaments of the pelvis and lower back is important to allow for the passage of the baby during labor. However, this can lead to some of the painful musculoskeletal conditions of pregnancy, such as low backache, sacroiliac strain and pain in the symphysis pubis. Progesterone also tends to increase the body temperature. The placidity of pregnancy is attributed to a calming effect of progesterone on the brain.

Other hormones important in pregnancy include prolactin (PRL) from the pituitary gland, adrenal corticosteroids and thyroid hormones. PRL stimulates the development of the milk-producing glands within the breast in the last ten weeks of pregnancy. The adrenal corticosteroids are important to help the body deal with the demands of pregnancy, but in excess may lead to weight gain, high blood sugar and high blood pressure. The thyroid hormones play a role in the regulation of increased growth. Under the influence of estrogen, the thyroid gland may enlarge to twice its normal size. Occasionally, if this enlargement is excessive, a goiter may develop.

The first symptoms of pregnancy

The first symptoms of pregnancy may be felt as early as the first two weeks after conception. Some women are aware of a different feeling even before the first missed period,

and some may experience nausea or breast tingling at this early stage. It is more usual that symptoms are experienced at around week six of gestation. The most common include breast tingling or tenderness, nausea, and sensitivity to certain smells or tastes. The missed period is not a universal experience. Some women may have a painless bleed at four weeks, and even at eight weeks of gestation, despite having a healthy pregnancy. As well as being a potential source of great anxiety, this form of bleeding can very much confuse the dating of the pregnancy, as the estimate of the length of the gestation normally relies on the date of the last menstrual period.

The effects of the enlarging uterus

As the embryo develops into a rapidly growing fetus, the uterus and the placenta enlarge to accommodate the growth and increasing nutritional requirements. At about 12 weeks of gestation, the amniotic sac is 10cm in diameter and the uterus can be felt just above the pubic bone. At 20 weeks of gestation, the top of the uterus is at the level of the umbilicus, and by 36 weeks the uterus has reached the level of the xiphisternum. Amazingly, the remaining abdominal contents continue to function relatively normally, despite their increasingly cramped conditions.

However, certain problems can arise from the compression of the abdominal organs. In particular, compression of the abdominal aorta can lead to discomfort and faintness when lying supine (on the back) in late pregnancy. Restriction of the free flow of blood in the deep pelvic veins can contribute to the development of varicose veins, hemorrhoids and ankle swelling. Heartburn can be very severe in late pregnancy, as the uterus presses on the stomach from below. Occasionally, nerve compression can cause areas of pain and tingling. The most common site for this problem is down the front of the thigh, a result of the compression of a nerve that runs down from the crease of the groin. Rapid growth of the uterus can also lead to stretch marks and itching of the skin of the abdomen. Both these problems are compounded by the excessive weight gain that can complicate some pregnancies.

Changes in the uterus, cervix and vagina

The uterine muscle fibers lengthen markedly during pregnancy, thus allowing for the elongation of the uterus. The natural tendency for these fibers to contract becomes more pronounced. Mild contractions of the uterus start to occur from very early in pregnancy. Some, but not all, women become aware of these contractions, known as Braxton Hicks contractions from about 20 weeks of pregnancy. The sensation is usually described as a painless tightening of the abdomen, which lasts for a few seconds. Some women do describe the sensation as painful, akin to period cramps, and for this reason Braxton Hicks contractions can sometimes be confused with the onset of labor. Braxton Hicks contractions increase in frequency and intensity as the time for the onset of labor approaches.

During pregnancy, the cervix and vagina respond to the increased levels of estrogen and progesterone. The cervix becomes softer in consistency, a change that can be detected by a skilled examiner at as early as eight weeks of gestation. This change occurs in preparation for the dilatation that has to occur during the first stage of labor. The vaginal walls also change in consistency to allow for the expansion that will be necessary to allow the birth of the baby. In addition, an odorless vaginal discharge is produced. This normal feature of pregnancy can be distressing for those women who are unprepared for its occurrence.

Changes in the maternal circulation

As pregnancy progresses, the blood vessels of the mother dilate, and an increased volume of blood circulates through them. These changes are to accommodate the increased requirements of the blood vessels in the placenta. Although the actual number of red blood cells is increased in a pregnant woman, the concentration of hemoglobin within them is usually slightly less than in the non-pregnant state. This can mean that a blood test will indicate anemia. If this finding is mild, it need not be treated. However, many women will be offered treatment with iron tablets if the anemia is severe, or if symptoms such as tiredness or dizziness develop.

The heart works much harder in pregnancy, as it has to pump up to 50 percent more blood than usual. The pulse is recognized to become more full and rapid in pregnancy, and this is accompanied by feelings of warmth. The slippery quality that is a characteristic of the radial pulse in pregnancy to a Chinese medicine practitioner is possibly equivalent to this conventionally recognized pulse change.

Many women become more aware of palpitations in pregnancy. Conventionally, this symptom is not usually considered to be serious.

Changes in the respiratory, urinary and digestive systems

After about week 30 of pregnancy, the downward movement of the diaphragm becomes more restricted, and this is compensated for by an increased expansion of the ribcage during breathing. Some women will easily become breathless on exertion as this change develops.

The kidneys are more active in pregnancy, as they have to deal with the extra waste products coming from the fetus.

More urine is produced. The muscles of the urinary system become more relaxed under the influence of progesterone. As previously mentioned, this can lead to an increased tendency to bladder infections. The risk of these infections spreading to involve the kidneys (pyelonephritis) is also increased in pregnancy.

The most common changes to affect the digestive system are spongy gums, heartburn and constipation. All these changes are results of the effect of progesterone. There is also an increased tendency to gum disease (gingivitis). For this reason, women are encouraged to make at least one visit to the dentist during pregnancy.

Weight gain

By the end of pregnancy, the fetus and the placenta together should weigh just over 4 kilograms. It is also normal for the mother to put on some weight as uterine muscle and breast tissue develop and also as fat stores are laid down around the abdomen, buttocks and thighs. These fat stores will be drawn on in the first few months after birth as the mother breastfeeds. Adding up these different elements, the ideal weight gain in pregnancy is estimated to be around 11 kilograms.

However, there can be enormous variations around this ideal. Sometimes this can be because the woman herself either loses or gains weight during the pregnancy. Less commonly, abnormal weight gain may be an indication of poor fetal or placental growth, or conversely, excessive accumulation of amniotic fluid. The most common problem with weight gain in pregnancy is that too much fat is laid down. The current advice is that a pregnant woman should eat a normal nutritious diet, and should not "eat for two."

Psychological changes in pregnancy

Ideally, the psychological changes of pregnancy are positive ones. Pregnant women often report feeling calm and happy in the later stages of pregnancy, an experience attributed to the effects of progesterone. However, 5–10 percent of women develop depression during their pregnancy. This seems to be more common in first pregnancies, and in women who have poor social support. Often in such cases there may be deep unaddressed fears about the labor, giving birth to a malformed child, or coping with caring for a baby. Also, many women grieve for the loss of their figure and freedom. Women who suffer from depression in pregnancy seem to be more likely to develop postnatal depression.

Information box 5.3a-I

Pregnancy: comments from a Chinese medicine perspective[39]

According to Chinese medicine, the Blood and Yin associated with menstruation accumulate after conception in the Chong and Ren Channels in order to nourish the developing fetus. As a consequence, the mother becomes relatively Blood and Yin Deficient, and so her Yang becomes relatively Hyperactive. Liver Yang Rising or Liver Wind Rising may develop (which can manifest as migraine headaches or pre-eclampsia in later pregnancy). Also Heat can easily accumulate during pregnancy (and manifest as rashes, palpitations and indigestion).

Depletion of energy in the lower aspect of the Chong Channel in the first trimester to nourish a healthy embryo is attributed to be the cause of the Rebellious Qi of nausea of pregnancy. Stagnation of Qi in the Chong Channel as the baby enlarges later in pregnancy may lead to breathlessness and fullness in the chest.

However, in some cases the stopping of the menses may actually mean the pregnant woman has more Blood energy available to her, and so she may feel more energetic and well, particularly in the middle trimester.

The Spleen and the Kidneys are particularly important in supporting the nourishment and growth of the fetus, and so there may be a tendency in the mother to developing Deficiency of Spleen and Stomach Qi, with Accumulation of Damp and Phlegm, and also Deficiency of Kidney Qi. The Liver is responsible for the smooth flow of Qi. As pregnancy is a time of accumulation of the Vital Substances in the lower Jiao, Liver Qi can easily stagnate as the normal flow of Qi in the middle Jiao is impaired.

All these syndromes are more likely in those women who have a pre-existing imbalance in one or more of these Organ functions. Most of the complications of pregnancy can be interpreted from a Chinese medicine perspective as consequences of these common underlying syndromes.

The physiology of childbirth

All the physiological changes of pregnancy so far described are gradual in development. In a healthy pregnancy, most women adjust well to these changes as they progress over the 40 weeks of gestation. The onset of labor is quite different. All of a sudden, the woman's body is thrown into a series of profound changes, which escalate rapidly and culminate in the birth of the baby and the placenta, usually within a timescale of 24 hours.

The initiation of labor

The precise trigger for the onset of labor is not clearly understood. It is known that the uterus becomes more sensitive to the pituitary hormone oxytocin during late pregnancy. It is likely that a surge in the release of oxytocin from the pituitary actually brings about the relentless wave of contractions that are characteristic of established labor. It may be that it is a hormonal factor released from the maturing fetus, such as an adrenal corticosteroid, that actually stimulates this surge. It is recognized that external factors, such as shock, injury and fever, can stimulate early labor, and anxiety and exhaustion can delay the progression of labor.

As the time for labor approaches, the Braxton Hicks contractions of the uterus become more frequent. Usually, at about two weeks before the onset of labor, the head of the baby drops into the bowl of the pelvis. This descent, known as engagement, often brings about a feeling of more comfort in the diaphragmatic area, as more space is created. In some pregnancies, engagement does not occur until after the onset of labor. In a few of these, this may be because the baby is not in the correct head-down, posterior-facing position.

Established labor is characterized by the onset of regular painful contractions that cause the tiny canal of the cervix to start to widen (dilate). In many women this transition between Braxton Hicks contractions and labor contractions is not clear-cut. In these women there may be a period of a few days in which the contractions are mildly painful and regular from time to time. Vaginal examination during this time will show that the cervix has not yet started to dilate. As cervical dilatation begins, a plug of mucus is released, which appears as an odorless blood-stained discharge sometimes called a "show."

Healthy established labor involves regular contractions, which gradually become more frequent and sustained. A typical pattern is that the contractions start to occur at intervals of over 15 minutes and last for only a few seconds. As the cervix gradually dilates, the interval between contractions shortens to less than 5 minutes, and the pain of the contraction lasts for 1–2 minutes. As this progression occurs, the contractions become more painful. Initially, the woman will be able to carry on usual activities between the contractions. The pain at this stage is often compared to that of period cramps. It is usually felt in the lower abdomen and low back.

In some women, the amniotic sac ruptures at this early stage, leading to a trickle or a gush of clear fluid. Occasionally, this rupture occurs before the onset of labor. This can then stimulate the onset of labor. If labor does not start within 24 hours of the breaking of the waters, there is a potential risk of infection, and so labor may have to be induced medically.

The first stage of labor

Labor is described in terms of three stages. The show and the onset of regular painful contractions herald the first stage of labor. This is the part of labor in which the canal of the cervix dilates to a diameter of about 10cm. In this stage there is only a small downward movement of the baby.

In first pregnancies, a normal first stage can last up to 36 hours, although less than 24 hours is more usual. For many women who have a prolonged first stage, for much of this period the initial dilatation of the cervix is slow and the contractions are bearable. Usually, it is only in the later part of the first stage that the contractions become very strong. In subsequent pregnancies the first stage lasts only a few hours, and the progression to very strong contractions is more rapid.

As the first stage of labor becomes established, the pain of the contractions increases markedly. As the cervix dilates to greater than 5cm, the pain causes the woman to go inward, stop talking and lose eye contact with the birth attendants. The respite between the contractions shortens down to only a few seconds as the contractions last for longer and become more frequent. If this painful stage is prolonged, the woman can become exhausted. For this reason, it is now common practice to encourage the woman to continue to eat light starchy food in the early part of the first stage of labor. Midwives often recommend glucose drinks in the later part of the first stage, to sustain the woman as she goes through this marathon.

The transition between the first and second stages of labor

The transition time is when the cervix reaches its maximal dilatation. It is at this time that contractions are at their most painful. Very often, the woman feels totally overwhelmed by what she is experiencing. Some women experience great fear or panic, believing that they are about to die. Other women become aggressive and abusive. Some may insist that they can no longer cope with the pain, and might demand medical pain relief. However, these behaviors are often signs that labor is progressing well. This transitional time usually lasts less than 30 minutes.

Occasionally, the woman has a desire to push during the transitional stage. If this occurs, she may be advised by the midwife to avoid pushing, until it is certain that the cervix is fully dilated. This is because a premature onset of pushing can cause the cervix to tear.

It is usually around the time of transition that the waters break if they have not done so already.

The second stage of labor

The second stage of labor is the stage in which contractions of the uterus are combined with the woman voluntarily pushing her abdominal muscles. This combined action forces the baby downwards through the pelvic canal. The second stage ends with the birth of the baby. It should last no more than 2 hours.

The second stage is characterized by the experience of the urge to push. Generally, the contractions are very frequent and strong, but may be more bearable than in the first stage. This means that if a woman can be supported through the transition without resort to medical pain relief, she may not need to request it for the second stage.

The forceful downward contractions encourage the head of the baby to descend down the pelvic canal, usually with the face directed backwards. The mother begins to feel an intense pressure as the head enters the vagina. Very commonly, women panic at this stage, fearing that they are going to open their bowels. This is because the feeling of fullness can also be sensed in the rectum. The downwards descent of the head can be seen by the birth attendant a few contractions before the baby is actually delivered.

Once the head has reached the perineum, the surrounding tissues become very tightly stretched. At this point the woman feels an excruciating bursting sensation. It is at this stage that the tissues of the vaginal wall and perineum may tear. Ideally, tearing can be prevented by controlling the force of the contractions. To enable this, the midwife will usually advise the women when to push and when to avoid pushing, by the use of breathing exercises. The midwife will also try to control the descent of the baby's head with manual pressure. However, the instinctive urge to push is often too great to be controlled, and tearing cannot be avoided. The practice of episiotomy, in which the midwife makes a cut in the perineum, is now becoming outmoded. It is recognized that most natural tears heal more efficiently than the surgical cut of the episiotomy.

Once the head has been delivered, the midwife checks that the umbilical cord is not tightly wrapped around the baby's neck. If it is, the midwife will free the cord before the rest of the baby's body is delivered. This is a common occurrence, which, if managed correctly, does not usually have serious consequences. Delivery of the rest of the baby's body usually occurs within another one or two contractions. A healthy newborn baby will make a cry within a few seconds. If there are no complications, it is common practice to hand the baby to the mother straight away to allow it to suckle. Ideally, time should be given (2–3 minutes) to allow the pulsation of blood in the vessels of the umbilical cord to stop before the cord is clamped and cut.

Once the baby has been delivered, there is usually a dramatic cessation of pain and discomfort for the mother. She often experiences a surge of renewed energy as she first sees and holds her new baby.

The third stage of labor

The third stage of labor involves the delivery of the placenta and the amniotic membranes (afterbirth). By the time of the labor, the placenta is a grapefruit-sized mass of soft tissue, with the color and consistency of fresh liver. After the umbilical vessels have stopped pulsating, the placental blood vessels contract, so allowing the placenta to come away from the wall of the uterus without excessive blood loss. After about 10–20 minutes, continued contractions of the uterus force the separated placenta, amniotic membranes and remaining umbilical cord out through the vagina. A smooth third stage is enabled by the midwife, who applies pressure to the uterus, and controlled traction to the cord as the placenta passes out of the uterus.

The uterus continues to contract after the expulsion of the placenta, so that its rich network of blood vessels is encouraged to shut down. These continued contractions are encouraged by the suckling of the baby, as this stimulates a natural release of oxytocin from the mother's pituitary gland.

To facilitate this process, it is very common practice to administer an injection of an oxytocin-like drug called syntometrine to the mother. This is intended to speed the contraction of the uterus so that blood loss is minimized. This injection is usually given into the mother's thigh just after the delivery of the baby's head. This treatment is believed to reduce the incidence of severe blood loss by half. However, if it is given, the umbilical cord needs to be clamped as soon as the baby is delivered to prevent the drug reaching the baby. Syntometrine may cause headaches and nausea in the mother. The significant complication of syntometrine use is that the uterus may contract prematurely around the placenta, so preventing its removal. If this occurs, a minor operation is required so that the placenta can be removed manually.

The contractions of the third stage are much less painful than those of the first and second stages. Often the mother may be unaware that this stage has taken place, as she is so involved with holding and suckling her newborn baby.

After the delivery of the placenta, the midwife inspects it to check that it is intact, and to estimate the approximate blood loss. The amount of blood lost in an average labor is around 400 milliliters. An amount greater than 500 milliliters is considered excessive, and replacement therapy, either by means of iron or blood transfusion, may be considered necessary. If there has been a tear, this is then stitched, either by the midwife or the doctor in attendance.

The effect of labor on the fetus

During labor, the head of the human fetus experiences much greater pressure than occurs during the birth of other mammals. The soft, immature plates of bone that form the skull are often molded into an elongated shape during the passage of the head through the pelvic canal. A more normal shape is reassumed over the course of the few days after birth. Severe molding can occur if the second stage is prolonged, or if assisted methods of delivery such as forceps have to be used.

The baby always suffers from a period of low oxygen supply during labor. This can affect the heart rate of the baby, which is monitored by the midwife. A prolonged period of abnormal fetal heart rate is taken seriously. If this occurs, it may lead to the use of medical interventions to speed up the labor, or the decision to proceed to a cesarean section.

Another response of fetal distress is that the fetus opens its bowels during the course of labor. The appearance of black, sticky meconium in the leaking amniotic fluid is a warning sign of fetal distress in labor. If meconium has been released, not only does this indicate possible distress in the fetus, but there is also a risk of the meconium being inhaled by the fetus. Therefore, the release of meconium is another reason why medical intervention may have to take over the course of the labor, so that the baby is delivered as soon as possible.

There is no doubt that even uncomplicated labor is stressful for the fetus. The fetal adrenal glands are stimulated to produce excessive amounts of adrenaline and corticosteroids in response to this stress. It is believed that high levels of these hormones are important in promoting the dramatic changes that occur in the cardiovascular and respiratory systems of the baby just after birth.

 Information box 5.3a-II

Labor: comments from a Chinese medicine perspective

In Chinese medicine, labor is believed to be a time when Yang expels Yin. After 40 weeks of relative Stagnation of Qi in the Lower Jiao, a powerful and smooth downward movement of Qi leads to the expulsion of the fetus. This has also been described in terms of Qi moving Blood. A healthy labor is dependent on healthy Blood and Qi. Healthy Spleen, Kidney and Liver Organs are particularly important in ensuring that a labor progresses smoothly through all three stages.

The physiology of the puerperium

The puerperium is defined as the six-week period that follows childbirth. During this time, the uterus slowly returns to its normal size and shape. At the end of the puerperium, any trauma to the vagina and perineum should have healed completely. The puerperium is also the time when the foundations of the relationship between the mother and the baby are established.

In many cultures across the world, ranging from a traditional Indian confinement of 10–40 days to the Chinese (30 days) and Eastern Orthodox (40 days), the time of the puerperium is a period when the woman is confined to house rest. This was also the practice in ancient China. This tradition allows the mother to divert all her attention into bonding with her child, to establish a pattern of breastfeeding, and to rebuild her own reserves of energy. However, in the developed world, this practice is not the norm. Many women now choose to be up and about on the day following labor, and, once home, may resume normal activities such as shopping or housework straight away. This is encouraged by modern healthcare systems that often discharge mothers with babies very shortly after delivery, and then request for them to attend medical appointments for infant health screening early after discharge.

Immediately following a normal birth, the pelvic area of the mother is in a bruised and torn state. It is usual for there to be considerable discomfort in this area for the next few days, which can make sitting, walking and going to the toilet painful. It is often difficult to pass urine for a few hours after labor because of pain and swelling in the region of the urethra. There is an increased risk of urinary infection at this time. Unless there has been a serious tear, these problems resolve rapidly.

For the first few weeks after birth, an odorless watery and blood-stained discharge, known as lochia, is usual. This discharge comes from the contracting uterus. It gradually diminishes with time, and should have stopped by the end of the puerperium.

Breastfeeding

Breastfeeding (lactation) is usually encouraged from the moment the baby is born. The suckling reflex does not have to be learned. As long as the baby is allowed to find the right position on the nipple, it will suckle efficiently. The correct positioning of the baby on the breast is believed to be absolutely essential if breastfeeding is to be problem-free. Sore and cracked nipples are a very common initial experience in the first few days of feeding. This problem is worse if the positioning of the baby is not correct. This potentially preventable problem is the most common reason why many women give up breastfeeding after only a few days.

Normal milk is not produced until a few days after the birth. Until this time, a yellowish, antibody-rich fluid, called colostrum, is produced. This fluid is believed to be highly beneficial to the digestive and immune systems of the baby. Even if the mother has made a prior decision not to breastfeed, she may be encouraged to do so at least for the first few days, so that the baby can receive the colostrum. When the normal milk comes in, the breasts become engorged and uncomfortable. This discomfort is relieved over the next few days as the baby continues to suckle, when a balance is achieved between milk production and feeding.

Suckling is a stimulus for the release of two pituitary hormones. Prolactin (PRL) stimulates the production of the milk from the lobules of the breast, and oxytocin stimulates the letdown of this milk into the lactiferous ducts, which open out into the nipple. Oxytocin also has a beneficial effect on maintaining the contraction of the uterus, which continues over the ensuing few weeks. For this reason, some women will experience mild period-like cramps in the early days of breastfeeding.

If the mother chooses not to breastfeed, it is normal for there to be period of one to two weeks of uncomfortable engorgement. The drug bromocriptine, which inhibits the production of PRL from the pituitary, may be prescribed to alleviate this discomfort. Because of the potentially severe side effects of this drug, it is usually given only in situations when it is considered very important to suppress lactation, such as following the death of a baby. There is also doubt about the clinical effectiveness of this medication, and whether it offers any benefit over no treatment at all.[40]

Milk is produced according to the demand of the baby. The more the baby feeds, the more milk is released by the glandular cells in the breast. However, some women manage to produce much more milk than others, and can experience problems from overflow of milk at inappropriate times. It is unusual for the baby to fail to thrive because of insufficient milk production. However, illness, stress and anemia can all contribute to poor milk supply.

Breast milk is rich in fat and sugars. It also contains all the vitamins and minerals the baby requires for at least the first six months. It may also contain traces of drugs and toxins that have entered the circulation of the mother. Some drugs enter breast milk more easily than others.

The breastfeeding mother requires more nutrients than a mother who chooses not to breastfeed. She will draw on her reserves of body fat, and will also require a diet rich in vitamins and minerals. It is particularly important that calcium and iron are available from the diet. If these are deficient, the mother will draw on her own reserves of these minerals. For this reason, weak teeth, thinned bones and anemia can develop during the weeks to months of breastfeeding. It is not uncommon for the skin to dry and the hair to become lusterless and thin in this time, a result of the cumulative depleting effect of pregnancy and lactation. Vitamin D is recommended as a supplement for feeding mothers.

Psychological changes in the puerperium

For the mother, the time following the birth is characterized by a roller coaster of emotions. There are a number of understandable reasons why these emotional changes might occur. First, a profound adjustment is necessary to the arrival of the baby and the prospect of life never being the same again. Second, in the first few days after childbirth, the body has to recover from an exhausting physical upheaval, and then may be expected to give more of its nutritional reserves in breastfeeding. In addition to this, there are dramatic changes in the hormone balance of the body, as the high levels of estrogen and progesterone suddenly drop with the delivery of the placenta. The effect of these natural changes may be compounded by additional factors such as the shock of suffering a traumatic delivery, recovering from a cesarean section, or the finding of congenital defects in the baby.

However, some women are elated after the birth, and this feeling may be sustained for days to weeks. Others experience a brief period of volatile emotions, often called the baby blues. This period occurs at around the third day after the birth. The mother may feel down, weepy or irritable. Normally this period of low mood should last for no more than a few days. If this state is prolonged it may be a warning sign of the more severe condition of postnatal depression.

The first six weeks after childbirth are characterized for most parents by periods in which the baby cries inconsolably, very disturbed nights, and anxiety for the baby's health. All these are bound to be draining, but by the end of a healthy puerperium, the mother should still feel hopeful, happy and that she is coping.

Lack of sexual interest is normal in the first few weeks after childbirth. This may be prolonged in the breastfeeding mother. This again is normal, and is thought to be a consequence of the hormones that maintain the state of lactation. The midwife or doctor may advise the mother to refrain from sexual intercourse for the first six weeks after childbirth in order to give the perineal tissues a chance to heal.

In women who are not breastfeeding, fertility may return very quickly, and so contraceptive measures are advised to be used from three weeks after the birth. Although breastfeeding is believed to inhibit ovulation, pregnancy has been known to occur in breastfeeding mothers. Therefore, contraceptive advice is given to all women at the end of the puerperium, irrespective of their choice of feeding method.

 Information box 5.3a-III

The puerperium: comments from a Chinese medicine perspective

In Chinese medicine it is expected that following childbirth the mother will be relatively depleted in Blood and Kidney Qi. Nevertheless, an uncomplicated labor can have very beneficial consequences, because it encourages a profound movement of Qi and so can clear Stagnation on many levels. If a woman can be supported through the puerperium so that her reserves of Blood and Qi are built up, she may actually experience an improvement in health and well-being through conceiving and giving birth to a child.

The mother's Blood and the Kidneys should be supported during the puerperium by good nutrition and rest. Any stressful factors in this time will adversely affect both the Blood and the Kidneys, and ideally should be avoided.

In Chinese medicine, breast milk is believed to be drawn from the mother's Blood and Essence (Jing). The possible negative effects of breastfeeding on the energy levels and calcium reserves of the mother align with this interpretation. In light of this, it is understandable why certain cultures consider the six-week confinement to be so important in protecting the mother's reserves of energy. The positive energetic effects of breastfeeding are that it enables a smooth movement of Liver Qi. In keeping with this interpretation, many women describe how breastfeeding has a calming effect. Breastfeeding can improve appetite, and yet promote the loss of the fat that was laid down in pregnancy. This suggests that breastfeeding also has a beneficial effect on Spleen Qi, and stimulates the Clearance of Damp.

After the puerperium

The puerperium is considered to be the time required for the body to return to its pre-pregnant state. Of course this is not the case for those women who continue to breastfeed. Even for those who do not breastfeed, the weeks to months following the puerperium are a time of continuing adjustment to the arrival of the baby. Most women do not feel back to their normal state for up to one year after the puerperium.

5.3b Routine care and investigation in pregnancy and childbirth

Routine antenatal (prenatal) care

Antenatal and prenatal are both terms that literally mean before birth. They are used conventionally to describe the time from conception to the onset of labor.

The rationale for routine antenatal care

The provision of routine antenatal care is believed to be a very important factor in the improvement of the health of both the mother and child in pregnancy. Following the introduction of routine antenatal care in the UK in the early part of the 20th century, the numbers of deaths at the time of childbirth in both women and newborn babies (the perinatal mortality rate) dropped markedly, although the most marked drop was between the 1950s and 1970s, 30 years after the institution of midwifery and antenatal care, and probably has a lot to do with the improved health of people in developed countries. Over the past 100 years the number of interventions offered as part of antenatal care has been pared down as evidence has revealed some of the older practices offer little benefit. For example, in the 1930s in the UK one antenatal practice was to X-ray the pelvis to estimate risk of vaginal delivery, a practice now known to be very harmful to the unborn baby.

The World Health Organization (WHO) has confirmed that of the 850 women who die across the world every day as a result of childbirth, only five of these (less than 1 percent) are from developed countries.[41] This is testimony to the benefits of the combination of good health in the mothers and the safeguards offered by structured antenatal care.

Antenatal care is structured so that the common problems that are known to develop in pregnancy can be detected at an early stage and remedial action taken at that early stage. The antenatal appointments are also opportunities to encourage those aspects of lifestyle change that are likely to have a great bearing on the health of the pregnancy and the unborn child.

Antenatal care can have an impact on factors over and above physical health. During the regular antenatal visits a pregnant woman will be encouraged to express her concerns and fears about the impending labor and the prospect of caring for a child. Good psychological and social support given in the context of the antenatal appointments may be very important in giving confidence, teaching parenting skills and reducing the incidence of postnatal depression.

The structure of antenatal care

Antenatal care in the UK is usually shared between a woman's family doctor, a team of midwives that is attached to her general practice, and a hospital maternity team headed by a consultant specialist in obstetrics. The emphasis should be on the fact that pregnancy is a healthy time, and so, if all is well, investigations are kept to a minimum. In an uncomplicated pregnancy there may be no need for the woman to make any contact with the hospital department until the time when labor begins (with the exception of visits for ultrasound scans and an introductory visit to the hospital maternity wards).

Antenatal care begins at around eight to ten weeks of gestation, when the pregnant woman is encouraged to make a first appointment with either her physician or midwife. Thereafter, she is encouraged to attend appointments, which are spaced at regular intervals and of increasing frequency as the expected date of delivery (EDD) approaches. For a healthy first pregnancy in the UK there are usually ten scheduled antenatal appointments, and seven for all subsequent pregnancies. To enable smooth communication between the different health professionals with whom she will be in contact, the mother is often encouraged to carry her own case records (maternity notes). The details of each appointment and the results of any investigations are recorded in these records.

The first antenatal appointment

The first appointment is made at a time when the greatest risk of miscarriage has passed (between eight and ten weeks). At this appointment, the general health of the mother is assessed. It is also important to clarify whether or not the pregnancy has been planned, and whether or not it is wanted. This is to gauge how happy the mother is for the pregnancy to proceed. Unplanned and unwanted pregnancies carry with them a higher risk of depression, and so in these cases the mother should receive particular support during the pregnancy.

Health factors that may adversely affect the pregnancy and labor are explored. For example, small size (reflected by height and shoe size) may be a predictor of difficult labor resulting from a small pelvis. Gynecological problems such as ovarian cysts and fibroids may require early surgical attention. Medical problems such as hypertension, diabetes and epilepsy need careful management in pregnancy, and so the woman can be referred for specialist advice at an early stage.

The history of previous pregnancies will be taken, including any obstetric complications experienced by close family members, as both these may point towards potential problems in the current pregnancy.

Blood samples are taken at this stage, and tests include a full blood count (FBC), assessment of the mother's blood group and a screen for antibodies to Rhesus factor. A blood test is also done to screen for antibodies to important infectious diseases that may affect the health of the fetus, including syphilis, hepatitis B and the human immunodeficiency virus (HIV). The mother is also tested for immunity to rubella (German measles).

The urine is tested for protein and glucose by means of a dipstick test.

All the information gathered at the booking appointment and the results of the blood tests are recorded in the case notes, which the mother usually is encouraged to carry. She may be instructed to take these notes to every antenatal appointment she attends from then on, so that a comprehensive record of her pregnancy can be maintained.

At each subsequent appointment the growth of the baby is assessed by palpation of the size of the uterus. The fetal heart beat is assessed and the weight of the mother is measured. The mother is questioned about the movements of the baby, which should be felt after about 18 weeks. In addition, the woman's blood pressure is checked and her urine tested for protein and glucose. At about two-thirds of the way through the pregnancy, simple blood tests for anemia and antibodies to the Rhesus factor may be taken for a second time. At each antenatal appointment the doctor or midwife will also explore the particular needs and concerns of the mother.

Other routine tests made in the antenatal period

Women will be offered ultrasound scans of the uterus during the pregnancy. In the UK these are most usually performed at 11–14 weeks and then at about 18–20 weeks of gestation. The purpose of these scans is to check for developmental defects in the growing fetus, and also to clarify the date of gestation. At 11–14 weeks, the scan will accurately confirm the age of the embryo and also reveal any gross abnormality of the spine or limbs. It will also, by means of assessment of nuchal fat (deposited at the back of the neck), suggest the possibility of Down syndrome (about 65 percent of Down syndrome pregnancies will be detected by means of this test, with a false-positive rate of 5 percent). At 20 weeks, structural problems of the fetal brain and spinal cord, heart, kidneys, genitalia, face, limbs and also the placenta can be detected.

If all appears to be well, the ultrasound scans can be a very encouraging experience for the parents-to-be, as they get their first opportunity to see their child, and in the later scans its movements, and also evidence of its sex.

Ultrasound scans are performed at later stages in a pregnancy if there are ongoing concerns about the health of the baby or the placenta. A decision to induce the labor prematurely may be made on the basis of a scan, if the baby is seen to be failing to thrive.

Ultrasound waves are believed conventionally to be totally harmless, but there are studies that suggest otherwise. Ultrasound is known to heat tissues, and heat (e.g. resulting from prolonged fever in the mother) is known to be potentially harmful to the fetus. One theory for the mysterious rise in preterm births and also in autism is that exposure to ultrasound in pregnancy has harmed fetal development. There is no doubt that ultrasound exposure has increased over the past 20 years, and particularly so in complicated pregnancies and IVF (in vitro fertilization) pregnancies, but the long-term outcome of this practice has not yet been clearly evaluated.[42] It is of note that national obstetric bodies such as the American College

of Obstetricians and Gynecologists and the US Food and Drug Administration (FDA)[43] do not support the practice of "keepsake ultrasound" in which private operators offer detailed 3D or 4D ultrasonic images of fetuses just for their photographic value. This surely indicates a concern that unnecessary exposure to ultrasound could be harmful.

Screening tests for genetic defects

There are a number of tests that may be performed to screen for genetic defects in the fetus. An ultrasound scan assessment of the physical form of the fetus, as described above, is one such screening test that is believed to have the benefit of not being very invasive.

Another relatively non-invasive test involves the assessment of proteins found in a sample of the mother's blood. This blood test can give an indication of the probability of certain conditions, including Down syndrome and spina bifida. A simple form of this test, which detects two proteins, HCG and pregnancy-associated plasma protein A (PAPP-A), may be performed after the nuchal scan to increase the detection rate of Down syndrome. The results of this simple test are not definitive. An abnormal result simply suggests an increased likelihood of Down syndrome, and the woman may then be recommended to have a more invasive sampling test to confirm or exclude a diagnosis of abnormality (see below).

The most definitive prenatal tests require a sample of fetal cells, so that the chromosomes can be analyzed. The two currently used methods of obtaining fetal tissue for genetic testing are chorionic villus sampling (CVS) and amniocentesis.

CVS is performed at weeks 9–11 of gestation. A needle is inserted into the mother's abdomen and guided to the placenta by means of ultrasound scanning. A sample of the placenta is sucked into a syringe from the needle. This tissue is then analyzed within 24 hours. CVS carries a risk of inducing miscarriage in 1 in 100 tests. Another concern is that some evidence suggests that it can cause limb defects.

Amniocentesis can only be performed at a later stage in pregnancy. The earliest time it can be used is at 15 weeks of gestation. In this test a needle is used to withdraw a sample of amniotic fluid from the abdomen. Amniotic fluid contains a few shed fetal cells, but not in sufficient numbers to be suitable for immediate testing. Therefore, the withdrawn sample has to be cultured for three weeks to allow the cells to multiply before testing can be performed. Although this may be more inconvenient for the parents, amniocentesis carries about half the risk of miscarriage as CVS.

Some genetic defects can be fairly simply detected by examining the form of the chromosomes in the fetal cells. A number of congenital conditions result from a gross defect in the shape of the chromosomes. These chromosomal defects very often lead to some degree of learning difficulty as well as characteristic physical defects. Down syndrome is the most common such chromosomal condition. The syndrome is recognized by the presence of an extra chromosome 21 (known as trisomy 21).

More recently, as the mapping of various genetic defects to particular places (loci) on the chromosome has advanced, increasing numbers of genetic conditions can be detected at an early stage in pregnancy. This form of genetic screening involves complex tests, which are costly to perform. Although technically it is now possible to screen for a range of conditions such as cystic fibrosis, polycystic kidney disease and hemophilia using tissue samples obtained by means of CVS or amniocentesis, these tests are only offered in special cases when the potential benefit is estimated to outweigh the risks and costs of the tests involved.

All these additional screening tests are only performed in those pregnancies in which there is considered to be an increased risk of fetal abnormality. However, as the risk of having a baby with Down syndrome increases dramatically in women over 35, tests such as amniocentesis are increasingly common choices.

Antenatal testing for fetal abnormality is presented to the mother as a health screen, when in fact the early diagnosis of abnormality in the fetus leaves the mother with the stark decision of whether or not to terminate the pregnancy. The usually unspoken and unquestioned belief in this process is that it is a good thing to be able to eliminate those early fetuses with a measurable abnormality before they have a chance to develop any further.

Some women choose to refuse all screening tests, as they would never opt to have a termination, and would rather not undergo the anxiety and risks that accompany the tests.

In an ideal situation, all women should be counseled by their doctor or midwife about the possible consequences of having screening tests before the tests are performed, so that they are able to make an informed decision about whether or not to go ahead with the pregnancy.

Antenatal classes

As the time of labor approaches, the parents may be encouraged to attend antenatal classes. These are often offered by the local midwifery team with the aim of preparing parents for the onset of labor, what is likely to happen in labor, and the choices available for pain relief. The prospective birth partner is also encouraged to attend these classes. Basic parenting skills may also be covered in these classes. In the UK, the National Childbirth Trust offers antenatal classes at a relatively low cost.

An added benefit of antenatal classes is that mothers to be can meet other women at a similar stage in pregnancy. It is not unusual for these meetings to lead to the formation of networks of local young mothers who continue to meet following the birth of their babies.

Routine care during labor

Assessment of the labor

The mother is encouraged to contact the midwife when she experiences the warning signs of the onset of labor. At this stage, a vaginal examination is performed to estimate the progression of labor. If a hospital delivery is planned, the woman should be in hospital once labor is well established (when the contractions are lasting more than 1 minute and are less than 5 minutes apart).

The conventional site for childbirth in most developed countries is the delivery suite of the local hospital. Here, the woman is ideally attended primarily by the midwifery team that has been overseeing her antenatal care. In most cases, doctors do not intervene unless the woman so desires, or if there are complications. The labor usually takes place in a private room, equipped with a bed, cushions and beanbags. A birthing pool may be available in some centers. Emergency resuscitation equipment and an operating theatre are always close at hand.

Throughout established labor, the role of the midwife is to check that the progression of labor is smooth, to ensure that the fetus remains healthy, to make adequate pain relief available to the mother, and to encourage the mother and her birth partner(s).

Progression of labor is assessed by the frequency of contractions and by the degree of dilatation of the cervix. The maternal blood pressure is recorded at regular intervals. The fetal heart rate is monitored by means of the Doppler probe, as used in antenatal care. This instrument also makes use of continuous ultrasonic waves.

If there are any concerns about the health of the fetus, the mother may be monitored more closely by means of a cardiotocograph (CTG). Taking a CTG involves placing a belt around the abdomen of the mother to assess the contractions, and electrodes on the descending head of the fetus to assess its heart rate. The CTG is used to assess whether or not the fetal heart rate responds normally to the contractions. Abnormal responses can be a sign of fetal distress. It is well known that CTG traces may indicate an abnormality when in fact all is well. This means that a woman being monitored with a CTG is more likely to have an unnecessary intervention to speed up the delivery (such as cesarian section or instrumental vaginal delivery).[44] The CTG should, therefore, be reserved for those cases in which the health of the fetus is a serious concern.

Pain relief during labor

Increasingly, the use of techniques such as aromatherapy, massage and water birth is being accepted in delivery suites as non-medical interventions that can reduce the need for pharmacological pain relief. TENS (transcutaneous electrical nerve stimulation) is another frequently used non-medical pain relief technique. This involves the passage of a low-intensity, high-frequency electrical current between two pads placed on the skin of the abdomen or the back. The frequency of most TENS machines is much higher than that used in electro acupuncture. TENS is believed to work by stimulating the large Aβ sensory nerve fibers, which, when stimulated, inhibit the thin C fibers that carry pain messages to the spinal cord (the gate mechanism of blocking pain).

Nevertheless, very few women go through normal labor without having some form of medical pain relief. The usual options of pain relief are inhaled nitrous oxide (gas and air), injected opiates and epidural anesthesia.

A mixture of inhaled nitrous oxide and oxygen, also known as gas and air or laughing gas, is very commonly used during labor. It can be self-administered by the mother, and so is only used when needed, which is usually during the peak of a contraction. The pain relief wears off within about 15 seconds of inhalation, and the gas does not appear to have any adverse effects on the baby. The side effects include nausea and drowsiness in some women.

Pethidine used to be the most commonly used injected opiate. The effects last about 3–4 hours. Side effects include nausea, a drop in blood pressure and sweating in the mother. More seriously, the newborn may be drowsy, and can have depressed breathing as a consequence of the pethidine. More recently, another opiate, meptazinol, has become increasingly used. This reportedly carries a lower risk of depression of respiration in the baby.

Epidural anesthesia involves the injection of a local anesthetic drug into the epidural space at the level of the third and fourth lumbar vertebrae. The epidural space lies outside the outermost (dural) lining of the spinal meninges. The roots of the motor and sensory nerves that supply the perineum, legs, low back and abdomen pass through this space. The anesthetic temporarily numbs these nerves, so providing pain relief both from contractions and during the delivery of the baby. An epidural may also be used as the sole anesthetic for a cesarean section. The injection is performed by an anesthetist by means of a tiny tube. This tube is left in place so that top-ups of anesthetic may be given when required.

There is no doubt that the use of epidural anesthesia can delay the progression of labor, and this may necessitate the need for further interventions to assist delivery, such as the use of forceps (see later). Complications in the mother include a drop in blood pressure, backache and headaches lasting up to one week after delivery. A misplaced epidural can have very severe consequences, but this is a very rare event.

Routine postnatal care

Postnatal care: the first two weeks

Routine postnatal care begins from the moment of the birth, when the mother is encouraged to bond with her newborn child. After the delivery of the placenta, the vagina and perineum are inspected for lacerations, and suturing of any episiotomy and any other significant tears is performed. It would be usual for women to stay in hospital for two to five days after delivery, although increasingly many women opt for an early discharge back to their home.

For the first few days after birth, ideal routine postnatal care involves at least daily visits from members of the midwifery team. In these few days it is important to ensure that a regular feeding pattern has been established, and that the baby is well nourished and hydrated. The umbilical stump is inspected, to check that it has dried up without any infection within about one week after birth.

In the first couple of days after the birth the baby is given an injection or three oral doses of vitamin K by the midwife. This is to minimize the risk of bleeding that can result from reduced levels of clotting factors from an immature liver (this is the rare condition known as hemolytic disease of the newborn). Between days 5 and 9 the baby is screened for some or all of the following nine inherited diseases: neonatal hypothyroidism, phenylketonuria, cystic fibrosis, homocystinuria, sickle cell disease and medium-chain acyl coenzyme A dehydrogenase (MCAD) deficiency (a rare metabolic disorder). This involves card-testing a drop of the baby's blood, which is withdrawn by means of a heel prick (known as the Guthrie test). The midwife will also examine the baby's skin for signs of neonatal jaundice in these few days.

Once it is clear that the baby is thriving, the mother is coping and the routine tests have been performed, the midwives no longer need to be involved in the future care of the mother and baby. From this stage on in the UK, postnatal care is provided by the woman's GP and a health visitor.

The 6–8 week postnatal check

The 6–8 week postnatal check marks the end of the routine postnatal care. It may be conducted by a physician or a specialist nurse. At this check-up, the mother is questioned about feeding patterns, the healing of her abdominal muscles and perineum, and the presence of lochia. She is advised about contraception, and her mood is assessed for early features of postnatal depression. The baby is given its second developmental check at this appointment. The mother may be reminded about the first infant immunization at eight weeks.

5.3c Abortion and bleeding in pregnancy

The complications of pregnancy are studied in this and the next section. This section explores those conditions that manifest in vaginal bleeding. Section 5.3d looks at some of the other important conditions that can give rise to unwanted symptoms and signs in pregnancy.

The definition of abortion

This section begins with a discussion about abortion. This term is used medically to describe the premature expulsion of an embryo or fetus. The term is not used if the fetus is expelled after the time at which it may survive outside the womb. This time has been defined by the WHO as any time after 22 weeks of gestation or after the fetus has achieved a weight of over 500 grams.

Although the term abortion is commonly used to describe medically or surgically induced removal of the fetus, it is also applied by physicians to the condition more usually described as miscarriage, when the embryo or fetus is expelled as a result of a spontaneous natural process (spontaneous abortion). Medically or surgically induced abortion is known as induced abortion. A more euphemistic term for induced abortion is therapeutic abortion.

Spontaneous abortion or miscarriage

It has been estimated that between 15 and 20 percent of diagnosed pregnancies end in miscarriage. This figure does not include those pregnancies that end at a very early stage before the pregnancy has been confirmed. If these are included, then possibly up to half of fertilized eggs do not progress to form an established pregnancy. It is recognized that miscarriage is also more common in older women and those who have had a previous miscarriage. Smoking, alcohol use and obesity are all risk factors.

Spontaneous abortion is considered to have two main causes:

- a congenital defect of the embryo or fetus (more common in the first 10 weeks of pregnancy or 12 weeks of gestation)

- factors relating to the health of the mother (more common at 11–20 weeks of pregnancy or 13–22 weeks of gestation) or structure of the womb.

By far the most common cause of miscarriage seems to be a failure in the healthy development of the embryo. In up to 75 percent of miscarriages the fetus is found either to be malformed or to have failed to implant successfully. For this reason, women who experience an early miscarriage may well be counseled that the miscarriage was probably for the best, as the fetus was very likely to have been not quite right in some way.

In conventional terms, miscarriage due to fetal malformation is generally seen as a quirk of nature, as it is so common, even in healthy women. After a first early miscarriage, a conventional practitioner is likely to reassure the couple that the chances are that the pregnancy will be healthy when they next conceive, particularly if they pay attention to routine preconception advice concerning lifestyle and diet. The woman might be counseled to try to lose weight if she is obese.

Symptoms of spontaneous abortion

The primary symptoms of early spontaneous abortion are abdominal pain and vaginal bleeding. The pain results from uterine contractions that follow the detachment of the early placenta from the uterine lining. As the placenta detaches completely, the contractions become more efficient and the cervical canal dilates slightly to permit expulsion of the placenta and the fetus (these together are described, rather unemotionally, as the products of conception). As the cervix dilates, the cramping pain can become very severe and the bleeding profuse, particularly if the miscarriage is occurring in an advanced stage of pregnancy.

There is a risk of serious blood loss in some cases of spontaneous abortion. However, in most cases, the pain and bleeding may not be too severe (comparable to a heavy menstrual period). Very often the bleeding is self-limiting over the course of a few days. Because of this, some early miscarriages may never be diagnosed. Instead, the symptoms are attributed by the woman to a late heavy period.

Complete and incomplete abortion

When all the products of conception are completely expelled, this is termed complete abortion. However, there is a risk that the placental tissue is not expelled completely, a situation described as incomplete abortion. The retained products of conception may lead to serious consequences, as they are a potential source of infection in the womb. Untreated incomplete abortions can result in a very severe form of acute pelvic inflammatory disease (PID). The symptoms of an incomplete abortion would include a persistent offensive discharge, vague abdominal pain, dyspareunia and fever, all following the first few days of abdominal cramps and bleeding.

In later pregnancies, the fetus is expelled first, followed by the placenta. The uterine cramps are more like labor pains in later miscarriages, as a wide dilatation of the cervix is necessary to expel the fetus. In later miscarriages there is also a risk of retained products of conception, as the placenta can be held in the uterus after the fetus has been expelled.

Threatened abortion

Sometimes the detachment of the placenta is partial. Although some bleeding and cramping pains may result, the pregnancy may actually continue to be viable. In this situation, the pain and bleeding associated with the partial separation of the placenta is not associated with dilatation of the cervical canal. This condition is known as threatened abortion.

Missed abortion

Sometimes, early death of the embryo or fetus does not stimulate uterine contractions, and so the mother may be unaware for some time that the pregnancy has terminated, as she continues to carry the non-viable products of pregnancy. This condition is termed missed abortion. It is believed that in these cases, despite the death of the embryo or fetus, the placenta continues to secrete progesterone, and this maintains the semblance of pregnancy. Most cases of missed abortion end in spontaneous abortion. However, some cases present with less marked symptoms of vague crampy pain and a brownish discharge.

Treatment of spontaneous abortion

As a general rule, all vaginal bleeding in pregnancy should be treated as a serious condition. The only exception to this rule is the painless bleeding that can occur in healthy pregnancies at or around four, eight or twelve weeks of gestation. In this case, the bleeding is usually very light, and lasts for no more than two or three days. If there are any doubts as to the nature of the bleeding, the patient should be referred on the same day to a conventional practitioner for further investigations.

A woman who is experiencing the symptoms of a threatened or spontaneous abortion will be referred by her GP to the hospital department of gynecology, where she will usually be examined solely by means of an ultrasound scan of the uterus. This investigation will reveal whether or not the fetus is still alive, thus distinguishing between threatened and inevitable spontaneous abortion. In established abortion, the scan will also indicate whether or not the expulsion of the products of conception is complete or incomplete.

If threatened abortion is diagnosed, the woman is advised to rest (although not necessarily in bed) until the pain and bleeding have ceased.

In the case of an inevitable abortion, the woman may be given medication or a vaginal pessary to promote efficient contractions of the uterus. If there are any doubts about the completeness of the abortion, the woman will be sent to the operating theatre, so that the retained products of conception can be removed by means of the surgical procedure of vacuum aspiration of the inside of the womb. Before this procedure, fine forceps may first be inserted into the womb through the cervix to remove the larger retained fetal and placental tissue. The remaining clots and tissue are then removed using a suction tube. After this operation, the bleeding usually ceases gradually over the course of ten days. Persistent bleeding or offensive discharge after surgically assisted spontaneous abortion both suggest the complication of an infection of the womb. This complication is treated with antibiotics.

If a missed abortion has been diagnosed, the usual procedure is to advise the woman to wait for up to 28 days until a spontaneous abortion has occurred, as this is considered to be a less traumatic procedure than removing the dead fetus and its placenta by medical or surgical means. If it is clear that the woman cannot bear to wait for this to happen, the expulsion of the products of conception is assisted. If the pregnancy is earlier than 12 weeks of gestation, surgical vacuum extraction is performed, as described above for incomplete abortion. If the gestation is later than 12 weeks, a medically induced labor is initiated by means of a gel inserted into the vagina. This medication contains a prostaglandin that is similar in structure to the natural prostaglandins that trigger a normal labor.

Prevention of recurrent abortion

In less than 1 percent of women, miscarriage is a recurrent problem. Recurrent abortion is a term used to describe three or more successive miscarriages. It is recognized that women who suffer from recurrent miscarriages are also at more risk of delivering a premature baby even if they do fall pregnant. In most women who have recurrent early miscarriages the underlying cause is not clear, although uterine abnormalities and infections account for a small minority of cases.

In women who tend to miscarry after 12 weeks of gestation, physical problems of the uterus and cervix are more common, accounting for over half of cases.

The prevention of recurrent miscarriage focuses first on the elimination of any underlying physical problem. For example, this may involve surgical removal of fibroids, or encircling a lax (incompetent) cervix with a removable suture. More general measures include advice on a healthy diet and lifestyle, and in particular, weight loss, cessation of smoking and intake of alcohol. Patients may be advised to abstain from sexual intercourse and travel during pregnancy. Some conventional authorities advocate acupuncture as one option that may help prevent recurrent miscarriage.[45]

Psychological effects of spontaneous abortion

A recent conventional medical study has estimated that over 90 percent of women experience a grief reaction following a miscarriage, and that this reaction persists for over a month in 20 percent of cases. It is believed that a healthy grief reaction is enabled by encouraging the woman to ask questions about why the pregnancy terminated, and what the risks are of a miscarriage happening again.

Although there is this acknowledgement that miscarriage is a disturbing event for most women, the prolonged impact on the physical and emotional state may be underestimated by many doctors. Many women feel physically drained for some weeks after a miscarriage, and may continue to suffer recurring feelings of grief or guilt about the loss of the pregnancy.

 Information box 5.3c-I

Miscarriage: comments from a Chinese medicine perspective

In Chinese medicine, a threatened miscarriage is described as "vaginal bleeding during pregnancy," whereas an early spontaneous abortion is termed "falling fetus." The symptoms of an early spontaneous abortion are termed "restless fetus." Spontaneous abortion in later pregnancy is described as "small labor." The situation in which painless bleeding occurs as part of a normal pregnancy at four, eight or twelve weeks is termed "swimming menses."

The conditions of "vaginal bleeding during pregnancy" and "falling fetus" are attributed to a weakness of the Directing and Penetrating Vessels, so leading to a Deficiency of Blood for nourishment of the fetus. The underlying pathologies are Deficiency of the Kidneys, Blood Deficiency, Qi Deficiency and Sinking of Qi, and Blood Heat. Blood Stagnation may be an additional pathology in recurrent miscarriage.

The important etiological factors for these conditions are considered to be overwork, chronic illness and fever, poor diet (especially hot and spicy foods), emotional problems, excessive sexual activity during pregnancy, and physical shocks and trauma. With the exception of emotional problems, all these factors are also recognized as risk factors in conventional medicine.

Maciocia (1998) advises that acupuncture treatment to rectify the pathology and to calm the fetus should be used in all cases of threatened miscarriage. He further offers the view that miscarriage of a seriously malformed fetus is inevitable, and will not be prevented by acupuncture.[46]

Miscarriage is considered to be very draining to the Blood and Kidneys, and so afterwards the woman needs to rest and build up her emotional and energetic reserves before trying to conceive again.

Induced (or therapeutic) abortion

Induced or therapeutic abortion is the term applied to an abortion that is initiated by medical or surgical means. The other very commonly used term for an induced abortion is termination of pregnancy, often abbreviated to termination. In many Western countries induced abortion is legal, but is only performed according to strict inclusion criteria. In the UK, these criteria were established through the 1967 Abortion Act. This Act was subsequently amended in 1991, during the passage of the Human Fertilisation and Embryology Bill. The amendment reduced the time limit by which most abortions could be performed, from 28 weeks of gestation to 24. This amendment was in acknowledgement of the fact that the majority of fetuses are viable at 28 weeks of gestation. Nevertheless, as has already been stated, the WHO has recommended that viability could be expected to be possible after the fetus has reached 22 weeks of gestation.

Prior to the Abortion Act, abortion was illegal in the UK. This meant that some women who had an unwanted pregnancy resorted to any one of a range of risky methods for inducing a miscarriage. Some women paid large sums of money to illegal operators to perform the so-called back-street abortions. As the number of unwanted pregnancies increased in the 1960s, the serious complications of these often unsterile procedures became of concern. The Abortion Act was passed primarily to protect women from the hazards of back-street abortions, as it permitted those women who had reasonable grounds for a termination of pregnancy to have the procedure performed by skilled operators in sterile surroundings.

According to the Abortion Act, abortion may be performed for a clearly specified range of reasons. These criteria are more limiting if the pregnancy has extended over 24 weeks of gestation. Also according to the Act, two medical practitioners have to be signatories to indicate that they are satisfied that the pregnancy in question meets the criteria for abortion as defined in the Act. These criteria for legal abortion as defined in the Abortion Act are as follows:

- if continuance of the pregnancy would involve risk to the life of the pregnant woman greater than if the pregnancy were terminated

- if termination is necessary to prevent grave permanent injury to the physical or mental health of the pregnant woman

- if the pregnancy has not exceeded its 24th week, and if continuance of the pregnancy would involve risk, greater than if the pregnancy were terminated, of injury to the physical or mental health of the woman

- if the pregnancy has not exceeded its 24th week, and if continuance of the pregnancy would involve risk, greater than if the pregnancy were terminated, of injury to any existing children of her family

- if there is a substantial risk that if the child were born it would suffer from such physical or mental abnormalities as to be seriously handicapped.

If a woman wishes to have an induced abortion, she has to be seen by two doctors. In the UK these doctors are often either her general practitioner (GP) or the family planning clinic doctor, together with the gynecologist who will perform or oversee the procedure.

Each doctor is legally required to complete a form indicating that they agree that the woman is entitled to a termination for one of the listed reasons. Ideally, as this process takes place, the woman is given an opportunity to think carefully about her decision to terminate the pregnancy. She should be informed about the possible physical and emotional consequences of an induced abortion, and be given time to consider her decision.

Despite the seemingly strict inclusion criteria, in the UK it is most unusual for a woman in early pregnancy to be refused a termination. The majority of early terminations are performed for the reason that the pregnancy has not exceeded its 24th week, and that continuance of the pregnancy would involve risk, greater than if the pregnancy were terminated, of injury to the physical or mental health of the woman. Many doctors would argue that any unwanted pregnancy would probably injure the mental or physical health of the woman. Therefore, most doctors would not hesitate in advocating a termination if the pregnancy was obviously not wanted.

There are fierce opponents to this apparent laxity of interpretation of the criteria of the Abortion Act, as in practice the Act places little or no barrier to a woman who sincerely desires to terminate her pregnancy before the 24th week of gestation. The anti-abortion (pro-life) lobby argument is that the inclusion criteria pay no reference at all to the rights of the unborn fetus before this time of gestation, despite the fact that the fetus may be viable from 22 weeks of gestation.[47] This is a just criticism, but is at odds with the general medical opinion that the rights of the mother to make this choice for her future outweigh those of an unviable or poorly viable fetus.

If the fetus is found to have a physical abnormality, the Abortion Act permits termination to be carried out even after 24 weeks and at any time up to the end of pregnancy. Terminations for conditions that are undoubtedly compatible with a long life, such as club foot, cleft palate and Down syndrome, are still occasionally performed at this late stage in pregnancy, as in some cases the condition doesn't become apparent until after the 20-week anomaly scan.

The procedure of induced abortion

Most induced abortions are performed before week 12 of gestation. If the abortion is performed at this early stage of pregnancy, the risk of complications is very low. It is estimated that less than 1 percent of women will develop an infection following an early induced abortion, whereas the complication rate rises to 3–5 percent for abortions performed later than week 12 of gestation. There is no evidence that an uncomplicated induced abortion compromises the health of future pregnancies.

Early abortions of fetuses up to 15 weeks of gestation can be performed by a surgical approach as is used in the case of miscarriage. The products of conception are evacuated under anesthetic by means of a suction tube inserted through the cervix. After this procedure, it is normal for bleeding to persist for up to ten days. Sometimes the woman may be given a course of antibiotics to prevent infection.

The medical approach can only be used if the pregnancy is earlier than nine weeks of gestation. This approach is considered to be the ideal because it avoids the potential risks of a general anesthetic. It involves the oral administration of the drug mifepristone, followed 36–48 hours later by the application at regular intervals of a prostaglandin gel (as used in cases of missed abortion) in the form of a pessary inserted in the vagina.

The combination of these medications stimulates contractions of the uterus and thus expulsion of the fetus. The pain of these contractions may be severe, so that the woman may also require opioid analgesic medication. Nausea and vomiting is a common occurrence with medically induced abortion. In 10 percent of cases a surgical procedure is necessary to evacuate retained products of conception.

If the pregnancy is more advanced (after week 15 of gestation), the uterus is stimulated to contract by means of a combination of prostaglandin-like drugs. The medical approach is far preferable to the surgical approach at a later stage in pregnancy, but as with earlier abortions, is not always successful. A failed late medical abortion has to be followed by a surgical removal of the products of conception, which, in a more advanced stage of pregnancy, is a bloody and prolonged procedure. Up to one-third of patients who have a late medical abortion will require this procedure.

After the termination has been performed, the gynecologist is obliged to notify the Chief Medical Officer that the termination has been performed within a defined length of time. This means that accurate data about the numbers of terminations performed nationally can be collated. For example, it is known from these data that over 184,000 terminations were performed in 2014 in the UK, and just over 3000 were on the basis, as specified in the 1967 Abortion Act, that the child would be "seriously handicapped." Of this subgroup, about half had a congenital malformation and about one-third chromosomal abnormalities; 662 fetuses with Down syndrome were terminated in this year.[48]

The large majority of these terminations are for pregnancies that could have been prevented by proper use of contraceptive methods. It is well known that the termination rate in the UK is one of the highest in Europe, a fact attributed to poor use of contraception, particularly amongst teenagers and young single women.

The psychological consequences of induced abortion

Medical research has indicated that many women do not suffer a prolonged period of grief or guilt following a termination. The American Psychological Association, on the basis of a seminal study by Adler *et al.* (1990), stated that "legal abortion of an unwanted pregnancy does not pose a psychological hazard for most women."[49] Nevertheless, the physical effects of feeling drained for up to a few weeks are comparable to those following a spontaneous miscarriage. The fact that this physical disturbance is likely to occur may not be recognized by the patient's doctor. There is no doubt that some women do suffer from prolonged deep regret about having undergone the procedure. It is known that those who do have negative feelings after an abortion are more likely to have been ambivalent about having the procedure at the time.

Ectopic pregnancy

Ectopic pregnancy, or extra-uterine pregnancy, is the term used to describe a pregnancy in which the fertilized ovum has implanted outside the body of the uterus. The most common site for an ectopic pregnancy is within the fallopian tube, but the zygote can also implant on the surface of the ovary, on the wall of the cervical canal and within the abdominal cavity.

It has been estimated that between 0.8 and 1.5 percent of all pregnancies are ectopic in location. An ectopic pregnancy is more likely to occur in women who have a condition of the uterus that might impair implantation in the uterine wall. Ectopic pregnancies are recognized to be rare complications of the use of the progesterone-only pill and the intrauterine device (IUD). This is because neither of these contraceptive methods prevents ovulation, but instead, they induce the lining of the uterus to be hostile to implantation. Pelvic inflammatory disease (PID) is also associated with an increased risk of ectopic pregnancy, presumably because damage to the fallopian tubes prevents the normal passage of the zygote into the uterine cavity.

Symptoms of ectopic pregnancy

The early weeks of an ectopic pregnancy are characterized by the same symptoms as a normal pregnancy. Despite its unusual location, the invasive placenta releases the same hormones as it would if correctly located in the uterus.

In about two-thirds of cases, the ectopic pregnancy spontaneously aborts between weeks 6 and 10 of pregnancy. At the time of the abortion, the woman may not be aware that she is pregnant. The canal of the fallopian tube, the most common site for an ectopic pregnancy, is very fine, and so complete abortion from this site is very rare. Usually, the accumulation of blood and detached products of conception in the fallopian tube cause abdominal pain, which can be very severe. The pain may or may not be associated with vaginal bleeding. In some cases the pain is not so severe initially, and thus there may be a delay before a correct diagnosis is made.

In one-third of cases, the zygote has implanted in the narrowest portion of the fallopian tube. The rapid growth of the embryo and its associated tissues causes first distension and then rupture of the fallopian tube. This may occur very early in the pregnancy, at around the time of the first missed period (weeks 4–6 of gestation). In these cases, the woman will most often be unaware of the fact that she is pregnant. Rupture of the fallopian tube is a devastating event for the woman, who experiences a sudden onset of severe abdominal pain as the torn fallopian tube hemorrhages into the abdominal cavity. Often the pain is so severe as to cause collapse with fainting. A ruptured fallopian tube is a surgical emergency, as there is high risk of continuing severe internal bleeding. Again, the diagnosis may be delayed because the possibility of pregnancy might not have been considered.

Very rarely, an ectopic pregnancy in the abdominal cavity may continue to progress to term, requiring delivery by surgical means. However, the most likely outcome of abdominal pregnancies is that the pregnancy aborts at an early stage, so causing abdominal pain due to blood in the peritoneal space. Rarely, the fetus dies at a later stage, and in these cases the fetal and placental tissue can gradually get reabsorbed by the body.

An ectopic pregnancy is diagnosed in the first instance from the clinical picture, and this diagnosis is then confirmed by an ultrasound scan. A pregnancy test will be positive, even after the onset of symptoms, so this may be the first investigation to be performed if the symptoms are inconclusive.

The treatment is always surgical. In acute cases an abdominal excision is performed so that the affected fallopian tube can be removed. If the fallopian tube has not ruptured, it may be possible to excise the ectopic pregnancy by means of a keyhole technique. This requires a laparoscope to visualize the fallopian tube. If the diagnosis is made early, an alternative technique is to inject the developing amniotic sac with a cytotoxic drug. This will destroy the developing tissue, which should then be reabsorbed into the fallopian tube. The woman is then tested on a weekly basis for blood levels of HCG (i.e. a pregnancy test) to check that the pregnancy has been terminated.

It is estimated that about one-quarter of women who suffer from an ectopic pregnancy become unable to conceive naturally. For those who remain fertile, there is an increased risk of a second ectopic pregnancy.

Information box 5.3c-II

Ectopic pregnancy: comments from a Chinese medicine perspective

In Chinese medicine the pain of an ectopic pregnancy is compatible with Blood Stagnation. The scarring caused by preceding pelvic inflammatory disease (PID) could be interpreted as Qi Stagnation resulting from Damp Heat in the Uterus.

The energetic consequences of an ectopic pregnancy might include Blood and Kidney Deficiency. These can be severe in some cases, and could contribute to the infertility that can follow an ectopic pregnancy.

Antepartum hemorrhage

Antepartum hemorrhage is the term used to describe bleeding that occurs in the second half of pregnancy. Very rarely, bleeding in late pregnancy is unrelated to the pregnancy itself, instead coming from a cervical condition such as a polyp. However, most commonly the bleeding originates from the placenta, and so is a threat to the health of the fetus. Therefore, antepartum hemorrhage is always a warning feature of serious disease. The two most common causes of antepartum hemorrhage are placenta previa and placental abruption. These are discussed in turn below.

Placenta previa

Placenta previa describes a placenta that is located over or close to the opening of the cervical canal. This condition is usually diagnosed from the ultrasound scan at 20 weeks before it is the cause of any symptoms. It is a relatively rare finding, occurring in about 1 in 200 pregnancies.

If the placenta is found to be low at the 20-week scan, a repeat scan at 30 weeks may show that there is no longer cause for concern, as the uterus has grown so that the placenta has become distanced from the cervical opening. However, if the placenta remains low, the risk of bleeding is significant.

The first symptom of placenta previa most often is slight, painless bleeding. If this occurs, the woman should be referred immediately to hospital, where the treatment involves bed rest and repeated assessment of the pregnancy by means of ultrasound scans. There is always a risk that the bleeding will suddenly become severe. In the event of severe bleeding, the only option is to deliver the fetus by cesarean section, irrespective of its stage in development, as there is grave risk to the life of the mother.

With continued mild bleeding the treatment is more expectant, with the mother kept on bed rest and under close supervision. If the placenta is so low that it completely covers the opening of the cervix, the baby will be delivered by cesarean section at 36 weeks of gestation, the time at which it is known that the chances of healthy survival outside the womb are high. If the placenta is just close to the cervical opening, normal labor may be possible, although this is likely to be induced before week 38.

Even if there has been no bleeding at all, a mother with a very low placenta should not be allowed to go into natural labor, as the dilatation of the cervix could cause catastrophic bleeding. In these cases a cesarean section is performed by week 37 or 38.

Any episode of placental bleeding is a potential risk to the fetus, but in most cases of mild bleeding, the fetus remains healthy, and perinatal mortality is low. There is an increased risk of postnatal hemorrhage for those mothers with placenta previa who undergo a natural labor.

Placental abruption

In other cases of antepartum hemorrhage the bleeding comes from a placenta that is normally located high in the uterus. This complication affects 4 in 100 pregnancies. In the majority of cases of bleeding from a high placenta the cause is unknown, and the bleeding stops spontaneously. This syndrome has been termed accidental hemorrhage. Less commonly, the bleeding occurs behind the placenta, and there is a risk that the placenta will become separated from the wall of the uterus. This is described as placental abruption. In these cases vaginal bleeding may be very slight, or even absent. However, the separation of the placenta from the uterine wall causes pain, which can be severe. In these cases, on examination the uterus is found to be tense and tender. If the bleeding is severe, even though it may not be apparent vaginally, the mother can go into a state of shock resulting from the blood loss internally. This condition is a surgical emergency.

Accidental hemorrhage and placental abruption are more likely to occur in women who have had at least one baby already, and also in cigarette smokers.

In accidental hemorrhage, the mother may be discharged from hospital once an ultrasound scan has demonstrated that the fetus and placenta appear healthy, and after the bleeding has settled down.

In placental abruption there is always grave risk to the health of the fetus and, in severe cases, to the mother also. The treatment usually involves giving a blood transfusion to the mother. In severe cases, the fetus will die from blood loss, and thus a cesarean section has to be performed. If the fetus is still alive, it is delivered either by rapid induction of labor or by cesarean section.

 Information box 5.3c-III

Bleeding in pregnancy: comments from a Chinese medicine perspective

In Chinese medicine, painless blood loss from a placenta previa may equate to Spleen Qi Sinking, with Spleen not holding Blood. This would accord with the finding of an inappropriately low placenta, which could be attributed to a combination of Deficient Spleen and Kidney Qi. In contrast, the intensely painful bleeding associated with placental abruption equates more closely to Blood Stagnation.

The red flags of bleeding and abdominal pain in pregnancy

The red flags of bleeding and abdominal pain are incorporated into Table 5.3d-I, which summarizes all the red flags of pregnancy. This can be found at the end of Section 5.3d.

5.3d Other complications of pregnancy

This section is divided into two parts, which are designed for study in separate sessions. Part I gives an overview of the most common minor disorders of pregnancy, while Part II is dedicated to the more serious conditions that can complicate pregnancy.

The conditions explored in this section are:

Part I: Minor disorders of pregnancy

- backache
- pubic symphysis diastasis
- heartburn
- nausea and vomiting (morning sickness)
- constipation
- hemorrhoids (piles)
- varicose veins in the legs
- leg cramps

- urinary frequency and incontinence
- edema
- carpal tunnel syndrome and other mononeuropathies
- palpitations and breathlessness
- anemia
- insomnia
- itch (pruritus)

Part II: More serious complications of pregnancy

- hypertension, pre-eclampsia and eclampsia
- maternal diabetes mellitus
- thromboembolism
- Rhesus disease
- infections in pregnancy
- abnormalities of the placenta and amniotic fluid
- problems in the timing of labor
- the at-risk fetus and high-risk pregnancy.

Part I: Minor disorders of pregnancy

Many of the minor disorders of pregnancy described in this first part are conventionally considered to be normal aspects of pregnancy. Very few pregnancies are not affected by at least one of these common conditions. It will be helpful to be familiar with the theoretical basis to the physiological changes of pregnancy as described in Section 5.3a for full understanding of these disorders.

Backache

Backache is a very common symptom, particularly in late pregnancy. The common sites of pain are around the lumbar spine and, most commonly, the sacroiliac joints. Pain may also be referred to the buttocks and down the distribution of the sciatic nerve (sciatica). The primary cause of this pain is believed to be increased levels of progesterone, which increases the laxity of the ligaments in the lumbosacral spine. Poor posture can contribute to the discomfort. The posture of the pregnant woman can worsen as she tries to accommodate the increasing weight of the uterus.

The conventional treatment for backache during pregnancy is usually supportive. The patient may be referred to a physiotherapist who will recommend specific exercises to relieve the discomfort. Sometimes a brace may be prescribed to give support to the lower back. In most cases the problem disappears after the birth of the baby, although some women continue to suffer from recurring back problems.

Information box 5.3d-I

Backache in pregnancy: comments from a Chinese medicine perspective

In Chinese medicine, lumbosacral back pain may be the result of Stagnation of Blood and Qi on a background of an underlying Deficiency of Kidney Qi. Cold and Damp may also contribute to the problem.

Pubic symphysis diastasis

Pubic symphysis can also be adversely affected by the relaxing effect of progesterone on the pelvic ligaments. In pubic symphysis diastasis, the fibrous joint between the pubic bones becomes excessively lax, leading to pain in the groin and pubic area. In some women, the pain can become so severe that they are obliged to rest in bed to obtain relief. The conventional treatment of pubic symphysis diastasis includes physiotherapy, painkillers and the prescription of a supportive brace.

Information box 5.3d-II

Pubic symphysis diastasis: comments from a Chinese medicine perspective

In Chinese medicine, the pain of pubic symphysis diastasis corresponds to Blood and Qi Stagnation. Kidney Deficiency is very likely to be an underlying factor.

Heartburn

The sensation of acid or burning in the upper chest or throat is a very common symptom of pregnancy. In many cases this discomfort is made worse after eating certain foods and by leaning forward or lying down. Heartburn during pregnancy is also believed to be the result of the action of progesterone, as this hormone relaxes the cardiac sphincter muscle that sits at the base of the esophagus. The condition may be exacerbated as the uterus enlarges and places upwards pressure on the contents of the stomach. Iron-containing preparations, which are very commonly prescribed in pregnancy, can also irritate the stomach lining, and so worsen the discomfort of heartburn.

Conventional treatments for heartburn include dietary advice, practical measures, such as raising the head of the bed by a few inches, and antacid medication such as suspension of sodium alginate with calcium carbonate

(e.g. Gaviscon). Although harmless to the baby, antacid medications may impair the mother's absorption of iron.

Information box 5.3d-III

Heartburn in pregnancy: comments from a Chinese medicine perspective

In Chinese medicine, heartburn during pregnancy corresponds to Stomach Heat, retention of food in the Stomach or rebellious Stomach Qi. There is usually an underlying Deficiency of Spleen Qi.

Nausea and vomiting (morning sickness)

Nausea and vomiting is an almost universally experienced characteristic of the first trimester (first 12 weeks) of pregnancy. It is believed to be a bodily reaction to rising levels of either estrogen or to HCG, and possibly a combination of both. A mild degree of nausea, beginning as early as week 4 of gestation, is a very common symptom affecting up to 90 percent of pregnancies. It is often worse in the morning, but the term morning sickness can be a misnomer, as for some women the nausea gets worse as the day goes on. Some women vomit in addition to feeling nauseated. In some, but not all, the vomiting can relieve the nausea temporarily. Morning sickness usually ceases to be a problem by weeks 12–16 of gestation.

Even without the symptom of vomiting, this condition can be extremely debilitating. The nausea can dominate the whole day, and can be accompanied by extreme aversions to everyday foods and smells. Other accompanying symptoms include extreme tiredness, food cravings and a strange taste in the mouth. In mild cases morning sickness is not believed to affect the health of the fetus. The conventional treatment of mild morning sickness is usually simply supportive. The mother is advised to eat small meals at regular intervals, and to avoid rich foods. Simple treatments such as drinking ginger tea or applying acupressure to acupoint PC-6 (Nei Guan) by means of Sea-Bands may be recommended. A regular dose of mild antiemetic drugs, such as metoclopramide or prochlorperazine, or an antihistamine, such as cyclizine, may be prescribed.

In some rare cases the vomiting can be so severe as to lead to dehydration and exhaustion in the mother. This condition, known as hyperemesis gravidarum, is a serious problem, as there is a risk that liver damage may ensue when dehydration occurs in pregnancy. When the mother is in a state of dehydration, the health of the fetus is also at risk. The conventional treatment might involve hospital admission for administration of fluids and powerful intravenous antiemetic medication, including corticosteroids and 5-hydroxytryptamine 3 (5-HT3) antagonists such as ondansetron.

Information box 5.3d-IV

Nausea in pregnancy: comments from a Chinese medicine perspective

In Chinese medicine, nausea in pregnancy may have a range of underlying causes. A Deficiency of Stomach and Spleen Qi is usually an important factor. Imbalances in the Liver and Kidney Organs will also contribute to the symptoms.

The Chong Channel is linked with the Stomach Channel at ST-30 (Qi Chong). If the Stomach Qi is weak, the accumulated Blood and Qi in the Chong Channel can counter flow upwards, so causing nausea and vomiting.

Deficient Kidney Yin can result in Rising Yang, which can also result in a counter flow of Stomach Qi. This effect might explain the increased incidence of morning sickness in older mothers, in multiple pregnancies and in pregnancies resulting from assisted conception.

Stagnant Liver Qi causing the Stomach Qi to rebel can also cause the counter flow upwards.

The presence of Heat, Damp or Stagnation will result in symptoms characteristic of excessive conditions, such as improvement after vomiting and worsening after eating.

Maciocia (1998) states that nausea of pregnancy may also be a result of failure of Heart Qi to descend. This is a possible reason why acupoint PC-6 (Nei Guan) can be a very effective point for this condition.[50]

Constipation

Constipation is a common symptom of pregnancy. It is believed to be the combined result of the action of progesterone on the smooth muscle of the bowel wall, and the physical obstruction caused by the enlarging uterus. The symptoms are not usually severe, and may just amount to a reduced frequency of bowel opening, dry stools and a slight degree of discomfort. Iron-containing preparations can also contribute to the symptoms.

The main treatment is the recommendation of a high-fiber diet. Non-stimulant laxatives, such as ispaghula husk and lactulose, may be prescribed.

Information box 5.3d-V

Constipation in pregnancy: comments from a Chinese medicine perspective

In Chinese medicine, constipation can result from Deficiency of Blood and Yin, Qi Stagnation and Heat. Iron-containing preparations are Heating in nature.

Hemorrhoids (piles)

Distension of the veins in the anus is an almost universal occurrence in pregnancy. Again, the combined effects of progesterone and pressure from the uterus on the large veins in the pelvis are believed to be responsible. If severe, the distension may manifest as a bulging of the flesh at the anal margin. This can cause uncomfortable symptoms, including a feeling of fullness in the anus after defecation, and anal itch. In some cases there may be a persistent ache or fresh bleeding from the anus after defecation.

Hemorrhoids may also result from the straining and distension of the pelvic tissues that occurs during labor. For this reason, the symptoms may take a few weeks to abate after childbirth. In a minority of cases the condition never fully resolves after childbirth.

Conventional treatment includes reassurance that the condition usually abates in the weeks following delivery of the baby. Constipation, which can aggravate the condition, should be treated. Topical soothing preparations containing zinc oxide and bismuth subgallate may be prescribed.

Information box 5.3d-VI

Hemorrhoids in pregnancy: comments from a Chinese medicine perspective

In Chinese medicine, hemorrhoids are usually attributed to Deficiency of Spleen Qi, with Spleen Qi sinking. Itch, discharge and bleeding may be manifestations of a combination of Damp and Heat. Blood and Yin Deficiency and Liver Qi Stagnation may contribute to the formation of Heat in the Lower Jiao.

Varicose veins in the legs

Varicose veins in the legs have the same underlying conventional medical cause as hemorrhoids. They tend to increase in size as pregnancy progresses, and may give rise to discomfort, which worsens as the day goes on.

Conventional treatment includes advice to raise the legs when resting and to wear support stockings.

Information box 5.3d-VII

Varicose veins in pregnancy: comments from a Chinese medicine perspective

In Chinese medicine, varicose veins may reflect an underlying weakness of Zong Qi and also Spleen Qi. Discomfort and inflammation indicate that Stagnation of Blood and Qi with generation of Heat may also be contributory.

Leg cramps

The conventional understanding of leg cramps is not clear. Cramps are certainly more common in pregnancy, occurring most commonly at night and increasing in frequency as the pregnancy progresses.

Gentle exercise that involves stretching the calf muscles, such as walking and yoga, may help to prevent cramps, as can massage of the muscles before bedtime. Some women obtain relief if the foot of the bed is raised a few inches. As this is the opposite of the advice for relief of the common heartburn, this practice may not be of value to those women who suffer from both conditions at night.

Information box 5.3d-VIII

Leg cramps in pregnancy: comments from a Chinese medicine perspective

In Chinese medicine, leg cramps reflect Blood and Qi Stagnation resulting from Liver Blood and Yin Deficiency.

Urinary frequency and incontinence

Frequency of urination is a characteristic feature of pregnancy. In early pregnancy the frequency is a consequence of increased urine production, but in late pregnancy it is the result of the decreased capacity of the compressed bladder.

A slight degree of urinary incontinence affects over half of all pregnant women, particularly in second or subsequent pregnancies. Like hemorrhoids, this symptom may also be worsened by the strain placed on the pelvic floor tissues during labor. Many women will complain of persisting incontinence of urine after childbirth, although in most cases this is relatively mild stress incontinence.

Pelvic floor exercises increase the tone of the external urethral sphincter, and so can reduce stress incontinence during pregnancy. If correctly and regularly performed, these exercises are believed to prevent long-term urinary problems after childbirth.

Information box 5.3d-IX

Urinary frequency in pregnancy: comments from a Chinese medicine perspective

In Chinese medicine, urinary frequency in pregnancy is a result of Deficiency of Kidney Qi. Incontinence in the long term after pregnancy is also likely to reflect an underlying Deficiency of Spleen Qi, leading to Spleen Qi Sinking, as the underlying problem is persisting weakness of the tissues of the pelvic floor.

Edema

A degree of accumulation of tissue fluid (edema) is not uncommon in pregnancy. It is particularly obvious around the ankles as pregnancy advances, but may be more generalized, giving rise to swollen fingers and a sensation of bloating or heaviness. If this symptom is mild and also not associated with a rise in blood pressure, it is not conventionally considered to be of concern. The cause is attributed to a combination of the effect of estrogen and the pressure of the uterus on the veins in the pelvis.

The conventional advice is that the woman should rest with her feet elevated as much as possible. There is no place for drug treatment in mild edema of pregnancy. However, if the blood pressure is found to be rising above the normal range, edema may be a warning feature of pregnancy-induced hypertension or pre-eclampsia, and is treated with seriousness (see Part II of this section).

Information box 5.3d-X

Edema in pregnancy: comments from a Chinese medicine perspective

In Chinese medicine, edema of pregnancy often results from a Deficiency of Kidney and/or Spleen Yang, and is a manifestation of Damp.

Carpal tunnel syndrome and other mononeuropathies

Carpal tunnel syndrome is a common mononeuropathy of pregnancy, which is believed to be caused by fluid accumulation around the wrist joint. The increased pressure within the carpal tunnel of the wrist affects the median nerve. This nerve follows the distribution of the Pericardium and Lung Channels in the wrist and hand. The symptoms include numbness and tingling of the radial side of the hand, thumb and index finger, with weakness of grip. The discomfort may be worse at night, and may be relieved by dropping the hand by the side of the bed.

Other neuropathies may occur in pregnancy as a result of a combination of fluid accumulation and pressure from the enlarging uterus. Another common neuropathy is of the lateral cutaneous nerve of the thigh, which follows the distribution of the Stomach Channel in the upper leg. When this nerve is compressed, a condition called meralgia paresthetica results. This is characterized by pain and numbness of the anterolateral aspect of the thigh.

Conventional treatment for these symptoms is supportive. Wrist splints, which prevent the wrist from flexing forward, may give relief in carpal tunnel syndrome.

Information box 5.3d-XI

Neuropathy in pregnancy: comments from a Chinese medicine perspective

In Chinese medicine, the numbness and tingling of a neuropathy may be due to Blood Deficiency and Accumulation of Damp. The site of the symptoms will give more information about imbalances in a specific organ and/or channel. For example, carpal tunnel syndrome suggests an additional underlying Deficiency in the Pericardium or Lung Channels.

Palpitations and breathlessness

Both palpitations and breathlessness on exertion are common as pregnancy advances. In the majority of cases the cardiovascular and respiratory systems will be found to be normal on examination. The patient can be reassured that these symptoms are normal features of pregnancy. In some cases treatment of anemia of pregnancy (see below) may help these symptoms.

Very occasionally, palpitations and breathlessness may be an indication of previously undiagnosed heart disease, and so it is advisable that the patient reports these symptoms to her midwife or doctor.

Information box 5.3d-XII

Palpitations and breathlessness in pregnancy: comments from a Chinese medicine perspective

In Chinese medicine, palpitations indicate a Deficiency in Heart Yin with Empty Heat, or Deficiency of Blood and/or Qi. The precise diagnosis depends on the time of onset and nature of the palpitations. Pregnancy predisposes to Deficiency of Yin, and overwork will exacerbate this.

Breathlessness in pregnancy is usually most apparent on exertion. This may be an indication of Stagnation of Qi of the Heart and Lungs and may result from Uprising of Qi as a result of relative Deficiency in the lower aspect of the Chong Channel. Thus Kidney or Blood Deficiency will be at the root of breathlessness in pregnancy.

Anemia

Anemia describes a condition in which the concentration of hemoglobin in the blood is below the normal range (below 11.5 grams/deciliter). Mild anemia is frequently diagnosed in pregnancy through routine blood testing. In borderline cases mild anemia can be attributed to the increased volume of the blood that circulates in pregnancy. As more fluid is held in the circulation, the red blood cells are diluted, and this gives rise to a measurable drop in concentration without any underlying deficiency of iron or folic acid (folate). However, depletion of iron and folic acid is not uncommon in pregnancy because of the increased demands of the growing fetus. For this reason, anemia of pregnancy is often a combined result of physiological dilution of the blood cells together with a deficiency of iron and/or folate.

Anemia resulting from deficiency is treated with seriousness, as it is known to be linked with increased susceptibility to infection, failure of the fetus to thrive, and increased risk of hemorrhage both before and during delivery.

The conventional approach is to treat anemia of pregnancy only if it is quite severe (less than 10 grams/deciliter) or if symptoms such as tiredness, palpitations or breathlessness are present. An iron supplement, such as ferrous sulfate, and folic acid may be prescribed. Iron supplements are well recognized to cause side effects such as heartburn and constipation, which can be problematic in pregnancy. Slow-release preparations of iron may overcome these potential problems. Herbal preparations of iron are often easier to digest but are less powerful sources of iron and folic acid.

Information box 5.3d-XIII

Anemia in pregnancy: comments from a Chinese medicine perspective

In Chinese medicine, anemia in pregnancy is a manifestation of Blood and Qi Deficiency.

Insomnia

Insomnia is another problem that increases in frequency as pregnancy advances. Concurrent symptoms such as heartburn, palpitations, cramp and backache may impair the quality of sleep. Some women feel very uncomfortable, and even faint, when lying down in advanced pregnancy. This effect is probably because the uterus is exerting pressure on the large blood vessels that run through the abdomen. Towards the end of pregnancy, many women are wakeful at night, even without these symptoms. Some attribute this to the fact that the baby is more active at night, or that they are woken with a need to eat in the early hours of the morning.

Information box 5.3d-XIV

Insomnia in pregnancy: comments from a Chinese medicine perspective

In Chinese medicine, insomnia in pregnancy may have diverse causes. Possible causes that are very common in pregnancy include Blood Deficiency and Deficiency of Heart and/or Kidney Yin. Spleen Deficiency and Liver Qi Stagnation may contribute to the problem.

Itch (pruritus)

Generalized itch in pregnancy is a common distressing condition affecting up to 20 percent of women. In most cases the cause is the changes in the skin that result from stretching and increased blood supply, and, although uncomfortable, it is benign in nature. In up to 1.5 percent of cases generalized itch can be an indication of obstetric cholestasis, a condition in which the mother's liver fails to clear the bile from the bile ducts (probably a result of an inherited susceptibility to estrogen). The buildup of bile salts in the blood is the cause of the itch, and if prolonged, may possibly increase the risk of stillbirth. Levels of bile can be tested simply by means of taking a blood sample. If a pregnant woman develops generalized pruritus, she should be referred to her doctor or midwife for further tests.

Benign itch in pregnancy may be relieved by simple measures to keep cool, such as turning off heating and applying ice packs to the hands and feet. Simple moisturizers can help.

Information box 5.3d-XV

Itch in pregnancy: comments from a Chinese medicine perspective

In Chinese medicine Liver Blood and Kidney Yin Deficiency are often at the root of itching. Blood and Yin Deficiency can predispose to dryness of skin and then Invasion of Wind Heat that will manifest as intense itching of acute onset or changing location.

Part II: More serious complications of pregnancy

The conditions discussed in the second part of this section are treated conventionally with seriousness as they pose a threat to the health of either the mother, the fetus or both.

Pregnancy-induced hypertension and pre-eclampsia

In a healthy pregnancy, the blood pressure may fall gradually by a few millimeters of mercury (mmHg) as the pregnancy progresses. However, if the blood pressure is found to be rising above the level of the measurement taken at the booking appointment, this may be a red flag of a serious condition known as pregnancy-induced hypertension (PIH). If protein is also found in the urine, the condition of pre-eclampsia is diagnosed.

PIH occurs in about 5–6 percent of all pregnancies. Pre-eclampsia is more common in first pregnancies, of which it complicates about 1–4 percent. It is also more common in women who already have a pre-pregnancy diagnosis of hypertension.

In PIH, the rising blood pressure is an indication of a disturbance of placental function, the cause of which is unclear. In this condition, the placental cells release chemicals that cause the mother's arterioles to constrict, and salt to be retained in the circulation. Both these factors tend to increase the blood pressure, and to reduce blood circulation to the placenta. Reduced circulation to the placenta then leads to a vicious cycle of events, in which there is an increased risk of blood clotting in the maternal circulation. In this situation, the circulation to the glomeruli of the kidneys can be seriously impaired.

Warning signs of kidney damage include the appearance of protein in the urine (proteinuria), rapidly worsening edema and rising blood pressure, all features of the syndrome of pre-eclampsia. The rising blood pressure tends to worsen the condition of the placenta further. This vicious cycle can precipitate a life-threatening condition called eclampsia (see below). Eclampsia can be prevented if the warning rise in blood pressure is monitored carefully, and if the blood pressure is treated as soon as it begins to rise above a certain level.

The most common time for these conditions to become apparent is during the third trimester (last 12 weeks) of pregnancy, although a rise in blood pressure and proteinuria may be first detected during the second trimester (from weeks 14 to 28).

A rise in blood pressure of 30mmHg systolic or 15mmHg diastolic is a serious warning feature of pre-eclampsia, even if the blood pressure remains in the normal range for a non-pregnant person. For example, it would be of concern if the blood pressure was measured as 100/70mmHg at the booking appointment, and was then found to be 125/85mmHg at a later appointment. In a case when the blood pressure remains in the normal range, the condition is described as potential PIH. If potential PIH is diagnosed, the women will be requested to return for repeated checks of her blood pressure and urine at more frequent intervals.

In mild PIH, the diastolic pressure is found to be 90–99mmHg, the systolic pressure is below 140mmHg and the urine is normal on testing for protein. This situation would be monitored closely, but is considered safe as long as the blood pressure rises no higher.

If hypertension is sustained above the level of mild PIH, the patient may be admitted to hospital for treatment. This involves bed rest, intensive monitoring of blood pressure and urine output, and oral antihypertensive medication. Drugs that may be used include atenolol, labetalol, nifedipine and methyldopa.

Pre-eclampsia is diagnosed if a significant quantity of protein is detected in the urine in a patient with PIH. PIH carries significant risks of widespread organ damage and is treated with seriousness. Often patients are admitted to hospital for bed rest, intensive monitoring and intravenous antihypertensive medication. The drug of choice is hydralazine. A decision may be made to perform a cesarean section if the pregnancy is at a sufficiently advanced stage.

The term eclampsia comes from the Greek word for flash of lightning, which hints at the rapidity of the development of the symptoms. Eclampsia is the condition in which damage to the maternal kidneys is in an established downward spiral. It is accompanied by the signs of pre-eclampsia, and also by severe headache, blurred vision and abdominal pain. Edema is usually present. These are severe warning features of a condition characterized by signs of serious damage to the brain cells, including twitching, disorientation, convulsions and coma.

The convulsions are similar in form to a grand mal epileptic seizure, except that rapid recovery to a state of consciousness is unlikely. This state may develop either just before labor, during labor or, in just over half of all cases, just after delivery. Death may occur from either cerebral hemorrhage or from heart failure due to overload of fluids in the circulation. In those who recover, some may have persisting damage to the kidneys.

Eclampsia is treated with drugs to reduce blood pressure and drugs such as intravenous diazepam or magnesium sulfate to inhibit convulsions. Delivery of the fetus is considered of paramount importance. This may be effected by either cesarean section or induction of labor, depending on the state of health of the mother. With recent advances in perinatal care, the maternal mortality rate in cases of severe PIH or eclampsia is very low in developed countries. This is in marked contrast to the experience of childbirth in developing countries, in which up to one-fifth of women who develop eclampsia may die.

However, even in developed countries, the risks to the fetus in established eclampsia are much higher. The stillbirth rate is up to 30 percent in a pregnancy complicated by eclampsia.

 Information box 5.3d-XVI

Hypertension in pregnancy: comments from a Chinese medicine perspective

In Chinese medicine, the raised blood pressure of pregnancy-induced hypertension may be attributed to Liver and Kidney Yin Deficiency with Liver Yang Rising. Liver Yang Rising is the cause of the rise in blood pressure. Liver Wind may then develop. This is the cause of severe dizziness, headache and convulsions. Poor diet and Spleen Qi Deficiency will contribute to the formation of Phlegm. This, too, will contribute to the hypertension, and, carried upwards by the Liver Wind, can obstruct the Orifices of the Heart, causing unconsciousness.

Essential hypertension

If a woman with essential hypertension becomes pregnant, the pregnancy carries particular risks. First, the blood flow to the placenta can be compromised, leading to poor fetal growth. Second, there is an increased risk of the blood pressure rising further (this occurs in up to 60 percent of women who are hypertensive at their booking appointment). In this situation the condition is indistinguishable from PIH, and is treated as such. In such cases there is a high risk of progressing to pre-eclampsia.

The blood pressure of a woman with essential hypertension will be treated with drugs including methyldopa, beta blockers and calcium channel blockers (CCBs). She may be advised to rest as much as possible to maximize the blood flow to the placenta. If the fetal growth is shown by ultrasound scan to be slowing down, premature labor may be induced.

Maternal (gestational) diabetes

Between 1.5 and 2.5 percent of all women demonstrate a temporary inability to maintain their blood glucose within a healthy range in pregnancy. This condition is called gestational glucose intolerance or, if the problem is more severe, gestational diabetes. It appears to be an excessive response to the hormones from the placenta, which tends to counteract the effect of insulin. Although this condition usually abates after delivery, it is recognized that women who have been diagnosed with gestational glucose intolerance are more likely to develop type 2 diabetes in later life.

One important problem with raised maternal blood glucose in pregnancy is that the fetus is exposed to raised levels of blood sugar. This will stimulate the fetal pancreas to secrete excessive amounts of insulin. High levels of insulin can severely affect the development of the fetus, causing excessive body growth (i.e. a large baby), impaired lung maturation and inability to control the salts in the blood. In later life, the child may develop obesity and a tendency to diabetes. Pregnancies in women who are known to be diabetic at the time of conception also carry risks to the fetus, but these risks are the same in those affected by gestational diabetes.

The condition is usually diagnosed in the mother when glucose is found in the urine on routine testing. The diagnosis is confirmed by a blood test (the glucose tolerance test) and, if confirmed, the mother is referred to an endocrinologist who, in conjunction with the obstetrician, will oversee the management of the woman's blood glucose levels for the remainder of her pregnancy. The treatment is by means of attention to diet and insulin injections. Fetal well-being is monitored by means of regular ultrasound scans.

If gestational diabetes has been diagnosed, the baby will need special attention after delivery, as there is a risk of it developing a very low level of blood sugar – a result of its own excessive secretion of insulin. Blood glucose levels may have to be monitored for up to two days after delivery, with treatment involving intravenous nutrition and glucagon injections, until the blood sugar level stabilizes.

 Information box 5.3d-XVII

Diabetes in pregnancy: comments from a Chinese medicine perspective

In Chinese medicine, the energetic interpretation of gestational diabetes is comparable to the description of diabetes as summarized in Section 5.1d. The underlying Deficiency is of Kidney Yin and Spleen Qi, together with Accumulation of diverse Pathogenic Factors, including Damp, Heat, Blood Stagnation and Phlegm. It was suggested in Section 5.1d that hyperglycemia is a possible manifestation of Damp Heat. The mother needs to take care not to eat sweet or starchy foods which are Damp Heat forming.

Thromboembolism

In pregnancy there is an increased risk of diseases that result from excessive blood clotting (thromboembolism). In particular, deep venous (vein) thrombosis (DVT) is well recognized, although this serious condition is rare. Even more rarely, a life-threatening pulmonary embolus or cerebral infarction can occur. The overall rate of thromboembolic conditions is approximately 5–6 pregnancies per 10,000. It is now recognized that certain women are more at risk due to an inherited condition of the clotting factors. The risk is also increased in those women who are unable to stop smoking during pregnancy.

 Information box 5.3d-XVIII

Thromboembolism in pregnancy: comments from a Chinese medicine perspective

The underlying process of thromboembolism in any part of the body would be interpreted as Blood and Qi Stagnation in Chinese medicine. The precise Chinese medicine diagnosis would depend on the part of the body affected by the blood clot. DVT has the features of Blood and Qi Stagnation with Heat affecting the region of the Bladder Channel in the calf. The much more serious condition of pulmonary embolus is a manifestation of Heart Blood Stagnation and can lead to Heart Yang Collapse.

Rhesus disease of the newborn

Rhesus disease of the newborn is the result of when the blood group of a pregnant woman is different to that of her unborn child. This problem is only clinically important when the mother has a Rhesus-negative blood group and the child is Rhesus-positive. Maternal antibodies to the Rhesus factor can cross the placenta and damage the Rhesus factor-containing fetal red cells. This can cause severe anemia, jaundice and sometimes death of the unborn baby.

It is recognized that maternal antibodies to the Rhesus factor develop particularly in women who have already had a Rhesus-positive baby, and seem to form just after the first baby is born. Usually the blood of the mother and fetus do not mix, but it is believed that a little fetal blood enters the mother's circulation during childbirth, and also during miscarriage. This can be sufficient to stimulate the mother's immune system to produce anti-Rhesus antibodies. The ability of the immune system to produce these antibodies tends to persist, and so antibodies can cause problems in subsequent pregnancies.

To anticipate the problems of Rhesus disease, the blood group of all women is tested in early pregnancy. In Rhesus-negative women the presence of antibodies to the Rhesus factor is also assayed, and this is repeated at intervals (at weeks 28 and 36 of gestation) during the pregnancy.

The development of Rhesus antibodies to fetal Rhesus-positive cells can be prevented. After childbirth or miscarriage, and sometimes at stages during a normal pregnancy, Rhesus-negative women are given an immunization with an antibody that can destroy any Rhesus-positive cells that may have entered their circulation. This allows the removal of the foreign blood cells before the mother can develop an immune memory to the Rhesus factor. This immunization has dramatically reduced the death and disability that can result from Rhesus incompatibility in the newborn.

However, not all cases can be prevented. If Rhesus incompatibility is suspected in pregnancy, the mother is referred to a specialist in the condition. Advanced techniques can be used to test for anemia in the fetus and actually transfuse blood while it is in the womb. The baby may require intensive care after birth, and treatment for the jaundice that can result from the damage to its red blood cells.

Infections in pregnancy

Although in general a pregnant woman is no more susceptible to infectious disease than anyone else (there are exceptions to this rule, influenza being a notable one), the effects of the infection on the fetus should always be of concern. For example, a prolonged high fever may induce spontaneous abortion or developmental abnormalities in the fetus in early pregnancy. As well as causing direct harm to the fetus, the blood and nutrient flow through the placenta may also be affected by a fever. These are non-specific effects of infections. Specific effects of infections depend on the nature of the individual infectious agent. The important infections of pregnancy are described in turn below.

VIRAL INFECTIONS IN PREGNANCY

Some viral infections seem to be particularly severe in the pregnant mother and are more likely to promote miscarriage. The recently prevalent H1N1 strains of influenza (flu) infection seem to have this characteristic. Hospital admissions and deaths were particularly marked in the 2009 Swine flu epidemic for pregnant mothers. For these reasons all pregnant mothers are currently encouraged to have the influenza vaccine at any stage in pregnancy.

Smaller organisms are able to invade the placenta from the bloodstream with ease. This means that the fetus is likely to be affected by the virus if the mother has a viral infection. Although most viruses (such as the rhinoviruses, which cause the common cold) are not so harmful to the fetus, there are five important droplet-borne viral infections that can have devastating effects on fetal development. The viruses that are well recognized to cause significant congenital disease are rubella, cytomegalovirus (CMV), varicella zoster (chickenpox), herpes simplex (HSV) and parvovirus B19.

The fetus can also develop chronic viral infections through the placental transfer of virus, and this can lead to deteriorating ill health in childhood. HIV and hepatitis B and C are three viruses that are an important cause of progressive ill health in babies born to infected women.

Rubella virus infection (German measles) used to be a very common mild childhood illness, which, before widespread vaccination, was contracted by just fewer than nine out of ten children. Although rubella infection usually leads to lifelong immunity to the disease, about one-tenth of those who contract rubella do not obtain lifelong immunity. From these figures it can be estimated that, before the introduction of widespread immunization to rubella, just less than 25 percent of women entered their childbearing years without immunity to rubella.

Rubella infection in the first trimester of pregnancy is known to cause damage to over 40 percent of fetuses. Depending on the precise stage of development, the rubella virus causes damage to the developing eye, ear, kidney and heart, as well as causing more general problems such as growth retardation and learning difficulties. This combination of abnormalities is known as congenital rubella syndrome (CRS). The incidence of CRS has dropped dramatically since the introduction of widespread rubella immunization.

Cytomegalovirus (CMV) causes a mild flu-like infection in most people, although in some it can take the form of a more prolonged state of debility akin to glandular fever. It is estimated that over half of women entering pregnancy are already immune to CMV. For those women who contract CMV during pregnancy, there is a small risk of the baby having a congenital abnormality, with 3–7 percent of babies affected in this way. CMV infection can lead to neurological problems such as deafness, epilepsy, cerebral palsy and learning difficulties. There is no way of preventing this infection.

Varicella zoster virus can affect the fetus either in the first 20 weeks of pregnancy or just before delivery. There is only a risk from this infection if the mother develops chickenpox at these stages in her pregnancy. Chickenpox during the first trimester can lead to skin, eye and neurological damage in the fetus in about 5 percent of cases. If the mother develops chickenpox just before or after delivery, the newborn is at risk of a severe blistering rash, which can be life-threatening. Moreover, in pregnancy chickenpox can be a particularly severe condition for the mother, with a high incidence of pneumonia. Preventive treatments for pregnant women exposed to the virus include immunization with zoster immune globulin for the mother and, if chickenpox develops, antiviral medication (aciclovir) for the mother and also the newborn at delivery if affected.

Herpes simplex virus (HSV) is the cause of cold sores and genital herpes. This infection is only problematic if it is active in the genital area at the time of delivery, when the baby is exposed to high levels of the virus during its passage through the birth canal. The consequences of neonatal infection with HSV are severe, with a high risk of neonatal death from widespread infection. For this reason, if active genital herpes is present at the time of delivery, it is recommended that the baby is delivered by cesarean section.

Parvovirus B19 (slapped cheek disease) is a cause of a mild childhood infection that causes fever, headache, and then, in the recovery phase, a rash like a flush appears on the cheeks. Although harmless to healthy children, if a pregnant woman contracts the infection, parvovirus can cause a serious life-threatening condition in the fetus, called hydrops. If a mother contracts slapped cheek disease in late pregnancy, the health of the fetus might be monitored by means of serial ultrasound scans.

Human immunodeficiency virus (HIV) infection appears to have no adverse effect on the pregnancy or the health of the fetus. However, without preventative treatment, the infection is transmitted to the fetus from an infected mother in 20–40 percent of cases. This risk is substantially reduced if the mother takes antiviral drugs such as zidovudine (AZT) from week 20 of pregnancy and if breastfeeding is avoided.

Hepatitis B virus infection is readily transmitted from an infected mother to the fetus. If not treated, these babies have a high risk of developing chronic liver disease and liver cancer in later life. This risk is substantially reduced if the babies are given antibodies to hepatitis B and also hepatitis B immunization at the time of the birth.

Hepatitis C virus, in contrast to hepatitis B infection, is only rarely transmitted to the fetus from the mother.

The long-term risks of infection are chronic liver disease and liver cancer.

BACTERIAL INFECTIONS IN PREGNANCY

Most bacterial infections in the mother do not infect the fetus. Some may have deleterious effects on the pregnancy because of fever and general maternal ill health.

Urinary tract infections are more common in pregnancy because of the relaxing effect of progesterone on the muscle tone of the ureters and bladder. Infections may give rise to no symptoms in pregnancy, but can still have serious consequences. This is one reason for the practice of regular dipstick testing of urine throughout pregnancy. The presence of bacteria in the urine in pregnancy is recognized to increase the risk of developing pregnancy-induced hypertension and also of having a low birth weight baby. In 30 percent of those women who are untreated, pyelonephritis will then develop. This severe kidney infection can cause high fever and rigors. In the long term, it can lead to reduced renal function due to chronic scarring of the kidneys. If bacteria are found in the urine in pregnancy, the mother is prescribed antibiotics such as amoxicillin, nitrofurantoin or cefalexin.

Vaginal infections can affect the health of the fetus. A flare up of *Candida* infection (thrush) is very common in pregnancy, but is harmless to the baby. In contrast, the condition of bacterial vaginosis (due to overgrowth of *Gardnerella*) is believed to increase the risk of premature birth. If this infection is diagnosed it may be treated with antibiotics, even if symptoms are minimal.

Syphilis is a rare infection in developed countries, because of readily available antibiotic treatment. Nevertheless, all pregnant women are screened for this infection early in pregnancy because of the devastating effect it can have on the developing fetus. Congenital syphilis, a condition that leads to failure to thrive in the infant, and abnormalities of the bone and teeth, can be prevented by treating the mother during pregnancy with penicillin.

Listeria is an organism that causes a mild, flu-like illness, and very occasionally can manifest as a form of meningitis in the immunocompromised. *Listeria* originates from cattle and poultry, and so can be contracted through contact with unpasteurized dairy products, pâtés and poorly cooked chicken. Infection in pregnancy can lead to miscarriage, premature delivery or *Listeria* infection of the newborn. *Listeria* infection in a newborn can result in septicemia, pneumonia or meningitis, and can be life-threatening. It carries a 30 percent mortality rate. The condition is prevented by the avoidance during pregnancy of those food products that may be contaminated with *Listeria*.

Toxoplasmosis is an infection that can be contracted from handling raw meat and from cat feces. It can lead either to no symptoms, or to a mild, flu-like illness, which in some people can be more prolonged and debilitating.

Infection in pregnancy can lead to miscarriage or to fetal deformities. In particular, the eyes and the nervous system may be seriously damaged. The condition is prevented by the avoidance of direct contact with raw meat, cat litter and garden soil during pregnancy.

TROPICAL DISEASES IN PREGNANCY

In terms of the risk it may pose to the fetus, the most important tropical disease is *malaria*. This is another infection to which a pregnant woman may have an increased susceptibility compared to a non-pregnant woman. The infection affects the fetus primarily by causing profound ill health in the mother. Occasionally, the infection is transmitted to the fetus. As many of the anti-malarial drugs are potentially harmful to the fetus, it is advisable for women to avoid travel to areas in which malaria is endemic while they are pregnant.

Abnormalities of the placenta and amniotic fluid

TUMORS OF THE PLACENTA (GESTATIONAL TROPHOBLASTIC DISEASE)

Placental tumors are believed to be the result of false pregnancies, which occur either when the sperm fertilizes an egg that has no nucleus, or when more than one sperm enters the ovum. The most common form of placental tumor is known as a hydatidiform mole. In this condition, after the abnormal conception and implantation of the embryo, a large tumor develops from the placental tissue. This can almost replace the placenta. In most cases a fetus does not develop at all. Most moles are benign, but 5 percent may become malignant, and can metastasize to other organs (choriocarcinoma).

The first sign of a mole may be vaginal bleeding. This can be followed by a miscarriage of the mole, resulting in the expulsion of fleshy, grape-like tissue. In other cases the tumor may grow without bleeding, but faster than a normal pregnancy would. In these cases diagnosis can be confirmed by means of an ultrasound scan, and the finding of very high levels of the placental hormone HCG.

Information box 5.3d-XIX

Hydatidiform mole: comments from a Chinese medicine perspective

In Chinese medicine, the development of a hydatidiform mole suggests Phlegm or Blood Stagnation.

Treatment of a benign mole is by means of surgical removal of the remaining abnormal tissue. The woman then will require follow-up at two-week intervals to check that the growth is not recurring. If a malignant growth is found to be developing, the woman is treated by means of combination chemotherapy.

OLIGOHYDRAMNIOS AND POLYHYDRAMNIOS

Oligohydramnios means too little amniotic fluid, and polyhydramnios means too much amniotic fluid. Both may be a reflection of an underlying problem in the fetus. Also, both can cause complications in pregnancy and fetal development.

In a healthy pregnancy, the amniotic fluid is secreted by the lining cells of the placenta. It is swallowed by the fetus, and this swallowed fluid is recycled back into the amniotic fluid as it is filtered and excreted by the fetal kidneys.

Oligohydramnios may be caused by defective placental cells, but can also be an indication of a kidney problem in the fetus. If it occurs early in pregnancy, miscarriage is the usual result. Later on in the pregnancy, the fetus may suffer from the lack of adequate space and lubrication, developing problems such as weak lungs, bony deformities and dry, leathery skin.

Information box 5.3d-XX

Oligohydramnios: comments from a Chinese medicine perspective

In Chinese medicine, the deficiency in fluids in oligohydramnios would suggest severe Deficiency of Kidney Yin or Jing.

Polyhydramnios is either due to a very large surface area of placenta, such as occurs in a multiple pregnancy, or may be an indication of an abnormality of the fetal nervous system or digestive tract (including spina bifida). Polyhydramnios can cause considerable discomfort to the mother, and can precipitate premature labor. Fluid may be removed from the amniotic sac by means of amniocentesis to relieve the discomfort. After delivery, the baby is examined carefully to exclude a poorly developed esophagus or duodenum (atresia of the gastrointestinal tract).

Information box 5.3d-XXI

Polyhydramnios: comments from a Chinese medicine perspective

In Chinese medicine, the excessive fluid of polyhydramnios would suggest an Accumulation of Damp, with an underlying Deficiency of Spleen and/or Kidney Qi.

Problems in the timing of labor

According to conventional medicine, the ideal time for the delivery of a baby is between 36 and 42 weeks after the date of the last menstrual period (LMP). The mother is given the date of the 40th week after conception as the estimated date of delivery (EDD), but in reality this date is somewhat arbitrary, as the precise length of her pregnancy depends on when she conceived, and not on the date of the LMP. Although the average date of conception is 14 days after the LMP, the actual timing of ovulation and conception can vary widely from just a few days after the last menstrual period to some weeks after that date in someone who is ovulating irregularly.

Nevertheless, pregnancies in which labor begins either before 36 weeks of gestation (preterm) or after 42 weeks of gestation (post-term) are considered to carry greater risk to the fetus. For this reason, efforts are made to avoid the occurrence of both preterm labor and post-term pregnancy.

Preterm labor

A preterm labor is defined as a labor that begins before the 36th week of pregnancy. The result is a preterm or premature baby. Also, by definition, a baby that weighs less than 2500 grams is also described as preterm or premature. This means that a preterm or premature baby might have been delivered at later than 36 weeks.

A preterm baby is at risk of a wide range of problems that result from immaturity. These problems are greater for those preterm babies who are small not because the labor started too early, but because their growth in the womb was insufficient for some other reason.

Preterm labor is associated with a wide range of risk factors, including low social class, young age of the mother, multiple pregnancy, smoking, eating disorders in the mother and fetal abnormalities. In addition, various medical conditions of pregnancy may increase the risk of preterm labor. These include any cause of placental bleeding in pregnancy, incompetent (lax) cervix, hypertension, anemia and bacterial vaginosis.

If preterm labor is demonstrated to be established with evidence of dilatation of the cervix, medical treatment can be given to protect the fetus and to attempt to slow the progression of labor. This may not be offered if the labor is after the 34th week, and there is a good facility for neonatal care, as a premature baby can be well cared for in an intensive care setting after this stage of development.

Otherwise the treatment given to a mother in preterm labor first involves an injection of corticosteroids. This treatment has been shown to enhance the production of a fluid called surfactant in the fetal lungs, and so prevent a serious condition called respiratory distress syndrome. This treatment has to be given more than 24 hours before the birth to be effective, and so, once it is given, the mother in some cases is treated with intravenous drugs (most commonly beta blockers) that inhibit the force of the contractions. This treatment can also buy time to enable the woman to be transferred to a unit that has neonatal intensive care facilities.

Cesarean section is more commonly used in the delivery of preterm babies than term babies, because it is believed to offer a far less physically stressful passage into the outside world.

Information box 5.3d-XXII

Premature labor: comments from a Chinese medicine perspective

In Chinese medicine, premature labor may be a result of Qi and Blood Deficiency. It is a manifestation of a premature descent of Qi, and so Spleen Qi or Kidney Qi Deficiency would be expected to predispose to premature labor.

Premature rupture of membranes

Ideally, the membranes surrounding the amniotic sac rupture during labor, either at its onset or, most commonly, around the time of transition from the first to the second stage of labor. If the membranes rupture before the onset of labor, amniotic fluid starts to leak out through the vagina, and a potential pathway for infection of the uterus is opened. In some centers it is the practice that, if natural labor does not start within 24–48 hours following premature rupture of membranes (PRM), labor is induced in order to minimize the time during which infection might enter the uterus. There is reasonable evidence to suggest that a labor that is delayed to over 24 hours after PRM is more associated with infection of the womb.[51]

There is much more of a concern with preterm PRM (occurring at less than 37 weeks), because the woman is less likely to go into labor so soon after the rupture. However, in these cases early labor is less than desirable. In such cases the risks that might result from infection and the loss of amniotic fluid have to be weighed against the potential problems of preterm labor.

In general, the treatment in preterm PRM is conservative. The woman is observed for signs of infection and only treated with antibiotics if these develop, or at the point when labor starts. If the membranes rupture before week 35, corticosteroids are given to the mother to protect the fetus from respiratory distress syndrome.

Post-term pregnancy

Post-term pregnancy is defined as a pregnancy that has extended past 42 weeks. This occurs in one in ten pregnancies. The concern is that the perinatal mortality rate starts to rise once the pregnancy has extended into the

43rd week. This is because there are risks from the fetus outgrowing the blood supply of the aging placenta, and also of difficult labor resulting from a large baby. These risks are most marked in older women and those with pregnancy-induced hypertension or diabetes mellitus.

The treatment of post-term pregnancy is induction of labor. This treatment can be initiated as early as the 10th day after the expected date of delivery. The onset of labor is encouraged by a stepwise introduction of treatments of increasing invasiveness. The order and range of induction techniques varies from center to center.

Often the first approach is one that can be performed by a midwife. This is the stretch and sweep, a manual procedure in which a finger is introduced into the cervix to stretch the membranes. This alone may be sufficient to initiate labor. Another manual technique is amniotomy, in which a sterile instrument is used to rupture the membranes artificially (ARM).

If these techniques are not successful, a medical approach is used. This involves the introduction of a pessary (a medication inserted vaginally) containing a hormone called a prostaglandin. This will soften the cervix in preparation for the uterine contractions. The woman is then given an intravenous infusion of a synthetic form of oxytocin, the uterine-stimulating hormone. As the levels of synthetic oxytocin build up in the mother's bloodstream, contractions become inevitable and will increase in intensity depending on the rate of infusion.

Medical induction is recognized to result in a labor that is rapid, more painful and, for some women, shocking in its intensity. The downward spiral resulting from induction is that the intensity of pain forces some women to choose opioid analgesics or epidural anesthesia at an early stage in labor. This then can increase the likelihood of the need for interventions such as forceps and cesarean delivery. The National Institute for Health and Care Excellence (NICE) (2008) state in their guideline on induction that after induction only one-third of women go on to have a natural labor.[52] Fifteen percent of women have instrumental deliveries and 22 percent cesarean sections after medical induction.

Information box 5.3d-XXIII

Delayed onset of labor: comments from a Chinese medicine perspective

In Chinese medicine, delayed onset of labor can be the result of Blood and Qi Deficiency, Kidney Deficiency and Stomach and Spleen Qi Deficiency.

The at-risk fetus and high-risk pregnancy

THE AT-RISK FETUS

The term at-risk fetus is used to describe a situation in which at any particular stage of gestation the fetus is much more vulnerable than is normal for a healthy fetus. An at-risk fetus is more likely to suffer from intrauterine death, distress during labor, death during delivery (stillbirth) and poor health in the neonatal period and early infancy. It is now recognized that this poor start to life may well be related to health problems that persist throughout childhood and even into late adulthood. A fetus may be at risk because of congenital abnormality, or because of factors that impair the environment in which it is developing. These include all the serious complications of pregnancy described above, and also the concurrent use of therapeutic or recreational drugs during pregnancy.

Intrauterine growth retardation (small-for-dates fetus)
Failure to achieve a predicted rate of growth (when the fetus is said to be small-for-dates) is the most common underlying factor that puts the fetus at risk. A wide range of risk factors is associated with a poor rate of fetal growth. For some of these the growth is slow or retarded throughout pregnancy, and for others (notably those that are to do with poor placental function) the growth rate starts off normally and then begins to decline towards the end of the pregnancy.

The factors associated with poor fetal growth throughout the pregnancy include a previous birth of a baby weighing less than 2500 grams, previous stillbirth or neonatal death, history of urinary tract infection or kidney disease, bleeding during the pregnancy, smoking during the pregnancy and fetal malformations.

The factors that tend to affect the ability of the placenta to provide sufficient nourishment include high blood pressure (pregnancy-induced hypertension), post-term pregnancy, eating disorders and severe anemia in the mother, and multiple pregnancy.

Poor fetal growth may only be detected relatively late in pregnancy because the rate of weight gain in the mother or the size of her bump may have little or no correlation with the size of the fetus, particularly in early pregnancy. In later pregnancy, a failure to put on weight in the later weeks together with a lower than normal increase in girth may be warning signs of poor fetal growth. The first accurate measurement of the growth of the fetus is usually made midway through pregnancy by means of the routine ultrasound scan.

The presence of one or more of the risk factors associated with poor fetal growth might alert the obstetrician to the possibility of poor fetal growth. If poor growth is then confirmed by ultrasound scan, the woman will receive more intensive antenatal care, particularly in the last trimester of pregnancy.

Although most at-risk fetuses demonstrate growth retardation, not all do. Some fetuses with congenital abnormalities may maintain normal growth rate, but still are more vulnerable to serious conditions than a healthy fetus. The large baby in a pregnancy complicated by diabetes is also more at risk of serious complications.

THE HIGH-RISK PREGNANCY

A pregnancy in which the health of the fetus is at risk is termed a high-risk pregnancy. High-risk pregnancies should be managed with much more attention to regular monitoring than would be normal in a healthy pregnancy. The care of a woman with a high-risk pregnancy in the UK will always be transferred from the local midwifery team and general practice to the specialist obstetric team at the local hospital.

During the last weeks of a high-risk pregnancy, tests are performed at regular intervals to assess the health of the fetus. These include counts of fetal movements, serial ultrasound scans, assessment of the blood flow in the umbilical cord and use of the cardiotocograph (CTG). As is true in labor, the use of the CTG, although very reassuring when normal tracings are obtained, may result in the use of unnecessary medical interventions when it produces an abnormal reading, when in fact all was well. This is because an abnormal pattern does not always accurately indicate that the fetus is in actual distress.

If the serial assessments of a high-risk pregnancy indicate deteriorating fetal health, delivery of the baby will be expedited, either by medical induction of labor or by cesarean section. In some cases, when the health of the fetus is considered to be very much at risk, this will mean inducing a preterm delivery.

THE AT-RISK FETUS DURING LABOR

Delivery of an at-risk fetus requires intensive monitoring, so that if any sudden deterioration in the health of the fetus is detected, delivery can be expedited (usually by cesarean section, and sometimes by forceps if the distress occurs during the second stage of labor). CTG monitoring is always used to assess changes in the fetal heart rate during contractions. As previously mentioned, the CTG may indicate a problem when there is no actual cause for concern. One consequence of a false-positive CTG trace result can be an unnecessary cesarean section. If there is doubt about how to proceed, a sample of blood may be withdrawn (via the vagina) from the scalp of the fetus. This is tested for increased acidity, which is a definite sign of fetal distress.

The at-risk fetus is more likely to require intensive care as a neonate. This need for intensive care is assessed by a pediatrician who is called to be present to examine the newborn at the end of the labor or the cesarean section.

Information box 5.3d-XXIV

The at-risk fetus: comments from a Chinese medicine perspective

In Chinese medicine, the precise energetic interpretation of the at-risk fetus and high-risk pregnancy would depend in part on the underlying causative conditions. However, it is likely that Kidney or Jing Deficiency is common to all cases.

The red flags of the disorders of pregnancy

Many women with symptoms of the minor conditions and all of those who have signs of the serious conditions of pregnancy will benefit from referral to a conventional doctor for assessment or treatment. Red flags are those symptoms and signs that indicate that referral should be considered. The red flags of the disorders of pregnancy are described in Table 5.3d-I. A summary of the red flags in a format designed for quick reference in clinical practice can be found in Appendix III. This gives advice on the degree of urgency of referral for each of the red flag conditions listed.

Table 5.3d-I A37: Red flags of the disorders of pregnancy

Red flag	Description	Reasoning
A37.1	Bleeding: any episode of vaginal bleeding in pregnancy	Refer all cases to the general practitioner (GP) to arrange investigation (ultrasound scan). Slight, painless bleeding occurring at four, eight or twelve weeks of gestation is most likely to be physiological (i.e. benign) in nature, but refer to exclude miscarriage
		Painless or painful bleeding at a later stage in pregnancy may result from placenta previa or placental abruption, both of which are a serious threat to the health of the fetus and the mother
		Refer as an emergency if there are any signs of shock (see A19.3), as internal bleeding may not be immediately apparent
A37.2	Abdominal pain: any episode of sustained abdominal pain in pregnancy	Gripy abdominal pains (like mild period pains) are common in early pregnancy, and if they do not prevent daily activities are not worrying
		Severe or worsening abdominal pain in early pregnancy may be the first indication of ectopic pregnancy, and needs to be referred on the same day
		Severe pain in later pregnancy may be a symptom of placental abruption, and likewise merits urgent referral. It also can be the first sign of pre-eclampsia
		Abdominal pain is particularly serious if any signs of shock are apparent (see A19.3), as internal bleeding may not be immediately apparent
		Periodic, mild, cramping sensations in later pregnancy (lasting no more than a few seconds) are likely to be benign Braxton Hicks contractions. If becoming regular and intensifying, these might signify premature labor (if before week 36 of pregnancy) or labor. If in any doubt, refer for an assessment
A37.3	Nausea and vomiting with dehydration for >1 day in pregnancy	Refer if unremitting (patient unable to drink freely for more than 1 day) or if there are any features of dehydration (see A3.5). The patient may need hospital admission for administration of fluids
A37.4	Edema in pregnancy	Mild swelling of the ankles and hands is common in middle to late pregnancy
		Refer if edema extends to >2cm above the malleoli, if there is facial edema, or if there is an associated rise in blood pressure of >15mmHg above the usual blood pressure, or any degree of hypertension (systolic >140mmHg, diastolic >90mmHg). All these signs suggest the possibility of pre-eclampsia
		Occasionally, edema can develop as a result of an undiagnosed cardiac abnormality
A37.5	Palpitations in pregnancy	Usually, when palpitations are experienced there is the occasional missed beat, and this is nothing to worry about. However, the increased cardiac output may lead to a previously undiagnosed heart abnormality becoming apparent
		Refer if the pulse rate is either rapid (>100 beats/minute) or irregular, or if there are frequent missed beats (more than 1 every 5 beats)
		Remember that palpitations may result from the added strain on the cardiovascular system that results from anemia in pregnancy
A37.6	Pubic symphysis pain in pregnancy	Refer for a medical assessment of the pain if it is not responding to treatment, and if it is affecting mobility (may benefit from expert physiotherapy advice and aids)

A37.7	Anemia (tiredness, depression, breathlessness, palpitations) in pregnancy	Anemia is common in pregnancy. The risks of bleeding during labor are higher in women with anemia, so medical wisdom is that if significant it should be treated with iron replacement
A37.8	Itching (severe), especially of the palms and soles, in pregnancy	May result from cholestasis, a condition that can damage the fetus. Refer as a high priority so that appropriate blood tests can be performed
A37.9	Potential pregnancy-induced hypertension (PIH)	Refer if you find that the blood pressure has risen to 30mmHg systolic or 15mmHg diastolic above any measurement taken previously
A37.10	Mild pregnancy-induced hypertension (PIH)	Refer if the diastolic blood pressure is 90–99mmHg, and the systolic blood pressure is <140mmHg
A37.11	Moderate to severe pregnancy-induced hypertension (PIH)	Refer as a high priority if the diastolic blood pressure is >100mmHg or the systolic blood pressure is >140mmHg
A37.12	Features of pre-eclampsia/HELLP syndromes: headache, abdominal pain, visual disturbance, nausea and vomiting, edema (in middle to late pregnancy)	Headache, abdominal pain and visual disturbances can presage eclampsia, even in the absence of raised blood pressure Nausea and vomiting, headache and edema together suggest the development of the HELLP syndrome (hemolysis, liver abnormalities and low platelets) Both these syndromes, which may overlap, are absolute emergencies
A37.13	Thromboembolism: pain in the calf, swollen or discolored leg, or breathlessness, with chest pain or blood in the sputum in pregnancy	Refer any features of a thromboembolic event, i.e. deep venous thrombosis (DVT) of the calf or pelvic veins (see A11.7), pulmonary embolus (see A17.10) or stroke (see A22.3) as an emergency The risks of these events are greater in pregnancy. Thromboembolism is the most significant cause of maternal death in pregnancy
A37.14	Fever: refer in pregnancy if high (>38.5°C) and no response to treatment in 24 hours	Refer for management of the underlying cause as high fever may affect the embryo/fetus
A37.15	Fever with rash in the first trimester of pregnancy	Refer suspected rubella or chickenpox so that the health of the embryo/fetus can be monitored
A37.16	Fever with rash in the last trimester of pregnancy	Refer if chickenpox or shingles is suspected, as there is a risk of fatal fetal varicella infection
A37.17	Outbreak of genital herpes (see A35.8) in the last trimester of pregnancy	Refer to GP or midwife for discussion of birth plan, as there is a risk of transmission of herpes virus to the baby during delivery
A37.18	Urinary tract infection in pregnancy	Always refer for urine testing for bacteria, as if present there is an increased risk of induction of miscarriage in the first trimester, and also chronic kidney infection in the mother
A37.19	Offensive, fishy-smelling discharge (possible bacterial vaginosis (BV)) in pregnancy	Refer for treatment, as BV leads to an increased risk of early labor and miscarriage
A37.20	Any watery vaginal leakage in middle to late pregnancy	A very watery discharge in middle to late pregnancy is amniotic fluid until proven otherwise. Premature rupture of the membranes (PRM) carries a risk of uterine infection, and needs to be assessed as a high priority. Even if the pregnancy has come to term, PRM without the onset of labor carries this risk, and conventional practice is to induce labor, if this has not started naturally, within 24 hours of PRM

5.3e Complications of childbirth and the puerperium

This section summarizes the problems that can complicate the process of childbirth, from the onset of the first stage of labor, to the completion of the third stage of labor, when the placenta is delivered. In preparation for this, it will be helpful to be familiar with the physiology of the three stages of childbirth and the puerperium, which is summarized in Section 5.3a.

The complications of childbirth discussed in this section are:

- Complications of the first and second stages of labor:
  - abnormal positioning of the fetus
  - umbilical cord prolapse
  - multiple pregnancy
  - prolonged and obstructed labor
  - rapid labor
  - perineal tears
  - episiotomy
- Complications of the third stage of labor:
  - postpartum hemorrhage and retained placenta
- Complications of the puerperium:
  - puerperal infection
  - thromboembolism
  - psychiatric problems.

Instrumental delivery

The term instrumental delivery is used to describe a delivery in which obstetric interventions are employed to assist the delivery of a baby when labor is not straightforward. There are two instrumental techniques used to encourage the downward movement of the fetus when labor is not progressing well in the second stage: forceps delivery and delivery by vacuum extraction (ventouse). These techniques can only be used when the cervix is fully dilated, and when the head of the fetus has started its descent through the pelvis. Both require local analgesia, either epidural anesthesia or an anesthetic that numbs the nerves that supply the perineum. Between 5 and 12 percent of all deliveries in the UK involve either forceps or vacuum extraction.

Forceps delivery

Forceps delivery involves the insertion of two curved metal instruments that are designed to cradle the head of the fetus and allow the obstetrician to apply downward traction on the head. The woman has to be positioned on her back with her legs held apart in stirrups to allow the forceps to be inserted. After the perineal area has been anesthetized, an episiotomy (surgical incision of the perineal tissues) is performed to widen the passageway for the descent of the head.

Although the most usual complication of forceps delivery is temporary molding of the head of the fetus, in rare cases it can result in severe physical trauma to the head of the fetus. There is also a risk of trauma to the vagina and the cervix of the mother.

Ventouse vacuum extraction

The ventouse is a cup-like instrument that is placed against the head of the fetus. Suction is then applied through the cup, so that traction on the cup will pull the head downwards. Ventouse extraction is less likely to result in vaginal and perineal damage than forceps delivery. It always leaves a temporary unsightly raised circle of swelling on the head of the baby (lasting up to 48 hours), and is more likely to damage the skin of the baby's scalp. More serious complications of ventouse extraction are considered to be rare.

Cesarean section

Cesarean section is the term used to describe the surgical operation to remove the baby from the womb via an abdominal incision. Planned cesarean section is performed before the natural onset of labor in order to prevent either the deterioration of the health of the fetus in the womb or the potential complications of labor. Planned cesarean section is considered to be a relatively safe operation for the mother, as there is an opportunity for her to be prepared for the procedure.

In contrast, emergency cesarean section is performed when labor has been allowed to start naturally, but then complications have arisen that threaten the health of the fetus or the mother. Emergency cesarean section is performed to expedite delivery in an ongoing labor. This is usually because labor is not progressing as smoothly as expected. Also, cesarean section may be performed if at any time the monitoring of the fetus suggests severe fetal distress. This is more likely to occur in an at-risk fetus. Emergency cesarean section is performed to enable a rapid removal of the fetus from the womb. It carries more risks to both the mother and the fetus because it is performed at a time when both are under the extreme physical stress of complicated labor.

Cesarean section is performed either under general or epidural anesthesia. It usually involves a horizontal incision just above the pubic bone. After the operation, the mother is encouraged to be up and about within one to two days. Usually recovery from a cesarean section is uncomplicated, and the mortality rate is extremely low.

Nevertheless, a cesarean section will necessitate a longer stay than normal in hospital after delivery (seven to ten days). As with all abdominal operations, pain from the healing wound will restrict normal activities including lifting and driving for the next few weeks. This can have a big impact on the experience of life with a newborn baby. Those women who have had to undergo an emergency cesarean section may take longer to recover from the physical and emotional shock of the procedure.

Between 3 and 12 percent of cesarean sections are affected by complications. Minor infections and bleeding from the scar are relatively common. A womb infection is a more severe complication, which will necessitate high-dose antibiotic treatment. There is a small increased risk of deep vein thrombosis (DVT) after cesarean section.

Complications of the first and second stages of labor

Abnormal positioning of the fetus in the uterus

If the fetus is in a less than ideal position at the onset of labor, the smooth progression of labor may be impeded. Ideally, the fetus should have found a head-down position in the few weeks leading up to labor. In the days leading up to labor, the head should have dropped (engaged) into the bowl of the pelvis. The occiput (the posterior aspect of the crown of the head) is ideally the part that presses on the cervix, and which descends through the cervix foremost. If the occiput presents foremost, the head presents its narrowest diameter to the constrained passageway provided by the pelvis, and birth will be less difficult. In addition, even pressure on the cervix from a well-positioned occiput will encourage efficient and even dilatation of the cervix.

OCCIPITO-ANTERIOR PRESENTATION

At the onset of labor the back of the fetus should be directed forwards and slightly to one side. This is termed the occipito-anterior position. In this position, the occiput is most likely to present foremost. A normally shaped healthy uterus and pelvis will encourage the fetus to find this position as it grows to fill the abdominal cavity. A healthy degree of uterine muscle tone will literally squeeze the fetus into this most natural position.

It is often possible for a skilled midwife to confirm the occipito-anterior position, as the body of the fetus can be palpated through the mother's abdominal wall. The smooth back of the fetus is felt to be facing outwards either to the left or the right. In addition, the shoulders can

be felt just above the pubic bone, indicating that the head has indeed engaged.

MALPRESENTATION

If the fetus is not in this ideal occipito-anterior position at the onset of labor, this is described as a malpresentation. A malpresentation means that the descent of the fetus is more likely to be restricted by the passageway of the pelvis, and also that the cervix is not exposed to the even pressure necessary to generate efficient contractions. The first stage of the labor is, therefore, more likely to be prolonged, the contractions more painful and the need for assisted delivery more likely. Occipito-posterior presentation and breech presentation are the two most common malpresentations. These are now discussed in more detail.

Occipito-posterior presentation

In one-tenth of pregnancies the fetus is head down, but its spine is lying against the mother's spine. This position is called the occipito-posterior position. This position may result either from deficient uterine tone, or from an unusually shaped pelvis. This position is commonly diagnosed before the onset of labor because of the characteristic shape of this fetal position when felt during palpation of the mother's abdomen. In this position the head is often unable to engage until the onset of labor, because the neck is not free to flex. Like an egg lying sideways on in an egg cup, the head can present a wider diameter to the pelvis, so that descent of the head becomes more difficult.

Because the head is not in the ideal position, the pressure it exerts on the cervix may be uneven, and this can result in inefficient contractions, which might start and stop. Nevertheless, the contractions can be very painful, and are often felt in the back. In about 70 percent of cases of occipito-posterior presentation normal delivery is possible, although additional analgesia is often necessary. In about 20 percent of cases instrumental delivery by means of forceps or ventouse extraction may be necessary. In fewer than 10 percent of cases the baby is delivered by cesarean section because labor becomes too prolonged.

Breech presentation

Breech presentation means that the baby has found a head-up position in the womb. This is commonplace earlier on in pregnancy, when the fetus has a lot of freedom of movement. However, by week 35 of gestation over 90 percent of babies have found a head-down position. Even after this time some babies will turn spontaneously, so that only 3 percent of all pregnancies are breech presentation at term (40 weeks of gestation). In some of these cases there is an obvious physical reason for the malpresentation, such as an unusually shaped pelvis in the mother or placenta previa.

If there are no obvious physical obstructions to an occipito-anterior position, it may be possible for a skilled obstetrician to turn a breech baby at around week 37 of gestation by means of a procedure called version. This involves manually shifting the baby's position by means of palpation through the mother's abdominal wall. The fetal heart rate is monitored throughout. There is a small risk of premature rupture of membranes or induction of labor when this technique is performed. Version is not always successful.

Breech presentation presents a problem during normal delivery because labor is inevitably more difficult. There is a 1 in 100 chance of a healthy fetus dying during delivery if it presents in a breech position, and this risk is greatly increased if the baby is premature or post-term. For this reason, 30–60 percent of breech presentations are managed by a planned cesarean section. Furthermore, if normal delivery is attempted, in up to 40 percent of cases an emergency cesarean section may be necessary.

Other malpresentations
Occipito-posterior and breech are the most common malpresentations. However, the fetus can present in a range of unfavorable positions at the onset of labor. These include transverse (horizontal) and oblique presentation and shoulder presentation. These malpresentations can also be diagnosed before the onset of labor by means of skilled abdominal palpation. With transverse and oblique presentations, the baby may be encouraged to find a head-down position by means of version. If this is not possible, or if there is a shoulder presentation, planned cesarean section is usually the chosen method of delivery.

Sometimes, just the position of the baby's head can greatly complicate the progression of labor. Problems with the position of the head may not be diagnosed until labor is established. In particular, face and brow presentations can cause problems, which may necessitate a cesarean section or instrumental delivery. Occasionally, these presentations occur because of the presence of a severe malformation of the baby's head or neck.

Information box 5.3e-I

Malpresentation: comments from a Chinese medicine perspective

In Chinese medicine, a malpresentation may represent a Deficiency in the Spleen or Kidney Qi of the mother. This is particularly the case when the underlying problem is a deficiency in uterine tone, placenta previa or an unusually shaped pelvis. If the problem is due to fetal malformation, this is more indicative of Jing Deficiency, which may, of course, have its foundation in a Deficiency of Kidney Qi in the parents.

Umbilical cord prolapse

In all the less common forms of malpresentation there is a risk that the umbilical cord will drop into the space in the uterus below the baby, and can then fall down into the vagina ahead of the baby during delivery. This complication, known as umbilical cord prolapse, can seriously threaten the health of the fetus because the cord can become compressed during delivery. Cord prolapse can also occur when the baby is presenting in the normal occipito-anterior position, but this is a rare event, as the tight application of the occiput against the dilated cervix usually prevents the cord from dropping downwards.

If cord prolapse is diagnosed (after vaginal examination during labor), the safest option is to deliver the baby by emergency cesarean section.

Information box 5.3e-II

Umbilical cord prolapse: comments from a Chinese medicine perspective

In Chinese medicine, a cord prolapse, itself a form of malpresentation, likewise may reflect an underlying Deficiency of Spleen and/or Kidney Qi.

Multiple pregnancy

Multiple pregnancy occurs as a result of two distinct physiological processes. It results either from a multiple release of egg cells (ova) from the mother's ovaries, or from an early division of the cells of an embryo. The former (multizygotic) process results in non-identical siblings and the latter process (monozygotic) in apparently identical siblings.

Twins are the most common form of multiple pregnancy, occurring in approximately 1 in 90 pregnancies that reach term. Triplets occur in approximately 1 in 8100 pregnancies. The rate of occurrence of triplets, quadruplets and even larger multiple pregnancies is increasing since the introduction of assisted-fertilization techniques.

The introduction of early ultrasound scanning has shown that twin pregnancy is more common than was previously thought. This investigation has demonstrated that it is not uncommon for one of the twins in a twin pregnancy to die in the first few weeks of pregnancy, and then to become reabsorbed into the mother's womb. This situation, described as vanishing twin syndrome, will then manifest as an apparently singleton pregnancy at later stages in gestation.

In a multiple pregnancy, multizygotic (non-identical) fetuses each develop with their own placenta and amniotic sac. In contrast, monozygotic (identical) fetuses share a common placenta and amniotic sac.

Babies born from a multiple pregnancy are generally smaller than average, presumably because they have to draw from a single and limited source of nutrients. Monozygotic fetuses in multiple pregnancies very commonly are markedly different in size. This is because they share one placenta, and often one gets a larger proportion of the blood supply flowing through its umbilical cord.

Multiple pregnancy is more likely to be associated with complications, and so, once diagnosed, the mother may be offered more frequent antenatal care from a specialist center. The complications that are more likely to occur in multiple pregnancies include:

- pregnancy-induced hypertension
- anemia (due to iron and folic acid deficiency)
- polyhydramnios
- premature labor
- death of the fetus around the time of the labor.

In addition, many of the minor complications of pregnancy, such as morning sickness, backache, heartburn, hemorrhoids and poor sleep, are exacerbated in multiple pregnancies. The greater the number of fetuses, the more common are all of these complications.

Labor poses an additional problem in multiple pregnancies, partly because the incidence of malpresentation is very high. Only in 45 percent of cases of twin pregnancies do both fetuses present head down. There is a five times greater risk of a fetus in a multiple pregnancy dying during a vaginal delivery. This is partly a result of the risk of malpresentation, and partly because the fetus is more likely to be underweight. For this reason, cesarean section is commonly advised for the delivery of multiple pregnancies.

 Information box 5.3e-III

Multiple pregnancy: comments from a Chinese medicine perspective

From a Chinese medicine perspective, multiple pregnancies are bound to Deplete the Blood and Kidney Qi of the mother. Deficient Kidney Qi in the mother may manifest as Jing Deficiency in the fetuses; this is reflected in the low birth weight of many babies born from a multiple pregnancy.

Prolonged and obstructed labor

A normal first stage of labor should take no more than 12–24 hours in first pregnancies, and no more than 12 hours in subsequent pregnancies. A normal second stage should last no more than 2 hours. If the labor is prolonged in either of the two stages, there are increasing risks of maternal exhaustion and death of the fetus. If the fetus becomes stuck on its way through the pelvic canal, this is termed obstructed labor. The end result of obstructed labor can be rupture of the uterus. Rupture of the uterus is much more likely if there is a scar from a previous cesarean section.

Prolonged labor will frequently result in the use of instrumental delivery or emergency cesarean section. This is always the case in obstructed labor. Rupture of the uterus is a complication that should be avoided if at all possible, as its treatment commonly involves emergency cesarean section followed by hysterectomy.

As has been described, prolonged and obstructed labor may be a result of the position of the fetus. In malpresentation, the fundamental problem is that the presenting part of the fetus is simply too wide to pass easily through the pelvic canal. Similarly, a pelvis that is too narrow to permit the passage of the head of the fetus, even when correctly presented, will result in problems in labor. This problem, rather clumsily termed cephalopelvic disproportion (CPD), is more likely to occur if the woman is of small stature, and particularly if the small stature is the result of illness or malnutrition in childhood. For this reason, CPD is much more common in developing countries than in developed nations. If it appears likely that CPD may be a problem, for example, if the pregnant woman is very short, or if she has a small shoe size, the dimensions of the pelvic canal can be measured by means of a pelvic scan. A decision can then be made about whether or not the baby should be delivered by planned cesarean section.

Occasionally, if the baby is large, the head may be delivered normally, but the shoulders become stuck in the pelvic canal. This problem, known as shoulder dystocia, poses a severe risk to the life of the fetus. The delivery in a case of shoulder dystocia requires considerable experience on the part of the obstetrician or midwife. In this situation, tearing of the perineal tissues of the mother is not uncommon, and the baby often suffers damage to the structures in the area of its neck, such as the clavicle or the brachial plexus of nerves.

Another common reason for prolonged labor is more functional in nature, in that the presentation of the fetus is normal and the size of the pelvic canal is adequate. In these cases, the problem is attributed to an abnormality of uterine action. In some cases of abnormal uterine action, the contractions are too weak and inefficient to lead to full dilatation of the cervix. In particular, the onset of dilatation of the cervix may be very slow to start. It is now increasingly recognized that a calm and restful environment helps to encourage efficient contractions.

Any stimulus that promotes anxiety in the mother can halt the contractions and may even reverse the progression of the dilatation of the cervix. It is believed that excessive release of adrenaline in the mother in the first stage of labor can counteract the effect of oxytocin, the natural uterine stimulant. Potential stressors include transfer to an alien hospital environment, excessive pain and an anxious birth partner(s). All these may be compounded by the mother having negative expectations of childbirth, as are commonly held by women in modern societies.[53]

Insufficient uterine activity may respond well to the provision of a calm environment for the mother. If the first stage of labor is prolonged, an infusion of synthetic oxytocin will be initiated, akin to the medical induction of labor. There is a greater than normal probability that this type of functional prolonged labor will end in instrumental delivery or a cesarean section because of failure of the labor to progress and maternal exhaustion.

In contrast, the uterus may be contracting with force, but the contractions are not coordinated, and so do not result in smooth dilatation of the cervix. In this type of functional prolonged labor, the pain of the contractions may be severe. Emotional factors also appear to play an important role in this abnormality of uterine action. Treatment of functional prolonged labor when the contractions are forceful but inefficient may also include artificial rupture of the membranes before the institution of an oxytocin infusion. There is a greater than normal probability of instrumental delivery and of emergency cesarean section with this type of prolonged labor.

In some cases the cervix ceases to continue to dilate significantly despite continued contractions. This is described as cervical dystocia. If previous scarring to the cervix is the cause of the problem, it is termed cervical stenosis. In this situation, there is a real risk of obstructed labor and fetal distress. If there is no response to an oxytocin infusion within a few hours, an emergency cesarean section will be performed.

Information box 5.3e-IV

Prolonged labor: comments from a Chinese medicine perspective

In Chinese medicine, prolonged labor is often a reflection of underlying Deficiency in the mother, notably of Blood and Qi. The Deficiency may have its root in Spleen and Stomach Qi Deficiency or Kidney Qi Deficiency. Stagnant flow of Liver Qi and Blood may also contribute to the problem, and this would seem likely in the case of forceful but uncoordinated contractions or cervical dystocia. Fear and tension will Sink and Stagnate the Qi, and so are likely to inhibit labor.

Of all the causes of prolonged labor, the problems of uterine function are those that may respond well to acupuncture treatment.

Rapid (precipitate) labor

A labor that is too rapid may also cause problems. A precipitate labor is defined as one that takes less than two hours. In such a labor the contractions are very intense. The fetus may suffer from lack of oxygen in the womb, and from compression injuries during delivery. Moreover, the delivery is more likely to take place in an unsuitable place, and without trained birth attendants. The mother may be in a state of exhaustion and shock after a precipitate labor.

Perineal tears

Vaginal and perineal tears are very common. They occur at the end of the second stage of labor as the head and then the body of the fetus pass through the vagina and then the stretched perineum. Ideally, tearing can be minimized by controlling the speed at which the head descends through the vaginal canal, although this degree of control is not always possible.

In the least severe cases, these injuries will simply be superficial grazes of the vaginal and perineal epithelium. These minor tears will heal very rapidly.

More severe tears are graded as follows:

- a first-degree tear involves damage to the superficial tissues only

- a second-degree tear involves damage to the superficial tissues and the perineal muscles

- a third-degree tear extends backwards from the vagina to also involve damage to the muscles of the anus

- a fourth-degree tear not only extends to the anal muscle, but also tears the lining tissues of the anal canal.

The vagina and perineum should always be inspected after delivery for tears. First-degree tears usually heal well with one or two sutures (stitches). Second- or third-degree tears require more care in their repair, but can usually be repaired well. Third- or fourth-degree tears are not common, and are most likely to occur during instrumental (forceps) delivery, delivery of a large baby or a delivery of a baby in the occipito-posterior position. With a fourth-degree tear the repair requires a skilled operator. The recovery from the repair may be slow, with many women suffering from persisting incontinence of wind, and some with fecal incontinence.

Even if there are only minor lacerations, it is common for many women to suffer quite severe perineal discomfort for the first few days after delivery. Ideally, this discomfort should largely have gone by one to two weeks after delivery. However, it has been estimated that up to 15 percent of women still suffer perineal discomfort by 12 weeks after the delivery. It is not uncommon for sexual intercourse to be uncomfortable for over 20 weeks after delivery. In some cases the trauma of a perineal tear can cause profound psychological damage, and this can continue to affect a sexual relationship adversely for a much longer period.

Episiotomy

Episiotomy is a deliberate incision of the perineum performed at the end of the second stage of labor. It is performed to ease the passage of the fetal head through the perineum. It is less commonly performed in uncomplicated labors than it used to be, because it is now appreciated that most naturally occurring tears heal just as well as an episiotomy, if not better. It is recognized that long-term complications, including perineal pain and difficult intercourse, appear to be more common in women who have had an episiotomy. Nevertheless, in cases when the perineum appears to be over-distending and threatening to tear in a particularly damaging way, an episiotomy may be performed. In some types of forceps delivery, an episiotomy is always performed.

Complications of the third stage of labor

Postpartum hemorrhage and retained placenta

Some blood loss during and following the third stage of labor is to be expected, but is considered excessive if it exceeds 500 milliliters within the first 24 hours after delivery of the baby. If the blood loss is estimated to exceed this amount, the term primary postpartum hemorrhage (primary PPH) is applied. If the blood loss occurs at some point after the first 24 hours after the birth, then the term secondary PPH is applied.

PRIMARY POSTPARTUM HEMORRHAGE (PRIMARY PPH)

In the majority of cases of primary PPH, the bleeding comes from a uterus that has failed to contract down sufficiently during the third stage of labor. Pre-existing conditions, including anemia and fibroids, can increase the risk of this form of PPH. Even with the use of synthetic oxytocin (ergometrine) injection at the end of the second stage of labor, this form of primary PPH still occurs following approximately 3 percent of vaginal deliveries. In an additional one-fifth of cases of primary PPH, the bleed originates from a cervical or vaginal laceration.

As blood loss from the womb is prevented by efficient shrinking down of the body of the uterus, any factor that prevents this from occurring will increase the risk of PPH. Inefficient postpartum contractions may occur if the mother is exhausted after a prolonged labor, or if the uterus has been over-distended by a multiple pregnancy. Any retained blood clots or pieces of placenta in the womb will also prevent the uterus from contracting down. Finally, failure of the placenta to separate from the uterus, a situation known as retained placenta, will also cause PPH. Together these causes account for 80 percent of cases of PPH.

If there are retained blood clots or retained placenta, these have to be removed. This is often impossible by natural means because the uterus has contracted down around the clot or placenta, thereby preventing their release. This particular problem is exacerbated by the administration of synthetic oxytocin (ergometrine) in the second stage of labor. In this situation, if massage of the uterus has no effect, the retained products have to be removed manually while the woman is under either general or epidural anesthesia. In this operation, the obstetrician removes the placenta from the womb using a gloved hand. After the procedure, an injection of ergometrine is given to facilitate further contraction down of the uterus.

If bleeding continues from an empty uterus, this can rapidly become an emergency situation. In such cases an intravenous drip is set up to replace lost fluids while the uterus is massaged. A continuous infusion of a synthetic oxytocin is then administered.

The principal treatment for PPH from cervical and vaginal laceration is careful location and stitching of these tears.

SECONDARY POSTPARTUM HEMORRHAGE (SECONDARY PPH)

Delayed hemorrhage from the uterus is also usually due to failure of contraction of the uterine lining and retention of blood clots. In this case, the diagnosis can be confirmed by ultrasound scan. Most cases respond to ergometrine injection.

Occasionally, infection in the womb will manifest as secondary PPH (see below).

Information box 5.3e-V

Postpartum hemorrhage: comments from a Chinese medicine perspective

In Chinese medicine, PPH is most likely to be a result of Spleen Qi Deficiency with Spleen Not Holding Blood. Excessive Heat may be contributory in some cases.

Retention of the placenta suggests Stagnation of Qi or Blood in the Uterus. Blood and Qi Deficiency may be the underlying causes of this failure to generate sufficient downward movement of Qi after delivery.

Complications of the puerperium

The puerperium is the time during which the mother's body recovers from the changes of pregnancy and the physical trauma of labor. For this reason, minor emotional and physical disturbances are common, and these are considered normal. The puerperium is also the time during which a feeding routine is established for the baby. The complications of breastfeeding, although they are most common during the puerperium, are described in Section 5.3f.

Serious complications of the puerperium are uncommon. These are summarized below.

Puerperal infection

Puerperal infection is defined as a rise in temperature to over 38°C for more than 24 hours occurring within the first ten days after childbirth. Such a rise in temperature is usually due either to a womb infection, a urinary infection or mastitis (inflammation of the lactating breast). Very rarely, a fever may result from thromboembolism (see below). Before the advent of hygienic midwifery techniques and antibiotic therapy, puerperal infection of the womb was common, and was a major cause of perinatal maternal mortality.

The treatment of puerperal infection is administration of appropriate antibiotic therapy.

Information box 5.3e-VI

Postnatal fever: comments from a Chinese medicine perspective

In Chinese medicine, the differentiation of postnatal fever depends on the nature of the symptoms. Full conditions include Invasion of Wind Cold or Wind Heat, Blood Stagnation and Food Retention. Blood Deficiency may be the underlying problem in a situation in which there is continuous low-grade fever after childbirth.

Thromboembolism

The problem of excessive blood clotting is a serious, but rare, problem during pregnancy. In fact, thrombosis is more likely to occur during the puerperium and in particular between days 5 and 15 after the birth of the baby. Nevertheless, less than 1 in 1000 births is affected by this complication.

The most usual site for a thrombosis to occur is in the deep veins of the leg (DVT). In 1 in 6000 births a pulmonary embolus results from a DVT. This has a one in five mortality rate.

Information box 5.3e-VII

Puerperal thromboembolism: comments from a Chinese medicine perspective

Thromboembolism represents Blood Stagnation in Chinese medicine. In the puerperium, Stagnation is most likely to result from an underlying severe Deficiency of Blood and Qi following childbirth. Pulmonary embolism is Acute Heart Blood Stagnation, which, if severe, may progress to Collapse of Yang.

Psychiatric complications of the puerperium

The two serious psychiatric complications of the puerperium are postnatal depression and postnatal psychosis.

POSTNATAL DEPRESSION

The brief period of low mood known as the "baby blues," first described as an aspect of normal puerperium in Section 5.3d, affects up to two-thirds of women on days 3–5 after birth. However, in up to 10 percent of women a more severe form of depression can be diagnosed during the postnatal period. This is termed postnatal depression.

Postnatal depression is recognized to be more common in certain groups of women. Risk factors include:

- young age at the time of the birth (<16)

- personal or family history of depression

- poor experience of childrearing during childhood

- lack of positive support from husband or partner

- lack of supportive network of family or friends after the birth

- complications during pregnancy or childbirth.

In recent years there has been increased awareness of the possibility of postnatal depression amongst physicians and midwives. Women may be asked specific questions during the 6–8 week postnatal check, the answers to which might point to a depressed state. It is believed that the best form of treatment is practical support rather than medication. In severe cases, medication or even admission to a psychiatric hospital may be necessary. Even with hospital admission, the current practice is to aim to ensure that the mother and baby are not separated. If possible, the mother is admitted to a dedicated mother and baby unit.

Information box 5.3e-VIII

Postnatal depression: comments from a Chinese medicine perspective

In Chinese medicine, postnatal depression is primarily attributed to Deficiency of Blood and the effect this has on the Heart Organ. The main patterns that can underlie postnatal depression include Heart Blood Deficiency, Heart Yin Deficiency and Heart Blood Stagnation.

POSTNATAL PSYCHOSIS

Psychosis is defined as a mental health disorder in which the patient loses contact with reality. It is considered to be a severe mental health condition, and is usually managed by means of a combination of hospital admission and medication with major tranquillizer drugs.

Postnatal psychosis affects 1–3 in 1000 women in the few weeks following delivery. The condition is often indistinguishable from an episode of bipolar disorder or schizophrenia. Initial symptoms include confusion, depression and anxiety. Delusions and hallucinations, often concerning the baby, are characteristic. There is a grave risk of neglect of the baby and of suicide in the mother.

Treatment usually involves hospital admission, ideally to a psychiatric mother and baby unit, where major tranquillizer medication is given. In most cases, the condition settles within weeks and the medication can be withdrawn. However, there is a significant risk that the problem will recur, either in a subsequent pregnancy, or in the form of a more chronic major mental illness. Approximately one-third of women who develop postnatal psychosis will have a recurrent form of psychosis at a later date.

Information box 5.3e-IX

Postnatal psychosis: comments from a Chinese medicine perspective

In Chinese medicine, psychosis can be attributed to Heart or Liver Blood Stagnation or to Phlegm Fire Harassing the Heart. Underlying imbalances that may contribute to the development of psychosis include Heart and Liver Blood Deficiency with Qi Stagnation, as these can predispose to Blood Stagnation. Spleen Qi Deficiency may contribute to the development of Phlegm.

The red flags of the disorders of the puerperium

Acupuncturists should not need to be familiar with the red flags of childbirth, as a trained midwife or doctor should be present to oversee the safety of a woman in labor. However, acupuncturists do need to be able to recognize the red flags of the disorders of the puerperium.

Some women suffering from disorders of the puerperium will benefit from referral to a conventional doctor for assessment or treatment. Red flags are those symptoms and signs that indicate that referral should be considered. The red flags of the disorders of the puerperium are described in Table 5.3e-I. A summary of the red flags in a format designed for quick reference in clinical practice can be found in Appendix III. This gives advice on the degree of urgency of referral for each of the red flag conditions listed.

Table 5.3e-I A38: Red flags of the disorders of the puerperium (the eight weeks that follow delivery)

Red flag	Description	Reasoning
A38.1	Fever in the puerperium	Refer any case of fever developing in the first two weeks of the puerperium (temperature >38°C for >24 hours) to exclude possible uterine infection
A38.2	Postpartum hemorrhage (PPH): refer if bleeding is any more than a blood-stained discharge	Blood-stained discharge (lochia) is normal in the early puerperium, but moderate to severe bleeding (like a heavy period or heavier) is not, and needs to be referred as it can herald a more serious bleed A profuse bleed of >500ml or the symptoms of shock (see A19.3) constitute an emergency
A38.3	Thromboembolism: pain in the calf, discolored or swollen leg, or breathlessness, with chest pain or blood in the sputum in the puerperium	Refer any features of a thromboembolic event, i.e. deep venous thrombosis (DVT) of the calf or pelvic veins (see A11.7), pulmonary embolus (see A17.10) or stroke (see A22.3) as an emergency The risks of these events are greater in the puerperium
A38.4	Postnatal depression	Refer any case of depression developing in the postnatal period, lasting for >3 weeks and not responding to treatment Refer straight away if the woman is experiencing suicidal ideas, or if you believe the health of the baby is at risk
A38.5	Postnatal psychosis	Refer straight away if you suspect the development of postnatal psychosis (delusional or paranoid ideas and hallucinations are key features), as this condition is associated with a high risk of suicide or harm to the baby
A38.6	Insufficient breast milk	Refer if the mother is considering stopping breastfeeding within the first few months after delivery because of apparently insufficient milk production. In the case of poor latching on of the baby, advice from an expert breastfeeding adviser, midwife or health visitor will often remedy the problem
A38.7	Sore nipples/blocked ducts during the time of breastfeeding	Refer to the midwife (early days) or health visitor for advice on breastfeeding technique and for treatment of possible thrush infection. Encourage the mother to keep feeding despite the discomfort, as a continued flow of milk can help with healing
A38.8	Mastitis during the time of breastfeeding not responding to treatment in two days	Refer if not responding to treatment within two days, or if you suspect the development of an abscess (a firm mass is felt in the affected breast, and the mother feels very unwell). Encourage the mother to keep feeding despite the discomfort, as a continued flow of milk can help with the healing

5.3f Lactation and disorders of the breast

This concluding section summarizes the normal physiology of the breast, and the disorders that can affect the breast. Although the principal function of the breast is to provide milk in the process termed lactation, for most of a woman's life the breast is not performing this role. Nevertheless, the quiescent breast tissue is vulnerable to a range of important medical conditions. It must not be forgotten that men also have a small amount of breast tissue, which can give rise

to some of the breast diseases that are more commonly recognized in women.

Usually, in conventional practice, disorders of the breast are referred not to an obstetrician but to a consultant surgeon. Problems with breastfeeding are usually overseen by the woman's GP and the midwife.

The important disorders of the breast described in this section are:

- The disorders of lactation:
  - poor milk supply
  - sore and cracked nipples

- blocked ducts and mastitis

- overflowing milk

• The disorders of the non-lactating breast:

- benign breast disease

- benign tumors of the breast

- breast cancer

- gynecomastia.

The physiology of the breast and lactation[54]

The breast is also known as the mammary gland. It is composed of numerous exocrine glands, called lobules, as illustrated in Figure 5.3f-I.

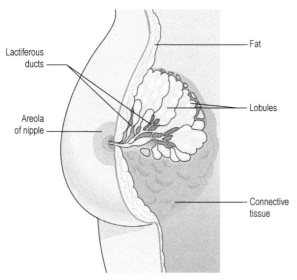

Figure 5.3f-I The structure of the breast

Estrogen and progesterone are important for the development of the breast tissue from puberty onwards. Estrogen is the hormone that is released from the developing ovarian follicle in the first half of the menstrual cycle, and progesterone is released from the corpus luteum in the second half of the menstrual cycle. It is probable that it is an imbalance in the level of progesterone that is responsible for the engorgement of breasts, which is such a common feature of the premenstrual phase of the cycle.

In pregnancy, estrogen and progesterone produced in both the ovary and the placenta are responsible for enlargement of the breast tissue and fat deposition around the breast. The lobules of the breast produce milk in response to prolactin (PRL), which is secreted by the pituitary gland. The milk produced in each lobule reaches the nipple by passing first through a lactiferous sinus and then a lactiferous duct. All the ducts converge at the nipple,

from where the milk will be ejected through tiny openings. The lobules are supported and protected by fatty tissue.

After childbirth, the stimulus of suckling causes release of both PRL and oxytocin from the pituitary. PRL continues to stimulate the production of milk in the lobules. Oxytocin stimulates a muscular contraction of the lining of the lactiferous sinuses, so causing a fine jet of milk to be released from the nipple (this is known as the let-down reflex).

Lactation ideally should begin within minutes of delivery of the baby. A newborn will reflexively search for a nipple when its cheek is stroked, and will then latch on to the nipple once it is found.

Once the baby has the nipple correctly inserted in its mouth, the pinching of its jaw will stimulate the let-down of milk, via the release of oxytocin. Directly after delivery, the first milk produced is a thin, watery fluid known as colostrum. This has some nutritional value, in particular being rich in vitamin K, and also contains maternal antibodies. Despite the production of PRL, the production of milk is inhibited during the latter part of pregnancy by estrogen from the placenta. As the levels of estrogen drop after delivery, and as the nipple is stimulated by the suckling baby, milk begins to be formed. This can lead to a sudden and tender engorgement of the breasts approximately two to three days after delivery. At this point the milk is said to have "come in." The discomfort is relieved by feeding the baby, and this is a clear incentive to continue feeding.

The production of milk draws on water and nutrients from the mother's blood. Breast milk is known to contain all the nutrients required to sustain a growing baby for the first six months of its life. It also contains antibodies from the mother, which continue to protect the newborn from disease, including gastroenteritis. The mother's reserves of glucose, calcium, iron and fat are drawn on in particular to supply the baby's needs. Therefore, a breastfeeding mother will need to ensure that her diet is rich in nutritious high-energy foods and calcium. It is well recognized that nutritional deficiencies manifesting in weak teeth, a reduction in bone density, anemia, thinning of hair and weight loss can affect a woman who is breastfeeding. Many women who are breastfeeding a baby of more than a couple of months of age will describe feeling drained after feeding.

The World Health Organization (WHO) now recommends that most babies should be exclusively breastfed for the first four months and ideally for six months, either before introducing formula milk or before solids are introduced. This is because breast milk is considered to have a number of advantages over bottle feeding with formula milks and early weaning (supplementation with solid foods). First, breast milk is recognized to be superior nutritionally to formula preparations. This is of particular significance in some developing nations in which the practice of giving over-diluted formula milks is known to be common among poorer communities. Breast milk is also protective against disease because it contains maternal antibodies, and is far less likely to be contaminated with bacteria than milk powder that has been mixed with water. Finally, early weaning with solid food may introduce food materials that are potentially allergenic.

However, it is recognized that although many women attempt breastfeeding after childbirth, by week 6 after the birth less than 60 percent are still breastfeeding. This figure is much lower for women from a low socio-economic class. The reasons for stopping breastfeeding are complex, and include socially driven perceptions of acceptable behavior and also about what is best for the baby. Also, some women are forced to stop feeding because the baby is not getting the nutrition it requires, or because the experience of breastfeeding is very difficult or painful for the mother. Both these problems are largely preventable, and are explored in the next section on the disorders of lactation.

Very few women in the UK will be exclusively breastfeeding by six months after the birth. Even for those who continue to breastfeed, many will have introduced occasional formula feeds and solid food by month 3 or 4. Women choose to supplement breastfeeding partly because it may be more convenient, but also because the baby may appear to be unsatisfied on breast milk alone.

Nevertheless, current medical advice is to avoid the introduction of solid food until the baby is six months old in order to minimize early contact with potential dietary allergens.

If breastfeeding is stopped suddenly, either because of choice, or because of illness in the mother or the baby, the breasts will rapidly become engorged and uncomfortable. This discomfort will settle within a few days as the milk production ceases, and the stored milk is reabsorbed. In cases in which the discomfort is very distressing, the mother may be prescribed a drug that inhibits the release of PRL (bromocriptine), although there is currently debate about its efficacy.

Breastfeeding is not always the best or safest option. Certain infections and drugs can be transmitted to the baby via the breast milk. In particular, HIV is known to be transmitted through the breast milk – 25 percent of HIV-negative babies who are breastfed by an HIV-positive mother will become HIV-positive. Recreational drugs such as nicotine, alcohol and cannabis pass readily into the breast milk. These may cause long-term developmental delay if the baby is exposed to these over a long period. Also, certain medications can pass into breast milk, and potentially harm the baby. If these drugs are considered necessary, the mother may be obliged to stop breastfeeding.

Information box 5.3f-I

The breast and lactation: comments from a Chinese medicine perspective

In Chinese medicine, the Organs that have particular significance in breast diseases are the Stomach and the Liver. The Liver, in particular, is believed to control the nipple. A combination of Deficient Stomach Qi and Stagnant Liver Qi is at the root of many breast disorders. Breast milk is dependent on Blood for its formation and on healthy Qi for a smooth flow from the lobule to the nipple. Deficiency of Blood and Qi and Liver Qi Stagnation can lead to problems in lactation.

The disorders of lactation

Poor milk supply

A baby who is not getting sufficient breast milk will, in general, be miserable, unsatisfied after feeding, and fail to gain weight as might be expected. If a baby is not contented at the breast, the mother may be too quick to assume that she has a poor supply of milk. A common consequence of this misconception is that she gives up breastfeeding and replaces breast milk with formula milk feeds.

However, a true inability to produce sufficient milk is considered only very rarely to be the underlying cause of an unsatisfied baby. Instead, most cases of problems with feeding are due to a failure in stimulation of the let-down reflex. In these cases, the milk flow can be encouraged to improve with advice about correct latching on of the baby to the breast. This is because the baby needs to have a large portion of the nipple in its mouth to stimulate an adequate release of oxytocin, and this correct positioning may not always be obvious to a new mother. It is also known that stress and cold inhibits the flow of oxytocin (this is also the case during childbirth). The mother should be encouraged to breastfeed in a calm and warm setting, and be reminded that holding fears about failure may actually make the milk flow slow down.

Occasionally, the baby never adequately manages to stimulate the let-down reflex. Although milk can be expressed by means of a manual pump, the baby remains unable to obtain the milk it requires by suckling. This is more likely to occur when the baby has a coexisting developmental disorder such as cerebral palsy. In this sort of case, the use of a manual or electric pump may be a helpful short-term method for obtaining milk for the baby, but may prove too difficult and time-consuming an approach to maintain in the long term.

If the mother is very run down, stressed or chronically ill, the milk may indeed be in short supply, because her body has a need, in a stressful or depleted situation, to hold on to its nutritional reserves. In such a case the breasts would not feel engorged. In this sort of situation, it may be for the best that the baby is fed largely on formula milk, to allow the mother to regain health.

 Information box 5.3f-II

Poor milk supply: comments from a Chinese medicine perspective

In Chinese medicine, poor milk supply due to maternal depletion corresponds to Blood and Qi Deficiency. Liver Qi Stagnation can also be contributory. In this case the breasts will feel slightly distended and uncomfortable.

Sore and cracked nipples

Sore and cracked nipples are a very common complaint early in the experience of breastfeeding. The problem is attributed to poor positioning of the baby at the breast such that the nipple is only partly inserted into the baby's mouth. It may also be the result of a particularly vigorous sucking action. The pain from sore nipples can be so severe as to prevent feeding. Treatment includes the use of soothing creams and a plastic shield placed around the nipple during feeding. These treatments do not always provide satisfactory relief from the problem.

 Information box 5.3f-III

Sore nipples: comments from a Chinese medicine perspective

In Chinese medicine, sore nipples are a manifestation of local Stagnation of Qi with Generation of Heat as a result of physical trauma. The Blood Deficiency that leads to dry skin, and in particular, of the Liver, may predispose to sore nipples.

Blocked ducts and mastitis

The lactiferous ducts can easily become blocked if the production of milk in the lobules exceeds the demand made by the baby. As milk lies stagnant in the lactiferous sinuses and ducts, it can solidify. Then, a backlog of milk can build up behind the blockage, leading to pain and inflammation in the region of the lobule. A blocked duct will lead to an acutely tender, localized area in the breast, which feels warm to the touch. The skin overlying the area

may appear red. A firm lump is felt in the region of the most tenderness. The treatment of a blocked duct is to encourage the baby to breastfeed as much as possible. This alone can resolve the problem. Alternatively, the mother can sit in a hot bath and massage the breasts towards the nipple. This also can encourage the flow of milk, and may even result in the extrusion of a fine worm-like cast of clotted milk as the blockage is relieved.

If not treated with speed, a blocked duct can rapidly lead to a very painful enlarging area of inflammation of the breast tissue. This condition is called mastitis. The more painful the breast becomes, the more difficult it is for the mother to bear either to continue feeding from the affected breast or to massage the breast. In severe mastitis, the breast is visibly swollen and the skin is tense, red and shiny. The mother can develop a high fever and feel very unwell.

Mastitis may also be caused by bacteria entering the breast tissue from the nipple. Infectious mastitis classically occurs at the end of the first week of breastfeeding. Occasionally, this can lead to a collection of pus in the affected breast, known as a breast abscess.

Mastitis is more likely to develop if the mother is tired or dehydrated. Also, a disturbance in the natural routine of feeding, such as might affect a working mother, can trigger an attack.

In all cases of mastitis the mother should be encouraged to breastfeed. In some cases the treatment as described for blocked ducts, together with bed rest, painkillers and plenty of fluids, may be sufficient to allow the condition to resolve. The conventional treatment usually includes a course of antibiotics (flucloxacillin is often given because it is believed to be harmless to the breastfeeding baby). If a breast abscess has developed, it is considered best that this is drained by means of a minor surgical procedure.

 Information box 5.3f-IV

Blocked ducts and mastitis: comments from a Chinese medicine perspective

In Chinese medicine, blocked ducts and mastitis are usually thought to correspond to Liver Qi and Blood Stagnation and the development of Full Heat. The pathology of severe mastitis and breast abscess is described as Heat and Toxic Heat affecting the Liver, Stomach and Gallbladder Channels.

Overflowing milk

Some women appear to produce milk in abundance. The milk flows not only during breastfeeding, but also at other times of the day. In particular, it may be triggered by the thought or sound of the baby, an indication that these emotional responses are also stimuli for the release of oxytocin. Overflowing milk can be very inconvenient, as the woman needs to wear pads over the nipple to prevent leakage, and may need to change her clothes frequently.

From a conventional perspective, overflowing milk is not seen as a problem. Women with excessive milk production may be encouraged to express the milk by means of a manual pump, so that it can be donated for use in special care baby units.

Information box 5.3f-V

Overflowing milk: comments from a Chinese medicine perspective

In Chinese medicine, overflowing milk is not a sign of health. In contrast, it may either be an indication of the failure of Qi to hold fluids or a result of Liver fire agitating the breast milk. The underlying imbalances are Spleen and Stomach Qi Deficiency, and Stagnation of Liver Qi, respectively.

The disorders of the non-lactating breast

Benign breast disease (lumpy breasts)

Breast tissue in a non-lactating woman undergoes a cyclical change corresponding to the consecutive peaks of estrogen and progesterone in the first and second halves of the menstrual cycle, respectively. It is normal for the breast to enlarge slightly under the influence of progesterone in the second half of the menstrual cycle. In some women, in particular in those over 30, this enlargement in the second half of the cycle is excessive. It has been suggested that this problem may be a result of an imbalance between the amount of estrogen and progesterone circulating in the second half of the cycle.

In benign breast disease, the woman experiences uncomfortable swelling of the breasts in the premenstrual phase, and in some the breasts can feel lumpy, particularly in the outer parts of the breast tissue. Sometimes the lumpiness is confined to one portion of the breast, so giving rise to a concern that the lump represents cancer. However, the fact that the lumps become enlarged and tender premenstrually is an encouraging sign that these changes are benign, and result from fluctuations in the sex hormones.

It is recognized that benign breast disease may have an emotional component. Sometimes another functional condition, such as irritable bowel syndrome, unexplained pelvic pain and premenstrual syndrome, may coexist with benign breast disease.

On examination, a tender irregular lump may be found, or there may be a general feeling of firm irregularity, with the breasts tender all over. If there is concern about the nature of the lumpiness, a sample of breast tissue cells may be withdrawn from the lumpy area by means of a fine needle and syringe (fine needle biopsy). In some cases clear or blood-stained fluid can be withdrawn from the area, indicating the formation of benign cysts. Although withdrawal of the fluid may bring about temporary relief of the problem, the cysts often refill with fluid over the next few weeks. This test is usually combined with a simple ultrasound scan of the lumpy area. If no evidence of cancer is found, the woman is reassured that the problem is common and related to hormonal changes.

Advice includes wearing a well-fitting bra, and reducing fat and caffeine in the diet. Some women are helped by vitamin B6 (pyridoxine) supplements and evening primrose oil (gamolenic acid). However, medical studies have suggested that these approaches have no benefit when compared to placebo treatments.

If the symptoms are very severe, drugs that suppress the release of follicle-stimulating hormone (FSH) may be prescribed (danazol or gestrinone). These drugs have a range of side effects resulting from a drop in the levels of estrogen and an increase in levels of testosterone, the male sex hormone. Alternatively, some women may be prescribed a synthetic preparation of progesterone in the second half of the cycle, as one theory is that the problem is due to a relative deficiency of progesterone.

Information box 5.3f-VI

Benign breast disease: comments from a Chinese medicine perspective

In Chinese medicine, benign breast disease is primarily a result of Stagnation of Liver Qi. This might explain how functional conditions such as irritable bowel syndrome and premenstrual syndrome can coexist with benign breast disease. If the discomfort is severe, this may reflect Blood Stagnation. Lumpiness and cyst formation might indicate the Accumulation of Phlegm.

Although hormonally related breast disease is benign, it is now believed that women who suffer from certain subtypes have a slightly increased risk of breast cancer. For this reason, a patient with this condition may be advised to have a regular mammogram examination from the age of 40.

Benign tumors of the breast

The finding of a painless, smooth and mobile lump in the breast in a relatively young woman (often this occurs in women less than 30 years old) is indicative of a benign tumor called a fibroadenoma. Sometimes the lump is extremely mobile, and may slip from under the examining fingers. For this reason it has also been described as a breast mouse. There is no link between this condition and the future development of cancer. Nevertheless, if a breast mouse is found, the woman is often advised to have it removed surgically. Removal of a breast mouse is a relatively minor operation.

Information box 5.3f-VII

Fibroadenoma of the breast (breast mouse): comments from a Chinese medicine perspective

In Chinese medicine, the development of a painless breast mouse is indicative of an accumulation of Phlegm. There may be an underlying Deficiency of Stomach and Spleen Qi and Liver Qi Stagnation that has led to Accumulation of Phlegm.

Breast cancer

Breast cancer used to be the most common form of cancer in women, although it has now been overtaken by lung cancer as a result of the increase in the incidence of smoking in women. Breast cancer affects 1 in 14 women, usually after the onset of the menopause. The cause of breast cancer is unclear, although it is recognized that it is more common in women of higher socio-economic classes, and in those who choose to have their families late in life. These factors may not be unrelated. Childbearing before the age of 30, which is more common in women from lower socio-economic classes, appears to be protective.

The risk of breast cancer is increased if there is a family history of breast cancer. In particular, one rare but particularly aggressive form of breast cancer is recognized to affect over 80 percent of first-degree female relatives. This form of cancer has been associated with a mutation in genes called BRCA1 and BRCA2, for which genetic tests are available.

It is also recognized that long-term use of the oral contraceptive pill is associated with a slightly increased risk of breast cancer, although this risk is usually not considered to be great enough to outweigh the perceived benefits of the use of the pill. Hormone replacement therapy (HRT) is also known to confer an extra risk of breast cancer.

If breast cancer is diagnosed early in its development, before any signs of spread to the axillary lymph nodes, it may be treated by a combination of surgery and radiotherapy. The aggressive approach of total breast removal, known as mastectomy, has now been found to be no more effective than simple removal of the tumor in early cancers. After surgery, adjuvant radiotherapy is directed at

the armpit, with the aim of eliminating any tiny metastases that may have formed in the lymph nodes.

If the tumor is small, but one or more of the lymph nodes is found to contain cancer cells, long-term survival is increased if the woman undergoes additional adjuvant treatment immediately after surgery. Chemotherapy, long-term treatment with anti-estrogen drugs such as tamoxifen and anastrozole, and, in premenopausal women, removal of the ovaries, are all forms of adjuvant therapy that have been demonstrated to have similar benefits in node-positive breast cancer. The choice of adjuvant therapy depends partly on whether or not the examining pathologist has classified the tumor as one that may grow in response to estrogen.

If the tumor spreads outside the breast tissue to involve either the subcutaneous tissue and skin or the underlying pectoralis muscle, it is described as advanced. In an advanced cancer there may be obvious distortion of the breast contour, or puckering and a color change of the skin over the lump. If the breast cancer is advanced, total breast removal, together with excision of the axillary nodes (radical mastectomy), is necessary. Adjuvant therapy is also used in advanced cases.

Breast cancer tends to metastasize most commonly to the bones, the brain and the liver. There is little hope of total remission once secondary spread has occurred.

An increasing number of genetically engineered antibodies are available that target and cause the destruction of the protein growth factors produced by tumors. These include trastuzumab (Herceptin), which was designed to counteract a growth factor known as Her2. Her2 plays a role in the maintenance of metastatic breast cancer, and so trastuzumab may be prescribed to control the symptoms of metastatic disease.

Survival after a diagnosis of breast cancer depends on the age of the woman and the stage of progression of the tumor at diagnosis. As a general rule, a breast cancer diagnosed before age 40 is more likely to be aggressive than one that is diagnosed after the menopause. Nevertheless, there is a possibility of prolonged remission if the tumor is diagnosed at a very early stage, whatever the age of the woman.

For this reason, early detection of breast cancer is considered to be very important. Public health campaigns focus on teaching women to examine their breasts, and to report any unusual changes quickly. Also, a program of X-ray imaging of the breasts (mammography) encourages women to undergo annual screening after the age of 40–50 (50 in the UK). If any abnormal changes are seen on the X-ray images, the woman is called for further tests, which may include a fine needle biopsy of the suspicious area.

A mammography is associated with the same problems as the cervical screening test, in that a worrying mammogram may not necessarily indicate a true cancer. After further tests the woman can sometimes be reassured that there is no sign of cancer. The mammogram is less helpful in younger women, as X-ray images of young breast tissue are much more difficult to interpret, which is why it is not usually preformed in women less than 45 years of age.

Information box 5.3f-VIII

Breast cancer: comments from a Chinese medicine perspective

In Chinese medicine, as with all cancers, breast cancer is an indication of Phlegm or Blood Stagnation on the background of underlying Deficiency of Yin or Yang. In particular, imbalance of the Stomach, Spleen, Liver and Kidney Organs might be expected to be contributory. Moreover Liver Qi Stagnation combined with Stagnant Heart and Lung Qi, all from emotional upset, can lead to impaired Qi circulation in the breast region and eventually Blood Stagnation and Phlegm. Poor diet and obesity are associated with Damp formation that will be contributory in the formation of Phlegm.

Lahans (2007) explains that deficiency in the lower aspects of the Chong and Ren meridians from Kidney Yang or Yin Deficiency may contribute to Stagnation and Fire in their upper portions and the development of Toxic Fire Poison. She states this is more likely after the menopause when the natural method for expulsion of toxins from these channels has been lost, and also in those who do not exercise.[55]

Gynecomastia

Gynecomastia is the medical term used to describe the development of breast tissue in men. It is a very common finding in pubescent boys, in up to 50 percent of whom a small amount of breast tissue may appear under one or both nipples. In most cases this tissue growth is not very visible, and will subside within a few months. If persistent, and a cause of embarrassment, it can be removed by means of a minor surgical procedure.

Gynecomastia developing in men has a wide range of recognized causes, including a response to certain prescribed medications and recreational drugs, in which case it is not serious. However, if it develops after puberty it should be taken seriously, as it can be a consequence of a hormone-secreting tumor or rarely it might indicate primary breast cancer. Once a significant amount of breast tissue has developed, it will not regress, and may need to be removed surgically.

Information box 5.3f-IX

Gynecomastia: comments from a Chinese medicine perspective

In Chinese medicine, the development of a painless lump in the region of the nipple in men would suggest accumulation of Phlegm consequent on an underlying imbalance in the Stomach, Spleen or Liver Organs.

The red flags of the disorders of the breast

Some patients with structural disorders of the breast will benefit from referral to a conventional doctor for assessment and/or treatment. Red flags are those symptoms and signs that indicate that referral should be considered. The red flags of the disorders of the breast are described in Table 5.3f-I. A summary of the red flags in a format designed for quick reference in clinical practice can be found in Appendix III. This gives advice on the degree of urgency of referral for each of the red flag conditions listed.

Table 5.3f-I A39: Red flags of the disorders of the breast

Red flag	Description	Reasoning
A39.1	Insufficient breast milk when breastfeeding	Refer if the mother is considering stopping breastfeeding within the first few months after delivery because of apparently insufficient milk production. In the case of poor latching on of the baby, advice from an expert breastfeeding adviser or midwife will often remedy the problem
A39.2	Lactation/nipple discharge but not breastfeeding	The production of milk or nipple discharge in someone who is not breastfeeding or during late pregnancy may be a sign of a pituitary disorder or breast cancer, and investigation is merited (see A33.5) However, in most cases inappropriate secretion of milk has a benign cause, or may be the response to medications such as the contraceptive pill
A39.3	Sore nipples/blocked ducts during the time of breastfeeding	Refer to the midwife for advice on breastfeeding technique and for treatment of possible thrush infection. Encourage the mother to keep feeding despite the discomfort, as a continued flow of milk can help with healing
A39.4	Mastitis during the time of breastfeeding not responding to treatment in two days	Refer if not responding to treatment within two days, or if you suspect the development of an abscess (a firm mass is felt in the affected breast, and the mother feels very unwell). Encourage the mother to keep feeding despite the discomfort, as a continued flow of milk can help with the healing
A39.5	Inflamed breast tissue but not breastfeeding	Inflammation of a portion of a breast is common in breastfeeding mothers (mastitis), but needs prompt assessment if it occurs in someone who is not lactating, as this may signify inflammation from an underlying tumor
A39.6	Pain in the breast but no inflammation or lump	Tenderness in the breast tissue is common and usually results from periodic premenstrual hormone stimulation. This symptom can be asymmetrical Pain is not a usual symptom of breast cancer, and an anxious patient can be reassured. The patient should be questioned to ensure that the pain is not actually chest pain, because angina can present with pain that may be described as pain in the breast
A39.7	Lump in the breast	When a breast lump is found, skin dimpling and fixity or irregularity of the lump are more sinister signs Tender lumps are more likely to be benign cysts Conventional medical practice in the UK is now to refer all suspicious lumps in the breast for prompt assessment, because it is known that one in ten breast lumps are found to be cancerous. For this reason, all cases of breast lumps should be referred to a general practitioner (GP) for further investigation
A39.8	Breast tissue development in teenage boys and adult men (gynecomastia)	Refer any case of gynecomastia in a teenage boy or adult male. A pubescent boy can be reassured that this problem (if confined to breast-bud development) is a common feature of puberty which should settle down, but refer nevertheless to exclude rare endocrine diseases. Adult men with this condition need investigations to exclude cancerous change and endocrine disorders
A39.9	Eczema of nipple region	A one-sided, crusty, non-healing skin disorder of the nipple may be a form of cancer (Paget's disease). This particularly affects middle-aged women. Refer for investigation

5.4

Children's Health

5.4a Introduction to children's health

Why do children have special health needs?

This last section of Stage 5 is dedicated to the special health needs of children and the disorders that can affect them. That children have particular health needs is reflected in the fact that in conventional medical practice the specialty of pediatrics requires further training over and above that required of a general physician. Although children may be vulnerable to many of the conditions that have already been described in this text, there is a wide range of conditions of childhood that can develop because the physiology and susceptibility of the child are different from that of the adult.

There are, of course, many conditions from which the child is protected because of its youth. These conditions are the chronic adult diseases that result from the cumulative effects of an unhealthy lifestyle and aging. For this reason, a child is usually not vulnerable to some of the most important adult diseases such as coronary heart disease, stroke, adult cancers and the degenerative diseases of old age, such as osteoarthritis and Alzheimer's disease.

Children have special health needs for two overarching reasons: first, the physiology of the child is immature; and second, the child is in a process of rapid growth and development. These factors combine to give a third reason why children need special focus, which is that any illness

becoming apparent in a growing child may cause setbacks in growth and development, which may then have lasting, even lifelong, consequences. These three reasons are now explored in more detail.

The physiology of the child is immature

Immaturity of the immune system in children means that a child may be more susceptible to conditions from which adults are relatively protected. These conditions include certain infections and allergies. Also, a child who is ill is more vulnerable to extreme fever. The small size of a child means that the child is more vulnerable to dehydration when unwell.

The immature nervous system of a child is more likely to be disturbed by fever or trauma, which can result in convulsions, confusion and loss of consciousness.

An immature digestive system is more likely to succumb to conditions such as colic, gastroenteritis and constipation.

Many of the common childhood cancers develop from the immature blast cells, which are present in developing tissue in a small child, damage to which may have even been sustained in the womb. Blast cells are the rapidly dividing fetal progenitors of adult cells.

The physical, emotional and mental faculties of a child are immature. This means that they are more vulnerable to extremes of temperature, accidents, physical abuse (non-accidental injury), and emotional and sexual abuse.

Because of the vulnerability that comes from immaturity, children require special protection from any noxious factors that might have the potential to damage their health.

The child is in a process of rapid growth and development

Growth requires a constant supply of adequate nutrients. Nutritional deficiencies in childhood can lead to lasting health problems.

Physical growth and the development of physical, mental and emotional skills also require a complex input of less measurable factors, including love, security, consistency, play, exercise, rest, access to education and a supportive social network. If any of these factors is deficient, the physical, mental and emotional health of the child may suffer, again, with long-term consequences.

Vulnerability to setbacks in growth and development

Any disturbance in health can affect growth and development. A child with a chronic childhood illness may suffer long-term consequences of impaired growth and development as a result of the illness. In particular, the impact of congenital disease can be very significant, as it can affect growth and development from the time of the birth of the child.

What are the special health needs of children?

The health needs of children are those factors that enable a child to remain healthy in the face of its immaturity and state of growth and development. Meeting these health needs is all the more important if the child has been born with a constitutional deficiency resulting from congenital disease and prematurity or if they should later develop a serious illness.

The special health needs of children include a balanced nutritious diet, protection from injury, toxins and extremes of climate, protection from infection, freedom to play and exercise, adequate rest, love, security, consistency of care and access to a social network, access to education and protection from physical, sexual or emotional abuse.

The importance of meeting these health needs at every stage in a child's development cannot be overestimated. It is well recognized that if a child falls behind in growing and developing as might be expected, it is often very difficult for the child to catch up at a later date. Therefore, failure to meet these basic health needs during childhood can have an impact on long-term health and well-being, and so might compromise health in adult life.

The special health needs of children are considered below in detail.

A nutritious diet

Children need an adequate supply of the basic nutrients in their diet to grow and develop healthily. The basic nutrients include protein, carbohydrate, fats, and a wide range of vitamins and minerals. All these nutrients are required to enable the tissues to form at the normal rate. If there are nutritional deficiencies, the child will fail to grow and to develop as would be expected.

Nutritional deficiency can cause problems in physical growth and development, such as the small stature and vulnerability to infection that results from protein-calorie deficiency. The high infant and childhood mortality from infection in developing countries is largely a consequence of protein-calorie deficiency. Those children who have had to subsist on too little food but who do survive to adulthood are likely to be smaller than average, and to continue to be prone to infection and problems of inadequate physical development, such as later difficulties in childbirth.

It is now recognized that the long-term effects of nutritional deficiency begin in the womb. Babies who are assessed as less well nourished at the time of birth are more likely to develop a severe chronic illness such as coronary heart disease in later life.[56]

Individual vitamins and minerals each play a role in the healthy development of the tissues. If there is a specific vitamin or mineral deficiency, this, too, can have a long-term bearing on health. For example, a deficiency of vitamin D in childhood can lead to the condition of rickets. Rickets leads to bony deformities, which are then set for life into the adult skeleton. Vitamin A deficiency leads to weak epithelial tissues and a vulnerability to infection, and is probably one of the most important reversible causes of infant mortality from measles in developing countries. Iron deficiency is now recognized to be common, not only in developing countries, but also in the more affluent Western nations, in which the food given to an infant may be plentiful, but unbalanced in nutrients. Inadequate iron in the diet of infants can have a lasting effect on mental development, leading to learning difficulties in later life.

Certain components of a child's diet may be harmful if given to the child too early or if in excess. The World Health Organization (WHO) recommends that all children should be exclusively breastfed for at least the first four months, and ideally for the first six months, of life.[57] It is increasingly recognized that certain nutrients may be harmful to the immature digestive system of the baby. It is possible that the early introduction of wheat, cows' milk, egg, nut and pulse proteins may induce long-term allergies or food intolerance. It is partly for this reason that late weaning after the sixth month is recommended, and advice is given that babies should avoid cows' milk products if possible for the first year of life. Whole foods are not considered to be so healthy for young babies and children, who may suffer from colic and diarrhea as a result of the excess dietary fiber.

An excess of fat and refined carbohydrate will lead to obesity in children. As well as affecting the ability to play and exercise, obesity in children can lead to a long-term reduction in health and well-being. Obese babies are known to be more likely to grow into obese and inactive adults. Obesity in childhood can lead to social exclusion and being bullied. Obesity is an increasing problem in children of affluent societies, and one that carries significant consequences to health in future life.

Protection from injury, toxins and extremes of climate

Many of the important health problems of childhood are preventable, as long as the child is given adequate physical protection. In affluent countries, childhood accidents, and in particular, head injuries, are the single most important cause of death in those under 14. Many of the accidents that are fatal might have been prevented by the appropriate use of car restraints, cycle helmets, smoke alarms and window locks.

Poisoning is another very common cause of illness and death in children. Contrary to popular belief, the most common poisons to cause harm in children are not wild berries and mushrooms, but those found in the home, such as alcohol, cleaning fluids and prescription medicines. Again, harm would be prevented if these substances were kept out of the reach of children.

A young child is very vulnerable to extremes of heat and cold, and also to radiation from the sun. It is now understood that sudden infant death syndrome (SIDS) can result from allowing a baby to become overheated or too cold. Children are more likely than adults to suffer from fever, dehydration, headache and confusion in very hot weather, a condition described as heat stroke.

A child's skin is vulnerable to burning with very little exposure to the sun's rays. Although the discomfort of sunburn may be temporary, there is a well-established link between the incidence of sunburn in children and the development of skin cancer, including melanoma, in adult life.[58] Sunburn is prevented by protecting the child's skin from direct sunlight by means of wearing long sleeves, sun hats and high-factor, ultraviolet light-blocking sun creams.

Protection from infection

Children can be protected from the serious childhood infections by the time-honored method of separating an infectious child from other children. This might mean ensuring that a child has a few days of convalescence at home during and after an illness. However, this practice is increasingly less prevalent, as the pressures on parents to return to work may oblige them to return their child to school sooner than would be advisable after an infectious illness. In such situations, medications such as paracetamol and ibuprofen are commonly used to enable a child to feel well enough to return to school, although these medications do not cure the underlying illness.

An important medical approach for managing the risk of infection is the practice of childhood vaccination. Children in the UK are currently offered immunizations to protect them against 16 strains of infectious diseases. The timing of the vaccinations in the UK immunization schedule is summarized in Table 2.4d-I.

However, vaccines are not available for many of the important childhood infections. These include the common cold, scarlet fever, tonsillitis, most forms of bronchitis and pneumonia, many forms of meningitis, herpes simplex virus (HSV), most forms of gastroenteritis, conjunctivitis and impetigo. For all these infections, exclusion of the infected child is the most important aspect of the protection of other children.

Freedom to play and exercise

A child needs to be in a stimulating environment from early babyhood. Psychological studies of babies in orphanages who were given little stimulation throughout the day indicate that the mental and physical development of these babies was delayed, despite the fact that the babies appeared contented and well nourished.[59]

If given a safe degree of freedom and stimulating objects, a child will naturally play, and through play will gradually develop physical and mental skills. A child will also naturally want to exercise. This tendency is apparent even in the womb. The routine ultrasound scan performed at 20 weeks of gestation demonstrates a fetus that is flexing its limbs and performing breathing movements. As well as helping to develop skills of balance and coordination, exercise stimulates muscle and bone development. It also aids the proper utilization of food and prevents obesity.

It is clear that children in affluent societies exercise far less than their parents did, and even less than their grandparents did as children. The reasons for this are multiple, and include the increased use of the car, a reduction in allocated time for physical activity in school curricula (many children in the UK are obliged to attend less than half an hour of physical education per week) and the almost universal availability of habit-forming and sedentary methods of entertainment such as television and computer games. The impact that this decline in physical activity in today's children will have is likely to be significant. It is well recognized that children who do not exercise are even less likely to exercise when they become adults.[60] The habit of exercise is apparently one that is most easily formed when young. Lack of activity in childhood may, therefore, contribute to problems such as heart disease, obesity and osteoporosis in adulthood.

Adequate rest

The value of adequate rest for children is emphasized in conventional guides to childcare. Overstimulation and lack of sleep in a child will lead to poor concentration and irritability in the day. It is conventionally recognized that the development of a child can be adversely affected as a result of inadequate rest alone.[61]

Love, security, consistency of care and access to a social network

Although very difficult to measure, it is also known that interpersonal factors, including love, a sense of security, consistency of care and access to a social network, are extremely important in the healthy mental, emotional and physical development of a child. Although it may make sense that the emotional development of a child deprived of one or more of these factors might be adversely affected, it may come as a surprise that mental and physical development can also be impaired by emotional deprivation. The effect of emotional deprivation can be so marked that the term psychosocial short stature has been coined to describe the phenomenon of otherwise unexplained stunted growth in children in whom there is evidence of emotional deprivation.[62] The conventional explanation for this phenomenon is that, through the effect of emotional deprivation on the brain, the release of the hormones that stimulate growth and the development of the brain in children (including growth hormone, the thyroid hormones, insulin and, after puberty, the sex hormones) is inhibited.

Access to education

The definition of what constitutes appropriate education will vary according to the society in which the child grows up. At the very least, education should allow a child to develop skills and the confidence to be able to function as an independent adult in their society. At best, education should also enable a child to develop the skills to continue to learn and develop throughout adult life.

Theories abound about when is the best time to begin to acquire skills such as reading, playing the violin or driving a car. What is generally understood is that there is an optimum time period in the life of a child during which a skill, such as learning to read, can be acquired. It is also believed that most children require a foundation of basic skills before they can progress on to learning more complex skills. For example, for most children reading will follow only after the skill of letter recognition has been mastered. A good educational system, whether it is at school or at home, will enable the child to concentrate on the skills that are most important to develop according to the child's particular stage in development. If the window of opportunity in childhood for learning a particular skill is missed, and reading is a good example, it may be very difficult for the adult ever to acquire the skill with proficiency. A child may miss out on an important stage in educational development because of a long period

of poor health, because of an unstable social setting or because of lack of parental support and encouragement.

Education has a significant impact on health. Not only can it enable the child to develop the skills and confidence to follow a healthy lifestyle as an adult, it also opens the door to a choice of professions. There is now no doubt that there is a strong correlation between professional status (by which the five socio-economic classes are defined) and health. For a wide range of diverse diseases, including most forms of cancer, heart disease, childhood asthma, pneumonia and type 2 diabetes, there is a very striking correlation between the incidence of the disease and socio-economic class (of the child or parent). A person who is classified by profession into a high socio-economic class (e.g. a judge would be classified as Class I) is more likely to enjoy better health and a longer life than someone who is classified by profession into a low socio-economic class. This correlation cannot be completely attributed to differences in lifestyle between people from different socio-economic groups. So it seems that, over and above the advantages an education might offer in terms of learning about healthy living (or possibly the wealth and security that tend to accompany it), it also appears to protect against disease in its own right.[63]

Protection from physical, sexual or emotional abuse

The deleterious effects that any form of abuse may have on a child are obvious. If the abuse is severe or occurs on a long-term basis, the child's growth and development will be affected adversely, probably by a similar mechanism as results from emotional neglect.

Physical abuse is also termed non-accidental injury (NAI). NAI may manifest as bruises, lacerations, cigarette burns or fractures. In some cases, NAI results in wounds or fractures that would be very unlikely to occur by accident (e.g. bruising within the pinna of the ear), and so should alert the examining doctor to the possibility of abuse. Rarely, a child may be deliberately poisoned by his or her parents with alcohol or prescription medicines. Munchausen syndrome by proxy is a very rare syndrome in which the parent or caregiver causes or feigns illness in the child as an indirect form of attention seeking.

Physical neglect is also a form of physical abuse, and may manifest in the child as failure to gain weight, inadequate hygiene with skin infections and infestations, poor speech development and failure to attend health check-ups.

Emotional abuse includes emotional neglect and withdrawal of love, but also malicious criticism, threats and scapegoating. The child may appear withdrawn and may have speech difficulties and other features of developmental delay.

Sexual abuse may result in the features of emotional abuse and also in precocious sexual awareness or behavior in a young child. Both physical and sexual abuse may cause the child to become vigilant and still when close to adults, a response described as "frozen watchfulness." A sexually abused child may present with the symptoms of a sexually transmitted disease, or may fall pregnant. There are some characteristic signs that may be found on examination of the genitalia of a sexually abused child, but the finding of these signs is not always conclusive.

Commonly, two or more of the forms of abuse may coexist. Apart from causing developmental delay, the long-term effects of child abuse on the individual's future relationships and care of future children may be serious and very difficult to remedy. It is recognized that abused children are more likely to abuse others in adulthood. Children who have been victims of sexual abuse are at great risk of suffering from psychiatric disorders and sexual dysfunction in adulthood.

The concept that parents or carers might abuse their children only began to be noted as a possible widespread problem in the 1950s. In recent years there has been an increased awareness that abuse may underlie the health problems of a child, and conventional health professionals are now given specific training in recognizing the warning features of abuse in a child.

If there is good reason to suspect the abuse of a child, a conventional health practitioner in the UK is expected to report the matter to the local children's social care team or to the police if urgent. In the first instance, after a report has been made, an assessment has to be made about the degree of risk. This assessment will involve a social worker interviewing the family and associated professionals such as teachers and medical staff. If the child seems to be at high risk, a decision may be made about whether the child should be separated straight away from the suspected abuser, either by admission to hospital or by placing the child into the care of a foster parent or children's home. Whether or not this is done, a multidisciplinary case conference is convened, which will have representation from a wide range of relevant professionals, including social workers, health visitors, the general practitioner (GP), hospital doctors and nurses, police officers, teachers and lawyers. The evidence relevant to the case will be discussed and a decision will be made about:

- whether to place the child on the Child Protection Register, so that the child continues to remain at home while under the surveillance of health visitors and social services

- whether to apply to the court for long-term protection of the child and prosecution of the possible abuser

- what sort of follow-up is required.

If, as a practitioner of acupuncture, there are any concerns about possible abuse of a child, it is necessary to seek further advice. In the UK it would be appropriate to contact either the NSPCC or local children's social care services[64] for advice. This is an example of a situation when it may be appropriate to breach the professional code of confidentiality.

 Information box 5.4a-I

Children's health: comments from a Chinese medicine perspective

In Chinese medicine, children are recognized as energetically different in nature from adults, and these differences become gradually less marked as the child grows older. Scott and Barlow (1999) expand on the principal differences that are summarized succinctly by seven aphorisms from Chinese medical pediatrics.[65] These are as follows:

"Children's Spleen is often insufficient"

This refers to the fact that the digestive system of a child has to work full time to ensure adequate growth and health of the Organs. For this reason, a young child is particularly vulnerable to digestive disorders. Late weaning and a balanced and regular diet consisting largely of Warm foods are extremely important for the health of the child. Accumulation Disorder (akin to the adult syndrome Retention of Food in the Stomach) and Spleen Qi Deficiency are syndromes very commonly found in young children.

"Children's Yin is often insufficient"

Although the nature of children is very Yang, the Yin is immature. This can result in the tendency to high fevers and dehydration that are characteristic of children. Scott and Barlow (1999)[66] suggest that the reason why Yin Deficiency is not seen more often in Western children is that their Heat symptoms have been treated too readily with antibiotics, which are, by nature, cooling and damaging to the Yang.

"Organs are fragile and soft; Qi easily leaves its path" and "Children easily become ill: their illnesses easily become serious"

These statements both refer to the fact that a slight insult from a Pathogenic Factor (such as the Heat of a hot day, or Damp Heat from over-rich food) can easily disturb the Qi and so cause illness. This can easily progress to a disturbance of the Qi of the whole body, and so lead rapidly to serious illness. Likewise, emotional disturbances can also lead to health imbalances, which can escalate into serious conditions.

"Yin and Yang Organs are clear and spirited. They easily and quickly regain their health"

As a counterpoint to the preceding maxims, despite the vulnerability that arises from immaturity of the organs, the clarity of the Spirit of the child's Organs means that, in many cases, a child can return very rapidly to good health even after a major illness. Also, emotional disturbance in a child is often very short-lived, as long as the stress that has caused the disturbance is not maintained for a long time.

"Liver often has illness"

This statement refers to the tendency of children to succumb to Liver Wind and so to suffer from convulsions. However, health problems that result from Stagnation of Liver Qi are not so prominent in children, presumably because small children in general have not learned the tendency to restrain their emotions.

"Treat the mother to treat the child"

Health and emotional imbalances in the mother may readily be transmitted to the child, and so treatment of the mother may be important in the management of a child health problem. Conversely, a mother may become unwell in response to the health problem of her child, and her condition may only get better when the health of the child starts to improve.

5.4b Assessment of child health and development

Why does the assessment of the health of children require a specialized approach?

The assessment of the health and development of children is different from the assessment in adults, in as much as the physiology of children is different from that of adults. The health of a child can only be assessed properly if there is a prior knowledge of the normal range of physiological variables in a child at that particular stage of development. Therefore, most of this section is concerned with what the acupuncturist can expect to be normal when examining a child at a particular age (stage of development).

Even without a specialized knowledge of how diseases manifest in children, a firm grasp of the normal physiology of childhood development will enable a more ready recognition of those situations when a child is becoming unwell.

This section introduces the main differences between normal children at various stages of development and adults. For the sake of clarity, the differences that might be found in the physical examination of a passive child are considered first. Then, the ways in which a child differs from an adult in terms of the child's interaction with their environment are discussed. These are considered within four domains: motor (movement) skills, language skills, hearing and vision, and social skills.

A child health surveillance program

The health of a child will always be assessed when the child presents to a conventional practitioner with a particular complaint. In addition to these unpredictable points of contact with health practitioners, most children in developed countries are also offered health checks at prescribed stages in their childhood. Considered together, these health checks comprise a program of child health surveillance.

In the UK the child health surveillance program involves health checks that are usually offered at birth, and at 6–8 weeks, 9 months and 18–24 months of age. The professionals who work together to provide this care include the hospital pediatrician, the general practitioner (GP) and the health visitor (a nurse with specialist training in community health issues). For most healthy children, the only point of contact with the hospital pediatrician is likely to be during the routine neonatal examination, which can take place within the first 24 hours after birth in hospital. Thereafter, the health surveillance is overseen by the GP and the health visitor. However, if a child has a serious congenital condition or chronic severe illness, the hospital or community pediatrician will be much more involved in the health surveillance for that child.

During these routine health checks important aspects (indicators) of the physical health of the child are assessed, together with certain indicators of the four domains of how the child is interacting with their environment. During these routine health checks the important aspects (indicators) of the physical health of the child are assessed, together with indicators of the four aforementioned domains of how the child is interacting with their environment.

Developmental milestones

Assessment of the domains of physical health, motor skills, language skills, hearing and vision, and social skills requires an understanding of how a healthy child might be expected to develop within each of these different domains as time goes on. A useful concept in the assessment of children's health over the course of time is that of the developmental milestone.

A developmental milestone is a measurable attribute or skill that is attained during the course of normal development in childhood. The first smile of a baby and the ability to reach out and grasp an object, to sit unaided, to walk and to say single words with meaning are all developmental milestones that are usually attained within the first two years of life.

All children are unique with regard to the precise time and order in which these milestones are attained. For example, a normal healthy child might first walk unaided at any time between 7 and 15 months of age. The age by which half of all children have taken a few steps is 12 months. This is the median age for the milestone. Outside the extremes of 7 and 15 months there may be unusually early or late walkers who nevertheless continue to develop normally. There is no known link between early walking and physical prowess, despite some parents' assumptions to the contrary. However, if a child is not walking by the age of 18 months, there is a significant possibility that this is an early indication of abnormality such as muscular dystrophy. Eighteen months is described as the "limit age" for the developmental milestone of walking unaided. If a child has not achieved a milestone by the limit age for that milestone, the child will be referred for specialist examination to exclude any possible underlying health problems. Median and limit ages for some of the important developmental milestones are listed in Table 5.4b-I.

Table 5.4b-I Median and limit ages for some developmental milestones

Developmental milestone	Median age	Limit age
Responsive smiling	6 weeks	8 weeks
Good eye contact maintained	6 weeks	3 months
Reaches for objects	3–4 months	5 months
Sits unsupported	6 months	10 months
Says single words with meaning	13 months	18 months
Speaks in phrases	24 months	30 months

Physical assessment of the passive child

Height, weight and head circumference

Height, weight and head circumference are measurements that are very commonly used in the assessment of the health of children. In young babies, head circumference and weight are the most frequently assessed health indicators, whereas in older children who are able to stand upright, the assessment of height replaces that of head circumference.

The concept of the normal range was introduced in Section 1.2a. By way of illustration, Figure 1.2a-I shows the normal range of birth weight according to stage of pregnancy. The normal range for a variable, such as weight, is the range of values of that variable into which the large part (usually between 80 and 96 percent for most normal ranges) of the population will fall. When the height, weight or head circumference of a child is measured, the value is compared to charted values that indicate the normal range of that variable in the population. The charts used by health professionals are prepared with such accuracy that the precise position of the child in terms of the variable as compared to the population as a whole can be determined.

For example, a four-year-old boy may be assessed as having a height that is on the 25th centile. This means that he just falls within the shortest quarter (25 percent) of the population. At the same assessment, his weight is found to be on the 33rd centile (meaning that he just falls within the lightest one-third (33 percent) of the population). Both these measurements are within the 94 percent normal range, and so would be considered unremarkable by a health professional. However, if the two measurements indicated that the child was on the 2nd centile for height and weight, this would mean that he is just on the bottom edge of the 94 percent normal range, and just falls within the shortest and lightest 2 percent of the population.

A health professional might then take more time to assess whether or not there might be an underlying health or social issue as a cause of the short stature in that child.

Monitoring variables such as height and weight relative to the normal range over the course of time can be very useful. If a child is seen to "drop in centiles" from, say, the 40th to the 10th centile over the course of time, this might indicate failing health. In this way a possible problem with growth can be detected long before the child can be assessed as falling outside the normal range of growth indicators.

However, problems can arise from repeated measurement of height, weight and head circumference. As is true for all measurements that fall outside a normal range, there remains uncertainty as to whether the measured abnormality is a valid indicator of lack of health. Many health professionals might testify to the anxiety that repeated measurement of a small baby can induce. It is understandable that a mother will be concerned if her baby is assessed as not gaining weight at the same rate as an average baby (as indicated by the weight chart). Even if this is actually a healthy pattern for that child (who is, of course, very unlikely to be an average baby in all respects), the concern may lead to lack of well-being in the mother (which can then be transmitted to the child) or to changes in feeding behavior, such as stopping breastfeeding in favor of formula milk.

For this reason it is important to place an abnormal measured value in context against other measures of health in the child. A contented baby who is well in all other respects is unlikely to have a serious underlying health problem, even if the baby's weight dips below the normal range. Although an abnormal finding must be followed up, every effort should be made to reassure the mother that it need not necessarily indicate that anything is wrong with their child.

Pulse rate

The pulse rate drops gradually over the first few years of life to assume the normal adult rate after the age of 12. The normal ranges for pulse rate in children are given in Table 5.4b-II.

Table 5.4b-II The normal ranges for pulse rate in children

Age (years)	Rate (beats/minute)
<1	110–160
2–5	95–140
5–12	80–120
>12	60–100

Respiratory rate and peak flow rate

Like the pulse rate, the respiratory rate drops as the child gets older. The normal ranges for respiratory rate in children are given in Table 5.4b-III.

Table 5.4b-III The normal ranges for respiratory rate in children

Age	Normal rate (breaths/minute)	Rate if breathless (breaths/minute)
Newborn	30–50	>60
Infant	20–40	>50
Young child	20–30	>40
Older child/ adult	15–20	>30

The peak flow rate is proportional to the height and age of the child, meaning that it increases as the child gets taller and older. The normal range for peak flow rate in children can be determined from the information that will accompany a good quality peak flow meter when purchased.[67]

Heart sounds

The heart sounds of children are routinely assessed in surveillance checks to exclude the possibility of congenital heart disease. When using the stethoscope, the doctor listens for the rushing noise of a heart murmur. A murmur can be a normal finding in very young children, but is unlikely to be normal if found in school-aged children. If there is any concern, the child will be sent for a non-invasive echocardiogram to exclude defects in the structure of the heart.

Mouth, palate and anus

The mouth and palate of the newborn baby are assessed at the neonatal check to exclude hare lip and cleft palate. The anus is examined to exclude the rare condition of imperforate anus.

Abdomen and testes

The abdomen and testes are examined in newborns and children up to the preschool years. The doctor examines the abdomen of newborns to exclude abdominal distension, enlarged liver or spleen, and abdominal masses. In this way conditions such as congenital bowel obstruction and abdominal tumors may be detected. The scrotum is palpated in boys up to the preschool years to check for complete descent of the testes.

Hips

The movements of the hips of newborns and babies up to the age of two are also routinely assessed to exclude the condition of congenital dislocation of the hip.

The skin

Benign birthmarks are common findings in newborn babies. In particular, reddened mottled patches at the nape of the neck or around the eyelids (stork marks), bluish areas of discoloration over the base of the spine and buttocks ("Mongolian" blue spots) and tiny white pimples on the cheeks and nose (milia) are findings that will resolve spontaneously.

The port-wine stain (a clearly demarcated, purplish patch on the face or scalp) and the strawberry nevus (a bright red, rounded lump, often the size of a strawberry) are two fairly common birthmarks that are more persistent. The port-wine stain can be very prominent on the face of a growing child, but can now be treated in later childhood by means of laser therapy. The strawberry nevus tends to increase in size for the first few months of life and then often shrinks down to a negligible size. For this reason treatment is not offered unless it is a cause of physical discomfort in early infancy. Cosmetic surgery can be offered if the nevus is unsightly by the time the child reaches school age.

Tufts of hair, skin lumps or other birthmarks are taken seriously if they are found around the base of the spine, over the spine or on the skull. Rarely, birthmarks in these regions can indicate a mild form of spina bifida known as spina bifida occulta.

General appearance

Finally, in the physical assessment of a passive child, the child's overall physical appearance may indicate to a trained eye that there is an underlying congenital condition or chronic illness. Many of the genetic conditions that manifest in childhood give rise to a characteristic cluster of physical features, which in themselves are diagnostic of the condition, for example, Down syndrome and achondroplasia.

Assessment of movement (motor skills) in a child

A newborn baby should be able to make symmetrical strong movements of all four limbs when lying on its back. If supported by a hand under the abdomen the baby will be unable to hold up its head unsupported, but will not be too floppy (i.e. the baby has good muscle tone). The baby has a strong grip, so much so that it can support its own weight when gripping the index fingers of the examining doctor. When held upright as if standing, a newborn will make reflex stepping moves with its legs. Within six to eight weeks the strong grip and walking reflex are no longer to be found. This is because the strong grip and walking reflex of the newborn are primitive reflexes, which later become overridden by motor nerve impulses from the developing brain.

Some of the major motor developmental milestones are listed in Table 5.4b-IV.

Table 5.4b-IV Some of the major motor developmental milestones

Milestone	Median age
Able to lift head when lying on abdomen	6 weeks
Sits without support	6 months
Can pass objects from one hand to another	6 months
Stands with support	7 months
Pulls to standing	9 months
Has good pincer grip of a small object	10 months
First steps unsupported	12 months
Scribbles with a pencil	14 months
Kicks a ball	20 months
Builds a tower of six cubes	24 months
Hops on one foot	3.5 years
Draws a man of three parts	4 years

Assessment of language skills in a child

A newborn has no language, but does have a characteristic cry, which is a very effective, albeit not very specific, method of achieving contact with its mother. Within the first few months the baby is able to recognize and quieten to the mother's voice. Some of the major developmental milestones of language are listed in Table 5.4b-V.

Table 5.4b-V Some of the major developmental milestones of language

Milestone	Median age
Babbles and says "mama," "dada," "baba," but without meaning	10 months
Can understand simple commands and say one or two words appropriately	13 months
Can combine two different words	20 months
Can say first and last name	3–4 years
Can say the name of colors	3 years
Speech fully comprehensible to strangers	4 years

Speech difficulties in young children have diverse causes. The problem may be seated in difficulties in understanding speech (receptive dysphasia), either because of deafness, a global learning disability, or a specific defect in the way in which the brain processes speech. Alternatively, the actual production of words may be impaired (expressive dysphasia), despite good comprehension. For this reason, the assessment of the root of problems in language development is a complex skill.

Assessment of hearing and vision in a child

A newborn should respond to sound, and will startle or blink in response to sudden noises. It will not show any preference at this stage to particular sounds, such as the mother's voice.

The eyes of a newborn are examined to exclude conditions that are the cause of blindness, including congenital cataract and a rare congenital tumor called retinoblastoma.

As the baby grows, the mother is questioned about whether or not she thinks her child reacts normally to sounds and visual images. The mother's opinion is considered to be an extremely sensitive indicator of whether or not there could be underlying hearing or visual defects.

Hearing is assessed in the newborn by means of objective electronic testing of the inner ear or brain to sounds focused into the baby's ear. This reliable test has in the UK largely replaced routine assessment by the distraction test, which, until recently, was performed by the health visitor on a baby aged six to nine months.

By six to eight weeks of age the eyes of the baby should be moving together (conjugate gaze), with no evidence of independent movement (squint). At every stage of child health surveillance the child should be assessed informally for the presence of a squint. If there is any concern about one eye not moving as far as it should in any direction, the child is referred for a formal diagnosis by an optometrist, because squint requires early treatment to prevent lifelong impairment to binocular vision.

Some of the major developmental milestones of hearing and vision are listed in Table 5.4b-VI.

Table 5.4b-VI Some of the major developmental milestones of hearing and vision

Milestone	Median age
Startles to a sudden noise	at birth
Looks at faces; responds to light	at birth
Stills to a sudden new noise	1 month
Eyes will follow a moving object, and will move together with no squint	6 weeks
Quietens or smiles to mother's voice	4 months
Turns to the sound of mother's voice	7 months
Searches for quiet sounds made out of sight	9 months
Shows response to his own name and some other familiar words	12 months
Can copy a circle	3 years

Assessment of social skills in a child

The developing child will display increasingly complex methods of interacting with the people around the child, and behaving according to expected norms. Even a newborn appears to respond to being picked up in a way that is different to its response to less social stimuli.

The assessment of the social skills domain includes the assessment of those skills, such as self-feeding and self-dressing, which are essential for the child to attain independent existence.

Some of the major milestones in social development are listed in Table 5.4b-VII.

Table 5.4b-VII Some of the major milestones in social development

Milestone	Median age
Smiles responsively	6 weeks
Can put solid food in mouth	6 months
Waves "bye-bye"	8 months
Becomes wary of strangers	8–10 months
Drinks from a cup	12 months
Shows symbolic play with dolls, chair, spoon, etc.	18 months
Can remove a garment	18 months
Feeds self with a spoon	18 months
Asserts own wishes	18 months
Washes hands and brushes teeth with help	3–4 years
Shows sympathy when appropriate	3–4 years
Vivid make-believe play	3–4 years
Will play independently with other children	3–4 years

What happens when a child fails to reach developmental norms?

In general, failure to fit into the normal range for a physical measurement such as weight or pulse rate, or failure to have attained a developmental milestone by its limit age, should be put into the context of the overall well-being of the child. If the child is otherwise well, then, as has been explained regarding weight gain in babies, the mother should be reassured that it is very possible that there is not an underlying health problem. Nevertheless, it is generally good practice to follow up a child who fails an aspect of the child health surveillance program with further tests or a referral for a specialist opinion.

5.4c Congenital disorders

Congenital diseases are those conditions that have existed in a person since birth. There are two broad categories of congenital diseases: genetic diseases and diseases of multifactorial inheritance. Genetic diseases are those that result entirely from a defect in the genetic makeup of the person. In genetic conditions, the defect has either been inherited from the parent or has arisen during the division and maturation of one or both of the gametes. The genetic condition is therefore usually present from the moment of conception, and so will affect the genetic material of every body cell of the child with the condition. Genetic diseases can be diagnosed by testing a sample of body cells for the genetic defect. Very rarely, the genetic defect can arise as a result of an error in the early divisions of the zygote, and so will affect many, but not all, of the cells of the developing baby (this is genetic mosaicism; see later). Genetic diseases can be further divided into two subcategories: those that result from chromosomal abnormalities and those that result from single-gene defects.

In contrast to genetic diseases, there is a broad range of congenital conditions that are described in this section as being of multifactorial inheritance. These conditions may have an underlying genetic susceptibility at their root, but can also result from a range of external factors that have in some way damaged the embryo or fetus during the time of its development in the womb, or during the time of labor. In these conditions, the genetic material in the cells of the body will appear to be grossly normal, and genetic testing is not usually helpful in the diagnosis of the condition, except that it may reveal an underlying susceptibility to the condition in some cases.

The most common congenital disorders are described in this section. It is beyond the scope of the text to go into detail about the features and management of all these conditions, many of which are very rare. The aim of this section is to illustrate the breadth of the range of congenital conditions, and the complex ways in which they can arise.

The problems that arise from prematurity are also described in this section. Although a preterm baby may be entirely healthy for its stage of development, the fact that it has been born before the ideal time for delivery means that it inherits at birth a number of particular health problems which, according to the definition above, are in themselves a form of congenital disease.

This section is divided into three, which you are advised to study in separate sessions. The conditions discussed in this section are:

Part I: Genetic conditions

- Chromosomal abnormalities:
  - Down syndrome
  - Turner syndrome
  - Klinefelter syndrome
  - fragile X syndrome
- Single-gene defects:
  - cystic fibrosis
  - sickle cell disease and thalassemia
  - phenylketonuria (PKU)
  - albinism
  - color blindness
  - muscular dystrophy (MD)
  - hemophilia
  - achondroplasia
  - osteogenesis imperfecta
  - familial hyperlipedemias

Part II: Conditions of multifactorial inheritance

- congenital heart disease
- hare lip and cleft palate
- esophageal atresia
- pyloric stenosis
- imperforate anus
- congenital liver disease and neonatal jaundice
- club foot (talipes equinovarus)
- congenital dislocation of the hip
- maldescent of the testes
- congenital hernia

- congenital blindness

- congenital deafness

- neural tube defects

- cerebral palsy

- congenital hypothyroidism

- inherited tendency to developing adult diseases

Part III: The premature (preterm) baby

- infant respiratory distress syndrome (IRDS)

- irregularities of breathing and heart rate

- temperature control

- problems with nutrition

- retinal damage

- brain damage

- jaundice

- problems after discharge from hospital.

These three parts are followed by a section on screening for congenital disease, which covers the following:

- the role of genetic counseling

- genetic screening of parents

- antenatal testing for genetic disease

- presymptomatic testing of children.

Part I: Genetic conditions

Chromosomal abnormalities

As first described in Section 1.1b, the genetic material in the human is found within the nucleus of almost all the cells of the body (the red cells and platelets are exceptions to this rule, as they lose their nucleus at a late stage in their development in the bone marrow). During the process of replication of body cells, known as mitosis, the nuclear material condenses into 23 pairs of elongated bodies known as chromosomes (see Figure 1.1b-VI). There are a total of 22 non-sex chromosomes (autosomes) and one pair of sex chromosomes (XX or XY), which make up the total complement of the non-dividing human cell. The autosomes are described by a number, from 1 to 22, and the sex chromosomes by the letters X and Y. Each chromosome consists of coiled and densely packed strands of DNA (deoxyribonucleic acid). Each DNA strand is made up of chains of separate genes, which are tiny sections of DNA that direct the formation of the millions of proteins that make up the human body. Together, these strands of DNA make up what is now termed the human genome.

The different genes that make up the human genome have now been mapped, and can be located to particular chromosome pairs. The function of many of these genes is now understood. For example, the gene that codes for part of the protein that forms hemoglobin is located on chromosome pair 11, and the gene that codes for the clotting factor that is deficient in hemophilia A is located on the X sex chromosome. As the chromosomes are in matching pairs, with the exception of those genes on the sex chromosomes, each gene is doubly represented within the nucleus.

A chromosomal abnormality is a structural problem affecting one (or more) of these 23 pairs of strands of DNA. Because a chromosomal abnormality is likely to affect a large number of the thousands of genes represented on the DNA of the chromosome, the diseases that result commonly involve multiple structural abnormalities and learning difficulties. Over 100 diseases arising from chromosomal defects have now been documented.

A chromosomal defect usually arises as a result of an error in meiosis, the process by which gametes are formed from the germ cells in the ovary or testis. In this case, the chromosomes of the parents are normal. More rarely, the defect is present in the chromosomes of one of the parents, albeit not in a form that would manifest in severe disease. In this more rare circumstance, the defect can be passed down directly to the child, and occasionally in a form that results in severe abnormalities of development of that child. In both cases the chromosomal defect may be in the form of an absent chromosome or an absent section of a chromosome (a deletion), or may involve the presence of an extra chromosome (a trisomy).

Rarely, a chromosomal defect develops after conception, during one of the first mitotic divisions of the zygote. This results in a baby who has some normal cells and some cells that carry the defect. This phenomenon is known as mosaicism, and often results in a condition that is a less severe form of the disease that would have arisen if all the cells had been affected.

Because chromosomal defects are often apparent simply from a study of the shape of the chromosomes (which can be seen using a simple microscope), these were the first form of genetic disease to be understood and described as such. The first three chromosomal abnormalities to be described included Down syndrome. The chromosomal defect of Down syndrome (trisomy 21) was first described in 1959, only three years after the normal chromosomal complement was first described.

DOWN SYNDROME (TRISOMY 21)

Down syndrome was first described by Dr J.L.H. Down in 1866, but was ascribed to a chromosomal defect just less than a century later. The syndrome arises as a result of a trisomy in the chromosome pair known as 21.

In 94 percent of cases, Down syndrome arises from an error in meiosis, and in nine out of ten of these cases the error has affected the ovum rather than the spermatozoon. This form of Down syndrome is more likely to arise with increasing maternal age (see Table 5.4c-I). As will be appreciated from the table, the risk of having an affected pregnancy rises sharply after the age of 35, but is nevertheless a relatively unlikely occurrence (affecting less than 1 in 100 pregnancies) in women who are under 40.

Table 5.4c-I Risk of Down syndrome according to maternal age at delivery

Maternal age (years)	Risk of Down syndrome occurring at birth
All ages	1 in 650 births
30	1 in 900 births
35	1 in 380 births
37	1 in 240 births
40	1 in 110 births
44	1 in 37 births

In a small number of cases of Down syndrome, the condition arises from a defect known as a translocation in the genetic material of one of the parents. If this is the case, there is risk of recurrence of the condition in a subsequent pregnancy of up to 15 percent.

In 1 in 100 cases of Down syndrome, mosaicism (see above) is found. This often manifests in a less severe form of the condition.

Down syndrome is currently the most common cause of severe learning difficulties, arising in 1 in 650 live births (see Table 5.4c-I). It is usually diagnosed at birth because of the characteristic cluster of physical features, which are apparent on examination of the newborn. These include a round characteristic face and a protruding tongue (see Figure 5.4c-I), and abnormal creases on the palms and soles. The diagnosis is confirmed by means of chromosomal analysis (requiring a blood test). This test takes several days to process. At a later stage the parents will be offered genetic testing to exclude the rare possibility of a translocation.

In addition to the external features found on neonatal examination, a baby with Down syndrome is likely to have floppy muscle tone. As the child grows, a delay in the attainment of the motor developmental milestones is likely. In addition, 40 percent of babies with Down syndrome have some form of congenital heart defect, often requiring surgery in infancy. Other problems that are likely to affect the child with Down syndrome include moderate to severe learning difficulties (in which difficulties in problem-solving are most prominent), a tendency to recurrent respiratory infections, glue ear and visual impairment from cataracts

or squints. In later life, a person with Down syndrome is at increased risk of developing leukemia, hypothyroidism and Alzheimer's disease.

Despite the cluster of physical and mental problems and the tendency to serious disease in middle age, a child with Down syndrome is often robust in general health and buoyant and sensitive in spirit.

Figure 5.4c-I Characteristic features of Down syndrome

 Information box 5.4c-I

Down syndrome: comments from a Chinese medicine perspective

In Chinese medicine, the underlying diagnosis in Down syndrome would be Jing Deficiency. This is manifest in cognitive impairment and tendency to early onset of Alzheimer's disease. The frequency of heart defects is an indication of a specific imbalance in the Heart Organ. This would accord with the observation that a joyful, open and warm nature is very often found in a person with Down syndrome.

A protruding tongue, and recurrent respiratory infections and glue ear, indicate that tendency to Phlegm Damp is an Excess problem in this condition, and this is a result of underlying Kidney Deficiency with difficulty in handling fluids. Scott and Barlow (1999) report that often the features of Phlegm Damp (including difficulties in learning) respond very well to acupuncture given at frequent intervals before the age of three. Once this Pathogenic Factor has been cleared, Full Heat may then become apparent.[68]

TURNER SYNDROME (45,X)

Turner syndrome is a condition in which there is only a single X sex chromosome. This means that there are only 22 complete pairs of chromosomes. Babies born with Turner syndrome are always girls, as it is the Y chromosome that directs the development of the male sexual characteristics in the fetus.

It has been estimated that 95 percent of embryos with Turner syndrome do not survive past eight weeks. Nevertheless, Turner syndrome is a relatively common chromosomal disorder, affecting approximately 1 in 2500 live-born baby girls. The features of the syndrome include short stature, a webbed appearance to the neck, widely spaced nipples and failure in the development of the ovaries. Intellectual development is normal. Occasionally, a congenital heart defect, coarctation of the aorta, is present. This may require surgical correction.

Diagnosis of Turner syndrome may be missed in the baby, and may only be made when it becomes apparent that the child is very short for her age, or at the time when it becomes obvious that her periods have failed to commence.

Treatment is with growth hormone (GH) therapy in childhood if short stature is a significant problem, and hormone replacement therapy (HRT) from puberty onwards. HRT will not reverse the problem of infertility, but will enable the development of the secondary sexual characteristics, and will aid in the maturation and strengthening of the bones.

Information box 5.4c-II

Turner syndrome: comments from a Chinese medicine perspective

In Chinese medicine, the underlying imbalance in Turner syndrome is Jing Deficiency manifesting in short stature and infertility. A specific deficiency of Heart Qi may be apparent, and can manifest in the form of cardiac malformations.

KLINEFELTER SYNDROME (47,XXY)

Klinefelter syndrome is the result of a trisomy in the sex chromosomes, involving the presence of an extra X chromosome (XXY). As with Turner syndrome, the abnormal complement of sex chromosomes leads to abnormalities of sexual development.

Klinefelter syndrome affects 1 in 1000 live-born males. The features of the syndrome include underdeveloped small testes, infertility, breast development in adolescence (gynecomastia) and tall stature. Intellectual development may be normal, but there is a higher than average incidence of educational and psychological problems in boys with Klinefelter syndrome.

The main treatment is with male sex hormones in puberty, although these are used with caution in individuals who manifest behavioral problems.

Information box 5.4c-III

Klinefelter syndrome: comments from a Chinese medicine perspective

In Chinese medicine, Klinefelter syndrome is a result of Jing Deficiency. The sexual and behavioral problems may indicate an additional imbalance in the Liver Organ.

FRAGILE X SYNDROME

Fragile X syndrome is the result of a multiplication of a small portion of the DNA in the long arm of the X chromosome. In girls, the impact of this defect can be overridden by the healthy chromosome in the pair of sex chromosomes (although there may be mild learning difficulties in one-third of girls who carry fragile X). However, in boys there is no additional X chromosome to perform this function. For this reason, fragile X syndrome primarily manifests in boys. The main features of fragile X syndrome are learning difficulty, large forehead, long face and protruding ears, and large testes (see Figure 5.4c-II).

Figure 5.4c-II Characteristic features of fragile X syndrome

Unlike Down syndrome, fragile X syndrome is almost always inherited from the mother, who is the carrier of the gene defect. As it affects 1 in 2000 live-born boys, this makes it the most common inherited form of severe to moderate learning difficulty (IQ ranges between 20 and 80). It is the second most common genetic cause of learning difficulty after Down syndrome.

Information box 5.4c-IV

Fragile X syndrome: comments from a Chinese medicine perspective

In Chinese medicine, fragile X syndrome is a form of Jing Deficiency.

Single-gene defects

In contrast to the chromosomal defects that can affect thousands of genes encoded within one strand of DNA, the single-gene defects are the result of a mutation in a tiny portion of DNA. A single-gene defect typically affects the production of only one of the millions of proteins that are manufactured as part of the healthy functioning of the body. Since the mapping of the human genome, gene defects can be localized to a specific area on a chromosome. For example, in 70 percent of cases of cystic fibrosis the condition can be attributed to a defect in a section of the DNA called δF508. This defect is located on the chromosomes in the chromosome pair 7.

A single-gene defect may arise spontaneously as a result of an error in the formation of the gametes during meiosis, or it may be transmitted from a parent who carries the defect in his or her genetic material via an affected gamete to the child.

The presence of a single-gene mutation need not manifest in overt disease. One reason for this is that a defect might affect a portion of the DNA which is not absolutely essential for the healthy balance of the body. In this case the mutation may either have no effect or instead might cause the individual to be different in some tiny way, but not necessarily less healthy.

Recessive gene defects

Some forms of genetic defect, even if present in a very important section of DNA, need not cause disease if the defect is not present in the corresponding chromosome of the pair. An example of this type of genetic defect is the one on chromosome 11 that leads to abnormal hemoglobin production in sickle cell anemia.

In the case of this type of genetic defect, if there is a normal gene present on the other chromosome of the pair, this normal gene can enable the formation of the essential protein in the person who carries the defect. In this scenario, the defective gene is described as recessive, because it does not lead to serious disease if counterbalanced by a normal gene on the partner chromosome.

Carriage of recessive genes

In the condition of sickle cell anemia, if only one-half of the chromosome pair 11 is affected by the genetic defect, only the mild condition of sickle cell trait manifests. However, in many of the recessively inherited conditions, the person who carries only one of the possible pair of defective recessive genes manifests no disease at all. The person who carries a single recessive gene is called a carrier for that condition. The carrier state is a very common one. For example, approximately 1 in 25 seemingly healthy people carry the defective gene responsible for cystic fibrosis. In fact, most people carry one or more recessive defective genes related to significant conditions, despite the absence of any manifest genetic disease.[69]

The fact that sickle cell anemia is a recessively inherited condition means that the disease only becomes fully apparent if a child has inherited the sickle cell genetic defect from each parent, meaning that both of the hemoglobin genes on chromosome 11 are affected. The parents of a child with sickle cell anemia are usually found to be carriers of the condition (if this is not the case, it implies that one or both of the gene defects in chromosome 11 of the child arose spontaneously during formation of the gametes). The fact that both hemoglobin genes are affected means that the child has no capacity to produce a normal balance of hemoglobin proteins, and so will manifest the features of sickle cell anemia early in life.

The inheritance of recessive conditions

Half of the gametes from a parent who carries a single recessive gene defect in one chromosome of a pair are likely also to carry that defect. This means that if the other parent does not also carry that defect, 50 percent of the children of those parents are likely to carry the defect. If the carrier state does not lead to manifest disease, all these children will appear as normal. The problem arises if both parents are carriers of the same defective recessive gene. This means that one-quarter of their children will inherit normal genes from their parents, half will inherit the carrier state (only one of the pair of genes is defective) and the remaining quarter will develop the recessive condition (both of the genes in the pair are defective).

The problem of "inbreeding"

Recessive conditions are more likely to become manifest if the parents of a child are closely related to one another. This is because relatives are more likely to carry a similar pattern of recessive defective genes. Inbreeding, medically described as consanguinity, therefore leads to an increased incidence of miscarriages of genetically abnormal embryos, and of children who have illness resulting from a matching pair of recessive genes.

DOMINANT GENE DEFECTS

In contrast to recessive gene defects, some genetic defects will lead to disease even if only present on one of the two chromosomes of the pair. Despite the presence of a normal gene on the partner chromosome, the defective gene produces a protein that acts as if it is "putting a spanner in the works," and leads to a recognizable syndrome. In this case, the gene defect is described as dominant. Huntingdon's disease is a condition that is the result of a dominant gene defect located on chromosome 4.

Dominant genes can also be transmitted from parent to child. In the case of one parent carrying a dominant defective gene (such as the one that causes Huntingdon's disease), half of the gametes produced by that parent will also carry that gene. This means that, even if the other parent is unaffected, half the children will manifest the dominantly inherited condition carried by a parent. Dominantly inherited conditions are more likely to result wholly from spontaneous mutation than recessively inherited conditions. This is because only one of the gametes needs to be affected to give rise to a dominantly inherited condition.

X-linked recessive conditions

X-linked recessive conditions are those recessive conditions that are the result of single-gene defects of the X chromosome of the sex chromosome XY pair (rather than on any one of the remaining 22 non-sex or autosomal chromosomes). In girls, X-linked recessive conditions behave as any other autosomal recessive condition, in that the presence of a normal gene on the corresponding X chromosome of the pair will counterbalance the defect and prevent the manifestation of serious disease.

However, in boys, a gene defect on the X chromosome behaves more like a dominantly inherited defect. This is because the stumpy Y chromosome actually contains very few of the genes that are represented on the X chromosome, and so does not carry a healthy matching gene for the defective one found on the X chromosome. Therefore, all boys who inherit the gene defect in an X-linked condition will manifest the disease.

Hemophilia is one of the most well known of the serious X-linked recessive conditions. In hemophilia the carriage of the defect is always through females, and the condition is usually manifested in boys. Color blindness is another, less serious, X-linked condition that is carried by females, and usually manifested in boys.

CYSTIC FIBROSIS

Cystic fibrosis is a condition of recessive inheritance. Approximately 1 in 25 people of north European ancestry are known to carry the defective cystic fibrosis gene on one of the chromosomes in pair 7. The probability of the parents of a child both being carriers of the cystic fibrosis gene is 1 in 625 (= 25 × 25). Such parents have a one in four chance of having a child with cystic fibrosis. Therefore, the incidence of cystic fibrosis is 1 in 2500 (= 25 × 25 × 4) births. Cystic fibrosis is described in more detail in Section 3.3d.

SICKLE CELL DISEASE AND THALASSEMIA

Both sickle cell anemia and thalassemia are conditions of recessive inheritance. The features of these inherited forms of anemia are described in Section 3.4c.

In homozygous sickle cell disease (meaning the same sickle cell defect is present on both chromosomes), the condition results from a mutation in a gene on chromosome pair 11. This leads to a defect in the structure of hemoglobin. Approximately 1 in 16 people of African or Afro-Caribbean ancestry is known to carry the defective sickle cell gene (i.e. sickle cell trait). Using the principles of probability described above for cystic fibrosis, this means that there is just less than a 1 in 1000 probability of a child with sickle cell anemia being born to parents who are both of African or Afro-Caribbean ancestry.

In thalassemia, there is a range of genetic defects that cause problems in the rate of production of hemoglobin. One in ten people of Mediterranean (or Asian) origin are estimated to be carriers of one of the forms of thalassemia.

It is not unusual in populations in the Middle East or North Africa for one person to inherit both a sickle cell and a thalassemia gene. This can lead to a condition of similar severity to homozygous sickle cell disease.

PHENYLKETONURIA (PKU)

Phenylketonuria (PKU) is a condition in which the amino acid phenylalanine cannot be handled by the body. This is the result of the absence of an essential enzyme. Without careful dietary exclusion of sources of phenylalanine (including milk), a child with PKU will develop brain damage. The excess phenylalanine in the body fluids is toxic to developing nervous tissue.

PKU can be detected at birth by means of the heel prick (Guthrie) test. Once PKU is diagnosed in a baby, the parents are given specific dietary advice to protect the child from permanent brain damage. Although the diet is less essential for PKU sufferers in adulthood, a woman with PKU should be strict about her diet in pregnancy; otherwise, the high levels of phenylalanine can damage the developing fetus.

PKU is a recessively inherited condition. The defective gene is fairly rare, being carried by 1 in 50–70 of the population. This means that the incidence of PKU is 1 in 10,000–20,000 births.

ALBINISM

Albinism is usually a recessively inherited condition (although there is a rare X-linked recessive form) in which there is absence of the gene that codes for the enzyme tyrosinase. Tyrosinase is essential in the manufacture of the dark-colored pigment melanin.

There are different forms of albinism, some that affect the eye only and some that also affect the skin and hair. The most important clinical consequence of albinism comes from the lack of pigment in the eye, which affects both the iris and also the choroid layer that lies behind the retina. In albinism the iris of the eye appears pale blue. The lack of protective pigment means that the eye is unable to fix on an object because the incoming light is too bright, and so the eye flickers from position to position, with a movement called nystagmus. The child learns to screw up their eyes to protect them from light. Without early intervention (tinted glasses or contact lenses), the sight can become severely impaired.

In the form of albinism that also affects the skin the child has very pale skin and fair hair and eyebrows. The skin is very vulnerable to sunburn, and so protection from the sun is always required.

Information box 5.4c-V

Albinism: comments from a Chinese medicine perspective

In Chinese medicine, the Liver is the Organ that opens into the eyes. The Liver Blood moistens and nourishes the eye, and gives it the capacity to see. However, as Maciocia (1989) explains, other Yin and Yang Organs affect the eye. In particular, Kidney Jing and the Heart Organ are important in maintaining the health of the eyes.[70] In the case of albinism, Jing Deficiency would appear to be the fundamental problem. Squinting and flickering eye movements might suggest Wind (possibly in the Liver and Gallbladder Channels), which has built up as a consequence of Kidney Deficiency.

COLOR BLINDNESS

Color blindness is an X-linked condition. The most common form of color blindness results in an inability to distinguish between red and green, and varying intermediate shades of brown. It is due to the absence of a particular pigment in the cone cells of the retina necessary for color discrimination. It is common, affecting up to 1 in 50 men, and is important in that its presence might affect eligibility for certain forms of employment (e.g. train driving).

MUSCULAR DYSTROPHY (MD)

Muscular dystrophy (MD) is a general term used to describe a group of congenital conditions in which the muscles undergo a process of progressive degeneration. The two most common forms of MD, Duchenne and Becker MD, both have X-linked recessive inheritance. The defective genes for these two distinct conditions are located on the short arm of the X chromosome.

Duchenne is the most common form of MD, affecting 1 in 4000 male infants. The clinical features of Duchenne MD are described in Section 4.2f.

HEMOPHILIA

Hemophilia is a term used to describe the range of disorders of blood coagulation that result from defective production of clotting factors. The three most common forms of hemophilia are hemophilia A, hemophilia B (Christmas disease) and von Willebrand's disease.

Hemophilia A is an X-linked recessive condition, affecting 1 in 5000 of the male population. The disorder results from defective production of clotting factor VIII. The gene that codes for the production of this factor is found on the X chromosome. The clinical features of hemophilia A are described in Section 2.1c.

Hemophilia B (Christmas disease) is clinically very similar to hemophilia A. It, too, is an X-linked recessive condition, but results from the absence of clotting factor IX. It affects 1 in 30,000 males.

Von Willebrand's disease results from a deficiency of a factor that aids in platelet adherence as well as in the action of factor VIII. This rare form of hemophilia is a recessive condition because the defective gene is found on chromosome pair 12, rather than an X chromosome.

In all three conditions, the severity of the condition depends on the precise nature of the genetic defect.

ACHONDROPLASIA

Achondroplasia is a dominantly inherited condition that leads to dwarfism in the person who carries the defective gene. In 50 percent of cases the condition arises as a result of a spontaneous mutation. In an adult, the condition manifests with marked shortening of the limbs, a pronounced curvature of the lumbar spine, a large head and a depressed nasal ridge (see Figure 5.4c-III). All these features develop as a result of defective maturation of cartilage into bone. Despite these very pronounced features in the adult, the diagnosis may not be made until early childhood.

Figure 5.4c-III Characteristic features of achondroplasia

 Information box 5.4c-VI

Achondroplasia: comments from a Chinese medicine perspective

In Chinese medicine, the underlying problem in maturation of bone in achondroplasia suggests Kidney (Jing) Deficiency.

OSTEOGENESIS IMPERFECTA (BRITTLE BONE DISEASE)

Osteogenesis imperfecta is a term that is applied to a group of genetic disorders that vary in their severity. In osteogenesis imperfecta, underlying genetic defects lead to disordered metabolism of collagen, resulting in weakness of bone.

The most common form of osteogenesis imperfecta is dominantly inherited and manifests in the occurrence of recurrent fractures in childhood. If there is no prior family history, a child with the condition may be mistaken for a case of non-accidental injury. Another characteristic feature of this most common form of osteogenesis imperfecta is that the sclerae (whites) of the eyes have a bluish coloration. There is also an increased incidence of the condition otosclerosis, which leads to progressive loss of hearing in adult life.

 Information box 5.4c-VII

Osteogenesis imperfecta: comments from a Chinese medicine perspective

In Chinese medicine, brittle bones, the blue color of the eyes and progressive deafness characteristic of osteogenesis imperfecta all suggest that Kidney (Jing) Deficiency is at the root of the condition.

FAMILIAL HYPERLIPIDEMIAS

The term hyperlipidemia simply refers to the fact that a raised concentration of fats (including cholesterol) has been found in the serum blood sample. There are over seven well-recognized forms of inherited hyperlipidemia. In these conditions, an underlying gene defect, or a number of gene defects, affect the way in which lipids are manufactured in the liver.

Hyperlipidemia is strongly associated with an increased risk of coronary heart disease (CHD). The risk of CHD associated with hyperlipidemia depends on the precise nature of the genetic defect. Some forms of hyperlipidemia confer a higher risk of CHD than others.

Familial hypercholesterolemia is a common, dominantly inherited form of hyperlipidemia, in which the most important imbalance is a raised level of cholesterol in the blood. Approximately 1 in 500 of the UK population is affected by this condition. Many adults who have familial hypercholesterolemia may only become aware of the diagnosis through routine blood testing. However, it has been estimated that over half of men with this condition will die of a heart attack before the age of 60. Some, but not all, people with this condition may develop the classic skin signs of hypercholesterolemia, the xanthoma (plural xanthomata) and xanthelasma (plural xanthelasmata). A xanthoma is a substantial cholesterol deposit that can appear as a yellowish nodule in the skin around bony prominences, in the tendons and on the palms. A xanthoma is a rare finding in childhood. Xanthelasmata are less substantial yellowish plaques of cholesterol, which can develop in the loose skin around the eyelids.

The treatment of most forms of hyperlipidemia is by means of a lipid-lowering diet together with high doses of one or more of the cholesterol-lowering drugs, including statins (e.g. simvastatin). It is known that the risk of CHD is reduced if the blood lipid levels can be reduced by this combined treatment approach.

If a person inherits a familial hypercholesterolemia gene defect from both parents, the condition is much more serious. In these cases there can be a hugely elevated cholesterol level from childhood. The natural history of this very rare condition is death from ischemic heart disease in late childhood or adolescence.

Familial combined hypercholesterolemia is another commonly occurring, dominantly inherited hyperlipidemia, in which raised levels of cholesterol and also of another class of lipid, the triglycerides, are found. This form of hyperlipidemia affects 1 in 200 of the population.

Familial hypertriglyceridemia involves elevated levels of triglycerides alone. This condition may respond very rapidly to abstinence from alcohol.

 Information box 5.4c-VIII

Hyperlipidemia: comments from a Chinese medicine perspective

In Chinese medicine, the finding of elevated blood lipids and the resulting development of atheroma and xanthomata suggest that Phlegm Damp is prominent in the manifestation of hyperlipidemia. Thus imbalance in the Kidney Spleen and Liver Organs is likely.

An underlying Deficiency of Jing is also a factor in the inherited forms of hyperlipidemia and in this case will predispose to a vulnerability to accumulating Phlegm Damp and to developing Stagnation and eventually Heat symptoms as a result of this. This vulnerability suggests an inherited weakness of Spleen or Kidney Yang (failure to transform fluids) and Liver Qi (failure to move obstructions). Poor diet, inactivity and negative emotions will compound these problems.[71]

Part II: Conditions of multifactorial inheritance

The genetic conditions discussed in the first part of this section all have an origin that can be clearly related to a defect in the structure of the genetic material. This defect will be found in the DNA contained in all the nucleated cells of an individual with the condition (with the very rare exception of mosaicism).

In contrast, the conditions of multifactorial inheritance tend to have a less clear genetic origin. In some of these conditions, it is well recognized that the cause is an external factor that has affected the growth of the fetus in the womb (e.g. congenital heart disease as a result of maternal rubella virus infection in the first trimester). However, in other cases of the condition there is no clear external factor. In these cases it may be concluded that the problem has arisen as a result of a combination of genetic defects (leading to a susceptibility), together with one or more of a whole host of diverse external factors that may have affected development of the embryo/fetus in the womb (e.g. malnutrition, smoking, alcohol, medication, stress). It is not unusual to find more than one congenital condition of multifactorial inheritance in the same child. For example, a child with esophageal atresia may also be found to have congenital heart disease or a kidney defect.

In general, the risk of recurrence of these conditions in another child in the same family is low, which does suggest that environmental factors play a strong part in their origin. However, the risk is greater than it would be for an unrelated child, thus suggesting that genetic susceptibility is also important for these conditions to arise. Without analysis of the genome, it may be very difficult to understand the degree to which genetic factors have impacted on the emergence of symptoms because environmental factors can also run strongly in families or cultural groups (e.g. disease-forming dietary habits, exposure to cigarette smoke, low levels of exercise and exposure to radiation might all be shared by children from the same family).[72]

Congenital heart disease

Congenital heart disease is the single most common group of structural disorders in children. Up to 2 in every 100 children are born with some degree of cardiac malformation, although in only less than half of these is the malformation of a severe nature. Congenital heart disease may also affect the ability of the fetus to survive outside the womb, evidenced by the fact that one in ten stillborn babies has a cardiac malformation.

Congenital malformations of the heart and aorta are more likely with certain chromosomal abnormalities such as Down syndrome and Turner syndrome.

In only a small proportion of cases can the cardiac abnormality be explained by an environmental factor that has impacted on fetal development. External factors that have been linked to congenital heart disease include maternal rubella infection in the first trimester, maternal antibodies in systemic lupus erythematosus (SLE), a high maternal intake of alcohol, and poorly controlled maternal diabetes mellitus.

It is likely in most cases that the causation of cardiac malformations is multifactorial inheritance.

For example, it is recognized that the risk of the condition recurring in a second child is higher than would be expected for the general population. This suggests that there is some, as yet unexplained, genetic factor that increases the susceptibility of the developing fetus to the condition.

The most common forms of congenital heart disease, septal defect, aortic stenosis (narrowing of the aortic valve), coarctation of the aorta (narrowing of the upper arch of the aorta) and the complex abnormalities that lead to cyanotic heart disease, are explained in more detail in Section 3.2g.

Information box 5.4c-IX

Congenital heart disease: comments from a Chinese medicine perspective

In Chinese medicine, congenital heart disease is a particular manifestation of Jing Deficiency. This makes sense because, if untreated, significant congenital heart disease will lead to continual ill health and poor growth and development in the child.

According to the particular defect, Deficiency of Heart Qi, Yang and/or Yin will also be present. Breathlessness is a common feature of untreated congenital heart disease indicating Deficiency of Lung and also Kidney Qi. The bluish color in cyanotic heart disease suggests that Qi or Blood Stagnation has developed as a consequence of severe Heart Deficiency.

Hare lip and cleft palate

Hare (cleft) lip and cleft palate affect just over 1 in 1000 babies. The problem is a failure in the normal fusion of the tissues of the lip and palate. These should grow together in the fetus in the first trimester of pregnancy. In a healthy baby the evidence of normal fusion lies in the two parallel ridges of skin that bridge the inner nostrils and the lip (the philtrum).

Most cases of cleft lip and palate arise spontaneously with no obvious external causative factor, although it is known that maternal smoking and alcohol intake increases the risk of a baby developing the condition. As with congenital heart disease, the inheritance is multifactorial and there is a slightly increased risk of relatives also having the condition. Palatal deformities can be diagnosed prenatally by means of the 20-week-of-gestation ultrasound scan.

Hare lip is the least severe of the abnormalities. In this situation the internal structure of the mouth is normal, but the philtrum is distorted and the baby has large gaps in the lip where the ridges of the philtrum should be. Although this is a very unsightly abnormality, and one that is often shocking for the parents, surgical repair of the lip can have very impressive results. Ideally, this surgery should be delayed for a few months to achieve the best outcome (see Figure 5.4c-IV).

Cleft palate leaves a gaping space between the mouth and the nasal spaces. It can make breastfeeding very difficult in some cases. Cleft palate frequently, but not always, coexists with hare lip. Diagnosis is made by inserting a finger into the mouth of the neonate. Affected babies are more prone to bouts of choking and frequent episodes of ear infections

(otitis media) because of distortion of the Eustachian tube. In later life speech can be affected, as the child develops a characteristic nasal quality to the voice.

Surgical correction of cleft palate is usually performed at several months of age. This also can have good results, but the child may still be left with some degree of cosmetic, auditory and speech problems.

Figure 5.4c-IV Cleft lip (a) before and (b) after surgery

 Information box 5.4c-X

Hare lip and cleft palate: comments from a Chinese medicine perspective

In Chinese medicine, the underlying cause of hare lip and cleft palate is Jing Deficiency. The involvement of the mouth and nose suggests a more specific Deficiency in the Spleen/Stomach and Lung Organs.

Esophageal atresia

Esophageal atresia is a rare abnormality in which the esophagus fails to develop normally. It may first present with the accumulation of amniotic fluid (polyhydramnios) in late pregnancy, as the developing fetus is unable to swallow the fluid as does a healthy fetus. After birth, the baby will very soon start to drool saliva and choke and vomit when feeding. Once the diagnosis is made, the baby is examined for other malformations, as almost half will have at least one other congenital abnormality. The condition is treated immediately by surgery.

Pyloric stenosis

Pyloric stenosis is another malformation that impairs the passage of nutrients through the gastrointestinal tract. In pyloric stenosis, the malformation is a thickening of the pyloric sphincter, the muscular valve that separates the stomach from the duodenum. The condition is four times more common in boys, and more common if one of the parents suffered from the condition.

The baby presents in the first days to weeks of life with vomiting of bile and undigested milk. The vomiting can be so forceful as to be projectile. The baby may be very unwell by the time of diagnosis because of loss of fluids and salts. Treatment is by means of surgery to the pyloric sphincter after the fluid and salt imbalance has been corrected.

Duodenal and small bowel obstruction is a similar, although less common, abnormality, in which the obstruction is a result of failure of the development of the passageway for food and fluids at one or more points along the bowel. These cases may take a few more days before symptoms become apparent, depending on how far down the bowel the obstruction is situated. An additional symptom is that the child may develop a much distended abdomen as the upper part of the intestine fills with wind and fluid.

 Information box 5.4c-XI

Esophageal atresia and pyloric stenosis: comments from a Chinese medicine perspective

In Chinese medicine, abnormalities of development of the gastrointestinal tract suggest Jing Deficiency with a specific Deficiency in the Spleen/Stomach and Liver Organs. The Liver Organ is implicated because, in all forms of gastrointestinal obstruction, the symptoms suggest failure of smooth movement of Qi in the Middle and Lower Jiao.

Imperforate anus

In this rare malformation, there is failure in the development of the rectum and anus. If this is not diagnosed at the neonatal check at birth, the child will eventually present with similar symptoms to small bowel obstruction. Again, the treatment is surgical.

Congenital liver disease and neonatal jaundice

Jaundice is a common finding in newborns. Over 60 percent of newborns become visibly jaundiced within the first few days of life. The potential problem with neonatal jaundice is that the raised bilirubin levels that cause jaundice can be very harmful to the developing nervous system, and can cause a permanent form of brain damage called kernicterus.

In most cases of neonatal jaundice, the problem arises as a combined result of immaturity of the red blood cells and the liver. This condition is termed physiological jaundice. Physiological jaundice becomes apparent at two to five days after birth, and usually resolves within two weeks without any need for treatment. In some babies, a temporary intolerance to breast milk may exacerbate physiological jaundice (breast milk jaundice). However, this complication is rarely so severe as to prevent continuation of breastfeeding.

The problem of raised bilirubin levels in physiological jaundice can be more severe in some babies, particularly if they are premature, in which case most will respond to phototherapy. Phototherapy involves exposing the skin of the newborn to blue light in an incubator. The light promotes the conversion of the bilirubin in the blood to a harmless pigment. In less severe cases, exposure to sunlight will perform this task. In very severe cases the baby may require a treatment called exchange transfusion, in which blood is withdrawn from the baby and replaced with donor blood.

Jaundice may also result from conditions that cause excessive damage to the red blood cells (hemolysis). Rhesus and other blood group incompatibilities are the most common causes of neonatal hemolysis.

In cases in which the jaundice persists for more than two weeks, congenital liver disease may be the underlying problem. In these cases the jaundice is usually accompanied by pale stools and dark urine. Biliary atresia and neonatal hepatitis are the two most common forms of neonatal liver disease.

Biliary atresia (bile duct obstruction) is a condition in which the bile ducts fail to develop normally, and so are obstructed. Surgical bypass of the bile ducts is performed ideally within two months after birth. Without this procedure, the baby will rapidly develop a fatal form of liver failure. Even when this operation is successful there is continued damage to the liver. The child will eventually require liver transplantation to avoid progression to cirrhosis. If the bypass operation is unsuccessful, liver transplantation has to be performed without delay.

Neonatal hepatitis refers to inflammation of the liver tissue at birth. The causes include congenital infections and a range of rare genetic diseases of metabolism, including cystic fibrosis. In many cases of neonatal hepatitis the cause cannot be clarified. Unlike in a typical case of biliary atresia, the child with neonatal hepatitis is unwell and jaundiced from birth. There may be a palpable enlarged liver and spleen. In all cases the treatment is largely supportive, and of course includes treatment to prevent rising bilirubin levels, as described above. In some cases the condition will resolve, but in others the child may develop progressive cirrhosis for which transplantation of the liver is the only treatment. There is a small risk of acute liver failure, which has a high mortality.

Information box 5.4c-XII

Jaundice: comments from a Chinese medicine perspective

In Chinese medicine, persistent jaundice would suggest that the underlying imbalance involves Jing Deficiency, with a specific Deficiency in the Spleen and Liver Organs.

Club foot (talipes equinovarus)

Club foot refers to abnormal positioning of the foot at the ankle joint. The medical term for this condition is talipes equinovarus. The entire foot is inverted and the forefoot is turned outwards so that the soles of the baby's feet tend to face each other (see Figure 5.4c-V). The problem is due to an imbalance in the tension of the muscles of the lower leg and foot, with consequent shortening of the tendons. A mild form of talipes is common, and results from compression of the feet in the womb. This will usually resolve naturally, and can be helped by simple stretching exercises.

Figure 5.4c-V Club foot (talipes equinovarus)

A more severe form of this condition can result in a permanent deformity of the foot, and so requires much more active management from the time of birth. Severe talipes equinovarus affects 1–2 in 1000 births, and is more common in boys. It may be a result of compression in the womb, but does also have a tendency to run in families, thus suggesting a genetic susceptibility.

The treatment of severe talipes involves stretching and strapping of the foot. Sometimes, serial plaster casts may be used to hold the foot in the correct position, so allowing the tendons to find their normal length. Corrective surgery to the tendons may be required at the age of six to nine months.

 Information box 5.4c-XIII

Club foot (talipes equinovarus): comments from a Chinese medicine perspective

The imbalance in the tension of the muscles and tendons at the root of club foot (talipes equinovarus) suggests that the underlying cause in Chinese medicine would be Jing Deficiency, with a specific Deficiency in the Liver and Gallbladder Organs.

Congenital dislocation of the hip

The term congenital dislocation of the hip (CDH) embraces a wide spectrum of disorders that involve the structure of the acetabulum, which is the cup-like depression in the pelvis that cradles the head of the femur in the hip joint. In less severe cases, the curvature of the acetabulum is slightly too shallow, meaning that the head of the femur easily clicks out of place. In these less severe cases, as the child grows, the acetabulum may enlarge to cradle the femur more neatly, and the problem resolves. In more severe cases the acetabulum is very distorted in shape and, without treatment, the hip joint may never develop normally. This condition is not obviously apparent in the newborn. Before the introduction of screening for CDH in the first few months of life, undiagnosed CDH would progress to a disabling permanent condition.

A skilled examiner can detect CDH by the occurrence of perceptible clunks from the hip joint when the thighs of the baby are moved in a certain way. The first time at which this test is performed is during neonatal screening. A specific abnormality of the hip is detected by this test in 6 out of 1000 newborns. However, most of these abnormalities will resolve spontaneously. The true incidence of a problem with the hip joint is probably only 1.5 in 1000 newborns. The problem rarely may be missed initially, but then can be picked up at the eight-week examination. If missed entirely, it may not be until the child starts to walk with a limp that the possibility of CDH becomes apparent.

The degree of the problem in the newborn can be assessed by means of ultrasound examination of the hip joints. If this confirms a moderate to severe abnormality, the baby may be placed in a harness or splint for several months to hold the hips in an abducted (frog-like) position. This encourages the acetabulum to develop in a normal way. In most cases this treatment is successful in preventing a permanent deformity. If this conservative approach is unsuccessful, or if the condition is diagnosed at a later stage, surgical treatment of the bones of the joint and application of a plaster splint may be necessary.

Information box 5.4c-XIV

Congenital dislocation of the hip: comments from a Chinese medicine perspective

In Chinese medicine, the focus of the abnormality of the hip joint suggests that Jing Deficiency, together with a specific Deficiency of the Liver and Gallbladder, may underlie CDH.

 Information box 5.4c-XV

Maldescent of the testes: comments from a Chinese medicine perspective

In Chinese medicine, failure of the testis to descend, with the consequent risk of reduced fertility, is suggestive of Jing Deficiency. As the Liver Channel passes through the area of the scrotum, it is likely that there is also a specific Deficiency in Liver Qi.

Maldescent of the testes

It is necessary for the testes to be suspended outside the abdomen in the scrotum for the production of healthy spermatozoa. Infertility may result if the testis is misplaced. It is also well recognized that a misplaced testis, either in the abdomen or the groin, is more likely to become cancerous.

The testis originates in the fetus from the same embryonic tissue as the ovary. Under the influence of male sex hormones, it then descends during the third trimester through a gap in the muscles of the groin area to find its correct position in the scrotum of the fetus. In 5 percent of male babies this descent is found not to have occurred normally, for either one or both testes. The diagnosis is made by the examining doctor at the neonatal check, when the testes (or testis) are either impalpable or felt higher up in the groin. The occurrence of maldescent of the testes is more common in babies born prematurely.

In some cases of maldescent of the testes the problem resolves spontaneously as the testes find their way into the scrotum during the first few weeks of life. In cases that persist beyond three months of age there may be little chance of spontaneous resolution. If by the age of one to two years the testes (testis) are completely impalpable, a laparoscopic examination is performed to assess whether the testes are either somewhere within the abdominal cavity or entirely absent.

Treatment for undescended testes is necessary to promote fertility and to prevent cancerous change. For testes that are situated in the groin area, the treatment is an operation called orchidopexy. This is performed after the age of one year, and before the child has reached his third birthday. It is usually a straightforward procedure, in which the testes are located via an incision in the groin, and then drawn into the scrotum. It is much more difficult to move a testis that is located in the abdomen. Because of the risk of cancer, a single intra-abdominal testis will be surgically removed, and an artificial testis implanted into the scrotum at a later date (as close to adulthood as is reasonable) for cosmetic purposes. If both testes are intra-abdominal, a much more complex microsurgical technique is required to transplant the testes to their correct position.

Congenital hernia

A hernia can be defined as the movement of an internal organ outside its usual anatomical position through an area of weakness in the surrounding supportive tissue. There are three common types of hernia that can develop in adulthood: inguinal, femoral and hiatus hernias.

In adulthood, hernias usually develop as a result of prolonged strain on the supportive tissues in the area of the hernia, although in some cases there may be an underlying congenital weakness in the herniated area. In contrast, congenital hernias develop because the supportive tissue in the area is underdeveloped in some way. The three important forms of congenital hernia are the inguinal, hiatus and umbilical hernias.

CONGENITAL INGUINAL HERNIA

Congenital inguinal hernia is related in origin to maldescent of the testes. This weakness of the muscle wall of the groin area is a result of a failure of the passageway formed in the third trimester of pregnancy by the testis (as it descends through the groin region) to close off completely. The resulting area of weakness is a site through which the abdominal contents can bulge outwards. In mild cases a lump can be felt in the groin, but in more severe cases the intestines can spill out through a gap in the muscle tissues to form a bulging mass in the scrotum (see Figure 5.4c-VI). Although inguinal hernias are more common in boys, they can also affect girls. A congenital inguinal hernia is initially painless, but there is a risk that abdominal contents can become trapped and damaged as they bulge out through the opening of the hernia. The treatment is surgical repair of the weakness in the muscle wall.

If undiagnosed at birth, the hernia can present in later life as a painful lump in the groin, which is an indication that the intestinal tissues, together with the spermatic cord, have become compressed in the tight space in the muscle tissue. It may be possible to give the baby a light anesthetic and push this lump back into the abdominal cavity. If this is not possible, immediate surgery is required, as there is serious risk that either the bowel or spermatic cords become obstructed, or that their blood supply becomes cut off (with the risk of infarction of the bowel and loss of the testis).

Figure 5.4c-VI Left-sided inguinal hernia (slightly swollen left groin area)

CONGENITAL HIATUS HERNIA

In some young babies, a weakness in the lower esophageal (cardiac) sphincter results in frequent regurgitation of partly digested milk. In mild cases this problem resolves with time, and, in the interim, may be helped by adding thickening agents to feeds. In more severe cases the repeated episodes of regurgitation can leave the child in a malnourished state. The child may be found on investigation to have a widening of the cardiac sphincter (a hiatus hernia), which is unlikely to resolve rapidly with time. Some of these cases may respond to drugs that enhance the emptying of the stomach, but in other cases surgery may be required to narrow the opening of the sphincter.

CONGENITAL UMBILICAL HERNIA

A small weakness between the two strap-like muscles that run from the anterior arch formed by the lower ribcage and xiphisternum down to the pubic bone (the rectus abdominis) is common in newborns, especially those of Afro-Caribbean descent. The result is a bulge in the area of the umbilicus. Although this is a true hernia of intra-abdominal contents, the risk of obstruction of bowel contents is very low. The condition usually resolves as the child gets older and abdominal muscle tone increases.

 Information box 5.4c-XVI

Congenital hernia: comments from a Chinese medicine perspective

In Chinese medicine, a congenital hernia might represent Jing Deficiency with specific Deficiency of the Spleen Organ and also the Liver and Gallbladder Organs, as it is Spleen Qi that is responsible for Raising Qi and the Liver and Gallbladder governs the sinews.

In inguinal hernia Deficiency/Imbalance of Liver Qi is also evidenced by the fact that symptoms of extreme Blood Stagnation (obstruction and/or infarction) are a possible consequence of such a hernia.

Congenital hiatus hernia presents with symptoms suggestive of Deficiency of Stomach Qi, as regurgitation is the most prominent symptom.

Congenital blindness

Severe visual impairment affects 1 in 3000 births. About 50 percent of these cases are genetic in origin (including albinism, congenital cataract and a rare inherited form of tumor, retinoblastoma). Many of the remaining cases arise as a result of congenital infection such as rubella or toxoplasmosis. Excess maternal alcohol intake is also a known cause of profound visual defects in babies, one aspect of fetal alcohol syndrome.

Another important cause of visual impairment is marked prematurity. In very premature babies (less than 32 weeks) there is a tendency for the retinal vessels to grow too rapidly, and so cause occlusion of the retina. This problem can be prevented in some cases by regular screening of the newborn baby, and by giving laser treatment to the retina if new vessel growth is detected.

Severe visual impairment is usually detected by the time the child is six months old as it becomes readily apparent to the parents. Early diagnosis by screening is of great value, as the parents of a visually impaired child will benefit from advice on how to give appropriate stimulation through speech and touch, and appropriate educational support can be arranged in advance for the child. The eyes are examined at the newborn and eight-week baby check for gross defects.

 Information box 5.4c-XVII

Congenital blindness: comments from a Chinese medicine perspective

In Chinese medicine, congenital blindness is a manifestation of Jing Deficiency. There may also be specific Deficiencies in the Liver and Heart Organs, as these Organs, together with the Kidney, are particularly important for clear vision.

Congenital deafness

Congenital deafness affects 1 in 1000 births. The causes include hereditary malformations of the structure of the inner ear and congenital infections such as rubella, toxoplasmosis, syphilis or the human immunodeficiency virus (HIV). In many children there is no obvious cause.

In many cases the deafness is not absolute, in that the child can perceive some ranges of sound. If this is the case, it means that there is hope of improving the child's ability to hear by means of a hearing aid. If deafness is absolute, a cochlear implant (a tiny device, which includes a microphone and an electrode, implanted surgically into the inner ear – the electrode stimulates the auditory (VIII) cranial nerve in response to incoming sounds; see Section 6.1e) may be of great help. Early diagnosis of deafness has been much improved in the UK by the introduction of the neonatal hearing screening program.

Electronic tools for assisted hearing work best if the diagnosis is made early so that the child becomes used to the transformed sound that they produce, and so parents and carers can be guided in the way in which they communicate with the child. It is most important that hearing aids are in use at the time when the child would be developing speech. If this window of opportunity is missed, the older child may never learn to speak clearly.

Information box 5.4c-XVIII

Congenital deafness: comments from a Chinese medicine perspective

In Chinese medicine, congenital deafness would suggest an underlying Deficiency of Jing and Kidney Qi, as it is the Kidney that is responsible for clarity of hearing.

Neural tube defects

In the early stages of its development, the nervous system begins as a flat plate of tissue, which then curves in on itself to form a tube. This tube will eventually form the brain and spinal cord. The hollow running through the center of this tube will develop into the ventricles of the brain and the central canal of the spinal cord. These are the spaces that contain the cerebrospinal fluid (CSF). The neural tube defects result from a failure in the fusion of the tissues of the brain and spinal cord in the first few weeks of development of the embryo.

The most important neural tube defects are anencephaly and spina bifida (including meningocele, myelomeningocele and spina bifida occulta). Together these defects used to be the most common serious malformations detected at birth (affecting 2–4 per 1000 births in the 1960s). In developed countries the incidence has now fallen, partly as a result of improved nutrition with supplementation of food (such as bread and breakfast cereals) with the vitamin folic acid and partly as a result of detection of the abnormality early on in pregnancy.

Anencephaly is an abnormality that always results in neonatal death or stillbirth. The baby suffers from a failure in the development of a large portion of the brain and skull bones. This abnormality is usually picked up early in pregnancy, in which case the mother will be offered a therapeutic termination of pregnancy. Nervous system defects accounted for almost half of all the terminations conducted as a result of physical defects found on screening in the UK in 2014.[73]

Spina bifida literally means that the spinal bones are divided in two (bifid). In all types of spina bifida there is failure of the two arms of the spinal arch of some of the vertebrae (usually in the lumbar area) to meet together.

In spina bifida occulta, deformity of the lumbar vertebrae may be the only defect. In some cases there are no other symptoms, and the diagnosis may only be made incidentally when an X-ray image is taken of the lower back for other reasons. In other cases of spina bifida occulta, the underlying spinal cord may be distorted in some way, and this may give rise to neurological problems of the bladder and lower limbs. Occasionally, a birthmark or unusual tuft of hair may be found on the skin overlying spina bifida occulta.

A meningocele is a fluid-filled outpouching of the spinal meninges through the gap formed by a spina bifida. The meningocele forms a rounded swelling overlying the lumbar spine. Despite its startling appearance, the meningocele can be repaired surgically, and may actually lead to little or no neurological deficit.

A myelomeningocele is a more serious problem. In this condition, the tube-like structure of the lumbar spinal cord does not form, and instead the spinal cord in this region develops into a flat plaque within a meningocele. This deformity may have little or no overlying skin, and so exposes the nervous system to infection. In addition to this gross defect, babies with myelomeningoceles also often have deformities at the level of the cerebellum that prevent a free flow of CSF out of the ventricles of the brain (see Section 4.1a). Without prompt treatment the result is a buildup of fluid in the ventricles, and stretching and distortion of the brain tissue. The soft plates of bone of the baby's skull are stretched, so that the head enlarges. This condition is called hydrocephalus.

Babies who are born with a myelomeningocele may suffer from severe problems, including paralysis of the legs (a spastic paraplegia), sensory loss of the buttocks and legs, impaired action of the bladder and bowel, and scoliosis. Those who also suffer from hydrocephalus may suffer from intellectual impairment.

Treatment includes immediate surgery to the back to close the defect and protect the spinal cord from infection. Also, a plastic shunt may be inserted at the level of the base of the brain to allow free fluid flow between the ventricles and the CSF that surrounds the brain and spinal cord.

Affected children require regular physiotherapy to prevent muscle contractures, and bladder catheterization to prevent buildup of the pressure of urine in the bladder and damage to the kidneys. The prognosis for affected children is much better now than it was even as recently as the 1970s because of advances in surgical techniques and specialized nursing care.

Prenatal screening and therapeutic abortion account for the fact that these defects are becoming less prevalent in the developed world.

 Information box 5.4c-XIX

Neural tube defects: comments from a Chinese medicine perspective

In Chinese medicine, all forms of neural tube defect would be regarded as profound manifestations of Jing Deficiency.

Cerebral palsy

Cerebral palsy is the result of brain damage that occurs either late in fetal development, during labor or in the neonatal period. This condition is described in Section 4.1f.

Congenital hypothyroidism

Congenital hypothyroidism used to be one of the most important causes of severe learning difficulties. Its impact is now minimal since the introduction of the neonatal heel prick (Guthrie) test. It is described in Section 5.1c.

Inherited tendency to developing adult diseases

Many of the most common adult chronic diseases, including coronary heart disease (CHD) and cancer, have their root in a susceptibility that is congenital in origin. Sometimes this susceptibility is inherent in the genes of the affected person. In these cases, a family history of the early onset of the condition (e.g. heart attack or breast cancer) would be typical. Sometimes the susceptibility can be attributed to a less than ideal fetal environment. It is now recognized that poor fetal nutrition may predispose to conditions such as high blood pressure, type 2 diabetes and heart disease in later life.[74]

Currently it is only in a very few chronic adult conditions (such as some forms of inherited breast cancer) that the susceptibility to that condition can be pinpointed early in life by means of a screening test. However, with rapid advances in genetic testing, it may be possible that our individual susceptibility to a whole host of conditions may be predicted. The benefits of such screening tests might appear to be considerable, in that both appropriate lifestyle advice and treatment for the established condition can be offered at an early stage. However, the disadvantages of early screening may, for many conditions, outweigh the benefits. Early diagnosis of susceptibility to conditions such as cancer or schizophrenia may cause anxiety, stigmatization and very practical problems in terms of reduced eligibility for work or life insurance.

Part III: The premature (preterm) baby

A preterm baby is one that is born before it has attained the maturity required for a healthy start in life. By definition, all babies born before 36 weeks of gestation are preterm. Also, whatever the stage of gestation at birth, all babies with a birth weight of less than 2500 grams are also described as preterm.

The health of the preterm baby depends on the degree to which it is of low birth weight or how much it is born before the normal time. Babies born before 24 weeks of gestation are very unlikely to survive. Babies born at 24–31 weeks of gestation experience the most problems, but with intensive neonatal care increasing numbers can survive the very fragile first few weeks. Nowadays, the prognosis is excellent for babies born after 32 weeks of gestation. The main problems experienced by preterm babies are described below.

Infant respiratory distress syndrome (IRDS)

Infant respiratory distress syndrome (IRDS) is a serious condition of the lungs that results from immaturity in the production of a substance called surfactant. This oily liquid is secreted by the lining cells of the lung, and is essential in enabling the full inflation of all the alveoli of the lung after birth. Without surfactant there is a tendency for the alveoli to stay in a collapsed state, thus impairing the ability of the lungs to exchange oxygen and carbon dioxide during breathing. The majority of babies born at 28 weeks of gestation have IRDS, but the incidence becomes progressively lower as the age of gestation at the time of birth increases.

A newborn with IRDS has a rapid breathing rate, and shows discomfort and strain when breathing. The baby may become cyanosed. Treatment is by means of oxygen at high pressure supplied to the baby by a ventilator, sometimes by mask, and sometimes by means of a tube inserted into the trachea. A recent advance is the injection of artificial surfactant into the lungs through the breathing tube. The use of artificial protein-free surfactant, together with continuous positive airways pressure (CPAP) ventilation, has lowered the death rate from IRDS by 40 percent, although carries the risk of life-threatening lung injury, pneumothorax and hemorrhage. The administration of corticosteroid drugs to a mother at least 24 hours before delivering a preterm baby can also reduce the severity of IRDS.[75]

Babies who require a prolonged period of ventilation may develop lung damage from a combination of the high pressure of ventilation, recurrent infections and accumulated secretions. Some of these babies may require oxygen therapy in the first few months of life, and thereafter may be more prone to respiratory problems in childhood. In such babies there is an increased risk of death from respiratory problems in the first few years of life.

Irregularities of breathing and heart rate

Irregularities of breathing and heart rate, including periods during which the breathing stops entirely (apnea), are common in babies born before 32 weeks of gestation. Therefore, the preterm baby requires constant monitoring. If episodes of apnea are frequent, ventilation may be required.

Temperature control

Tiny babies have a relatively large surface area compared to body weight, thin skin and low body fat. These all contribute to the problem of difficulty in maintaining body temperature. It is very important to control the external temperature of the baby at an ideal level. This is achieved by means of an incubator. The humidity of the environment within the incubator is also controlled in order to prevent excessive fluid loss from the skin.

Problems with nutrition

Babies born before 35 weeks of gestation will not be able to suck and swallow milk. Feeding has to be by means of a tube inserted into the stomach via the nose or mouth. Even in very preterm babies, breast milk from the baby's own mother is the ideal source of food, although it may need to be supplemented with vitamins, protein, calories and minerals. If the baby is very sick, a highly specialized form of nutrition may be given by vein. Blood transfusions may be required to replace blood removed for laboratory tests, to compensate for low iron stores and the immature production of blood cells.

Episodes of low blood sugar (hypoglycemia) are more common in preterm babies. This has to be taken seriously, as prolonged episodes of low blood sugar can lead to permanent damage to the developing nervous system. Prevention involves regular blood testing and infusion of intravenous glucose solution.

A very serious complication of the gastrointestinal tract in preterm babies is necrotizing enterocolitis. This condition, in which the bowel becomes inflamed and then suffers tissue death, is thought to be a combination of poor blood supply to the bowel wall and invasion of the bowel tissue by bacteria. The baby develops a distended abdomen, vomits feeds and has bloody stools. Surgery for a perforated bowel may be required. About 20 percent of babies who develop this condition will die from shock or overwhelming infection.

Retinal damage

It has been mentioned earlier that one of the causes of congenital visual impairment is marked prematurity. The problem of new retinal vessel growth (retrolental fibroplasia or retinopathy of prematurity) is found to some degree in one-fifth of babies at 32–38 weeks of gestation. However, because of advances in screening for the condition and the use of laser treatment, the condition only causes severe visual impairment in less than 1 percent of preterm babies.

Brain damage

Intracranial hemorrhage is a common severe problem of prematurity affecting up to 45 percent of very tiny preterm babies. Babies born at less than 30 weeks of gestation will be screened for this problem by means of an ultrasound scan. Most episodes of hemorrhage occur shortly after the birth of the baby as the new circulation pattern settles down. Brain hemorrhages are also more common in babies who suffer from respiratory distress syndrome (RDS) or a pneumothorax. The bleed commonly affects a small area of tissue around the ventricles of the brain.

Surprisingly, many babies do not seem to be affected seriously by these bleeds. However, in some cases the bleed can extend. The blood can clot and prevent drainage of the cerebrospinal fluid (CSF) in the ventricles, thus bringing about hydrocephalus. Widespread multiple areas of hemorrhage are associated with a poor developmental outcome.

Jaundice

Jaundice is a common problem of prematurity, and carries a risk because high levels of bilirubin are toxic to the developing nervous system. Premature babies will very often require phototherapy treatment to reduce the circulating levels of bilirubin. In some cases exchange transfusion will be required.

Problems after discharge from hospital

In general, preterm babies, even when they have reached the time at which the delivery should have taken place, are thinner and have shorter bone length than babies who are born at term. This discrepancy in height and weight may remain throughout childhood.

Those who have had respiratory problems may develop recurrent chest infections and wheezing episodes. Readmission to hospital in the first year of life is four times more likely in a baby who has been born prematurely.

Very low birth weight infants may develop a wide range of developmental problems. Conditions such as visual impairment, cerebral palsy, hearing loss and learning difficulty are more common in children who were born before 32 weeks of gestation. There is an increased incidence of specific learning difficulties, such as delayed language development, poor attention span and poor fine motor skills. Behavioral problems are also more common. All these problems are more marked the earlier the week of gestation at birth.

The burden on the parents of having a preterm baby in hospital for some weeks cannot be overestimated, particularly if there are older children at home to be cared for. The neonatal intensive care unit may be many miles away, and thus many hours each week may be dedicated to visiting the baby. Until the last couple of decades, close contact and handling of the very preterm baby had to be minimized. However, increasingly neonatal intensive care units are recommending episodes of "kangaroo care" in which mothers are encouraged to give the preterm baby long periods of skin-to-skin contact and breastfeeding if possible. Kangaroo care has shown remarkable benefits in terms of not only bonding but also physical and neurodevelopmental outcomes.[76]

 Information box 5.4c-XX

Preterm birth: comments from a Chinese medicine perspective

In Chinese medicine, the foundation of all the problems of prematurity would be regarded as Jing Deficiency.

The gynecologist Chen Jia Yuan wrote during the Qing Dynasty that each lunar month of pregnancy was associated with the development of a different Chinese Organ (West 2008).[77] Weeks 24–32 are associated with the development of the Lungs and Large Intestine, and weeks 32–40 with development of the Kidney and Bladder.

This would very much accord with the observation that the preterm baby, by missing out on the opportunity for protected development in the womb during the period from 24 weeks of gestation onwards, carries a particular weakness in the development of the lungs, the bowel and the nervous system.

Screening for congenital disease

The role of genetic counseling

If there is any concern about the possibility of congenital disease, either before conception or during pregnancy, the couple may be referred to a clinical geneticist for specialized genetic counseling. The geneticist is knowledgeable about the different modes of inheritance of the genetic congenital diseases, and will be able to advise the couple on the risks that their child (or potential child) might be carrying any one congenital disease. Potential parents are usually referred for genetic counseling if there is a personal or family history of possible congenital disease.

As techniques of DNA analysis are becoming more sophisticated, the number of disease-causing gene defects that can be detected in potential parents, and also the developing fetus, is ever increasing. The results of these tests will increase the specificity of the advice given by the geneticist.

Genetic screening of parents

Genetic screening through DNA analysis may be offered to parents for whom there appears to be a significant possibility that a genetic disease might be transmitted to their children. At present, there is not a specific DNA test available for all the known genetic mutations that underlie the carriage of genetic diseases. However, there are many mutations that can be detected directly from a sample of bodily cells from the parent. For example, tests are possible for the carriage of thalassemia, muscular dystrophy, cystic fibrosis, sickle cell disease and Huntingdon's disease. Use of more sophisticated techniques, such as the polymerase chain reaction (PCR), can allow the detection of a genetic abnormality from a tiny sample of bodily fluid, such as is obtained in the neonatal heel prick (Guthrie) test.

If one or both parents are found by DNA analysis to be carriers of a specific mutation, they can be given very clear unequivocal information about the risk of conceiving a child with the condition related to the carriage of that mutation.

Antenatal testing for genetic disease

In addition to testing for chromosomal abnormalities and neural tube defects, the fetal cells obtained by means of amniocentesis and chorionic villus sampling may also be tested for specific genetic defects such as cystic fibrosis or muscular dystrophy. Testing for disease in the fetus at this stage in pregnancy provides information that might lead parents to make the difficult choice of terminating the pregnancy.

Presymptomatic testing of children

DNA analysis may be used to confirm the diagnosis of a genetic disease in a child. Alternatively, the presence of a particular disease may be confirmed by means of a specific biochemical test (e.g. the amino acid assay used to diagnose phenylketonuria) or physical test (e.g. the examination of the eyes that is used to conform or exclude retinoblastoma).

Many genetic diseases vary in their severity from individual to individual. The progression of the disease in the individual may be monitored by means of repeated tests as the child grows up (e.g. repeated ultrasound scans of the kidney are performed in people who are known to carry the dominant gene for polycystic kidney disease). In this way, the more severe cases of the disease may be offered early treatment, and the less severe cases be given reassurance that their own form of the disease appears to be running a more benign course.

There is an ethical dilemma around whether or not a presymptomatic test should be performed on an apparently healthy child, who has no say in the matter about whether or not they want to know the result of the test. For those conditions in which there is no obvious benefit of knowing the diagnosis (e.g. Huntingdon's disease), it is generally accepted that children should not be tested until the time at which they are able to give informed consent.

5.4d Infectious disease in childhood

Infections are the most common form of acute disease in children, both in developed countries and in the developing world. In the developing world, infections are by far the most important cause of death in young children, just as they used to be in more developed countries prior to the middle of the 20th century. In developed countries, childhood mortality from infection has dropped markedly over the last 100 years in parallel with improvements in nutrition, sanitation, housing and advances in medical care, and latterly, the introduction of antibiotic therapy and vaccination. The infant mortality rate in the US dropped by 90 percent from 1915 to 1995, and 60 percent of this drop had occurred by 1940, before widespread access to antibiotics and the implementation of vaccine programs.[78] This drop in mortality is attributed to improved survival from infectious diseases. Since the 1990s the infant mortality rate in the US has dropped further by about 50 percent in 30 years,[79] but in this time period the main causes of death (congenital disease, sudden infant death syndrome, accidents, preterm birth and maternal complications in pregnancy) were non-infective.

In the first months of life, the immune system of the newborn is immature. Moreover, the newborn has yet to encounter the thousands of antigens that will, in time, allow its immune system to build up an immunological memory for many of the common infectious agents that will form part of its everyday environment.

For the first few weeks of life an infant relies on maternal antibodies as a protective barrier against infectious disease. These antibodies entered its bloodstream during the pregnancy, but by three to four months of age the antibody levels will have declined to an insignificant level. From just before the time of the birth, the fetus is able to produce its own antibodies. After birth, these will be produced in increasing quantities as the newborn is introduced to a wide range of foreign antigens, including those found on the structure of infectious agents. Gradually, the gap left by the decline in the maternal antibodies will be filled by the infant's own antibodies. However, there is a period of a few months in the first year of life when the infant's blood carries relatively low levels of antibodies compared to an older child. It is during these few months that the infant is particularly vulnerable to succumbing to infection. Breast milk is one natural source of antibodies that can be transferred to the infant during this vulnerable time.

These facts inform the rationale for the introduction in the UK of the childhood vaccination program, in which the first vaccinations are administered to babies at eight weeks of age. Vaccination presents to the young baby a range of antigens derived from infectious agents. These are intended to stimulate the production of protective antibodies to replace, in part, the declining levels of maternal antibodies.

Even after the levels of circulating antibodies in the child have reached normal adult levels (which happens, for the large part, by the end of the second year of life), children still remain particularly vulnerable to succumbing to certain infections and, in some cases, to suffering from debilitating consequences of these infections. In many childhood infections the child's response to the disease is strong because it is the first time it has encountered the infectious agent. It also appears to be in the nature of the child's response to infection that a high fever often develops. It is not unusual for this fever to be accompanied by mental changes such as drowsiness or confusion. A febrile convulsion (fit) is a potentially serious complication of a childhood fever that affects 3 percent of children at some point in childhood.

This section begins with a description of the more serious complications of fever in childhood, and then looks at some of the more important infectious diseases of childhood. The conditions discussed here are:

- Complications of febrile infections:
  - febrile convulsions
  - dehydration
- Congenital infections (see under "Infections in pregnancy," Section 5.3d)
- Common respiratory infections of childhood:
  - the common cold
  - sore throat and tonsillitis
  - sinusitis
  - acute otitis media
  - viral croup
  - epiglottitis

- bronchitis and whooping cough
- bronchiolitis and viral-induced wheeze
- pneumonia
- Other common viral infections of childhood:
  - measles
  - mumps
  - rubella
  - herpes simplex virus (HSV) infection
  - chickenpox and shingles
  - infectious mononucleosis (glandular fever)
  - cytomegalovirus (CMV) infections
  - roseola infantum
  - slapped cheek syndrome
  - enterovirus infections
  - poliomyelitis
  - viral gastroenteritis and rotavirus
  - viral hepatitis
  - warts and molluscum contagiosum
  - HIV infection and AIDS
- Staphylococcal and streptococcal infections:
  - impetigo
  - boils
  - scarlet fever
  - scalded skin syndrome
  - toxic shock syndrome
  - Kawasaki disease
- Urinary tract infection in childhood:
  - cystitis
  - vesico-ureteric reflux disease and pyelonephritis
- Fungal infections and infestations of the skin (see under "Fungal infections" and "Skin infestations," Section 6.1c)
- Notifiable diseases.

Complications of febrile infections

Children have a tendency to develop a high fever when their immune system is dealing with infectious agents. Fits (febrile convulsions) and dehydration are serious consequences of the effect of fever on the immature nervous system, and of fluid loss, respectively. Conventional medicine recognizes that prolonged fever can take its toll, leading to a state of exhaustion after the illness has passed.

Information box 5.4d-I

Fever in children: comments from a Chinese medicine perspective

In Chinese medicine, fever corresponds to Heat. The Heat may result from an invasion of Wind Heat or Summer Heat, or may originate from internally lodged Heat, or may be a combination of both. Scott and Barlow (1999)[80] suggest that fevers, particularly in spring time, are one way of discharging either Accumulated Heat from the winter period or from Latent Pathogenic Factor. Either way, they serve a useful purpose and should be welcomed. The child with fever is at risk of Depletion of Qi or Yin, and so needs to be looked after carefully when unwell, and encouraged to rest and drink fluids, but not eat. Frequent use of antibiotics and antipyretics prevent fever from running its course, and may predispose to prolonged Qi Deficiency and Lingering Pathogenic Factors. In Scott and Barlow's opinion, Yin Deficiency, a common complication of fever in Eastern children, is actually very uncommon in the West, a finding they attribute to the frequent use of antibiotics. They disagree with the use of flu vaccination in children except for the child whose constitution is so weak it might make contracting flu a life-threatening condition.

Febrile convulsions

The word febrile comes from the Latin word for fever. The term febrile convulsion therefore describes a fit that accompanies a fever. This phenomenon is most common in children between six months and three years of age, but can affect children up to the age of six. It has been estimated that over 3 percent of children will suffer from this condition before they are six years old. A febrile convulsion appears to be most common in a viral infection in which there is a rapid rise in fever. The convulsion tends to occur in the phase during which the fever is rising most rapidly. In 10–20 percent of cases a first-degree relative has a history of either febrile convulsions or epilepsy, suggesting that there may be an inherited susceptibility.

The usual pattern of events is that the febrile child suffers a brief seizure, akin to a tonic-clonic seizure in generalized epilepsy. This usually lasts no more than 1–2 minutes. There is a risk of recurrence in the same illness, and overall about one in three children who have suffered a febrile convulsion will have at least one other in the future.

In a small percentage of cases (2–4 percent), the child will later be diagnosed with epilepsy, the febrile convulsion being the first manifestation of this chronic condition. This is more likely to be the case if the child has suffered a prolonged seizure, or has suffered recurrent fits. However, it is not believed that the febrile convulsion is a cause of epilepsy, but rather that in some cases the fact that a child has a convulsion is an early sign of underlying epilepsy.

Convulsions may be prevented by strict attention to reducing fever in early infections. The advice that is currently given to parents of the febrile child has changed in recent years. Attempts to cool the child with sponging and fans are not recommended. Moreover, paracetamol and ibuprofen are not recommended as readily as they used to be. The advice is now only to use them if the child is in distress.

In the event of a brief convulsion the same advice applies. In all cases, even if the fit has settled down, a doctor should be called. If the convulsion is not settling down within 1–2 minutes, the airway of the child should be protected and the emergency services summoned, as a prolonged fit can lead to lasting brain damage.

After a seizure it is important for the doctor to assess the child to exclude a more serious underlying infection, such as meningitis, and to give the parents clear advice on controlling the child's temperature and the first aid management of a future seizure. The child may be prescribed the tranquillizer medication diazepam in suppository form for the parents to administer in the case of a recurrent prolonged seizure.

that the surface area of a child is much greater relative to the child's body weight than that of an adult. This means that fluid loss through the skin when sweating will be more likely to affect the body's fluid balance adversely. Moreover, a febrile child is more likely than an adult to suffer from a disturbance of consciousness. Confusion and drowsiness are common in otherwise benign fevers, and may mean that it is difficult to encourage the child to keep on drinking. Dehydration is of particular concern in babies and children who are suffering from vomiting or diarrhea.

Dehydration may develop insidiously in a child. Its features include dry mouth and skin, infrequent urination and, in more severe cases, a sunken fontanel in babies, mottled skin, cool extremities and drowsiness or confusion. As these latter two features are also characteristic of fever, it may mean that the dehydration may pass unnoticed for some time. Severe dehydration in a child can affect the function of the brain and lead to the development of acute renal failure.

Prevention of dehydration requires vigilant attention to the fluid intake in a febrile or vomiting child. If fluid intake is impossible, hospital admission may be prudent so that the child can receive intravenous fluids.

Information box 5.4d-II

Febrile convulsion: comments from a Chinese medicine perspective

Infantile convulsions are one of the four great pediatric diseases, according to Chinese medicine, because they are potentially life-threatening.

In Chinese medicine, a febrile convulsion is the result of two Pathogenic Factors, Heat and Phlegm.

Wind Heat alone may impair the movement of Qi and Blood in a child with immature Yin, and the resulting dryness of Sinews and Vessels can lead to stirring upwards of Liver Wind. Liver and Kidney Yin Deficiency will predispose to acute convulsions.

The convulsion may also be complicated by Phlegm. This may be apparent in the form of a cough in the time leading up to the fever. Chinese medicine considers that Phlegm and Heat together can cause Wind, which rises up rebelliously to cause loss of consciousness, stiffness and physical convulsions. Scott and Barlow (1999)[81] consider that fright or shock may also be an underlying factor, which leads to disturbance of the Shen, and thereby enables the turbid Phlegm more easily to cloud the sensory orifices.

Information box 5.4d-III

Dehydration in infants: comments from a Chinese medicine perspective

In Chinese medicine, dehydration is seen to deplete Yin. If it occurs rapidly it can also injure both Yin and Yang. Treatment would be directed first at rehydration and then at supporting the Kidney function.

Congenital infections

The important infections in pregnancy that can lead to infection or developmental disorder of the unborn child include rubella, cytomegalovirus (CMV), chickenpox, herpes simplex, parvovirus, human immunodeficiency virus (HIV), hepatitis B and C, syphilis, listeriosis and toxoplasmosis. These are all discussed in detail in Section 5.3d.

Common respiratory infections of childhood

Respiratory infections are common in children. A preschool child in the West suffers from, on average, six to eight respiratory infections per year, most of which are

Dehydration

A child is more prone to dehydration when unwell because of the child's small size. A consequence of small size is considered to be mild and self-limiting. Overall, 80 percent of respiratory infections in Western children involve only the nose, throat, ear or sinuses. By definition, these are the upper respiratory tract infections (URTIs), and include the common cold, sore throat, tonsillitis, sinusitis and otitis media.

It is recognized conventionally that certain environmental factors may render a child more susceptible to developing a respiratory infection. Low socio-economic status is strongly linked to an increased risk of infection in children. This may be at least partly attributed to the fact that being poor exposes the child to independent risk factors for infection, which include large family size, exposure to cigarette smoke and atmospheric pollution, poor housing, damp environments and poor nutrition.

The health of the child is also an important factor that may determine susceptibility to respiratory infection. Respiratory infections are more common in premature infants, children with congenital heart or lung disease, and those with immunodeficiency.

The majority (80–90 percent) of childhood respiratory infections are attributed to viruses. The five major classes of respiratory viruses are the respiratory syncytial virus (RSV), rhinoviruses, parainfluenza, influenza and adenoviruses. Within each class there are many different strains, which can cause several different patterns of illness. This means that a child who has developed immunity to one strain of RSV infection following an infection such as a cold may still be prone to succumbing to another pattern of infection, such as croup, when exposed to another strain of RSV. For this reason, with the exception of the influenza vaccination, effective vaccinations for these viral infections have not yet been developed.

Viral infections do not respond to antibiotic treatment. In viral infections, antibiotics will only be effective if the infection has been prolonged and has permitted a bacterial infection to supervene. This would not be the norm in a healthy child. For this reason, the parents of children who have symptoms that are characteristic of a viral URTI in its early stages (short history of one to four days, clear discharges, sneezing, fever and aches) should, in general, be advised to withhold antibiotic treatment.

If the respiratory tract, including the larynx and below it, is affected, this is termed a lower respiratory tract infection (LRTI). In general, LRTIs are more serious infections in children because the swelling induced can rapidly lead to life-threatening obstruction of the airways. These infections include croup, bacterial epiglottitis, bronchitis, bronchiolitis and pneumonia. Warning features suggesting that an infection is an LRTI include the development of a coarse barking cough and/or stridor and/or breathlessness.

Viral LRTIs may exacerbate an underlying tendency to asthma (see Section 5.4e). In this case, the cough and breathlessness may not be entirely due to infection, but instead to the bronchoconstriction of asthma. The diagnosis is crucial here. A child with virally triggered asthma may require treatment with bronchodilators and inhaled steroids, not with antibiotics.

Information box 5.4d-IV

Respiratory infections: comments from a Chinese medicine perspective

In Chinese medicine, the Lungs of a child are particularly fragile and may easily suffer from exposure to impure air (including cigarette smoke), stuffiness, dryness, too much heat or too much cold. An attack of Wind Cold can easily develop into a cough as the Lung Qi is Depleted, and the resulting impairment of dispersal of body fluids leads to Phlegm Accumulation.

The common cold

The common cold is the most common infection of childhood. As in adults, the symptoms involve a clear nasal discharge, sneezing, nasal blockage and, in some cases, a mild fever. A phlegmy (wet-sounding) cough is also a frequent additional symptom in children. Well over 100 strains of virus are known to cause the common cold syndrome. This explains why a single child with apparently normal immunity may suffer from recurrent colds.

A child with a common cold should be treated only symptomatically. Paracetamol or ibuprofen are commonly given to children for colds or fever, but are not now medically recommended unless the child is in pain or distress with the fever. Aspirin should never be given to a child under 12 because of the extremely low risk of inducing Reye's syndrome, a severe form of liver inflammation.

Information box 5.4d-V

The common cold: comments from a Chinese medicine perspective

In Chinese medicine, the common cold corresponds to an Invasion of Wind Cold or Wind Heat. A child with Lung Qi Deficiency or Spleen Qi Deficiency is more prone to these syndromes. Accumulated Phlegm or Internal Heat may become apparent when an affected child catches a child and will manifest as phlegm in nose and chest and high fever.

Sore throat and tonsillitis

The features of a sore throat (pharyngitis) include a reddened pharynx, discomfort in the throat area, and sometimes some of the more general features of infections such as fever, malaise and headache. In most cases the cause is viral. The most common bacterial cause is a penicillin-sensitive bacterium, the *Streptococcus*. This is more likely to be the pathogen in older children. In past decades, streptococcal infection carried a high risk of precipitating the serious post-infectious complications of rheumatic fever and acute nephritis (Bright's disease). For this reason, a ten-day course of penicillin was commonly recommended in the case of a sore throat. Nowadays, these complications are extremely rare, and doctors are advised not to prescribe antibiotics in an uncomplicated infection, not least because in most cases the infection is of viral origin. In most cases the infection is self-limiting and resolves within three to five days.

Tonsillitis is a manifestation of viral or bacterial invasion of the tonsils. In severe cases the tonsils become inflamed and enlarged, and may have yellowish patches on their surface. It is impossible to distinguish between viral and bacterial tonsillitis, although if the patient becomes more constitutionally unwell with headache, enlarged cervical lymph nodes and joint pains, this is more suggestive of a bacterial infection. Bacteria are considered as the cause of tonsillitis in 15–50 percent of cases (depending on the age of the child), with *Streptococcus* being the most common pathogen. One common viral cause of tonsillitis is Epstein-Barr virus (EBV), the virus that may also cause glandular fever (see later).

Doctors are more likely to prescribe antibiotics in tonsillitis than if the diagnosis were pharyngitis. This is despite the appreciated fact that these drugs will be totally ineffective in those cases (the majority) that are of viral origin.

The tendency to prescribe is because tonsillitis can become a more debilitating condition. The malaise that accompanies tonsillitis can be profound in some cases, and the symptoms may persist for five to seven days or more. Penicillin or erythromycin are two commonly used antibiotics. It is not good practice to prescribe amoxicillin as there is a risk of inducing a rash if the infectious agent is EBV.

In some children, attacks of tonsillitis are recurrent. If a pattern of over four severe infections a year is emerging, particularly in an older child or teenager, the operation of tonsillectomy is considered to be a reasonable choice of treatment. Another indication for this operation is if the tonsils (and adenoids) have become so enlarged as to cause mouth breathing and disturbed sleep at night. This problem can have marked repercussions on daily life, as it may cause the child to be sleepy in the day. In some children the difficulty in breathing at night may be so severe as to put the heart under strain.

Tonsillectomy will often result in a marked reduction in throat infections, and almost always has beneficial results at least in the short term, when the tonsils have impaired the ability to breathe with ease. In some cases the child who has suffered from recurrent episodes of tonsillitis might continue to suffer from repeated episodes of pharyngitis after the operation, but these are usually less severe than the original infections.

Most children make a rapid recovery from tonsillectomy, although there is a risk of severe bleeding from the root of the tonsils in the immediate postoperative period. For this reason the child requires an overnight stay in hospital, so that they can be carefully observed after the operation. Long-term studies conducted in the past decade suggest correlations with obesity and heart disease in those who have had childhood tonsillectomies, but these links are neither proven nor understood fully.

 Information box 5.4d-VI

Sore throat and tonsillitis: comments from a Chinese medicine perspective

In Chinese medicine, acute sore throat and tonsillitis are often manifestations of Wind Heat. In some cases of severe tonsillitis there are features to suggest that the Heat has progressed to the Yang Ming (Bright Yang) stage, with "big fever, big thirst, big sweating and big pulse." In some cases, Stomach Heat may be the underlying syndrome, in which case frontal headache may be prominent. Severe cases of tonsillitis, in which the tonsils are enlarged with yellow patches on them, indicate the development of Fire Poison.

In Chinese medicine, chronic tonsillitis may be a consequence of a lingering Pathogenic Factor (Interior Heat) that has never become dislodged since the first attack. The Pathogenic Factor obstructs the Qi and Blood flow in the throat area. This can lead to Phlegm Accumulating in the tonsils, together with Stagnation and more Heat. Scott and Barlow (1999)[82] suggest that suppression of emergence of Interior Heat from infections by antibiotic treatment and also the introduction of Toxic Heat in the form of immunizations can contribute to the persistence of lingering Pathogenic Factor in the throat.

From this perspective, the operation of tonsillectomy removes a route of expression of the imbalance of lingering Pathogenic Factor, but does not attend to the underlying imbalance. This means that the underlying imbalance might recur in a different form.

Sinusitis

Sinusitis is most usually a complication of a viral infection such as the common cold, influenza, measles or whooping cough. It is described in more detail in Section 3.3c.

Acute otitis media

Otitis media literally means inflammation of the middle ear. In its acute form it is common, affecting up to 20 percent of all children under four years of age at least once a year. The middle ear, as described in Section 6.1a, is, from an anatomical viewpoint, an extension of the respiratory tract. It is linked to the nasopharynx by means of the Eustachian tube, and is lined by mucus-secreting respiratory epithelium. In viral URTIs it is not uncommon for the respiratory epithelium of the middle ear to also become affected. Early symptoms may include ear pain and deafness, as excessive mucus discharge is unable to drain via the inflamed Eustachian tube. These symptoms are more common in young children. This is because blockage of this route of drainage from the middle ear is more likely to develop, a result of the anatomy of the small child's Eustachian tube.

When the middle ear cannot be drained of mucous secretions in the early stages of a viral infection, bacterial infection (often by the usual bacterial inhabitants of the healthy respiratory tract) can easily supervene, and the infection can become prolonged. In both bacterial and viral cases this can lead to severe pain in one or both ears, high fever and a red, bulging eardrum on examination. In small children, otitis media may present only with fever and confusion, and so the ears should always be examined in a child with an unexplained fever.

In some cases of otitis media the inflammation resolves through natural perforation of the eardrum. Perforation is surprisingly painless. Instead, it often results in a dramatic cessation of symptoms, as the pus is drained through the external auditory canal. A perforated eardrum usually heals within days of the resolution of the middle ear infection.

Before the advent of antibiotic therapy, severe complications of otitis media were common. It is very likely that the poor nutritional status of children also contributed to the susceptibility of these complications, which included chronic discharging ears (chronic otitis media), local bone infections (mastoiditis), meningitis and brain abscess. Although it is accepted that most cases of bacterial otitis media nowadays would resolve fully without the need for antibiotics, the specter of this past association with severe complications has meant that until recent years it was usual practice to prescribe antibiotics (most commonly amoxicillin) in a case of acute otitis media. Current medical wisdom is that antibiotics should not be prescribed in simple cases unless the ear has perforated and is discharging pus.[83]

The resolution of acute otitis media may be complicated by the persistence of a non-inflammatory mucous discharge in the middle ear cavity. This condition is known as chronic secretory otitis media or glue ear. This sticky fluid can impair the transmission of sound waves from the eardrum to the inner ear. The tendency to develop otitis media and glue ear runs in families.

Information box 5.4d-VII

Otitis media: comments from a Chinese medicine perspective

In Chinese medicine, otitis media may correspond to an External Invasion of Wind Heat or Wind Cold. Damp is sometimes an additional Pathogenic Factor. Also, in older children Heat can enter the Liver and Gallbladder Channels and then rise up to manifest as pain and Heat in the ear. In these children, constraint of Liver Qi might be a predisposing factor. Recurrent attacks of otitis media might suggest a lingering Pathogenic Factor.

Viral croup

Croup is the most common form of LRTI in children. It is understood to be caused by a viral infection that leads to inflammation of the larynx, trachea and bronchi (also known as laryngotracheitis). The affected child is usually aged 12–24 months, and suffers from symptoms that include fever, runny nose, a barking cough, and a harsh noise on inspiration (stridor), which indicate narrowing of the trachea. In severe cases there is marked obstruction of the trachea, and the child may demonstrate a rapid pulse and respiratory rate, cyanosis, and the appearance of a sucking in of the sternum and intercostal muscles on breathing in.

In mild cases the child with croup can be managed at home. Exposure to steam is believed to ease the obstructed breathing, and is often recommended, although current medical evidence has put the value of this practice in doubt. In more severe cases oral or inhaled steroids may help to reduce inflammation. In a severe case the child is admitted as an emergency to hospital, and in extremely rare cases it may be necessary to insert a stiff tube into the trachea (tracheal intubation) to keep the airway patent while the inflammation resolves.

Recovery from croup may be prolonged, with many children suffering from a recurrent coarse cough, particularly at night. In these cases it is considered important to exclude the diagnosis of virally induced asthma.[84]

Information box 5.4d-VIII

Croup: comments from a Chinese medicine perspective

In Chinese medicine, croup may be a result of one or more of the following: Invasion of Wind Heat with Lung and/or Spleen Qi Deficiency, Phlegm and lingering Pathogenic Factor.

Information box 5.4d-IX

Epiglottitis: comments from a Chinese medicine perspective

In Chinese medicine, the rapidity of the development of epiglottitis suggests invasion of Wind Heat leading to obstruction of the Descent of Lung Qi.

Epiglottitis

Epiglottitis refers to acute inflammation of the epiglottis. In children this is almost always due to the bacterium *Hemophilus influenzae* type B (HiB). This incidence of epiglottitis has declined dramatically since the introduction of the HiB vaccine in developed countries in the 1980s and 1990s. In 2010 only 30 invasive cases of HiB were reported, and there were no deaths in that year at all from the disease.[85]

The epiglottis is a flap of cartilage-containing tissue that protects the larynx from the inhalation of food during swallowing. In epiglottitis the swelling of this tissue can threaten to block the opening of the larynx, an event that can be provoked by asking the child to stick out the tongue. The affected child sits upright, is breathless, drooling saliva, reluctant to speak or swallow, and may have a harsh inspiratory stridor (see Figure 5.4d-I). A child with this clinical picture should be treated as an emergency and taken to intensive care facilities so that there is access to tracheal intubation. Intravenous antibiotics are given. With this intensive support, most children recover from this life-threatening condition within three to five days.

Figure 5.4d-I Child sitting upright with acute epiglottitis

Bronchitis and whooping cough (pertussis)

Bronchitis in children, unlike acute bronchitis in adults, is usually the result of a viral infection. It leads to persistent cough and fever, and does not usually respond to antibiotics.

Whooping cough is a highly infectious form of bronchitis caused by the bacterium *Bordetella pertussis*. Infections by this bacterium tend to appear in epidemics once every three to four years in the UK. The symptoms begin with two to three days of runny nose and cough, which then becomes paroxysmal (meaning involving exhausting bouts of recurrent coughing). After a paroxysm of coughing, which is usually worse and more frequent at night, a child with whooping cough characteristically will draw breath with a "whoop." The paroxysms may cause the child to be unable to draw breath, and may result in him or her going blue in the face. Vomiting during a paroxysm is common.

The symptoms of whooping cough can last for up to 12 weeks, during which time the child can become very drained and unwell. Complications of whooping cough include bacterial pneumonia, and long-term lung damage in the form of bronchiectasis. There is a significant risk of death from whooping cough in babies under 12 months old.

Although the infection is bacterial, antibiotic treatment does not seem to affect its course. However, antibiotics may be prescribed to prevent spread of the infection. Immunization is strongly recommended by the medical establishment to prevent the infection. Immunization for whooping cough (usually given as part of the infant vaccination schedule) appears to provide protection against infection in 80–90 percent of those children who are immunized. Immunization campaigns have resulted in a marked drop in the incidence of whooping cough in the community, so providing evidence for its effectiveness in preventing severe infections. Nevertheless, vaccinated individuals can still contract a muted form of the condition, and this can become apparent in the form of a chronic cough.

Information box 5.4d-X

Bronchitis and whooping cough (pertussis): comments from a Chinese medicine perspective

In Chinese medicine, bronchitis corresponds to Phlegm Heat in the Lungs. The onset of whooping cough (pertussis) is a result of an Invasion of Wind Heat/Cold, which leads to impaired descent of Lung Qi. If it develops to a serious condition, it suggests that the child had a predisposition in the form of blocked Spleen Qi (Phlegm or Accumulation Disorder). The Pathogenic Heat and Phlegm can lead to Rising of the Lung Qi, resulting in paroxysmal coughing, expectoration of phlegm and vomiting. Damage to the Lungs can lead to nosebleed and coughing up of blood. Phlegm Heat can obstruct the orifices of the Heart, and so cause collapse and delirium. In the long term, the condition can Deplete Qi and Yin.

Scott and Barlow (1999)[86] propose that whooping cough may be a condition in which the child is trying to throw off a Phlegm pathogen that has been present since the time of birth (akin to the way in which the febrile diseases of childhood are seen to allow the clearance of Heat Toxin). They suggest, with the use of alternative treatment such as acupuncture and herbs early in the infection, that a child genuinely may be strengthened through suffering from the infection. However, they do make the caveat that a child under three years old is at more risk from long-term damage from the copious Phlegm that is produced in the infection. They comment that many children who have recovered from whooping cough have much improved appetites as a result of clearance of Phlegm.

Bronchiolitis

Bronchiolitis is a term used in the UK to describe a viral infection that primarily affects babies under the age of one year. It is common, and affects 2–3 percent of babies to such a degree that they have to be admitted to hospital. The causative virus is the respiratory syncytial virus (RSV) in the majority of cases. In the US the term is also used to describe a condition known in the UK as viral-induced wheeze (see below).

The symptoms of bronchiolitis begin with runny nose and cough, and then progress to breathlessness, wheeze, over-inflation of the chest and a rapid pulse rate. The breathlessness is due to inflammation of the tiny airways of the lungs, the bronchioles.

Most babies have mild symptoms, can be cared for at home and will recover fully within seven to ten days.

A baby with severe bronchiolitis is unable to feed, and is at risk of periods of apnea (cessation of breathing). The baby should be treated in a pediatric intensive care unit with humidified oxygen, and will be monitored for attacks of apnea. Fluids and feeds may be given by means of a nasogastric tube.

Most infants recover fully from the attack, although as many as 50 percent will suffer from recurrent episodes of cough and breathlessness in the few years following the initial episode of bronchiolitis.[87]

Viral-induced wheeze

Bronchiolitis has a clear definition in the UK as describing viral-induced infection of the lower airways. Viral-induced wheeze is a syndrome recognized to affect older children up to the age of three and, in contrast to bronchiolitis, the children do not have the signs that indicate that the lowest parts of the airways have been compromised.

Viral-induced wheeze differs from asthma in that episodes of wheeze seem exclusively linked with coughs and colds and get better after the infection has been cleared. In approximately 50 percent of these children, episodes of viral-induced wheeze presage asthma in later childhood, but others tend to grow out of the vulnerability.

The treatment is supportive or with inhaled beta agonist medication (see "Asthma" in Section 5.4e) in severe cases.

Information box 5.4d-XI

Bronchiolitis and viral-induced wheeze: comments from a Chinese medicine perspective

In Chinese medicine, bronchiolitis and wheeze in young children corresponds to Phlegm or Phlegm Heat in the Lungs following on from an Invasion of Wind Heat or Wind Cold. The Phlegm obstructs the descent of Lung Qi and leads to cough and shortness of breath. Children are vulnerable to Phlegm Damp because of excess Damp-forming foods in a typical Western child's diet (cheese, milk, cold food, orange juice, peanut butter, bananas, sweet foods and bread-based meals). Also, antibiotics predispose to Damp. Lung and Kidney Qi Deficiency resulting from inherited weakness, too little exercise and emotional stress can make the Lungs vulnerable. Latent Pathogenic Heat may be present in the system from previous infectious diseases and the Heat Toxins from vaccination. Invasion of Wind Heat or Wind Cold will exacerbate these imbalances and allow their expression in the Lungs.[88, 89]

Pneumonia

Pneumonia results from infection reaching the air spaces of the lungs, the alveoli. In infancy, pneumonia is most commonly viral in origin, RSV being the most frequent cause. In older children, bacteria and bacteria-like organisms are the most likely pathogens. Common organisms include *Streptococcus pneumoniae, Hemophilus influenzae* and *Mycoplasma pneumoniae.*

The symptoms of pneumonia are similar to those experienced by an adult. Fever, cough and breathlessness, together with marked constitutional malaise, are common. All these may follow on from a mild URTI. In some cases, particularly viral and *Mycoplasma* pneumonia, the symptoms may not be very severe. A child with severe symptoms of pneumonia should be nursed in hospital.

The diagnosis can be confirmed by X-ray examination of the chest. It may be difficult to obtain sputum for bacterial and viral analysis. Blood tests and fluid aspirated from the back of the nose may be required to confirm the cause of the infection.

Antibiotics are always prescribed before the results of the analysis of the infectious agent are known. Usually, a broad-spectrum antibiotic is prescribed to treat a wide range of potential organisms.

Information box 5.4d-XII

Pneumonia: comments from a Chinese medicine perspective

In Chinese medicine, pneumonia is most closely associated with the syndrome of Phlegm Heat in the Lungs (see also Information box 5.4d-XI). Invasion of External Wind is an important etiological factor. In extreme cases Stagnation of Qi in the chest can lead to symptoms and signs of Blood Stasis. Scott and Barlow (1999) suggest that an underlying Deficiency of Qi or Jing is also likely to have predisposed the child to such a serious condition. After recovery, lingering Pathogenic Factor, Yin Deficiency and Lung and Spleen Qi Deficiency may all persist to affect the health of the child.[90]

Other common viral infections of childhood

There is a range of viral infections that more often manifest in a young child rather than an adult. In many of these infections the symptoms are more severe in older children or adults. With the exception of HIV infection, all the infections described below are endemic in Western communities (or used to be before the advent of vaccination). Many of these infections follow a course that is characteristic of the infecting virus, and so can be diagnosed on the basis of signs and symptoms alone. In most of them the disease follows a relatively mild course, and the child recovers with lasting immunity to the infection. This is not necessarily the case if the child is weakened by a condition such as poor nutrition or congenital disease. Much of the infant mortality in some developing countries is the result of viral infections that run a relatively benign course in healthy children. In populations with high levels of malnutrition, up to one in ten unvaccinated children who develop measles die from it.[91]

Measles

Measles (rubeola) is the result of infection by the measles virus. Before the widespread introduction of the measles vaccine in the 1970s, measles used to be a very common infection. However, the reported incidence of measles has dropped dramatically over the past three decades. Measles is a notifiable disease (see below). Doctors should confirm a suspected diagnosis by means of taking saliva samples for analysis.

Measles is contracted by inhalation of infected droplets. Symptoms begin ten to fourteen days after exposure to an infected child. The first symptoms include inflamed eyes, cold symptoms, fever and a cough. The child is infectious from this stage until the cold symptoms have abated. After about two days, characteristic white dots, known as Koplik spots, appear on the inside of the cheek. It is only after three to four days from the onset of the cold symptoms that the measles rash appears. This blotchy, flat, non-itchy, red rash spreads downwards from behind the ears and lasts about seven days (see Figure 5.4d-II). The skin may become scaly towards the end of this time. The fever of measles peaks at around five days after the onset of the symptoms, and may become very high. Most children make a full recovery from measles.

Figure 5.4d-II Blotchy appearance of rash in measles

Other complications of the infection have been reported to occur in 1 in 15 infections. These complications include progression to pneumonia, otitis media, febrile convulsions, diarrhea, ulceration of the cornea of the eye and liver inflammation. All these complications are more likely in poorly nourished and chronically ill children.

In 1 in 5000 reported cases in the West a serious inflammation of the brain called encephalitis occurs.

Over one in ten children who develop measles encephalitis will die as a result. In 1 in 100,000 cases a devastating degenerative condition of the nervous system, known as subacute sclerosing panencephalitis (SSPE), can develop after a delay of up to seven years after an initial infection in a small child. SSPE is believed to be the result of delayed immune-mediated damage. It culminates in total paralysis, dementia and, eventually, death.

Conventional advice is that the child should rest in a darkened room. Vitamin A might be recommended for children who are malnourished. This is known to reduce the severity of the condition.

Measles vaccination is advocated conventionally because of the known risk of serious complications. These are recognized to affect preferentially those children who are seriously ill, such as those with leukemia. There is no doubt that the incidence of serious complications has dropped since the introduction of the vaccination program for measles.

The measles vaccine is a live vaccine, and is recognized to induce a mild form of measles in some recipients. It is generally only available as part of the combined live vaccine (MMR) which contains measles, mumps and rubella vaccines.

 Information box 5.4d-XIII

Measles: comments from a Chinese medicine perspective

Scott and Barlow (1999)[92] state that in Chinese medicine measles is considered to be the result of both Internal and External factors. The view that measles is the result purely of release of Womb Toxin is an ancient belief, dating back to the Song Dynasty (960–1279). By the Ming Dynasty (1368–1644), measles is described as a result of "Womb Toxin combined with seasonal change," and since the Qing Dynasty (1644–1911), measles has been described as "from Womb Toxin, change of season, warm weather and infection."

Measles is currently viewed as a Yang Heat Toxin, which transforms into Heat and Fire deep in the Interior and which readily damages Yin and Fluids. According to Chinese medicine this Toxin enables the expression and clearance of the Internal Pathogenic Heat known as Womb Toxin. The Toxin of measles is described as affecting a range of Yin Organs, including Lung, Spleen, Heat, Pericardium and Liver. This explains the diversity of possible complications of infection. The rash is seen as a good sign, indicating that the Heat has reached the Exterior, and also that Womb Heat is being cleared.[93]

A child will be initially much depleted after an episode of measles, and needs to be encouraged to rest for a few days and eat nourishing warm foods to build up Qi and Yin. In the long run, the child would be expected to be healthier after recovery from an uncomplicated bout of measles as a result of Clearance of Womb Toxin.

Mumps

Mumps also used to be a very common childhood infection in the West, before the introduction of vaccination. Like measles, mumps is a viral infection spread by infected droplets. The incubation period is two to three weeks after exposure. The affected child then develops fever, malaise and swollen, tender parotid salivary glands. The child might complain of earache or difficulty swallowing. In most cases the symptoms subside after three to four days. In some children a prolonged state of tiredness and depression (lasting six to eight weeks) can follow an attack of mumps.

In some cases the pancreas may become inflamed, and this very rarely can lead to frank acute pancreatitis. In boys, the testes may also become inflamed (orchitis). This carries a risk of the very rare complication of infertility in adulthood. In about one in ten cases there are symptoms of a mild form of meningitis. As is the case in measles infection, only in 1 in 5000 cases does a more serious nervous infection, encephalitis, develop.

 Information box 5.4d-XIV

Mumps: comments from a Chinese medicine perspective

In Chinese medicine, mumps is seen as deriving in part from Womb Heat Toxin and in part due to External Wind Heat Toxins invading the Foot Shao Yang (Gallbladder) Channels. The Pathogenic Factor is considered to be Wind Damp Heat. It is a less severe disease than measles, in that it is seen as residing in the Channels rather than the Organs. The Gallbladder Channel has an internal–external relationship with the Liver Channel, thus explaining the possibility of spread to the genitals.

Rubella

Rubella is a mild childhood disease. It is transmitted by infected droplets, and has an incubation period of two to three weeks. It begins with a mild fever, which is followed by the development of a fine rash that starts on the face and body and then spreads to involve the limbs. The rash is non-itchy and fades after three to five days. Swollen lymph nodes are common, and may be found in the sub-occipital region in particular.

Complications of rubella are rare in childhood. They include persistent joint pains and encephalitis. The major concern about the infection is its profound effect during the first trimester of pregnancy, and the fact that it very often leads to the constellation of congenital defects known as congenital rubella syndrome (CRS). Widespread rubella vaccination has been followed by a significant reduction in CRS.

Information box 5.4d-XV

Rubella: comments from a Chinese medicine perspective

In Chinese medicine, rubella in the child is usually a mild condition, the manifestation of which might be considered to exclude the expulsion of Womb Heat Toxin. The Toxic nature of the pathogen is most apparent in maternal infection in which profound damage to the Essence of the unborn child may be engendered. Thus the rubella infection might be seen as a trigger for Womb Toxin that has the power to cause great Deficiency in the unborn child.

Herpes simplex virus (HSV) infection

The most common herpes simplex virus (HSV) infection in childhood is the cold sore. HSV can also cause more widespread infection of the mouth (gingivostomatitis), and can cause a serious complication of skin diseases in which there are broken areas of skin such as eczema (eczema herpeticum). Infection of the eye can lead to severe ulceration of the cornea. In adults, genital infection can lead to genital herpes (see Section 5.2d). The diagnosis of genital herpes in a child should always raise the suspicion of sexual abuse.

Very rarely, HSV can cause a very severe form of encephalitis, which has a mortality of 70 percent, and carries a high risk of permanent memory loss and disturbance of brain function in those who recover.

There are two main types of HSV, namely, HSV1 and HSV2. HSV1 is mainly transmitted through saliva and HSV2 through a wide range of genital secretions. HSV1 is the class of HSV that is most commonly found in childhood infections. It is transmitted by close physical contact. In most children the primary infection is in the mouth. This infection may be without symptoms. In some children this primary infection can lead to the

severe condition of gingivostomatitis, in which there is widespread ulceration of the lining of the mouth (see Figure 5.4d-III). In a severe case the child has a high fever and is reluctant to eat or drink. In some cases hospital admission is necessary to provide intravenous fluids.

Figure 5.4d-III Primary infection with herpes simplex virus (HSV) (gingivostomatitis)

Cold sores are recurrent outbreaks of the virus that appear on the lips or the nose following a primary infection of the mouth. They are more likely to appear when the child has a fever, is run down or following exposure to intense sunlight.

In early severe cases of HSV infection the symptoms may be less severe if the patient is given the antiviral drug aciclovir. In usual practice, oral aciclovir is given only in cases of encephalitis or infections in immunocompromised children. Topical aciclovir may be prescribed for recurrent cold sores.

Information box 5.4d-XVI

Gingivostomatitis and cold sores: comments from a Chinese medicine perspective

In Chinese medicine, gingivostomatitis corresponds to Full Heat in the Stomach and Spleen. Cold sores represent Wind Damp Heat.

Chickenpox and shingles

Chickenpox and shingles result from infection by the varicella zoster virus, a virus that is related to HSV. Chickenpox is contracted by inhalation of infected droplets that originate from the mucous membranes of an infected individual, and also from the fluid-containing spots (vesicles) of the rash of chickenpox or shingles. Children are infectious up to two days before the onset of the rash, which usually starts on the scalp or the trunk, only later spreading to involve the limbs. In severe cases, the mucous membranes of the mouth and genitalia can be affected.

The rash is typically slightly raised (maculopapular) and consists of crops of sometimes intensely itchy, fluid-filled vesicles that enlarge, burst and then crust over. In young children severe generalized illness is unusual. However, adults can become very unwell, with fever, cough and, in severe cases, pneumonia. In both adults and children, the rash can become complicated by bacterial infection, in which case scarring of the infected vesicles is more likely. Most children recover fully from the infection, and then usually have lasting immunity to the disease.

Chickenpox encephalitis is an extremely rare complication that occurs three to six days after the onset of the rash.

One important medical concern relating to children with chickenpox is that they are infectious and may confer a risk to vulnerable or pregnant individuals with whom they have close contact. All carers of children with chickenpox should be advised of the risk of transmission of chickenpox in pregnancy, which is believed to be greatest from two days before the onset of the rash to five days after its first appearance. Chicken pox in pregnancy is potentially a very serious condition. A pregnant woman is more vulnerable to a severe form of the disease, with a higher risk of pneumonia and encephalitis. The unborn baby is vulnerable to fetal varicella syndrome if exposed to the virus in the 1st and 2nd trimesters in particular. This can lead to limb, eye and skin deformities and impaired brain development. If the mother has active disease at the time of labor, the baby may be born with an overwhelming chickenpox infection that has a high risk of fatality.

The treatment of chickenpox is usually supportive, although in severe adult cases, aciclovir may be prescribed. A vaccination does exist for chickenpox, but in the UK it is not currently routinely recommended in children. However, in other Western countries, chickenpox vaccination forms part of the routine childhood schedule of vaccinations, and is mandatory for school entry in all 50 states of the US.[94]

If a pregnant woman who is not already immune to chickenpox (and most women are immune in the UK) is exposed to a child with chickenpox, she needs to be medically assessed to discuss whether she should be given a form of immunization called varicella immune globulin. A patient needs to be referred for advice without delay after possible exposure so treatment may be given as soon as possible.

After infection, the varicella zoster virus can reactivate after lying dormant in the nervous system for some years. In its reactivated form, the rash of varicella zoster is usually limited to the distribution of a sensory dermatome on one side of the body. This gives rise to the localized strip of redness and crusting that is characteristic of shingles (see Figure 5.4d-IV). Shingles is unusual in childhood.

Figure 5.4d-IV Shingles scattered on the back of the leg along the distribution of the first sacral nerve (S1) dermatome

 Information box 5.4d-XVII

Chickenpox and shingles: comments from a Chinese medicine perspective

In Chinese medicine, chickenpox corresponds to an Invasion of Wind Heat Damp. Shingles corresponds to an Invasion of the Channels by Wind Heat or Wind Damp. When developed in pregnancy, the transmitted Heat Toxin has the potential of damaging the Essence of the unborn child.

Infectious mononucleosis (glandular fever)

Glandular fever is a disease that results from infection by the Epstein-Barr virus (EBV). This virus is a relation of the herpes simplex and varicella zoster viruses. The infection is contracted by droplet spread, and requires close physical contact. Most infections that are contracted through childhood and adolescence lead at most to a mild flu-like illness from which the child fully recovers. Over 90 percent of children will have developed antibodies to EBV by the end of their adolescence, and most of these will not have suffered from glandular fever, which is described below.

In some children the infection leads to a syndrome involving fever, malaise, tonsillitis and widespread enlargement of the lymph nodes. This is the syndrome that is diagnosed as glandular fever or "infectious mono." In some cases the tonsils may become so enlarged as to obstruct swallowing and threaten the airway. In severe infections the liver and spleen may also enlarge and become tender. Jaundice may develop if the liver becomes significantly inflamed. There may be a fine rash of reddened spots. If the child is given amoxicillin during this period (to treat suspected bacterial tonsillitis), the chances of the rash developing are greatly increased. Glandular fever is more common in older children and adolescents. It may affect a child during a time of stress, such as when taking examinations.

In severe cases the symptoms may persist for some weeks, and the child may become very tired. Glandular fever is one of the most well-recognized precursors of the prolonged syndrome currently described as chronic fatigue syndrome (CFS) (formerly described as myalgic encephalomyelitis (ME)). Symptoms of chronic fatigue, by definition, must have persisted for more than six months before the description of CFS is used.

Glandular fever is diagnosed by means of examination of a blood film, and by testing for characteristic antibodies (relying on the Monospot test and Paul Bunnell reaction, respectively). Treatment of glandular fever is usually supportive. Rest during the symptomatic phase is recommended. Occasionally, corticosteroids may be given to reduce the inflammation of grossly enlarged tonsils. Antibiotics should only be given if a throat swab demonstrates the presence of *Streptococcus*, but amoxicillin should always be avoided.

Information box 5.4d-XVIII

Infectious mononucleosis (glandular fever): comments from a Chinese medicine perspective

In its acute form, infectious mononucleosis presents like an uncomplicated upper respiratory disease such as flu or tonsillitis, and may actually not be recognized as any different from these conditions. It would be seen as a Wen Bing or epidemic fever, and is the result of exogenous Wind Heat or Wind Cold leading to emergence of Heat Toxin in the body. In severe cases the Heat Toxin can consume Yin and Blood and cause severe acute disease and chronic exhaustion.

Scott and Barlow (1999)[95] list three syndromes that may underlie glandular fever: Liver Qi Stagnation, lingering Pathogenic Factor and Yin Deficiency. They suggest that Stagnant Liver Qi may exacerbate the Heat and Stagnation of Fluids, and thus the formation of Phlegm in the Channels. This is the etiology of the swollen lymph nodes and tonsils. Lingering Heat, Pathogenic Factor and Yin Deficiency may all coexist to promote the formation of Phlegm and recurrent lymph node swelling. They add that, in some cases, and particularly those in which a rash is evident, the condition may also serve a function in the expulsion of Womb Heat Toxin.

Cytomegalovirus (CMV) infections

Cytomegalovirus (CMV) is a virus from the same family as HSV, varicella zoster virus and EBV. Like EBV, CMV is a very common pathogen in children, usually leading to a very mild, flu-like illness. In rare cases it can lead to a glandular fever-like syndrome, with widespread enlargement of the lymph nodes and malaise. It, too, can be the precursor of CFS.

CMV can cause much more serious disease in immunocompromised children and adults. It is also very harmful in pregnancy when it leads to fetal infection. This results in inflammation of a wide range of internal organs, leading to encephalitis, hepatitis, esophagitis, colitis and inflammation of the retina. Serious CMV infection can be treated with antiviral medication.

 ### Information box 5.4d-XIX

Cytomegalovirus infection: comments from a Chinese medicine perspective

In Chinese medicine, the glandular fever-like syndrome that may follow CMV infection follows a similar pattern to that of glandular fever. Unlike infectious mononucleosis, CMV is a very harmful Heat Toxin in pregnancy, in some cases leading to damage to the Essence of the unborn child.

Roseola infantum

Roseola infantum (exanthem subitum) is a common cause of fever and rash in children caused by the human herpes virus 6 (HHV6). The main symptom of infection is high fever lasting two to three days, followed in some children by a generalized red rash. Most children recover fully from the infection, although it may be the cause of febrile convulsions in some. Very rarely, the virus can cause a mild form of meningitis and encephalitis.

Information box 5.4d-XX

Roseola infantum: comments from a Chinese medicine perspective

In Chinese medicine, the fever and rash of roseola infantum corresponds to an Invasion of Wind Heat. Like rubella, it may serve a function in the expulsion of Womb Heat Toxin.

Slapped cheek syndrome (parvovirus infection)

Slapped cheek syndrome (erythema infectiosum) is a condition that results from infection by parvovirus B19. Infection usually leads to a very mild illness, but in some children gives rise to a syndrome involving fever, headache, muscle aches and malaise for a few days. This is followed by a characteristic facial rash during the recovery period. The rash can progress to form a lace-like reddening of the skin of the trunk and the limbs. Most children will recover fully from this infection. A minority may develop a persistent syndrome of symmetrical joint pains that might take a few weeks to resolve.

Up to 60 percent of adults in the West are immune to this prevalent virus.

Parvovirus in non-immune pregnant women is a serious infection, which can cause the death of the fetus (fetal hydrops). For this reason, children with slapped cheek syndrome should be kept at home until they recover from the infection, and women who develop a rash in pregnancy should be referred promptly to have investigations to exclude parvovirus.

Information box 5.4d-XXI

Slapped cheek syndrome (parvovirus infection): comments from a Chinese medicine perspective

In Chinese medicine, the energetic interpretation of slapped cheek syndrome is similar to that of rubella and roseola infantum. Like rubella, parvovirus can be a harmful Heat Toxin in pregnancy, and lead to the death of the unborn child.

Enterovirus infections

The enteroviruses are a group of viruses that include coxsackie viruses A and B and echovirus. They are common causes of childhood infections, most of which are mild and non-specific. The viruses are spread by the feco-oral (hand to mouth) route rather than by droplet spread. Infections are most common in the summer and autumn. This is in contrast to the viral infections described above, which are transmitted by droplet spread, and most of which peak in the winter months.

Common specific conditions that result from enterovirus infections include herpangina, hand, foot and mouth disease and Bornholm disease.

Herpangina is a syndrome of small painful ulcers in the mouth, which may cause loss of appetite, pain on swallowing and fever. Clinically it is indistinguishable from a mild primary infection with HSV (see above).

Information box 5.4d-XXII

Herpangina: comments from a Chinese medicine perspective

In Chinese medicine, painful oral ulcers (herpangina) correspond to a diagnosis of Heat or Damp Heat in the Stomach and Spleen. Ulcers on the tongue tip correspond to Heat in the Heart.

Hand, foot and mouth disease is not the same as foot and mouth disease. It is a mild condition in which painful, fluid-filled spots erupt on the hands, feet, mouth and tongue. It usually subsides within a few days.

Information box 5.4d-XXIII

Hand, foot and mouth disease: comments from a Chinese medicine perspective

The generalized vesicular rash of hand, foot and mouth disease has some similarities to mild chickenpox. In the same way, this would be diagnosed as an Invasion of Wind Heat Damp. The mouth ulcers correspond to Heat or Damp Heat in the Stomach and Spleen. Ulcers on the tongue tip correspond to Heat in the Heart.

Bornholm disease (pleurodynia) is an inflammation of the joints between the sternum and ribs (costochondritis). The child will have a fever and complain of chest pain, which may be worse on deep inspiration (pleuritic pain). It is important to distinguish this mild condition from the more serious conditions that can also cause pleuritic pain – pericarditis and pleurisy. The child will usually recover fully within a few days.

>
> ### Information box 5.4d-XXIV
>
> **Bornholm disease: comments from a Chinese medicine perspective**
>
> In Chinese medicine, Bornholm disease may correspond to Heat and Stagnation in the Channels that have their course in the region of the pain (Kidney and Stomach, usually).

Poliomyelitis

Poliomyelitis (polio) is also caused by an enterovirus. The condition is very rare in developed countries, as a consequence of widespread immunization. Poliomyelitis is discussed in Section 4.1g.

Viral gastroenteritis and rotavirus

Gastroenteritis is described in detail in Section 3.1c. In children, the most common cause of gastroenteritis is viral infection, rotavirus being the most common infectious agent. Viral gastroenteritis in children is highly contagious, not least because it is difficult with children to minimize close physical contact with other people, and also to maintain scrupulous hygiene. Prior to the introduction of the rotavirus oral vaccine, studies showed that 100 percent of children aged five had already developed immunity to the virus through infection.

Although usually a self-limiting illness in the West, worldwide rotavirus is the cause of 5 percent of deaths in children younger than five.

The rotavirus vaccine was introduced in the UK in 2013 to prevent the serious disease that can be caused by rotavirus gastroenteritis in vulnerable children and infants. Prior to the vaccine being introduced, there were approximately 18,000 hospital admissions per year of young children for the treatment of dehydration resulting from rotavirus infections. The vaccine is thought to prevent between 85 and 100 percent of severe infections in the West.[96]

Symptoms include vomiting, diarrhea, abdominal pain and fever. Dehydration is the most serious concern with children, and in particular, with babies. In most cases the symptoms resolve spontaneously, but in severe cases children may need to be admitted to hospital to receive intravenous fluids.

>
> ### Information box 5.4d-XXV
>
> **Gastroenteritis: comments from a Chinese medicine perspective**
>
> In Chinese medicine, the symptoms of gastroenteritis usually correspond to an Invasion of Damp or Damp Heat in the Intestines. In children, imbalances such as Stomach and Spleen Deficiency, Cold in the Stomach or Accumulation Disorder may cause the child to be susceptible to a severe episode of gastroenteritis.

Viral hepatitis

Viral hepatitis is discussed in detail in Section 3.1d. Infectious hepatitis (hepatitis A), which is now uncommon in the UK, is transmitted by the feco-oral route. Children tend to suffer from a much more mild form of the disease, and then develop lasting immunity.

Hepatitis B is usually contracted in childhood either from an infected mother during pregnancy and breastfeeding, or by close physical contact with an infectious family member. Although many infections contracted in childhood do not lead to inflammation of the liver, development of the carrier state puts the child at risk of chronic liver disease and liver cancer in later life. Hepatitis B infection in childhood is rare in the UK, but is relatively common in countries such as Indonesia and Taiwan, in which a high proportion of the general population are carriers of the hepatitis B virus.

Hepatitis C is not as readily transmitted during pregnancy and breastfeeding as hepatitis B. In the UK, most cases of childhood hepatitis C result from receiving contaminated blood products. However, this risk has been minimized since the development of screening tests for the hepatitis viruses in blood products.

EBV infection (see under "Infectious mononucleosis (glandular fever)" above) may also be a cause of hepatitis.

> ### Information box 5.4d-XXVI
>
> **Hepatitis: comments from a Chinese medicine perspective**
>
> In Chinese medicine, the symptoms of hepatitis may correspond to an Invasion of Damp Heat in the Liver, Gallbladder and Spleen.

Warts and molluscum contagiosum

Warts are the result of a local infection by the human papilloma virus (HPV). Usually, bodily warts are caused by different strains of HPV to those that cause genital warts, and in particular, to the strain that is implicated in the genesis of cervical cancer. Warts in children are common in areas such as the palms, soles and knees, where the skin is repeatedly exposed to minor trauma. A wart is a virally induced overgrowth of the cells of the epidermis.

A verruca is a wart that has developed on the pressure-bearing part of the sole. Weight bearing causes the verruca to become pressed flat into the skin of the sole. Like a stone in the shoe, the ingrowing verruca can be painful.

A wart or verruca may grow rapidly over the course of a few weeks, or may be indolent in growth, appearing slowly over a period of a few years. Warts can appear as solitary growths or in crops. They can disappear suddenly without treatment, which may be the reason for the magical qualities with which they have been attributed in folklore. This phenomenon, which can be seen to affect a whole crop of warts at the same time, is believed to be a result of an immune response that may have been triggered following minor damage to the warts.

Warts are infectious, but it is doubtful whether their removal actually reduces the transmission of the virus, as it is endemic in the community. The exception to this may be transmission in swimming pools, at which there is a general expectation that verrucae should be covered to prevent transmission of the virus.

As treatment can be inconvenient and painful, and because warts usually resolve spontaneously, medical treatment for warts is usually restricted to those children for whom the wart is causing pain or has become a cosmetic problem. Warts and verrucae can be treated daily by the application of salicylic acid (aspirin) paint or glutaraldehyde. They can also be damaged by a freezing spray of liquid nitrogen, but this is a painful (burning) treatment. It is likely that both these approaches work by causing sufficient damage to the wart to stimulate the natural immune response of the body. Occlusion of the wart 24 hours a day with waterproof tape is another effective treatment that requires perseverance.

Molluscum contagiosum is another contagious wart condition, which causes crops of pearly lumps on the skin (see Figure 5.4d-V). It usually affects a very young child. The spots will usually disappear within a year. Lasting immunity is likely to follow the disappearance of the spots, as they rarely recur. Molluscum spots can also be treated by means of damage; this can be in the form of injection with phenol or the application of a spray of liquid nitrogen. However, this is not a very practical approach in the treatment of a small child with multiple molluscum spots. Most doctors recommend parents to leave well alone, and to let the condition take its natural, albeit prolonged, course.

Figure 5.4d-V Pearly papules of molluscum contagiosum on the chest and upper arm

 Information box 5.4d-XXVII

Viral warts: comments from a Chinese medicine perspective

From a Chinese medicine viewpoint, Scott and Barlow (1999) suggest that warts will only grow in the presence of Damp.[97] This fits with the observation that they are commonly contracted at swimming pools. The position of the warts is an indication of the location of the Damp. Warts on the hand suggest Damp in the Spleen and Lungs, and verrucae suggest Damp in the Spleen and Kidneys. Chinese medical treatments can include local burning of the wart by moxibustion or topical herbs such as aloe and calendula, but also with treatment to boost the Upright Qi, as it is recognized that it is Deficiency, particularly of Spleen and Lung, which has allowed the Pathogen to invade. Flaws (2006) suggests that the form of the wart can inform more about the pathology. A dry, cracked surface can suggest underlying Blood Deficiency as well as Spleen Deficiency, and marked nodularity the presence of Phlegm. Occlusion of warts will tend to cause inflammation of the wart as the Damp is exacerbated and turns to Heat.[98] In children warts tend to disappear as the Spleen matures.

HIV infection and AIDS

Like hepatitis B, HIV infection in childhood is usually contracted from an infected mother, either during pregnancy or through breastfeeding. In Europe, approximately 15 percent of babies born to infected mothers will become infected. The infection rate has been estimated as being much higher in those developing countries in which HIV infection is endemic. In contrast to hepatitis B, transmission of HIV from an infected parent to a non-infected child is less likely to occur at a later stage.

It is now well recognized that transmission to a baby is potentially preventable if the HIV infection is diagnosed during pregnancy and the mother is first treated with antiviral medication, and does not then breastfeed the baby. HIV testing in pregnancy is now performed routinely in the UK.

Infected children may remain without symptoms for many months or years before progressing to the acquired immune deficiency syndrome (AIDS). First symptoms of AIDS include lymph node enlargement, recurrent bacterial infections, oral thrush, diarrhea and respiratory infections. Opportunistic infections and involvement of the nervous system are features of severe disease.

Children with HIV infection are treated in a similar way to adults with the disease (see Section 5.2d). They require early treatment with combined antiretroviral medication and regular medical review, even before the development of AIDS. The management of the condition is often complicated by the fact that one or both of the parents are also HIV-positive.

In established AIDS, aggressive treatment of infections is considered essential.

The use of combined antiviral drugs will delay the progression of the disease, but it is not known yet for how long this control of the infection can be sustained.

 Information box 5.4d-XXVIII

HIV infection and AIDS in children: comments from a Chinese medicine perspective

The Chinese medicine interpretation of HIV infection, as a modern disease, cannot be drawn from the classic texts, but established AIDS has many of the features of cancer.

The initial infection in adults has the features of an Invasion of Wind Heat Damp. The development of AIDS suggests that this Toxic Heat Pathogen has penetrated into the Interior to damage the Organs. Immune deficiency resulting from the deterioration of the function of the white blood cells (T leukocytes) in the marrow corresponds to severe Kidney Deficiency, which is presumably a result of this initial insult. The lymph node enlargement, infections and tumors that characterize AIDS correspond to a combination of Phlegm, Damp, Heat and Blood Stagnation, all of which may have accumulated as a consequence of the Kidney Deficiency and also Spleen Deficiency.

Treatment principles in HIV infection in infants and children would be the same and so would include clearance of Heat and Damp-Phlegm, movement of Stagnation and support of the Upright Qi and Spleen and Kidney function.

Staphylococcal and Streptococcal infections

The *Streptococcus* and the *Staphylococcus* are families of bacteria from the class of bacteria known as *cocci*, which is characterized by a spherical shape when viewed under the microscope. Both types of bacteria are potentially pathogenic when they develop an ability to penetrate the bodily tissues, and because they can release substances that are toxic to the tissues. They both readily induce the formation of pus, which can complicate infections, as its presence in excess may impair the full resolution of inflammation. Nevertheless both families can be found as significant contributors to the human microbiome. It is not clear how certain strains of *cocci* are pathogenic in one individual and remain harmless to another. Certain strains are more associated with disease and these include *Staphylococcus aureus*, *Staphylococcus epidermidis* and Group A *Streptococci*.

The complications of infections by the *cocci* are usually readily treated because most strains of both types are sensitive to certain antibiotics. However, there is increasing concern that the overuse of antibiotics for both medical and agricultural reasons has promoted the development of antibiotic-resistant strains of the *cocci* (and, of course, other types of bacteria). Methicillin-resistant *Staphylococcus aureus* (MRSA) is an example of a strain of *Staphylococcus* that is able to multiply in the presence of all the commonly prescribed antibiotics. Colonization by this strain usually does not harm a healthy individual, but can be the cause of a life-threatening and untreatable condition in someone who is immunocompromised.

The Group A *Streptococcus* bacteria can be the cause of tonsillitis and pharyngitis. Streptococcal infections may rarely be followed within three to four weeks by a damaging immune response to the infection. Rheumatic fever and Bright's disease are two now very rare conditions that are recognized to be post-streptococcal.

Invasive group A streptococcal (IGAS) infections can be particularly severe in vulnerable individuals, and are causative in two potentially life-threatening conditions – necrotizing fasciitis and streptococcal toxic shock syndrome. Both these conditions are a result of toxins released by the multiplying IGAS bacteria.

Impetigo

Impetigo is a crusting infection of the skin that may be caused by strains of *Streptococcus* or *Staphylococcus*. It is common in children in whom close physical contact and minor injuries are features of everyday life. In many cases it presents as a small area of yellowish crusting affecting an area of cracked or damp skin (e.g. in eczema). The skin around the mouth and nostrils is a common site for impetigo (see Figure 5.4d-VI). Although it can resolve without treatment, impetigo can spread to cause an enlarging area of crusting and new areas of infection on other parts of the body. It can be highly contagious.

Small areas of impetigo may be treated by means of topical antibiotic creams, but a child with more extensive disease might be prescribed oral antibiotic therapy.

Figure 5.4d-VI The crusting rash of impetigo

Information box 5.4d-XXIX

Impetigo: comments from a Chinese medicine perspective

In Chinese medicine, impetigo corresponds to Damp Heat. Spleen Deficiency with Damp and Heat (Accumulation Disorder of childhood) may predispose to the development of impetigo.

Boils

Boils are usually the result of multiplication of a strain of *Staphylococcus* that is found in the normal skin microbiome. Recurrent boils suggest that the child is run down in some way. A diagnosis of diabetes mellitus or immune deficiency should be considered and excluded.

Large boils may be treated by lancing to remove the pus, and then by means of oral antibiotics.

Information box 5.4d-XXX

Boils: comments from a Chinese medicine perspective

In Chinese medicine, boils correspond to Damp Heat or Fire Poison.

Scarlet fever (scarlatina)

Scarlet fever is an unusual consequence of a streptococcal infection such as sore throat or tonsillitis. It develops two to four days after the initial infection, as a result of the formation of a particular toxin by the *Streptococcus*. Scarlet fever used to be a common childhood disease, and carried

the risk of being complicated by rheumatic fever and glomerulonephritis (Bright's disease). However, it is far less common nowadays, and when it does develop, it does not usually lead to serious complications. Doctors may call this less severe presentation of scarlet fever scarlatina to make it clear to patients that this is a mild disease.

In the severe form of disease the scarlet fever toxin leads to a syndrome of enlarged lymph nodes, high fever and severe malaise. Headache and vomiting are common, and so the illness may initially be suspected to be meningitis. After a day or so of these symptoms, a characteristic red rash of tiny spots appears, spreading down from the neck to involve most of the whole body, with the exception of the region around the mouth and nose, the palms and the soles. During this time the tongue develops a thick white coating, with prominent red spots on the body (strawberry tongue). Later on in the illness the white coating disappears to leave a bright red, raw appearance (raspberry tongue). After a few days, the skin starts to peel extensively. The treatment is with a ten-day course of penicillin. A patient with scarlet fever is highly contagious for up to three weeks after the initial infection. For this reason, children with this erstwhile dreaded disease used to be nursed in conditions of strict isolation.

In scarlatina the child may have a high fever and sore throat and develop the characteristic rash, but otherwise may not be too unwell. Scarlet fever and scarlatina are notifiable diseases (see below).

Information box 5.4d-XXXI

Scarlet fever: comments from a Chinese medicine perspective

In Chinese medicine, the symptoms of scarlet fever correspond to an epidemic fever, and symptoms result from acute Invasion by Wind Heat or Wind Damp Heat together with emergence of Fetal Toxin. Scaling of the skin is suggestive of Damp. The peeled, red tongue and scaling of the skin that appear at the end of the condition suggest that the Heat has depleted Yin. In severe cases there can be meningitis or myocarditis, both indications of severe Damage to Qi and Yin. The rare long-term complications of rheumatic heart disease and glomerulonephritis likewise suggest damage to Qi and Yin resulting from Lingering Pathogenic Factor. It is therefore very important that a child with scarlet fever is encouraged to rest and recover from the infection.

Scalded skin syndrome

Some strains of *Staphylococcus* release a toxin that causes rapid separation of the layers of the epidermis of the skin, causing the skin to appear scalded (see Figure 5.4d-VII). This serious infection affects babies and infants. There is a risk of dehydration from the exposed areas of dermis. The affected child should be nursed in hospital, where the child can receive intravenous antibiotics and fluids.

Figure 5.4d-VII Blistering in scalded skin syndrome

 Information box 5.4d-XXXII

Scalded skin syndrome: comments from a Chinese medicine perspective

In Chinese medicine, scalded skin syndrome equates to an Invasion of Wind Damp Heat.

Toxic shock syndrome

This syndrome became notorious when a number of cases resulted from the use of infected tampons in the 1970s. However, it was first described in children. It is the result of a release of a toxin from a strain of IGAS. The primary infection may be situated anywhere in the body, including the skin. In a severe infection, the toxin causes severe systemic illness, involving fever, rash, shock and organ failure. The patient should be treated as an emergency and given intravenous antibiotics and fluids. On recovery, the skin of the palms, soles, fingers and toes can be seen to peel.

 Information box 5.4d-XXXIII

Toxic shock syndrome: comments from a Chinese medicine perspective

In Chinese medicine, toxic shock syndrome corresponds to Pathogenic Heat that has penetrated to the Interior so that it damages the Yin and the Organs. The peeling of the skin that occurs in the recovery stage is a sign of the Heat and Damp moving outwards to the Exterior.

Kawasaki disease

Kawasaki disease is a serious modern non-contagious disease of children, first described in the 1960s. Its cause is still unclear, although it does have some similarities to toxic shock syndrome, suggesting that it might result from an unusual immune reaction to a bacterial toxin. Kawasaki disease is more common in children of Asian background, and it mainly affects young children between six months and four years of age. This incidence of Kawasaki disease continues to rise in Japan. It has overtaken rheumatic fever in being the most significant infective cause of heart disease.

The disease begins with high fever, dry inflamed mucous membranes, conjunctivitis and enlarged lymph nodes. After a few days, a vague, blotchy rash may be seen, and then after a few further days, peeling of the skin on the hands and feet occurs, as is seen in toxic shock syndrome (see Figure 5.4d-VIII). More seriously, inflammatory changes affect the large blood vessels of the body during the course of the disease. In particular, the coronary arteries can become affected, and can develop both aneurysms and areas of narrowing. Death can then result from thrombosis and ischemia of the cardiac muscle.

Figure 5.4d-VIII Red cracked lips and conjunctivitis in Kawasaki disease

Treatment includes injections of gamma globulin, a drug that modulates the immune response. This seems to prevent the deterioration in the structure of the coronary arteries. Aspirin is given to prevent thrombosis.

The recovery period is very long and drawn out for this potentially devastating illness, but after two years vascular damage has recovered in the majority of children who have survived the acute illness. Medical treatment with immunoglobulin has dramatically improved the outlook of this disease by inhibiting the formation of vascular aneurysms.

Information box 5.4d-XXXIV

Kawasaki disease: comments from a Chinese medicine perspective

The energetic interpretation of this rare condition corresponds to that described for toxic shock syndrome. The Heat Toxic is extremely pathogenic; vascular aneurysms and myocardial infarction correspond to Qi and Yin Deficiency and Blood Stagnation. Individual susceptibility is key to the development of the disease that indicates that Deficiency of Essence plays a role in etiology.

Urinary tract infection in childhood

Urinary tract infections in childhood are to be taken seriously, as they may point to a serious underlying abnormality of the urinary tract, and can also be the cause of progressive kidney disease (chronic pyelonephritis) (see Sections 4.3c and 4.3d).

Cystitis

It is estimated that up to 3 percent of girls and 1 percent of boys have an episode of urinary infection (cystitis) before the age of 11. Over half of these have recurrent infections. It is considered important that children with urinary symptoms are referred for investigation, as up to half of these may have a structural abnormality of the urinary tract (leading to vesico-ureteric reflux disease (VUR)). VUR can allow bacteria in the bladder to ascend the ureters, and damage the delicate structure of one or both of the kidneys. Cystitis is described in detail in Section 4.3d.

Vesico-ureteric reflux disease (VUR) and pyelonephritis

VUR is a result of a relatively common congenital abnormality of the vesico-ureteric junction. This abnormality tends to run in families. VUR becomes a problem in small children when the urine in the bladder is infected, as it permits passage of bacteria to the kidneys. Chronic infection of the kidneys can lead to the progressive condition of chronic pyelonephritis. Many children will grow out of the problem of VUR as their bladder enlarges with normal growth, and so early treatment in childhood can prevent long-term kidney damage. This condition is described in detail in Section 4.3c.

 Information box 5.4d-XXXV

Acute cystitis and vesico-ureteric reflux disease: comments from a Chinese medicine perspective

In Chinese medicine, acute cystitis corresponds to Invasion of Damp Heat or Damp Cold into the Bladder. Once in the Bladder, the Pathogen appears to transform into Damp Heat.

Scott and Barlow (1999) suggest that the Pathogen may originate from the External environment, but may also originate from Heat in the Liver and Gallbladder or Damp Heat in the Stomach and Intestines.

Recurrent or chronic urinary infections (including those resulting from VUR) may have one or both of Spleen and Kidney Yang Deficiency or Kidney Yin Deficiency as the underlying imbalance.

Lingering Pathogenic Factor can manifest in the form of urine infections.

Jing Deficiency would, of course, be at the root of these conditions in children with a congenital abnormality.[99]

Notifiable diseases

Notifiable diseases (see also Section 2.4d) are those infections that doctors are obliged professionally to report for the purposes of nationwide disease surveillance. This requirement, which is considered to transcend any obligations on the doctor to maintain confidentiality about a diagnosis, exists because of the significant impact the notifiable diseases are believed to have on the health of the community.

Disease notifications allow the incidence of a disease and its impact to be assessed year by year. They can be very useful in the management of an outbreak of a potentially serious disease such as food poisoning. They can also help to assess the success, or otherwise, of a vaccination program. The notifiable diseases in the UK include all those diseases that are targeted by the current childhood immunization program. Many of the remaining notifiable diseases are not endemic in the UK, and these include serious tropical diseases such as malaria, typhoid fever and the viral hemorrhagic fevers.

Unlike doctors, complementary therapists are not bound by a professional code of conduct to report notifiable diseases. However, it is reasonable to propose that all healthcare workers should become aware of the features of those notifiable diseases that they are likely to encounter in their practice. If a child is demonstrating features of a notifiable disease, the practitioner could then advise a visit to their physician for a confirmation of the diagnosis (accompanied by an appropriate referral letter). In this way the diagnosis would be confirmed, and the episode reported. It is arguable that to refer for this reason would be in the best interests of the community at large.

See Table 2.4d-II for a list of the notifiable diseases in the UK.

5.4e Other common disorders of childhood

This section is a summary of those common conditions of childhood that have not been described either in the earlier sections of this stage or elsewhere in this book.

The section begins with a review of the common disorders of babies and children. Although most of these conditions are not serious in terms of their impact on the long-term health of a child, they can be a source of great concern to parents. Together, they account for a significant proportion of the consultations made by parents of small children with community pediatricians and child health nurses. For many of these conditions, great benefit can result from a combination of careful explanation, reassurance and simple advice. There follows a summary of some of the more serious conditions of childhood. Note that a few of the most important childhood conditions, such as meningitis, diabetes and congenital heart disease, which are very significant in terms of their impact on children's health, are not listed here simply because they have been described in sufficient detail in other sections.

This section is divided into two parts that are designed to be studied in separate study periods. The conditions discussed here are:

Part I: Other common disorders of childhood

- Common minor problems of babies and children:
  - colic and crying
  - feeding problems in babies
  - teething
  - toddler diarrhea
  - constipation and soiling
  - sleep problems
  - bed-wetting
  - tantrums and disobedience
  - minor skin disorders in babies and small children
- Disorders of growth and puberty:
  - failure to thrive (FTT)

- short stature
- tall stature
- precocious puberty
- delayed puberty
- intersex disorders

- Disorders of the digestive system:
  - recurrent abdominal pain
  - mesenteric adenitis
  - intussusception
  - appendicitis
  - gastroenteritis
  - celiac disease
  - inflammatory bowel disease

Part II: Other common disorders of childhood continued

- Disorders of the respiratory system:
  - asthma
  - sudden infant death syndrome (SIDS)
- Disorders of the urinary system and genitalia:
  - inherited malformations of the urinary tract
  - balanitis and phimosis
  - torsion of the testis
- Disorders of the eyes, ears and nervous system:
  - squint
  - glue ear
  - epilepsy
- Cancer in childhood:
  - leukemia and lymphoma
  - brain tumors
  - neuroblastoma
  - Wilms' tumor
  - bone and muscle tumors
  - retinoblastoma
  - germ cell tumors
- Skin disorders (see Section 6.1c)
- Psychiatric developmental and behavioral disorders:
  - autism spectrum disorder (ASD)
  - dyslexia
  - attention deficit hyperactivity disorder (ADHD)
  - tics.

Part I: Other common disorders of childhood

Common minor problems of babies and children

COLIC AND CRYING

Crying is the means by which a baby communicates its needs and in a well baby may indicate hunger, physical discomfort from a wet diaper, being cold or overheated, or a need for human contact. In these cases the crying should cease when the underlying needs of the baby are met. However, all babies may cry for apparently no reason, and some do this more vigorously and more persistently than others.

An inconsolable baby can be a great source of stress to already tired parents. It is not easy for most parents, having developed a normal bond with their newborn, simply to let their baby cry, even when all obvious reasons for the crying have been excluded. The natural parental instinct is to keep on trying to find a way to settle the baby. When all attempts to provide comfort are unsuccessful, and also when this occurs frequently day after day, some parents can be driven to near breaking point. It is important for the health practitioner to be aware of the potentially serious impact that a crying baby can have on the baby's family.

If the crying of a baby is unexplained, it is important first to check that there is no underlying illness causing the distress. This is particularly important if the crying appears as a new phenomenon in a previously settled baby. It may be wise to refer the baby for a medical opinion in this situation.

Inconsolable crying may be related to the emotional atmosphere of the baby's home. Anxiety or irritability in the parents is very easily transmitted to the baby, and may result in unsettled behavior. However, as an inconsolable newborn can itself be a cause of anxiety and irritability in the parents, it may be difficult to untangle which problem came first.

Infant colic is the term given to a common condition affecting babies from two weeks to up to four months of age. It is very often diagnosed as the cause of inconsolable crying. In medical terminology, the word colic literally refers to the waves of pain that result when the passageway through a tube-like organ (bowel, biliary tree or ureter) is obstructed. However, in the case of colic in young babies, there is no firm medical evidence that babies with these symptoms are actually suffering from true colic of the bowel or any other organ. The true physical cause of the symptoms is poorly understood. In some cases the symptoms may be attributed to gastro-esophageal reflux of acid via an immature esophageal sphincter.

The classic presentation of colic is that from a few days to weeks after birth the baby starts crying as if in pain. This pattern commonly appears particularly after feeds and towards the end of the day. The baby may draw up its knees during the bouts of crying. Sometimes, if the baby is enabled to bring up some wind, this brings temporary relief. Some breastfeeding mothers find that eating particular foods such as dairy products, spicy foods or oranges make the symptoms worse for their baby. Babies who are fed formula milk may be more settled after the type of formula has been changed, and occasionally if cows' milk formulas are excluded.

Conventional advice is that the baby should be allowed to feed in a calm environment and should be allowed to bring up wind at regular intervals during the feeds. Thickening of food, which has the aim of preventing reflux of acid into the esophagus, can be of benefit in some cases. Simeticone is a silicon-based medication described in the *British National Formulary* (BNF) as an antifoaming agent. It is commonly used for colic, despite a lack of firm evidence that it is of true benefit. In more serious cases, a preparation such as Gaviscon Infant may be prescribed, again to mitigate the effects of acid reflux. Parents should be reassured that the symptoms rarely persist beyond six months of age, and have usually subsided within three months.

 Information box 5.4e-I

Infant colic: comments from a Chinese medicine perspective

In Chinese medicine, the symptoms of colic may be ascribed to Cold. This can be either External in its origin (e.g. from foods that have a cold energetic nature or cold weather), or it may result from Deficiency of the Organs, in particular, the Stomach and Spleen. Cold stagnates Qi, and this causes intense pain.

Another cause of colic is irregular feeding and overfeeding, which can then lead to Accumulation Disorder, a very common Full condition of childhood. Too much food blocks the Middle Burner, obstructs the flow of Qi, and thus causes pain.

Regular feeding and avoidance of External Cold, Cold or Spicy foods in the breastfeeding mother's diet and overfeeding may help in the case of colic. It is important to maintain a calm stress-free environment for the child.

FEEDING PROBLEMS IN BABIES

Ideally, according to guidance from the World Health Organization (WHO), babies should be fed entirely on breast milk at least until six months of age. However, over and above the cultural forces that might act against the continuation of breastfeeding, potentially preventable difficulties in producing milk or discomfort in feeding can often lead a mother to choose to stop breastfeeding and switch to formula (powdered) milk.

Formula milk feeding is the medically recommended alternative to breastfeeding. Unmodified cows' milk is not suitable for babies under one year. A cows' milk formula powder is based on cows' milk protein (casein), but has a more appropriate balance of salts, added nutrients and whey protein. Soya protein formulas are available for babies who demonstrate intolerance to cows' milk protein. It is not advisable for these to be used unless there is proven cows' milk intolerance, as soya itself is quite allergenic in young babies. Also, the regular use of soya formula is associated with lower levels of protective antibodies in the baby.

As formula milk is heavier in nature than breast milk, a formula-fed baby may appear more satisfied after a feed, and may fall into a deeper sleep after feeding. Formula-fed babies tend to have a greater weight gain than breastfed babies. This factor should be taken into account when interpreting predicted weight gain for a breastfed baby from charts that demonstrate average predicted weights. It should be remembered that these averages will have been calculated from a population of babies of whom the large majority would have been formula fed.

Current medical advice is that solid foods should not be introduced before the age of six months. The baby can then be given small amounts of pureed simple grains and vegetables, such as baby rice, carrots and cooked fruit. Added salt and sugar are not necessary, and should be avoided for as long as possible in the child's life. More lumpy foods, and also meat and eggs, can be introduced soon after when the baby begins to be able to chew.

New foods should be introduced one day at a time, so potential intolerances to a particular food can be isolated. Currently, it is advised that cows' milk is not introduced as a drink until 12 months of age, because of its indigestible and potentially allergenic nature. However, it is considered acceptable when mixed with other foods or in the form of cheese or yogurt.

Vitamin drops containing vitamins A, C and D are recommended to be given daily to all babies and children up to the age of five from six months onwards, and are available free of charge to those families with low incomes.[100]

Although many parents will experience difficulties of one sort or another in feeding their babies and small children, feeding should only be considered a medical problem if the child is failing to receive the nutrition the child requires for healthy growth and development. In many cases of apparent feeding difficulties it is evident that the child is well, and is gaining sufficient weight for the child's stage in life. In these cases the parents should be reassured that, although the child may appear to be refusing milk or fussing at the breast, the child is obviously getting sufficient nutrition for its needs.

However, there are cases in which difficulties with feeding do lead to nutritional deficiency and poor weight gain. A small baby, and particularly one that is premature, is particularly vulnerable to the effects of a poor dietary intake. This is because a small baby has not had the opportunity to build up sufficient reserves of fat, proteins, minerals and vitamins to tide it over lean times.

The measurements of weight in babies and height in older children are very frequently used indicators of healthy development. Sometimes it is when a baby or a small child is found to be consistently dropping below a previously satisfactory centile measurement for weight or height that problems with feeding are exposed.

Infant colic is one cause of problematic feeding. The unsettled baby may be reluctant to take feeds, or may start feeding with willingness, only to stop after a few minutes apparently because of pain or discomfort. This problem usually subsides by the time the baby is three months old.

Vomiting part of a feed (also known as posseting) is a normal phenomenon and affects most babies, often towards the end of a feed. In most cases, the baby brings up a small proportion of the feed, usually together with some wind. Usually, this form of vomiting in otherwise healthy babies is effortless, and does not seem to cause them distress. Formula-fed babies may tend to vomit larger amounts of more strong-smelling milk than breastfed babies. Posseting does not lead to nutritional deficiency. If posseting is very frequent, thickening of the milk may be helpful, but in breastfed babies this will require the mother first to express the milk.

Vomiting that appears as a new phenomenon in a previously easily fed baby suggests that either an infection or intolerance to a new food may be the underlying problem. Infection that has its focus anywhere in the body, such as otitis media or cystitis, can lead to vomiting in an infant. If the cause is not clear, and the vomiting is persisting, the baby should be referred to a doctor for investigation.

Forceful (projectile) vomiting in a small baby is a serious warning feature, and may be an indication of pyloric stenosis. Projectile vomiting can lead rapidly to an imbalance of the salts and fluids in the blood in small babies, and should be referred for medical diagnosis and treatment.

Refusal of feeds is a problem that is much more prevalent in toddlers than in smaller babies. A common pattern is that a child who previously accepted a wide range of solid foods when a baby becomes very fussy after the age of 18 months and refuses all but the smallest range of foods. This problem can persist well into the school years, and can be very trying for parents. The general approach of health practitioners is to reassure parents that most children, despite having bird-like dietary tendencies, do seem to manage to put on weight and develop well.

Children tend to respond adversely to emotional issues at mealtimes, and so parents should be advised to try not to make the food refusal an issue, which can easily escalate into a three-times-a-day losing battle.

Vitamin and iron supplements may be encouraged if there are concerns that the child who is refusing food is not receiving the basic nutrients that they require.

 Information box 5.4e-II

The infant digestive system: comments from a Chinese medicine perspective

The aphorism "the child's Spleen is often insufficient" expresses the Chinese medical view that the child's digestive system has to work full time to provide the nutrients required for growth and development, and so can easily become taxed by inappropriate food, lack of food, excessive food, eating at the wrong times and eating when surrounded by an unhelpful emotional atmosphere.

Accumulation Disorder (comparable to the adult syndrome of Acute Retention of Food in the Stomach) and Spleen Qi Deficiency are syndromes very commonly found in young children.

Accumulation Disorder is a Full condition, which results from stagnation of food in the child's system. It results from a combination of overfeeding at a time when the Spleen function is still immature. Stagnating food leads to Heat, which manifests as irritability, insomnia, foul-smelling stools and red cheeks. Fluids can then dry up to form Phlegm, and so lead to thick nasal discharge, glue ear and a phlegmy cough.

Spleen Qi Deficiency is an Empty condition, and is a very common imbalance in Western children. It can also be a consequence of long-term Accumulation Disorder, and so can present as a mixed condition. The features of Spleen Qi Deficiency include a pale complexion, and a weak, lackluster disposition. The child might be sleepy in the day, but then does not sleep well at night (because Qi and Blood are weak). The stools may not smell bad but can be loose, or alternate with constipation. The child is prone to Phlegmy illnesses and is picky about its food.

Scott and Barlow (1999) advise that, from a Chinese medicine perspective, babies ideally should be fed breast milk and offered solids at no earlier than two months of age. The child should not be demand fed, but instead an interval of two hours should be left between feeds. The breast milk can be affected by the mother's emotions, and can cause abdominal pain if the mother is not relaxed. They state that cows' milk protein formulas are Phlegm-forming in newborns. Overfeeding of any type of food can lead to diarrhea and digestive disturbances.

The nature of the food given to the baby is very important. Wholefoods (such as wholemeal bread) might be too indigestible for a baby, even though they are considered healthy foods as part of an adult diet. Cold energy foods (e.g. bananas and yogurt) can cause particular problems in a child of a cold disposition, and hot foods (red meat and spices) can cause problems in one who tends to heat. Physically cold foods straight from the refrigerator can be particularly damaging.

Poor or picky appetite in babies or small children suggests Spleen Qi Deficiency.

Vomiting in small children might simply be a result of Retention of Food and Milk as a result of overfeeding a healthy child. If it is recurrent, it might suggest the development of Accumulation Disorder. In less healthy children who suffer from recurrent vomiting, Deficiency of the Stomach and Spleen is usually the underlying problem. The Deficiency may be complicated by Interior Cold, Phlegm or Heat.[101]

Teething

Teething is the term used to describe the process of the eruption of the milk teeth in babies. The first teeth to appear are the lower incisors (cutting teeth), which erupt at the front of the mandible. These are usually "cut" after the age of five to six months. By nine to ten months all eight incisors (four upper and four lower) have appeared in most babies. The four canines (tearing teeth) and the first four molars (chewing teeth) do not usually appear until after the first birthday. The second molars make their appearance after another delay, at some time between 20 and 24 months of age.

A child can become quite unsettled just before a new tooth appears. This is more common with the appearance of the molars, and in particular, the second molars. Before the eruption of the tooth, the child may be irritable, and may even have a slight fever. A common sign is reddening of the cheek on the affected side of the mouth. Also, during teething the stools may become loose, and diaper rash can develop. All these symptoms indicate that teething can lead to a temporary generalized constitutional upset in the child.

The teething child may obtain some comfort from chewing on a hard toy or food, such as a rusk. Some parents find that anesthetic gels or oil of cloves rubbed onto the gums can be of help, although rubbing of the gum alone may in itself be therapeutic. An infant preparation of paracetamol is commonly used to ease the distress of teething.

Information box 5.4e-III

Teething: comments from a Chinese medicine perspective

Teething is not a recognized pattern in Chinese medicine. Flaws (2006) explains, however, that times of growth and change are associated with extra Heat, by means of a process termed Bian Zheng, meaning "change and steaming," and the Heat is a result of increased activity by the Ming Men Fire or Kidney Yang[102] (a similar process accounts for some of the Heat in adolescent acne).

Scott and Barlow (1999) suggest that cultural and dietary factors could be just as important in explaining the fact that Chinese babies do not seem to suffer from this common Western problem. They suggest that teething is primarily a digestive problem, which develops only if Accumulation Disorder is already present.[103]

The eruption of teeth is dependent on Kidney Qi. However, as teeth push through the gums, they influence the flow of Qi through the Stomach and Intestines. This can cause stagnation of Qi in these Channels, and can cause the manifestation of the Full symptoms of a previously mild case of Accumulation Disorder. For this reason, it would make sense to advise the parents to lighten the baby's diet when teething, to offer only simple foods, and especially to avoid meat and high-protein foods.

TODDLER DIARRHEA

Toddler diarrhea is the most common cause of persistent loose stools in young children. As its name suggests, it is a functional condition that primarily affects otherwise well children. The stools vary between being soft but formed, and explosive and loose. Undigested food may be seen in the stools (peas and carrots syndrome), suggesting that the food has made a very rapid transit through the gastrointestinal tract.

From a medical viewpoint, toddler diarrhea is usually not serious. As long as food intolerances (e.g. celiac disease), other causes of malabsorption (e.g. cystic fibrosis) and chronic infection (e.g. *Giardia*) have been excluded by means of stool tests, the parents will be reassured that their child should grow out of this condition.

In older children, the passage of loose stools and slight fecal incontinence may be a manifestation of overflow diarrhea, a problem that paradoxically results from constipation. It is very important in these cases that the correct diagnosis is made (see below).

Information box 5.4e-IV

Chronic diarrhea: comments from a Chinese medicine perspective

In Chinese medicine, chronic diarrhea in a small child suggests that either Accumulation Disorder or Deficiency of Spleen Qi is an underlying problem. The precise diagnosis depends on the symptom pattern in the child.

CONSTIPATION AND SOILING

Difficulty passing stools is a common problem in young children. In some, the passage of a hard stool after a period of straining can lead to pain, and even a shallow anal tear. This is more likely to occur after a short period of illness during which the child has taken in much less food or drink than usual, so causing the stools to become dry. Pain during the passage of a stool can in some cases lead to a vicious cycle, as fear inhibits the passing of later stools. Negative emotions associated with defecation, perhaps a result of forceful toilet training, can also cause this vicious cycle to be set up.

In most children, a change in diet, increased fluids and sometimes a dose of a mild laxative can relieve the problem. In more serious cases the rectum can become impacted with a hard stool. Involuntary soiling of a stool may then occur, as liquid feces seep past this solid mass and leak out. This can generate a social problem for the child, who is usually of preschool or early school age, as they then become vulnerable to embarrassment and teasing.

It is important in a case of constipation to exclude medical causes, such as hypothyroidism and a rare congenital abnormality of the bowel called Hirschprung disease. In this condition the autonomic nerve supply to the bowel is not sufficient. For this reason, children with constipation and overflow diarrhea may be referred to a pediatrician for correct diagnosis and management.

In cases in which impacted feces have accumulated, it is important to manage the child with care. Ordinary laxatives may only serve to worsen the problem of overflow diarrhea. The child is first treated for a fortnight with stool-softening laxatives (lactulose or docusate), and only then is given a large dose of a stimulant laxative over the course of the next few days. This regimen should induce expulsion of the impacted stools in liquid form. Some children may require brief hospital admission so that an enema can be given to aid bowel emptying.

However, the treatment is not complete at this stage. The child often then needs to relearn the habit of regular bowel emptying, as the normal bowel-emptying reflexes are commonly disrupted during the period of impaction. This can be a laborious process, often requiring prolonged treatment with reducing doses of laxatives and a reward system (such as a "star chart") to encourage daily bowel opening.

Soiling of the underpants or bed with feces (encopresis) is most commonly an involuntary result of stool impaction. However, it can occur in children who are not constipated and who were previously continent. In these cases the problem is often one of emotional distress. For those children who soil despite having an empty rectum, psychiatric advice may be sought.

 Information box 5.4e-V

Constipation: comments from a Chinese medicine perspective

In Chinese medicine, constipation may be a manifestation of Accumulation Disorder or Spleen Qi Deficiency. As is the case for diarrhea, the precise diagnosis depends on the symptom pattern in the child.

SLEEP PROBLEMS

A healthy newborn baby will wake between two and four times a night to be fed and changed. Usually one of these feeds is before midnight, and the others spread between midnight and 5.30 am. Each feed, together with a diaper change, may take up 20–60 minutes until the baby is settled again, and this is even if the child does not start crying for some inexplicable reason. It is no wonder that parents of newborns can become exhausted so rapidly.

Many babies lose this pattern of regular nocturnal waking after a short time, some sleeping through the night from as early as two months of age. However, others continue to wake and demand food or comfort for over a year, with some persisting well into the preschool years. This means that some parents, and particularly those who go on to have more children, may continue to have recurrent broken nights for a period of a few years. The impact on the health and the emotional state of the parents, not to mention the child, can be significant.

Getting the baby to fall asleep can also become a big problem. Most young babies will initially require to be held and to be comforted while they drop off to sleep in the early evening. This is normal. Many will later settle down very quickly after being put down in the cot following a bedtime routine. However, others loudly continue to demand the presence of a parent if left in the cot. The parent's choice is either to stay with the child to keep the peace, or to let the child cry itself to sleep. The latter is an option that is not the most natural one for many modern parents. The problem is that staying with the child until it falls asleep can become an ingrained habit. Bedtime can thus become a grueling marathon, involving reading stories, getting drinks, stroking a small head for half an hour, and then creeping out of a darkened room only to be called back in within minutes by agonized cries from the abandoned child.

Most doctors and health visitors will advise behavioral methods described as "sleep training" to help with the problems of getting off to sleep and nocturnal waking. The basic principle behind sleep training is that the child is educated in a gradual way that crying at night will not generate the rewards of unlimited comfort that it previously did.

The advice given to the parents of a child who cannot fall asleep on their own is that, after a brief but consistent bedtime routine (e.g. pajamas on, teeth brushed, one story, cuddle), the parent says a clear goodnight and leaves the child. The child is allowed to cry for a short time (say 2 minutes), and then the parent returns to reassure the child that they are still there, but that they are going to leave them to sleep again. Then the child is allowed to cry for a little longer (say 5 minutes) before the parent returns. This process of returning for reassurance after increasingly longer intervals is repeated until the child falls asleep. The first few nights of sleep training may be grueling, but a surprisingly high percentage of babies and children respond very rapidly (within days) to this approach, so that within one to two weeks they no longer cry when left at bedtime. A similar approach is used for nocturnal waking. The parent appears to give reassurance, but neither stays with the child nor offers a sweet drink or food. After leaving with a clear goodnight they should only reappear after allowing increasing time intervals for crying.

These simple techniques are pleasing in theory, but actually require strong willpower on the part of the parents in practice, particularly in the early hours of the morning. Some doctors might prescribe the child sedatives to give the parents a couple of nights of respite before they tackle sleep training.

Some children wake at night having suffered from nightmares. If this is the case, sleep training is not appropriate. The child will require comforting. As long as the nightmares are not occurring more than once a week, most doctors would be reassuring about their occurrence.

Night terrors can be a disturbing experience for parents of children aged three to six. In a night terror, the child appears to wake suddenly in a disorientated or terror-struck state, but does not respond to being comforted. The child might push the parents away or seem to look right through them. They will often then fall back off to sleep after a few minutes. In some cases the child may actually get out of bed and sleep walk. In the morning the child has no recollection of the episode. Night terrors tend to recur at the same time in the night. They can indicate, in some cases, that the child has been shocked or unsettled in some way in their day-to-day life.

Information box 5.4e-VI

Difficulty in sleeping in children: comments from a Chinese medicine perspective

In Chinese medicine, digestive disturbance is common in children who have difficulty sleeping. Spleen and Heart Deficiency may underlie a pattern of Qi and Blood Deficiency in a child who is not sleeping well. These children will wake frequently in the night. Cold foods, in particular, can lead to a Cold Spleen and a colicky pain, which can cause the child to wake at night in a disturbed state. Also, Heat in excess can cause restless sleep and early waking.

Excessive overstimulation by computer games, television or strong parental emotions and unexpressed fright can be held in a child's body, and can then lead to disturbed sleep. In these cases the child can wake with nightmares or night terrors.

BED-WETTING (ENURESIS)

Children usually become dry by day a little earlier than they become dry by night. Most children learn to use the potty by day at some point during their third year of life. Girls often become potty trained a little earlier than boys.

However, most children will not be dry by night until at least some point during their fourth year. For a few months after a child has learned to be dry by night, the occasional wet bed is still to be expected, particularly if the child's daily routine has been disrupted or if the child is under stress in some way. Occasional bed-wetting continues to affect a few children as they enter their school years. It is estimated that 15 percent of five-year-olds, 7 percent of seven-year-olds and 1 percent of young adults still wet the bed on occasion. A preschool child is usually unconcerned about bed-wetting, but as a child enters the school years the problem can become an increasingly potent source of shame and embarrassment.

An established pattern of bed-wetting (enuresis) is more common in boys and first-borns. It also seems to run strongly in families. It is very rare for there to be any underlying physical abnormality, such as spina bifida occulta or recurrent urinary infections, which might account for the problem, but these causes need to be considered. Coexistent constipation is a more common treatable cause, and if this is a problem it needs to be addressed by dietary change, increasing fluids and possibly prescription of gentle laxatives. It is also not unusual to find that the child who continues to wet the bed is suffering from emotional distress of one form or another, and this possibility needs to be explored and addressed.

Parents may try a range of simple treatments for the problem, most of which are not considered in current medical practice to be very effective. Fluid restriction can help in those cases in which the child was drinking excessively before bedtime, but this is not the case for most bed-wetters. Lifting the sleeping child to the potty in the night prevents the consequences of bed-wetting on the bedding, but does not treat the problem. Bribes and punishment of the child do not work.

Other treatments need not be offered before the child has reached five years of age, as the majority of bed-wetters will stop spontaneously before their fifth birthday. For older children, a simple reward system such as a star chart (praise and a star given in the morning after every dry night) can be a very effective behavioral technique. Over 50 percent of bed-wetting children will become dry by using this method alone. In children over the age of seven, a bed-wetting alarm is considered to be the most effective method. A moisture-sensitive pad is placed under the child's bedding. This sounds a bell when the child begins to urinate in the bed. Although a positive response may take up to eight weeks, most children are deterred from the habit of bed-wetting by this apparatus. The alarm is kept in use until there has been at least one month of dry nights, and is then removed. Success is more likely if there are no underlying psychological triggers for the problem. If the child relapses from this treatment more than twice (as occurs in 20–40 percent of cases), the child may be referred to a psychologist so that any underlying emotional factors can be explored more carefully.

Drugs are available to prevent bed-wetting, but these suppress rather than cure the problem. They should be restricted to those occasions, such as overnight visits, when the bed-wetting might become problematic socially. The drugs that are currently used include a low dose of the antidepressant imipramine, and a synthetic form of antidiuretic hormone (ADH), known as desmopressin. Desmopressin is administered via nasal spray.

Information box 5.4e-VII

Bed-wetting (enuresis): comments from a Chinese medicine perspective

In Chinese medicine, there are four main patterns associated with bed-wetting (enuresis). These are Kidney Qi Deficiency ("weakness in the lower gate"), Spleen and Lung Qi Deficiency, Damp Heat in the Liver Channel, and Lingering Pathogenic Factor. In the last three of these patterns there will also always be some underlying Kidney Deficiency.

TANTRUMS AND DISOBEDIENCE

A tantrum is an expression of fury, which becomes more prevalent from the age of two. It is believed that by the age of two the child begins to want to exert their independence, but at the same time has to be very much under the control of their parents. This paradox is the cause of the frustration, and the mounting extreme anger that is experienced can induce great fear in the child.

Typically, a child who is having a tantrum is consumed by the rage, and enters a state of screaming, hitting out and kicking, which can persist for some minutes. When in the state of a tantrum, it can be very difficult for the child to be calmed down. It sometimes seems as if any approach to the child simply exacerbates the anger. Some children can scream so much in a tantrum that they may actually vomit or go blue in the face. Some hold their breath until they almost lose consciousness. Although these behaviors can be disturbing for the parents to witness, they are very rarely a cause of physical harm to the child.

Some children resort to this route of expression of their anger more readily than others. Many parents find the third year of their child's life an exhausting time, as they struggle with the management of a child who might explode into uncontrollable anger whenever thwarted. This is why this period has been termed the "terrible twos," although some children may continue to have tantrums well past their third birthday. In contrast, some children never really experience explosions of anger that are not readily soothed by appropriate parental responses.

Current advice is that a child having a tantrum cannot be reasoned with. Rewards or appeasements offered during a tantrum may simply reinforce the behavior. Parents may be advised either calmly to walk away from the child (as long as it is safe) to let the tantrum burn out, or to take the child to a particular room or corner where they are left to have "time out." Neither of these techniques is very practical if the tantrum begins by the checkout queue at the supermarket, but can be helpful in reducing the occurrence of tantrums if practiced with calmness in the home.

A child who is willfully disobedient can be a source of extreme frustration to the parents. The temptation to hit a child who is ignoring all other forms of control can be very strong. Smacking is absolutely not advocated as a valid method of control of a disobedient child. Although it can be effective in the short term, it is now believed that it can reinforce in the child the idea that violence is the way by which things can be achieved.

Current advice for dealing with disobedience centers on some basic principles. First, the parent should not display or react with emotion that is out of control (e.g. extreme anger), and second, the parent should be consistent with regard to any rules that may have been set. If a rule (such as "You do not throw food") is broken, the child should be treated in the same way every time this occurs.

In the case of food throwing, the response might be a reprimand and removal of the plate of food. If there is a repeat performance, the next step might be to remove the child and calmly place them in the bedroom for 5 minutes of "time out." If this occurs every time, most children will learn that it is not worth their while breaking the rule. However, if a few episodes of the behavior are overlooked (and this usually occurs because of parental exhaustion), this inconsistency can strongly erode the potential effectiveness of the method.

In summary, with difficult behavioral patterns in children, the basic principles are the same: make rules, stick to them, keep calm and cool, do not give in (i.e. be consistent once the rules have been established), and take the child to a separate place to have "time out" if necessary.

 Information box 5.4e-VIII

Tantrums: comments from a Chinese medicine perspective

From a Chinese medicine viewpoint, excessive tantrums are not considered to be a healthy expression of anger. Perhaps surprisingly, the underlying patterns that are described to be associated with anger outbursts do not relate to Stagnation of Liver Qi, which is not usual in small children. Instead, the extreme physical manifestations of anger in children can be attributed to patterns of underlying Heat, Phlegm Heat and Hyperactive Spleen Qi Deficiency.

MINOR SKIN DISORDERS IN BABIES AND SMALL CHILDREN

There are a number of common skin complaints of young children that are not related to infection and which tend to resolve as the child gets older. These include neonatal urticaria, milia, cradle cap and diaper rash.

Neonatal urticaria is a painless rash that can appear in newborns within a few days of delivery. The spots are tiny white pimples (papules) surrounded by a reddened halo, and come and go from different sites, particularly on the trunk. This rash usually resolves after a few days.

Milia are tiny painless pimples that appear on the face of a newborn and can persist for some weeks. The name comes from the Latin word for millet seed, and this very much describes their appearance. Milia also resolve spontaneously without any need for treatment.

Many small babies will develop transient blotchy red patches, particularly on their face, which can come and go with surprising rapidity. In some cases their occurrence may be related to feeding. The cause is poorly understood. Most children will grow out of this skin reaction as they reach toddler age. In some children these blotches can be a precursor of the development of eczema (see later).

Cradle cap is the popular name for a condition medically described as seborrheic dermatitis. This first appears on the scalp of babies at about eight weeks of age, when it appears as a non-irritating scaling of the scalp. In mild cases moisturizing creams can be sufficient to treat the scaling. In more severe cases the scales heap on top of each other to form the waxy thickened layer described as cradle cap.

In some babies, the rash can spread to the skin behind the ears and to the skin creases of the limbs. This may appear like eczema, but the rash of seborrheic dermatitis is not itchy. However, it can be very unsightly. Although this problem will always resolve within a few months, most parents will want treatment for cradle cap. If moisturizing creams are insufficient, olive oil can help to dissolve the waxy coat of the cradle cap, and the scales can then be removed by gentle friction. Some doctors will prescribe a corticosteroid cream or a mixture of topical sulfur and salicylic acid, both of which are effective treatments.

Information box 5.4e-IX

Minor skin disorders in children: comments from a Chinese medicine perspective

From a Chinese medicine viewpoint, the fact that these mild skin complaints resolve spontaneously suggests that many of them are manifestations of Pathogenic Factors, such as Heat and Damp, which are being cleared. Some of these factors may have been present from before the time of birth (i.e. Womb Toxin), and in other cases they may result from inappropriate dietary constituents. This implies that their presence should be welcomed and, particularly as the child is not distressed by them, they should not be treated with topical suppressive creams unless absolutely necessary.

Diaper rash affects most babies at some point in the first year of life, but some are afflicted more seriously and persistently than others. This problem has been less prevalent since the introduction of disposable diapers. The most common cause of the rash is irritation of the skin that is in prolonged contact with urine and/or feces. The rash usually affects the buttocks, perineum and the top of the thighs, and is often absent from the skin creases. In severe cases the skin can appear scalded and ulcerated. Most children tend to stop succumbing to diaper rash after the first year of life, presumably because the skin matures and becomes less sensitive to the effect of external chemicals, including those found in urine.

The severity of the problem can be reduced by the regular use of barrier creams and frequent changing of diapers. If it is possible to leave the child without a diaper, this can also help allow the rash to heal. In very severe cases the doctor might prescribe a short course of a topical corticosteroid cream.

Candida infection (thrush) can complicate severe diaper rash. In this case, the rash may appear more brick red, and often spreads to involve the skin creases. The treatment for *candida* infection is a topical antifungal cream such as clotrimazole.

Information box 5.4e-X

Diaper rash: comments from a Chinese medicine perspective

In Chinese medicine, the symptoms of diaper rash correspond to Heat, or Damp Heat. External Pathogenic Factors originating from the diet or the climate are often the cause. Diaper rash can become a problem at the same time as teething, suggesting a similar underlying pathology, in this case, the rising up of Heat from Ming Men Fire. Accumulation Disorder may underlie the problem.

Disorders of growth and puberty

FAILURE TO THRIVE (FTT)

Failure to thrive (FTT) is a term used to describe a case in which the child is consistently failing to achieve the expected developmental milestones for weight and growth. In addition, the child who is failing to thrive will not appear to be in full health, although any features of illness may be non-specific. Typical non-specific features include an irritable disposition, a poor appetite and loose stools. The plotting of serial measurements of weight and height is crucial in the diagnosis of FTT. FTT is a very common reason for referral to a pediatrician. In all cases the treatment should be directed at treating the underlying cause, whether it be organic (physical) or non-organic (psychosocial).

There is a wide range of physical (organic) causes of FTT. These include those disorders that prevent the child from obtaining the nutrients required for normal growth, such as feeding problems, diarrhea and vomiting, malabsorption and food intolerances. Chronic illness can also be a cause of FTT, even if the diet is adequate and the digestive processes of the child are normal. Conditions such as severe eczema, asthma, cystic fibrosis, congenital heart disease, chronic renal failure, hypothyroidism and childhood cancer may all result in poor growth and development in a child.

Non-organic FTT is the poor growth and development that occurs in a child exposed to psychosocial deprivation. This might be the result of, for example, maternal psychiatric illness, parental learning difficulties or chronic child abuse. Psychosocial short stature is a term used to describe the poor growth apparent in non-organic FTT.

Information box 5.4e-XI

Failure to thrive: comments from a Chinese medicine perspective

In Chinese medicine, failure to gain weight and to grow can reflect a Deficiency in Kidney Qi and, more particularly, the Essence. This would be the case for some of the children who have chronic illness and also in congenital disease.

A lingering Pathogenic Factor (which can contribute to a condition such as chronic cough or eczema) can also impair the production of Qi, and so may also be the cause of FTT in chronic illness.

A previously healthy child may fail to thrive if they are unable to produce the Qi required from their environment. This would be the case if the diet is poor or if the child is emotionally deprived in some way. In both cases the Spleen Qi in particular will be weak, and the child can benefit from Tonification of Qi.

SHORT STATURE

Short stature is usually defined as height below the 2nd or 3rd centile. However, because of the vagaries of defining normality (as discussed in Section 5.4b), most of the children so labeled will actually have no other health problems. They are short simply because that is the height that has been determined by their genetic constitution. However, in a small proportion of short children an underlying physical or emotional problem may be found as a cause of poor growth. FTT is an all-embracing term for the various pathological conditions that can result in short stature. FTT usually manifests with additional features of ill health (see above).

Chromosomal disorders such as Down syndrome or Turner syndrome are often associated with short stature. As the child is often otherwise well, failure to grow to a height that is within the normal range would not be classified as FTT.

There are endocrine causes of short stature in which the child may otherwise be in good health. This is in contrast to the child who is failing to thrive. Growth hormone (GH) deficiency is the most important of these disorders. This can occur with no other apparent physical problem. It may result from pituitary damage (e.g. from birth trauma or a brain tumor). Diagnosis is problematic, as GH deficiency

is notoriously difficult to distinguish from constitutional growth delay (a "normal" cause of short stature). Even if the underlying cause cannot be established for certain, the affected child can respond well to regular injections of genetically engineered growth hormone. Before 1985, GH was extracted from human pituitaries at post-mortem examinations. The use of nervous tissue from cadavers is now known to increase the transmission of prion diseases, including Creutzfeldt-Jakob disease. Unfortunately, the use of cadaveric GH before 1985 did result in a few cases of this fatal condition.

Information box 5.4e-XII

Short stature: comments from a Chinese medicine perspective

In Chinese medicine, short stature, if not associated with any other form of ill health, is not in itself a sign of energetic imbalance. Any underlying physical cause, such as a chromosomal disorder or GH deficiency, would point to a relative Deficiency in Kidney Essence.

TALL STATURE

Tall stature is less commonly considered to be a medical problem, as in Western cultures it is socially more acceptable to be relatively tall. In most cases of tall stature the underlying cause is the genetic constitution of the child. It is only in rare cases that a physical abnormality is the cause. The most notorious cause of tall stature is the very rare endocrine condition of gigantism, in which there is excess GH secretion as a result of a pituitary tumor. In this case the affected child can, by adulthood, reach a height of over 2.10 meters (7 feet). Other causes include hyperthyroidism and Klinefelter syndrome.

PRECOCIOUS PUBERTY

Precocious puberty is defined as the premature development of secondary sexual characteristics before the age of eight in females and nine in males. It is most common in females. As in most cases of short stature, the most common cause in females is familial tendency, and the condition is therefore not associated with any other form of ill health. However, as puberty heralds the final stages of bone growth and the ossification of the epiphyses, a child with precocious puberty may only attain a relatively short stature by adulthood. In boys, the most common cause is a pituitary hormone-secreting brain tumor. This serious problem can also affect girls. There are also rare congenital conditions that can lead to precocious puberty in both sexes.

A child with precocious puberty should be investigated for the rare possibility of a physical cause, which should then be the focus of treatment. Drugs to suppress the effect of the sex hormones may be used to reduce the speed of skeletal maturation. The child may need specialized psychological support to enable them to adjust to the potentially stigmatizing bodily changes that result from precocious puberty.

Information box 5.4e-XIII

Precocious puberty: comments from a Chinese medicine perspective

In Chinese medicine, although premature puberty manifests in early development of sexual characteristics, the end result is short stature because of premature bone maturation (even in familial cases). The underdevelopment of the bones as a result of the premature puberty suggests that in such cases there is Deficiency of Kidney Essence.

DELAYED PUBERTY

Delayed puberty is defined as the absence of pubertal development by the age of 14 in females and 15 in males. Delayed puberty is more common in boys, and is usually a result of a familial tendency, rather than any underlying physical cause. An affected child will have delayed growth relative to their peers, and may be the focus of teasing, but is likely to catch up in height once they enter puberty, albeit at a late stage.

Other underlying causes that can affect both boys and girls include chronic physical disease and emotional deprivation (akin to the syndrome of FTT). Causes that more specifically affect the release of the pituitary hormones, luteinizing hormone (LH) and follicle-stimulating hormone (FSH) include anorexia nervosa, excessive physical training, hypothyroidism, pituitary tumors and Klinefelter syndrome.

Information box 5.4e-XIV

Delayed puberty: comments from a Chinese medicine perspective

Although it depends on the cause, in most cases delayed puberty is very likely to suggest a relative Deficiency in Kidney Essence.

INTERSEX DISORDERS

There is a range of intersex disorders that result in a child in whom the external sexual characteristics do not match the child's genetic sexual identity. In general, these disorders result from a failure in the sexual differentiation of the genitals and gonads that occurs in the fetus during the first trimester of pregnancy. These disorders are mentioned briefly in Section 5.2g.

Disorders of the digestive system

Many of the childhood digestive disorders correspond directly to their adult counterparts. The following conditions are either characteristic conditions of childhood, or follow a different course to that which is usually followed in adulthood.

RECURRENT ABDOMINAL PAIN

Recurrent abdominal pain of sufficient intensity to interrupt day-to-day activities is a very common complaint affecting children of school age. Episodes of pain, recurring over a period of at least three months, are estimated to affect up to one-tenth of all school-age children. In the bulk of these cases there will be no clearly definable physical cause. In other words, the pain is non-organic or functional. For those children in whom no obvious physical cause can be identified, the nature of the recurrent pain may have some typical features: it is often located around the umbilicus, it is worse on waking, and may be associated with a family history of migraine, travel sickness or irritable bowel syndrome (IBS). In many of these children the symptoms are worse with stress.

In the management of recurrent abdominal pain, first, it is important to exclude the more common physical causes of abdominal pain, which can explain about 10 percent of cases. The physical causes of functional abdominal pain include mesenteric adenitis (see below), appendicitis (see below), inflammatory bowel disease (see below), peptic ulceration, urinary tract infection or urinary stones (see below), and, in pubescent girls, gynecological disorders.

Once a physical cause has been excluded, a doctor is likely to reassure the parents and the child that the pain is most likely to be due to an abnormality of the sensitivity of the bowel to normal bowel movements. This explanation, which is akin to the conventional explanation for the pain of IBS, is supported by scientific evidence. This evidence, based on studies that correlated pain with the pressure within the contracting bowel, also suggests that anxiety increases the pain by increasing the frequency of bowel movements.

In about one-half of children with non-organic recurrent abdominal pain, referral to a pediatrician and reassurance can result in rapid resolution of the pain. Of the remainder, one-half have partial resolution and the other half go on to experience IBS in adulthood.

Information box 5.4e-XV

Abdominal pain in children: comments from a Chinese medicine perspective

In Chinese medicine, abdominal pain in children can be a feature of a wide range of patterns, of which External Cold (usually from Cold foods), Accumulation Disorder, Interior Cold from Deficiency, Retention of Phlegm Damp, and Lingering Pathogenic Factor are the most common. Qi Obstruction and Stasis can explain some of the more serious forms of abdominal pain, which would be more frequently seen in children admitted to hospital departments.

MESENTERIC ADENITIS

Mesenteric adenitis is a term used to describe abdominal pain that arises from inflammation of the abdominal lymph nodes. In small children, this cause of abdominal pain can accompany upper respiratory tract infections and other more generalized illnesses.

On examination, there may be tenderness on palpation, which can be localized to one particular region of the abdomen, most commonly the umbilical region. Clinically, if the pain is severe it can be difficult to distinguish mesenteric adenitis from appendicitis (see below). Although mesenteric adenitis is not a serious condition, the child might eventually undergo surgical exploration to exclude appendicitis if the pain is severe and persistent.

Information box 5.4e-XVI

Mesenteric adenitis: comments from a Chinese medicine perspective

In Chinese medicine, the pain of mesenteric adenitis might correspond to any of the patterns listed above for recurrent abdominal pain.

INTUSSUSCEPTION

Intussusception is the most common cause of bowel obstruction to affect young children, particularly those under the age of one. The obstruction is the result of one segment of the bowel folding inside itself, so obstructing the flow of feces, and causing compression of the blood vessels that supply that segment. There is often no obvious underlying cause of this problem. The most popular explanation is that viral infection has caused swelling of the lymphoid tissue of the bowel lining, which can then form the lead point of the infolding of the bowel tissue. If intussusception occurs in an older child, a more substantial physical cause may be found (e.g. a polyp or bowel tumor).

The obstruction causes severe pain, which causes a baby to draw up its legs and scream. The baby may vomit or pass small amounts of blood-stained stool. The abdomen distends and a sausage-shaped mass may be felt in the abdomen. The child, if not too shocked, may be treated by means of pumping air gently into the rectum. In many cases this can help the bowel to unfold. If the child is very unwell, surgical treatment is required.

Information box 5.4e-XVII

Intussusception: comments from a Chinese medicine perspective

In Chinese medicine, the acute abdominal pain of the intussusception corresponds to Qi and Blood Obstruction, and Stasis.

APPENDICITIS

The appendix is a blind-ended, worm-like tube that projects outwards from the first part of the large intestine (the cecum). It sits in the region of the abdominal cavity described as the right iliac fossa. The lining wall of the appendix contains a dense concentration of lymphoid tissue.

Appendicitis is a term that refers to the fact that the appendix has become inflamed. This is a relatively common occurrence in children aged three to sixteen. In children, the lymphoid tissue in the gastrointestinal system readily swells in reaction to exposure to new antigens found within the intestinal contents. Because the hollow of the appendix is very narrow, just a slight swelling of its lining wall will cause the passageway to become blocked, thus causing fecal material to become retained within the appendix. This situation can then rapidly lead to inflammation, as the stagnant feces start to irritate the lining of the appendix.

The early stages of inflammation of the appendix first become apparent as deep pain in the center of the abdomen. The child may be reluctant to move, and may vomit. A low-grade fever is common. In some cases this pain can fluctuate in intensity over the course of days to weeks, and may even settle down. This is the so-called grumbling appendix.

In more severe cases, the pain can intensify as the inflammation spreads to affect the complete width of the appendix wall. Then, as the lining layer of the peritoneum becomes involved, the pain can move downwards and to the right, becoming localized in the right iliac fossa. If this progression occurs, the child can become very unwell, with severe pain and vomiting. If the progression is very rapid, the appendix may rupture and so lead to the serious condition of peritonitis. In this case, the child's condition will deteriorate rapidly and shock can ensue. This is a surgical emergency.

Diagnosis of an early case of appendicitis is not straightforward. Functional abdominal pain is common in children, and also mesenteric adenitis can readily mimic the classical features of appendicitis. In very young children the features of appendicitis can be very non-specific, sometimes only becoming apparent in the form of fever and irritability. If the diagnosis appears obvious, there may be no need for further investigations, but ultrasound and computed tomography (CT) scans may be used to confirm a diagnosis in an atypical case.

CT scanning is the best test by far in terms of accuracy for confirming diagnosis, but ultrasound tends to be a preferred test in children as CT involves high exposure to X-radiation.

Even if diagnostic uncertainty remains, because the complication of peritonitis is so devastating, early surgical exploration of suspected cases may be necessary practice, particularly as the operation is a simple and relatively safe one to perform. The operation of an appendectomy involves locating the appendix via a small incision in the right iliac fossa, and then removing the whole of the appendix, whether or not it is obviously inflamed. In conventional practice it is not believed that the loss of the appendix is detrimental to the health of the child. The child would be expected to make a rapid recovery over the course of the next few days. In between 10 and 20 percent of appendectomy operations the appendix is found to be healthy, and the complication rate from the surgery is reported at just over 6 percent.

Surprisingly there is still uncertainty over whether the introduction of preoperative CT scanning actually reduces the rate of unnecessary appendectomies. It may be that clinical judgment is the most reliable indicator of the true diagnosis and need for surgery.[104]

Information box 5.4e-XVIII

Appendicitis: comments from a Chinese medicine perspective

From the conventional understanding of the pathology of appendicitis, it would be expected that the Chinese medicine interpretation might embrace Qi and Blood Stagnation and Heat. This obstruction could be preceded by Exterior Cold or Accumulation Disorder. Early cases of appendicitis may be resolved by acupuncture treatment alone, although referral to a conventional practitioner would be advised in all suspected cases.

GASTROENTERITIS

Gastroenteritis is described in detail in Section 3.1c. The most important point to bear in mind with a case of gastroenteritis in a small child is that the risk of dehydration is much greater than that in a previously healthy adult.

CELIAC DISEASE

Celiac disease is described in detail in Section 3.1e as one of the most common causes of the malabsorption syndrome. Celiac disease in children will often present with failure to thrive (FTT). Although loose stools are one of the cardinal features of malabsorption, this symptom may not be a prominent feature, even in a case of sufficient severity to cause delayed attainment of developmental milestones in a child. For this reason, celiac disease should always be considered in a case of unexplained poor growth in a child (see Figure 5.4e-I).

Figure 5.4e-I Celiac disease, causing muscular wasting together with distension of the abdomen

INFLAMMATORY BOWEL DISEASE

Inflammatory bowel disease, a term that embraces Crohn's disease and ulcerative colitis, is described in detail in Section 3.1e.

Crohn's disease is a condition which, for a reason that is unclear, has been increasing in incidence since the 1950s. This increase has been particularly marked in children, and there is no clear understanding about why this should be. About one-quarter of patients with Crohn's disease first become apparent in childhood or adolescence. However, Crohn's disease is rare in children under the age of ten. Suggestions that this increased incidence may be attributed to the introduction of the measles, mumps, rubella (MMR) vaccination are hotly contested by the medical establishment. The scientific evidence that has been used to support this possible link with the MMR vaccine is not at all conclusive when considered from a conventional viewpoint.

In children, Crohn's disease can present with the characteristic features of diarrhea, weight loss and the passage of mucus. FTT and delayed onset of puberty are common. In some children, loss of appetite and weight may be more prominent than the symptom of loose stools, so much so that the condition may be confused with anorexia nervosa. In general, the long-term outlook for children with Crohn's disease is good, with most being able to lead a normal adult life, albeit with occasional bouts of recurrent disease.

In contrast to Crohn's disease, the incidence of ulcerative colitis has not altered over the past few decades. The presentation of ulcerative colitis in children is similar to that in adults. As with Crohn's disease, FTT and delayed puberty are common features in severe cases in children.

Part II: Other common disorders of childhood continued

Disorders of the respiratory system

The most common disorders of the respiratory system in children are the infectious diseases of the respiratory tract, described in detail in Section 5.4d. This section describes asthma, the most common non-infectious respiratory disease of childhood, and the relatively rare but very important condition of sudden infant death syndrome (SIDS). All the other important respiratory disorders of childhood, such as cystic fibrosis, are discussed elsewhere in this text.

ASTHMA

Asthma is the most common chronic respiratory disorder to affect children. Recent studies suggest that up to 15 percent of school children in the UK have been given the diagnosis of asthma at some point in their lives. Moreover, asthma now accounts for up to 20 percent of acute pediatric hospital admissions. Although the condition is rarely of a very severe nature in children, nevertheless asthma accounts for a great deal of restricted activity and school absenteeism in affected children. The incidence of asthma in children has been increasing in recent decades for reasons that are unclear. Young boys are affected twice as commonly as girls, but by adolescence equal numbers are affected.

The pathology of asthma is described in detail in Section 3.3d. Children almost always develop the extrinsic form of asthma, in which there is a tendency for the child to be oversensitive (allergic) to a wide range of environmental allergens, and in which a family history of atopy is common. One-third of children with asthma suffer also from eczema, and up to one-half have the features

of allergic rhinitis, including a persistently stuffy nose and nasal discharge. Common triggers for childhood asthma include animal dandruff, house dust mite feces, pollen and molds, and certain foods, including wheat, milk and eggs. It is well known that other environmental factors, such as damp living conditions, atmospheric pollution and cigarette smoke, can exacerbate the symptoms of asthma in children.

The diagnosis is based on a history of wheeze, cough and breathlessness or, in preschool children, nocturnal cough. The diagnosis can be confirmed in children over the age of five by means of serial peak-flow measurements. In some children the symptoms may only occur in brief bouts, sometimes precipitated by a respiratory infection. Less commonly, the symptoms are more chronic. Unless the asthma is very severe, the health of the affected child is usually otherwise unaffected. However, in severe cases there may be evidence of FTT, with poor attainment of developmental milestones.

The aim of treatment is to enable the child to lead a normal life, and to prevent deterioration of the symptoms to a serious, potentially life-threatening condition. The management of asthma by means of inhaled and oral bronchodilators and prophylactic (preventive) medication is similar in principle to the management strategy that conventional practitioners are advised to follow for adults (as described in Section 3.3d). The main difference to adult treatment is that in young children either an oral anti-inflammatory medication, called montelukast, or a form of theophylline may also be prescribed in addition to a corticosteroid such as beclometasone. Even small babies can be administered inhaled medication by means of a plastic "spacer" device, with a mask or a nebulizer pump if large doses are required. From the age of five many children become competent in the use of dry powder inhalers.

Most asthmatic children (about 70 percent) have less than four episodes a year. In these children the symptoms can be controlled by means of intermittent use of a bronchodilator inhaler such as salbutamol. Severe episodes may require the additional use of nebulized bronchodilators or a brief course of oral steroids, but with the expectation that the child can be weaned off these medications after a few days.

About 25 percent of children have asthmatic symptoms at least once every two to four weeks, but also have some periods of complete respite from symptoms. These children will be prescribed a regular dose of a prophylactic medication, such as beclometasone.

The remaining 5 percent of asthmatic children have persistent symptoms. Most of these will be prescribed regular doses of inhaled corticosteroid and bronchodilators. These are children who may also be prescribed oral theophylline or montelukast. In severe cases, oral corticosteroids may also be prescribed. These children may be supervised by

625

a hospital consultant, and will require regular monitoring of their general health and growth, particularly if they are on oral steroid medication. Because of judicious use of preventive medication, severe uncontrollable exacerbations of asthma are uncommon in children; in the UK, 20–30 children die of status asthmaticus per year.

Information box 5.4e-XIX

Asthma: comments from a Chinese medicine perspective

In Chinese medicine, asthma is known as Xiao Chuan (meaning wheezing and breathlessness or gurgling). In general, the underlying patterns found in children are Deficiency of Lung, Spleen and Kidney Qi, together with Accumulation of Damp and Phlegm. Invasion of External Pathogenic Factors or a Lingering Pathogenic Factor can exacerbate these patterns. In the acute attack Liver Qi insulting the Lungs, Phlegm or Heat are the principal causes of the difficulty in breathing.

Scott and Barlow (1999) propose that medication, including repeated prescriptions of antibiotics, will only serve to worsen these imbalances in the long term. Inhaled bronchodilator and corticosteroid medication tend to weaken the Qi of the Lungs and Kidneys, and corticosteroids can cause accumulation of Damp and Heat in the Lungs.

Predisposing factors in the etiology of asthma include an inherited Deficiency, repeated infections with prescription of antibiotics, Phlegm-forming foods and additives in the diet, and weakening of the Spleen from irregular and inappropriate feeding of the small child. Excessive use of television and computer games, lack of exercise, poor posture and emotional trauma (particularly when a state of fear or panic is induced) are also believed to be very important contributors to the development of asthma.[105]

SUDDEN INFANT DEATH SYNDROME (SIDS) (COT DEATH)

Sudden infant death syndrome (SIDS) is defined as the sudden and unexpected death of a child for which no adequate cause is found at post-mortem examination. This tragic event most commonly occurs in babies aged between two to four months. In affluent societies SIDS is the most common cause of death in babies aged between one and twelve months. It is believed that the underlying cause of death is cessation of breathing (apnea), primarily as a consequence of immature respiratory reflexes. It is believed that the small baby is relatively insensitive to the buildup of carbon dioxide in its bloodstream, which is normally a potent trigger for more rapid and deeper respirations.

It is recognized that an ongoing respiratory infection and environmental cigarette smoke both increase the risk of SIDS.

The incidence of SIDS in the UK has fallen dramatically over the past few years since the introduction of a national campaign that advocated three cardinal principles. These were:

- the child should not be laid to sleep on its front (i.e. not face down)
- the child should not be allowed to overheat when sleeping
- the child should not be exposed to cigarette smoke.

Advice about bed sharing has been added to these principles – bed sharing and especially sleeping with a baby on a sofa is linked with increased risk of SIDS and especially if the parent has used drugs or alcohol. In contrast, if parents share a bedroom with the baby, this is protective against SIDS. The current advice is that babies should sleep in their own cot or Moses basket in the parents' bedroom.

In the event of SIDS, the family will require sensitive support to enable them to comprehend what has happened and to move on from their bereavement. It is believed that it is very important for the family to be allowed to hold the dead child. In all cases the coroner has to be informed of the death and a post-mortem performed. The family will have to be interviewed by the police in all cases, and their homes may be the subject of an investigation, which will, of course, only add to the shock and distress of the death. The family needs to be prepared for this, and it is essential that it is explained to them that this routine practice does not imply that they are under any suspicion. Written information about the nature of SIDS should be given to the parents, together with the details of bereavement support agencies such as Child Death Helpline or CRUSE. When the results of the post-mortem are known, the parents should be offered an explanatory interview and, when relevant, genetic counseling.

Disorders of the urinary system and genitalia

The most important conditions to affect the urinary system in children include the inherited malformations of the urinary tract, urinary infections (which are often associated with inherited abnormalities), glomerulonephritis and tumors of the kidney. Of these, only the inherited deformities are discussed below, as urinary infections and glomerulonephritis have already been discussed in detail earlier in this section and also in Sections 4.3c and 4.3d. Tumors of the kidney are described later.

The most important disorders of the genitalia in children are those that affect boys. Of these, maldescent of the testis and congenital inguinal hernia have been discussed in Section 5.4c. Germ cell tumors of the testis are described later in this section. Only the important disorders of the foreskin, phimosis and balanitis, and torsion of the testis are discussed below.

INHERITED MALFORMATIONS OF THE URINARY TRACT

The widespread use of antenatal ultrasound screening of the 20-week-old fetus can demonstrate all of the gross abnormalities of the urinary tract. These abnormalities are detected in 1 in 400 of fetuses, indicating that a malformation of the urinary system is a relatively common occurrence. However, not all these malformations will lead to manifest disease in the child.

Abnormalities that do not often lead to serious symptoms include horseshoe kidney, in which the two kidneys are fused together to form the resulting horseshoe-shaped organ, and duplex kidney system, in which one or both kidneys give rise to two ureters. In some cases both these abnormalities may give rise to an obstruction of the flow of urine through the unusually situated ureters. This can lead to back pressure of urine in the kidney, and thus progressive kidney damage, increased risk of repeated kidney infections, and chronic pyelonephritis. Vesico-ureteric reflux (VUR) is also more common with a duplex system, and is an important cause of chronic pyelonephritis.

Obstruction to the flow of the urine in one or both ureters, usually due to a malformation of the ureter itself, can also be detected by means of ultrasound scans. Obstruction to flow can also occur at the neck of the bladder in boys, as a result of a flap of tissue known as a posterior urethral valve. In cases of severe obstruction, the affected kidney may appear dilated or shriveled, even at this early stage of fetal development. Both kidneys will be affected if a posterior urethral valve is the cause of the obstruction. In severe cases the child can be born with permanently damaged renal function, which will then lead to chronic renal failure in early childhood. Detection of bilateral kidney damage would be a reason to induce labor as early as possible (35 weeks) so that the obstruction can be relieved by means of immediate surgery, and the progression of damage to the kidneys halted.

Information box 5.4e-XX

Urinary tract malformations: comments from a Chinese medicine perspective

In Chinese medicine, inherited malformations of the urinary tract would normally indicate Deficiency of Kidney Essence.

BALANITIS AND PHIMOSIS

The foreskin of a baby boy is usually prevented from retracting and exposing the glans of the penis by fibrous adhesions that join its inner surface to the surface of the glans. As the child gets older these adhesions break down, so that in the majority of six-year-old boys the foreskin has become retractile. By the age of 16, only 1 percent of boys are unable to retract their foreskin.

Phimosis is the term used to describe a non-retractile foreskin. Phimosis is normal in very young boys. Phimosis that persists, but causes no symptoms, is not usual, but is not necessarily a cause for concern. Phimosis only becomes a problem if the foreskin becomes inflamed or damaged. This can occur if there have been repeated forceful attempts of retraction of the foreskin, or if there have been episodes of infection of the space between the foreskin and the glans, a condition known as balanitis. An episode of balanitis is usually treated by means of oral antibiotics.

A damaged foreskin can become scarred and thickened. This can restrict the normal flow of urine, and can predispose to recurrent bouts of balanitis. A scarred and thickened foreskin is considered to be an indication for circumcision. This operation, when necessary for health reasons, is performed under general anesthetic (in contrast to religious circumcision).

Information box 5.4e-XXI

Balanitis and phimosis: comments from a Chinese medicine perspective

From a Chinese medicine perspective, asymptomatic phimosis probably does not represent any underlying imbalance. However, in cases in which balanitis and scarring occur, this suggests the Pattern of Damp Heat in the Liver with an underlying Kidney Deficiency or Liver Disharmony, as both these Organs relate to the penis.

TORSION OF THE TESTIS

Torsion of the testis is a condition that primarily affects the young child or adolescent, but it may occasionally occur in young men. It is believed that the problem, which involves the testis twisting around the root that provides its blood and nerve supply, is much more likely if there is a slight congenital abnormality of one or more of the position, orientation or shape of the testis. The ovary can also undergo torsion, although this problem almost always occurs in women of childbearing years. In women, the presence of an ovarian cyst will predispose to torsion of the ovary.

A testicular torsion will present as a sudden onset of severe pain in the lower abdomen and scrotum. The affected scrotum becomes swollen and inflamed. The child may vomit with the pain. If the torsion affects an undescended testis, the pain will be localized to the abdomen and groin, and may mimic a strangulated hernia. In some cases, the acute episode may have been preceded by a few episodes of partial torsion, in which less severe warning pains in the groin region were felt for short periods of time.

Torsion requires emergency surgery to prevent gangrene of the testis. This has to be performed within a few hours, at most, of the onset of the symptoms if the function of the testis is to be preserved. If the testis can be saved, it is anchored surgically to the surrounding tissues. This procedure is usually repeated for the unaffected testis. A gangrenous testis has to be removed (orchiectomy), and the unaffected testis is surgically anchored in place. When the child reaches late adolescence, he will be offered an operation to implant a prosthetic testis in the empty side of the scrotum.

Information box 5.4e-XXII

Torsion of the testis: comments from a Chinese medicine perspective

In Chinese medicine, acute pain in the scrotum might correspond to Stagnation of Blood and Qi or Cold in the Liver Channel. As there is a congenital predisposition to torsion of the testis, this suggests that there is an underlying Deficiency of Kidney Essence.

Disorders of the eyes, ears and nervous system

The conditions of the eyes and ears will be studied in detail in Sections 6.1d and 6.1e. This section introduces only the two most important of these conditions that primarily affect children, namely, squint (strabismus) and glue ear (chronic secretory otitis media).

SQUINT (STRABISMUS)

Squint, or strabismus, is primarily a disorder of the external ocular muscles (the muscles that control the coordinated movements of the eyeballs within the orbits of the skull) rather than an internal problem of the eye itself. However, if uncorrected, a squint can lead to a long-term underdevelopment of the nerve pathways that are responsible for depth (or stereoscopic) vision, a condition known as amblyopia. For this reason, squint is one of the conditions that should be excluded through the routine child health surveillance checks of the preschool years.

In health, the eyes should both be directed towards the object that is the focus of the gaze. If the object moves, the eyeballs move so that they each remain directed towards the object. Because the eyes are not in exactly the same place in relation to the object, each receives a slightly different image. As the nervous system develops during the preschool years, the brain learns to use the differences in these images to perceive how far away the object is in relation to other objects in the field of vision. This is stereoscopic vision. Stereoscopic vision is an important faculty that enables the judgment of distance and the controlled and accurate movement of the limbs or body. It is of particular importance for the correct performance of delicate manual tasks, such as needlework, and also for all forms of sport that require the judgment of distance, such as ball games.

In the form of squint that is most common in childhood, the direction of the eyes in relation to each other is misaligned so that the eyes do not receive corresponding images of the viewed object. In some children this misalignment is obvious, in that one eye always appears to be gazing slightly in the wrong direction. In other children, the misalignment is more prominent when the child is tired.

If this sort of misalignment were to occur suddenly in an adult (most commonly as a result of a mononeuropathy of one of the cranial nerves that supply the eye muscles), the result would be unremitting double vision. One way for the adult to cope with this problem is to place a patch over one eye in order to suppress the confusing image from the affected eye.

However, in the developing nervous system of the small child, double vision does not occur. Instead, the image from one of the eyes is suppressed internally by nerve impulses from the brain. This means that far less confusing information is received, and a clear image of the object can be generated, albeit without the added information required to judge its distance. If this suppression occurs for long enough, the ability of the nervous system to perceive a clear image from the affected eye is permanently lost. Although the child does not become blind in the affected eye, when both eyes are used it is as if only one eye is active in generating the image that is perceived by the brain. This is amblyopia, or, as it is more commonly known, "lazy eye." In a case of established amblyopia, if the good eye is covered, it is evident that the affected eye is able to receive only very vague visual information compared with the good eye. This is a problem that cannot be corrected by wearing glasses.

Squints are relatively common. They are even more common in children who have other neurological problems that have been present from birth. In rare cases, the inability to focus one eye on the object may be due to a very severe refractive error (a problem in the ability to focus the lens of the eye), a congenital cataract (clouding of the lens) or an intraocular tumor (retinoblastoma). For this reason, when a squint is detected, the child should be referred for expert ophthalmological diagnosis.

Once serious underlying causes have been excluded, the child is treated by means of glasses to correct any refractive error, and by the use of patches to cover the good eye for defined times of the day. This stimulates the affected eye, and enables the nerve pathways that radiate from the eye to the visual centers of the brain to continue to develop. This treatment should be initiated as long as possible before the child's seventh birthday, after which there is little hope for further improvement. In cases when there is very obvious divergence or convergence of the eyes, the child may be offered a surgical operation to correct the squint. This is of value for cosmetic reasons, but is recognized not to be an effective treatment for the prevention of amblyopia.

 Information box 5.4e-XXIII

Squint (strabismus): comments from a Chinese medicine perspective

From a Chinese medicine perspective, Scott and Barlow (1999) suggest that the manifestation of a squint may be the result of Womb Heat. This has become lodged in the channels that relate to one or more of the extraocular muscles (Liver, Gallbladder and Bladder). In this case the squint is present from birth, and is often quite pronounced in appearance.

Alternatively, if the squint develops after the time of birth, it may be the result of the Depletion in energy of the eye muscles resulting from an Invasion of Full Heat or a lingering Pathogenic Factor in the channels. It is possible that the internal (Empty) Heat generated from overstimulation or overexcitement of a child can, in the same way, deplete the Qi in the channels that relate to the eye muscles. These forms of squint may vary in severity according to the nervous state or level of tiredness of the child.

Treatment principles include Clearing of Heat from the Liver, Gallbladder and Kidney Channels, and Tonification of the Kidney Qi.[106]

GLUE EAR

Glue ear is the aptly descriptive common term for the condition of chronic secretory otitis media (CSOM) (also termed otitis media with effusion). CSOM can be a long-term outcome of an attack of acute otitis media, the infectious inflammation of the middle ear that is known to affect up to one-fifth of all children under four within any one year. The tendency to develop a persistent, thick but non-infective discharge in the middle ear runs strongly in families. It is believed that it is a combination of a particular anatomical structure of the Eustachian tube in children (inherited) and susceptibility to upper respiratory tract infections that causes the susceptibility to this condition. CSOM affects up to one-third of children at some point in their lives. The condition is most common in children between the ages of two and nine.

There need not be a history of acute otitis media for CSOM to develop. Secretions in the middle ear originate from the respiratory epithelium that lines this cavity. Normally these secretions drain away to the throat via the Eustachian tube. Anatomical abnormalities of the Eustachian tube, the presence of enlarged adenoids, and a cleft palate are all recognized to be associated with CSOM, because they lead to impaired drainage of the middle ear. Factors that lead to increased secretions in the middle ear, such as infections, allergic rhinitis, damage to the eardrum during air travel and cigarette smoke, can also promote the development of CSOM.

The primary symptom of CSOM is deafness in one or both ears. This conductive deafness is a result of the fluid in the middle ear impairing the transmission of sound waves from the eardrum through to the nerve endings in the inner ear. If the deafness is not recognized, the child may appear to be dreamy, or in a world of their own. The child may also develop low-grade discomfort in the affected ear, tinnitus or unsteadiness, but these complications are relatively rare. CSOM is a significant problem in young children, because it can have a marked impact on their interactions with the people around them, and on their development of speech and language.

CSOM gives rise to a characteristic appearance of the eardrum, and so its presence may be suspected by a physician after simple visualization of the eardrum (otoscopy). The diagnosis can be confirmed by an audiologist by means of a non-invasive test called impedance audiometry. This test assesses the degree to which sound is absorbed by the eardrum, and also the springiness of the membrane of the eardrum.

Most cases of CSOM will resolve spontaneously. However, if there is a susceptibility, the condition may recur several times in the early life of the same child. Current medical opinion is that a period of watchful waiting should be allowed before treatment is offered for CSOM. The decision to treat should be based not on test results, but on how the condition is affecting the child. Simple medical treatment includes the prescription of short courses of antibiotics if infection is suspected, antihistamines in cases of allergic rhinitis, and mucolytics (drugs intended to reduce the thickness of secretions, the benefit of which is very uncertain). Surgical treatment is considered if hearing loss persists for some months, if the child is demonstrating negative social or educational consequences of intermittent deafness, or if there are symptoms such as pain or dizziness.

The surgical treatment of CSOM involves piercing the eardrum, aspiration of the fluid from the middle ear and the insertion of a tiny tube-like structure known as a grommet into the hole formed by the piercing. The tube of the grommet has a widened margin at each of its ends, and stays in place as a result of this structure. However, the grommet will eventually be pushed out of the eardrum into the outer ear canal as the epithelium of the eardrum turns over. This takes an average of six months. The grommet is intended to permit free drainage of fluid from the middle ear. It should not adversely affect hearing, and the eardrum usually appears completely normal after its extrusion. Insertion of grommets is conventionally considered to be a relatively non-invasive operation.

In some children the CSOM recurs after the extrusion of the grommets, and in these cases it may be considered necessary to repeat the operation.

 Information box 5.4e-XXIV

Glue ear (chronic secretory otitis media): comments from a Chinese medicine perspective

In Chinese medicine, otitis media is considered to be a channel problem, and thus CSOM can respond well to acupuncture treatment. It may correspond to Lingering Pathogenic Factor. This can result in the buildup of Phlegm and the Obstruction of Qi in the ear cavity. The child may also suffer from a pre-existing depletion of Spleen Qi. This can contribute to the accumulation of Damp and Phlegm.

Alternatively, and less commonly, Depletion of Liver and Kidney Yin may lead to undernourishment of the ear. This would lead to a sticky fluid on the eardrum rather than a profuse phlegmy discharge. In these cases the Depletion may be a result of overstimulation, and may appear in a slightly hyperactive child.

Epilepsy

The various forms of epilepsy are described in detail in Section 4.1f.

Childhood epilepsy is fairly common, affecting 5 in 1000 school-aged children. In 70–80 percent of cases of childhood epilepsy there is no obvious underlying cause. Intrauterine infections, brain damage from birth trauma, intracerebral bleeds in prematurity and brain tumors are the most common of the known structural causes in children.

In addition to tonic-clonic epilepsy, which usually presents in later childhood, there are some particular syndromes that are characteristic of childhood epilepsy. These are considered briefly here.

West syndrome is a form of epileptic spasm that affects children from the age of about four to six months. The diagnosis may be delayed, as the spasms may not be recognized as such for some time. In many cases there is an underlying physical abnormality of the brain. In later childhood, many affected children show developmental delay and can suffer from forms of epilepsy more characteristic of adulthood, such as tonic-clonic epilepsy.

Absence (petit mal) seizures affect 1–2 percent of children with childhood epilepsy. The age of onset is four to twelve years. The affected child will momentarily go pale and stare for up to about 30 seconds. The child will regain consciousness as if nothing has happened, but may look puzzled if they become aware that they have missed something during the absence. In most children the absences cease before adulthood. Frequent absence attacks may interfere with concentration, and so can affect school performance.

Benign rolandic epilepsy is a partial epilepsy of childhood in which the seizures almost always stop by the mid-teens. Seizures often affect one side of the body only, but may become generalized tonic-clonic in form if they occur during sleep.

As in adult epilepsy, diagnosis is established by means of electroencephalogram (EEG) examination. Computed tomography (CT) or magnetic resonance imaging (MRI) may be used to exclude focal brain pathology if the age of onset is less than five years.

Seizures in children may be provoked by diverse factors, including deep sleep, lack of sleep, excitement, anxiety, menstruation and rapid withdrawal of anticonvulsant medication. In some cases seizures may be provoked by exposure to rapidly flashing light sources (photosensitive epilepsy). Children with photosensitive epilepsy will be advised to watch television only in a brightly lit room, and to avoid stroboscopic lighting.

Children who are prone to unpredictable seizures in the daytime are in need of protection against injury. They are advised to avoid swimming unless under very close supervision, and also other activities such as cycling or climbing, during which a seizure could place them in great danger.

Anticonvulsant medication is prescribed with caution in children, and may not be used at all in some cases. The anticonvulsant drugs that are prescribed are the same as those prescribed in adult epilepsy. In a very few cases the seizures may be relieved by surgical removal of the physical focus of the seizures from the brain.

Information box 5.4e-XXV

Epilepsy: comments from a Chinese medicine perspective

A grand mal seizure is seen in Chinese medicine as Liver Wind stirring upwards and causing Phlegm to Obstruct the Orifices of the Heart. Other seizures that manifest in muscular twitching would also be diagnosed in terms of Liver Wind. In absence seizures, the prominent pathology would appear to be Phlegm impeding the functions of the Shen.

The sudden onset is again indicative of Wind. There is usually an underlying Deficiency in all forms of epilepsy, including Deficiency of Liver and Kidney Yin, which predispose to the Stirring of Liver Wind, and Spleen Deficiency, which predisposes to the Accumulation of Phlegm.

Scott and Barlow (1999) suggest that epilepsy that suddenly becomes apparent in childhood does so as a progression from an earlier deeply rooted imbalance. They suggest that three primary factors may underlie the development of epilepsy in children: weak Yuan (source) Qi, Phlegm Obstructing the Orifices and Blood Stasis (brain injury). They go on to describe that weak Yuan Qi will predispose to Liver and Kidney Yin Deficiency, and also instability of the Qi of the Heart and the Liver.[107]

They explain that the external factors that may contribute to the development of childhood epilepsy include repeated febrile convulsions, sudden shock, Latent Pathogenic Heat from immunizations, brain injury, a severe attack of diarrhea and inappropriate (Cold) medication. The first two of these factors contribute to Depletion of Yin, and the last three promote the development of Phlegm by Combination of Heat with Damp resulting from Depletion of Spleen Qi.

Flaws (2006) explains that factors affecting the fetus in the womb including maternal shock or inappropriate diet may lead to inherited predisposition to epilepsy which is deeply rooted and difficult to treat. However, treatment is essential to prevent progression as each seizure is likely to further deplete the Yin and Qi and also lead to more entrenched Phlegm binding.[108]

Medical treatments for epilepsy tend to have a wide range of profound side effects including drowsiness, clumsiness and dizziness, with confusion and loss of balance, if drugs are taken in excessive dose. These side effects all suggest that these drugs are Phlegm Forming and possibly Cold in nature. The drugs clearly prevent Stirring up of the Wind and Pacify Heat (their physical action is to increase the action of the inhibitory nerves of the brain), but do not seem to address the main root cause of the problem, which is, of course, the Accumulation of Phlegm.

The various additional side effects are due to drug-induced disease. Swollen gums indicate Heat and Phlegm in the Stomach, and rashes indicate Heat in the Blood. Most of the drugs are toxic to some degree to the liver, and this would be in terms of damage to Liver Yin.

The fact that the medication can worsen the Chinese medical pathology of epilepsy goes some way in explaining how difficult it can be to withdraw from the medication once it has been taken for some years.

Cancer in childhood

Cancer affects 1 in 650 children under the age of 15. Over one-third of these cancers are forms of leukemia, the cancerous growth of the immature white blood cells. Lymphomas, cancers of the mature white blood cells, account for a further 10 percent of childhood cancer. The other important childhood cancers, in order of frequency of occurrence, are brain tumors (the cause in over 20 percent of childhood cancer cases), kidney (Wilms') tumors (7 percent), nerve cell tumors (7 percent), bone tumors (6 percent), muscle tumors (5 percent) and tumors of the retina of the eye (3 percent).

The range of cancers known to affect children is different to that recognized in adults. The hopes for survival in childhood cancer are greater than in most forms of adult cancer. Over 60 percent of children diagnosed with cancer will still be alive five years after diagnosis, and many of these can be considered cured. The survival rate in childhood cancer has improved dramatically over the past 30 years. Much of this improvement can be attributed to modern approaches in chemotherapy and radiotherapy.

It is believed that in most cases of childhood cancer the underlying cause is a combination of individual susceptibility and exposure to adverse environmental factors such as radiation or viruses. In many childhood cancers, a structural change in the genetic material of the cancer cell can be detected, and some of these changes can be linked to an inherited chromosomal or genetic abnormality. In childhood cancer, the condition may present either as a localized growth, or with features of more generalized disease, such as recurrent infections, or bruising and bleeding, or both.

When cancer is diagnosed in a child, the treatment should ideally be managed from a dedicated cancer center at which multidisciplinary supportive care can be offered to the child and the family. Children need particular support in dealing with the side effects of treatment and its long-term effects. Both the child and the family need to be supported as they struggle with the prospect of a potentially fatal illness. Practical issues that need to be surmounted include education and social stimulation for the sick child, and finances for the family to cover the expenses of transport to numerous hospital appointments, time off work for the parents and childcare for siblings.

It has been estimated that currently about 1 in 1000 young adults in the UK are survivors of treatment for childhood cancer. These young people are likely to have residual problems resulting from recurrent cycles of chemotherapy and radiotherapy, including poor growth and infertility, and the consequences of reduced access to education. There is also an increased risk of secondary tumors in children who have been exposed to cancer therapies.

LEUKEMIA AND LYMPHOMA

Leukemia and lymphoma have been described in detail in Section 3.4e. Although leukemia and lymphoma are rare in adults, they are two of the most common forms of cancer in children and young people.

Leukemia accounts for about 35 percent of childhood cancer. In four-fifths of these cases the cause is a form of acute leukemia known as acute lymphoblastic leukemia (ALL). As is the case in adults, affected children present with symptoms of rapidly worsening bone marrow failure (susceptibility to infections, bruising and bleeding, and anemia). The treatment depends on the precise diagnosis of the leukemia. Nowadays, up to 65 percent of cases of ALL will be cured by chemotherapy regimens, the success depending in part on how extensive the tumor is at diagnosis. Treatment for ALL may often extend over a course of over two years. For the remaining forms of leukemia, the prognosis is less favorable (e.g. the cure rate is below 50 percent in acute myeloid leukemia).

Lymphoma can be categorized into various types according to the type of white blood cells involved. Hodgkin lymphoma is the form that is particularly frequent in young adults and teenagers. However, in young children, the other forms of lymphoma (generally termed non-Hodgkin lymphoma (NHL)) are more common.

The treatment for NHL depends on the nature of presentation. Some forms present very similarly to ALL and are treated in the same way as ALL. The prognosis for survival is similar. The form of NHL that most often presents in the form of enlarged head or neck lymph nodes is treated with relatively short courses of chemotherapy and has a very good prognosis. However, the types of NHL that present with nodes in the abdomen are often at an advanced stage at diagnosis, and the prognosis is less good.

The treatment for Hodgkin lymphoma depends on the stage of the disease. Localized disease (in one lymph node site) can often be cured by radiotherapy alone. Otherwise, combined chemotherapy and radiotherapy is used. Hodgkin lymphoma has a relatively very good prognosis, with 80 percent of children who are treated being cured.

BRAIN TUMORS

In children, brain tumors are almost always primary (rather than metastatic, as is the case for many brain tumors in adults). The most common childhood brain tumors are malignancies of the glial cells. They most often develop in the cerebellum or the brainstem, and can present with symptoms such as headache, vomiting, squint, double vision and dizziness.

The outcome of the treatment of a childhood brain tumor depends very much on the type of the tumor and on how closely the tumor is located to vital areas in the brain. Treatment usually involves surgery and radiotherapy, together with chemotherapy in some cases. The combination of damage from the growing tumor, surgery to a delicate area of the brain, and the effect of radiotherapy can mean that the very few surviving children may suffer from long-term complex difficulties, such as poor growth, physical disability, epilepsy and educational problems.

NEUROBLASTOMA

Neuroblastoma is a tumor of primitive nerve cells. It most commonly arises in the adrenal medulla or in the chain of sympathetic nerves that run either side of the spinal cord. It usually presents in a child of less than five years of age as an abdominal mass. Often, by the time of diagnosis, the disease has metastasized to the bones or bone marrow.

Non-metastatic disease has a relatively good prognosis, with many children being cured by surgery alone. However, if the disease has metastasized, the prognosis is not at all good. The disease is then treated with a combination of surgery and high-dose chemotherapy. Less than 30 percent of children with metastatic disease will be cured.

WILMS' TUMOR (NEPHROBLASTOMA)

Wilms' tumor is a tumor of primitive kidney cells. It is a tumor that is associated with a genetic susceptibility. Its development has been linked to a deletion in chromosome 11. In most cases the disease presents in a child less than five years of age as an abdominal mass.

In 15 percent of cases of Wilms' tumor, metastases are found, most commonly, in the lung. Other problems that can complicate treatment result from the tumor bulk, particularly if it is compressing the major vessels of the abdomen, such as the renal arteries or the inferior vena cava.

Treatment is by means of surgical removal of the mass, followed by chemotherapy. In advanced disease, radiotherapy may also be given. Overall, about 80 percent of children will be cured of the disease.

Bone and muscle tumors

Malignant bone tumors are rare in children before puberty. Malignant osteosarcoma is the most common form of childhood bone tumor. This tumor primarily affects the long bones of the limbs. Ewing sarcoma is a less common bone tumor that also mainly affects the limbs.

Both forms of bone tumor are difficult to treat. However, the prognosis has improved in recent years as a result of the use of combination chemotherapy before surgery. Radiotherapy can also be of value in controlling the growth of Ewing sarcoma.

The rhabdomyosarcoma is a tumor that originates from primitive muscle tissue. It most commonly arises in the head and neck region or the genital region. In 15 percent of cases metastatic spread to the lung, liver, bone or bone marrow has occurred by the time of diagnosis. Only in the minority can the tumor be excised completely, in which case the prognosis is favorable. Otherwise, the disease requires treatment with combination chemotherapy and radiotherapy, and has a poor prognosis.

Retinoblastoma

Retinoblastoma is a tumor of primitive retinal cells that arises within the posterior chamber of the eye. It is usually first detected in a child under the age of two through routine eye checks, when it manifests either as a squint or in difficulty of the examiner in obtaining a view of the retina.

In about one-third of cases the condition arises as a result of an inherited mutation of a gene on chromosome 13. This gene is known to control retinal differentiation. In some cases of inherited retinoblastoma, tumors are found to be developing in both eyes. In the non-inherited cases, the mutation of the gene has occurred in one of the cells within the developing embryonic retina.

Treatment by means of radiation or laser therapy may be sufficient to treat small tumors, but in advanced cases the eye needs to be removed (enucleation). In hereditary cases there remains a significant risk of a second tumor developing (osteosarcoma being the most common form). For this reason, in hereditary cases there should be regular screening of affected children and their siblings for retinal and other tumors.

Germ cell tumors

Germ cell tumors arise from the immature germ cells that in the fetus are destined to mature within the gonads. These rare tumors develop either in the sacro-coccygeal region, and so become apparent as a mass close to the anus, or in the gonads themselves.

Even the malignant forms of these tumors are very sensitive to chemotherapy, and there is generally a good prognosis with treatment.

> **Information box 5.4e-XXVI**
>
> ## Childhood cancer: comments from a Chinese medicine perspective
>
> Most of the childhood tumors arise from primitive cells that were present in the embryo. In health, these rapidly dividing primitive cells are destined to be the basis of more mature cells in the growing child. The fact that these growing and developing cells are defective suggests that, from a Chinese medicine perspective, Deficiency of Kidney Essence is likely to be a prominent imbalance in childhood cancer. As in all forms of cancer, the substantial manifestation of the disease corresponds to Stagnation of Blood and/or Accumulation of Phlegm. In cancer, both these imbalances develop as a consequence of a severe underlying Deficiency.

Skin disorders

The most important skin disorders of children, including infantile eczema, will be described in detail in Section 6.1c.

Psychiatric developmental and behavioral disorders

Section 6.2b describes how mental health disorders are classified. The two classification systems that are widely used by psychiatrists across the world are the WHO's 1993 International Classification of Diseases, tenth revision (ICD-10),[109] and the more recently updated 2013 American Psychiatric Association's (APA) *Diagnostic and Statistical Manual of Mental Disorders*, fifth revision (DSM-5).[110] There is now very close correspondence between the diagnostic criteria listed in these systems. Both order all the known psychiatric diagnoses within major groupings that include the neurodevelopmental disorders, anxiety disorders, schizophrenia, eating disorders, substance misuse disorders and sexual dysfunctions.

There are subtle differences in categorization, and these reflect both the rationale behind the compilation of these systems and also the changing approach of psychiatry between the different decades in which they were drawn up.

Both systems define autistic spectrum disorder and the language, speech and reading disorders (including the dyslexias) as developmental disorders.

According to ICD-10, hyperkinetic disorders (including attention deficit hyperactivity disorder, ADHD) and tic disorders (including Tourette's syndrome) are classified as behavioral disorders, whereas in DSM-5 these are also classified as neurodevelopmental disorders.

Likewise, in ICD-10 children with learning difficulties would be classified in the "mental retardation" category, whereas in the more recent DSM-5, the term "mental retardation" is replaced by the more currently accepted term of "intellectual disability," and is also classified as a neurodevelopmental disorder.

This section considers only the following important psychiatric conditions of childhood: autism spectrum disorder (ASD), the disorders of spelling and reading (dyslexias), ADHD and tics. Anxiety disorders of childhood and eating disorders are described in Section 6.2d.

AUTISM SPECTRUM DISORDER (ASD)

Autism is a diagnosis that falls in the ICD-10 under the broader diagnosis of pervasive development disorder (PDD). PDD, as defined in ICD-10, is a relatively uncommon spectrum of disorders (affecting up to 15 children per 10,000 births), and is characterized by disturbance in communication skills, difficulties in social interactions, and problems in imaginative and play activities and behavior. It is often associated with impaired intellectual capacity.

Autism as defined by ICD-10 is the most common form of PDD. Asperger syndrome is defined as a separate form of PDD in which language and intellectual skills are better developed. Both these forms of PDD are 4–8 times more common in boys than in girls.

In DSM-5 autism and Asperger syndrome are not separated diagnostically but are classed together as autism spectrum disorder (ASD).[111]

ASD classically presents before the age of three. Features that are noticeable at this age include impaired speech development, poor eye contact, aloofness, treatment of people as objects, ritualistic behavior, intolerance of change and limited creative play. In some children odd movements, such as flapping of the hands, spinning or walking on tiptoe, may also appear by this age.

There is evidence that in some cases there is a genetic predisposition to ASD, suggesting a biological basis for the condition. In some cases it is thought that stressors such as oxygen deprivation around the time of birth may be linked with persisting subtle changes in brain function. In up to 20 percent of cases epilepsy is a concurrent problem, which is further evidence of a structural biological basis. Occasionally, the condition can follow on from episodes of organic brain disorders such as encephalitis. MRI studies in young children who later turned out to have ASD suggest that a disordered growth of key areas in the brain between the ages of 6 and 18 months is then followed by impaired function, and altered circuitry of the neurons in the brain.

Claims that autism can result from the MMR vaccine are not substantiated by conventional analyses of the statistics of the incidence of autism. There is no evidence to suggest that the condition results from emotional trauma or poor parenting.

The long-term outlook for a child with ASD is improved if the child can be integrated into a specific educational and behavioral program from an early age, sometimes within the setting of a special school. Such a setting should also become an invaluable source of support for the families of affected children. Although ASD cannot be cured, about 10 percent of children will develop a capacity for independent living. A further 50 percent might be able to achieve semi-independent supported community living. The prognosis is better for those children who, from an early age, have higher scores on IQ (intelligence quotient) testing and more advanced development of speech.

Information box 5.4e-XXVII

Autism spectrum disorder: comments from a Chinese medicine perspective

In Chinese medicine the Heart Spleen and Kidney overrule reason and awareness, and so ASD might be understood in terms of an imbalance in the function of these three Organs. Phlegm and Phlegm Fire can lead to confusion, dullness, impaired interactions and agitation, and may be the result of inherited deficiencies of these organs that have later been compounded by poor diet, External Pathogenic Factors and also emotional disturbance in early life.

Scott and Barlow (1999) emphasize that autism can respond well to acupuncture. They describe the common patterns that underlie autism as extreme Qi Deficiency, Lingering Pathogenic Factor (particularly Heat and Phlegm), Kidney Weakness and Disturbances of the Spirit. They also describe brain damage as a separate pattern. They explain that in some cases an extreme fever or immunization can cause the Shen to be unable to rest in the Heart, either because of extreme Depletion of Qi, or because of Residual Heat in the Heart. In contrast to the conventional view that the social influences on a child have no impact on the development of autism, Scott and Barlow believe that both shock and the imploded anger that can follow abuse or neglect can also lead to an autistic state.[112]

It would make sense in Chinese medical terms that very careful attention to diet with avoidance of Damp-forming and Hot foods would be crucial in the long-term management of ASD.

DYSLEXIA

Dyslexia is a term used to describe a range of distinct conditions, all of which have the consequence of difficulty in learning to read despite adequate intelligence and teaching. It is classified by DSM-5 and ICD-10 as a developmental disorder.

Disorders of reading are common, affecting up to 10 percent of children, and are up to four times as common in boys than in girls. Dyslexia is strongly inherited, suggesting a genetic basis in some cases, and certain genes have been recently associated with dyslexia. Environmental factors are also significant – reading disorders are more common in children from disadvantaged families. They are also associated with disruptive behavior and other psychiatric disturbance, although these problems may be a result of the educational difficulties and stigmatization that the child with a disorder of reading very often experiences. Dyslexia can also develop following a brain injury, suggesting that there is a physical basis to the disorder within the structure of the brain. If dyslexia is acquired in this way, it is more correctly termed alexia.

In some children, the main problem appears to be a problem in processing language, or the sound of language, and in others the problem lies more in the realm of visual perception. In some cases there may be other developmental problems, such as clumsiness (motor dyspraxia) or hyperactivity.

However, there is no agreed classification system for dyslexia, and no proven medical treatment. The general approach for a child with a disorder of reading is to offer intensive reading support. In most cases the child will learn to read by adulthood, but reading speed will be slow and difficulties with spelling may persist.

 Information box 5.4e-XXVIII

Dyslexia: comments from a Chinese medicine perspective

It is not clear if dyslexia was recognized in ancient China. Dyslexia certainly exists in China, and seems to be of a more and intractable complex form as a consequence of the ideographic language having no direct relationship to the sounds of words.

Scott and Barlow (2009) suggest there are four imbalances, each of which may be a factor underlying dyslexia. These are: Heat, Phlegm, Qi Deficiency and Kidney Weakness. They explain that with Heat the words all come tumbling out too fast, whereas with Phlegm it seems as if there is a fog inside the head. In the deficient conditions it is as if the child has no energy to string the words together in the correct way.[113]

There are points that are used for dyslexia in the more recent acupuncture systems of scalp and ear acupuncture, but little has been published on their effectiveness.

ATTENTION DEFICIT HYPERACTIVITY DISORDER (ADHD)

Attention deficit hyperactivity disorder (ADHD) is a disorder of disruptive behavior, which usually presents in children aged five to twelve. It is up to four times more common in boys than in girls. Overall, it may affect up to 5 percent of children, depending on exactly how the condition is defined.

ADHD is characterized by inappropriate degrees of inattention, impulsiveness and over-activity. On questioning, parents will often say that the child has been restless and a poor sleeper ever since he or she was a small baby. Children with ADHD are accident-prone. They become notorious in the nursery or at school for their inability to complete set tasks and their ability to disrupt other children. Language delay and learning difficulties often accompany ADHD. Over 30 percent of children with ADHD also have dyslexia.

A family history of ADHD, problems in childbirth, inconsistent parenting, unrealistic parental expectations and poor housing are all associated with the development of ADHD.

Treatment might involve meetings with a child psychologist, who might work around family issues and behavior modification. Reduction of sugar, caffeine and other additives from the diet may be helpful in some cases, but are not routinely recommended by doctors. Increasingly, children over the age of seven are referred to a child psychiatrist for consideration of the prescription of a stimulant drug (most commonly methylphenidate) that may be taken until adulthood and beyond. The stimulant drugs paradoxically help the child to focus his or her energies, and can very much improve behavior and compliance at school. They can help the child to benefit from the behavior modification as advised by the child psychologist. However, the stimulant drugs do have serious potential side effects, including growth retardation, insomnia, irritability, headache, thought disorders and the development of tics. On withdrawal of the medication, depression and worsened hyperactivity can develop. There is also a high risk of abuse with stimulants, and it appears that their use in teenagers is associated with abuse of illicit drugs. This is thought to be a result of the impulsivity that is part of the ADHD condition rather than a result of the stimulants.[114]

The long-term outlook for children who have been prescribed stimulants to support them in behavior modification programs is as yet not well understood. Before the introduction of such regimens, affected children tended to continue to do poorly at school and could drift into truancy and antisocial activities, and studies support the idea that use of stimulants is associated with better performance in school and less unhelpful behavior such as truancy. However, it is known that regular stimulant use increases the number of dopamine reuptake receptors in the brain, so it certainly induces long-term changes. The consequences of these changes are as yet not understood.

Information box 5.4e-XXIX

Hyperactivity: comments from a Chinese medicine perspective

From a Chinese medicine perspective, hyperactivity in a child might be the result of deficiency or excess, and usually a combination of the two if the symptoms are so entrenched. Kidney, Heart and Spleen Deficiency might predispose to the condition and Phlegm and Phlegm Heat are suggested by impulsive restlessness. Clumsiness suggests Liver Disharmony. Heat might originate from childhood infections, immunizations, food additives and Toxic Womb Heat and Phlegm from diet or overuse of antibiotics.

Dharmananda explains that ADHD is understood in terms of Essence Deficiency leading to a primary Deficiency in Kidney Yin and corresponding Hyperactivity of Yang. Phlegm complicates the condition and treatment is used to Nourish Yin, Clear Phlegm and Sedate Yang.[115]

The stimulant medications used in ADHD calm the system by powerful moving of Phlegm. However, their action as stimulants in the long term is likely to be depleting to the Heart and Kidneys.

Tics

A tic is a repetitive movement of a part of the body, usually the head or neck. The tic apparently appears to be purposeful, in that the child has a degree of control over the movement, and the child can repeat it on request. However, if the child is asked to refrain from the movement, this can result in mounting discomfort. Common tics include blinking, frowning, sniffing and head flicking. Tics appear to be more frequent when the child is inactive, and can also become more prominent when the child is anxious. They tend to disappear if the child is busy concentrating on performing a task. In most cases the tics are minor and will pass with time. The parents should be reassured, and advised not to draw too much attention to the tic.

A more serious tic disorder is Giles de la Tourette syndrome (Tourette's disorder), in which the child is rarely free of performing a diverse variety of tics and involuntary vocalizations, including hoots, grunts and swear words. This disorder can be extremely embarrassing and socially disabling. Tourette's disorder is very strongly associated with obsessive-compulsive disorder, and there is often a family history of the disorder.

The tics may respond to cognitive behavioral therapy. In a severe case the child may be prescribed major tranquillizer medication or in extreme cases stereotactic brain surgery.

In adulthood one-third of patients will have grown out of the problem, and one-third will remain severely affected by them.[116]

Information box 5.4e-XXX

Tics: comments from a Chinese medicine perspective

A possible Chinese medicine interpretation of muscular tics could be Wind arising as a result of a Liver imbalance such as Liver Yin Deficiency. In Tourette's disorder, the imbalance is more profound. The involuntary vocalizations suggest that, in addition to Wind and Liver imbalance, a disturbance involving obstruction of the Heart Orifices such as Phlegm or Heat might also be a factor.

The red flags of the diseases of childhood

Some children who become unwell will benefit from referral to a conventional doctor for assessment or treatment. Red flags are those symptoms and signs that indicate that referral should be considered. The red flags of the diseases of childhood are described in Table 5.4e-I. A summary of the red flags in a format designed for quick reference in clinical practice can be found in Appendix III. This gives advice on the degree of urgency of referral for each of the red flag conditions listed.

Table 5.4e-I A40: Red flags of the diseases of childhood

Red flag	Description	Reasoning
A40.1	Maternal concern	Any condition in which the parent is very concerned about the health of the child is worth referring for a second opinion. The parent is the person who will know best if something is not right with the child, even if it is not very specific. It is wise to respect this instinct, as small children sometimes do not generate very specific symptoms even when seriously unwell
A40.2	Inconsolable baby: for >3 hours	Although this feature is very common and usually benign, consider referral if inconsolable and unexplained crying (for at least 3 hours) starts in a previously settled baby
A40.3	Childhood cancer: red flags include progressive symptoms – loss of weight, sweats, poor appetite, an unexplained lump or mass or an enlarged unilateral lymph node (>1.5cm in diameter), recurrent infections, bruising, anemia and bleeding	Refer any case in which there is a short history of unexplained symptoms that have arisen within the past weeks to months and which are progressive. Also, refer as a high priority if there are red flags of bone marrow failure (see A1.4)
A40.4	Infections in infants (aged between 0 and 6 months)	Infections in infants can become serious conditions very quickly because of the immature immune system, poor temperature control and small size. They lead easily to high fever and dehydration. The infant is at increased risk of convulsions and circulatory collapse

Fever of >38.0°C (>100.4°F) in a child 0–3 months needs to be referred as a high priority

Fever of >39.0°C (>102.2°F) in a child 3–6 months needs to be referred as a high priority |
| A40.5 | High fever in an older child that does not respond to treatment within 5 days | Although risk of convulsions is low in this group of patients, a high fever of >38.0°C (>100.4°F) is very depleting and can lead to dehydration. If a high fever in an otherwise well hydrated (see A40.8) and alert child is not responding to treatment in 5 days, this suggests the possibility of a serious condition which merits further investigations

If the child with fever is distressed or shows any other red flags refer as a high priority

Otherwise, fever in a small child who is not otherwise distressed may be of no cause for concern, but the child will need vigilant attention to ensure no deterioration |
A40.6	Febrile convulsion in child: ongoing	Refer a case in which the convulsion is not settling within 2 minutes as an emergency. Ensure the child is kept in a safe place and in the recovery position while help arrives
A40.7	Febrile convulsion in child: recovered	Refer all cases in which the child has just suffered a first febrile convulsion (the parents need advice on how to manage future fits, and the child should be examined by a doctor)
A40.8	Dehydration in a small child (less than 5 years): signs include dry mouth and skin, cold extremities, gray or mottled complexion, loss of skin turgor (firmness), drowsiness, sunken fontanel (soft spot on the crown of the head in region of acupoint DU-24, Shen Ting) and dry diapers	A dehydrated infant is at high risk of circulatory collapse because of its small size and immature homeostatic mechanisms. Infants who are dehydrated may lose the desire to drink, and so the condition can rapidly deteriorate. High priority or urgent referral is required

A40.9	Dehydration in older children if severe or prolonged for >48 hours. Signs include: dry mouth and skin, loss of skin turgor, low blood pressure, dizziness on standing and poor urine output	Although not as unstable as an infant, a dehydrated child or adult still needs hydration to prevent damage to the kidneys. Referral should be made if the patient is unable to take fluids or if the dehydration persists for >48 hours. Refer elderly people as a high priority, as the ability to take in fluids is often reduced and the kidneys and brain are more vulnerable to damage
A40.10	Confusion in older children with fever	Confusion is common and usually benign in young children (<8 years) when a fever develops. However, it is not usual in older children, who should be referred to exclude central nervous system involvement (e.g. meningitis or brain abscess)
A40.11	Any features of a notifiable disease*	All the immunizable diseases are notifiable diseases. Consider referral of these cases so that the doctor can report the episode to the local Health Protection Agency
A40.12	Vomiting: refer if persistent, and either a cause of distress to the child (i.e. not posseting), a cause of dehydration, or if projectile	Vomiting is common in children, and usually self-limiting. In babies regurgitation of milk is normal (posseting) and not a cause for concern if the child is contented and continuing to gain weight Refer if there are features of dehydration, or if the vomiting is projectile (a feature of pyloric stenosis in newborn babies) Food poisoning and infectious bloody diarrhea are notifiable diseases*
A40.13	Diarrhea: if persistent, and associated with either dehydration, poor weight gain, weight loss or chronic ill health	Chronic loose stools in a child may signify the presence of an infectious organism, celiac disease or inflammatory bowel disease Refer as a high priority if dehydration is present (see A40.8–A40.9) Food poisoning and infectious bloody diarrhea are notifiable diseases*
A40.14	Soiling with feces (in underwear or bed)	Always refer for diagnosis if persistent and appearing in a previously continent child (could signify constipation with fecal overflow, a developmental problem of the bowel, or emotional disturbance)
A40.15	Recurrent or constant intense abdominal pain: if pain is associated with fever, vomiting, collapse, and rigidity and guarding on examination	All these features are signs of the acute abdomen (see A6.8), which in children is most commonly due to appendicitis or a form of bowel obstruction (from a twist or obstruction in a hernia). Urgent surgical assessment is required. All these conditions can spontaneously resolve, but a recurrence is likely. Refer for treatment or assessment
A40.16	Recurrent mild abdominal pain	Features of abdominal pain in children that suggest a more benign (functional) cause include mild pain that is worse in the morning, location around the umbilicus, and pain is worse with anxiety. Refer only if child is not responding to treatment
A40.17	Jaundice (yellowish skin, yellow whites of the eyes, and possibly dark urine and pale stools)	Jaundice is always of concern in children and babies with the exception of the mild form of jaundice that can affect the newborn. Refer all cases to ensure serious liver disease is excluded

A40.18	Any new onset of difficulty breathing (i.e. increased respiratory rate,** nocturnal wheeze or noisy breathing) in a small child (<8 years) Also if there is unexplained sudden blockage of one nostril	Always take a new onset of difficulty breathing in a child seriously, and refer for medical assessment to exclude serious disease. Common causes include lower respiratory tract infections, asthma, allergic reactions, inhalation of foreign bodies and congenital heart disease A nostril may suddenly block after the unwitnessed insertion of a foreign body. This is a serious situation, as the foreign body (e.g. a pea) is at risk of becoming inhaled
A40.19	Complications of tonsillitis: severe constitutional upset not responding to treatment within 5 days	Tonsillitis is common and usually self-limiting in children. The child should be back to their usual self within 3–4 days, so only refer if there is no improvement after this time period
A40.20	Complications of tonsillitis: a single grossly enlarged infected tonsil (quinsy) in an unwell and feverish child	Quinsy is the development of an abscess in the tonsil. It carries a serious risk of obstruction of the airways and requires a same-day surgical opinion. Refer urgently if the child is experiencing any restriction in breathing (stridor may be heard (see A40.21))
A40.21	Stridor (harsh noisy breathing heard on both the in breath and the outbreath)	Stridor is a noise that suggests upper airway obstruction. It is a serious red flag if it develops suddenly. It suggests possible swelling of the air passages due to laryngotracheitis, quinsy or epiglottitis. If restriction to breathing is significant, the patient with stridor will be sitting very still It is important not to ask to see the tongue, as this can affect the position of the epiglottis, and may worsen the obstruction
A40.22	Features of severe asthma: at least two of the following – rapidly worsening breathlessness, increased respiratory rate,** reluctance to talk because of breathlessness, need to sit upright and still to assist breathing; cyanosis is a very serious sign (see A17.12)	Severe asthma is a potentially life-threatening condition and may develop in someone who has no previous history of severe attacks Urgent referral is required so that medical management of the attack can be instigated Keep the child as calm as possible while you wait for help to arrive Cyanosis describes the blue coloring that appears when the blood is poorly oxygenated. Unlike the blueness from cold, which affects only the extremities, central cyanosis from poor oxygenation can be seen on the tongue
A40.23	Bedwetting: if persisting over the age of 5 years	Consider referral if the child is >5 years, so that physical causes can be excluded and the parents can have access to expert advice
A40.24	Features of vesico-ureteric reflux disease (VUR) in a child: any history of recurrent episodes or a current episode of cloudy urine or burning on urination should be taken seriously in a prepubescent child	Urine infections are common in young children but need to be taken seriously, particularly if there is a history of recurrent infections. The small child is more vulnerable to VUR, which means that when the bladder contracts some urine is flushed back towards the kidneys In the case of infection of the bladder, VUR can lead to infectious organisms causing damage to the delicate structure of the kidney. Sometimes this damage occurs with very few symptoms, but if cumulative and undetected can lead to serious kidney problems and high blood pressure in later life For this reason it is wise to refer all prepubescent children with a history of symptoms of urinary infections to exclude the possibility of VUR Refer children with current symptoms as a high priority, and those who are currently well non-urgently

A40.25	Acute testicular pain: radiates to the groin, scrotum or lower abdomen	Refer any sudden onset of severe testicular pain (radiates to the groin, scrotum or lower abdomen). This could signify inflammation of the testicle (orchitis) or a twist of the testicle (torsion). If the pain is very intense (with collapse and vomiting), refer as emergency
A40.26	Precocious puberty: secondary sexual characteristics appearing before age 8 in girls and 9 in boys	Refer if secondary sexual characteristics begin to appear before age 8 in girls and 9 in boys so that an endocrine cause can be excluded
A40.27	Delayed puberty: secondary sexual characteristics not apparent by age 15 in girls and 16 in boys	Refer if secondary sexual characteristics have not started to appear by the age of 15 in girls and 16 in boys. Refer if menstruation has not begun by the time of a girl's 16th birthday (primary amenorrhea)
A40.28	Epilepsy: refer any child who has suffered a suspected blank episode (absence) or seizure (see A24.5)	Epilepsy most commonly first presents in childhood, and is more common in children who have experienced febrile convulsions. Early diagnosis is important as early management can help prevent deleterious effects on education and social development
A40.29	Squint or double vision: in any child if previously undiagnosed	Refer any child who demonstrates a previously undiagnosed squint. In young children this usually results from a congenital weakness of the external ocular muscles, but needs ophthalmological assessment to prevent long-term inhibition of depth vision. If appearing in an older child it may signify a tumor of the brain, pituitary gland or orbital cavity
A40.30	Complications of acute otitis media in a child: persistent fever/pain/confusion for >3–4 days after the onset of the earache (may indicate spread of the infection, e.g. mastoiditis or brain abscess)	Otitis media is an uncomfortable but self-limiting ear infection that commonly affects young children. It is now considered good practice not to prescribe antibiotics in a simple case, which will generally settle within 1–3 days, sometimes after natural perforation of the eardrum. This is a beneficial healing process (so some sticky discharge for 1–2 days after an earache is not a cause for concern)

However, persisting high fever, confusion or intense pain is not usual, and the child should be referred to exclude the rare possibility of infectious complications |
| A40.31 | New onset of difficulty hearing in a child: lasting for >3 weeks | Refer if prolonged, if interfering with social interactions and education, or if associated with pain in the ear or dizziness. The most likely cause is glue ear, a chronic accumulation of mucoid secretions in the middle ear |
| A40.32 | Persistent discharge from the ear in a child | Chronic discharge from the ear for >1 week after the infection of otitis media has settled down may indicate the development of chronic otitis media, and this needs further investigation as there is risk of permanent damage to the middle ear |
| A40.33 | Features of autism: slow development of speech, impaired social interactions, little imaginative play, obsessional repetitive behavior | Mild degrees of autism may not be diagnosed until the child reaches secondary school age

Refer if you are concerned that the child is demonstrating impaired social interactions (aloofness), impaired social communication (very poor eye contact, awkward and inappropriate body language) and impairment of imaginative play (play may instead be dominated by obsessional behavior such as lining up toys or checking). Early diagnosis can result in the child being offered extra educational and psychological support |

| A40.34 | Sexual or physical abuse: unexplained or implausible injuries, miserable, withdrawn child, still, watchful child – "frozen watchfulness," overtly sexualized behavior in a prepubescent child, vaginal or anal discharge or itch | All the listed features may have a benign explanation, but if you have any concerns you should take the situation very seriously

In the UK you can start by seeking confidential advice from the NSPCC helpline or from the local Safeguarding Board, the statutory organization responsible for dealing with child protection. In the UK Safeguarding Boards operate from the local county councils

Suspected child abuse is a situation in which you might have to break your professional obligation of confidentiality

If you have any concerns about doing this, first discuss the case with the ethics adviser from your professional body |
|---|---|---|

* Notification of a number of specified infectious diseases is required of doctors in the UK as a "statutory duty" under the UK Public Health (Infectious Diseases) 1988 Act and the Public Health (Control of Diseases) 1988 Act.
Public Health England (PHE) collates details of each case of each disease that has been notified. This allows analyses of local and national trends.
This is one example of a situation in which there is a statutory requirement for a doctor to breach patient confidentiality.
Diseases that are notifiable include:[117] acute encephalitis, acute infectious hepatitis, acute meningitis, acute poliomyelitis, anthrax, botulism, brucellosis, cholera, diphtheria, enteric fever (typhoid or paratyphoid fever), food poisoning, hemolytic uremic syndrome (HUS), infectious bloody diarrhea, invasive group A streptococcal disease, Legionnaires' disease, leprosy, malaria, measles, meningococcal septicemia, mumps, plague, rabies, rubella, scarlet fever, severe acute respiratory syndrome (SARS), smallpox, tetanus, tuberculosis, typhus, viral hemorrhagic fever (VHF), whooping cough, yellow fever.

** *Categorization of respiratory rate in children*
The normal range for respiratory rate in children varies according to age.
The following rates indicate moderate to severe breathlessness:
Newborn (0–3 months) >60 breaths/minute
Infant (3 months to 2 years) >50 breaths/minute
Young child (2–8 years) >40 breaths/minute
Older child to adult >30 breaths/minute

Notes

1   Waugh, A. and Grant, A. (2014) *Ross and Wilson: Anatomy and Physiology in Health and Illness.* Twelfth Edition. Edinburgh: Elsevier, Chapter 9.

2   Flaws, B. and Sionneau, P. (2010) *The Treatment of Modern Western Medical Diseases with Chinese Medicine.* Boulder, CO: Blue Poppy Press, pp.241–244.

3   Tidy, C. (2015) 'Hypothyroidism.' Available at http://patient.info/doctor/hypothyroidism, accessed on 3 August 2016.

4   Flaws, B. and Sionneau, P. (2010) *The Treatment of Modern Western Medical Diseases with Chinese Medicine.* Boulder, CO: Blue Poppy Press, p.281.

5   Newson, L. (2015) 'Hyperthyroidism.' Available at http://patient.info/doctor/hyperthyroidism, accessed on 3 August 2016.

6   Tidy, C. (2016) 'The management of type 2 diabetes.' Available at http://patient.info/doctor/management-of-type-2-diabetes, accessed on 3 August 2016.

7   Flaws, B. and Sionneau, P. (2010) *The Treatment of Modern Western Medical Diseases with Chinese Medicine.* Boulder, CO: Blue Poppy Press, pp.207–216.

8   Flaws, B. and Sionneau, P. (2010) *The Treatment of Modern Western Medical Diseases with Chinese Medicine.* Boulder, CO: Blue Poppy Press, p.203.

9   Waugh, A. and Grant, A. (2014) *Ross and Wilson: Anatomy and Physiology in Health and Illness.* Twelfth Edition. Edinburgh: Elsevier, Chapter 18.

10 O'Grady, K. (2008) 'Early puberty for girls: The new "normal" and why we need to be concerned.' *Canadian Women's Health Network* *11*(1). Available at www.cwhn.ca/en/node/39365, accessed on 4 August 2016.

11 International Menopause Society (2016) 'Menopause terminology.' Available at www.imsociety.org/menopause_terminology.php, accessed on 3 August 2016.

12 Harding, M. (2014) 'Cervical screening (cervical smear test).' Available at http://patient.info/doctor/cervical-screening-cervical-smear-test-pro, accessed on 3 August 2016.

13 Harding, M. (2016) 'Polycystic ovary syndrome.' Available at http://patient.info/doctor/polycystic-ovary-syndrome-pro, accessed on 3 August 2016.

14 Harding, M. (2016) 'Menorrhagia.' Available at http://patient.info/doctor/menorrhagia, accessed on 3 August 2016.

15 Maciocia, G. (1998) *Obstetrics and Gynecology in Chinese Medicine.* Edinburgh: Churchill Livingstone, p.197.

16 Payne, J. (2015) 'Premenstrual syndrome.' Available at http://patient.info/doctor/premenstrual-syndrome-pro, accessed on 7 August 2016.

17 Schellenburg, B (2001) 'Treatment for the premenstrual syndrome with agnus castus fruit extract: Prospective, randomized, placebo controlled study.' *British Medical Journal 322,* 134.

18 Maciocia, G. (1998) *Obstetrics and Gynecology in Chinese Medicine.* Edinburgh: Churchill Livingstone, Chapter 18.

19 Maciocia, G. (1998) *Obstetrics and Gynecology in Chinese Medicine.* Edinburgh: Churchill Livingstone, Chapter 14.

20 Newson, L. (2016) 'Menopause and its management.' Available at http://patient.info/doctor/menopause-and-its-management, accessed on 8 August 2016.

21 Pote, K. (2015) 'Menopause around the world.' Portland, OR: Women in Balance Institute, National University of Natural Medicine. Available at https://womeninbalance.org/2014/09/17/menopause-around-the-world, accessed on 8 August 2016.

22 The North American Menopause Society (2016) 'Decreased desire.' Available at www.menopause.org/for-women/sexual-health-menopause-online/sexual-problems-at-midlife/decreased-desire, accessed on 8 August 2016.

23 Newson, L. (2016) 'Hormone replacement therapy including benefits and risks.' Available at http://patient.info/doctor/hormone-replacement-therapy-including-benefits-and-risks, accessed on 8 August 2016.

24 Maciocia, G. (1998) *Obstetrics and Gynecology in Chinese Medicine.* Edinburgh: Churchill Livingstone, Chapter 58.

25 AVENwiki (2013) 'Research relating to asexuality.' Available at www.asexuality.org/wiki/index.php?title=Research_relating_to_asexuality, accessed on 8 August 2016.

26 Shen-Nong Ltd (2006) 'Impotence.' Available at www.shen-nong.com/eng/exam/specialties_menimpotence.html, accessed on 8 August 2016.

27 Herpes Virus Association (2016) 'Frequently asked questions.' Available at http://herpes.org.uk/frequently-asked-questions/#9, accessed on 8 August 2016.

28 Wang, Y. and Prodoehl, C. (2016) 'Herb formulas and dietary therapy for human papilloma virus (HPV).' *Vitality.* Available at http://vitalitymagazine.com/article/herb-formulas-and-dietary-therapy-for-human-papillomavirus-hpv, accessed on 8 August 2016.

29 Maciocia, G. (1998) *Obstetrics and Gynecology in Chinese Medicine.* Edinburgh: Churchill Livingstone, Chapter 61.

30 Knott, L. (2015) 'Human immunodeficiency virus.' Available at http://patient.info/doctor/human-immunodeficiency-virus-hiv, accessed on 17 August 2016.

31 Rosenberg, Z. (2000) 'A Chinese look at Western pharmaceuticals.' Available at www.acupuncture.com/herbs/pharma.htm, accessed on 9 August 2016.

32 Maciocia, G. (1998) *Obstetrics and Gynecology in Chinese Medicine.* Edinburgh: Churchill Livingstone, p.66.

33 Cancer Research UK (2014) 'Prostate cancer risk factors: Medical conditions: Vasectomy.' Available at www.cancerresearchuk.org/health-professional/cancer-statistics/statistics-by-cancer-type/prostate-cancer/risk-factors#heading-Fourteen, accessed on 9 August 2016.

34 United Nations Department of Economic and Social Affairs Population Division (2006) *Levels and Trends of Contraceptive Use.* Available at www.un.org/esa/population/publications/wcu2002/WCU2002_Report.pdf, accessed on 15 December 2016.

35 Population Reference Bureau (2002) *Family Planning Worldwide.* Available at www.prb.org/pdf/FamPlanWorldwide_Eng.pdf, accessed on 9 August 2016.

36 British Fertility Society (2012) *In Vitro Fertilisation: Perinatal Risks and Early Childhood Outcomes.* Scientific Impact Paper 8. Available at www.rcog.org.uk/globalassets/documents/guidelines/scientific-impact-papers/sip_8.pdf, accessed on 10 August 2016.

37 Cancer Research UK (2016) 'Cervical cancer screening.' Available at www.cancerresearchuk.org/about-cancer/type/cervical-cancer/about/cervical-cancer-screening, accessed on 9 August 2016.

38 Maciocia, G. (1998) *Obstetrics and Gynecology in Chinese Medicine.* Edinburgh: Churchill Livingstone, p.66.

39 Maciocia, G. (1998) *Obstetrics and Gynecology in Chinese Medicine.* Edinburgh: Churchill Livingstone, p.443.

40 Cochrane Collaboration (2012) 'Treatments for suppression of lactation.' Available at www.cochrane.org/CD005937/PREG_treatments-for-suppression-of-lactation, accessed on 10 August 2016.

41 WHO (World Health Organization) (2015) 'Maternal mortality.' Available at www.who.int/gho/maternal_health/mortality/maternal_mortality_text/en, accessed on 10 August 2016.

42 Rodgers, C. (2006) 'Questions about prenatal ultrasound and the alarming rise in autism.' Available at www.midwiferytoday.com/articles/ultrasoundrodgers.asp, accessed on 10 August 2016.

43 US FDA (United States Food and Drug Administration) (2014) 'Avoid fetal "keepsake" images, heartbeat monitors.' Available at www.fda.gov/ForConsumers/ConsumerUpdates/ucm095508.htm, accessed on 10 August 2016.

44 Cochrane Collaboration (2013) 'Comparing continuous electronic fetal monitoring in labor (cardiotocography, CTG) with intermittent listening (intermittent auscultation, IA).' Available at www.cochrane.org/CD006066/PREG_comparing-continuous-electronic-fetal-monitoring-in-labour-cardiotocography-ctg-with-intermittent-listening-intermittent-auscultation-ia, accessed on 10 August 2016.

45 For example, Betts, D., Smith, C.A. and Hannah, D.G. (2012) 'Acupuncture as a therapeutic treatment option for threatened miscarriage.' *BMC Complementary and Alternative Medicine 12,* 20. Available at www.ncbi.nlm.nih.gov/pmc/articles/PMC3342918, accessed on 10 August 2016.

46 Maciocia, G. (1998) *Obstetrics and Gynecology in Chinese Medicine.* Edinburgh: Churchill Livingstone, Chapter 43.

47 Life (2014) 'There's no such thing as a potential human being is there?' Available at https://lifecharity.org.uk/news-and-views/there-is-no-such-thing-as-a-potential-human-being-is-there, accessed on 10 August 2016.

48 DH (Department of Health) (2014) *Abortion Statistics England and Wales 2014.* Available at www.gov.uk/government/uploads/system/uploads/attachment_data/file/433437/2014_Commentary__5_.pdf, accessed on 10 August 2016.

49 Adler, N., David, H.P., Major, B.N., Roth, S.H., Russo, N.F. and Wyatt, G.E. (1990) 'Psychological responses after abortion.' *Science 248*(4951), 41–44. Available at http://155.97.32.9/~bbenham/Phil%207570%20Website/aAdler1990.pdf, accessed on 10 August 2016.

50 Maciocia, G. (1998) *Obstetrics and Gynecology in Chinese Medicine.* Edinburgh: Churchill Livingstone, Chapter 29.

51 Jazayeri, A. (2016) 'Premature rupture of membranes (at term).' Available at http://emedicine.medscape.com/article/261137-overview#a2, accessed on 11 August 2016.

52 NICE (National Institute for Health and Care Excellence) (2008) *Inducing Labour.* NICE Guidelines CG70. Available at www.nice.org.uk/guidance/cg70/chapter/introduction, accessed on 11 August 2016.

53 Buckley, S. (2011) 'Undisturbed birth.' Available at www.aims.org.uk/Journal/Vol23No4/undisturbedBirth.htm, accessed on 11 August 2016.

54 Waugh, A. and Grant, A. (2014) *Ross and Wilson: Anatomy and Physiology in Health and Illness.* Twelfth Edition. Edinburgh: Elsevier, Chapter 18.

55 Lahans, T. (2007) *Integrating Conventional and Chinese Medicine in Cancer Care.* Edinburgh: Elsevier, p.91.

56 WHO (World Health Organization) (2002) *Programming of Chronic Disease by Impaired Fetal Nutrition.* Available at www.who.int/nutrition/publications/programming_chronicdisease.pdf, accessed on 10 August 2016.

57 WHO (World Health Organization) (2016) 'Breastfeeding.' Available at www.who.int/topics/breastfeeding/en/, accessed on 11 August 2016.

58 Dennis, L.K., VanBeek, M.J., Beane Freeman, L.E., Smith, B.J., Dawson, D.V. and Coughlin, J.A. (2008) 'Sunburns and risk of cutaneous melanoma: Does age matter? A comprehensive meta-analysis.' *Annals of Epidemiology 18*(8), 614–627. Available at www.ncbi.nlm.nih.gov/pmc/articles/PMC2873840, accessed on 11 August 2016.

59 Van Ijzendoorn, M.H. *et al.* (2011) 'Children in institutional care: Delayed development and resilience.' *Monographs of the Society for Research in Child Development 76*(4), 8–30. Available at www.ncbi.nlm.nih.gov/pmc/articles/PMC4130248, accessed on 12 August 2016.

60 Telama, R., Yang, X., Laakso, L. and Viikari, J. (1997) 'Physical activity in childhood and adolescence as a predictor of physical activity in young adulthood.' *American Journal of Preventive Medicine 13*(4), 317–323. Available at www.ncbi.nlm.nih.gov/pubmed/9236971, accessed on 12 August 2016.

61 Dahl, R.E. (2007) 'Sleep and the developing brain.' *Sleep 30*(9), 1079–1080. Available at www.ncbi.nlm.nih.gov/pmc/articles/PMC1978403, accessed on 12 August 2016.

62 Sirotnak, A. (2015) 'Psychosocial short stature.' Available at http://emedicine.medscape.com/article/913843-overview#a4, accessed on 12 August 2016.

63 WHO (World Health Organization) (2003) *Social Determinants of Health: The Solid Facts.* Chapter 1, 'The Social Gradient.' Available at www.euro.who.int/__data/assets/pdf_file/0005/98438/e81384.pdf, accessed on 12 August 2016.

64 Gov.UK (2016) 'Report child abuse.' Available at www.gov.uk/report-child-abuse, accessed on 12 August 2016.

65 Scott, J. and Barlow, T. (1999) *Acupuncture in the Treatment of Children.* Seattle, WA: Eastland Press, Chapter 1.

66 Scott, J. and Barlow, T. (1999) *Acupuncture in the Treatment of Children.* Seattle, WA: Eastland Press.

67 Clement Clarke International (2004) *Predictive Normal Values (Nomogram EU Scale).* Available at www.peakflow.com/top_nav/normal_values/index.html, accessed on 12 August 2016.

68 Scott, J. and Barlow, T. (1999) *Acupuncture in the Treatment of Children.* Seattle, WA: Eastland Press, Chapter 32.

69 ScienceDaily (2015) 'Hidden burden: Most people carry recessive disease mutations.' Available at www.sciencedaily.com/releases/2015/04/150408100522.htm, accessed on 12 August 2016.

70 Maciocia, G. (1989) *The Principles of Chinese Medicine.* Edinburgh: Churchill Livingstone, p.89.

71 Flaws, B. and Sionneau, P. (2010) *The Treatment of Modern Western Diseases with Chinese Medicine.* Boulder, CO: Blue Poppy Press, Chapter 32.

72 Lobo, I. (2008) 'Multifactorial inheritance and genetic disease.' *Nature Education 1*(1), 5. Available at www.nature.com/scitable/topicpage/multifactorial-inheritance-and-genetic-disease-919, accessed on 12 August 2016.

73 DH (Department of Health) (2014) *Abortion Statistics, England and Wales 2014.* Available at www.gov.uk/government/uploads/system/uploads/attachment_data/file/433437/2014_Commentary__5_.pdf, accessed on 10 August 2016.

74 WHO (World Health Organization) (2002) *Programming of Chronic Disease by Impaired Fetal Nutrition.* Available at www.who.int/nutrition/publications/programming_chronicdisease.pdf, accessed on 10 August 2016.

75 Tidy, C. (2016) 'Infant respiratory distress syndrome.' Available at http://patient.info/doctor/infant-respiratory-distress-syndrome, accessed on 20 August 2016.

76 Jefferies, A. (2012) 'Kangaroo care for the preterm infant and family.' *Paediatrics & Child Health 17*(3), 141–146. Available at www.ncbi.nlm.nih.gov/pmc/articles/PMC3287094, accessed on 18 August 2016.

77 West, Z. (2008) *Acupuncture in Pregnancy and Childbirth.* Edinburgh: Churchill Livingstone, p.27.

78 CDC (Centers for Disease Control and Prevention) (1999) 'Achievements in public health 1990–1999.' Available at www.cdc.gov/mmwr/preview/mmwrhtml/mm4838a2.htm, accessed on 18 August 2016.

79 Child Trends Databank (2015) *Infant, Child and Teen Mortality.* Available at www.childtrends.org/?indicators=infant-child-and-teen-mortality, accessed on 12 August 2016.

80 Scott, J. and Barlow, T. (1999) *Acupuncture in the Treatment of Children.* Seattle, WA: Eastland Press, Chapter 14.

81 Scott, J. and Barlow, T. (1999) *Acupuncture in the Treatment of Children.* Seattle, WA: Eastland Press, Chapter 14.

82 Scott, J. and Barlow, T. (1999) *Acupuncture in the Treatment of Children.* Seattle, WA: Eastland Press, Chapter 23.

83 Lowth, M. (2016) 'Acute otitis media in children.' Available at http://patient.info/doctor/acute-otitis-media-in-children, accessed on 12 August 2016.

84 Knott, L. (2015) 'Croup.' Available at http://patient.info/doctor/croup-pro, accessed on 16 August 2016.

85 Ladhani, S. (2012) 'Two decades of experience with the Haemophilus influenza serotype b conjugate vaccine in the United Kingdom.' *Clinical Therapeutics 34*(2), 385–399. Available at www.ncbi.nlm.nih.gov/pubmed/22244051, accessed on 16 August 2016.

86 Scott, J. and Barlow, T. (1999) *Acupuncture in the Treatment of Children.* Seattle, WA: Eastland Press, Chapter 22.

87 Knott, L. (2013) 'Bronchiolitis.' Available at http://patient.info/doctor/bronchiolitis-pro, accessed on 17 August 2016.

88 Scott, J. and Barlow, T. (1999) *Acupuncture in the Treatment of Children.* Seattle, WA: Eastland Press, Chapter 18.

89 Flaws, B. (2006) *A Handbook of TCM Pediatrics.* Boulder, CO: Blue Poppy Press, p.166.

90 Scott, J. and Barlow, T. (1999) *Acupuncture in the Treatment of Children.* Seattle, WA: Eastland Press, Chapter 17.

91 WHO (World Health Organization) (2016) 'Measles.' Fact sheet. Available at www.who.int/mediacentre/factsheets/fs286/en, accessed on 17 August 2016.

92 Scott, J. and Barlow, T. (1999) *Acupuncture in the Treatment of Children.* Seattle, WA: Eastland Press, Chapter 20.

93 Flaws, B. (2006) *A Handbook of TCM Pediatrics.* Boulder, CO: Blue Poppy Press, p.243.

94 CDC (Centers for Disease Control and Prevention) (2012) 'Childcare and school chickenpox vaccination requirements.' Available at www.cdc.gov/vaccines/vpd-vac/varicella/basic-school-daycare-req.htm, accessed on 17 August 2016.

95 Scott, J. and Barlow, T. (1999) *Acupuncture in the Treatment of Children.* Seattle, WA: Eastland Press, Chapter 44.

96 Tidy, C. (2014) 'Rotavirus and rotavirus vaccination.' Available at http://patient.info/doctor/rotavirus-and-rotavirus-vaccination, accessed on 17 August 2016.

97 Scott, J. and Barlow, T. (1999) *Acupuncture in the Treatment of Children.* Seattle, WA: Eastland Press, p.598.

98 Flaws, B. (2006) *A Handbook of TCM Pediatrics.* Boulder, CO: Blue Poppy Press, p.207.

99 Scott, J. and Barlow, T. (1999) *Acupuncture in the Treatment of Children.* Seattle, WA: Eastland Press, Chapter 42.

100 NHS Choices (2015) 'Your baby's first solid foods.' Available at www.nhs.uk/conditions/pregnancy-and-baby/pages/solid-foods-weaning.aspx, accessed on 18 August 2016.

101 Scott, J. and Barlow, T. (1999) *Acupuncture in the Treatment of Children.* Seattle, WA: Eastland Press, pp.13–14.

102 Flaws, B. (2006) *A Handbook of TCM Pediatrics.* Boulder, CO: Blue Poppy Press, p.111.

103 Scott, J. and Barlow, T. (1999) *Acupuncture in the Treatment of Children.* Seattle, WA: Eastland Press, Chapter 9.

104 Khairy, G. (2009) 'Acute appendicitis: Is removal of a normal appendix still existing and can we reduce its rate?' *Saudi Journal of Gastroenterology 15*(3), 167–170. Available at www.ncbi.nlm.nih.gov/pmc/articles/PMC2841415, accessed on 18 August 2016.

105 Scott, J. and Barlow, T. (1999) *Acupuncture in the Treatment of Children.* Seattle, WA: Eastland Press, Chapter 18.

106 Scott, J. and Barlow, T. (1999) *Acupuncture in the Treatment of Children.* Seattle, WA: Eastland Press, Chapter 37.

107 Scott, J. and Barlow, T. (1999) *Acupuncture in the Treatment of Children.* Seattle, WA: Eastland Press, Chapter 40.

108 Flaws, B. (2006) *A Handbook of TCM Pediatrics.* Boulder, CO: Blue Poppy Press, p.252.

109 WHO (World Health Organization) (1993) *The ICD-10 Classification of Mental and Behavioral Disorders. Diagnostic Criteria for Research.* Available at www.who.int/classifications/icd/en/GRNBOOK.pdf, accessed on 18 August 2016.

110 APA (American Psychiatric Association) (2013) *DSM V Table of Contents.* Available at https://www.psychiatry.org/File%20Library/Psychiatrists/Practice/DSM/APA_DSM-5-Contents.pdf, accessed on 18 August 2016.

111 Autism Speaks (2013) 'DSM-V diagnostic criteria.' Available at www.autismspeaks.org/what-autism/diagnosis/dsm-5-diagnostic-criteria, accessed on 18 August 2016.

112 Scott, J. and Barlow, T. (1999) *Acupuncture in the Treatment of Children.* Seattle, WA: Eastland Press, Chapter 33.

113 Scott, J. and Barlow, T. (1999) *Acupuncture in the Treatment of Children.* Seattle, WA: Eastland Press, Chapter 34.

114 Tidy, C. (2014) 'Attention deficit hyperactivity disorder.' Available at http://patient.info/doctor/attention-deficit-hyperactivity-disorder-pro, accessed on 18 August 2016.

115 Dharmananda, S. (1996) 'Chinese herbal treatment for attention deficit disorder.' Available at www.itmonline.org/arts/add.htm, accessed on 18 August 2016.

116 Imm, N. (2015) 'Tourette's syndrome and other tic disorders.' Available at http://patient.info/doctor/tourettes-syndrome-and-other-tic-disorders, accessed on 18 August 2016.

117 Public Health England (2010) 'Notifiable diseases and causative organisms: How to report.' Available at www.gov.uk/guidance/notifiable-diseases-and-causative-organisms-how-to-report#list-of-notifiable-diseases, accessed on 6 June 2016.

THE SKIN, EYE AND EAR, MENTAL HEALTH AND CONCLUSIONS

6.1

The Skin, the Eye and the Ear

6.1a The physiology of the skin, the eye and the ear

This section focuses on the physiology of three of the sensory organs of the body: the skin, the eye and the ear.

The skin is considered as a physiological system in its own right, also known as the integumentary system (a term derived from the word integument, which means skin). In conventional practice, diseases of the skin are managed within the medical specialty of dermatology.

The eye and the ear are, technically speaking, complex sensory organs that form part of the nervous system. However, in conventional practice the diseases of the eye and the ear are managed within distinct specialties. Eye diseases are managed within the medical specialty of ophthalmology, and ear diseases are managed within the surgical specialty of otorhinolaryngology (meaning the study of the ear, nose and throat). This specialty embraces diseases that relate to two overlapping systems: the nervous system and the respiratory system.

In this section the diseases of the skin, the eye and the ear are considered separately, as if each is an individual system.

The physiology of the skin (the integumentary system)

The functions of the skin[1]

The skin is often described as the largest organ of the body. It may not be immediately obvious that the skin, like many of the deep organs, has a range of complex functions. The functions of the skin include:

- Protection of the body: the skin provides a mechanical barrier that protects the deeper tissues from mechanical injury, toxins in the environment and radiation from the sun.

- Regulation of body temperature: the skin contributes to the homeostasis of body temperature by means of mechanisms including sweating in the heat and erection of body hair in the cold (goose pimples). The blood vessels in the skin also are very responsive to body temperature – they dilate in the heat and contract in the cold.

- Formation of vitamin D: the skin is the main source of vitamin D, which is essential for the maintenance of the health of the bones. Vitamin D prevents rickets and osteomalacia. It is manufactured in the skin (from a steroid precursor chemical) as a response to the action of sunlight.

- Sensation: the skin forms the boundary between the external environment and the internal environment of the body. The nerve endings in the skin are adapted to sense light, touch, deep pressure, pain and temperature. In this way the skin can communicate to the internal tissues what is going on in the outside world.

- Excretion: the skin is able to excrete unwanted substances through the sweat. It is also able to secrete aromatic chemicals, which act together with the extensive and unique community of microbes on the surface of the skin to give each person a unique smell that contributes to the non-verbal communication between individuals.

- Absorption: although this function is conventionally believed to be limited, the skin can absorb substances from the external environment. This can be interpreted as another aspect of the sensory role of the skin, allowing the body to respond to what is happening in the outside world.

The structure of the skin

The skin is composed of two thin layers known as the epidermis and the dermis. Throughout the body these two layers rest on a deeper layer of subcutaneous fat. The fascia, considered part of the musculoskeletal system, is the silvery fibrous connective tissue layer that underlies the subcutaneous fat and separates it from underlying muscles and bones. This is the glistening surface tissue that is seen surrounding the carcass when the skin of animals, for example, has been removed in the process of food production.

The epidermis is an example of stratified squamous epithelium, whereas the thicker dermis is made up of loose (areolar) and fatty connective tissue. Figure 6.1a-I illustrates the structure of these two delicate layers of the skin and how they rest on the underlying fat. The upper part of the dermis forms folds called papillae, and it is these that give rise to characteristic skin markings such as the fingerprint. The bumpiness prevents easy separation of the epidermis and dermis.

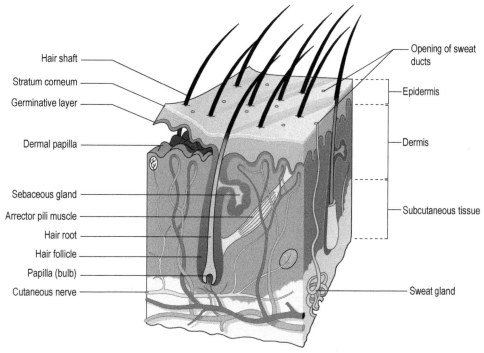

Figure 6.1a-I A section of the skin, showing how the epidermis rests on the dermis, which in turn rests on a layer of subcutaneous fat

Figure 6.1a-II is a more detailed image of the stratified structure of the epidermis. The cells of the epidermis continually multiply from the germinative layer and grow upwards in layers. As they progress upwards the cells become progressively more hardened with the protein keratin. The uppermost layers, the stratum corneum and lucidum, consist of lifeless keratin-stuffed cells, which have a vital protective function. This layer thickens in response to repeated trauma, such as that which continually happens to the palms of the hands and soles of the feet. As dead epithelial cells are shed from the skin they are replaced by new cells growing upwards from the germinative layer.

The pigment called melanin (dark brown), also produced by the cells of the epidermal layer, gives the skin its color. Clusters of deeply pigmented germinative cells form moles and freckles.

The sweat glands and the sebaceous glands originate in the looser areolar tissue of the dermis. The sweat glands are shaped like a coiled tube. They excrete a watery fluid onto the skin via a duct that passes through the epidermis. The watery fluid contains waste products. However, the most important function of the sweat is temperature control rather than excretion of wastes.

The sebaceous glands secrete an oily substance into the hair follicles and thence onto the skin. The sebum has a protective role in that it waterproofs the skin and hair, and helps to keep them soft and pliable. It is also believed to prevent penetrating skin infections.

Stratum corneum

Stratum lucidum

Stratum granulosum

Germinative layer

Epidermis

Dermis

Figure 6.1a-II The epidermis, illustrating the stratified squamous epithelial nature of this tissue

The hair follicles are specialized tubules of germinative epithelium that generate the cells and the protein keratin, which form the strand of hair. A hair develops at the base of a hair follicle, where numerous keratin-containing skin cells are compacted together. As the skin cells die, the keratin remains and this is pushed out of the follicle to form a single hair. The arrectores pilorum muscles are tiny smooth muscle structures that attach the base of a hair follicle to connective tissue fibers in the dermis. When the arrectores pilorum muscles contract, the hairs become erect and stand on end.

The nails are also composed of keratinized dead skin cells. They grow out of the nail bed, which is an area of tissue lined with the rapidly dividing epidermal skin cells of the germinative layer.

The dermis is also richly supplied with nerve endings and blood capillaries. A healthy blood supply gives the skin a reddish pink glow. Bile salts (yellow/green) from the liver and carotenes (red/yellow) obtained from the diet also contribute to skin color.

The role of the skin in the control of temperature

It is vital that the body maintains a steady temperature because the complex metabolic processes of the body work optimally within a very narrow temperature range. If the temperature rises, the metabolic processes speed up, and if it drops, they slow down. If the metabolic rate becomes too fast or slow, the fine balance between the different chemical reactions in the body can be lost and ill health will result, as evidenced in someone suffering either from a prolonged high fever or from hypothermia.

The skin plays only a minor role in heat production. The main heat-producing tissues are the skeletal muscles, the liver and the digestive organs. Nevertheless, the contraction of the arrectores pilorum muscles in the skin does also generate a certain amount of heat. These tiny but numerous muscles also cause the body hair to stand on end, a response that will tend to conserve heat in a furry animal.

However, the most important physiological mechanism for heat conservation in the human is the constriction of the capillary network in the skin. This is mediated by the sympathetic nervous system. When vasoconstriction occurs, the blood is held deep in the body, and the skin will start to feel cold, and look pale or even blue. A similar response occurs in acutely frightening or stressful situations.

The role of the skin in the loss of heat is also very important. By far the largest proportion of body heat is lost from the skin. This heat loss is minimized by vasoconstriction and the erection of body hair. Body fat and layers of clothing also reduce this loss of body heat. In contrast, the loss of heat is increased by the physiological responses of vasodilatation and sweating.

Dilatation of the blood vessels in the skin raises the surface temperature of the skin, and so heat loss to the outside environment is increased. Vasodilatation is mediated by the parasympathetic nervous system, and is controlled by the hypothalamus. Sweating, which occurs when the body temperature rises by a fraction of a degree, causes the skin to become moist. Moisture requires energy (heat) to evaporate, and thus in hot, dry weather the evaporation of the sweat has a cooling effect.

 Information box 6.1a-I

The skin: comments from a Chinese medicine perspective

In Chinese medicine, the skin and body hair are considered to be controlled by the Lungs, and sweating by the Heart. Other Chinese Organs play a part in the healthy function of the skin as it is conventionally understood. The Spleen is attributed to the control of healthy flesh and muscles. Temperature control depends on a healthy balance of Yin and Yang. This function of the skin might be attributed to the Kidney (in particular, the Ming Men) and Triple Burner Organs. The production of vitamin D in that it is essential for strengthening the bones would correspond to a function of the Kidney Organ.

The physiology of the eye[2]

The eye and the optic nerve pathways in the brain

The eyes are sensory organs that are specialized to respond to the stimulus of light. The eyes contain the cell bodies and nerve endings of the sensory nerves known as the optic nerves (second cranial nerves). Optic nerve fibers carry visual messages to the brain to a control center in the thalamus. From here the information is taken further back via connector neurons to the visual areas in the occipital lobe at the back of the brain. Here the complex processing necessary for visual perception takes place. Before the optic nerve fibers reach the thalamus, some of the fibers cross to the opposite side. This crossing point, known as the optic chiasm, is adjacent to the site of the pituitary stalk (overlying the sphenoid bone of the skull). This explains why pituitary tumors often result in visual disturbance. Figure 6.1a-III illustrates the optic nerves and their pathways from the eyes, which cross before they reach the occipital lobe of the brain.

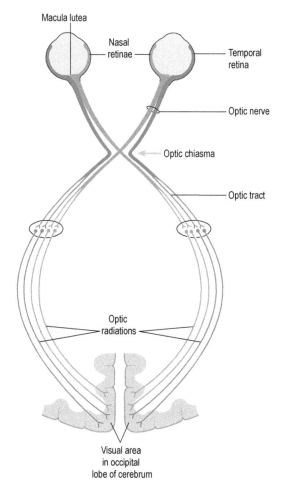

Figure 6.1a-III The optic nerves and their pathways

Although the eyes are situated at the front of the head, the information that they sense is processed at the back of the brain. Because of the optic chiasm, information from each eye is sent to each half of the occipital visual area. This allows for the binocular vision, the facility that gives what we see an appearance of depth.

The structure of the eye

The eye has a very specialized structure that allows it to perform the function of focusing and sensing visual images. This structure is illustrated in simplified form in Figure 6.1a-IV.

The outer lining of the eye is composed of three distinct layers. The outermost layer, the sclera, is dense and glistening white in color. The sclera becomes transparent anteriorly; this clear area is called the cornea. The next layer, the choroid, is dark in color. This blends into the ciliary body and the iris at the front of the eye. The deepest layer is the light-sensitive retina. The retina is not present anteriorly, as it stops at the border of the ciliary body. The lens in the eye is responsible for focusing the light that enters the cornea so that it forms an image on the retina, akin to the way a camera lens focuses light onto a film. The space that lies between the lens and the cornea is called the anterior chamber. This chamber contains a watery fluid called the aqueous humor (in this situation the term humor means fluid). The space in the body of the eyeball behind the lens is called the posterior chamber. This chamber contains a jelly-like fluid called the vitreous (glass-like) humor.

The ciliary body is responsible for suspending the lens in the correct position in the eye. The smooth muscle of the ciliary body controls the stretching and relaxation of the lens. This muscle control of the curvature of the lens enables the eye to alter its focus so that both distant and close objects can be seen clearly.

The iris controls the amount of light that enters the eye, in a similar way to the aperture of a camera. The smooth muscle fibers in the iris contract and relax to vary the diameter of the pupil, the central hole in the iris. The pupil tends to contract in response to bright light, and also when the eye is required to focus on a close object. The color of the iris depends on the amount of brown and green pigment it contains. The amount and composition of these pigments is genetically determined.

The retina contains specialized sensory nerve cell bodies called rods and cones. These contain a light- and color-sensitive pigment that alters in structure in response to light of different wavelengths. Each rod and cone has a long nerve axon, which sweeps backwards and leaves the eye within the optic nerve. The rods play an important role in the vision of low-intensity light, and it is thus the rods that enable night vision. They are not sensitive enough to distinguish between lights of different wavelengths (i.e. of different color).

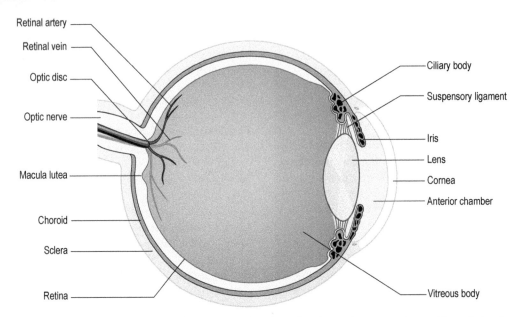

Figure 6.1a-IV Cross-section of the eye, showing the three layers to its wall and the lens

The cones are sensitive to different colors of light, but do not respond to light of low intensity. This is why it is not possible to distinguish colors in a darkened room.

The blind spot (optic disc) is the point at which all these nerve fibers converge to form the optic nerve. It is a tiny area of the retina that is devoid of rods and cones. Therefore, it is literally a blind spot, as it cannot respond to the light that falls on it. The macula lutea (yellow spot) is the region of the retina that holds the densest concentration of sensory cell bodies, and is the region that responds to light coming from the center of the field of vision. It is at the macula where fine detail and bright clear colors are distinguished.

The globe of the eye sits embedded within fatty tissue in the bony orbit. The optic nerve extends from the back of each eye to pass posteriorly through the sphenoid bone towards the optic chiasm (optic nerve crossing) within the skull. Six strips of muscle extend from the walls of the orbit to attach to the sclera of each eye. These are the extrinsic or extraocular muscles of the eye. All these structures hold the eye in place (see Figure 6.1a-V).

In thyroid eye disease, the eyes become pushed forward so that the eyelids appear to retract. In severe cases, the eyelids can no longer fully close. This is the result of excessive growth of the supportive fatty tissue in the orbit, which is stimulated by an autoantibody that appears in some cases of Graves' disease (see Section 5.1c).

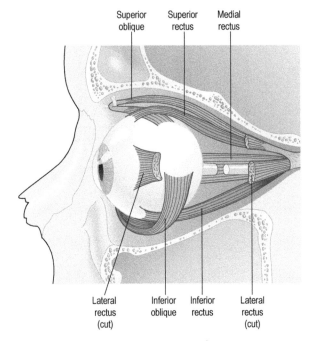

Figure 6.1a-V The extrinsic muscles that hold the eye in the bony orbit

The physiology of sight

The lens enables an image of the outside world to fall on the retina. For this to be possible for all objects in the field of vision, whether they are close or distant, the lens has to alter in shape to allow a clear image of the viewed object to be formed at the retina. Simply speaking, the lens needs to be fat (bulging) in shape to focus on a near object and thin (stretched) to focus on a distant object. In a healthy eye, when the ciliary muscle is relaxed, the lens is stretched so that it can focus on distant objects without any effort. The ciliary muscle has to work to contract so that the bulging lens can allow the eye to focus on close objects, and this is partly why close work can tire the eyes.

The eye has to make two other adjustments to enable close vision. First, constriction of the pupils takes place. This reaction enables only a thin beam of light to pass through the lens. This aids the focusing of the image because a narrow beam of light is easier to focus. This principle is used in a pinhole camera. Second, the eyeballs converge inwards when viewing a close object. When extreme, convergence causes the viewer to appear cross-eyed. Convergence allows the image of the object being viewed to fall onto the center of each retina. Without convergence the viewer would experience double vision.

In distance vision (objects more than 6 meters away) constriction of the pupils and convergence are not necessary, and also, as mentioned, the ciliary muscle becomes fully relaxed. It follows from this that the most restful aspect of vision is distance vision (e.g. when gazing on a countryside scene), as none of the three adjustments for close vision is required.

Each eye receives slightly different images, and the differences are more pronounced for close objects. The visual center of the occipital lobe of the cerebrum is the location for the interpretation of the two slightly different images that come from each retina, thereby giving the viewer an appreciation of the distance of a viewed object. The ability to visually appreciate distances is called stereoscopic vision.

The extraocular muscles and accessory organs of the eye

The six strips of skeletal muscle that form the extrinsic muscles of the eye guide the coordinated movements of the eyeballs (see Figure 6.1a-V). These movements, which are upwards, downwards, sideways and rotatory, are usually coordinated so that the two eyes move together.

Figure 6.1a-VI illustrates the extrinsic muscles of the eye in the orbit and the muscles that control the movements of the eyelids. One of these muscles, the levator palpebrae, lifts the eyelid when it contracts, while the other muscle, orbicularis oculi, because its fibers run circularly around the eyelids, closes the eyelid when it contracts. Figure 6.1a-VI also shows how the conjunctiva forms a protective sac behind the upper and lower eyelids.

The eyebrows, eyelids and conjunctiva are adapted to provide mechanical protection for the eye. The lacrimal gland is a specialized organ for producing the tears. Tears are constantly produced by this gland (see Figure 6.1a-VII) to lubricate the conjunctiva. Tears drain away via tiny channels called canaliculi to the nasolacrimal duct (tear duct), and thence to the nose. This is why a watery discharge from the nose frequently accompanies an episode of crying.

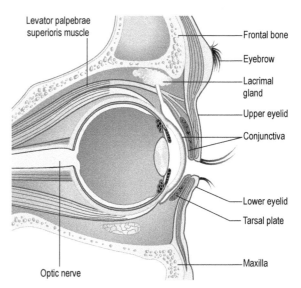

Figure 6.1a-VI The position of the eye in the orbit and the accessory structures of the eye

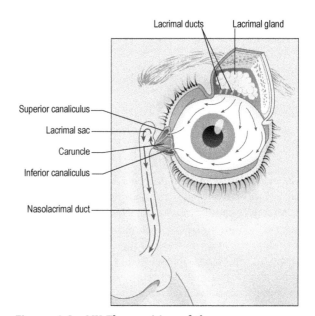

Figure 6.1a-VII The position of the lacrimal gland and the tear duct

 Information box 6.1a-II

The eye: comments from a Chinese medicine perspective

In Chinese medicine, the Liver is the Organ that opens into the eyes. The Liver Blood moistens and nourishes the eye and gives it the capacity to see. However, as Maciocia (1989) explains, many other Yin and Yang Organs affect the eye. In particular, Kidney Essence and the Heart Organ are important in maintaining the health of the eyes.[3]

The physiology of the ear[4]

The functions of the ear

The ear is the sensory organ responsible for hearing. The ear is also an important sensory organ in the control of balance. The nerve impulses leave the ear via the auditory or vestibulocochlear nerve (eighth cranial nerve), which passes from the ear to the brain through a tiny hole in the temporal bone of the skull. Impulses from this nerve are transmitted via control centers in the brainstem and the mid-brain to the auditory area of the cerebral hemispheres (for the perception of sound) and the cerebellum (for the control of balance).

The structure of the ear

The structure of the ear can be considered in three parts: the outer, or external, ear, the middle ear and the inner ear. This structure is illustrated in Figure 6.1a-VIII.

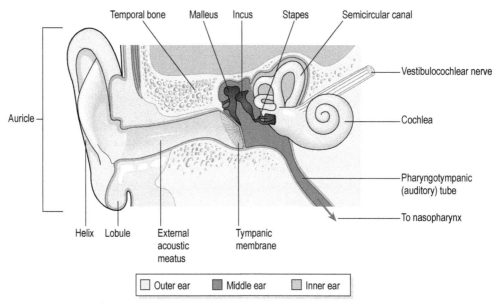

Figure 6.1a-VIII The structure of the three parts of the ear

The external ear consists of the pinna (auricle), the auditory canal (acoustic meatus) and the tympanic membrane (eardrum). The main purpose of the external ear is to provide a protective opening for the delicate inner structures of the ear. The hair- and wax-lined auditory canal protects the eardrum from trauma, foreign bodies and infection. The pinna also plays a role in directing sound waves into the auditory canal, although it is more obviously adapted for this purpose in species such as dogs, cats and rabbits.

The middle ear is a chamber lined with respiratory epithelium, which contains three tiny interlinked bones (ossicles) known as the malleus (hammer), incus (anvil) and stapes (stirrup). The ossicles provide a link between the eardrum (tympanic membrane) and another membrane that separates the middle from the inner ear (the oval window). The purpose of the ossicles is to transmit the sound vibrations that strike the eardrum through to the cochlea of the inner ear. Tiny movements of the oval window lead to vibrations within the fluid (perilymph) that bathes the membranous cochlea (see Figure 6.1a-IX). The largest ossicle, the malleus, can be seen through the eardrum when the eardrum is visualized by means of the hand-held otoscope (see Figure 6.1a-X).

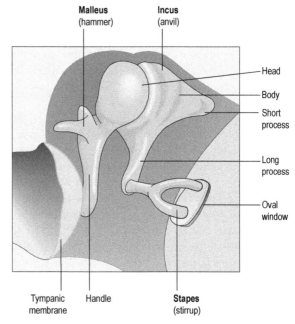

Figure 6.1a-IX The structure of the middle ear

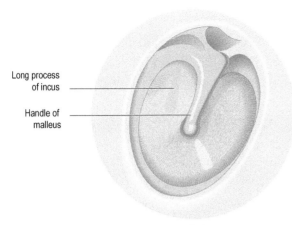

Figure 6.1a-X Otoscopic view of the eardrum, showing the handle of the malleus and a shadow formed by the incus

Long process of incus

Handle of malleus

From the perspective of the development of the ear in the embryo, the link that the middle ear has with the respiratory system becomes clearer. In the embryo, the middle ear forms from an upward pouching of the nasopharynx, whereas the inner ear develops outwards from the primitive nervous tissue. The middle ear and the interlinked mastoid air cells are lined with ciliated respiratory epithelium. The air and the surface microbes that they contain are in direct communication with the air and the surface microbes in the nasopharynx. This explains why respiratory infections can so readily involve the middle ear and lead to deafness and earache.

The spaces of the inner ear contain two interlinked fluid-filled membranous sacs which, like the middle ear, are safely protected, being bathed in fluid (perilymph) within bony cavities in the temporal bone of the skull. The first chamber, the cochlea, is spiral in form and contains fluid called endolymph. The cochlea is responsible for the interpretation of sound vibrations (see Figure 6.1a-XI).

Anterior membranous semicircular canal

Temporal bone

Lateral membranous semicircular canal

Posterior membranous semicircular canal

Cochlea

Cochlear duct

Bony labyrinth

Membranous labyrinth

Figure 6.1a-XI The structure of the inner ear

Within the cochlea, the spiral organ of Corti lies along its length and is fully immersed in the fluid of the endolymph. This tiny structure consists of a side-by-side arrangement of sensory nerve bodies, which are able to respond to sound vibrations. Messages are sent via nerve axons to auditory centers in the brain, where they can be interpreted as sound. Sound waves of different frequencies (corresponding to sounds of different pitch) stimulate different cells, and so pitch can be distinguished by the ear. Therefore, the organ of Corti is to the ear and hearing as the rods and the cones are to the eye and sight.

The second chamber of the inner ear consists of three semicircular canals, which sit in three different planes at right angles to each other. The semicircular canals are in direct communication with the cochlea, and, like the cochlea, also contain a membranous sensory organ, which is bathed in perilymph fluid. Movement of the head leads to fluid waves in the endolymph within the semicircular canals that are interpreted to allow perception of the head's position in space.

The semicircular canals provide important sensory information to aid the maintenance of balance. This information is processed, together with visual information and sensory information from the large joints of the feet and leg, in the cerebellum. As the head moves into a new position, particular waves of fluid movement are set up in the three canals, which are then sensed by sensory cells in the dilated ends of the semicircular canals. This sensory information can be interpreted in the brain in terms of the position and rate of movement of the head.

Information box 6.1a-III

The ear: comments from a Chinese medicine perspective

From a Chinese medicine perspective, the Kidney Organ opens into the ears. Maciocia (1989) states that, if the Kidneys are weak, hearing may be impaired and there may be tinnitus (ringing in the ears). He also describes that the Heart has an influence on hearing, with some types of tinnitus resulting from Heart Qi Deficiency.[5]

6.1b The investigation of the skin, the eye and the ear

The diseases of the skin, the eye and the ear are managed within the distinct specialties of dermatology, ophthalmology and otorhinolaryngology (ear, nose and throat), respectively.

Investigation of disorders of the skin includes:

- a detailed inspection of the skin rash, including exposure to a Wood's light

- culture and examination of samples taken by swab from the area of the rash

- examination of skin scrapings and nail clippings

- examination of a skin biopsy

- patch or prick testing for allergies

- a physical examination to exclude underlying medical conditions

- blood tests to exclude underlying medical conditions.

Investigation of disorders of the eye includes:

- examination of visual acuity using Snellen charts

- examination of the visual fields

- examination of color vision

- examination of the eye movements

- examination of the structure of the eye by means of a hand-held ophthalmoscope

- examination of the structure of the eye by means of a slit lamp

- examination of the intraocular pressure by means of a slit lamp and tonometry

- examination of the blood flow to the retina using fluorescein angiography

- imaging tests, including ultrasound, computed tomography (CT) and magnetic resonance imaging (MRI)

- electrophysiological tests

- culture and examination of samples taken by swab from the eye.

Investigation of disorders of the ear includes:

- visual inspection of the external ear and eardrum

- clinical assessment of hearing

- testing of hearing by means of audiometry

- testing of the flexibility of the middle ear by means of impedance tympanometry

- electrophysiological tests.

These investigations are considered below briefly in turn.

Investigation of disorders of the skin

Inspection of the skin rash

Pattern recognition is crucial in the assessment of skin disorders. A skilled dermatologist will be experienced in the recognition of the variety of ways in which skin disorders can manifest. Some skin disorders have such a characteristic appearance that once the rash is seen the doctor can be sure of the diagnosis. A physical sign that points to only one possible diagnosis is described as pathognomic (meaning that the sign itself leads to the knowledge of the underlying pathology).

Inspection of the skin should be thorough and systematic. All parts of the body might be examined to look for aspects of the rash that may not have been discovered by the patient. The skin may then be viewed under a hand-held microscope called a dermatoscope, which can reveal subtle changes to the skin markings not clearly visible to the naked eye. The rash may also be illuminated using ultraviolet light from a Wood's lamp. This light causes some rashes to fluoresce, and can allow pigmented rashes to be viewed with more clarity.

Culture and examination of samples taken by swab

If the cause of the rash is believed to be infective, the rash, or its discharge, may be swabbed, and the swab sent for microbiological analysis.

Examination of skin scrapings and nail clippings

Skin scrapings and nail clippings are samples that can be obtained painlessly. Microbiological examination of these samples can reveal fungal infection and infestation by scabies mites.

Examination of a skin biopsy

Skin biopsy is a very useful technique in the diagnosis of skin disorders. If the problem is small and localized (e.g. a worrying mole) then a biopsy can both treat the condition by removing it, and also generate a sample for examination. This approach, known as excisional biopsy, is ideally performed in such a way that the diseased area is completely removed, with no portion left remaining. A wide excision may be required to ensure full removal of a suspected skin cancer such as a melanoma. If only a small ellipse of skin is removed, the wound can be sutured so that the resulting scar is almost invisible. However, a wide excision may require a graft of skin from another part of the body (usually the outer thigh) to permit full healing of the area from which the section of skin was removed.

If the skin rash is more extensive, an incisional biopsy can be performed to remove a long ellipse of skin from the edge of the rash. As is the case with excisional biopsy, the resulting wound will require closure by sutures. Examination of the incisional biopsy should reveal both normal and affected skin, and thus allow comparison of the two.

A punch biopsy removes a fine column of affected skin by means of a tubular sampling blade. This leaves a tiny hole, which may require a single stitch to stem bleeding.

Patch or prick testing for allergies

Patch testing is used to test for sensitivity to various allergens that can result in contact dermatitis (contact eczema). The test involves holding diluted samples of a battery of common allergens against a flat area of skin (usually of the back) for up to 48 hours by means of an adhesive strip of patches. The development of a thickened red area of skin under one of the patches is indicative of sensitivity to that allergen. Allergens that commonly cause positive reactions in the patch test include nickel, rubber and colophony (a common constituent of sticking plasters).

Patch testing is a specific test for contact eczema. The aim is to exclude a delayed allergic reaction (type 4 hypersensitivity) that manifests in dermatitis/eczema (redness, localized swelling and itch) after two days or more of exposure to the allergen.

Prick or scratch tests are allergy tests that are aimed at excluding the more immediate allergic reaction that leads to urticaria, edema and asthma (type 1 hypersensitivity). In prick or scratch testing, a diluted sample of allergen is allowed to penetrate under the epidermis via the prick or the scratch, and the skin is examined for the appearance of a characteristic wheal. This reaction tends to develop within seconds to minutes if the test is positive. Allergens that are commonly found to lead to positive reactions in prick or scratch testing include animal dandruff, pollen and dietary constituents such as egg and nuts.

Physical examination to exclude underlying medical conditions

Dermatologists have a thorough grounding in clinical medicine. If a rash is found that indicates a possible medical condition as the underlying cause, the dermatologist will proceed to examine the patient for other features of that disease.

Blood tests to exclude underlying medical conditions

Blood tests may be ordered to exclude a suspected underlying medical diagnosis. For example, the blood may be tested for autoantibodies if an autoimmune condition such as systemic lupus erythematosus (SLE) is suspected as the cause of the rash.

Investigation of disorders of the eye

Eye disorders are often first picked up during examination by an optometrist (also known as optician). The optometrist routinely tests for clear, unrestricted sight by means of tests for visual acuity, the integrity of the visual fields, color vision and eye movements. The optometrist will also examine the internal structure of the eye by means of a hand-held ophthalmoscope. The optometrist may also check the visual fields and also the internal pressure of the eye by means of tonometry (see below), and also take a high-resolution photograph of the retina to check for signs of disease.

A hospital ophthalmologist will also perform these investigations, but has access to other powerful tools of examination, including the slit lamp, fluorescein angiography and imaging tests.

Examination of visual acuity

Visual acuity (acuteness) is the medical term used to describe the ability of the eye to see a clear image of the viewed object. A normal level of acuity depends on the health of the cornea, lens, vitreous humor, retina and the optic pathways. However, even in a healthy eye, acuity is always limited by the size of the image that lands on the retina. It makes sense that the smaller the image, the less clearly its features can be seen. The different aspects of an image that falls on the retina simply cannot be distinguished if they are smaller than the size of single cones on the retinal surface.

Acuity can be tested simply by means of the Snellen chart, probably the most familiar test associated with the optometrist. The Snellen chart consists of rows of letters (or pictures for those patients who are unable to read) of progressively decreasing height. The patient is placed at a fixed distance from the chart and is asked, for each eye in turn, what is the smallest size of letter that they can read with confidence. This is then compared with what is known to be a normal and healthy level of acuity.

The optometrist will then proceed to explore to what extent correcting the vision by means of a lens will improve the acuity. The degree to which a lens can correct the vision depends on the exact cause of the impairment in acuity. If the impairment is due totally to a problem in the focusing of the image by the lens in the eye, a perfectly suited lens should be able to offer the patient a return to normal visual acuity. If, however, the problem is a result of, for example, cataract or retinal damage, a lens may not be able to improve vision very much.

Examination of the visual fields

The visual field is the term used to describe the width and height of the view from each eye when the person is looking straight ahead. In health, even when looking straight ahead, movement that occurs almost to the side of the head can be detected because of the extent of the visual field. The visual field is less extensive to the medial side of the eye because the bridge of the nose gets in the way. However, objects can be seen when they are held almost at a right angle to the direction of the gaze on the lateral side of the eye.

There is a small area of the visual field, slightly lateral to the area on which the eye focuses, in which the image of the object becomes less distinct. This area is the blind spot, and corresponds to the area on the retina overlying the origin of the optic nerve, known as the optic disc.

Mapping of the visual fields and the blind spot is performed by means of asking the patient to register when they have seen tiny lights on a screen. This test can reveal restrictions that are characteristic of certain diseases, including chronic simple glaucoma and damage to the optic nerve chiasm by pituitary tumors.

Examination of color vision

Color blindness can be diagnosed by means of pictures that are made up of many dots of different colors. Color blindness will prevent an observer from distinguishing certain aspects of the pictures.

Examination of the eye movements

The eye movements are assessed by asking the patient to follow a moving object in the field of vision while keeping the head still. During the test the examiner watches for divergence or convergence of the eyes, and questions the patient about any episodes of double vision. This examination can reveal the presence of a squint (strabismus).

Examination of the structure of the eye by ophthalmoscope

The ophthalmoscope is a hand-held instrument through which the examining practitioner can focus on the various internal structures of the eye, ideally with the patient in a darkened room. The ophthalmoscope should allow inspection of the cornea, the iris and lens, the vitreous and aqueous humors, the pattern of vessels on the retina, and the optic nerve head (the disc).

Ophthalmoscopic examination of the retina is the only means by which a doctor can make a direct, but non-invasive, inspection of part of the nervous system. In addition to visualization of the optic nerve head, examination with an ophthalmoscope can reveal the characteristic changes that occur in a wide range of eye diseases, including cataract, vitreous detachment, retinal detachment, diabetic retinopathy and the changes that result from high blood pressure.

Examination of the structure of the eye by means of the slit lamp

The slit lamp (or bio-microscope) allows the examining practitioner to obtain a high-quality view of the external and internal structures of the eye. Prior to a slit lamp examination, a few drops of a mydriatic (a drug that causes widening of the pupils) are placed into the patient's eyes. This can have the effect of causing blurred vision until the drug wears off, and so the patient is advised not to drive until this side effect has faded. Once the mydriatic has taken effect, the patient sits in a chair in a darkened room and, to ensure immobility, places their head against a headrest attached to the slit lamp. The magnifying lens of the slit lamp can then be focused on the various structures of each eye in turn. A fluorescent dye called fluorescein can be instilled into the eye to reveal scratches and ulcers on the corneal surface. These damaged areas fill up with fluorescein, and will fluoresce green when viewed through the slit lamp.

Examination of the intraocular pressure by means of the slit lamp and tonometry

The fluid contents of the healthy eye are maintained at a steady level of pressure, which ensures that the tension of the lining of the eye is of a sufficient degree to maintain its spherical shape, but is not so high that the delicate nerve endings of the rods and the cones are damaged. Glaucoma is the name of the sight-threatening condition that results from excessively high intraocular pressure.

The intraocular pressure can be assessed by means of a sensitive pressure gauge called a tonometer. The measurement of the pressure can be made during a slit lamp examination during which the tonometer is held against each of the corneas in turn. This non-invasive examination, which takes a matter of seconds, is uncomfortable but not painful.

Examination of the blood flow to the retina using fluorescein angiography

Fluorescein angiography is a more invasive technique, which involves the injection of fluorescein into the circulation. The retina is then illuminated with blue light, which causes the fluorescein flowing through the retinal arteries to fluoresce with a bright green light. A photograph of the fluorescing vessels is then taken by means of a specialized camera. This examination can reveal more detail about the damage to the retinal circulation that can result from conditions such as chronic diabetes mellitus or atherosclerosis.

Imaging tests including ultrasound, CT and MRI scans

The ultrasound scan is a frequently used tool in ophthalmology to assess the health of the vitreous humor, the retina and the posterior coats of the eye. It is particularly useful when a cataract in the lens prevents slit lamp examination of the structures behind the lens.

CT and MRI are of value in assessing the shape of the orbit and the pathways of the optic nerves as they pass from the optic nerve head to the brain.

Electrophysiological tests

Specialized electrophysiological tests can be used to assess the responses of the nerves in the retina, optic nerve pathways and the visual cortex (at the back of the brain) to visual stimuli (such as flashing lights) presented to the eyes.

Culture and examination of samples taken by swab from the eye

Infections of the conjunctiva can be investigated by means of culture and examination of samples taken by means of swab from the conjunctival secretions.

Investigation of disorders of the ear

Visual inspection of the external ear and eardrum

The external ear (the pinna), the external ear canal and the outer aspect of the eardrum can be assessed by means of a hand-held instrument called an auriscope (or otoscope). The auriscope provides illumination of the external ear canal by means of a fiber-optic light source. The auriscope is inserted painlessly into the outer ear by means of a plastic conical speculum. The examining practitioner places gentle traction on the pinna of the ear to enable straightening of the external ear canal and so to permit visualization of the eardrum (see Figure 6.1a-X).

Examination of the external ear and external ear canal can reveal the changes caused by otitis externa and the excessive accumulation of earwax. Visualization of the eardrum will demonstrate certain problems affecting the middle ear, including acute otitis media, chronic secretory otitis media (glue ear), perforated eardrum and cholesteatoma.

Clinical assessment of hearing

As deafness is one of the major symptoms that accompany diseases of the middle and inner ear, clinical assessment of hearing can provide very useful diagnostic information. Voice and whisper tests are rough and ready methods of assessing the hearing in each ear. While simple to perform, they can be very useful in certain patient groups, young children in particular.

A more specific test involves the use of a tuning fork. A large tuning fork is used, which when percussed will produce a note of low pitch. The vibrating tuning fork is placed close to the external ear canal, and then held with its foot touching the central area of the forehead (close to the acupuncture point Yin Tang). The patient is asked to compare the volume of sound produced by both positions, and to say where they hear the sound when it is placed against the forehead. If the hearing problem is located in the middle ear (e.g. in glue ear), the sound conducted by the bones of the head, when the fork is placed on the forehead, will be louder than that produced when it is held close to the affected ear (in health the tuning fork will be loudest when placed close to the external ear canal). This is because bone conduction of sound bypasses the blocked middle ear, and will be heard by a healthy inner ear.

If the hearing in the inner ear on one side is compromised, the sound of the tuning fork when placed against the forehead will sound as if it is closer to the unaffected side.

Testing of hearing by means of audiometry

The audiometer is a machine that produces pure tones of sound at varying frequencies and varying intensities. The sound is fed to the patient either through earphones or via a microphone held against the mastoid process (the prominence of bone that sits postero-inferiorly to each ear). In this way air conduction of sound (to the middle ear) can be compared against bone conduction (directly to the inner ear).

The audiogram is a chart of hearing produced as a result of audiogram testing. This chart reveals the threshold of hearing for varying intensities of sound at different frequencies for each ear. Different hearing problems result in characteristic audiograms. For example, the damage to hearing that results from exposure to excessive noise results in impairment of hearing at high frequencies (high-pitched sound).

Speech audiometry is a variant of audiometry in which a recorded word list, rather than pure tones, is presented to each ear.

Testing of the flexibility of the middle ear by means of impedance tympanometry

Impedance tympanometry is a less patient-dependent non-invasive test which assesses objectively the degree to which the eardrum reflects the pure tones with which it is presented by an audiometer. This is a very useful test in assessing the degree to which glue ear is compromising hearing in babies and young children.

Electrophysiological tests (electric response audiometry)

The nerve responses to a sound wave that reaches the inner ear can be tested by means of a similar method to that used to test the nerve responses in the visual pathways. In electric response audiometry, a sound stimulus is applied to the outer ear. The response to this stimulus in the nerves that originate in the inner ear, and which travel via the auditory nerve to the auditory cortex in the brain, can be assessed by means of sensory electrodes placed against the bones of the middle ear, the base of the neck and the skull.

Because this non-invasive technique requires no response from the patient, it can be used in babies and young children, and also, by dint of its objectivity, to provide evidence in cases involving litigation for industrial deafness.

6.1c Diseases of the skin

The skin is able to react rapidly to a very wide range of environmental and internal factors, and in some cases this leads to disease. Known triggers for skin disease include genetic susceptibility, degeneration from aging, infectious agents, physical trauma, allergic reactions, light, heat, cold, psychological stress and self-harm. However, in many cases of skin disease the underlying cause is never clarified. Any one trigger can lead to a diverse range of manifestations of skin disease and it is often not very clear exactly why one person under stress develops itch and another psoriasis, or why antibiotics in one person will cause a painful blistering reaction and in another a rash of red spots.

From a more holistic perspective, it is generally appreciated that the skin, as it is the most superficial organ, might readily express symptoms and signs as an indication of a deeper imbalance. These would be the result of a combination of both internal and external factors, which would begin to explain the diversity of skin diseases.

The aim of this section is to introduce the wide range of ways in which the skin can manifest symptoms, and also the common treatment approaches used in dermatology. This section is split into two parts, which are designed to be studied in separate study sessions.

Generalized diseases in which the skin can be involved include peripheral vascular disease, diabetes mellitus, thyroid disease, Cushing's syndrome, Addison's disease, rheumatoid arthritis, chronic liver disease and a wide range of infectious diseases. As all these diseases have already been described in some length in earlier sections, their skin manifestations (with the exception of some of the important infectious skin diseases) are not mentioned further here.

The conditions discussed in this section are:

Part I: Skin infections, acne and scaling conditions

- Bacterial infections:
  - cellulitis and erysipelas
  - boils, abscesses and folliculitis
  - impetigo
  - scalded skin syndrome
  - leprosy
- Viral infections:
  - warts
  - molluscum contagiosum
  - rashes in generalized viral infections
  - herpes simplex infections
  - herpes zoster infections
  - hand, foot and mouth disease
- Fungal infections:
  - tinea (athlete's foot and ringworm)
  - candidal (yeast) infections
  - pityriasis (tinea) versicolor
- Skin infestations:
  - scabies
  - head, pubic and body lice
  - fleas and papular urticaria
- Acne:
  - acne vulgaris
  - acne rosacea

- Eczema (dermatitis):
  - exogenous eczema
  - endogenous eczema
- Psoriasis:
  - plaque psoriasis
  - scalp psoriasis
  - guttate psoriasis.
- Erythroderma

Part II: Moles and tumors, connective tissue disorders and other common skin conditions

- Moles and other nevi:
  - freckles and melanocytic nevi (common moles)
  - stork marks and blue spots in newborns
  - strawberry nevi
  - port-wine stains
  - Campbell de Morgan red spots
  - spider nevi
- Skin tumors – benign lumps:
  - seborrheic warts (senile keratoses)
  - skin tags
  - dermatofibromata
  - epidermal cysts (sebaoceous cysts), lipomas and milia
  - keloid scars
- Skin tumors – malignant skin tumors:
  - solar keratoses
  - basal cell carcinoma (BCC)
  - squamous cell carcinoma (SCC) and Bowen's disease
  - Paget's disease of the nipple
  - malignant melanoma
  - Kaposi's sarcoma
  - lymphoma and the skin
- Connective tissue disorders:
  - systemic lupus erythematosus (SLE) and discoid lupus erythematosus (DLE)
  - dermatomyositis
  - scleroderma and morphea
- Disorders of hair growth:
  - excessive hair growth

  - abnormal scalp hair loss
- Other common skin conditions:
  - urticaria and angio-edema
  - prickly heat (miliaria)
  - polymorphic light eruption (PLE)
  - chilblains
  - xanthelasmata and xanthomata
  - lichen planus
  - pityriasis rosea
  - pruritus
  - skin ulcers
  - reactions to drugs.

Part I: Skin infections, acne and scaling conditions

Bacterial infections

CELLULITIS AND ERYSIPELAS

Cellulitis is a rapidly spreading streptococcal or staphylococcal infection of the subcutaneous and deeper tissues. Erysipelas is a term given to the most superficial forms of cellulitis, but clinically there is no clear distinction between the two conditions. Both manifest as a spreading redness and swelling of the skin and underlying tissues, and are accompanied by fever, malaise and enlarged local lymph nodes.

Cellulitis is not usually a contagious condition and appears to be the result of a breakdown in the usual barrier of the skin to its own microbes. It is a known complication of needle puncture. The risk of infection as a result of acupuncture is minimized by preparation of a clean field, use of sterile single use needles and scrupulous hand washing.[6, 7]

The conventional treatment is with oral or systemic antibiotics (penicillin in most cases).

 Information box 6.1c-I

Cellulitis and erysipelas: comments from a Chinese medicine perspective

A Chinese medicine interpretation is that the cellulitis or erysipelas is a manifestation of Wind Heat. The infection is more likely to become apparent if there is Depletion of Blood/Yin and/or Internal Heat.

BOILS, ABSCESSES AND FOLLICULITIS

The pathology and energetic interpretation of boils and their treatment are described in Sections 2.2b and 5.4d.

Furuncle is another term for a boil. A carbuncle is a large boil (a collection of pus within inflamed subcutaneous tissue), which is often centered on a hair follicle. Folliculitis is a condition in which a number of tiny boils develop, each also centered round a hair follicle (often on the anterior thighs). An abscess is the medical term for a collection of pus anywhere in the body, and when a carbuncle is significant in size it may be described as an abscess.

Antibiotics may also be prescribed in minor cases. Folliculitis is treated with oral antibiotics and prevented with topical antibacterial preparations. A large carbuncle or abscess will require surgical drainage so that the pus can be cleared from the affected area. The wound may be packed and left open to permit continued drainage whilst the base of the wound heals by "secondary intention" (see Figure 2.1b-II).

As with cellulitis, boils and furuncles tend to develop in individuals who are unwell or run down in some way, and are not contagious.

Hidradenitis suppurativa describes a chronic condition in which there is a particular tendency to develop recurrent boils in the armpits and the groins. There is an inherited tendency to this condition, but it is also more likely to develop in obese people and also if there is recurrent hair removal of these bodily areas.

The medical treatment may involve antibacterial skin cleansers, acne creams and recurrent treatments with antibiotics. In severe cases surgical removal of the cysts may have to be performed.

 Information box 6.1c-II

Boils and abscesses: comments from a Chinese medicine perspective

In Chinese medicine, a boil represents Damp, Damp Heat, or Fire Poison. Internal factors are important in the causation of the accumulation of these Pathogenic Factors. A person who has a tendency to Damp and Phlegm and Heat as a consequence of Spleen Qi Deficiency and Yin Deficiency with Liver Qi Stagnation may be more likely to develop recurrent boils.

IMPETIGO

The pathology and energetic interpretation of impetigo (see Figure 6.1c-I) and its treatment are described in Section 5.4d.

Figure 6.1c-I The crusting rash of impetigo

SCALDED SKIN SYNDROME

The pathology and energetic interpretation of scalded skin syndrome and its treatment are described in Section 5.4d.

LEPROSY

The pathology and energetic interpretation of leprosy and its treatment are described in Section 4.1g.

Viral infections

WARTS

The pathology and energetic interpretation of warts (see Figure 6.1c-II) and their treatment are described in Section 5.4d.

Figure 6.1c-II A viral wart

MOLLUSCUM CONTAGIOSUM

The pathology and energetic interpretation of molluscum contagiosum and its treatment are described in Section 5.4d.

RASHES IN GENERALIZED VIRAL INFECTIONS

A number of generalized viral infections can manifest with a rash of pink blotches or flat spots (macules). These so-called viral exanthems (see Figure 6.1c-III) are common in childhood, and are not usually serious. The well-described viral infections that present with a rash include measles (rubeola), German measles (rubella), slapped-cheek disease and roseola infantum (exanthem subitum). The pathology and energetic interpretation of all these infections are described in Section 5.4d.

Figure 6.1c-III The rash of rubella (German measles), a typical viral exanthem

Many respiratory and feco-orally transmitted viruses can lead to the development of a rash. It is not uncommon for a child to suffer from a mild rash accompanied by features of a generalized viral infection such as fever and/or runny nose and sore throat and/or diarrhea and/or joint aches, while the precise diagnosis remains unknown.

The common viral infections that cause a vesicular rash (fluid-filled blisters), rather than macular rash (flat pink spots), are summarized below.

HERPES SIMPLEX INFECTIONS

The pathology and energetic interpretation of herpes simplex infections and their treatment are described in Section 5.4d.

HERPES ZOSTER INFECTIONS (CHICKENPOX AND SHINGLES)

The pathology and energetic interpretation of chickenpox and shingles (see Figure 6.1c-IV) and their treatment are described in Section 5.4d.

Figure 6.1c-IV The rash of shingles affecting a thoracic dermatome

HAND, FOOT AND MOUTH DISEASE

The pathology and energetic interpretation of hand, foot and mouth disease and its treatment are described in Section 5.4d.

Fungal infections

In a healthy person it is rare for fungal infections to cause symptoms anywhere else in the body other than the skin, nails and hair. Although deep fungal infections are rare, fungal infections of the skin and mucous membranes of the mouth and genitalia are very common. In some cases they are believed to be the result of overgrowth of fungi that might normally live as part of the skin commensal organisms without causing disease.

TINEA (INCLUDING ATHLETE'S FOOT AND RINGWORM)

The fungi that cause disease of the epidermis of the skin are known as dermatophytes. The word tinea means gnawing worm, and is a general term used to describe dermatophyte overgrowth.

The manifestation and description of tinea infections is based on the site. Tinea pedis is disease of the foot, more commonly known as athlete's foot. Tinea corporis is disease of the body skin, more commonly known as ringworm. Tinea cruris (see Figure 6.1c-V) is disease of the inguinal region, a problem that is more common in men than women.

Figure 6.1c-V Tinea cruris: ringworm of the groin

The main symptoms of tinea are itch, scaling of the affected skin and very often a red, well-demarcated border to the infected area. The infection is often asymmetrical, a feature that is not so common in other skin diseases.

Tinea unguium (see Figure 6.1c-VI) is a fungal infection that has penetrated the nail bed. The affected nail becomes yellowed and thickened, and may split into flakes at its distal margin.

Figure 6.1c-VI Tinea unguium: fungal infection of the toenail

The diagnosis of these tinea infections can be confirmed by the microscopic examination of skin scrapings and nail clippings, although most infections have a characteristic appearance, which means that this investigation usually is unnecessary.

Treatment of tinea pedis, corporis and cruris involves the regular application of local antifungal drugs such as clotrimazole. For more persistent infection, oral antifungal medication such as terbinafine and itraconozole may be prescribed for up to four weeks in skin infections, and for as long as 12 weeks in toenail infections. These medications carry a risk of headaches, digestive disturbance, rashes and disturbed liver function.

 Information box 6.1c-III

Tinea: comments from a Chinese medicine perspective

In Chinese medicine, a tinea infection would suggest Damp or Damp Heat. The location of the infection would be significant in making a more precise energetic interpretation of the condition.

The antifungal medications evidently clear Damp Heat, but the side effects suggest that they can induce Spleen/Liver Disharmony and perhaps Accumulation of Toxic Heat.

CANDIDAL (YEAST) INFECTIONS

Candida is a yeast that is a normal resident of the gastrointestinal tract and the vagina, and can be found in 30–70 percent of individuals at any one time. One individual may carry more than one strain of *candida*, and studies suggest that different strains are adapted to thrive in different anatomical locations.[8] The candidal infections of oral thrush, genital thrush and a certain form of nappy rash are a result of abnormal overgrowth of strains of this yeast.

The term *Candida* syndrome is used to describe a constellation of symptoms that are attributed to overgrowth of *candida* in the gastrointestinal and reproductive tracts. This syndrome is not recognized as an organic (as opposed to functional) condition in conventional medicine (see Section 2.4b).

The common presentations of *Candida* are described in Section 2.4b (*Candida* syndrome), 3.1c (oral thrush), 5.2d (genital thrush) and 5.4e (candidal nappy rash). Opportunistic infection with *candida* is described in Section 5.2d (HIV and AIDS).

Candida tends to only cause problems on the skin in healthy people in areas in which the skin is perpetually moist (e.g. the nappy region in babies and between folds of flesh in obese people). Candidal infection of the skin is much more common in people on long-term antibiotic therapy (where it tends to appear in the ano-genital areas), in those with immune deficiency and people with diabetes mellitus (when it is more likely to affect the mouth, upper digestive tract and airways). Skin infection is characterized by a brick-red rash with a clearly demarcated border. There may be tiny circular satellites of rash clustered close to the margins of the affected area (see Figure 6.1c-VII). Often the moist rash will have a yeasty or offensive odor.

Figure 6.1c-VII Candidal rash of the groin, showing satellite lesions

---

 Information box 6.1c-IV

Candida: comments from a Chinese medicine perspective

In Chinese medicine, *Candida* of the skin is a manifestation of Damp Heat. Candidal nappy rash in babies might indicate Accumulation Disorder.

Pityriasis (tinea) versicolor

Pityriasis versicolor is an overgrowth of a yeast called *Malassezia* that is also a normal resident of the hair follicles of the skin. Under certain conditions the yeast multiplies to cause scattered, light-brown macules on the trunk and upper arms. The cause of this overgrowth is unknown, but as it is not contagious, it is presumably due to an alteration in the host skin defenses. In pigmented skin, in some patients the affected areas may become depigmented, and in others, more pigmented. It is understood that the yeast in some way affects the production of melanin by affected skin cells.

The medical treatment of pityriasis versicolor involves application of a selenium sulfide shampoo or an antifungal cream. Oral antifungal agents may be prescribed in resistant cases.

Information box 6.1c-V

Pityriasis versicolor: comments from a Chinese medicine perspective

In Chinese medicine, the development of pityriasis versicolor is a manifestation of Damp.

Skin infestations

Skin infestations are infections by parasites that inhabit the surface of the skin. In the majority of infestations occurring in the developed world, the symptoms result from biting and burrowing by the parasites (usually lice, ticks, insects or mites), and the problem that results is primarily one of discomfort rather than a serious threat to health.

However, the invading parasites can be carriers of disease. Typhus is a serious disease of undernourished populations that is transmitted via body louse infestation. The features of typhus include high fever, headache, meningitis and a bruising rash. Lyme disease is a generalized infection that can lead to a range of symptoms, including fever, arthritis, meningitis and a skin rash. This disease is transmitted via tick bites (from sheep and deer ticks), and is well recognized to occur in temperate climates.

Scabies

Scabies is an infestation by the scabies mite. Transmission occurs by close physical contact, and it is therefore more common in children and young adults. The infestation often begins in the hands or genital regions, from where the mite burrows into the skin. After a few weeks, sensitivity to its feces builds up, and this results in intense itch in the skin, which is characteristically worse at night. The rash of scabies consists of clusters of tiny red bumps (papules), particularly in the armpits, on the thighs and on the abdomen. Tiny tracks, which are the burrows of the mite, may be found on the fingers, in the web spaces, and on the wrists, palms, soles and genitalia (see Figure 6.1c-VIII).

Figure 6.1c-VIII Typical scabies rash around the web spaces between the fingers

Scabies is usually diagnosed from the clinical appearance, but can be confirmed by examination of the mites and eggs obtained by taking scrapings of a burrow.

The treatment of scabies involves painting the whole body of the patient (from the neck down) with a preparation of an insecticide such as benzyl benzoate, lindane or permethrin, and then repeating this treatment in two weeks. Close contacts and family members should be treated in the same way. All these chemicals are toxic, and should be used with caution. Itching will resolve two to three weeks after successful treatment.

Information box 6.1c-VI

Scabies: comments from a Chinese medicine perspective

In Chinese medicine, scabies could be interpreted as an Invasion of Wind Heat. It is more likely to occur in undernourished or chronically ill people, which suggests that an underlying Deficiency (of Wei Qi or Kidney Qi) is likely to be present in severe cases.

Head, pubic and body lice

There are three types of lice that use humans as their host. The head louse favors head hair, eyebrows and eyelashes, the pubic louse (crab louse) lives in the pubic regions, and the body louse lives on unwashed clothing. All three forms of human louse derive their nourishment from human blood, and cause itching when they bite through the skin.

The head louse is about 2–3mm long and is transmitted by close head contact with an infected person. Children are the most usual hosts in developed countries, although they can readily pass on their lice to adult family members. The female louse lays eggs that firmly adhere to the hair roots. These eggs are what are commonly called nits. These are diagnostic of an established infestation, and herald the emergence of increasing numbers of lice. Head louse infestation can be prevented by regular combing with a fine-toothed comb. Once eggs have been laid, twice-daily combing for at least two weeks is necessary to remove the lice as they emerge from the eggs.

The pubic louse is transmitted by sexual contact. It cannot colonize scalp hair, but can affect eyelashes, beards and armpits, as well as the genital region. As is the case for head lice, when the eggs are laid they adhere to the shafts of the body hair.

Both head and pubic lice can be treated by chemical means. The insecticides carbaryl, malathion and permethrin in a lotion or shampoo preparation may be prescribed. Two treatments are recommended. The second treatment should be given one week after the first in order to eliminate any lice newly hatched from the more resistant egg cases.

The body louse is only really seen in conditions of poverty or poor hygiene. It lays its eggs in clothing or bedding. Both the body lice and its eggs are killed readily by laundering.

Information box 6.1c-VII

Head lice: comments from a Chinese medicine perspective

In Chinese medicine, the itch and inflammation from louse infestation would be described as an Invasion of Wind Heat in the Channels. Internal Heat might also be a contributory factor in the severity of the reaction to the infestation.

FLEAS AND PAPULAR URTICARIA

In healthy populations the flea does not use the human as its host, but fleas resident on pets or birds can lay their eggs on furnishings and multiply within the home. Flea bites are characteristically found below the knee, an indication of how high the fleas can jump from floor level. In most people the bites are insignificant, and may result only in transient itch. Some individuals develop sensitivity to the flea proteins injected into the skin through biting, and so can become prone to developing firm, itchy, red papules at the site of flea bites. In some people, sensitivity can be of such a degree that the papule can enlarge to form a significant blister. A number of bites can lead to a rash-like appearance (usually on the lower legs), a condition termed papular urticaria.

The most appropriate treatment for papular urticaria is to de-flea the offending host and its surroundings.

Information box 6.1c-VIII

Papular urticaria: comments from a Chinese medicine perspective

In Chinese medicine, papular urticaria might be described as Wind Heat with an underlying Deficiency of Wei Qi or Kidney Qi. Internal Heat and Damp may also be a contributory factor in a severe case with fluid-filled vesicle or blister formation.

Acne

The term acne (a corruption of the Greek word meaning point) is used to describe the skin condition in which the formation of papules (firm, red spots) and pustules (papules that have come to a head with a point of yellow pus) is prominent. There are a number of variants of acne, but the most common by far is acne vulgaris, which is experienced in some form by up to 80 percent of adolescents in the UK. Acne rosacea is the term used to describe a flushing condition of the facial skin in which pustules can occur.

ACNE VULGARIS

Acne vulgaris is characterized by papules, pustules and blackheads (comedones), often on the background of greasy skin (see Figure 6.1c-IX). As the pustules involve some inflammation, scarring of the skin may occur as they resolve. In a severe case, multiple scarred pits are permanent reminders of adolescent acne. Acne vulgaris most commonly affects the most sebum-rich areas of skin, including the nasal region, the chin and the forehead. In severe cases, wider areas of the face, neck, shoulders and chest can be affected.

Figure 6.1c-IX Blackheads and pustules in acne vulgaris

Acne vulgaris most commonly first appears as the sebum of the skin alters its composition at the time of the pubescent surge in male sex hormones (androgens). A surge in the levels of androgens affects girls as well as boys, but is obviously more pronounced in boys. One theory is that excessive sebum leads to blockage of the sebaceous ducts, and the formation of blackheads, and also to the small bumpy papules known as whiteheads. This results in inflammation of the duct associated with a normal skin commensal, *Propionibacterium (P.) acnes*, overgrowing within the sebaceous gland. The blackhead then becomes a papule, and ultimately a pustule. In severe cases, deep cyst-like areas of inflamed tissue and pus can develop at the site of a blocked sebaceous duct. A recent study has demonstrated that whilst all people have a similar proportion of *P. acnes* on their skin compared to other bacteria, those patients with acne had less diversity of *P. acnes* strains within this population of the microbiome. It appears that in the patient with acne, a single and inflammatory strain has overgrown, possibly in response to the change in amount of sebum of the skin that occurs in puberty.[9]

Most conventional doctors would disagree with the commonly held view that factors such as diet, poor hygiene or sexual behavior play any role in the development of acne.

Acne vulgaris is a cause of intense emotional distress for many teenagers. Doctors are well aware of this, and a wide range of powerful treatments may be prescribed to alleviate the anguish that is a very common accompaniment to the development of spots in adolescence.

The first stage of treatment is with topical lotions containing benzoyl peroxide, an irritant, or retinoic acid, a derivative of vitamin A, both of which cause the core of the blackheads to break down. Benzoyl peroxide has antibacterial and anti-inflammatory activity. The retinoid drugs are both inflammatory and also known to act directly at the cells that produce sebum and hasten their early death, and so deal with a key factor in the development of acne, the overproduction of sebum.

These lotions need to be applied regularly for optimal effect. Topical antibiotic preparations may also be prescribed. In more resistant cases, oral antibiotics (tetracycline, oxytetracycline or erythromycin) may also be prescribed for a period of at least three months, and often longer. Some girls can respond positively to a particular preparation of the oral contraceptive pill that contains an anti-androgen called cyproterone acetate that influences the production of sebum. In very severe cases, an oral derivative of vitamin A called isotretinoin may be prescribed.

Isotretinoin carries a risk of causing quite marked dryness and inflammation of the skin, joint aches and liver toxicity, and carries a high risk of damage to an embryo in the event of pregnancy. For this reason, it is generally only prescribed under the supervision of a hospital clinic. A course of over four months of isotretinoin will often have a positive effect on symptoms and, in the majority of cases, can lead to a long-term improvement in the symptoms of acne.

Information box 6.1c-IX

Acne vulgaris: comments from a Chinese medicine perspective

In Chinese medicine, the symptoms of acne would normally be regarded as a manifestation of Damp Heat. The redness is an indication of Heat and the white pustule Damp. In severe cases the Damp transforms to Phlegm and leads to painful Blood Stagnation.

Flaws and Sionneau (2010)[10] suggest that the Heat is in part a result of the flaring upwards of the Fire of Ming Men as the adolescent passes through puberty. This aggravates any tendency there might be to the development of Heat in the Lungs, Liver and Stomach. Frustrated emotions causing Liver Fire, smoking causing Heat in the Lungs, and poor diet leading to Stomach Heat and Damp will all contribute to the symptoms. Heat in the Stomach and Lungs is likely to manifest in the facial region (via Stomach and Large Intestine Channels). Contrary to conventional wisdom, modification of diet would appear to be crucial in the treatment of acne according to Chinese medical wisdom.

The anti-acne treatments evidently serve to clear Heat and Damp. Side effects suggesting Heat and Depletion of Yin (skin irritation and dryness) are common with both topical and oral treatments. The serious potential side effects of isotretinoin suggest that Liver Disharmony and damage to the Blood can result from this long-term medication

ACNE ROSACEA (ROSACEA)

In contrast to acne vulgaris, acne rosacea is a condition that usually first appears in middle age, and is more common in women than men. The initial symptoms are that the skin of the cheeks, forehead and nose tends to flush, a feature that is more prominent after alcohol consumption or exposure to the sun. In long-standing cases, broken veins can appear and pustules can develop (see Figure 6.1c-X). The skin takes on a permanent flushed appearance. In men, overgrowth of the tissues around the sebaceous glands can lead to a coarseness and thickening of affected areas of skin, particularly the nose. In severe cases the nose can appear bulbous and malformed, a condition known as rhinophyma. Blackheads are not a feature of acne rosacea. Some patients report that they also suffer from migraine.

Treatment is by means of long-term oral antibiotics. Topical antibiotic or salicylic acid creams may also be prescribed.

Figure 6.1c-X Papules and pustules in acne rosacea

 Information Box 6.1a-I

Acne rosacea: comments from a Chinese medicine perspective

In Chinese medicine, the symptoms of rosacea could represent Stomach and/or Lung Heat and Damp, although the effect of Damp is less prominent than in acne vulgaris. The increased incidence of migraine in sufferers, together with the worsening with alcohol consumption, would suggest that Liver Stagnation/Yang Rising may also have a part to play in the aetiology. The development of rhinophyma is suggestive of Phlegm.

Eczema (dermatitis)

Eczema is a general term used by dermatologists to describe a skin reaction in the acute stages of which itching, redness, some swelling, damp oozing of the skin, and tiny fluid-filled areas (vesicles) may be seen. The itching can be so intense as to provoke scratching that leads to bleeding. In more chronic cases, dryness and thickening of the skin is more prominent. In a severe case of chronic eczema painful fissures may develop in the skin close to joints. Eczema is typically symmetrically distributed.

The prevalence of eczema seems to be increasing in both children and adults, and seems to develop most commonly in children under the age of five. It is estimated that 20 percent of children in the developed world suffer from some form of eczema.

Eczema is a term derived from the Greek word meaning to boil over. The term dermatitis, meaning inflammation of the skin, is used interchangeably with the word eczema. It is important to appreciate that the terms eczema and dermatitis both describe a reaction of the skin, and not a disease in its own right. There is actually a wide range of

factors that can trigger eczema including imbalances in the bacterial balance of the skin, skin irritants, dietary factors, inhaled allergens, emotional stress and environmental damp and cold. In some individuals there is a clear genetic disposition to eczema.

When eczema is associated with a general tendency to skin allergy it is described as atopic eczema (see below). This is the most common form of eczema to affect children.

TREATMENT OF ECZEMA

The treatment of eczema first involves identifying any triggers of the problem. These may be external irritants or allergens, or may be dietary in origin. The diagnosis of the triggers is described below according to the type of eczema. Once identified, the triggers should be avoided if at all possible. This may mean that the person has to make a significant change in lifestyle, such as leave a current job, get rid of a pet or follow an exclusion diet.

Emollient preparations

The first and most basic treatment of eczema is the use of emollient (moistening and softening) preparations. Skin that is already dry and cracked will be more vulnerable to irritation by external triggers, and so regular use of an emollient can help keep eczema at bay. Preparations that are commonly prescribed include aqueous cream and emulsifying ointment, both of which contain white soft paraffin. These provide a waxy layer on the skin surface and so prevent further drying. Some emollients may contain potential allergens such as lanolin (derived from wool) and peanut oil, and so the response to the emollient must be monitored carefully.

Zinc, icthammol and coal tar all have anti-scaling and anti-inflammatory properties, and may be combined with emollients in a case of chronic eczema.

Topical corticosteroids

If the eczema is severe, it is generally considered wise practice to apply a corticosteroid cream to the affected areas. Corticosteroid creams are produced in a range of potencies, of which hydrocortisone (0.5 and 1 percent) is the least potent, clobetasone butyrate is moderately potent, and betametasone valerate and clobetasol propionate are very potent.

It is well recognized by doctors that corticosteroids simply suppress symptoms, and that very often symptoms can recur rapidly after discontinuing use of the cream. It is also well known that long-term high doses can have adverse effects on the skin structure, the balance of the skin microbiome and general health. Corticosteroids can cause general thinning of the skin and subcutaneous tissues, and can precipitate a reddening of the skin (especially of the face) akin to acne rosacea. They should not be used alone in infective conditions and acne, because they can inhibit the local immune response to infection, and so worsen the condition (although combined corticosteroid and antibiotic/antifungal preparations may be prescribed if an infection has led to an eczematous-type response). It is also known that corticosteroids applied over the long term to large areas of skin will lead to the general side effects of systemic steroids, and may suppress growth in young children.

For these reasons, the decision to prescribe a corticosteroid cream should not be made lightly. The risk of potential side effects should always be balanced against the adverse effects of the eczema. Moderate- to high-potency creams should never be applied to the delicate skin of the face. Nevertheless, it is conventionally understood as good practice to apply a high-potency cream from the outset to a moderately severe case of eczema in order to get control of the symptoms, and then to rapidly reduce the dose once control has been gained. This is similar in principle to the guidance given to doctors about the management of an attack of acute asthma.

In very severe cases of eczema, emollients and corticosteroid creams may be held in place against the skin by means of overnight bandaging (wet wraps).

The calcineurin inhibitors tacrolimus and pimecrolimus are newer steroid-sparing drugs that may be introduced for the treatment of eczema in severe cases. They work by inhibiting the immune cells of the skin and are used in place of steroids. Side effects include rashes, and they also carry the risk of permitting bacterial and viral skin infections to take hold.

Antibiotics
Antibiotics may be used in a flare-up of atopic eczema because it is known that the skin bacterium *Staphylococcus aureus* can be implicated in eczema outbreaks.

Other treatments used for eczema
Antihistamine medications may be prescribed at night for sedation and inhibition of itch. Exposure to ultraviolet light can be helpful in some cases. Oil of evening primrose may inhibit eczema, although the clinical evidence for this is not strong.

THE DIFFERENT FORMS OF ECZEMA
Atopic eczema
Atopy describes an inherited tendency to be susceptible to allergic conditions such as asthma, eczema and seasonal rhinitis (hay fever). Atopic eczema is a very common condition of childhood, which often first presents in the first year of life. In most cases the eczema resolves before the onset of puberty, but it may persist into adult life.

In early childhood the eczema may be generalized over the body, but later on in childhood takes on a characteristic distribution in which it can be found on the neck, the flexural skin creases of the elbow and knees (antecubital and popliteal fossae), the wrists and the dorsum of the feet (see Figure 6.1c-XI). In many cases, environmental triggers (e.g. animal dandruff, grass pollen), dietary constituents (e.g. egg, cows' milk) and also emotional stimuli (especially anxiety and frustration) are well recognized to cause a rapid flare-up of symptoms.

Information box 6.1c-XI

Eczema: comments from a Chinese medicine perspective

In Chinese medicine, the redness, vesicles and oozing of eczema correspond to Wind Damp Heat. The root of this is commonly internally generated Damp Heat, and the Wind may be external or internal in origin. Itch may be a result of Wind or Stagnation of Qi (due to Heat, Phlegm Damp under the skin, or suppressed emotions). Underlying Wei Qi (and/or Jing) Deficiency will predispose the patient to Wind Invasion.

The thickened and dry skin in chronic eczema is an indication of underlying Blood Deficiency, as Blood nourishes the skin. Blood Deficiency can predispose to the accumulation of Wind Damp Heat on the surface of the body.

Dry flaky skin in atopic eczema in children may be a manifestation of Phlegm (and Accumulation Syndrome).

Most of the medical approaches to eczema are suppressive in nature, in that they target the symptoms rather than the root cause of Deficiency of the Wei Qi, Kidneys and/or Blood. One exception might be oil of evening primrose, which may act by nourishing the skin, and so might be interpreted to work by strengthening one of the root deficiencies. This plant, which originates from South America, is also a herb recognized in Chinese medicine.

Figure 6.1c-XI Cracked and thickened skin in atopic eczema

Secondary infection of the eczema is a common complication. Impetigo is more likely to occur in a child with eczema. Children with eczema are also more likely to suffer from viral warts and molluscum contagiosum.

Eczema herpeticum is a very serious manifestation of herpes simplex virus (HSV) infection that can spread rapidly across the skin of a child with severe generalized eczema.

The life of a child with generalized atopic eczema can be severely disrupted by chronic itch, disturbed sleep, associated conditions such as asthma, and also the stigma that comes with a disfiguring skin condition. It is recognized that severe eczema can inhibit the growth and general well-being of the child. In a severe case, the routine of the whole family will be adversely affected by having repeatedly to apply topical treatments, avoid environmental triggers and the experience of broken nights' sleep.

For these reasons, the symptoms of eczema in children are often treated aggressively, meaning that strong treatments are used from the outset. Emollients should always be used, but potent steroid creams may also be prescribed to inhibit symptoms, although the duration of the course is limited to the absolute minimum possible. Medicated bandages (wet wraps) containing zinc, icthammol or coal tar can be applied to areas of severe eczema on the limbs. Sedative antihistamine tablets may enable uninterrupted sleep in some children.

 Information box 6.1c-XII

Atopic eczema: comments from a Chinese medicine perspective

From a Chinese medicine viewpoint, atopic eczema in children has been described as a result of Accumulation of Phlegm and Damp under the skin, Heat obstructing the flow of Blood to the skin, Qi and Blood Deficiency, Accumulation Disorder and Lingering Pathogenic Factor. Damp, Phlegm, Heat and unbalanced emotions can all lead to Stagnation of Qi under the skin and so to intense itch.

Atopic eczema very often first appears at the time when the child is introduced to formula milk or solid foods, which is a time when the Spleen is being overtaxed and when Damp and Phlegm can accumulate. It may also erupt after an infectious disease or immunization, suggesting in these cases that Lingering Pathogenic Factor is a cause.

Dietary advice is crucial in the management of eczema. This might involve the elimination of Phlegm-forming foods in all cases (e.g. cows' milk, peanut butter, oranges, bananas), and a careful consideration of possible food allergies.

Primary irritant eczema (dermatitis)

In contrast to atopic eczema, primary irritant and allergic contact dermatitis result from direct contact with environmental triggers. The terms primary irritant and allergic contact describe whether or not the resulting reaction is mediated by an allergic response to the contact. However, a patient who suffers from atopic eczema can be more prone to both these forms of exogenous eczema, so in clinical practice it can be challenging to be specific about the cause of a case of eczema.

Primary irritants physically damage the skin. Irritants that are well recognized to cause eczema include acids, detergents and petroleum products, and also exposure to extremes of cold and wind. The hands are a very common site for this form of eczema. Primary irritant eczema can become a significant problem in many occupations in which the person is continually exposed to an irritant. For example, a hairdresser might develop primary irritant eczema as a result of repeated hair washing with detergent-containing shampoos and conditioners.

In most cases the offending trigger is clear. The main treatment for primary irritant eczema is to avoid the trigger. The use of barrier creams and gloves may be sufficient to protect from primary irritant eczema, but in severe cases, the patient may be forced to change occupation.

Allergic contact eczema

Allergic contact eczema is a delayed immune reaction to exposure to an environmental allergen. The range of potential allergens is very wide. The allergens that are most commonly implicated in allergic contact eczema include nickel (in cheap jewelry, watches, studs in clothing and metal clips on bra straps), colophony (a component of sticking plasters), rubber (in gloves and shoes), chromate (in cement), hair dye, topical medications and plants (particularly the primula family in the UK).

Allergic contact eczema is diagnosed primarily on the basis of the history and distribution of the rash, although often, because of the delay in the development of the rash, the cause may not be clear (see Figure 6.1c-XII). Patch testing using a standard battery of the most usual allergens will expose which are the primary triggers for the eczema. If the eczema is severe, it may be treated first with potent steroids, as the test can in itself trigger a generalized attack of eczema.

Figure 6.1c-XII Dry inflamed eczematous skin resulting from contact with perfume

This form of eczema is treated by means of avoidance of the triggers and, if severe, with emollients and steroid creams.

Discoid eczema (nummular eczema)

Discoid eczema is a condition in which scattered circular patches of eczema develop on the trunk and limbs. The cause is unknown, but it can erupt after an episode of stress, shock or serious illness. There is also an association with alcoholism.

There is an association with increased colonization with the skin microbe *Staphylococcus aureus*.

Discoid eczema is usually treated with potent steroid creams and can resolve spontaneously after months to years.

Varicose eczema

This term applies to areas of eczema in the skin overlying varicose veins and areas in which the circulation is poor. It usually affects the sides of the legs in elderly people. It is probably the result of chronic accumulation of toxins in the regions where the blood flow away from the tissues is less than efficient. Interestingly, secondary spread of the eczema to the forearms is well recognized in varicose eczema.

Asteatotic eczema (eczema craquelé)

Asteatotic eczema is a form of eczema seen in old age. It develops when the oil content of the skin decreases and the surface layer of the epidermis becomes more dehydrated. It will be exacerbated in dry climates and with the excessive use of detergents on the skin.

When this state is advanced, the skin can develop an appearance like shiny "crazy paving." Itching usually begins on the legs, but may also affect the trunk and arms. Emollients are usually the mainstay of treatment. In severe cases topical steroids may be prescribed.

Seborrheic eczema (dermatitis)

Seborrheic dermatitis is usually classified as a form of eczema, although it is currently theorized that the cause may be an allergic response to and overgrowth of yeast (*Malassezia furfur*) that is a normal inhabitant of the skin. The condition presents usually in young men, with patches of itchy diffuse redness and scaling of the skin in the region of the scalp, forehead, eyebrows, nasolabial folds and beard area (see Figure 6.1c-XIII). Patches can also develop on the chest and upper back.

In infancy, seborrheic dermatitis is very common, and patches mostly appear on the scalp, although the neck and trunk can also be affected. If severe, a waxy layer can develop over the whole scalp, a condition termed cradle cap. However, the child remains symptom-free, and the parents should be reassured that this condition will resolve

as the child grows older. In old age, seborrheic eczema can progress to affect widespread areas of the body.

Current treatments for seborrheic eczema in adults involve the use of emollients, mild steroid creams and tar shampoos. Antifungal creams and shampoos may also be of help. In infancy, the patches can be treated by washing off the scales with baby shampoo, and then moisturizing with olive oil.

The development of seborrheic dermatitis is a common complication of acquired immune deficiency syndrome (AIDS), which is evidence that the cause is related to the immune system. It is also more common in patients with Parkinson's disease, and this is thought to be a result of increased sebum production in this condition.

Figure 6.1c-XIII Seborrheic eczema affecting the cheeks and nasolabial folds

 Information box 6.1c-XIII

Seborrheic eczema: comments from a Chinese medicine perspective

The Chinese medicine interpretation of seborrheic eczema would be similar to that of eczema, with Heat and Phlegm/Damp as a prominent aspect of the diagnosis. Itch is a less prominent aspect of the condition, and so Wind might be a less significant pathogenic factor in this condition compared to eczema.

Psoriasis

Psoriasis is an inflammatory condition of the skin that affects about 1.5 percent of the Western population. For most people affected, the most significant symptom of psoriasis is distress because of its cosmetic appearance, although excessive skin scaling and itch can also become severe problems. As psoriasis is a condition which, once it has appeared, often remains in some form for the whole of the patient's life, it is a significant cause of disease in the population.

The microscopic examination of psoriasis indicates that the epidermal layer of the skin undergoes marked thickening, and inflammatory cells accumulate in the affected areas. These cellular changes manifest in patches of skin that are thickened and have an underlying redness, but which are covered in a layer of silvery scales that flake off very readily.

Psoriasis is classified according to the pattern in which these patches appear. Plaque psoriasis is the most common form, in which large rounded areas of affected skin develop, primarily on the extensor surfaces of the limbs, the trunk and the scalp. In scalp psoriasis the affected skin is confined to the scalp. Guttate psoriasis frequently develops after a respiratory infection. In this form of psoriasis, there are numerous tiny patches on the affected areas of skin that first appear as a bodily rash. All forms of psoriasis have a tendency to develop at the sites of trauma or scarring.

A form of generalized inflammatory arthritis develops in up to 8 percent of cases of psoriasis. The most common presentation is of pain and deformity in the distal interphalangeal joints. In severe cases this arthritis is aggressively deforming, and can affect the large joints and also the sacroiliac joints. In many ways, psoriatic arthritis is akin to rheumatoid arthritis.

Like eczema, psoriasis is usually treated by application of creams and pastes. Emollient creams containing white soft paraffin may be sufficient to control scaling in mild cases. Preparations containing salicylic acid and/or tar can also reduce scaling.

Corticosteroid creams will suppress the formation of plaques, but are not recommended by all dermatologists because of the risks of long-term use, and also because in some cases they can trigger a change of plaque psoriasis into a more unstable scaling condition called brittle psoriasis.

Calcipotriol is a drug derived from vitamin D that can be effective when applied regularly to the plaques, and is generally free of side effects.

Dithranol is a potent suppressor of the plaques of psoriasis, although the mechanism of this action is unknown. It is applied in paste form to plaques on a daily basis, and can completely clear the skin within three weeks. However, it can burn the skin and cause staining of both the skin and clothing.

Ultraviolet B (UVB) light therapy can be very effective in reducing the formation of plaques. The patient is exposed two to three times a week to a dose that is sufficient to cause mild redness, but not full sunburn. Although there is a theoretical concern about the risk of skin cancer, in reality very few patients with psoriasis develop this complication from UVB therapy.

In severe cases of psoriasis the patient may be prescribed oral medication. Psoralens are drugs that cause inhibition of plaques on the skin when it is exposed to ultraviolet A (UVA) light. The treatment, known as PUVA, therefore involves oral psoralen medication together with regular exposure to UVA. Unlike exposure to UVB alone, PUVA carries a significant risk of inducing cancerous skin changes.

Other oral drugs prescribed in very severe cases include cytotoxic medications, retinoids (similar in structure to isotretinoin, which is used in acne), systemic corticosteroids and the immunosuppressants such as methotrexate, leflunomide and ciclosporin. All these drugs have a wide range of potentially toxic side effects, and so are prescribed as part of specialist management.

PLAQUE PSORIASIS

Plaque psoriasis is characterized by large, rounded areas of thickened skin that are symmetrically distributed on the extensor surfaces of the body, the scalp, the trunk and back. Elbows and knees are very commonly affected (see Figure 6.1c-XIV). The most effective first-line treatment for the majority of people is calcipotriol cream.

PUVA and the other potent oral treatments are reserved for cases when the plaques are extensive, or when there is significant emotional distress resulting from the cosmetic appearance.

Figure 6.1c-XIV Plaque psoriasis affecting the knees

SCALP PSORIASIS

In scalp psoriasis, the thickening and scaling is confined to the hairy portion of the scalp and its borders. In severe cases there may be temporary hair loss.

Tar shampoos can work well in keeping scalp psoriasis at bay. Tar gels and corticosteroid lotions are also used if thick plaques develop.

GUTTATE PSORIASIS

Guttate psoriasis involves the rapid development of a number of tiny plaques (about 1cm in diameter) scattered symmetrically over the body. The rash often appears in young people as a response to a streptococcal infection. These slightly itchy plaques can resolve very rapidly, but a few may persist and enlarge to develop into chronic plaque psoriasis.

Guttate psoriasis may respond well to a combination of a tar-based ointment and UVB therapy.

Information box 6.1c-XIV

Psoriasis: comments from a Chinese medicine perspective

In Chinese medicine, it would appear that Phlegm and Heat are important Pathogenic Factors in the development of psoriasis. Heat leads to Blood Dryness or Blood Heat. The thickened plaques and scaling and redness are evidence of Phlegm and Heat, respectively. Local Qi Deficiency and Qi Stagnation may play a role in the etiology, particularly in view of the fact that psoriasis can develop at the sites of trauma or scarring. The deforming arthritis is also suggestive of Damp/Phlegm and Heat with Qi/Blood Stagnation.

Heat can originate from the damaging effect of Pathogenic Wind Heat or Wind Cold, and its persistence will be predisposed to by longstanding Kidney or Liver Yin Deficiency. Emotional frustration can also lead to internally generated Heat as a result of its effect on the Liver.

The common location for psoriatic arthropathy at the distal interphalangeal joints is also suggestive of Accumulation of Heat, as these joints are close to the location for the Jing-Well (Heat clearing) points on the channels of the limbs.

Nails are also commonly involved, and can develop widespread pitting. These nail changes are almost always present if arthritis has developed. Nail involvement suggests Liver Disharmony.

Heating foods and alcohol and smoking should be avoided.

The conventional treatments for psoriasis appear to Moisten Dryness, Clear Heat or Clear Phlegm. They are all suppressive in nature.

Erythroderma

Erythroderma (exfoliative dermatitis) describes a generalized condition of the skin in which the whole skin surface is inflamed, and so the whole body surface appears red, hot and scaly. It results most commonly either from an extreme allergic reaction to a medication, or from severe extensive eczema or psoriasis. Rarely, it can be a manifestation of lymphoma of the skin.

Erythroderma is a medical emergency, because when the skin is inflamed in all parts, it loses its heat- and water-retaining properties. In addition, the metabolic rate rises and the body rapidly consumes its stores of energy. The patient becomes vulnerable to dehydration, heart and kidney failure, and hypothermia.

A person with erythroderma will require intensive nursing and fluid replacement. The underlying cause has to be treated with systemic drugs (corticosteroids in the case of eczema, and anti-psoriatic drugs in the case of psoriasis).

Information box 6.1c-XV

Erythroderma: comments from a Chinese medicine perspective

Erythroderma is a condition of Heat leading to collapse of Yin.

Part II: Moles and tumors, connective tissue disorders and other common skin conditions

Moles and other nevi

Mole is a commonly used term that describes a discrete area of the skin in which there is a concentration of altered but benign growth of the skin cells. In many moles there is an excess of melanin-producing cells, and in some there is thickening from excessive fibrous tissue in the dermis. The term nevus literally means birthmark, but is used more broadly in dermatology to embrace moles and other localized benign changes in the skin, as well as birthmarks.

FRECKLES AND MELANOCYTIC NEVI (COMMON MOLES)

A freckle consists of a benign cluster of epidermal skin cells that contain a higher concentration of the pigment melanin than in surrounding cells. It is believed that these cells in freckled skin are over-responsive to ultraviolet radiation, and so freckles become more apparent after sun exposure. The structure of the skin within a freckle is otherwise normal. In the area of the freckle the skin retains its usual texture and smooth surface. Freckles are common in people who have pale skin, and particularly in those of Celtic origin. The most common sites for freckles are the face, upper body and arms.

A mole (melanocytic nevus) is different to a freckle in that it consists of a cluster of melanin-producing cells, either in the deeper layer of the skin (the dermis) or at the junction between the dermis and the epidermis. The life history of most moles is that they originate at the dermo-epidermal junction and then migrate downwards in the dermis. They tend to emerge as deeply pigmented circular spots, after which they then can grow in size, sometimes significantly. Growth can cause the mole to be palpable as a smooth bump in the skin. Then, in later life (after 40 years of age) moles gradually lose the depth of the pigmentation as they mature and migrate downwards. This explains why elderly people have relatively few visible moles of this type.

The clinical significance of moles is that, very rarely, malignant change can occur in the melanin-producing cells, and so lead to the development of a malignant melanoma (see below). Rapid growth of a mole is not usually an indication of malignant change, as long as the growth is regular (i.e. maintaining a circular or ovoid contour). In some cases deep moles can take on a slightly bluish appearance. In other cases an immune response to the mole can cause a halo of pale skin to develop around the mole, which may then become red and then disappear. Both these developments in moles are benign in nature.

A congenital mole is found in about 1 percent of newborns. In some cases a large area of skin is affected, over which there may also be increased body hair growth. Congenital moles are clinically significant because the risk of malignant change, particularly in giant hairy congenital moles, is higher than for acquired moles. For this reason, parents might be advised that a large congenital mole is removed surgically.

Stork marks and blue spots in newborns

A stork mark is a flat area of pink skin commonly seen in newborns. One of the most common sites for these regions of dilated capillaries is at the nape of the neck, hence the name. Usually the pinkness of these patches fades over time, and so they are rarely a cosmetic problem for the child.

A Mongolian blue spot is another common benign finding in newborns, and in this case is usually located at the base of the spine. The blue spot is a diffuse blue-black patch resulting from an excess of melanin-producing cells in that area of skin. The appearance of the patch may be confused with that of bruising.

Strawberry nevi

A strawberry nevus becomes apparent very shortly after birth, and may enlarge rapidly over the first few months of life (see Figure 6.1c-XV). The principal underlying abnormality is a cluster of enlarged capillaries in the area, which means that the nevus can bleed profusely if damaged. The nevus is often a deep red in color and has a raised spherical or ovoid border. It is usually perceived as very unsightly, and so the parents have to be reassured that very often the lump becomes paler and less prominent over the first few years of childhood. In about half of cases there is total resolution of a strawberry nevus by the age of five. Only if the nevus is close to the eye, or if it is persistent beyond the age of ten, is surgical removal advised.

 Information box 6.1c-XVI

Moles and nevi: comments from a Chinese medicine perspective

From a Chinese medicine perspective, the fact that a nevus of one form or another has developed may reflect a degree of deficiency in that particular region of the body, as most nevi reflect abnormal development of the skin and subcutaneous tissues. This means that the precise location of nevus may hint at a specific energetic imbalance. For example, a large mole on the anterolateral border of the shin might suggest an Imbalance or Deficiency in Stomach Qi.

Moles are understood to be a manifestation of Stagnation of Qi in the Channels and, according to Maciocia (2004),[11] may represent Liver Blood Heat, Damp Heat or Blood Stasis. The color of the mole (from pale brown or red to dark black) is important in the differentiation.

Multiple nevi scattered over diverse regions of the skin might indicate an underlying imbalance of Lung and/or Jing, as the Lungs dominate the skin and Jing is the foundation of the healthy development of tissues. The tendency to develop multiple nevi is commonly inherited.

Figure 6.1c-XV A strawberry nevus in an infant

 Information box 6.1c-XVII

Strawberry nevi: comments from a Chinese medicine perspective

A Chinese medicine interpretation of a strawberry nevus might be that there is an underlying Deficiency of Jing, together with Heat in the Organ associated with the site of the nevus.

Port-wine stains

A port-wine stain is a flat region of deep violet coloration of the skin resulting from dilated capillaries deep in the dermis. The surface of the port-wine stain can be bumpy because of irregularities in the pattern of the enlarged capillaries. Although the nature of the underlying problem is similar to that of the stork mark, port-wine stains are much more of a cosmetic problem, and also do not tend to fade with time.

Rarely, a port-wine stain may be associated with vascular abnormalities in the brain, and in these cases a mental health disorder, fits and paralysis may become apparent.

Port-wine stains can now be treated cosmetically by means of laser therapy to the skin. Prior to the development of this expensive technique, the only treatment was the use of camouflaging cosmetic creams.

Information box 6.1c-XVIII

Port-wine stains: comments from a Chinese medicine perspective

The Chinese medicine interpretation of a port-wine stain might be similar to that as described for strawberry nevus. The deeper color might suggest that Blood Stagnation as well as Heat is more prominent in the diagnosis.

CAMPBELL DE MORGAN RED SPOTS
Campbell de Morgan red spots are the cherry-red, mole-like spots that are very commonly found on the limbs and body of adults, particularly after the age of 40. These are benign, and are the result of a cluster of abnormal blood vessels in the dermis or subcutaneous tissues, known as an angioma.

SPIDER NEVI
A spider nevus is more correctly termed a telangiectasia. A telangiectasia is a cluster of thread-like vessels that appear to radiate from a central vessel in the skin, akin to legs from a spider's body. The usual spider nevus (which is not really a nevus at all) is less than 5mm in diameter, although they can reach sizes of up to 1cm.

Spider nevi are of clinical significance, as they can be associated with an underlying medical condition, particularly if more than five are found. The most common underlying problem is chronic liver disease, in which the spiders commonly form on the face, neck, upper limbs and upper body.

Skin tumors – benign lumps
A nevus has been defined as a mole, birthmark or other benign minor skin change. All the other benign conditions that present as lumps in the skin can be categorized as skin tumors. The various forms of benign skin tumors are described below.

SEBORRHEIC WARTS (KERATOSES)
A seborrheic wart is an almost universal finding on the body of an elderly person. In some cases there can be over 100 of these brown, patch-like areas of skin, scattered particularly over the back, abdomen and chest (see Figure 6.1c-XVI). The usual size of a seborrheic wart is 0.5–3cm in diameter. The color varies from pale to deeply pigmented, and the surface has a slightly greasy and warty texture.

Figure 6.1c-XVI Seborrheic warts on the skin of the back

Seborrheic warts appear to be the result of a benign overgrowth of the deep cells of the epidermis. In some cases, friction (e.g. from a bra strap) seems to stimulate their development.

The main clinical problem with seborrheic warts is that they can be perceived as unsightly, and in some cases they may be confused with malignant growths. They can be removed by surgery, cautery or cryotherapy.

Information box 6.1c-XIX

Seborrheic warts: comments from a Chinese medicine perspective

From a Chinese medicine perspective, the thickened, waxy appearance of seborrheic warts suggests that Phlegm Damp may be an underlying Pathogenic Factor.

SKIN TAGS
Skin tags are tiny fleshy outgrowths of the skin that commonly appear to be on a stalk. They form around the neck, inner arms and armpits, particularly in obese and elderly people. Skin tags are entirely benign and can be easily removed by means of cautery.

Information box 6.1c-XX

Skin tags: comments from a Chinese medicine perspective

In Chinese medicine, the structure of skin tags would suggest that they are manifestations of Phlegm.

DERMATOFIBROMATA

A dermatofibroma appears as a painless, lentil-sized lump in the dermis, with a slightly pigmented appearance. Dermatofibromata are usually found on the legs, and may result from minor trauma such as an insect bite. They consist of fibrous tissue and blood vessels.

Dermatofibromata cause concern because they may be confused with a melanoma. For this reason doctors may be very ready to excise them, although this procedure is unnecessary in most cases.

Information box 6.1c-XXI

Dermatofibromata: comments from a Chinese medicine perspective

A dermatofibroma may well be a manifestation of Phlegm.

EPIDERMAL CYSTS (SEBACEOUS CYSTS), LIPOMAS AND MILIA

Epidermal cysts and lipomas can both present as large, smooth lumps under the skin. They can cause considerable concern to the patient when they are first discovered, but both are benign in nature.

Epidermal cysts (which include sebaceous cysts) contain a broken-down form of keratin that is cheesy in consistency. They are attached to the overlying skin and so move with it when palpated. They usually feel smooth, and the larger ones have a rubbery texture. They are common on the scalp, neck and trunk.

A lipoma is an overgrowth of adipose (fat) tissue and is found in the dermis and subcutaneous layers. It is readily distinguished from an epidermal cyst because it is not usually attached to the overlying skin (it moves freely over the underlying muscle) and because it has a very soft consistency.

Milia are tiny, millet-seed-sized keratin cysts that most commonly appear around the eyelids. They are no cause for concern.

Information box 6.1c-XXII

Epidermal cysts and lipomas: comments from a Chinese medicine perspective

Both epidermal cysts and lipomas suggest the presence of Phlegm Damp.

KELOID SCARS

The pathology and energetic interpretation of keloid scars are described in Section 2.1b (see also Figure 6.1c-XVII).

Figure 6.1c-XVII A keloid scar resulting from ear piercing

Skin tumors – malignant skin tumors

Although the term malignant describes the disordered pattern of growth that is characteristic of cancer, many malignant skin tumors are slow growing. For this reason, the majority of malignant skin tumors are readily treatable if diagnosed at an early stage in their development.

Information box 6.1c-XXIII

Skin cancer: comments from a Chinese medicine perspective

In Chinese medicine, the development of skin cancer suggests a marked underlying Deficiency of Vital Substances (in particular, Lung Qi and Jing) and the Accumulation of Phlegm (and/or Blood Stagnation). Exposure to sun and other environmental toxins is common in the history of skin cancer. It would make sense that sun exposure, as it involves burning, is likely to contribute to local Yin and Blood Deficiency, so participating in creating the background deficiency recognized in the pathology of cancer. Heat may also be important in the etiology of sun-related skin cancers.

SOLAR KERATOSES

Solar keratoses are reddened, scaly patches of skin that occur in chronically sun-exposed areas such as the scalp, bridge of the nose and forearms (see Figure 6.1c-XVIII). They consist of regions of the skin in which there is chaotic growth of epithelial tissues. Their size can wax and wane over time, and they may even regress fully. However, they can progress to a more established form of skin cancer, and so may be removed by cryotherapy or treated by means of a cream containing 5-fluorouracil (a chemotherapeutic agent) if they seem to be persistent or are growing relentlessly.

Figure 6.1c-XVIII Solar keratoses on the sun-exposed forehead

BASAL CELL CARCINOMA (BCC) (RODENT ULCER)

The basal cell carcinoma (BCC), or rodent ulcer, is a slow-growing tumor that tends to develop in sun-exposed regions of the skin (e.g. scalp, nose, behind the ear) in elderly people (see Figure 6.1c-XIX). It usually first appears as a smooth, raised nodule that then grows outwards with rolled edges, leaving a slight central depression. If the growth is unchecked, the central area can ulcerate (i.e. lose its epithelial surface layer). Fine, thread-like vessels can be seen on the edges and surface of the tumor, and these cause it to bleed readily with minor trauma. Although growth is slow, the BCC can extend downwards into bony tissue, at which stage it is much more difficult to halt its destructive growth pattern.

Figure 6.1c-XIX A basal cell carcinoma on the cheek

Small tumors are treated with cryotherapy or topical cytotoxic creams, and large tumors with excision and/or radiotherapy.

SQUAMOUS CELL CARCINOMA (SCC) AND BOWEN'S DISEASE

A squamous cell carcinoma (SCC) is another epidermal skin cancer that has a predilection for sun-exposed areas. The least invasive form of this cancer, known as Bowen's disease, involves a spreading of cancerous cells in the epidermis. This leads to a flat, red, scaly patch with an irregular border, and is a fairly common finding in elderly people.

Treatment for Bowen's disease is given to prevent progression, although this eventuality is fairly rare. Treatment involves topical cytotoxic creams or local cryotherapy to small areas, and radiotherapy if the skin changes are extensive.

Invasive SCC can take on a range of appearances, from an irregular, scaly lump (akin to a large solar keratosis), a fleshy tumor, or a non-healing ulcer (see Figure 6.1c-XX). Physical trauma or chemical trauma, such as a burn or repeated exposure of the lips to cigarettes, can promote the development of an invasive SCC.

Figure 6.1c-XX A squamous cell carcinoma on the earlobe

Treatment of SCC is by means of surgical removal or radiotherapy.

PAGET'S DISEASE OF THE NIPPLE

This is a specific variant of Bowen's disease, which develops in the region of one nipple. It should be treated as a high priority, as Paget's disease often reflects the presence of an underlying breast tumor.

MALIGNANT MELANOMA

The malignant melanoma is the most dangerous of the malignant skin tumors and, in contrast to the BCC and SCC, tends to affect a younger population. The incidence of malignant melanomas is rising rapidly, and this is believed to be attributable in part to increased sun exposure in sun-seeking Westerners on holiday, and also to a general increase in the levels of solar radiation reaching the Earth because of changes in the composition of gases in the atmosphere. A history of sunburn of the skin is of particular relevance in the development of melanoma, and it is known that the cumulative effects of episodes of sunburn in childhood are particularly dangerous.

The malignant melanoma has a range of appearances, of which the superficial, spreading form carries the best prognosis. In this form, the tumor appears as a fairly flat, brown-black patch with irregular areas of depth of pigmentation and also irregular borders. In contrast with the BCC and SCC, common locations are the upper leg and trunk. Unlike a melanocytic nevus, the surface of the malignant melanoma is unstable, and so it may itch or bleed easily. These are all warning features of its potential invasiveness. The rarer and rapidly growing nodular melanoma tends to have a more full growth both outwards and also inwards to deeper tissues.

In both forms of melanoma the prognosis depends on the depth to which the tumor has penetrated. Good prognosis (over 90 percent cure rate) is associated with a depth of less than 1.5mm. However, if the tumor has extended to a depth of over 3.5mm, the cure rate drops to below 40 percent. This is because the malignant melanoma very readily metastasizes, and the chances of this are increased as the tumor grows deeper into the dermis.

The most effective method of preventing deaths from malignant melanoma (after minimization of sun exposure) is public education. Ideally, suspicious-looking moles are brought to medical attention as soon as possible. Suspect tumors should be removed immediately and sent for pathological analysis. The cure rate for removing a small and non-invasive melanoma is very high.

In the case of a large malignant melanoma, surgery is still the preferred treatment, and a wide excision may be advised. To date, radiotherapy and chemotherapy seem to have very little effect in malignant melanoma that has metastasized.

KAPOSI'S SARCOMA

Kaposi's sarcoma is a once rare tumor of blood vessels that has been more widely reported in recent decades as it appears in an aggressive form in people with AIDS and other forms of immunosuppression. Kaposi's sarcoma presents as a number of purplish plaques and nodules in the skin. It is treated by means of radiotherapy.

 Information box 6.1c-XXIV

Malignant melanoma: comments from a Chinese medicine perspective

From a Chinese medicine perspective, the development of a malignant melanoma, as with all skin tumors, suggests chronic Depletion of Vital Substances, in particular, Lung Qi and Jing. The dark black color might indicate that Blood Stagnation as well as Phlegm is important in the diagnosis.

Maciocia (2004) subdivides the patterns that might underlie melanoma into the categories of Blood Heat and Blood Stasis. He explains that "the darker their color, the more Blood Stasis there is. The differentiation is also made on the basis of the nature of the skin lesion. Macules always indicate Blood Heat with Blood Stasis, plaques indicate Blood Heat with Damp Heat and nodules indicate Blood Stasis."[12]

LYMPHOMA AND THE SKIN

Lymphoma rarely can either spread to the skin, or may originate in the skin. It leads to red, scaly irregular patches, which may be confused with psoriasis or eczema. It is also the rarest cause of erythroderma. Treatment includes radiotherapy, chemotherapy and PUVA (see under "Psoriasis" above).

Connective tissue disorders

Connective tissue disorders are a form of multisystem (or rheumatic) autoimmune disease, where diverse tissues are affected by an autoimmune disease process (see also Section 2.2c). Connective tissue diseases are so called because the autoimmune damage is focused on various types of connective tissue. For this reason the skin is very often involved.

SYSTEMIC LUPUS ERYTHEMATOSUS (SLE) AND DISCOID LUPUS ERYTHEMATOSUS (DLE)

Systemic lupus erythematosus (SLE) is a multisystem connective disuse disorder that can cause arteritis, glomerulonephritis and arthritis. Psychiatric disorders are also common in SLE as a result of arteritis of the vessels in the brain. SLE typically affects women of childbearing age. It usually progresses in a series of relapses separated by remissions. In most cases the outlook is good, but in severe cases, SLE can be fatal. The most common cause of death in SLE is glomerulonephritis and consequent kidney failure. Discoid lupus erythematosus (DLE) is a variant of SLE in which the skin only is affected.

A butterfly-shaped rash affecting the cheeks and bridge of the nose is common in SLE (see Figure 6.1c-XXI). Sunlight provokes the development of this butterfly rash. Additional skin problems result from arteritis in the vessels of the dermis, and can manifest as itching and purpura (tiny areas of bruising).

Figure 6.1c-XXI The butterfly facial rash in systemic lupus erythematosus

In DLE the skin changes are slightly different. Light-exposed areas are affected principally, most usually presenting with a reddened, scaly appearance. In severe cases, large areas of the skin can become disfigured by scarring. The scalp can be affected, leading to areas of permanent hair loss (see Figure 6.1c-XXII).

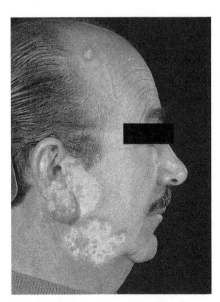

Figure 6.1c-XXII The scarring rash of chronic discoid lupus erythematosus

SLE is confirmed by means of assays of the serum for autoantibodies. DLE is diagnosed by means of skin biopsy.

Mild SLE can be treated with non-steroidal anti-inflammatory drugs (NSAIDs) or disease-modifying antirheumatic drugs (DMARDs). Severe relapses may require steroid injections and immunosuppressant medication. DLE is treated with corticosteroid creams and sunscreens.

 Information box 6.1c-XXV

Systemic lupus erythematosus: comments from a Chinese medicine perspective

In Chinese medicine, the features of SLE, in common with all multisystem autoimmune diseases, suggest that Heat and Phlegm might account for the most florid symptoms of rash, arthritis and psychosis. The underlying problem is autoimmune, indicating that a profound Deficiency in Kidney Qi and Essence is the basis of the accumulation of Heat and Phlegm. Flaws and Sionneau (2010)[13] explain that in susceptible individuals, the external invasion of Heat Toxins (e.g. exposure to sunlight) or internal engenderment of Heat Toxins (diet and emotional frustration) contribute to the development of SLE via scorching and burning the Yin and the Blood. Joint pain is due to Wind Damp Heat.

DERMATOMYOSITIS

Dermatomyositis is an autoimmune condition of the skin and muscles that can occur in both childhood and adult life in slightly different forms. In the adult form of the disease there may be an association with an underlying cancer.

The skin is affected by a purple-red rash affecting the face, neck and hands, together with puffiness of the skin around the eyes. There can be profound muscle weakness in some cases, typically of the thighs and upper arm muscles.

The treatment involves exclusion of cancer and treatment of this if it is found to be present. Oral corticosteroids and immunosuppressants are used to control the inflammatory symptoms.

Information box 6.1c-XXVI

Dermatomyositis: comments from a Chinese medicine perspective

From a Chinese medicine perspective, the violaceous rash in dermatomyositis might suggest that Stagnation of Qi is an additional Pathogenic Factor to Heat. The weakened muscles also are suggestive of an imbalance of Liver Qi. All these have occurred against a background of Deficiency of Kidney Qi and Essence. Flaws and Sionneau explain that the trigger for dermatomyositis might be the invasion of Wind Cold or Damp into the Lung and Spleen where the Qi is depressed and manifests as Heat in the skin and muscles, and can also, in the long term, damage the Qi and Blood.[14]

SCLERODERMA AND MORPHEA

Scleroderma literally means thickening of the skin, and is used to refer to a process of uncertain cause in which there is progressive formation of fibrous tissue in the skin. If scleroderma develops without any other medical features, it is called morphea. In systemic sclerosis, scleroderma occurs as part of a multisystem disorder.

In morphea, rounded areas or strips of skin undergo a process of thickening, which begins with the appearance of patches of a purplish hue. These then become white, shiny and inelastic. Impairment of limb movement and breathing can develop in severe cases. In most cases morphea will gradually resolve. There is no known treatment.

In systemic sclerosis the scleroderma results from a vasculitis of the skin. Thickening and tightening of the skin of the digits leads to reduced circulation to the fingers and toes. This can manifest in Raynaud's phenomenon (white finger). Ulceration of the fingertips can develop. Other features of systemic sclerosis include pinching of the facial skin, difficulties in swallowing and digestion (due to thickening of the lining of the esophagus and bowel), respiratory impairment, mild kidney failure, biliary cirrhosis, cardiac muscle impairment, arthritis and leg ulcers. It can be appreciated that systemic sclerosis is a true multisystem disorder. However, the progression of the condition is usually slow, and so the prognosis is fairly good in most cases.

There is no satisfactory disease-modifying treatment for either morphea or systemic sclerosis. Symptomatic treatment is the mainstay of medical therapy.

 Information box 6.1c-XXVII

Systemic sclerosis: comments from a Chinese medicine perspective

In Chinese medicine, the main features of thickening and loss of elasticity indicate Damp-Phlegm and Deficiency of Qi and Yin. Qi and Blood Stagnation are suggested by the impairment of the normal peristaltic action of the bowel and the severity of the Raynaud's phenomenon. Because of the similarity to the autoimmune multisystem disorders, a profound Deficiency of Kidney Qi and Essence may underlie the development of these diverse imbalances, although the cause is not obviously autoimmune in nature. Flaws and Sionneau explain that Invasion of Wind Cold or Damp when Qi and Blood is depleted is the initial pathogenesis of scleroderma. The Cold and Damp then obstruct the proper function of the skin and sinews. Obstruction of the free flow of Qi leads to worsening depletion of Yang and Qi primarily relating to the Spleen and Kidneys.[15]

Disorders of hair growth

EXCESSIVE HAIR GROWTH

Excessive hair growth is a problem because of its cosmetic consequences. For this reason, the problem mostly affects women. It has to be remembered that the development of excessive facial or body hair does not usually constitute a medical problem, but rather a distortion of what Western society has come to appreciate as normal or beautiful.

It is normal for many Western women to have visible body hairs on the legs, lower back, the pubic region and the skin close to these regions (the bikini line), around the nipples, and on the upper lip and chin. The density and thickness of these hairs can increase throughout the childbearing years. The visibility of body hair varies greatly with family patterns of hair growth and also racial origin. It can be particularly marked in women of Mediterranean or Middle Eastern origin.

It is also normal for there to be a great variation in the density of body hair in men, and again, for this to be related to family patterns of hair growth. Hairiness in men has formerly been seen as a marker of Samson-like manliness and strength. However, in some Western cultures excessive body hair in men has become less desirable.

There is also a marked variation of the degree of distress experienced by a person with a particular density of body hair growth. This can strongly reflect the cultural influences to which the person has been exposed. If the distress appears to be out of proportion to the actual amount of hair growth (when put into the context of the patient's culture), this can be a manifestation of dysmorphophobia, a condition in which the person perceives a normal body feature to be grotesque in some way.

Most Western women and men who perceive their body-hair pattern to be unacceptably excessive in some way will seek methods of removing the hair. Shaving, depilation creams and waxing are commonly used techniques, all of which lead only to a temporary cessation of the problem. Electrolysis, a technique in which the hair follicle is damaged by a combination of heat and electricity delivered by a pinpoint probe, is a method for bringing about a more permanent reduction in body hair.

In some cases excessive body hair may indicate an underlying medical problem. If the body hair distribution in women is in the usual distribution seen in men, the term hirsutism is applied. If the hair growth is more generalized,

it is termed hypertrichosis. The most common underlying causes of hirsutism in women are disturbances in the production of the sex hormones. Polycystic ovary syndrome is the most well recognized cause of secondary hirsutism in women. Anorexia nervosa can also lead to an increased density of very fine body hair (lanugo). Cushing's disease is a far less common, but more sinister, cause of excessive facial and bodily hair.

Some medications, including those that contain one of the steroid family of drugs, can lead to excessive body hair growth. The drug minoxidil, developed for the treatment of severe hypertension, was found to have the side effect of hirsutism. This property has since been utilized for benefit, as minoxidil is now marketed in the form of a topical fluid that can be applied to prevent male pattern baldness.

Information box 6.1c-XXVIII

Excessive body hair: comments from a Chinese medicine perspective

From a Chinese medicine perspective, distribution of body hair in the normal range, even if unacceptable to the patient, would not indicate an energetic imbalance. Generalized excessive body hair growth might indicate a specific imbalance in Lung Qi, as the Lung is the Organ that manifests in the body hair. Hirsutism which follows a male pattern of hair distribution might, in women, represent an excess of Yang. As the Liver and Kidney Organs are associated with sexuality, one might expect imbalances in the Qi of these Organs to also be present.

The treatments of shaving, depilatory creams and waxing may induce side effects. Depilatory creams (which literally dissolve the protein of the hair) can be toxic to the skin. They can cause temporary redness and dryness of the treated skin, and so are Heating

in nature. It might be expected that waxing may lead to a degree of shock to the skin (Qi Depletion and Stagnation) as numerous hair follicles are stripped of their hairs simultaneously. It is noteworthy that the recurrent infective condition of the armpits and groins, hidradenitis suppurativa, is more likely after depilation, so suggesting that this practice impairs the immune balance of the treated skin (possibly by interfering with the normal microbiome).

Electrolysis is obviously Heating, as it produces its effects by burning and scarring of the hair follicles. This is bound to cause Qi and Blood Stagnation locally and ultimately Deplete the Yin of the skin substance. Chronic scarring and tendency to dry skin and skin infections are known side effects of electrolysis.

ABNORMAL SCALP HAIR LOSS (ALOPECIA)

The diagnosis of scalp hair loss (alopecia) depends on whether or not the pattern of loss is diffuse or patchy. Scalp hair loss may be accompanied by a more generalized loss of body hair, but this feature is very rarely seen to be a problem by the patient.

Male pattern baldness

The most common pattern of diffuse scalp hair loss is male pattern baldness (androgenetic alopecia), in which the hair thins progressively from the temples and the crown, so leading to the very commonly seen receding hairline and bald pate. In most cases this is a normal response to male sex hormones in genetically susceptible individuals. Normal male pattern baldness runs very strongly in families,

and the extent and pace of the developing baldness is also strongly familial.

As is the case with normal visible body hair growth, male pattern baldness can be a cause of acute distress because of its perceived cosmetic effects, and so can lead the patient to seek a solution to the problem. Male pattern baldness can also affect a minority of women, in which case the cosmetic effects are usually much more significant for the patient.

The available treatments for male pattern baldness include minoxidil lotion, finasteride (an anti-androgen medication normally used to treat benign prostate disease) and surgical transplant of tiny portions of hair-producing scalp into the balding regions. Minoxidil appears to have some effect in slowing the progression of the baldness.

Information box 6.1c-XXIX

Male pattern baldness: comments from a Chinese medicine perspective

In Chinese medicine, the scalp hair is the manifestation of flourishing Kidney Essence. Shiny, strong and springy hair suggests healthy Kidney Qi and Essence, and weak, brittle, lackluster hair would indicate depletion in these substances. Male pattern baldness does not necessarily indicate a problem in Kidney Qi, as long as the remaining hair is healthy in nature.

Diffuse alopecia

Hairdressers recognize that flourishing hair growth is an indication of health, and thin, lackluster, brittle hair can mean that the individual is run down in some way. More specifically, gradual thinning of hair over time can indicate a nutritional deficiency (especially iron deficiency), a generalized medical problem such as thyroid disease, SLE or a response to certain drugs (e.g. corticosteroids and cytotoxic drugs).

Information box 6.1c-XXX

Diffuse alopecia: comments from a Chinese medicine perspective

According to Chinese medicine the hairs are an extension of Blood and Ying Qi (Nutritive Qi), so healthy hair is a marker of healthy Blood and Qi. If the supply of Blood and Qi is deficient, then local Wind can be generated, and this is thought to lead to hair loss. Internal Heat can contribute to this process by causing generation of Wind, as can Liver Qi Stagnation by impeding the flow of Qi and Blood to the hair.

Diffuse alopecia can result from a Depletion of Kidney Qi and Essence, which then causes Blood Deficiency. Shock is particularly damaging to the Kidney Qi and Essence, and it makes sense that it can result in telogen effluvium.

The patterns underlying hair loss can be summarized as Blood Heat giving rise to Wind, Deficiency of Yin and Blood, Deficiency of Qi and Blood, and Blood Stasis.[16]

The hair, or a large amount of it, can literally fall out overnight (or at least over the course of a few days) approximately three months following an experience of emotional or physical stress (e.g. childbirth, an operation, a car accident or major illness). This dramatic reaction is called telogen effluvium, and is a delayed response to the sudden cessation of the growth of many hairs. In the natural pattern of hair growth, when the growth of a hair has ceased it takes some weeks before the hair actually falls out, hence the delayed response. If the patient already has some gray hairs, a preferential loss of dark hairs can cause the appearance of going gray overnight. The normal consequence of telogen effluvium is that new hairs begin to grow immediately, but may temporarily have a different texture to the lost hairs.

Alopecia areata

Alopecia areata is the consequence of an immune reaction in the skin, leading to patches of total hair loss that expose a normal-appearing, rounded area of scalp skin. Most patches regrow after a few weeks, but not always. In severe cases the scalp might acquire a moth-eaten appearance, or the alopecia may be total (and also include body hair).

There is no satisfactory treatment for alopecia areata, although steroid injections might be used.

Information box 6.1c-XXXI

Alopecia areata: comments from a Chinese medicine perspective

In Chinese medicine, the pathogenesis of alopecia areata will be similar to generalized alopecia. The sudden onset and rapidly changing pattern of hair loss characteristic of alopecia areata is in keeping with the nature of Wind as a Pathogenic Factor.

Hair loss with abnormal scalp skin

Diseases that affect the scalp skin, such as psoriasis, seborrheic dermatitis and tinea capitis (all mentioned earlier), can manifest in patchy hair loss from the affected areas.

Other common skin conditions

URTICARIA AND ANGIO-EDEMA

The term urticaria is derived from the Latin word for stinging nettle. It is used to describe the skin reaction in which there is a rapid development of wheals, akin to the rash that develops after a nettle sting. A wheal is an area of raised skin that initially appears paler than the surrounding skin. It may itch or sting. Wheals always resolve within minutes to hours, but may be replaced by the formation of successive wheals in different body sites (see Figure 6.1c-XXIII).

Figure 6.1c-XXIII Wheals on the arm in urticaria

Urticaria develops from a rapid dilatation of the dermal blood vessels, which permit excess fluid to pass from the blood into the surrounding skin tissue (edema). The chemical histamine, released from the mast cell (a form of tissue-based lymphocyte), stimulates this reaction. In the case of the stinging nettle, a histamine-like chemical is introduced into the dermis from tiny prickles on the nettle leaf and stem.

Angio-edema is a term that describes the extension of the edema of urticaria to the subcutaneous tissues. This can result in an alarming swelling of the loose tissues around the eyes, lips and the airway in the pharynx. Angio-edema can also be accompanied by asthma, which is another histamine-mediated allergic reaction.

Both urticaria and angio-edema can be the result of a generalized anaphylactic reaction as a result of exposure to an allergen. Common causes of acute urticaria and angio-edema include skin contact with plants, animal fur or foods (e.g. milk, egg white), ingestion of certain foods (e.g. milk, shellfish, egg, nuts) and ingestion of drugs (e.g. penicillin). People with atopy are more prone to allergic urticaria and angio-edema.

Urticaria can also develop in response to pressure to the skin, heat, sweating, sunlight and cold, in which case its course is often chronic. In some cases of chronic urticaria there is no obvious trigger.

Acute urticaria often responds well to antihistamine tablets. If the allergic response is acute and severe, intravenous steroids, adrenaline and inhaled bronchodilators may also be used to control the reaction and prevent worsening of the airways obstruction. Chronic urticaria is less responsive to medication, and the treatment often depends on avoidance of the triggers, if these can be identified.

 Information box 6.1c-XXXII

Urticaria: comments from a Chinese medicine perspective

In Chinese medicine, the symptoms of urticaria correspond to Wind Heat Invasion, and angio-edema to Wind Water Invading the Lungs. In both there will be an underlying Deficiency of Wei Qi. Wei Qi Deficiency results from Lung Qi Deficiency and/or Kidney Deficiency.

PRICKLY HEAT (MILIARIA)
Prickly heat (miliaria) is the medical term used to describe the tiny, itchy heat bumps that develop as a result of obstruction of the sweat ducts in hot, humid conditions. The condition is aggravated by anything that stimulates sweating. Prickly heat can contribute to heat stroke because it inhibits the cooling benefits of sweating.

The treatment is avoidance of triggers to sweating, and application to the skin of emollient lotions.

 Information box 6.1c-XXXIII

Prickly heat (miliaria): comments from a Chinese medicine perspective

In Chinese medicine, prickly heat is a manifestation of brewing Summer Damp that inhibits sweating. It is described in terms of a specific Prickly Heat Toxin (Fei Du).[17]

POLYMORPHIC LIGHT ERUPTION (PLE)
Polymorphic light eruption (PLE) is a common disorder that is commonly misdiagnosed as prickly heat. It is an abnormal reaction to sunlight, not heat, and so primarily affects light-exposed areas. The manifestation of PLE is as tiny red spots, and sometimes blisters.

Sunscreens and sun avoidance will prevent PLE in most cases.

 Information box 6.1c-XXXIV

Polymorphic light eruption: comments from a Chinese medicine perspective

In Chinese medicine, PLE is a manifestation of Heat (and underlying Deficiency).

CHILBLAINS

Chilblains are painful areas of inflammation that develop in response to cold. They can develop on the fingers, toes and the fleshy aspect of the upper legs. Treatment of chilblains is simply avoidance of extremes of temperature.

Information box 6.1c-XXXV

Chilblains: comments from a Chinese medicine perspective

In Chinese medicine, chilblains are a result of Cold Stagnation leading to Heat. Zong Qi Deficiency can underlie the development of chilblains, as it is Zong Qi that is responsible for the even flow of Qi and Blood to the extremities.

XANTHELASMATA AND XANTHOMATA (CHOLESTEROL DEPOSITS)

Xanthelasmata (singular xanthelasma) are small (1–5mm in diameter), yellowish plaques (the name is derived from the Greek word for yellow) that form in loose areas of skin, in particular, around the eyelids. They sometimes develop in association with some of the various forms of hyperlipidemia.

Xanthomata (singular xanthoma) are a less common finding. These are more substantial cholesterol deposits, which appear as nodules in the skin around bony prominences, in the tendons and on the palms. Xanthomata are much more closely associated with hyperlipidemia, and so they are a warning feature of atherosclerosis.

Treatment is not usually offered for these cholesterol deposits, as they are rarely a cosmetic problem.

Information box 6.1c-XXXVI

Xanthelasmata: comments from a Chinese medicine perspective

In Chinese medicine, cholesterol deposits are a physical manifestation of Phlegm Damp.

LICHEN PLANUS

Lichen planus is an immune-related skin reaction of unknown cause, in which the skin erupts with numerous itchy, purplish, flat-topped papules. The papules most commonly appear on the wrists, ankles and small of the back (see Figure 6.1c-XXIV). Changes can also be found in the mucous membranes of the mouth and genitalia.

Figure 6.1c-XXIV Papules on the forearm in lichen planus

In most cases the eruption settles within a few months, although some cases can be persistent. If the rash and itching are severe, steroid creams and even corticosteroid tablets may be prescribed.

Information box 6.1c-XXXVII

Lichen planus: comments from a Chinese medicine perspective

The purplish color and the itch are suggestive that lichen planus is an expression of Heat and Stagnation of Qi.

PITYRIASIS ROSEA

Pityriasis rosea is a mysterious self-limiting condition that primarily affects apparently otherwise well children and young adults. It may well be a delayed response to a viral infection. The rash begins with a so-called herald patch of red, scaly skin on the trunk or upper arm. Then, within a few days, this is followed by an eruption of small, pink, oval patches on the back, abdomen, upper arms and thighs.

The patches in pityriasis rosea are slightly scaly and may be a cause of slight irritation. The rash clears up spontaneously within six to eight weeks. Usually no treatment is needed.

Information box 6.1c-XXXVIII

Pityriasis rosea: comments from a Chinese medicine perspective

In Chinese medicine, this rash would appear to result from an Invasion of Wind Heat. The scaling is suggestive of Phlegm Damp.

PRURITUS

Pruritus is a general term used to describe itching in the absence of an underlying skin disorder. Any cause of pruritus will lead the patient to scratch, and so will initially lead to the appearance of excoriated or bleeding skin. Chronic pruritus can cause the skin to become thickened and dry (lichenified), as can also occur in chronic eczema. Lichenified skin is more likely to itch, and so a vicious cycle of itch–scratch–itch is set up. If severe and chronic, pruritus can be a very distressing condition.

Itching has a wide range of causes, many of which have already been described in this section. Any possible underlying skin disease (e.g. scabies) has to be excluded before a diagnosis of pruritus can be made.

Localized pruritus may manifest in the form of a patch of lichenified skin, often in an overstressed or anxious individual. Common sites are the back, neck, shins and, distressingly for the patient, the perianal and vulval regions. Itchy skin nodules can also develop in addition to the thickened itchy patch of skin. Good hygiene, especially of the perineum, is important in the treatment of pruritus. Ideally, the patient's level of stress should be addressed. High-dose topical steroids may be used to inhibit the inflammation, and so break the cycle of itching and scratching.

Generalized pruritus is a very unpleasant disorder that is recognized to occur in a wide range of generalized medical conditions (e.g. iron deficiency, obstructive jaundice, chronic renal failure, thyroid disease and cancer). In pregnancy, generalized itch can in some cases be a serious indication of obstetric cholestasis, a condition in which the mother's liver fails to clear the bile from the bile ducts (probably a result of an inherited susceptibility to estrogen). The buildup of bile salts in the blood is the cause of the itch, and is a warning feature of serious damage to the unborn baby. If a pregnant woman develops generalized pruritus, she should be referred to her doctor or midwife for further tests.

In the management of generalized pruritus, first, the underlying cause should be treated, and then, symptoms may be controlled by use of topical steroids and oral sedative antihistamine tablets. In elderly people, pruritus

of an unknown cause may simply be the result of dry, poorly nourished skin. In this case, emollient creams can be of help.

Information box 6.1c-XXXIX

Pruritus: comments from a Chinese medicine perspective

In Chinese medicine, itch may be the result of Wind that arises because Blood in the Channels is Deficient. The Wind may be External in origin or may arise as a result of Internal Liver Disharmony. Treatment principles would therefore involve nourishing the Blood, Pacifying the Liver, and Clearing Wind.

SKIN ULCERS

Skin ulcer is the term used to describe any breach in the epithelial lining of the skin. Chronic skin ulcers are areas of skin in which this breach persistently fails to heal over (see Figure 6.1c-XXV). The cause, features and Chinese medicine interpretation of chronic skin ulcers have been described in some depth in Section 2.1b.

Figure 6.1c-XXV A chronic venous skin ulcer on the lower leg

REACTIONS TO DRUGS

The skin can generate diverse symptoms and signs as side effects to prescribed medication. Many drugs will have rash listed as one of their common side effects, but there are many other possible skin reactions to drugs including itch, urticaria, pigmentation and dryness with scaling. The drugs that are most commonly implicated in adverse skin reactions include antibiotics, non-steroidal anti-inflammatory drugs (NSAIDs) and tranquillizers (see Figure 6.1c-XXVI).

Figure 6.1c-XXVI A typical rash resulting from penicillin allergy

The commonly recognized skin reactions to drugs are:

- itchy red rashes (exanthems)
- urticaria and anaphylaxis (see earlier)
- inflamed scaliness (exfoliative dermatitis)
- vasculitis (inflammation of the tiny blood vessels that supply the skin)
- lichen planus
- acne-like rashes
- abnormalities in hair growth

- changes in pigmentation
- blistering
- light sensitivity
- SLE-like reactions
- worsening of pre-existing skin disease.

It can be appreciated that drugs can induce all manner of skin disease, and so, when a skin disease suddenly appears, it is prudent to take a good drug history. The ideal treatment for all these reactions is to withdraw the medication. Sometimes additional medication such as corticosteroids, antihistamines or emollients may be required to treat drug-induced skin disease.

The red flags of diseases of the skin

Some people with diseases of the skin will benefit from referral to a conventional doctor for assessment or treatment. Red flags are those symptoms and signs that indicate that referral should be considered. The red flags of the diseases of the skin are described in Table 6.1c-I. A summary of the red flags in a format designed for quick reference in clinical practice can be found in Appendix III. This gives advice on the degree of urgency of referral for each of the red flag conditions listed.

Table 6.1c-I A41: Red flags of diseases of the skin

Red flag	Description	Reasoning
A41.1	A rapidly enlarging patch(es) of painful, crusting or swollen red skin	Crusting, spreading skin disease suggests erysipelas or severe impetigo. If spreading rapidly, antibiotic treatment should be considered
		Refer with some urgency if this occurs in someone with eczema, as it can rapidly become a serious condition (or it may indicate herpes virus infection of the broken skin)
A41.2	A rapidly advancing region or line of redness tracking up the skin of a limb (following the pathway of a lymphatic vessel)	This suggests the deep spread of infection from a distal site (cellulitis and/or lymphangitis), and should be considered for antibiotic treatment
A41.3	Pronounced features of candidal infection (thrush) of the skin or mucous membranes of the mouth	Widespread candidiasis suggests an underlying chronic condition such as immunodeficiency or diabetes mellitus
		Refer to exclude underlying disease

A41.4	The features of early shingles: intense, one-sided pain, with an overlying rash of crops of fluid-filled reddened and crusting blisters. The pain and rash correspond in location to a neurological dermatome. The pain may precede the rash by 1–2 days	Shingles is an outbreak of the chickenpox virus (varicella zoster) that has lain dormant within a spinal nerve root since an earlier episode of chickenpox. It tends to reactivate when the person is run down and exposed to intense sunlight, and is more common in elderly people Warn the patient that the condition is contagious, and advise that immediate treatment (within 48 hours of onset of the rash) with the antiviral drug aciclovir has been proven to reduce the severity of prolonged pain after recovery of the rash. For this reason it is necessary to refer as a high priority to a doctor for advice on medical management
A41.5	Generalized itch	Generalized itch (not eczema) suggests an underlying medical cause (e.g. cholestasis), iron deficiency or cancer. It may also result from scabies. Refer for diagnosis if persisting over a few days
A41.6	Itching (severe), especially of the palms and soles, in pregnancy	May result from cholestasis, a condition that can damage the fetus. Refer as a high priority
A41.7	Large areas of redness affecting most (>90%) of the body surface (erythroderma): refer because of the risk of dehydration and loss of essential salts	Erythroderma can develop in severe cases of eczema and psoriasis and as a reaction to some medications. It can become a medical emergency, as the cardiovascular system can become under strain from the massively increased blood flow to the skin that results from the generalized inflammation
A41.8	Generalized macular rash (flat, red spots)	Refer if you suspect the possibility of a notifiable disease (i.e. rubella, measles or scarlet fever) Note: Chickenpox is not a notifiable disease, and there is no need to refer if there are no other red flags. A patient with chickenpox needs to be advised about the risk of contagiousness that is significant within the first five days of developing the rash
A41.9	Purpura or bruising rash (non-blanching)	A rash that contains areas of non-blanching or bruising suggests a bleeding disorder or vasculitis. Refer as an emergency if the patient is also acutely unwell with headache/fever or vomiting (possible meningococcal infection; see A23.4)
A41.10	Any lumps/moles with features suggestive of malignancy: recent change in shape, irregularity, a tendency to bleed, crusting, >5mm in diameter, irregularities in pigmentation, intense black color	Skin tumors include basal cell carcinomas (BCCs), squamous cell carcinomas (SCCs) and malignant melanomas Premalignant skin tumors are often associated with changes due to sun damage (on the scalp, temples and the backs of the hands), and appear as spreading, flat areas of dark pigmentation, or irregular scabs that never seem to heal Seborrheic keratoses are benign, waxy, darkened warty growths found on aging skin that are no need for concern, but may be confused with tumors If you have any doubt, it is worth referring for an early diagnosis
A41.11	Progressive swelling of the soft tissues of the face and neck (angio-edema) and/or urticaria (nettle rash)	Angio-edema can result from an acute allergic reaction and can precede life-threatening asthma. Refer urgently if there are any features of respiratory distress (itchy throat/wheeze)
A41.12	Hirsutism (unexplained hairiness)	Refer any unexplained increase in body hair in middle life, as this may indicate an endocrine disease or, in women, polycystic ovary syndrome

6.1d Diseases of the eye

Eye diseases are managed medically within the discipline of ophthalmology. However, many people with eye disorders may never encounter an ophthalmologist, and instead will rely on the diagnosis and treatment offered by an optometrist. Optometrists are non-medical specialists who are trained in the field of optics, and in the appropriate correction of problems in focusing. Problems in focusing are by far the most commonly experienced eye conditions in adults.

The optometrist is also trained to recognize and refer on any eye conditions that may merit specific medical treatment (e.g. chronic glaucoma or acute conjunctivitis) or that may be red flags of serious underlying medical disease (e.g. diabetes or hypertension).

The conditions discussed in this section are:

- Optics – problems in focusing:
  - myopia (short-sightedness)
  - hypermetropia (long-sightedness)
  - astigmatism
  - presbyopia (long-sightedness of old age)
- Conditions of the conjunctiva, cornea and sclera:
  - infective conjunctivitis
  - allergic conjunctivitis
  - infections of the cornea (keratitis)
  - episcleritis and scleritis
  - corneal surgery
- Conditions of the orbit, extraocular muscles, eyelids and tear duct system:
  - orbital cellulitis
  - chalazions and styes
  - blepharitis
  - dry eyes and Sjögren's syndrome
  - blocked tear ducts
  - ptosis (drooping eyelid) and paralysis of the lid
  - exophthalmos
  - squint and double vision
- Conditions of the internal structures of the eye (lens, ciliary body and retina):
  - cataract
  - uveitis
  - glaucoma
  - age-related macular degeneration (ARMD)
  - diabetic retinopathy
- Conditions of the optic nerve:
  - optic neuritis.

Optics – problems in focusing

Optics is the science of the behavior of light. With regard to clinical medicine, the term clinical optics refers to the study of how light is refracted (focused) by the eyeball to produce a clear image of the viewed object on the sensitive screen of the retina at the back of the eyeball. The cornea and the lens are the two parts of the eyeball that contribute most significantly to its refractive power (ability to focus).

Short-sightedness (myopia) and long-sightedness (hypermetropia) are both conditions in which the ability of the eye to focus on an image normally is impaired. In refractive conditions such as these, either the lens of the eye is not structured or functioning correctly, or the position of the retina with respect to the lens is not ideal (the eyeball is too long or too short).

Myopia (short-sightedness)

In myopia the lens of the eye tends to focus an image too far in front of the retina. In other words, for the patient's length of eyeball, the focusing power of the lens is too high. A patient with myopia will find it easier to focus on an object that is held very close to the eye, whereas all objects at a distance from the eye will be blurred. It is conventionally understood that the most usual cause of myopia is an inherited tendency for the eyeball to be too long in shape. This theory is used to explain why there can be a marked exacerbation of short-sightedness during the growth spurt in the mid-teens.

It is also now recognized that myopia seems to be more common in those children who don't spend much time outside. It is believed that excessive use of the eyes in close-up activities such as reading, use of computer and mobile phones will lead to strain of the ciliary muscle of the eye, and habitual over-compensation of the lens and possibly eye ball shape to meet the needs of regular close-sighted work. The result of this adaptation is that whilst very close clear vision is possible in the short-sighted person, distance vision will always result in blurred images.

The conventional approach to dealing with myopia is to prescribe corrective concave (negative) lenses. These diverge the rays of light coming from distant objects so that they can be focused on the retina by the over-compensated lens in the short-sighted person. Therefore distant objects can be seen clearly (see Figure 6.1d-I).

approach can be beneficial not just for myopia, but also for all types of refractive error. This method does not appear to have any conventionally accepted supporting evidence.[19]

Refractive surgery is a more permanent approach to the treatment of myopia. In this approach, the ability of the cornea to contribute to the focusing of light is modified. Radial keratotomy and laser keratoplasty are procedures that lead to flattening of the central cornea by means of surgery and laser therapy, respectively.

Hypermetropia (long-sightedness)

In hypermetropia (long-sightedness), the eye fails to focus the image on the retina. It is most usually a result of a relatively short eyeball. It can also result from the removal of the lens, which is part of a cataract extraction, which results in an extreme form of hypermetropia. A patient with hypermetropia will find it easier to focus on objects at a distance than on those that are close to the face.

Hypermetropia can be corrected by means of concave lenses (see Figure 6.1d-I) and also by laser keratoplasty.

Astigmatism

Astigmatism is a term used to describe a condition of the lens or the cornea in which there is an uneven (cylindrical) curvature of the lens, rather than the even curvature that would be akin to a section from a sphere. This means that only part of an image might be focused with clarity. A patient with astigmatism might have particular problems in focusing on an image that consists of lines at right angles to each other, such as a grid or a musical score.

Astigmatism often coexists with either myopia or hypermetropia, and is corrected by means of cylindrical concave or convex lenses, respectively.

Presbyopia (long-sightedness of old age)

The long-sightedness that develops in old age (but which may become apparent as early as the mid-40s) is not, strictly speaking, hypermetropia. Rather, it results from a weakening of the ability of the lens to accommodate for near objects (i.e. to fatten in response to constriction of the ciliary muscle).

The patient with presbyopia is still able to focus objects at a distance, but has trouble in seeing close objects with clarity. In presbyopia reading is aided by holding the book at arm's length.

Presbyopia is corrected by means of convex lenses within bifocal spectacles that are designed specifically for the condition. Bifocals have a stronger lens inserted at the bottom of the field of vision so that reading (when looking down) is aided, but usual vision (when looking ahead) need not be modified at all. The lenses in varifocal spectacles have a more gradual transition of power from the usual vision to the reading section of the lens. However, many

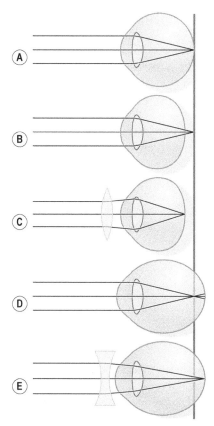

Figure 6.1d-I The common refractive errors of the eye with and without corrective lenses

The images illustrate how light is focused by the lens of the eye. In the normal eye (A) the light is focused on the retina. In the short-sighted (myopic) eye (D) the light is focused in front of the retina, and in the long-sighted (hypermetropic) eye (B) the light is focused behind the retina. Corrective lenses (C) and (E) enable the light to be focused in the correct place for clear vision.

There are critics of this approach who believe negative lenses will exacerbate the problem, as they permit a child to continue to use the eyes in excessive close work while the accommodating muscles are under strain. According to this theory, the answer to the prevention of myopia lies in reducing the amount of close-up work that is done in childhood, and using visual aids such as pinhole glasses to minimize the degree to which the eye muscles have to accommodate during close visual work. Whilst a compelling argument, the avoidance of corrective lenses may not be a practical solution to the demands of modern living. Also, current research suggests that children who are not prescribed corrective lenses may suffer in their early years learning and visual development.[18]

The Bates method, which was proposed by Dr William Bates over a century ago, is another alternative approach to myopia. The method is based on exercises that teach the eye to move while maintaining relaxation of the external eye muscles. Proponents of the Bates method claim that the people with presbyopia prefer to have two pairs of glasses, one for usual vision and one for reading.

 Information box 6.1d-I

Refractive errors: comments from a Chinese medicine perspective

From a Chinese medicine viewpoint, all the refractive errors might be explained in terms of Deficiency of Liver and/or Kidney Qi, or a general Deficiency of the Qi and Essence that flow in the Yang Channels that nourish the eye.

In children, eye strain, illness, rapid growth and emotional distress may cause insufficient flow of Qi to the eyes and thus lead to myopia. Outdoor play will invigorate and help move the Qi.

Presbyopia, appearing as it does very often at the end of the fifth decade of life, is very likely to be the result of decline in Kidney Essence.

Conditions of the conjunctiva, cornea and sclera

The conjunctiva is the protective epithelial membrane that lines the inner surface of the eyelids and the anterior portion of the eyeball (the anterior sclera and cornea).

Infective conjunctivitis

The conjunctiva is very commonly involved in minor infections caused either by bacteria or viruses. Conjunctivitis is diagnosed very often in children. The infections are transmitted either by droplet spread or by direct contamination with infection-laden discharges from an affected eye. Hand-to-eye contact is very common, and particularly so in children, so conjunctivitis is very contagious. A particular form of conjunctivitis can be contracted by the newborn during childbirth, a result of infection with the sexually transmissible organisms *Chlamydia* and *Gonococcus*.

The symptoms of conjunctivitis are redness and slight swelling of the conjunctiva, discomfort and itch of the eye, and discharge. The discharge is more likely to be thick and sticky in bacterial infection, and watery in viral infections. Usually both eyes are infected, but one may become symptomatic up to a few days before the other. (If there is severe pain, conjunctivitis is not a likely diagnosis, and another explanation such as episcleritis or iritis should be excluded.)

Trachoma is the consequence of recurrent conjunctival infections, and occurs almost exclusively in developing countries. Trachoma takes a much more serious course in

that the surface of the eye can become permanently scarred. Trachoma is the most common cause of blindness in the world. The infectious agent is the bacteria-like organism *Chlamydia*, which is transmitted by hand-to-eye contact and also possibly by flies. The tragedy is that infections can be entirely prevented by means of an appropriate prescription of antibiotics.

Most cases of conjunctivitis will settle down spontaneously with gentle cleansing with salt water. Conventional treatment includes exclusion of the affected child from their peers for the course of the infection and the regular application of antibiotic drops (in the UK most often chloramphenicol). Treatment with antibiotics is advisable in the newborn, and those who are immunocompromised or undernourished.

 Information box 6.1d-II

Infective conjunctivitis: comments from a Chinese medicine perspective

In Chinese medicine, infective conjunctivitis might correspond to an Invasion of Wind Heat. It can also be attributed to a Rising of Heat and Damp in the Channels local to the eye, or to Liver and Gallbladder Heat. Other organs can also express imbalance via the eye and so Heart, Stomach and Kidney Pathology may also underlie eye infections.

Allergic conjunctivitis

The eye can also become inflamed as a result of an allergic reaction to particles that have entered the eye. Common allergens in susceptible people include grass and tree pollen (in hay fever), animal dander, house dust mite and foods such as egg, milk and wheat.

The symptoms are similar to those of viral conjunctivitis, although itch and periorbital swelling may be much more prominent. In severe cases the conjunctiva can become so congested with fluid that its (temporary) appearance is that of a mass of clear jelly.

The allergic reaction can become chronic if exposure to the allergen is repeated. In this case, a characteristic appearance of seed-like bumps of inflammatory tissue may be seen on the inner surface of the conjunctiva.

Treatment of allergic conjunctivitis is by means of antihistamine or sodium cromoglicate eye drops. Both these drugs act to inhibit the excessive immune response to the offending allergens. Oral antihistamine may be prescribed for chronic allergic conjunctivitis, or in cases in which there are other symptoms of hay fever (allergic rhinitis).

Information box 6.1d-III

Allergic conjunctivitis: comments from a Chinese medicine perspective

In Chinese medicine, the syndromes in allergic conjunctivitis would be similar to those described for infective conjunctivitis (see above), although Heat may be more prominent and Damp less prominent. An underlying Kidney imbalance may also be part of the etiology of the condition.

Infections of the cornea (keratitis)

Normally the conjunctiva and the tears protect the deeper portions of the eyeball from infectious organisms. Infection of the cornea (keratitis) is serious because it can lead to scarring, and thence to permanent impairment of sight.

The cornea can become infected by bacteria if the protective barriers to disease are deficient, as can occur in eye trauma, or if the production of tears is impaired, as can occur in autoimmune diseases such as rheumatoid arthritis (see below). Bacterial keratitis first presents with redness around the cornea, dislike of light (photophobia), discharge and intense pain. Intensive treatment with antibiotics is required to prevent progression of the condition. The lid may be taped over the affected cornea to aid healing.

Information box 6.1d-IV

Keratitis: comments from a Chinese medicine perspective

In Chinese medicine, the initial infection of keratitis may be described as an Invasion of Wind Heat, although, as this is a deep condition, an underlying imbalance of any of the organs associated with moistening and nourishing the eye, namely, Liver, Kidney, Heart or Stomach, may be considered to have predisposed a person to the condition. The sclera is associated with the Lung in Chinese medicine, and so some Lung Pathology may also be evident.

Viral keratitis can occur without prior damage to the conjunctiva or the lacrimal system. Herpes simplex virus (HSV) keratitis can be contracted by hand-to-eye contact or droplet spread from an infected person. Herpes zoster virus keratitis can develop if shingles erupts from the branches of the trigeminal nerve that supply the conjunctiva. In both cases, the symptoms are similar to those found in bacterial keratitis, although the risk of permanent scarring is not as great. The treatment is with antiviral creams and closure of the lid over the affected cornea.

Episcleritis and scleritis

Episcleritis is a superficial inflammation of the sclera that presents as persistent patchy redness and discomfort of the white of the eye. There is no discharge, and so episcleritis should be easy to distinguish from conjunctivitis. Episcleritis is rarely serious, but when present, the deeper condition of scleritis should be excluded (see below).

In scleritis there may be an underlying autoimmune disease such as rheumatoid arthritis. Scleritis is a penetrating inflammation of the sclera in which there is patchy, deep redness and weakening of the sclera, accompanied by intense pain. The sclera is at risk of perforation. Perforation of the eye is an ophthalmic emergency. The iris may also be involved (uveitis; see below), in which case there is a risk of scarring of the lens of the eye (cataract).

The condition is treated by means of high doses of steroid or immunosuppressant medication.

Information box 6.1d-V

Scleritis: comments from a Chinese medicine perspective

From a Chinese medicine perspective, the intense pain and seriousness of scleritis indicates a deep condition of Full Heat in the Liver with underlying Imbalance of the organs associated with moistening and nourishing the eye, namely, Liver, Kidney, Heart or Stomach. Pain is indicative of Local Stagnation of Blood. Episcleritis is also an indication of Heat. The sclera is associated with the Lung in Chinese medicine, and so some Lung Pathology may also be evident.

Corneal surgery

Scarring of the cornea can result from the chronic inflammatory conditions of trachoma, keratitis and scleritis, and if severe, may lead to impairment of vision and even blindness. The scarred cornea can be replaced by a donor graft by means of a relatively straightforward operation. In most cases the donor graft is not rejected because this part of the eye is relatively protected from the immune system.

Unlike all other transplant operations, in which long-term immunosuppressant medication is necessary, the patient does not usually require any more than a short course of steroid eye drops in order to prevent rejection.

Donor corneas are obtained from the cadavers of people who have permitted their eyes to be used for donation, and can be stored in controlled sterile conditions in corneal banks until the time when they can be used.

Conditions of the orbit, extraocular muscles, eyelids and tear duct system

Orbital cellulitis

Orbital cellulitis is a spreading infection of the tissues that surround the eye, and originates most commonly from a sinus infection. The symptoms are a swollen and painful eye socket and lids and difficult eye movements in a very unwell patient. There is serious risk of the infection spreading inwards to form a brain abscess, and so the patient should be referred immediately for intravenous antibiotic therapy.

Chalazions and styes

A chalazion is a blocked meibomian gland (oil gland) in the eyelid, which usually appears as a painless, rounded swelling of the lid margin (see Figure 6.1d-II). This cyst, which comprises accumulated sebaceous secretions, can become infected, in which case the lump will enlarge and become painful. A chalazion can be treated by surgical excision if unsightly or infected.

A stye is an infected eyelash follicle. It appears like a boil, the head of which is on the lid margin. When examined carefully, it can be seen that a lash is protruding from the center of the head of a stye. Most styes will discharge or settle down spontaneously. Conservative treatment involves bathing the affected area with hot salty water. Nevertheless, antibiotic creams (and sometimes oral antibiotics) are commonly prescribed.

Figure 6.1d-II A chalazion of the eyelid

Blepharitis

Blepharitis describes a longstanding inflammation of the eyelids that manifests as crusting of the lids and consequent irritation of the eyes. There may be scaling of the lid margins. In severe cases the eyes themselves can become inflamed.

Blepharitis is associated with seborrheic dermatitis, atopic eczema and acne rosacea, and is believed to result from an imbalance of the formation of the waxy secretions from the meibomian glands in the eyelids together with a disturbance in the balance of the fungal and bacterial flora in the region of the lids.[20] It is a difficult condition to treat, although topical antibiotics and gentle cleansing of the scales with warm salty water may relieve the symptoms.

 Information box 6.1d-VI

Chalazions and styes: comments from a Chinese medicine perspective

From a Chinese medicine perspective, an uncomplicated chalazion would suggest Damp/Phlegm and also an imbalance of the organs that nourish and moisten the eyes, namely, Spleen, Liver or Kidneys. The Spleen and Stomach dominate the eyelids in Chinese medicine.

Infection of a chalazion could be described as Damp Heat. A stye has a similar interpretation, although, as it can appear rapidly, a possible diagnosis would be Wind Damp Heat.

The development of an infected chalazion or a stye (although these are considered to be minor conditions) is an indication that the patient may be quite run down or stressed (the Heat developing as a result of Yin Deficiency or Stagnation of Liver Qi).

 Information box 6.1d-VII

Blepharitis: comments from a Chinese medicine perspective

In Chinese medicine, the symptoms and signs of blepharitis correspond to Damp Heat with an underlying imbalance of the organs that nourish and moisten the eyes, namely, Spleen, Liver or Kidneys. The Spleen and Stomach dominate the eyelids in Chinese medicine.

Dry eyes (kerato-conjunctivitis sicca) and Sjögren's syndrome

The medical condition of dry eyes or kerato-conjunctivitis sicca (KCS) results from disease of the tear-forming lacrimal glands. The usual cause of KCS is a poorly understood degenerative process of aging, although it is well recognized as a feature of autoimmune diseases such as rheumatoid arthritis. KCS associated with dry mouth (xerostomia) is suggestive of Sjögren's syndrome, a connective tissue disease.

The symptoms of KCS include grittiness and tiredness of the eyes and dislike of light (photophobia). These symptoms are often worse in the evening. The eyes may become reddened and prone to attacks of conjunctivitis and keratitis (see above).

KCS is treated by means of artificial tears, which can be instilled into the eyes by the patient whenever needed. Shielded spectacles can ensure that the environment around the eyes stays as humid as is possible.

Information box 6.1d-VIII

Dry eyes: comments from a Chinese medicine perspective

In Chinese medicine, dryness of the eyes suggests Liver Blood and Yin Deficiency.

Blocked tear ducts (epiphora)

The nasolacrimal tear duct of the eye drains from the inner canthus of the eye. If this is blocked, tears cannot drain into the tear duct, and so will accumulate and eventually spill over (epiphora). The duct is commonly blocked in newborns, a result of the fact that the developing tear duct normally achieves patency only very close to the time of delivery. In this case, the problem almost always resolves with time. If blocked tear ducts are persistent up to the end of the first year of life, a surgical probing of the duct can be performed to clear the blockage.

In adults the passageway through the tear duct can become blocked by an inflammatory or degenerative process (see Figure 6.1d-III). The main symptom of blockage is epiphora, but also a persistently sticky eye may result. The symptoms are usually on one side only, and the sclera of the eye remains white, so distinguishing the problem from conjunctivitis. Treatment is by surgically opening the upper portion of the tear duct into the nasal cavity (dacrocystorhinostomy). This operation involves the removal of a small portion of the intervening nasal bone.

Information box 6.1d-IX

Blocked tear ducts (epiphora): comments from a Chinese medicine perspective

From a Chinese medicine perspective, an interpretation of epiphora appearing as it does at the extreme ends of a lifespan probably would be one of general Deficiency, and in particular, of Kidney Essence.

Figure 6.1d-III Acute inflammation of the lacrimal sac: dacrocystitis

Ptosis (drooping eyelid) and paralysis of the lid

A drooping eyelid (ptosis) can be a congenital abnormality. If uncomplicated, ptosis usually causes little other than a cosmetic problem, as it rarely leads to occlusion of the pupil. In those congenital cases that cause cosmetic or visual problems the lid can be slightly lifted by means of a minor surgical operation.

A ptosis that develops in later life may be a warning feature of nerve damage. In very rare cases and as a consequence of the complex anatomy of the nerves that supply the eyelid, this damage may result from a developing tumor of the apex of the lung or of the brain. Ptosis can also develop as part of myasthenia gravis, the disorder of muscle fatigability. For this reason the patient with a recent onset of ptosis should be referred for further investigations.

A one-sided (unilateral) paralysis of the lid can occur in Bell's palsy, in which case it appears as part of a generalized paralysis of the facial nerve. In a facial nerve paralysis, the nerve can be so severely affected that the lid cannot close at all, in which case the eyeball is at risk of damage (ulceration of the conjunctiva) through drying out. In the majority of cases the paralysis recovers fully within three months, but in longer-standing cases the lid may need to be partially closed by means of a minor operation (tarsorrhaphy) so that the eyeball can remain lubricated and protected.

Information box 6.1d-X

Ptosis: comments from a Chinese medicine perspective

In Chinese medicine, a weakness of the eyelid muscle in ptosis might indicate a Spleen or Liver Blood Deficiency that has become manifest in the channels of the face. This is because the Spleen and Stomach are associated with the eyelids in Chinese medicine and the Liver dominates the muscles. Facial palsy is considered to be the result of a Wind Invasion of the facial channels.

Exophthalmos

Exophthalmos (also known as proptosis) is the medical term used to describe the bulging outwards of an eyeball from the orbit. It is most commonly observed in Graves' disease (when it is described as thyroid eye disease) as a result of an antibody-stimulated accumulation of fatty tissue behind the eye. In Graves' disease, exophthalmos usually affects both eyes, although very often it can be more prominent in one eye. Exophthalmos can also develop on one side only (unilaterally) as a result of a tumor in the orbit, although this is very rare.

Exophthalmos becomes apparent as a staring look in the eye(s). If severe, the white of the eye can be seen both above and below the sclera. This is not a usual feature of a relaxed face.

Even in the early stages of exophthalmos, an examining doctor will be able to confirm that the movement of the lid is slowed over the eye as the patient is asked to look down (a sign known as lid lag). As the condition progresses, the patient may develop sore, red eyes, double vision or loss of clear vision.

The primary risk to the eye from exophthalmos is that the eye will eventually be unable to close fully and so will suffer the results of dryness in the same way as the eye affected by facial paralysis (see above). In thyroid eye disease there is added danger to the eye, as the accumulating soft tissue can start to compress and damage the optic nerve. The soft tissue can also affect the external muscles of the eye and lead to squint (see below). Treatment of the underlying thyroid disease may slow the progression of the exophthalmos, but cannot reverse the process. The main medical treatment is corticosteroid injections. Surgical treatments include removal of the accumulated soft tissue and, as is used to treat paralysis of the eyelid in Bell's palsy, partial closing of the eyelid (tarsorrhaphy).

 Information box 6.1d-XI

Exophthalmos: comments from a Chinese medicine perspective

From a Chinese medicine perspective, the staring look seen in exophthalmos (the four whites) is a feature of extreme Kidney Deficiency. In hyperthyroidism the primary Deficiency is of Kidney Yin (with Full Heat). The inflammation of the eye (also suggestive of Heat) and muscle paralysis of the external ocular muscles suggests that Liver, Gallbladder or Bladder Pathology is a factor to be considered.

Squint (strabismus) and double vision

Congenital (non-paralytic) squint is described in Section 5.4e. In infancy, the brain suppresses the images received from a divergent or convergent non-dominant eye so that the child can see clearly without double vision. If not treated before the age of seven at the latest, this developmental response has the deleterious consequence of amblyopia (permanent loss of depth vision).

Congenital squint is usually the result of an inherited imbalance in the functioning of the external muscles of the eye. More rarely it may follow from an inability of the eye to receive clear visual information, such as can occur in congenital cataract. The effects of the squint may be subtle, and so it may remain undetected until it is too late for treatment.

In contrast, the development of a squint in an adult becomes very obvious very quickly, as the patient develops disabling double vision. The most usual cause of a squint in an adult is a paralysis of one or more of the cranial nerves that supply the external muscles of the eye. For this reason, this form of squint is termed paralytic strabismus. Orbital tumors and the accumulation of the soft tissue that occurs in thyroid eye disease can also hinder the action of these muscles and so lead to the double vision of paralytic strabismus, although these are much less common causes of double vision.

Any cause of a mononeuropathy can lead to a paralytic squint resulting from damage to the third, fourth or sixth cranial nerves. Common causes of cranial mononeuropathies include diabetes, vascular disease and compression by brain tumors. Head injuries and raised intracranial pressure can also be complicated by damage to the cranial nerves that supply the eye muscles. For these reasons the development of double vision should be treated as a warning feature of serious disease.

Ideally, the cause of the paralytic squint can be treated rapidly to reverse the double vision, but often the damage that has occurred to the cranial nerves is irreparable. Urgent diagnosis and treatment of the underlying cause of the paralysis is always necessary.

If a permanent paralytic squint cannot be prevented by early treatment, the simplest treatment is to patch the affected eye. Spectacles containing prism lenses may also be used to realign the images of viewed objects that fall on the two retinas. Surgical correction of the extraocular muscles may also prevent double vision in cases in which the paralysis is permanent.

Information box 6.1d-XII

Squint: comments from a Chinese medicine perspective

A congenital squint may be the result of Womb Heat that has become lodged in the channels that relate to one or more of the extraocular muscles (Liver, Gallbladder and Bladder). In this case, the squint is present from birth, and is often quite pronounced in appearance.

Alternatively, if a congenital squint becomes apparent after the time of birth, it may be the result of the Depletion in the Qi of the Channels relating to the eye muscles. In a child this might result from either an Invasion of Full Heat or a Lingering Pathogenic Factor in the Channels or from the Internal (Empty) Heat generated from overstimulation or overexcitement.

A sudden onset of paralytic squint in an adult suggests that Wind is an underlying Pathogenic Factor that has triggered the condition. Again, the Gallbladder, Liver and Bladder Channels are those that are affected. Underlying vascular disease, diabetes or cancer might indicate that Phlegm and Heat are also lodged in the Channels, which may have become vulnerable because of longstanding deficiency in the associated organs.

Conditions of the internal structures of the eye (lens, ciliary body and retina)

Cataract

Cataract is the medical term used to describe opacification of the lens of the eye. It is the commonest cause of treatable blindness worldwide. In the West, aging is the most common cause of cataract (age-related cataract), and a long history of sun exposure is known to increase the risk of its development. Medical causes of cataract include diabetes mellitus and long-term use of corticosteroid medication.

A patient with significant bilateral cataracts will experience increasing difficulty in focusing that cannot be corrected with glasses. Bright light can make the symptoms worse for some patients who are troubled by glare.

The principal treatment for cataract is surgery. Surgical treatment is usually offered in the UK as soon as the cataract is recognized to be significantly affecting the patient's quality of life. There are two surgical techniques. The first involves an incision at the edge of the cornea and then removal of the clouded lens from its supporting capsule. The second surgical technique (phacoemulsification) involves liquefaction of the lens induced by an ultrasound probe inserted into the eye via a similar incision. In both

cases the lens is replaced by an artificial lens implant, which is designed to allow the eye to focus for distance viewing. Usually only one eye is operated on at a time.

Cataract extraction is considered a minor procedure, and carries very few risks, even for frail elderly people. After the operation the patient is prescribed a short course of steroid and antibiotic drops to reduce inflammation and minimize the risk of infection. In the vast majority of patients there is a significant improvement in visual acuity.

However, in approximately 20 percent of patients clouding of the remaining lens capsule can lead to a reduction in acuity over the months following the operation. This complication can be treated by means of laser therapy as an outpatient procedure.

Information box 6.1d-XIII

Cataract: comments from a Chinese medicine perspective

In Chinese medicine, a gradual deterioration in vision such as occurs with the slow development of a cataract is understood as failure in the Nourishment of the eyes. Patterns associated with cataract include Deficiency of Liver and Kidney Yin and Deficiency of Spleen Qi with Damp.[21]

Uveitis

Uveitis describes inflammation of the iris, ciliary body and the choroid layer of the eye (also known as the uveal tract). Depending on which of these three structures is predominantly affected, uveitis may also be termed iritis, cyclitis, choroiditis or posterior uveitis.

Uveitis can develop for no obvious reason, but in approximately half of cases it is associated with a more generalized disease, the most common of these being ankylosing spondylitis, juvenile arthritis, inflammatory bowel disease and chronic infections including those of cytomegalovirus (CMV), toxoplasmosis and human immunodeficiency virus (HIV).

Uveitis can flare up and then settle down (a relapsing-remitting condition), but there is a significant risk of permanent damage to the eye during an attack as a result of the inflammation. For this reason, a case of uveitis is treated with urgency in conventional medicine.

The patient with uveitis will experience intense pain in one eye, and the eye may appear red, with the redness particularly marked around the iris. This is in contrast with the redness and discomfort of the more benign condition of conjunctivitis, in which the redness is usually bilateral and affects the whole of the conjunctiva. In uveitis there will be blurring of the vision and a dislike of bright light.

The patient with uveitis will be examined by means of slit lamp. In an established case this will reveal inflammatory cells collecting in front of the iris, and may indicate that the iris is distorted, as there is a tendency for it to adhere to the lens as a result of the inflammation. If this is the first attack, the patient may well be offered a number of investigations to exclude a more generalized underlying condition.

The treatment of uveitis involves dilatation of the pupil by means of mydriatic eye drops (containing a drug such as atropine or cyclopentolate). This treatment prevents the iris from adhering to the lens, and so prevents scarring of these delicate tissues. Corticosteroids are applied in drop form to reduce the inflammation.

The risks of uveitis are that recurrent attacks can promote the development of cataracts and glaucoma (see below).

 Information box 6.1d-XIV

Uveitis: comments from a Chinese medicine perspective

From a Chinese medicine perspective, an attack of uveitis might correspond either to an Invasion of Wind Heat or to Rising of Liver Fire.

Glaucoma

Glaucoma is a term used to describe any condition in which the pressure of the fluid within the eyeball (intraocular pressure) is raised. The problem with glaucoma is that, over time, the increased pressure will damage the retina and the head of the optic nerve, and so will affect visual acuity. If the rise in pressure is sudden (acute glaucoma), the condition can be very painful.

The intraocular pressure depends on the production of the aqueous humor, the fluid inside the body of the eye, and also on the rate of its removal. In glaucoma, the pressure becomes raised because the fluid is not removed at the same rate at which it is produced. Aqueous humor normally drains from the eye through a meshwork of tissue situated in the angle between the iris and the cornea in the anterior chamber of the eye.

In those people who have an inherited tendency to glaucoma, this meshwork appears to become increasingly resistant to the outflow of fluid, and so the pressure in the eye rises slowly and painlessly. This is known as primary open angle glaucoma. It is a relatively common condition, being present in 1 in 200 people over the age of 40. The prevalence of the condition rises with age, so that 10 percent of those who are over 80 are known to have developed this form of glaucoma.

In some people the meshwork becomes blocked because of a condition that has developed in later life, such as uveitis or a traumatic bleed in the anterior chamber of the eye. In this case the condition is known as secondary glaucoma, and may develop fairly suddenly or slowly, depending on the cause.

Acute closed-angle glaucoma results from a sudden blockage of the angled area in which the meshwork is situated, and tends to occur in people who have a naturally narrow angle to the anterior chamber of their eyes. The acute attack is triggered in such people by administration of pupil-dilating medication (mydriatic drops).

In slowly developing chronic glaucoma of whatever cause, the patient will initially be unaware of the presence of the condition. Unless it is picked up early by an optometrist, undiagnosed glaucoma can lead to progressive damage to the optic nerve, and ultimately to loss of visual acuity. Classically, a patient with untreated chronic glaucoma will experience tunnel vision as it is primarily the periphery of the field of vision that is affected.

Chronic glaucoma is diagnosed and assessed painlessly by means of slit lamp tonometry. During this procedure both the intraocular pressure and the angle of the anterior chamber of the eye can be measured, and the optic nerve head can be examined.

Treatment for chronic glaucoma includes medication to reduce the production of aqueous humor. For example, beta blockers such as timolol are commonly prescribed in drop form to be administered twice daily on a long-term basis. Laser treatment to the meshwork may offer temporary relief of the intraocular pressure, but it often starts rising again after a short respite. Surgical opening of the anterior chamber to the space that lies under the conjunctiva (trabeculectomy) may be a preferred option.

Acute closed-angle glaucoma presents as an emergency, with excruciating pain in the tense eyeball. The pain is often so severe as to be associated with vomiting. The patient may also complain of distorted or lost vision. Urgent treatment is required, not only to reduce the pain, but also to prevent permanent damage to the vision. In an acute attack the eye is red and the cornea may appear cloudy. The pupil may be fixed and dilated.

Treatment involves the administration of painkillers, drugs that inhibit the formation of the aqueous humor (intravenous acetazolamide and topical beta blocker drops), and a drug to constrict the pupil and so open the angle of the anterior chamber of the eye (topical pilocarpine drops). Subsequent attacks are prevented by the surgical operation of iridectomy, in which a small hole is made in the iris.

Information box 6.1d-XV

Glaucoma: comments from a Chinese medicine perspective

From a Chinese medicine perspective, acute glaucoma is clearly a Full condition. The intensity of pain suggests Heat. Possible diagnoses include Liver Fire and Liver Blood Stagnation.

Chronic glaucoma presents in a similar way to cataract, in the form of steady loss of visual acuity, and so the Chinese diagnoses may include patterns that might lead to lack of nourishment of the eye such as Liver and Kidney Yin Deficiency. The fact that fluid is accumulating does, of course, suggest that Damp may be an additional Pathogenic Factor.

Age-related macular degeneration (ARMD)

The macula lutea, also known as the yellow spot, is the name given to the part of the retina on to which the center of the field of vision is focused. If the macula is damaged, the affected eye will never be able to generate a clear image of a viewed object.

Degeneration of the delicate cells of the retina with old age is a well-recognized phenomenon, and is the most important cause of irreversible visual loss in the West. An affected patient will experience blurring of vision and may also describe distorted vision. As peripheral vision is retained, the condition will not progress to total blindness. Cigarette smoking is a known risk factor for age-related macular degeneration (ARMD), and zinc and antioxidants (such as might be obtained from tomatoes, peppers and leafy vegetables) are thought to be protective.

ARMD can be diagnosed on the basis of the reduction in vision and the characteristic retinal changes that can be detected by means of the ophthalmoscope.

For most patients there is no known curative treatment. In a minority, with the more rapidly progressive wet form of ARMD, laser therapy can help impede the progression of the degeneration. Injections directly into the eye of a monoclonal antibody drug (ranibizumab), which prevents overgrowth of epithelial cells, have also been shown to slow the progression of wet ARMD. All patients can be helped by means of magnifying aids.

Diabetic retinopathy

The retina is dependent on a rich and consistent blood supply for optimal function. In diabetes, because of sugar-related damage to the retinal capillaries, there are three important ways in which the retina can become damaged. First, tiny leaks of blood and fat-containing fluid can be deposited outside the vessels and progressively damage the retina. Second, clots in the vessels can lead to infarcts in the retina. Although these are also tiny, as they accumulate, more and more of the field of vision becomes impaired. Finally, as the retina is starved of a rich supply of oxygen, its vessels are stimulated to sprout new branches. Although this is a healthy response in most of the body, in the eye this neovascularization crowds the retina with branching capillaries that literally block out the field of vision.

The first warning features of retinopathy can be detected by ophthalmoscopic examination even before the patient experiences any visual loss. If the characteristic changes are detected, the patient can be referred for preventive laser treatment to the retina. This outpatient procedure prevents leaks and also reduces neovascularization. The patient will also be counseled about the need to be very attentive to blood sugar levels, as the progression of diabetic retinopathy appears to be directly related to how often the blood sugar is poorly controlled. Smoking and poor control of blood pressure are also risk factors.

Diabetes is also associated with the development of cataract and glaucoma. Because of the seriousness of retinopathy and the other ocular complications, all patients with diabetes should undergo an ophthalmoscopic examination at least once a year.

Conditions of the optic nerve

Optic neuritis

Optic neuritis is the term used to describe inflammation of the optic nerve and optic nerve head, the point at which the optic nerve meets the retina. In many cases the cause of an episode of optic neuritis is unclear, although such an episode very often (in 40–70 percent of cases) turns out to be the first in a series of neurological episodes in a case of multiple sclerosis.

Optic neuritis is characterized by a sudden deterioration of vision, and pain on movement of the eyes (as eye movements lead to traction of the optic nerve). The deterioration in vision can then progress over the course of the next few days.

On ophthalmoscopic examination, the blind-spot area (optic disc) of the retina may appear swollen (papilledema), and tests of acuity will demonstrate impairment in both acuity and color vision.

No treatment is usually offered, although in a severe attack a short course of intravenous corticosteroids may be prescribed. After a period of days to weeks normal vision is resumed, although acuity is often never as sharp as it was before. A skilled examiner will notice that after the attack the optic disc appears paler than it should.

Information box 6.1d-XVI

Optic neuritis: comments from a Chinese medicine perspective

Optic neuritis manifests with a sudden deterioration of vision, which very commonly occurs in the context of multiple sclerosis (MS). In Chinese medicine, MS is a form of Atrophy Syndrome. Maciocia (1989) attributes the visual symptoms of MS to the Kidney–Liver Deficiency that is characteristic of the condition.[22] The sudden onset of optic neuritis is an indication of Wind Invading the Channels of the eye, presumably on a background of more longstanding Deficiency.

The red flags of diseases of the eye

Some people with diseases of the eye will benefit from referral to a conventional doctor for assessment and/or treatment. Red flags are those symptoms and signs that indicate that referral should be considered. The red flags of the diseases of the eye are described in Table 6.1d-I. A summary of the red flags in a format designed for quick reference in clinical practice can be found in Appendix III. This gives advice on the degree of urgency of referral for each of the red flag conditions listed.

Table 6.1d-I A42: Red flags of diseases of the eye

Red flag	Description	Reasoning
A42.1	An intensely painful and red eye	A painful red eye could result from iritis, choroiditis, acute glaucoma, corneal ulcer or keratitis. All these are serious conditions, and the patient should be advised to attend either their doctor or the nearest eye emergency department for early assessment
A42.2	A painful, red and swollen eye and eyelids: patient (often a child) is very unwell	If the eye and the surrounding tissues are intensely painful and swollen, this could be a spreading infection of the soft tissues of the eye (orbital cellulitis). Refer urgently to the emergency department
A42.3	A painful eye with no obvious inflammation: eye movements are painful	Deep, intense pain exacerbated by eye movement is characteristic of optic neuritis or choroiditis. Refer as a high priority to the nearest emergency department
A42.4	Discharge from the eye: if severe, prolonged and painful, or if seen in the following vulnerable groups: the newborn, those who are immunocompromised, those who are malnourished	Discharge from the eye(s) is usually the result of acute allergic, bacterial or viral conjunctivitis, and as such is usually self-limiting, and will not necessarily require antibiotic treatment. Advise the patient that they may be very contagious while the eye is discharging Only consider referral if the discharge continues for >5 days or if there is any pain
A42.5	Sudden onset of painless blurring or loss of sight in one or both eyes	Loss of sight or blurring in one or both eyes may be due to thromboembolic disease, optic neuritis, retinal tear or corneal ulcer. Some of these conditions require high-priority treatment to prevent blindness, so refer as a high priority to nearest emergency department Floaters and blurring alone in middle age is usually the result of the benign condition of vitreous detachment. Nevertheless, referral is advised to exclude the more serious possible causes
A42.6	Sudden onset of painless blurring or loss of sight in one or both eyes accompanied by one-sided headache	Loss of sight accompanied by a headache in an older person (>50 years) may represent temporal arteritis. This is more likely to occur in someone who has been diagnosed with polymyalgia rheumatica (see A28.3). Urgent treatment with corticosteroids may prevent progression to blindness. Refer urgently to the nearest emergency department
A42.7	Gradual onset of painless blurring or loss of sight in one or both eyes	Refer for assessment, as treatment of the causes of gradual loss of sight may prevent progressive deterioration of the sight Causes include refractive error, cataract, glaucoma and macular degeneration

A42.8	Squint: in any child if previously undiagnosed	Refer any child who demonstrates a previously undiagnosed squint. In young children this usually results from a congenital weakness of the external ocular muscles, but needs ophthalmological assessment to prevent long-term inhibition of depth vision. If appearing in older children, it may signify a tumor of the brain, pituitary or orbital cavity
A42.9	Recent onset of double vision in an adult	Double vision suggests a physical distortion of the orbital cavity or damage to a cranial nerve. Refer as a high priority
A42.10	Recent onset of drooping eyelid (ptosis)	Ptosis suggests damage to a nerve due to a tumor, or muscle-wasting disease. Refer for investigation
A42.11	Features of thyroid eye disease: staring eyes, whites visible above and below pupils, inflamed conjunctivae, symptoms of hyperthyroidism (tremor, agitation, weight loss, palpitations)	Thyroid eye disease results from specific antibodies that are generated in Graves' disease. If severe it can threaten the health of the eyes, as soft tissue builds up in the orbit, pushing the eye forward and putting pressure on the optic nerve
A42.12	Inability to close the eye	The eye may not close fully in thyroid eye disease and also in Bell's palsy. This can rapidly lead to serious damage to the conjunctiva and cornea (which rely on the moistness of tears to remain healthy) A simple first aid treatment is to keep the affected eye shut with a pad held in place with medical tape until medical advice has been sought
A42.13	Foreign body in the eye	If there is a foreign body that cannot be removed, gently keep the lid closed by means of a pad and medical tape and arrange urgent assessment at the nearest eye emergency department

6.1e Diseases of the ear

Most of the important diseases of the ear are managed within the conventional surgical specialty of otorhinolaryngology, which is the Latinized term for the study of the ear, nose and throat. This specialty falls into the domain of the surgeons, because much of the management of the serious disease of the ear, nose and throat requires surgical treatment of one form or another.

Those conditions of the nose and throat that require medical management are managed within the broader specialty of respiratory medicine, or within general practice if fairly minor (e.g. chronic sinusitis and pharyngitis). Most of the medical management of ear conditions occurs within general practice in the UK (e.g. treatment of otitis externa or otitis media).

The conditions described in this section are:

- Deafness
- Conductive deafness:
  - obstruction by wax
  - acute otitis media (AOM)
  - chronic secretory otitis media (CSOM) (glue ear)
  - chronic otitis media
  - otosclerosis
  - otitis externa and furunculosis
- Sensorineural deafness:
  - congenital deafness
  - deafness of old age (presbycusis)
  - noise-induced deafness
  - Ménière's disease
  - acoustic neuroma
  - deafness due to drugs and infections
- Earache:
  - dental and mandibular causes
  - pharyngeal and laryngeal causes
  - cervical spondylosis
- Tinnitus – local causes:
  - wax and serous otitis media
  - Ménière's disease
  - presbycusis (see under "Deafness")
  - otosclerosis (see under "Deafness")
  - noise-related

- Tinnitus – general causes:
  - fever
  - disease of the nervous system
  - anemia
  - drugs and alcohol abuse
- Vertigo:
  - vestibular neuritis
  - benign paroxysmal vertigo
  - central causes of vertigo.

Deafness

The causes of reduced hearing and deafness can be broadly categorized into two groups: those that result from disease of the external and middle ear, and those that result from damage to the sensory apparatus in the inner ear and the neural pathways that conduct nervous impulses resulting from sounds to the auditory centers in the brain.

Deafness resulting from the first group of causes is described as conductive, so called because it is the result of a problem in the conduction of sound waves to the inner ear. Deafness resulting from the second group of causes is termed sensorineural, because in this case it is the sensory apparatus or the neural pathways that are at fault. A simple tuning fork test can be used to distinguish between the two causes of deafness, although a more accurate assessment can be made by means of audiology tests.

If the cause of the deafness cannot be treated, for example, in deafness of old age, a hearing aid will be considered. Most hearing aids currently prescribed are worn behind the ear, and are attached to a tiny speaker device fitted into the patient's ear. A more sophisticated form of this sort of aid has all the electronics built into the device that is inserted directly into the auditory canal, so obviating the need for a behind-the-ear component to the aid. Some patient groups, for example, children, will be more suited to an aid that is held in a pocket attached to the clothing, and linked to the speaker by means of a flexible wire. In all these forms of aids the principle is simple amplification and then redirection of the amplified sounds directly into the auditory canal. This is a less than perfect solution for sensorineural forms of deafness, as there can be a very narrow threshold between sound that can be heard and sound that is too loud to be tolerated. Many modern hearing aids are fitted with a loop inductance system to facilitate the use of the telephone.

More recently, bone-anchored hearing aids have been developed that direct amplified sounds via a surgically implanted titanium screw through the temporal bone towards the inner ear. These aids are of value in patients who have disease of the outer or middle ear, which would prevent the use of the usual forms of hearing aid.

The cochlear implant involves the insertion of a range of electrodes directly into the cochlea (inner ear). The electrodes receive sound information from an externally situated microphone, and convert this information into impulses within the auditory nerve. This technically very complex device is only suitable for those who have absolute hearing loss, as the information that they generate in the auditory nerve is of a different quality to that generated by sound. Nevertheless, for those who are profoundly deaf, the brain can learn to process the nerve impulses to enable lip reading, speech and, in some cases, the ability to converse by telephone. Cochlear implants are now available for small children.

Lip reading is a valuable skill for the hearing impaired, and one that can be taught by skilled instructors. It is easier to acquire this skill while there is some residual hearing, so in a case of progressive hearing loss the patient should be urged to get instruction in lip reading as early as possible.

 Information box 6.1e-I

Deafness: comments from a Chinese medicine perspective

From a Chinese medicine viewpoint, impairment of hearing may be the result of a Full condition or a Deficient condition, or a combination of the two. Possible Full conditions include Phlegm and Damp obstructing the Shao Yang Channels (Gallbladder and Triple Heater), and Liver and Gallbladder Fire Rising. Deficient conditions include Kidney Qi Deficiency and Heart Qi Deficiency. As Deficiency of Kidney Yin can predispose to the Flaring Up of Liver Yang and Fire, it may be appreciated that deafness can be a mixed condition.

Conductive deafness

Obstruction by wax

Earwax is a protective secretion that is produced by modified sweat glands in the outer ear canal. It contains antibodies and is sticky, which enables the trapping and removal of dirt and foreign bodies from the canal. Some people produce more wax than others and so are more likely to develop obstruction by wax. Also, misguided attempts to clean the ear by the insertion of a hard object such as a cotton bud very often lead to impaction of the wax deep in the ear canal. Frequent immersion of the ears in water can also precipitate impaction by wax, as saturated wax tends to expand as it absorbs water.

Impacted wax can be the cause of pain, vertigo and deafness, but can easily be removed by syringing. If the wax is likely to be hardened, the application of olive oil or sodium bicarbonate drops nightly for one week can facilitate the syringing process. The syringing procedure involves the direction of a jet of warm salt water along the roof of the auditory canal, by means of either a manual syringe or an electric pump-powered water jet.

Information box 6.1e-II

Obstruction by wax: comments from a Chinese medicine perspective

In deafness resulting from obstruction by wax, a possible Chinese medicine diagnosis is Phlegm Damp obstructing the Shao Yang Channels.

Acute otitis media (AOM)

Acute otitis media (AOM) is the result of bacterial or viral infection of the middle ear. It can cause temporary deafness, and can predispose to the development of glue ear or chronic secretory otitis media, an important cause of hearing impairment in children under ten (see Section 5.4d).

Information box 6.1e-III

Acute otitis media: comments from a Chinese medicine perspective

In Chinese medicine, AOM might be a manifestation of an External Invasion of the Shao Yang Channels by Wind Heat or Wind Cold. Damp is sometimes an additional Pathogenic Factor. In older children Heat can also enter the Liver and Gallbladder Channels, and then rise up to manifest as pain and heat in the ear. In these children constraint of Liver Qi leading to Heat might be a predisposing factor. Recurrent attacks of otitis media might suggest a Lingering Pathogenic Factor.

Chronic secretory otitis media (CSOM) (glue ear)

Chronic secretory otitis media (CSOM) (also termed otitis media with effusion) is a very important cause of conductive deafness in children (see Section 5.4e).

Information box 6.1e-IV

Chronic secretory otitis media: comments from a Chinese medicine perspective

In Chinese medicine, CSOM may correspond to Lingering Pathogenic Factor. This can result in the buildup of Phlegm and the Obstruction of Qi in the ear cavity. The child may also suffer from a pre-existing Depletion of Spleen Qi. This can contribute to the accumulation of Damp and Phlegm.

Alternatively, and less commonly, Depletion of Liver and Kidney Yin may lead to undernourishment of the ear. This would lead to a sticky fluid on the eardrum rather than profuse phlegmy discharge. In these cases the Depletion may be a result of overstimulation, and may result in a slightly hyperactive child.

Chronic otitis media

Chronic otitis media (also known as chronic suppurative otitis media) is a confusingly named, long-term consequence of AOM. It has to be distinguished from CSOM, which is the non-infective condition of childhood also known as glue ear (see above). Chronic otitis media is much more common in undernourished or immunocompromised children.

In chronic otitis media there has been failure of resolution of the infectious process of acute otitis media. This means that there is an ongoing infective process with the production of damaging pus. Although the eardrum normally heals over after the perforation that can occur in AOM, in chronic cases the continued production of pus prevents this healing process, the eardrum retains its perforation and the ear continues to discharge pus.

If the infection simply affects the lining of the middle ear and the eardrum, there is a good chance of healing with the combined treatments of meticulous cleaning of the ear by means of delicate suction and mopping, along with appropriate antibiotic therapy.

The condition is much more serious if the infection has spread to the tiny bony structures within the ear or into the bony walls of the middle ear and the mastoid process. In this sort of case, surgery is required to clear away any infected material and bony regions. A mastoidectomy is one of the operations performed for bony chronic otitis media. The surgery required for middle ear damage is extremely delicate, and may involve refashioning of the eardrum and ossicles in order to preserve hearing.

The presence of chronic infection in the middle ear can also predispose to other deep serious conditions, including meningitis, acute mastoiditis (an acute pus-forming infection of the air cells in the mastoid process), brain abscess and paralysis of the facial nerve (this presents like Bell's palsy).

Information box 6.1e-V

Chronic otitis media: comments from a Chinese medicine perspective

From a Chinese medicine perspective, the chronic production of pus indicates Damp Heat against a background of chronic Deficiency, and in particular, of the Spleen and Kidneys. Progressive erosion of the bony walls of the middle ear as a consequence of chronic infection suggests Phlegm and Kidney Yin Deficiency.

Otosclerosis

Otosclerosis is a hereditary condition in which there is a progressive development of deafness as a result of abnormal bone growth around the base of the stapes, the stirrup-shaped ossicle of the middle ear. This growth can be worsened in pregnancy, and so the condition is more common in women. The operation of stapedotomy involves replacing the affected end of the stapes with a steel implant, but carries a small risk of total loss of hearing. If successful, and performed early in the progression of the condition, normal hearing can be regained.

Information box 6.1e-VI

Otosclerosis: comments from a Chinese medicine perspective

Because of its progressive and hereditary nature, otosclerosis would suggest a Chinese medicine diagnosis of Jing Deficiency.

Otitis externa and furunculosis

Otitis externa is the term given to any condition in which there is inflammation of the epithelium that lines the external ear canal. Common causes include fungal and bacterial infections, and contact eczema resulting from sensitivity to environmental substances. The symptoms and signs include itching, crusting and sometimes intense discomfort of the ear canal and the pinna of the ear. It is important to ensure that the crusting and discharge do not, in fact, originate from a discharging middle ear infection, so an otoscopic examination is advisable.

The condition can be triggered by persistent dampness of the ear canals, such as might affect frequent swimmers, sensitivity to environmental substances, such as shampoo, and medical treatments, such as antibiotic ear drops. Trauma to the ear canal as a result of attempts to scratch or clean the affected area can exacerbate the condition.

Treatment would include avoidance of immersion of the ears and of any potential skin sensitizers. A piece of cotton wool coated in Vaseline can prevent water entering the ears when showering, and ear plugs are recommended for swimming. Medical treatments include careful cleaning of the ears (dry mopping) and syringing. In severe cases dressings soaked in antibacterial, antifungal and corticosteroid medication can be inserted into the ear on a daily basis, and if less severe, the patient can self-administer a combination of antibiotic and steroid ear drops.

Furunculosis describes the tendency for small boils to form at the base of hair follicles in the external ear canal. Because the skin in this area is tightly apposed to the bony cavity through which the ear canal passes, furunculosis can be extremely painful. It is more common in people who suffer from diabetes, so this diagnosis should be excluded. Medical treatment includes insertion of a wick soaked in icthammol to help the boil come to a head, and antibiotics by injection if the condition is severe.

Both conditions can be a cause of deafness resulting from occlusion of the ear canal.

Information box 6.1e-VII

Otitis externa and furunculosis: comments from a Chinese medicine perspective

In Chinese medicine, otitis externa could represent an Invasion of Wind Damp Heat, or simply Damp Heat if the condition is chronic. Likewise, furunculosis would seem to be consistent with a manifestation of Damp Heat.

Sensorineural deafness

Congenital deafness

Congenital deafness is recognized to affect 1 in 1000 children. Early diagnosis is considered essential, and so in the UK there is now a routine neonatal hearing screening program (see Section 5.4c).

Deafness of old age

Deafness of old age, also termed presbycusis, is the most common cause of sensorineural deafness. In this case the deafness is simply the result of a gradual degeneration of the delicate structure of the cochlea and the vestibular nerve. The onset is characteristically gradual, and the deafness is more marked for sounds of high frequency (the range of female voices). The usual treatment for presbycusis is the prescription of a hearing aid.

A sudden onset of deafness in old age would be most likely the result of a vascular stroke or a viral infection on the vestibular nerve.

Information box 6.1e-VIII

Deafness of old age (presbycusis): comments from a Chinese medicine perspective

In Chinese medicine, presbycusis is a manifestation of declining Kidney Qi failing to nourish the ears.

Noise-induced deafness

Noise-induced deafness can be a component of presbycusis. In this case the deafness to high-frequency sounds is more marked because of trauma to the sensory cells of the cochlea from exposure to high-intensity sounds. Usually, for the deafness to be long term, the exposure to the sounds has to have been repeated over a prolonged period.

Noise-induced deafness is a recognized risk in some occupations, such as in the construction industry, and in this case it is the duty of the employer to ensure that exposed employees are provided with suitable protective ear muffs. Affected employees may be eligible for compensation.

Ménière's disease

In Ménière's disease, the fluid-filled labyrinth of one or both cochleas becomes waterlogged with excessive fluid. Onset is usually after the age of 40. The cause is unknown.

The symptoms of Ménière's disease include disabling vertigo, deafness and tinnitus, each of which typically appear in bouts, although the tinnitus and slight deafness can become persistent. In an acute attack the vertigo often will cause prostration and vomiting, and emergency treatment with an injection of a sedating antiemetic medication such as prochlorperazine can be helpful.

Advice for the prevention of attacks includes fluid and salt restriction, and avoidance of coffee, alcohol and smoking. Betahistine hydrochloride and cinnarizine are commonly prescribed drugs to be taken on a regular basis to reduce the frequency of attacks.

Surgical options for Ménière's disease are available but carry the risk of inducing deafness on the operated side, and so are usually only offered in severe cases or in those cases in which deafness is already established.

Information box 6.1e-IX

Ménière's disease: comments from a Chinese medicine perspective

Ménière's disease has the characteristics of a Full condition. A possible Chinese medicine interpretation would be Phlegm and Damp obstructing the Rising of Qi on a basis of underlying Depletion of Kidney Qi.

Acoustic neuroma

An acoustic neuroma is a benign, slow-growing tumor of the vestibular (acoustic) nerve. The tumor typically presents with the gradual onset of one-sided deafness and/or loss of balance. The diagnosis can be confirmed by a magnetic resonance imaging (MRI) scan. Early diagnosis can maximize the chances of a safe operative removal of the tumor, although surgery is unlikely to restore normal hearing on the affected side.

Information box 6.1e-X

Acoustic neuroma: comments from a Chinese medicine perspective

As it is a tumor, in Chinese medicine the symptoms of an acoustic neuroma will correspond to Phlegm and/or Stagnation on the basis of an underlying state of Depletion of Kidney Qi.

Deafness due to drugs and infections

Some prescribed medications, including certain antibiotics, aspirin, some diuretics and beta blockers, can, in rare cases, lead to deafness. In most cases the hearing impairment will abate on the withdrawal from the medication.

Certain infections can cause inflammation of the vestibular nerve, and so cause sudden deafness. This is a medical emergency that merits immediate referral. Mumps, herpes zoster virus, meningitis and syphilis are all recognized to be causes of deafness.

Earache

Earache can result from a number of the diseases of the ear already discussed. These include otitis externa and furunculosis, mastoiditis and acute and chronic otitis media. There is also a range of other conditions that lead to referred pain in the ear. This is because branches from four of the facial nerves and also the nerves emerging from the C1 and C2 levels of the cord also lead to the ear. Even though in these conditions the seat of the pain is elsewhere, acupuncture or electro-acupuncture focused on points close to the ear, the site of the pain, can be effective.

Dental and mandibular causes

Impacted wisdom teeth and dental caries of the molars (back teeth) can lead to pain in the ear. Excessive tension or arthritis of the temporomandibular joint (TMJ) can also lead to referred ear pain. With TMJ dysfunction, there is commonly also a trigger point in the masseter muscle that is worth treating by means of massage or acupuncture.

Pharyngeal and laryngeal causes

Pain from tonsillitis, quinsy and disease of the base of the tongue may also refer to the ear because a branch of the glossopharyngeal nerve also supplies the eardrum. Cancer of the larynx or pharynx can lead to sustained unexplained earache, and so if this is mentioned by a patient, it should be referred for investigation.

Cervical spondylosis

Rarely, pain from cervical spondylosis can be felt in the ear.

 Information box 6.1e-XI

Earache: comments from a Chinese medicine perspective

From a Chinese medicine perspective, pain felt in the ear is in all cases a reflection of Stagnation of Qi in the Channels associated with the ear. The underlying cause of this Stagnation will relate to the underlying cause of the pain.

Tinnitus

Tinnitus is the term used to describe the sensation of noises in the ears. Tinnitus may be unilateral or bilateral, high pitched or low pitched, intermittent or constant. Tinnitus is generally more troubling in quiet environments, as external noise can serve as a distraction from the internally generated sounds. Tinnitus, if persistent, can markedly affect quality of life. If the cause is unknown or cannot be treated, then hearing aid-like tinnitus maskers, which are designed to produce white noise, can make the tinnitus less obtrusive. Sometimes a radio playing in the background can provide the patient with relief from the noise.

In many cases the cause of tinnitus cannot be explained. Tinnitus may be the result of disease within the ear itself or can result from more general disease.

Local causes of tinnitus

Tinnitus can result from wax in the external ear canal and fluid in the middle ear, such as develops in CSOM (glue ear). It is also a well-known complication of Ménière's disease and otosclerosis. It is also associated with the development of presbycusis and noise damage to the ears.

General causes of tinnitus

Tinnitus can also result from more generalized conditions. For example, it is well recognized as a transient symptom of fever. It may also accompany a diagnosis of anemia and some degenerative diseases of the nervous system (e.g. MS). Certain medications (including aspirin) and alcohol abuse are toxic causes of tinnitus.

Vertigo

The medical definition of vertigo is the experience of movement, often manifesting as a spinning sensation. When patients describe a sensation of dizziness this need not mean vertigo, as this term is often used to describe a feeling of faintness or light-headedness. Vertigo can only be ascribed if the patient describes a moving sensation (as if they had just got off a boat or a roundabout).

Sustained vertigo is most unpleasant, and is often accompanied by sweating and vomiting. It is an absolute contraindication to driving. Patients who suffer from vertigo should be advised not to drive until they are free from episodes of dizziness.

Tranquillizing drugs such as prochlorperazine, chlorpromazine and cinnarizine can all be effective in reducing the severity of the symptoms of vertigo. These are the same type of drugs that are prescribed to prevent motion sickness.

Vertigo originates either from a disorder of the semicircular canals of the inner ear, or from the brainstem.

 Information box 6.1e-XII

Vertigo: comments from a Chinese medicine perspective

In Chinese medicine, the symptom of vertigo is a manifestation of Liver Wind Rising and/or Turbid Phlegm. Wind is implicated if the episodes are sudden in onset.

Vestibular neuritis (labyrinthitis)

Vestibular neuritis is probably the most common cause of sustained vertigo in young people. This presumed viral infection often accompanies the onset of a cold, and leads to a sudden onset of severe vertigo, which may then be episodic. In most cases there is full recovery, although this can be very gradual and may take a few weeks.

Benign paroxysmal vertigo

This episodic form of vertigo manifests in brief episodes of dizziness, which are triggered by a postural change to the head. It is the result of a mild degenerative change in the semicircular canals of the ears.

Central causes of vertigo

Damage to areas of the brainstem, such as can occur in strokes or the demyelination of MS, can result in loss of balance and vertigo. In such cases the vertigo is usually fairly short-lived (lasting no more than a few weeks), but if the damage is significant, the loss of balance may persist.

The red flags of diseases of the ear

Some people with diseases of the ear will benefit from referral to a conventional doctor for assessment and/or treatment. Red flags are those symptoms and signs that indicate that referral should be considered. The red flags of the diseases of the ear are described in Table 6.1e-I. A summary of the red flags in a format designed for quick reference in clinical practice can be found in Appendix III. This gives advice on the degree of urgency of referral for each of the red flag conditions listed.

Table 6.1e-I A43: Red flags of diseases of the ear

Red flag	Description	Reasoning
A43.1	Vertigo in a young person: lasting for >6 weeks, or if so severe as to be causing recurrent vomiting, or if patient may be at increased risk of stroke (e.g. in pregnancy, or previous episode)	The most likely cause of a sudden onset of dizzy spells in a young person is an inflammation of the inner ear (labyrinthitis). This usually settles down completely within six weeks. Medical treatment is to prescribe anti-sickness medication, so only refer if the sickness does not respond to treatment. Rarely, a sudden onset of dizziness is the consequence of a stroke or multiple sclerosis (MS). Consider referral if there has been any previous episode of neurological disturbance (e.g. blurred vision or numbness) or if there is an increased risk or history of thromboembolic disease
A43.2	Vertigo in an older person (>45 years)	Refer so that the patient can have investigations to exclude the possibility of stroke (dizziness can result from brainstem or cerebellar stroke). See A22.3
A43.3	Complications of acute otitis media: persistent fever/pain/confusion for >3–4 days after the onset of the earache (may indicate spread of the infection, e.g. mastoiditis or brain abscess)	Otitis media is an uncomfortable but self-limiting ear infection that commonly affects young children. It is now considered good practice not to prescribe antibiotics in a simple case, which will generally settle within 1–3 days If there is discharge following natural perforation of the eardrum, medical advice is for antibiotics to be prescribed to prevent persisting or deepening infection, and this should be discussed with the parents of the child Persisting high fever, confusion or intense pain is not usual, and the child should be referred as a priority to exclude the rare possibility of infectious complications
A43.4	Persistent discharge from the ear	Chronic discharge from the ear for >1 week after the infection of otitis media has settled down may indicate the development of chronic otitis media, and this needs further investigation, as there is risk of permanent damage to the middle ear
A43.5	Features of mastoiditis: fever, with a painful and swollen mastoid bone (the bony prominence of the skull immediately behind the ear)	Mastoiditis is a now rare complication of otitis media, and usually affects children. It is a serious condition, as it is a bone infection and so can be difficult to treat with antibiotics Refer as a high priority
A43.6	New onset of hearing difficulty in a child: lasting for >3 weeks	Refer if prolonged, if interfering with social interactions and education, or if associated with pain in the ear or dizziness. The most likely cause is glue ear, a chronic accumulation of mucoid secretions in the middle ear

A43.7	Sudden onset of absolute deafness (one-sided or bilateral)	Absolute deafness suggests damage to the acoustic nerve or auditory centers of the brain, and requires high-priority assessment
A43.8	Gradual onset of relative deafness in an adult for >7 days	A degree of hearing loss is common after a cold, but has usually subsided within a week. If hearing loss is slow and progressive, referral for audiometric assessment is advised to exclude the rare, but treatable, slowly growing acoustic neuroma
		Earwax is one of the common causes of relative hearing loss, so it is useful to possess an otoscope to check for this treatable possibility (earwax can be softened by administering five drops of warmed olive oil in each ear, every night, for a week)
A43.9	Tinnitus if progressive or if associated with hearing loss	Tinnitus (ringing or buzzing in the ear) is usually a benign finding, and remains fairly constant, or may increase in times of stress. It is not normally progressive or associated with hearing loss, and if it is, this may suggest a progressive disorder of the ear or the auditory nerve. Refer to the general practitioner (GP) for audiometric assessment
A43.10	Earache in an adult for >3 weeks	Earache is common after a cold, but should subside within a week or so. If persistent (>3 weeks) and unexplained, referral is merited as this is a red flag for cancer of the nasopharynx

Mental Health

6.2a Introduction to mental health

This chapter is dedicated to the study of the mind and its related diseases. Unlike all other physiological systems, the physical structure and functioning of the mind cannot be scientifically measured and described. This is in stark contrast to the measurability of anatomy and physiology of a system such as the skin or the blood. Despite this profound difference, in many ways the mind and its related diseases are categorized and studied within conventional medicine by means of a very similar approach to that used in the study of the more physically defined systems.

In conventional medicine the diseases of the mind are termed mental health disorders. The mental health disorders are managed within the medical specialty of psychiatry and the non-medical clinical specialty of psychology.

The medical specialty of psychiatry is a relatively young discipline in the history of conventional medicine. The term is derived from the Greek words *psyche* (meaning mind) and *iatros* (meaning doctor). Psychiatry is the specialty dedicated to the medical treatment of mental health disorders.

Psychology is a term used to describe the academic and clinical disciplines that are based on the study of the workings of the mind. A clinical psychologist is a therapist who has gained a degree in psychology, and then undergone further training in the practical application of psychology in the clinical situation.

Psychotherapy (literally meaning treatment for the mind) is a term that describes any approach that involves the use of the formal and systematic clinical relationship between the therapist and the client as a therapeutic tool. Psychotherapy may be utilized by psychiatrists and clinical psychologists, but also by practitioners who have undergone specific training in one (or more) particular form(s) of therapy. The different types of psychotherapy are explored in more detail in Section 6.2c.

The aim of this section is to introduce the general approach by which mental health disorders are understood conventionally. Psychiatrists and psychologists classify these disorders in a quasi-systematic way, but, unlike most of the diseases studied within the other medical specialties, the two classification systems currently used are in large part based on the manifestation (symptoms and signs) of the disorder rather than on its physical cause(s).

The section begins with a brief exploration of how the mind is generally seen from a medical perspective as a distinct entity with respect to the other physiological systems. This is despite increasing scientific evidence that the mind is inextricably linked with (and may well even be rooted in) the function of these other systems. The section then goes on to consider the conventional understanding of the causation of mental illness.

Mental health and the mind-body divide

The very existence of the disciplines of psychiatry and psychology indicates the depth to which the mind has, in recent medical history, been perceived as a separate entity to the other physical systems of the body, such as the cardiovascular or the urinary systems, and even the central nervous system.

Doctors would generally assent to the understanding that the mind emanates from the workings of the brain. It is commonly believed that the neural pathways, synapses and neurochemicals that are clearly the foundation for the electrical activity of the brain are also the basis for thoughts, memories and emotions. However, this neuropsychiatric perspective is a relatively recent phenomenon, and historically the mind would not have been so absolutely located within the space of the cranium. For example, the *Oxford English Dictionary* defines the mind as "the seat of awareness, thought, volition and feeling...concentration [and] memory." The full dictionary description does not mention the brain, but instead describes the mind as if it were a distinct and free-floating entity. Moreover, even in medicine there seems to be a division between the mind and the brain. The structure and known workings of the brain are embraced within the medical specialty of neurology, and yet neurologists are not necessarily expert in the psychiatric diseases. The mind is managed within a totally different specialty. This reflects the fact that as yet the precise links between the workings of the physical brain and many mental health disorders have not been adequately explained.

The idea that the mind springs from the physical workings of the brain is a relatively recent development in Western culture. In contrast, the theory that the emotional and mental disorders were rooted in the bodily humors and their imbalances was described by the Greek physician Galen (circa 200 BC). The belief in the four humors and their expression in personality and emotional balance persisted throughout Europe well into the third and fourth centuries AD. Thereafter, in the West, the influence of the monasteries strengthened the ancient concept that mental illness resulted from a possession of the spirit by evil forces and was something that could afflict even the righteous.

With the intellectual revolution of the Enlightenment in the 17th and 18th centuries came an increasing appreciation of the physical world as something that could be understood by means of reason and scientific method. Mind and spirit were believed to be distinct from this physical domain. As church and state diverged, the care of those with mental ill health became the province of the medical profession, and illness of the mind was recognized as different from the biological illnesses that required physically based treatments. The practice of psychiatry as we recognize it today emerged out of the 19th-century phenomenon of asylums. These institutions were a response to the management of mental illness in the overcrowded industrial cities. In these settings doctors, and notably the German neurologist Emil Kraepelin, started to classify mental illness on the basis of common features, and conditions such as manic-depressive illness and schizophrenia (dementia praecox) were distinguished. The concept that there was possibly a biological basis for mental illness became more prominent in this time. This was despite the fact that very often there were no obvious signs apparent in the physical structure of the brains of those with mental ill health. Later in the early 20th century biological treatments such as electroconvulsive therapy and lithium and antidepressants (derived from medication first used to treat tuberculosis) were trialed on patients in asylums and found to have profound effects.[23]

These discoveries presaged the current psychiatric biopsychosocial model as the theoretical basis of psychiatric practice. This model proposes that psychiatric conditions arise as the result of a combination of biological, psychological and social factors. In this way their origin is seen as linked not only to the mind, but also to physical changes in the body and to factors in the social environment of the patient.

There is now an increasing body of scientific evidence that strongly links some mental health disorders with certain chemical imbalances of neurotransmitters in the brain, and, more controversially, with levels of the hormones that circulate throughout the whole body. This is the realm of neuropsychiatry, a rapidly expanding discipline in which the focus is on how disease of the chemical structure of the brain might manifest as mental illness.

Neuropsychiatry offers a conventional description of an undeniable link between mind and body (i.e. the physical structure of the brain). Moreover, as it is increasingly recognized that there is a significant overlap between the diverse neurotransmitters of the central nervous system and the hormones of the endocrine system, it becomes possible that this mind-body link need no longer be confined strictly to the brain. Instead, as a product of the subtleties of hormone expression, the changes that appear to spring from the mind might have their origin in diverse sites throughout the body.

Exciting though the potential for holism in these conventional explanations may be, the mind-body divide that first became apparent in the Enlightenment does not seem to have been eroded significantly in conventional medical practice. Currently, many patients of conventional hospital practitioners will experience their mental and physical problems being treated as if they have no relationship to each other (with the exception of those well-described diseases of the nervous system that are recognized to result in mental health dysfunction, such as multi-infarct dementia).

The definition of a mental health disorder

The American Psychiatric Association (APA) offers a definition of mental health disorder in the *Diagnostic and Statistical Manual of Mental Disorders*, 5th edition (DSM-5).[24]

This describes a mental health disorder in terms of it being a collection of symptoms and signs (a "syndrome") that is the result of a dysfunction of either the psychological, biological or developmental processes which underlie the workings of the mind. A mental health disorder according to DSM-5 would be expected to be a cause of distress for the patient. The definition also makes it clear that an expected and culturally understandable response such as grief does not constitute a mental illness, and neither does socially deviant behavior.

It is clear that both parts of this definition, the features of the syndrome and also what constitutes distress, would be difficult to define with objectivity. What might appear as distress or a disturbance in cognition or emotion regulation to the diagnosing doctor might not be so interpreted by the patient or within their culture of origin.

This definition is useful in explaining how mental health professionals interpret mental health states, and also what they believe to be the root cause of mental health disorders (i.e. a dysfunction in the psychological, biological or developmental processes underlying mental functioning). The definition reflects the biopsychosocial model of thought, which has been increasingly embraced within modern psychiatry.

The causation of mental health disorder: the biopsychosocial model

As implied by the APA definition of mental health disorder, the diverse mental health disorders are generally considered to have a multifactorial basis for their origin. Many psychiatrists would subscribe to this biopsychosocial model of mental illness. The term biopsychosocial refers to the understanding that a combination of inherited and acquired physical factors (biological factors), factors related to the emotional development of the individual (psychological factors) and factors related to the cultural environment of the individual (social factors) are all relevant in the development of a mental health disorder in an individual. Ideally, in every case presenting to a psychiatrist or psychologist, biological, psychological and social causes need to be considered.

Biological factors in mental health disorders

A biological theory of the causation of mental illness proposes that physical changes in the body are at the root of any illness. The biological perspective is supported by the fact that many diseases or conditions that are known to involve physical changes in the brain can manifest with mental disturbance (e.g. Alzheimer's disease, traumatic head injury, alcohol intoxication). Moreover, the fact that certain conditions tend to run in families is strongly suggestive of a genetic inheritance, and thus physical basis, of a condition.

Adoptive studies, which demonstrate that children who have been adopted shortly after birth appear to carry the risk of developing mental health disorders apparent in their blood relations, are very strongly suggestive of the genetic inheritance of mental illness. Studies of twins who have been separated at birth and adopted by different families offer even more powerful evidence of inheritance of disease. Conditions such as schizophrenia, manic depression, simple depression, anxiety and panic disorder, obsessive-compulsive disorder and alcoholism have all been shown by these sorts of studies to have an inherited component in their causation. This means that a child of someone with one of these conditions is more likely than the average person to develop that condition.

The neuropsychiatric explanation offered for an inherited tendency to mental health disorders is usually given in terms of an inherited neurochemical makeup. For example, it is recognized that in schizophrenia there is increased activity of those brain systems that involve the release of the neurotransmitter dopamine. It is possible that the increased tendency for schizophrenia to run in families is due, in part, to an inherited tendency for these physical systems to be over-activated. This chemical basis for the genesis of schizophrenia is further supported by the fact that dopamine-stimulating drugs, such as amphetamines and cannabis, can trigger a psychosis similar in form to schizophrenia. Moreover, the drugs discovered originally by chance to be of benefit in schizophrenia, the major tranquillizers (first developed as anesthetic agents), are now known to act by blocking the action of dopamine.

Similarly, the tendency to develop depression may be, in part, a result of an inherited reduction in the expression of monoamine neurotransmitters such as noradrenaline and serotonin (5HT). This is supported by the fact that the various classes of antidepressant drugs all seem to increase the levels of monoamines in the brain. It is increasingly recognized that some of the addictive recreational drugs (e.g. nicotine, ecstasy) may induce a release of serotonin after their use, which is then followed by a more long-term depletion of this neurotransmitter in the brain. Because of this, use of the drug forces the user to face a long-term state of low mood if they choose to withdraw from the drug, particularly if the use of the drug has been prolonged over a period of months to years.

However, an inherited tendency to a condition does not in itself destine a child to develop that condition. It is clear that other factors are usually required to force the expression of a condition such as schizophrenia or depression. These other factors are considered to be either psychological or social in nature.[25]

Psychological factors in mental health disorders

The psychological explanation of mental illness rests on the principle that experiences during childhood and early adulthood can have a profound bearing on a person's mental and emotional health. This is such a commonly accepted principle that few would argue against the suggestion that a shocking experience or a period of deprivation in childhood would have long-term psychological repercussions. However, it is only in fairly recent years that studies of traumatic events in childhood have clearly demonstrated a link between certain forms of childhood deprivation and long-term mental ill health. The studies performed by the psychologist John Bowlby in the 1940s and 1950s demonstrated that prolonged or recurrent absence of a consistent mother figure in early life was associated with difficulties in forming emotional bonds and a tendency to criminality and emotional problems in later life.[26]

Since that time, psychological studies have shown that diverse factors in the family environment, including expressed angry discord, maternal depression, divorce, bereavement, overprotection, lack of parental authority, physical and sexual abuse, unremitting criticism, and taunting and inconsistent discipline, can all be risk factors for misbehavior in children and mental health disorders in later life.

The theories that propose psychological mechanisms for the causation of mental illness are only just over a century old. Sigmund Freud, now considered the founder of psychoanalysis, first proposed in 1905 that there are both conscious and unconscious aspects to the mind. He developed this theory over the next 20 years, and postulated that unconscious forces deriving from deeply ingrained value systems originating from parents or society (the superego), or instinctive drives (the id), could, together with pressures in one's external life, challenge and cause conflict with the conscious self (the ego).

The conscious self was considered by Freud to develop to its healthy adult form in distinct stages throughout childhood. Freud proposed that the healthy child has to progress appropriately through oral, anal, phallic, latent and genital phases in order to mature as a healthy adult, and problems encountered in any of the stages could result in lasting psychological disorder. For example, he proposed that the anal stage was when the toddler ideally achieves a sense of separateness and becomes independent in terms of toilet training. Problems in this phase might appear in adulthood as a fear of losing control, obsessional traits or depression because of not living up to expectations.

Freud's theories and their rigid distinctions are less accepted nowadays, but his beliefs that the psyche undergoes progressive development throughout childhood, and that unconscious material originating from episodes scattered along the course of that development can persist to lead to mental illness, still very much influence modern psychotherapeutic practice.

The concept of defense mechanisms, proposed first by Freud and later developed by his daughter Anna Freud, is one that is still very much recognized in modern psychology. A defense mechanism describes any mental response used by a person to protect themselves from psychological pain such as guilt, anxiety or shame. The naming of the various defense reactions has entered common usage. Commonly described defense reactions include denial, repression, regression, rationalization, displacement, projection, introjection, sublimation and reaction formation.

Defense mechanisms can be healthy, and responses such as distraction (e.g. looking for the positive or use of humor) are likely to be used by people who enjoy good mental health. However, mechanisms such as repression of unpleasant feelings (such as might follow an episode of severe abuse), or denial of what has really happened (e.g. an inability to take in a diagnosis of cancer), may actually lead to long-term problems in mental health. The theory is that these sorts of defense mechanisms simply shift conscious mental pain into the unconscious, where the pain may still be felt in the form of depression or anxiety, but from where it is much harder to treat the pain at its root. With this perspective on causation, a psychotherapist works to enable the patient to arrive at a place where this unconscious material is made conscious and the roots of the pain can be understood, and so transformed.[27]

The cognitive behavioral psychological perspective developed from practical therapies such as Albert Ellis' "Rational Emotional Behavior Therapy" and Aaron T. Beck's "Cognitive Therapy" after the 1960s. According to cognitive behavioral theory the causation of disease is based on the idea that the patient has learned inappropriate responses to the world around them because of negative past experience. The cognitive behavioral model interprets unhelpful behaviors in the light of the incorrect thoughts that underlie them. For example, a child who was shocked by the barking of a dog might then tend to be fearful whenever a dog comes close. A behavioral response of avoidance, and maybe even a physiological response of palpitations and sweating, might then persist into adulthood. The cognitive behavioral interpretation of this problem (termed a simple phobia) is that, because of the childhood experience, the belief that "dogs will make me frightened" has been learned, and the inappropriate reaction to dogs has become ingrained as a result of that belief.

Anxiety disorders, eating disorders and depressive disorders are examples of disorders that can be analyzed according to cognitive behavioral theory. The negative responses to the world expressed in these disorders can be related in cognitive behavioral theory to unhelpful learned patterns of thought.

Social factors in mental health disorders

A social perspective on the causation of mental illness necessarily overlaps with the psychological perspective, because it sees factors in the social environment as impacting on the developing psyche. Social theories of the causation of mental illness are particularly bound up in the studies of cultural factors common to communities. Studies on the incidence of mental illness in communities have identified that mental illness can relate to variables such as gender, age, marital status, social support and economic status. For example, there is a recognized link between depression in men and being divorced, a link that is far less pronounced in women who are divorced.[28]

The study of the effect of life events, such as marriage, birth, divorce, emigration and bereavement, falls into the remit of understanding the social causation of mental illness.

Predisposing, precipitating and perpetuating factors in mental illness

A psychiatrist or psychologist seeks to understand the evolution of mental illness in terms of three factors of causation: predisposing, precipitating and perpetuating factors. Ideally, the factors that have predisposed to the condition, those that have precipitated the condition and those that might be perpetuating the condition need to be clarified if the most appropriate treatment is to be chosen.

Predisposing factors in mental illness

Predisposing factors are those that might have led a person to have become more at risk of developing a mental illness before the illness became apparent. For example, if one looks at the case of schizophrenia appearing for the first time as the sudden onset of a paranoid psychosis in a 22-year-old male student, the predisposing factors might include a family history of serious mental illness (grandfather was in an asylum for ten years and mother had an episode of postnatal psychosis after the birth of his younger brother). There might also be a volatile emotional environment in the family home (mother and father have frequent arguments, and mother often breaks down in tears when stressed). As a child, this student was recognized to be withdrawn and awkward socially.

Precipitating factors in mental illness

Precipitating factors are those that have actually triggered a particular episode of illness. In this case these might include the stress of leaving home for the first time, and the inability to fit into a supportive network of people at college. A recent history of experimenting with ecstasy and frequent use of cannabis could also be included as precipitating factors.

Perpetuating factors in mental illness

Perpetuating factors are those that might prevent the resolution of the mental illness. In this case these could include the lack of social support, continued drug use and self-neglect.

The biopsychosocial model and the choice of treatment

Although there is a general appreciation amongst conventional practitioners that there are diverse factors at play in the generation of mental illness, psychiatrists and psychologists may vary in their treatment approaches as a consequence of the way in which they understand the causation of the disease. For example, for a patient with a mental health issue, a hospital psychiatrist who has expertise in neuropsychiatry and the biological basis of mental illness might favor medical drug treatments. In contrast, a psychoanalyst who is educated in the psychological causation of mental illness might treat the same patient by encouraging them to explore unhelpful emotional reactions that first started to emerge in childhood. The diverse approaches to the treatment of mental health disorders and their relationship to the perceived underlying cause of the disorder are explored in more detail in Section 6.2c.

Information box 6.2a-I

Mental health disorders: a Chinese medicine perspective

There are many terms used in Chinese medicine texts associated with the mind, but Shen (Spirit) and compound terms that include the term Shen, such as Jing Shen (Spirit Essence), are those that are used most commonly. In Chinese medicine the Shen with Qi and Jing (Essence) are described as the three treasures. These three substances are the interdependent manifestations of Qi.

Therefore, in Chinese thought there is no duality between the mind and body as is so evident in Western thought. Instead, the mind (Shen) is understood as a less substantial aspect of Qi and Essence. All three together comprise the body-mind (Xing-Shen).

Any imbalance or disturbance in the flow of Qi in any of the Organs will have a manifestation at the level of the Shen. All Chinese medicine patterns may therefore include signs and symptoms of a mental and/or emotional nature.

Unlike conventional medicine, in Chinese medicine mental health is not seen as a distinct specialty, but instead as one aspect of health as a whole, and may be treated by experts in "internal medicine" with herbs and acupuncture and methods for relaxation. Psychiatric or psychological diseases are described in Chinese medicine as Jing Shen Bing (Essence Spirit diseases). This term again pays reference to the unity of the substantial body with the less substantial mind.

The Shen is classically the most insubstantial and rapidly moving form of Qi, and is specifically associated with the mind. Shen is also associated with Heart Qi, and the Heart is said to house the Shen. Spirit, in the Chinese sense, has many layers of meaning, but when used from the perspective of the psychological diseases, it embraces the outward manifestation of life, together with consciousness, thinking and feeling.

The five Shen

The Chinese considered the Shen to consist of the five spiritual aspects of a human being, each of which is associated with a Yin Organ. The five aspects are the Hun (Liver), the Yi (Spleen), the Zhi (Kidney), the Po (Lung) and the specific spiritual aspect of the Heart Organ, also given the name Shen. To minimize confusion, in this text this last particular aspect of the Shen will be called Heart Shen.

Each of the five aspects of the Shen is recognized to have particular characteristics, as described below.

The mind/spirit (Heart Shen)

The Heart Shen is that aspect of the spirit which specifically resides in the Heart, but which also embraces the other four Shen. It is considered to be responsible for consciousness, intelligence, thought, insight, the generation of ideas and memory.

The Heart Shen is also important for the ability to fall asleep easily and to have sleep that is deep and refreshing. Shen is also used to describe the quality of liveliness that is inherent in someone who is emotionally very healthy.

The Heart Shen gives the capacity to have insight and to feel the emotions. The ability to form healthy relationships and to feel love and joy is a characteristic of the Heart and Pericardium, which must, in turn, be related to their spiritual aspect, the Heart Shen.

A healthy Heart Shen also confers wisdom, which is the ability to respond to knowledge and challenges with discernment.

The ethereal soul (Hun)

The Hun was thought to be that part of the spirit that leaves the body after death. It is rooted in the Liver Yin, from where it enables a sense of purpose, vision and direction in life. It is also linked with the courage required to face life's challenges, and the ability to make decisions.

If the Hun is well rooted, sleep is normal and dreams are few. However, the ability to gain inspiration, be intuitive and have dreams is a characteristic of the Hun. The Hun can make images, archetypes and symbols accessible to the conscious mind, and has a link with the universal mind (comparable to the collective unconscious as described by Jung).

The ability to move easily between introspection and relationships with other people has been attributed to the Hun. A balanced Hun prevents the emotions from becoming excessive, so underlying a healthy emotional life.

The corporeal soul (Po)

The Po was thought to be that part of the spirit which is linked to the body, and which remains with the body after death. The Po enables the body to move, and gives the skills of agility, balance and coordination.

The Po was also seen to be very important in enabling appropriate movement of the Jing (Essence), and so is involved in the first physiological processes after birth (such as the perception of the senses and the onset of breathing).

The Po is also important for the acuity of the senses. The Po is responsible for the experience of grief and for crying. It is also closely linked to breathing, and so can be calmed if the breath is regulated.

While the Hun is important for relationships with other people, the Po is more important for the establishment of internal integrity and protection from external psychic influences.

The intellect (Yi)

The Yi was thought to reside in the Spleen, and is responsible for clear thought. The ability to study, to concentrate, to assimilate new ideas, to retain facts and to work things out are all functions of the Yi. Memory will be good if the Yi is healthy, and this particularly relates to the memory of facts and ideas.

The will (Zhi)

The Zhi was thought to reside in the Kidneys, and is also important in the function of memory. The Zhi appears to be linked with long-term retention of facts and ideas, whereas the Yi is related to the laying down of memory of facts and ideas.

The Zhi is also linked to the drive and determination required to follow through with an idea. It also has the characteristic of tenaciousness in following an idea through to its conclusion. The Zhi is also characterized by the courage required to stand up to the challenges that life presents and which threaten to prevent success in one's endeavors.

The causation of mental illness in Chinese medicine

Just as is true for bodily illness, mental illness in Chinese medicine will result from the six climatic excesses, the seven emotions and the miscellaneous causes.

The six climatic factors of heat, summer heat, damp, dryness, wind and cold are less prominent in the etiology of mental illness, but each may cause organ damage, and in particular Stagnation of Qi, which will, in turn, engender mental and emotional symptoms.

The seven emotions of joy, overthinking, anger, fear, sorrow, fright and anxiety are well recognized in Chinese medicine to directly damage the organs when in excess. Whilst the seven emotions are normal expressions of the ebb and flow of Qi through healthy-functioning Organs and the interaction of a person with the ever-changing environment, if in excess each emotion can directly damage a particular Organ or Organs. For example, anger will damage the Liver and anxiety the Heart and the Spleen. Conversely, unhealthy organs will lead to unhealthy emotional expression, and so a damaged Liver will express itself in anger, and injury to Heart and Spleen might be manifest in anxiety. There is a bi-directional relationship between the organs and their corresponding emotions.

The miscellaneous causes of disease include faulty diet, lack of regulation between activity and stillness, unhealthy sexual activity, and the effects of medications and drugs. All these can conspire to cause Organ depletion, Stasis of Qi and Accumulation of Damp Phlegm and Heat. Very often it is this combination of Depletion, Fullness and Stagnation that is causative in mental illness. Each of these pathologies affects the Shen in characteristic ways.

The pathology of the Shen

There are three general patterns described in Chinese medicine that result from imbalance of the Shen: Deficient Shen, Disturbed Shen and Obstructed Shen.

The general patterns of these pathologies of the Shen are:

Deficient Shen	Dullness
	Apathy
	Lack of spirit or vitality
	Lack of joy
Disturbed Shen	Insomnia and dream-disturbed sleep
	Forgetfulness
	Anxiety and propensity to startle
	Poor memory
Obstructed Shen	Confusion and dull depression
	Clouded consciousness
	Unconsciousness

These patterns describe general imbalances that are seen in all manner of mental illness. However, each one of the five Shen has its own characteristics, which, when out of balance, may be discerned in mental illness. The characteristics of imbalance of the five Shen are:

Aspect of the Shen	Associated Organs	Characteristics of imbalance
Shen (mind/spirit)	Heart, Small Intestine, Pericardium, Triple Burner	Low intelligence, unclear thought, lack of clarity of ideas Poor memory for events Difficulty falling asleep and disturbed sleep Dull and lifeless personality and lack of joy Confusion and lack of consciousness Lack of experience of emotions or oversensitivity to emotions Problems in interpersonal relationships Unwise life decisions
Hun (ethereal soul)	Liver, Gallbladder	Lack of purpose, vision and direction Timidity and indecisiveness Dream-disturbed sleep and out-of-body experiences Lack of inspiration and intuition, and a sterile inner life Marked emphasis on the intuitive and second sight (e.g. connection with the spirit world, seeing ghosts, clairvoyance) Excessive emotional outbursts, in particular, anger
Po (corporeal soul)	Lung, Large Intestine	Difficulties with movement, clumsiness and lack of coordination Weakening of the senses and uncomfortable sensations (e.g. itching) Excessive grief and crying, or inability to feel grief Breathing difficulties, hyperventilation and shallow breathing A poor sense of self, and vulnerability to external influences and vibes
Yi (intellect)	Spleen, Stomach	Dull intellect, slow thinking, poor memory for facts
Zhi (will)	Kidney, Bladder	Overthinking Difficulty in concentration Poor long-term memory Lack of drive and initiative; ideas and dreams do not reach fruition Excessive fearfulness

The organ syndromes and mental-emotional problems

As described earlier, the Shen is simply an aspect of Qi or Essence. If Qi is out of balance when an Organ pattern is being expressed, it is to be expected that there will be some accompanying imbalance of the Shen. For example, in a state of Qi Deficiency one might expect Shen Deficiency, and in Qi Stagnation one might expect some degree of Shen Disturbance. As Qi is a Yang substance, the same applies to any pattern in which Yang is out of balance. In Yang Deficiency one might expect Shen Deficiency, and when Yang is Rising one might expect Shen Disturbance.

Similarly, a disorder of the Shen can be expected if there is an imbalance of Blood, as Blood is not only directly related to Qi as the mother of Qi, but is also said to House the Shen. If Blood is Deficient, Shen might be expected to be Deficient, but also Disturbed as it can no longer be properly rooted. As Blood is a Yin Substance, a Deficiency of Yin might also be expected to be accompanied by a Deficiency and Disturbance of the Shen.

In Full patterns it is also possible to predict the effect that certain Pathogenic Factors might have on the Shen. One might expect Heat and Wind to Disturb the Shen, and Phlegm and Damp to Obstruct it. Empty Heat simply Disturbs the Shen, but Full Heat can affect consciousness and thus can Obstruct as well as Disturb the Shen.

The disorders of the Shen and their overlap with the main pathologies in Chinese medicine are as follows:

Shen pathology	Chinese medicine pathologies
Deficient Shen	Qi Deficiency Blood Deficiency Yin Deficiency with Empty Heat Yang Deficiency
Disturbed Shen	Blood Deficiency Yin Deficiency with Empty Heat Empty Heat Qi Stagnation Blood Stagnation Full Heat Phlegm/Fire Wind
Obstructed Shen	Blood Stagnation Phlegm Full Heat Phlegm/Fire Damp

It is possible to use these correspondences to understand more about the mental-emotional disturbances described in the particular organ syndromes. Even more insight will be gained if the mental-emotional correspondences of the five Shen are also used to inform an interpretation of a particular organ syndrome.

For example, in the syndrome of Spleen Qi Deficiency, some features of Deficient Shen and also some features of Imbalance of the Yi might be expected. It is no surprise, then, that tiredness, lassitude and overthinking are features of this pattern, which reflect Shen Deficiency, but with a particular flavor associated with Imbalance of the Yi. On this basis, difficulties in thinking, generation of ideas and memory for facts might also be expected to be features of Spleen Qi Deficiency, and these are indeed familiar symptoms seen in patients in clinical practice.

Using the approach described above it is possible to describe what sort of mental-emotional features might be apparent in a presentation of any particular Chinese medicine syndrome. This aspect of the Chinese medicine interpretation of mental health symptoms and signs has been elaborated in some detail, as it will provide a foundation for the Chinese medicine interpretation of conventional descriptions of mental illness in subsequent sections in this chapter.[29, 30]

6.2b Classification of mental health disorders

In conventional medicine, the mental health disorders are classified in a systematic way. Superficially, this is comparable to the classification of diseases of any one of the more readily measurable physiological systems. However, the diseases of the mind are largely classified according to their symptoms and signs, rather than according to the underlying pathological process. For example, the various phobias are classified according to the nature of the phobia, rather than what precisely is going on in the nervous system in these disorders. This is in contrast to the basis on which the diseases of systems such as the cardiovascular or gastrointestinal systems are classified.

The process of classification in psychiatry involves sorting episodes of mental illness into diagnostic groups on the basis of common clinical features. For example, two episodes of depression might appear to be very different, in that one might be triggered by bereavement, and so be characterized by extreme sadness, and the other might occur in the postnatal period, and be characterized by feelings of guilt. However, both episodes will be recognized by a psychiatrist as cases of depression because of the common features of pervasive low mood, poor sleep, altered appetite and the presence of suicidal ideas.

The systematic classification of psychiatric diseases is considered to be of benefit for the purposes of communication about the condition, for facilitation of research and also for developing treatment protocols. This is because once a condition can be assigned a category, it can be compared readily with other cases diagnosed to fall within the same category. The responses to different treatments for people with the same sort of condition can be compared. Moreover, a new patient suffering from a condition that can be placed in an already specified category can be offered treatment that has been shown to benefit other people diagnosed with the same sort of condition.

Potential problems with classification of mental health disorders

However, the benefits of psychiatric classification and its corollary, the labeling of patients with a diagnosis of mental illness, are the subject of debate. The psychiatrist Robert Kendell, when writing about the role of diagnosis in psychiatry, stated that "in the last resort, all diagnostic concepts stand or fall by the strength of the diagnostic and therapeutic implications they embody."[31] What Kendell means is that a classification system is only of value if the diagnostic categories actually enable a truly therapeutic outcome for the majority of people who fall into each of the categories.

It can be argued that the diagnostic categories used in modern psychiatry are too simplistic. Each person has a unique makeup and is exposed to unique and diverse stressors. At a point of crisis they may have a mental breakdown, which likewise has its own very unique characteristics. No other person has ever before experienced the same pattern and range of troubling thoughts and disability as this person, and yet a psychiatrist is likely to focus in on a few key characteristics of the disorder and make a diagnosis such as paranoid schizophrenia or acute depression.

First, we need to question whether a diagnostic category such as schizophrenia is appropriate for this patient. Although the patient may share some clinical features in common with other patients, is it really right to group the patient together with these patients for the purpose of choosing treatment? On the basis of the diagnosis, this patient might be hospitalized against their will, and forced to be treated with the most widely accepted therapeutic option for acute schizophrenia, drugs from the major tranquillizer group. These drugs may lead to a wide range of side effects, including sedation, confusion, weight gain, Parkinsonian symptoms (i.e. akin to the stiffness seen in Parkinson's disease), muscle stiffness and restless movements (tardive dyskinesia). It is important to be sure that these side effects are worth the hoped-for benefit of improved mental health.

The problem of choosing one treatment to fit all members of a diagnostic category is not just an issue in the realm of psychiatry; it is also relevant in general medicine. Just because the majority of people in a clinical trial of treatment for, say, hypertension respond positively to a given drug, this does not guarantee that every individual with hypertension will respond positively. One drug does not necessarily fit all cases of hypertension. It is arguable that this issue is of even more significance in psychiatry, in which the clinical presentations of two people with the same diagnosis can be very different. Is it reasonable to expect one drug to fit all cases of depression or panic attack?

In the case of schizophrenia, it is not always clear whether or not the therapeutic option has conferred a benefit. In many cases, after a first episode of schizophrenia there is a prolonged period of up to a few years in which the patient may not regain their previous level of functioning in society. Some of this disability may well result from the side effects of hospitalization and drug treatment. Can we be sure that this treatment option was the best for this patient in their unique situation?

The diagnosis of schizophrenia is undoubtedly one that is stigmatizing in Western culture. The label provokes the memories and images that Western culture associates with the term. Most of these will not be positive, and importantly may not be relevant to the person's individual situation. The label carries consequences, not just in terms of the treatment that is offered, but may also affect the person's self-image and the way in which they will be able to integrate back into their community.

To summarize, the classification of mental health disorders, as well as offering benefits in terms of communication, and aiding in research and the design of treatment protocols, can also carry some negative consequences. Being assigned to a diagnostic category may oversimplify an individual case of mental illness. Being assigned to a category may imply that only a certain recommended treatment path is suitable for a particular patient (e.g. antidepressants in diagnosed depression), when this might not be the case at all. Moreover, categorization may actually lead to harm as a result of the application of a label that is perceived to be stigmatizing to a patient.

There are two widely accepted systems of the classification of mental health diseases: the International Classification of Diseases (ICD),[32] a system drawn up by the World Health Organization (WHO), and the *Diagnostic and Statistical Manual of Mental Disorders*, 5th edition (DSM-5),[33] designed by the American Psychiatric Association.

The International Classification of Diseases (ICD-10)

The most recent revision of the International Classification of Diseases, ICD-10, was published by the World Health Organization in 1992. ICD-10 consists of a number of chapters, each dedicated to a different physiological system or disease group. By means of this system, each disease category can be ascribed a unique numerical code, which can be useful for the purposes of studying the epidemiology of disease. Chapter 5 of ICD-10 is dedicated to mental health disorders.

In ICD-10, the mental health and behavioral disorders are subdivided into ten categories, as summarized in Table 6.2b-I.

Table 6.2b-I The ten categories of mental health disorder according to the Tenth International Classification of Diseases (ICD-10) (Chapter 5)

Organic, mental disorders

Mental or behavioral disorders due to psychoactive substance use

Schizophrenia, schizotypal and delusional disorders

Mood (affective) disorders

Neurotic and stress-related and somatoform disorders

Behavioral syndromes associated with physiological disturbances

Disorders of adult personality and behavior

Mental retardation

Disorders of psychological development

Behavioral and emotional disorders with onset usually in childhood or adolescence

Definitions of some of the terms used to describe these ten categories are as follows.

Organic: definition

This is a term that is used in all aspects of conventional medicine to describe a condition that has a measurable physical basis. From a psychiatric perspective, the organic mental health disorders include Alzheimer's disease and other forms of dementia, and any mental health disorders that result from brain damage, brain tumor or generalized disease.

Psychoactive: definition

Psychoactive describes something that has an effect on the functioning of the mind, and in the context of ICD-10 refers to substances such as alcohol, sedatives, recreational drugs and caffeine.

Affective: definition

Affective literally means relating to the mood. In psychiatry, the term affect is used almost interchangeably with the word mood. This category includes all the depressive disorders and also the condition of mania that manifests as periods of elevated mood.

Neurotic: definition

Neurotic is an adjective that is derived from the term used in psychiatry to describe a minor mental health disorder, a neurosis. By definition neuroses are those conditions in which there is mental health disturbance but that the patient's insight into the fact there is a mental health disturbance is maintained. By this definition, any person with a neurosis would readily admit that that was their problem. For example, minor depression and phobias are examples of neuroses in that the patient suffering from these conditions would be prepared to agree with the doctor about the nature of their problem.

The formal definition of a neurosis given in ICD-10 is as follows: "a mental disorder in which the patient may have considerable insight and has unimpaired reality testing, in that he does not easily confuse his morbid subjective experiences and fantasies with reality."

In contrast psychoses (singular psychosis) are those mental health conditions in which the patient has lost insight into the fact they have a mental illness. A psychosis is characterized by a degree of denial that there is anything wrong, and possibly by a reluctance to admit that treatment is necessary. Broadly speaking, this technical term corresponds to the commonly used words insanity and madness. Psychotic is a term that in psychiatry describes a state of mental health in which insight is lost. It might be used, for example, to describe a case of acute schizophrenia. It does not in any way imply dangerousness, which is the unfortunate common misunderstanding of the term.

The formal definition of a psychosis given in ICD-10 is as follows: "a mental disorder in which impairment of the mental function has developed to such a degree that interferes grossly with insight, ability to meet some ordinary demands of life or to maintain adequate contact with reality."

Somatoform: definition

Somatoform literally means a condition in which a mental health disorder is largely experienced as physical discomfort and attributed by the patient to a bodily problem. Somatization is the term used to describe the tendency to experience recurrent functional disease (such as headache, irritable bowel disease and dysmenorrhea)

when the medical interpretation of the root of the problem is a mental illness such as depression or anxiety.

Personality disorder: definition

Personality disorder is a term defined in ICD-10 as "deeply ingrained and enduring behavior patterns manifesting as inflexible responses to a broad range of personal and social situations." What this means is that a person diagnosed with a personality disorder has emerged from childhood as an adult with what the psychiatrist would consider an abnormal and often unhelpful way of responding to the world.

A tendency to mood swings (cyclothymia), to low mood (dysthymia) and to negatively interpreting the intentions of others (paranoia) are all examples of ways of responding to the world, which, if extreme, could be classed as personality disorders. Using these examples, a person markedly exhibiting these tendencies might be diagnosed as having, respectively, a cyclothymic, dysthymic or paranoid personality disorder.

The *Diagnostic and Statistical Manual of Mental Disorders,* 5th edition (DSM-5)

The APA's fifth revision of the *Diagnostic and Statistical Manual of Mental Disorders* (DSM-5) classifies mental health disorders in a way that is helpful for the coding of disorders within the US healthcare system. It contains a much more up-to-date classification of the rapidly evolving system of mental health disorder. The DSM-5 development website explains the rationale for having both an ICD-10 and DSM-5 system as follows: "DSM-5 and the ICD should be thought of as companion publications. DSM-5 contains the most up-to-date criteria for diagnosing mental disorders, along with extensive descriptive text, providing a common language for clinicians to communicate about their patients."[34]

This system explicitly avoids classification on the basis of known pathology, but rather categorizes purely on what can be gleaned from the clinical features (symptoms and signs) of the condition. This system also introduces lists of diagnostic criteria, which are lists of features that have to be present in order for a diagnosis to be made. These criteria were designed to increase the reliability of forming a psychiatric diagnosis.

The mental health disorders in DSM-5 are listed under 21 headings. Table 6.2b-II lists these clinical categories.[35]

Table 6.2b-II The 21 categories of mental health disorder listed in the APA's Fifth *Diagnostic and Statistical Manual* (DSM-5)

Neurodevelopmental disorders (including intellectual disability, autistic spectrum disorder, attention deficit/hyperactivity disorder, Tourette's syndrome)

Schizophrenia spectrum and other psychotic disorders

Bipolar and related disorders

Depressive disorders

Anxiety disorders

Obsessive-compulsive and related disorders

Trauma and stressor-related disorders

Dissociative disorders

Somatic symptom and related disorders

Feeding and eating disorders (including anorexia nervosa and bulimia nervosa)

Elimination disorders

Sleep wake disorders

Sexual dysfunctions

Gender dysphoria

Disruptive, impulse control and conduct disorders

Substance-related and addictive disorders

Neurocognitive disorders

Personality disorders

Paraphilic disorders

Other mental disorders (including mental disorders resulting from a general medical condition)

Medication-induced movement disorders and other adverse effects of medication

There are significantly more categories in DSM-5 than ICD-10, which allow for more precise definitions of mental health disorder. There has been much criticism of the exhaustive lists of diagnoses embraced by DSM-5; however, some of this is directed towards its apparent tendency to medicalize what might be considered part of the spectrum of normal human behavior and responses to stress into categories of disease. For example, depression resulting from bereavement, attention deficit disorder and transvestism are all included within the DSM-5 list of diseases.[36]

6.2c Assessment and treatment of mental health disorders

The assessment of mental health disorders

The assessment of mental health disorders in conventional medicine usually begins with a formal psychiatric examination. Ideally, the assessment will be in the form of an interview with the examining psychiatrist, lasting for about an hour. As is the case for the other physiological systems, the assessment follows the stages of questioning (history taking), examination and clinical investigations. However, in psychiatry, although physical examination may be relevant in the case of organic disease, the most important aspect of the examination is of the mental state. The mental state is also assessed primarily by questioning.

The psychiatric history

In psychiatry the questioning to elucidate the history of the mental disorder includes not only the development of the presenting problem, but also the family history of mental disorder, a detailed history of childhood development and family relationships, an educational, occupational, medical and psychiatric history, and details of the patient's current social situation. In this way, the psychiatrist builds up a picture of all the factors that may have contributed to the development of the current condition. By questioning in this way, the psychiatrist is displaying their training in the biopsychosocial model of the causation of mental illness.

The mental state examination

As with the routine of the physical examination, the examination of the mental state is structured and follows clearly defined stages. These stages are:

- assessment of appearance and behavior

- assessment of speech (especially rate, articulation, quantity and form)

- assessment of mood

- assessment of the content of the patient's thoughts

- assessment of abnormal beliefs

- assessment of abnormal experiences

- assessment of cognitive state (i.e. orientation, memory, attention, concentration and intelligence)

- assessment of insight.

Systematic examination of all the aspects of mental functioning reflected in the mental state stages is intended to reveal patterns of thought, mood and behavior that are characteristic of particular mental health disorders.

Physical examination and investigations

The psychiatrist may conduct a brief physical examination and perform relevant investigations to exclude any possible organic causes of mental health problems (e.g. hypothyroidism, substance misuse or withdrawal, or raised intracranial pressure).

The treatment of mental health disorders

Having formed an initial diagnosis through the history, mental state examination, physical examination and investigations, the psychiatrist will then consider the treatment options. As is the case for the diseases of the other physiological systems, a precise diagnosis is central to the process of choosing treatment. As is also true in general medicine, treatment is ideally chosen on the basis of high-quality research or well-established professional medical opinion.

Although in the majority of cases of minor mental health disorders drug treatment may be unnecessary, for many psychiatric diagnoses there are recognized pharmacological treatments for the condition. Drugs exert their effects primarily in the physical realm, and so might be expected to modify the biological factors that are associated with mental ill health. Other physically directed treatment options include electroconvulsive therapy and psychosurgery. Both these physically based forms of treatment are also known to lead to improvements through the placebo effect.

In accordance with the biopsychosocial perspective, many patients will also be recommended a treatment that is intended to exert its effects in the psychological domain, such as cognitive therapy, behavioral therapy or psychodynamic psychotherapy.

In addition, referral for social support, or a recommendation for couple counseling or grief counseling, might be chosen to ameliorate any social factors that are seen to be perpetuating the mental health disorder.

An important added aspect of the choice of treatment is whether or not treatment should be offered to the patient within a hospital setting or as an outpatient. Hospital may be appropriate for some patients, as their mental illness may be preventing adequate self-care or attention to treatment plans. Ideally, the patient will be willing to be admitted to hospital for psychiatric assessment and treatment, and fortunately this is usually the case. At best, in hospital a patient with a mental illness will have all their bodily needs attended to, constant supervision of their mental state, supervised regular drug therapy if necessary, and be offered easy access to other therapies and social support.

In the situation in which a patient is not willing to be admitted to hospital for assessment or treatment of a mental health disorder, in the UK the psychiatrist may choose to exert powers as specified under various of the sections of the England and Wales Mental Health Act 1983 (as amended in 2007) to make admission to hospital compulsory.[37] Separate legislation applies in Scotland and Northern Ireland. There is significant variation across the developed world with regards to the legal basis for enforced commitment to hospital for receiving hospital care. However, in all cases the legal constraints embody the tension there is between medical needs (as perceived by the medical team) and the human right to liberty and freedom of choice.

The legislation is designed to ensure that these powers should only be exerted in cases when such treatment would be considered necessary either to protect the patient's own well-being or for the safety of others.

Biological therapies for psychiatric disorders

The six most commonly prescribed medications used in mental health disorders are hypnotics, anxiolytics, antipsychotics, mood stabilizers, antidepressants and drugs used in Alzheimer's disease.

HYPNOTIC DRUGS

Hypnotic drugs are prescribed to induce a state of sedation or to treat insomnia. They generally have duration of action in the region of a few hours, and this is suitable for the purpose of enabling a full night's sleep.

The hypnotics include benzodiazepines (e.g. temazepam) and the benzodiazepine-like drugs that are believed to act on the same receptor in the brain as benzodiazepines (e.g. zopiclone), antihistamines (e.g. promethazine) and the drug chlormethiazole. All these drugs cause sedation and drowsiness, and in excess would lead to unconsciousness.

The benzodiazepine-like hypnotics are known to act at a receptor in the brain which, when bound by the drug, affects the action of a neurotransmitter known as GABA (gamma-aminobutyric acid). GABA is known to be an inhibitory neurotransmitter, and its action includes the calming of overactive nerve pathways in the brain.

Side effects include prolonged drowsiness the next day, confusion and unsteadiness, and in some cases inhibition of breathing. Rarely, in some people, these drugs can lead to an unstable mental state, with aggression and thought disorder. An important complication of benzodiazepine use is that dependence on the drug easily develops, and this is more pronounced if used for a long time. This means that the patient will experience a withdrawal syndrome involving restlessness, anxiety, sleeplessness and possibly aggression on stopping a regular dose of medication. For this reason, the UK Committee on Safety of Medicines (CSM) recommends that benzodiazepines are only used for insomnia if the insomnia is "severe, disabling or subjecting the individual to severe distress."[38]

The antihistamines are chemically related to the drugs that are used for the control of psychosis (see later, under "Antipsychotic drugs"). They are known to affect the action in the brain of a range of neurotransmitters, including dopamine, acetylcholine, histamine, serotonin and noradrenaline. It is thought that the action of inhibition of dopamine contributes most significantly to the sedating action of these drugs. Promethazine is the antihistamine used most widely for sedation because it has a relatively low risk of adverse side effects, and does not usually induce dependence. Side effects of promethazine include prolonged drowsiness, difficulty in urination, dry mouth, blurred vision and digestive disturbances.

Clomethiazole is a sedating drug that is used in the care of elderly people and to help with the management of the state of acute alcohol withdrawal. However, if used over a prolonged period, it is well recognized to induce a state of dependence, and so should be prescribed with care.

Barbiturates are a class of drug once used widely for sedation, but are now not recommended for use in the management of psychological conditions. Phenobarbital is a barbiturate used principally in the control of epilepsy.

The older antidepressants, such as amitriptyline, may also be prescribed in low doses, principally for their sedating effects. They are of particular use when insomnia is accompanied by low mood or chronic pain.

 Information box 6.2c-I

Hypnotic drugs: comments from a Chinese medicine perspective

From a Chinese medicine perspective, the induction of drowsiness and sedation could be described in terms of Obstruction of the Shen. The side effects of these drugs are manifest primarily in the realm of the mind and spirit, and the obfuscation that results might be described in terms of Turbid Phlegm that Obstructs the Orifices of the Heart.

Flaws and Lake (2001) are reluctant to specifically define the actions of the sedating drugs in Chinese medical terms, and quote the Chinese authors of the 1989 Chinese language text *Chinese Medical Psychiatry*, Li and Lui, who explain that their action can be explained when "the drugs' toxins flow into the viscera and bowels which result in the spirit mind becoming befuddled."[39]

Rosenberg (2000)[40] explains that benzodiazepines have a Hot Dispersing nature and Sedate Liver Fire, but by suppressing the rising of Liver Yang, this consumes Liver Yin and leads to side effects of irritability, restlessness, tremor and vertigo on withdrawal. He explains that they act in a similar way to alcohol, which is also very Heating. The initial response of both is relaxation because its Heat disperses Stagnant Qi. He doesn't explain how these drugs lead to loss of consciousness, but it is presumably the toxic effect of a large amount of the drug acting in a way that would be described as Phlegm Misting the Heart Mind.

Flaws and Lake do explain that Hot Western drugs that powerfully "up bear and out thrust" Yang Qi will give an experience of relaxation as Qi is moved, but ultimately this drains Yang Qi and dries Yin Qi, so leading to Rising Empty Heat that agitates the Shen. There is now a situation of a Depleted Lower Burner and an Agitated Upper Burner. Damp and Heat can result from this imbalance, and so Phlegm can be formed.

Antihistamines are principally used to suppress the histamine-caused features of allergic reactions. They therefore suppress itch, swelling and redness. The therapeutic action is to Clear Wind and Heat, presumably also by Dispersing Qi. The side effects of the antihistamines include dry mouth, headache, blurred vision and difficulty in urination, and suggest that these drugs may be Heating and ultimately Stagnating of Qi and may damage Kidney Yin. Sedation implies that the action is also obstructive to the Heart and so is akin to Phlegm.

ANXIOLYTIC DRUGS

Anxiolytic drugs are prescribed for the purpose of reducing anxiety.

Short- to medium-acting benzodiazepines (described above under "Hypnotic drugs"), which include diazepam and lorazepam, are the most commonly prescribed anxiolytics in the UK. As described above, these are believed to act by promoting the action of the inhibitory neurotransmitter GABA in the brain. The action of these drugs is fairly rapid and short-lived, which makes them appropriate for treating anxiety that might be short-lived (e.g. the fear of a plane flight) and to control a panic attack or a reaction to acute trauma. Long-term prescription of these highly addictive drugs is not considered to be appropriate, according to current medical guidelines.

Side effects of the short- to medium-acting benzodiazepines include drowsiness, confusion, unsteadiness, increase in aggressiveness and, occasionally, headache, digestive disturbances, urinary problems and blood disorders. As described for the hypnotic drugs, benzodiazepines readily induce a state of dependence, and so are highly addictive. After withdrawal from a long-term prescription an unpleasant withdrawal syndrome may become apparent.

Buspirone is a non-benzodiazepine anxiolytic that is considered to be a less-addictive alternative to the benzodiazepines. It is believed to act at the serotonin (5HT1A) receptor. The response to buspirone is delayed and may take up to two weeks to take effect, which means it is less likely to be prescribed in cases of acute overwhelming anxiety. Side effects of buspirone include nausea, dizziness, palpitations and dry mouth.

Beta blocker drugs, such as propranolol, may also be prescribed for their anxiety-reducing action. The beta blockers act by blocking the action of the neurotransmitter hormones adrenaline and noradrenaline. For this reason, they may be particularly effective if physical symptoms such as palpitations and tremor are the primary problems for the patient (such as might affect stage performers or musicians).

Side effects of beta blockers include slow heart rate, cold extremities, impotence and dream-disturbed sleep.

 Information box 6.2c-II

Anxiolytic drugs: comments from a Chinese medicine perspective

From a Chinese medicine perspective, anxiolytic drugs have a similar action as hypnotic drugs. The reduction in anxiety can be described as a Calming of the Shen. Hot medicinals may initially be calming because of their dispersing effect (see Information box 6.2c-I). In the long term, anxiolytic drugs induce dependence, and when they are suddenly withdrawn the resulting agitation and risk of seizures indicate a severe imbalance has developed. This might be described in terms of Depletion of Yin, Empty Heat Harassing the Heart, Stagnation of Liver Qi, Stasis of Liver Blood and sometimes Generation of Wind.

In contrast, the side effects of beta blockers suggest they have a Cooling action and manifest in Depletion of Heart Yang, as they slow the pulse, and cause cold extremities and low libido. However, side effects of rashes, diabetes, fatigue and increased tendency to allergies suggest that that they also redirect Heat into the Interior and also Deplete Qi. Presumably they are anxiolytic because they reduce the Harassing Effect of Heat on the Heart, but at the same time they are ultimately depleting. Greenwood (2007)[41] argues that their action further separates Yin and Yang and increases any original imbalance. He suggests that beta blockers place a block between Wood and Fire, meaning that the excess Yang that was previously manifesting in the circulatory system is now manifesting in Stagnant Qi and resultant Heat that impacts on other organ systems.

Confusion or drowsiness is a manifestation of Obstruction of the Shen (possibly indicating Phlegm-like action).

ANTIPSYCHOTIC DRUGS

Antipsychotic drugs are also known as neuroleptics and major tranquillizers. They may be used to manage patients who are acutely disturbed for a range of underlying causes. In the long term they are prescribed to manage the symptoms of thought disorder, hallucinations and delusions, which are characteristic of psychoses (including schizophrenia and bipolar disorder). They may also be prescribed in the long term for patients who manifest long-term symptoms of mental disturbance as a result of an underlying chronic mental health disorder (such as can develop in Alzheimer's disease).

Antipsychotic drugs are usually administered in tablet or liquid form, but may be given by intramuscular injection for rapid sedation in an acutely disturbed patient. For some antipsychotics a slow release form of the drug (depot medication) is available. Depot medication may be offered to patients in the community who are considered to be less likely to take tablets on a regular basis. A community psychiatric nurse usually gives the depot injections every two to four weeks.

Antipsychotic drugs are recognized to block the dopamine D2 receptors. They may also act on a range of other peptide receptors, including the acetylcholine, adrenaline, histamine and serotonin (5HT) receptors. The mechanism that underlies the antipsychotic action of these drugs is believed to be interference with the dopamine systems in the brain. However, for some of the older antipsychotic medications, this interference carries the well-recognized negative consequence of a Parkinsonian syndrome, including muscle stiffness, poverty of spontaneous movement and coarse tremor.

The important side effects of antipsychotic medications are summarized in Table 6.2c-I.

Table 6.2c-I Side effects of antipsychotic drugs (major tranquillizers)

Category of side effect	Specific side effects
General side effects	Drowsiness and sluggishness: these are very common and can contribute to the state of dullness or vacancy that can be characteristic of a person on antipsychotic medication
	Confusion and agitation
	Weight gain: this is very common, particularly with the newer major tranquillizers
	Raised blood sugar and diabetes (in association with weight gain)
	Acne and rashes: acne is common and sensitivity to sunlight is well recognized
	Drop in blood pressure and arrhythmias
	Disturbances in temperature control (rarely, life-threatening hyperthermia)
	Jaundice (disturbed liver function)
Antimuscarinic side effects (resulting from the effect of the drug in inhibiting the action of acetylcholine)	Dry mouth
	Constipation
	Difficulty in urination
	Blurred vision
Extrapyramidal symptoms (movement disorders resulting from neurochemical changes in the extrapyramidal nerve pathways in the brain)	Parkinsonian symptoms: muscle stiffness and tremor can appear gradually after a few days, but can progress to become both disabling and stigmatizing. These symptoms will reverse if the drug is withdrawn. Drugs such as trihexiphenidyl (Benzhexol) may be prescribed concurrently to counteract the Parkinsonian side effects
	Dystonia and dyskinesia: these terms describe acute states of muscular tension and bodily distortion that are rare but tend to affect young people after just a few doses of the drug
	Akathisia: this term is used to describe a state of muscular restlessness in which the patient feels an irrepressible urge to shift position, move their limbs and walk around. All these manifestations can add to the visual stigma associated with major mental illness
	Tardive dyskinesia: this is a state of abnormal muscle movement that usually appears after long-term treatment with antipsychotic medication. The patient will experience involuntary movements that particularly affect the muscles of the face (e.g. lip smacking, pouting and chewing movements). Again, these side effects are stigmatizing, and of the four muscle-associated side effects of the antipsychotic drugs are considered the most serious as they may not resolve on withdrawal of treatment

There are many antipsychotic drugs, each of which has its own characteristic range of side effects. For example, the more sedating drugs (such as chlorpromazine) may have less pronounced neuromuscular side effects than the less sedating drugs (such as fluphenazine).

The more recently developed antipsychotics (atypical antipsychotics), which include risperidone and olanzapine, are currently more widely prescribed than their predecessors such as chlorpromazine and haloperidol because they are associated with a reduced range of side effects. However, the newer drugs do have the unfortunate tendency of inducing metabolic syndrome (weight gain, raised blood sugar and lipids, and hypertension) and also delays in the conduction of the electrical charge in the heart in many people. This means people on antipsychotics will need regular healthcare checks including blood tests and an electrocardiogram (ECG).

The National Institute for Health and Care Excellence (NICE) guidelines (2014) for the management of psychosis and schizophrenia in adults[42] recommends that these new drugs should be the first or second choice of medication for new episodes of schizophrenia. However, one of these atypical antipsychotics, clozapine, carries a significant risk of depleting the white blood cells (agranulocytosis), and so is only prescribed if the patient can have regular blood tests and if two other antipsychotics have not proved acceptable.

Because of the range of disabling and stigmatizing side effects, the prescription of antipsychotic medication should be one that is made only after deep consideration. Ideally, the prescription and monitoring of these potent and potentially dangerous drugs should be supervised by a consultant psychiatrist.

Sudden withdrawal from antipsychotic medication is not advised because a recurrence of psychosis is a possible serious consequence. Ideally, withdrawal is supervised and gradual, and the patient is supported throughout the withdrawal process.

Information box 6.2c-III

Antipsychotic drugs: comments from a Chinese medicine perspective

To attempt a Chinese medicine interpretation of antipsychotic drugs is challenging. The principal therapeutic action is sedation and calming of agitated thoughts. The condition treated with these drugs is often the form of mental disorder known in Chinese medicine as Dian Kuang (see Section 6.2e). This is, in very general terms, a manifestation of Phlegm, and Heat Obstructing the Orifices of the Heart, often on the background of long-term Deficiency of, for example, Spleen, Heart and/or Lung Qi.

Because of this, the effect of the antipsychotic drugs might be interpreted as Cooling, in a similar way as the hypnotics and anxiolytics are seen as Cooling, in that they appear to Clear agitating Heat. It could also be said that these drugs Clear Phlegm. However, the drowsiness, confusion, sluggishness and dullness that result from these drugs all suggest that they cause a marked Obstruction of the Shen. Weight gain and acne imply the generation of Damp Heat and Phlegm, and rashes, dry mouth, constipation and hyperpyrexia all imply Heat. The extrapyramidal side effects of stiffness, tremor and involuntary muscle movements imply Stagnation of Liver Qi and Liver Wind. Jaundice suggests Damp Heat in the Liver.

The wide range of side effects is testimony to the potency of these drugs, and from an alternative perspective would speak very strongly of Suppression of the expression of Pathogenic Factors characteristic of psychosis (Heat and Phlegm) so that they manifest instead in the physical form of these sometimes very severe side effects.

MOOD STABILIZERS

Mood stabilizers (sometimes called anti-mania drugs) are medications that have been found to prevent the profound swings of mood that are characteristic of bipolar disorder (manic-depressive psychosis). The most commonly prescribed mood stabilizer is lithium carbonate (usually known as lithium), but some of the antiepileptic preparations may also be used with some effect if lithium is not helpful. Antiepileptic drugs that are used are carbamazepine, sodium valproate and lamotrigine. Atypical antipsychotics, such as olanzapine, may also be prescribed for their mood-stabilizing effects.

The action of lithium was discovered entirely by chance in the late 1940s. Even now the mechanism of the mood-stabilizing drugs is not clearly understood, although it has been recently clarified that lithium seems to damp down the activity of secondary messenger systems within nerve cells. These systems are those that are set in action within a cell when a peptide binds to a membrane receptor.

Lithium is a toxic drug, and its levels have to be monitored carefully (every three months), even when the patient is on a steady dose. Because lithium is particularly toxic to the kidneys and may induce hypothyroidism, both renal and thyroid function blood tests should be performed before the patient commences treatment. Side effects include digestive disturbances, weight gain, thirst, excessive urination, tremor and fluid retention. If the levels of lithium become too high, the patient can experience confusion, severe tremor, slurred speech and vomiting. This is a life-threatening situation and requires rehydration and hospital management.

In the long term, lithium has been associated with impairment of memory, thinking and thyroid disorders.

Although the side effects in the short term are less disabling and stigmatizing than those associated with antipsychotics, nevertheless, mood-stabilizing drugs are powerful preparations. They should not be prescribed without careful consideration of the balance of the potential risks and benefits.

Information box 6.2c-IV

Mood stabilizers: comments from a Chinese medicine perspective

From a Chinese medicine perspective, the primary action of lithium for stabilizing mood might also be interpreted as Cooling and Clearing of Phlegm and Stagnation. However, the side effects of lithium are very different to those of antipsychotic drugs. Thirst and excessive urination suggest Depletion of Kidney Qi, with Separation of Yang and Yin becoming manifest. Hypothyroidism is primarily a condition associated with the features of Kidney Yang Deficiency and Accumulation of Damp Phlegm. Long-term damage to thinking, memory and thyroid function all suggest Kidney and Jing Deficiency. Tremor suggests Liver Wind. Weight gain suggests Damp Phlegm, and digestive disturbances suggest Disorder of the Spleen/Stomach Qi.

Some of these diverse side effects can be explained in terms of Suppression of Heat (thus damaging Kidney Yin) and Phlegm formation.

ANTIDEPRESSANTS

Antidepressants are used to treat episodes of moderate to severe depression and also states in which there is chronically depressed mood. Ideally, brief periods of mild depression should not be treated with antidepressants.

There are four broad classes into which most prescribed antidepressants fall: tricyclics (amitriptyline and clomipramine), monoamine oxidase inhibitors (MAOIs), selective serotonin reuptake inhibitors (SSRIs) and the newer serotonin and noradrenaline reuptake inhibitors (SNRIs).

MAOIs are far less frequently used since the advent of the SSRIs because they can cause a dangerous syndrome when the patient consumes food containing the substance tyramine (e.g. cheese, pickled fish and yeast extract). However, these drugs may still be prescribed in a specialist setting in the case of severe intractable depression.

Tricyclics and SSRIs appear to have a similar profile of effectiveness in depression, but differ in terms of their side effects. The side effects of dry mouth, constipation, difficulty in urination and blurred vision are all more common with tricyclics, but the safety of these drugs is well established. The far more widely used SSRIs may have fewer long-term side effects than tricyclics, but concern about safety (in terms of increasing the risk of aggressive outbursts and suicide) may affect prescribing choices. SSRIs are also more associated with nausea and other digestive disturbances, although these side effects often diminish after a few weeks of treatment.

Antidepressants take two to six weeks to exert an effect on mood, although side effects will become apparent straight away. The patient needs to be informed of this so that they do not give up on the treatment before it has had the time to take effect. After this time interval, the patient often feels more optimistic and able to get on with life in a way that may have formerly seemed impossible. Observant onlookers may report that the personality of the patient may appear slightly blunted, as if a degree of sensitivity to the vagaries of life has been lost.

Sometimes the dose needs to be increased gradually for the optimum effect on mood to be obtained. In some cases a change in the type of antidepressant may effect a more beneficial change. The general recommendation is that the minimum length of prescription is six months.

Antidepressants are not addictive in the way in which hypnotic and anxiolytic drugs are. A patient will not crave a dose should they have to miss one or two. However, it is becoming increasingly recognized that antidepressants do induce a form of dependence in that a risk of relapse to a state of depression is more likely if withdrawal from the drug is abrupt. Also, some patients experience a withdrawal syndrome that includes symptoms such as anxiety, nausea, vomiting, diarrhea, dizziness and headache on abrupt withdrawal from the drug. For this reason it is advised that if a long course of treatment is followed, the withdrawal should be gradual and carefully monitored by the prescribing doctor.

St John's wort (*Hypericum perforatum*) is a herbal preparation that has established benefits in mild to moderate depression, although there is no proven benefit in major depression. The mode of action is unclear, but it is considered likely that it acts in the body in a similar way to SSRIs. For this reason it is not recommended that St John's wort is taken concurrently with any other antidepressant. Furthermore, because there are known interactions of St John's Wort with a range of prescribed medications, it should not be commenced by someone on other medication without first consulting the prescribing doctor. St John's wort is not currently available in the UK on National Health Service (NHS) prescription.

Dietary supplements such as tryptophan and 5-hydroxytryptophan (5-HTP) are also claimed to improve mood in some people, and demonstrate a rapid rather than delayed effect on mood. These supplements are both precursors of the manufacture of serotonin in the body, and so it would make sense that they could, in theory, help to lift mood by leading to a rise in serotonin levels. Tryptophan is an amino acid that is found in a range of high-protein foods, including warmed milk products, turkey, beef, chicken, eggs, yeast, nuts, seeds and bananas. It was banned by the US Food and Drug Administration (FDA) after 1989 because of fears about possible contamination. 5-HTP is a naturally occurring relative of tryptophan that is prepared from the African herb *Griffonia simplicifolia*. Neither of these supplements is available in the UK on NHS prescription, but like St John's wort, both are freely available from health food outlets.[43]

Information box 6.2c-V

Antidepressants: comments from a Chinese medicine perspective

In lifting depression, the primary Chinese interpretation of the therapeutic effect of antidepressants would be that they help to move the Liver Qi Stagnation that is often very apparent in depression. The brighter outlook, ability to act on plans and feelings of hope that can result from treatment are all testimony to a movement of Liver Qi. The return of feelings of emotional warmth would also relate to a Movement or Boosting of Heart Qi. These drugs are considered by Rosenberg (2000), Flaws and Lake (2001), and Greenwood (2004)[44] to be Warm in nature and they act by Dispersing and ultimately Depleting Yang Qi. This movement is perceived as relaxation and lifting of the mood by the patient, although this comes at an energetic cost. The Warming nature of these drugs not only Disperses Yang, but also Dries Up Yin and leads to Generation of Internal Heat.

Tricyclic antidepressants often cause dry mouth, thirst, constipation and rapid pulse rate, which could all be attributed to Internal Heat. On rare occasions they can cause heart arrhythmias and rashes, and are also recognized to trigger episodes of mania, confusion or psychosis. Rapid arrhythmias may be a manifestation of Heat in the Heart, and the mental complications may be due to Heat and/or Phlegm Obstructing the Orifices of the Heart.

Side effects of SSRIs include initial digestive disturbances, dry mouth, rashes and problems in sexual function. They can also trigger aggressive outbursts, suicidal ideas and episodes of mania. The digestive disturbances can be described in terms of Liver Qi Invading Stomach and Spleen (nausea, vomiting, diarrhea and abdominal pain). Sexual dysfunction (commonly an inability to achieve orgasm) can also be described in terms of an Imbalance of Liver function, as can aggressive outbursts. The risk of mania might be related to the tendency of the drugs to lead to Obstruction of the Orifices of the Heart by Stagnation, Heat or Phlegm.

The side effects of common antidepressants indicate that there is a possibility that these drugs might be shifting the imbalance of depression to a different level of expression in the body. The side effects of tricyclics speak strongly of release of Heat, perhaps created as a consequence of long-standing repressed emotions, whereas the side effects of SSRIs suggest that these drugs have led to a re-expression of an Imbalance in the flow of Liver Qi.

Withdrawal from antidepressants leads to a syndrome of low mood, agitation and anxiety that can be long-standing. The loss of the outward-moving action of these medicinals is likely to lead to Liver Qi Stagnation, and the patient's true state of Depletion and Disharmony of Yin and Yang is revealed.

DRUGS USED IN THE TREATMENT OF ALZHEIMER'S DISEASE

One class of drugs has been demonstrated to show modest benefits in terms of memory and concentration in up to about half of patients with mild to moderate Alzheimer's disease. These drugs, which act by affecting the function of a brain enzyme called acetyl cholinesterase, should only be prescribed under specialist supervision. They should be reviewed after three months of treatment to see if the benefit of taking the drug outweighs the problems that might have resulted from the side effects of the drugs (these include digestive disturbance, fatigue and dizziness). The drugs include donepezil, galantamine and memantine.

Information box 6.2c-VI

Drugs used in Alzheimer's disease: comments from a Chinese medicine perspective

From a Chinese medicine perspective, the action of the drugs used in Alzheimer's disease could be interpreted as Boosting Kidney Jing (Essence), but very possibly at the expense of Depleting Qi at a deeper level. Side effects are diverse and include abnormal dreams, aggression, agitation, fatigue, muscle cramps, nausea, depression and rash. These suggest potential to deep internal imbalance. Liver Qi Stagnation and Liver Yin Deficiency with Spleen Qi Deficiency and Depressive Heat could be associated with many of these symptoms.

Other physically directed treatments for psychiatric disorders

ELECTROCONVULSIVE THERAPY (ECT)
(ELECTRIC SHOCK THERAPY)

Seizure therapy was first developed in Hungary in 1934 when the erroneous observation was made that the incidence of schizophrenia appeared to be low in people who suffered from epileptic fits. For this reason, the practice of inducing epileptic fits in schizophrenic patients (initially by intravenous administration of a stimulant drug called cardiazol, and later by application of an electric current to the temples) was begun. It was first performed in the UK in 1939. Within 20 years, electroconvulsive therapy (ECT) was being used to treat a wide range of psychiatric conditions. Despite the link between epilepsy and schizophrenia being later discredited, ECT was found to bring about an improvement in mood in some patients. It is now almost exclusively to treat severe intractable mood disorders. Studies have demonstrated that ECT is effective in terms of relieving mood, sometimes strikingly so, but its use carries a high cost in terms of causing memory loss. The degree of memory loss is proportional to the number of treatments.

The administration of ECT prior to the 1950s was very basic, and patients frequently suffered from severe complications. Anesthetics were not given, and so the patient had to be strapped down prior to the shock. Poor control of the fit meant that severe injuries could be sustained. In current practice, the patient is given an anesthetic and a muscle relaxant prior to the treatment, so that the induced fit is less traumatic and dangerous. It has been discovered that application of the electrode to one temple only, rather than both, maintains the effectiveness of the treatment, but reduces the incidence and severity of memory loss and confusion afterwards. With the exception of memory loss the risks of the procedure are now similar to those of giving a general anesthetic alone.[45]

ECT is administered by a psychiatric doctor with an anesthetist in attendance in a hospital setting. Usually a course of six to ten treatments is given over the period of two to three weeks, each of which is expected to lead to a stepwise improvement in mood.

Information box 6.2c-VII

Electroconvulsive therapy: comments from a Chinese medicine perspective

From a Chinese perspective, an epileptic fit is described as a Stirring of Phlegm by Liver Wind. This term embraces the loss of consciousness and the tonic-clonic muscle contractions that occur in a generalized fit. This is possibly how one could describe the immediate action of the controlled ECT convulsion. The lifting of the state of profound low mood would suggest that this extreme stimulus has led to the movement of Phlegm and Liver Qi. However, as has been suggested in the interpretation of the electric shock of cardioversion, the shock is a Yang stimulus, and as such will be inherently Depleting of Yin. The cumulative memory loss that results from this treatment may be evidence of an insidious Depletion of Kidney Qi, and possibly Jing.

PSYCHOSURGERY

Brain surgery is now only a very rarely recommended treatment for psychiatric disease, although it was an option chosen much more often in the 1930s to 1960s. The operation of a lobotomy, which involves the severing of the fibers that link the frontal lobes to the other parts of the brain, was first introduced in the late 1930s in an attempt to treat schizophrenia. A marked change in personality and the development of epilepsy were serious outcomes of this crude procedure.

Information box 6.2c-VIII

Psychosurgery: comments from a Chinese medicine perspective

By its very nature, the removal of a portion of the brain has to be interpreted as Depleting of Qi and Jing. A positive outcome from the perspective of obsessive-compulsive disorder or depression would have to correspond to a movement of Liver Qi and/or Phlegm, but this will have been at the expense of a Depletion of Vital Substances.

Nowadays, psychosurgical approaches are far less crude, and involve surgical destruction of very tiny and precisely located areas of the brain. These operations are exclusively used to treat severe intractable obsessive-compulsive disorder and depression.

Psychological therapies for psychiatric disorders

A number of talking therapies have emerged for treating the psychological roots of mental health disorders. Most of these therapies involve the patient undergoing change as a result of talking with a therapist, or as part of a therapist-guided group. Talking therapies are also described as psychotherapies, and range in approach from simple supportive counseling to intensive psychoanalysis.

Talking therapies are characterized by some common features:

- the therapist–patient relationship is the therapeutic tool

- rapport and trust are essential for the effectiveness of the therapy

- change often occurs because the interaction provides the patient with new knowledge that helps them to make sense of their situation

- the interaction between therapist and patient enables new ways of thinking and behaving that are ideally beneficial for the patient.

Talking therapies differ from the help that might be offered by a supportive friend in that the therapist maintains a distinct role as a compassionate but detached professional, rather than an equal, and the therapist works in a systematic way from a series of previously defined psychological principles.

Counseling is a term that is often used interchangeably with psychotherapy, but strictly speaking refers to an approach in which the explicit aim is to help the patient through the development of increased insight into their situation. With increased insight the patient is enabled to make important decisions about specific aspects of their lives. Counseling may be tailored to diverse situations such as marriage guidance, grief management, dealing with terminal illness and making career choices.

Other therapies focus on encouraging the patient to make positive changes through certain activities, for example, art therapy, music therapy and participation in exercise programs. Talking therapies are summarized in Table 6.2c-II.

Table 6.2c-II The different forms of psychotherapy

Therapy type	Description
Behavioral therapy	Focuses primarily on helping the patient to create changes in unhelpful behaviors. It is based on the theory that, because all behavior is learned, maladaptive behaviors can be unlearned and new, more helpful, behaviors can be acquired. Different forms of behavioral therapy can be used to treat phobias, obsessional behavior, poor social skills and sexual deviance. Techniques used in behavioral therapy include: • graded exposure to an object of fear (e.g. a spider) in the treatment of phobias • flooding – the sudden exposure to an object of fear to enable the patient to realize that the anxiety will not overwhelm them (also for the treatment of phobias) • modeling – the patient is encouraged to model the therapist's behavior in order to learn new patterns of acting (used to treat phobias and obsessional behavior such as excessive hand washing) • social skills training
Cognitive therapy	Focuses primarily on helping the patient to modify unhelpful thought patterns. It can be used to treat depression, anxiety, phobias and eating disorders. The psychologist Aaron Beck proposed that negative patterns of thought may actually cause and maintain the state of depression, and so developed techniques to challenge these thought patterns and encourage more positive ways of thinking. The techniques used by a cognitive therapist include helping a patient to recognize and name their negative thoughts and then to challenge them. For example: "Do you think that it is really true that you get things wrong all the time?" or "Is it really possible that everybody hates you?" The therapist will also explore with the patient the roots of these thought patterns (often by uncovering negative experiences and relationships experienced in childhood) in order to help the patient understand their origin. The patient may be prescribed exercises to do at home, such as keeping a diary of negative thoughts and repeating positive affirmations
Individual analytical psychotherapy	Focuses on uncovering the deep psychological roots to a psychological problem. Often individual psychotherapy involves regular sessions one or more times a week, and may continue for several years. Ideally, the insight gained by the patient is the trigger for positive change. Techniques such as free association, dream analysis and recognition of projected feelings between the therapist and the patient (counter-transference and transference) are used to help point to the underlying psychological issues. There are a number of approaches to individual psychotherapy that reflect their underlying psychological theories (e.g. Freudian, Jungian, Rogerian, Reichian and transactional analysis)
Brief focal psychotherapy	Uses a range of approaches to meet a clearly defined goal (e.g. the management of anger outbursts) within a defined number of sessions
Group psychotherapy	Used to uncover deep psychological roots to problems, particularly problems that may manifest in the patient's interpersonal interactions. In group therapy the therapist facilitates the social interactions that occur within a safe group of people in order to help the individuals arrive at a deeper insight about themselves and the way in which they interact with other people. Safety is achieved by stressing the importance of confidentiality and clear boundaries for the group (e.g. group members will be advised against meeting socially outside the time of the sessions while the therapy is in progress)
Family therapy	Used to facilitate insight into the nature of the dynamics between the members of a family unit. The intention is to deal with dysfunctional family patterns or difficult behavior in one of the family members
Couples therapy	Focuses on the particular issues that can develop within intimate relationships. Ideally, both individuals involved in the relationship attend for most of the sessions with the therapist
Sex therapy	A particular form of couples therapy focused on sexual problems rather than relationship problems. It is not appropriate in those cases where the sexual problem is a manifestation of an underlying relationship problem. The sex therapist is likely to use a combination of cognitive and behavioral techniques to help deal with problems in the formation of a satisfying sexual relationship between partners

Art and music therapies	Often used in a group context to allow patients to express more unconscious aspects of their thought processes. The therapist can then, if it seems appropriate, enable the patient to learn to interpret what they have expressed, and so gain insight into deep psychological issues. The expression of unconscious material through music and art can be seen as cathartic and therapeutic in itself. Both music and art therapy can be of particular help in working with children and people with intellectual difficulties
Supportive psychotherapy	Involves therapy sessions that enable the patient to manage life issues that would otherwise overwhelm them. If the issues are acute in onset (e.g. following a sudden trauma or bereavement), the term crisis intervention may be used. If the issues are longstanding, the supportive psychotherapy can be compared to a medication used to control a chronic medical condition. In some situations the psychological problems are so longstanding and disabling that the patient requires regular supportive input literally to keep going. In such cases, dealing with the deep roots of the problem may be an unrealistic or, at the least, only a very long-term goal

Most of these therapies, and in particular short courses of cognitive behavioral therapy, are accessible to patients in the UK through the National Health Service (NHS), but provision can be sporadic and does not often meet demand. Faced with long waiting lists, patients may self-refer for private counseling or psychotherapy, without a clear understanding of their particular needs, or whether or not the approach of their therapist is one that is suited to these needs.

Information box 6.2c-IX

Psychotherapy: comments from a Chinese medicine perspective

From a complementary medical perspective, any therapy that enables the patient to move towards a more balanced and less dependent state could be described as curative in nature. In an ideal world all therapies would deal with the root causes of psychological imbalance, and so by definition would be effecting cure.

However, the root cause is not always immediately apparent, and many therapies, for pragmatic reasons, are not designed to target the root of the problem. For example, the behavioral therapies focus on modification of behavior, and so may not directly address the root causes of the unhelpful behavior patterns. If they do so, they may actually be suppressive in nature and, although symptoms may improve, a deep imbalance may persist after the therapy has been concluded. The problem of long-term dependence on therapy is well recognized (and can, of course, also apply to Chinese medicine consultations), a clear indication that whatever is being offered is not actually attending to the root cause.

Greenwood (2004)[46] argues that if any treatment is directed at the level of moving of Liver Qi Stagnation, very often understood in Traditional Chinese Medicine to be the root of depression or anxiety, even this will not be treating the deep roots of the problem. He suggests that Liver Qi Stagnation itself is a manifestation of a deeper existential crisis, one that springs from man's perceived separation of himself from the cosmos. Therefore, until the fundamental illusions at the heart of the perceived split are attended to, all treatments designed to smooth Liver Qi will be ultimately suppressive, and so the patient will remain dependent upon them.

In chronic severe psychological problems, a state of dependence on the therapy, as would apply in cases of supportive psychotherapy, could be the most that may reasonably be expected to be achieved. For this reason, a state of dependence on the therapist must not be seen as necessarily negative, particularly if it is enabling a patient to cope from day to day in a way that would have been impossible without the support offered by the therapy.

However, when dependence is recognized, the question needs always to be asked whether the patient could be offered something different that might enable them to move from their static position. Sometimes the addition of an entirely different approach to healing, such as hypnosis, acupuncture or other forms of body work, may be what is required. This may then move the patient on from a place of dependence to a place from where they can allow the insights gained in therapy to generate significant internal changes.

Therapies can, of course, also carry the risk of side effects. An unhelpful therapeutic relationship may actually compound emotional problems or, at worst, if abusive in some way, may even cause new imbalances.

Social interventions for psychiatric disorders

Occupational therapy in the treatment of psychological problems involves teaching patients skills of daily living such as cooking, shopping and organizing daily activities. Finding a satisfying recreational activity is also an aim of occupational therapy, and so arts and crafts workshops and yoga classes may fall under the remit of the provision of occupational therapy in hospitals and outpatient clinics. Skills such as word processing or gardening can be taught, which might enable a patient to find employment. Sheltered workshops are establishments in the community that preferentially employ people who have experienced mental health problems in order to enable them to develop skills that would be relevant to more independent employment in the future.

Rehabilitation is a term used to describe the process whereby a patient is enabled to return to as normal a life as possible after an episode of illness, be it physical or psychological. In the context of mental health problems, the process of rehabilitation of a patient requires multidisciplinary support from psychiatric nurses, occupational therapists, social workers and the patient's doctors. In the UK this multidisciplinary approach is mediated by community mental health teams (CMHTs), which support the patients who live in a particular locality.

Sheltered and supported housing ideally provide a supportive home in the community, where a person with mental health problems can find both social support and a sense of community. Often this is in the context of a group home, which is either overseen by a trained member of staff or regularly visited by members of the local CMHT.

Psychiatric social workers play a crucial role in the support of a person with severe mental illness, both in hospital and in the community. The social worker can advise the patient on their legal rights and also on access to financial support, such as housing and sickness benefits. As part of the CMHT, the social worker will function as a member of the team supporting the patient in the process of rehabilitation into the community.

The approved mental health professional (AMHP) is a social worker or mental health nurse who has been recognized to have the training appropriate for making recommendations that patients be admitted to hospital for assessment and/or treatment according to the various sections of the England and Wales Mental Health Act 1983 (amended in 2007). The AMHP plays a key role in relation to the practical application of the sections of the Mental Health Act as they apply to individual patients, as will be explored presently.

The England and Wales Mental Health Act 1983 (amended in 2007)[47]

The England and Wales Mental Health Act (MHA) 1983 summarizes the legislation that has been designed principally to protect the rights and enable the safe treatment of people suffering from specific mental health disorders. Section 1 of the Act, which was amended in 2007, attempts to provide a legal definition of those mental health problems that the MHA is intended to cover (i.e. mental health disorders), and also specifies that the term mental health disorders should not be applied by reason of dependence on alcohol or drugs.

Sections 2–5 of the MHA specify the conditions under which a patient can be compulsorily admitted to or held in hospital for assessment and/or treatment. The verb to section, as it applies to patients with mental illness, derives from these sections of the Act, and is often used to describe this process of admitting patients to psychiatric hospital against their will. Statistics from the charity Mind reveal that in a single year (2000–01) over 40,000 people in England and Wales were detained in hospital under one of these sections of the MHA.

Section 2 of the MHA describes the conditions for admission for assessment. This applies to a period of no longer than 28 days. For a patient to be compulsorily admitted to hospital under Section 2 of the Act they need to have a recognizable mental disorder as specified under Section 1. In addition, the admission has to be formally recommended by two medical practitioners, one of whom has been previously approved (according to Section 12 of the Act) to make psychiatric assessments.

An AMHP or the nearest relative in the patient's family is entitled under the terms of the Act to apply for the admission of the patient. It is usually best for the AMHP to make this application rather than the relative, in order to protect the relative from the implications of being the one who caused the admission to hospital.

Section 2 of the Act may be applied to a patient in whom the actual diagnosis of the mental disorder is unclear and where there is a need for an inpatient assessment of the mental health condition. Once in hospital under a Section 2 assessment order, the patient is not permitted to leave the ward at will. If the patient is considered to be at risk of absconding they may be placed in a locked unit, and if they are considered at risk of self-harm they may be placed under close nursing supervision.

Section 3 of the MHA describes the conditions for admission for treatment. This applies for a period of no longer than six months. In the case of Section 3 of the Act, the patient needs to have a recognizable mental health disorder that would be expected to respond to treatment, and that requires inpatient admission for the treatment to be administered.

Section 3 can be renewed by formal application by the responsible psychiatric doctor, and thereafter at yearly intervals. The patient has a right to appeal against the decision to a Mental Health Review Tribunal within six months of admission.

The responsible psychiatric doctor, the hospital managers and the patient's closest relative all have powers under Sections 2 and 3 of the Act to discharge the patient, although the responsible doctor can override any decision to discharge if they feel the patient or those around them would be put at risk if discharge were permitted.

Once in hospital under a Section 3 treatment order, a patient is not permitted to leave the ward at will and is obliged to comply with prescribed treatment. If the patient refuses treatment, the doctors and nursing staff are legally entitled to enforce the treatment on the patient. This might involve the use of control and restraint techniques, during which the patient might be held down whilst an injection is administered.

Section 117 of the MHA specifies that the medical team has a responsibility to set up adequate aftercare arrangements for patients discharged from an admission to hospital under Section 3 of the Act. In this Section a multidisciplinary approach to care is emphasized. The Mental Health (Patients in the Community) Act 1995 follows this Section of the Act, and controversially describes the conditions for supervised discharge for certain patients. In supervised discharge, the patient is obliged to follow certain requirements after discharge, which include living at an agreed place and attending for the administration of recommended treatment such as medication and occupational therapy. The patient also has to agree to permit access to a doctor or approved social worker when this is requested. This Act stops short of requiring patients to take medications against their will.

6.2d Anxiety, depression, somatoform disorders and eating disorders

This section is dedicated to those mental health disorders in which it is generally agreed that personality is intact and a degree of insight into the condition is retained by the patient. In all these disorders it would be possible to say that normal communication could be maintained between the patient and another person, and in general the patient would be seen as troubled rather than mad. The term neurosis can be used to describe a mental health disorder such as these in which a degree of insight into the condition is retained by the patient.

With the exception of bereavement, all the disorders described below are diagnoses described within the International Classification of Diseases 10 (ICD-10), and can be found in the sections entitled "Neurotic, stress-related and somatoform disorders," "Mood [affective] disorders" and "Disorders of adult personality and behavior."

The conditions discussed in this section are:

Part I: Anxiety disorders

- panic disorder and agoraphobia
- social phobia
- simple (specific) phobia
- obsessive-compulsive disorder (OCD)
- post-traumatic stress disorder (PTSD)
- generalized anxiety disorder (GAD)

Part II: Depression, somatoform disorders and eating disorders

- Depression:
  - the syndrome of depression
  - bereavement and grief
- Disorders manifesting in bodily functions:
  - malingering and factitious disorder
  - conversion disorder
  - hypochondriasis
  - somatization disorder
  - neurasthenia
  - dissociative disorders
  - psychosomatic disorders
- Eating disorders:
  - anorexia nervosa
  - bulimia nervosa.

Part I: Anxiety disorders

The syndrome of anxiety

The term anxiety, derived from the Latin word for choking, is used to describe a very commonly experienced syndrome. The term syndrome is appropriate for anxiety, as the full experience of anxiety is not just a fearful emotion but also involves a cluster of physiological changes and characteristic changes in thinking. Most people will be more than familiar with these features, as anxiety is one of the normal human responses to frightening situations. In the short term, anxiety serves a useful purpose in preparing the body for the fight-or-flight response to a threat. It is when anxiety becomes overwhelming or ingrained as a chronic (i.e. long-standing) response that it becomes debilitating and disabling. Here we explore what the syndrome of anxiety entails in terms of symptoms and signs, and then describe the different forms in which maladaptive anxiety can manifest.

The clinical features of anxiety

As mentioned above, the syndrome of anxiety has three distinct components: the emotional experience, characteristic changes in thinking, and physiological symptoms and signs.

The emotion associated with anxiety is a sense of foreboding or dread, and can be as extreme as a fear of impending doom.

In the state of anxiety the thoughts might appear to speed up or slow down, and there can be unusual perceptions of light, sound and reality. The anxious person can become over-vigilant and irritable, and very commonly sleep is disturbed.

The physiological changes associated with anxiety include a rapid heartbeat, raised blood pressure, chest pain, rapid breathing, tremor, muscle tension, dizziness, tingling, sweating, a sensation of choking, nausea, loss of appetite, altered bowel movements, frequency of urination and tendency to a pronounced startle response.

Not everyone who experiences anxiety will experience all these symptoms and signs, although in severe chronic cases it is not uncommon for a person to experience a large proportion of these clinical features.

If the degree of anxiety intensifies, it can develop into an overwhelming syndrome known as panic or a panic attack. In panic the emotion is one of intense fear, and often specifically a fear of dying. The physical symptoms intensify, leading to symptoms such as a racing heartbeat, thumping palpitations, pressure in the head, chest pain, difficulty breathing and shaking.

The rapid breathing or hyperventilation that develops in panic can lead to reduced levels of carbon dioxide in the blood. This causes a biochemical change that triggers involuntary muscle spasm and numbness of the extremities. Hyperventilation can also lead to dizziness and confusion.

The experience of these intense symptoms is, in itself, a trigger for more fear, and a vicious cycle of fear–symptom–fear develops, and this prevents the panic attack from subsiding rapidly.

In all forms of anxiety, the patient very often becomes absorbed in complex behavioral patterns in which the trigger for the anxiety is avoided. When this occurs, as it very commonly does, not only is the anxiety unpleasant and disabling, but the behavior that results from its avoidance can seriously impact on the patient's well-being and freedom.

The causation of anxiety

The causation of anxiety can be considered using the biopsychosocial model of disease.

Biological theories of the generation of anxiety are increasingly popular, and are supported by the fact that the tendency to develop anxiety disorders runs very strongly in families. It is known that a tendency to anxiety is associated with abnormalities in serotonin levels, and that serotonin-modulating antidepressants (such as the SSRI antidepressant paroxetine) are of specific benefit in certain anxiety disorders. This supports a physical basis of the condition.

However, commonly a trigger event or situation can be traced as the cause of a case of anxiety. This indicates that psychological and social factors are also important in the development of maladaptive anxiety. For example, it is not uncommon for chronic anxiety to develop after a sudden shocking episode of illness such as a heart attack. The high level of anxiety in populations who have survived the trauma of living in a war zone or in groups who have experienced chronic abuse is clear evidence that chronic anxiety can be induced by extreme adverse events impacting on individuals or even whole communities.

Anxiety is a feature of a number of distinct conditions known as the anxiety disorders. These are considered below in turn.

The conditions of anxiety
PANIC DISORDER AND AGORAPHOBIA

Panic disorder is a condition is which panic attacks are common. The attacks may appear to develop without an obvious trigger, although there may be a background level of generalized anxiety present for most of the time. In some cases the panic is very specifically associated with leaving a safe place, usually the patient's home. In this case the condition is known as agoraphobia (from the Greek meaning fear of the marketplace). This pattern may have originated with the experience of a particularly disabling or embarrassing panic attack in a public place, and this has then led to the development of fear of a repetition of this event. The affected patient might thereafter prefer to stay at home whenever possible, and become acutely anxious when having to leave home. In agoraphobia, anxiety might become particularly acute in crowded places such as cinemas, supermarkets or tube trains, where the escape route is not always close by.

In agoraphobia the avoidant behavior is one of withdrawal, although not necessarily into a hermit-like state. In mild cases, the affected person may simply avoid crowded places, or situations in which they are hemmed in. In a more severe case the person with agoraphobia becomes housebound and may be dependent on friends or family to run errands.

In all cases, when panic attacks are recurrent the treatment is first one of education about the bodily changes that occur in anxiety and panic attacks. The patient commonly feels that the symptoms are warning features of serious mental illness or heart disease, and very often can be reassured by a clear explanation of the vicious cycle of symptom–fear–symptom. There should also be an explanation of how hyperventilation leads to muscle spasm, numbness and dizziness. The patient can then be taught practical methods of relaxation, how to calm the breath and the use of rebreathing into a paper bag, all of which can help to abort a developing panic attack.

Ideally, cognitive behavioral therapy is offered to help the patient address the excessive fear of losing control in a public place, and the patient can be given graded exercises that help them face a seemingly fearful situation rather than avoid it. The idea is that, if the patient can learn that they can prevent a panic attack occurring in a public place, the fear of that situation will become extinguished over time.

In some cases, anxiolytic medication is prescribed for use only in acute situations, with the rationale that it can offer the patient the security of knowing that they will be able to get the situation within their own control.

Social phobia

Social phobia is a syndrome in which the patient is less concerned about crowds but instead with social encounters. In social phobia there may be fear of talking, shaking, blushing or vomiting in a social situation. The patient demonstrates excessive concern about what other people might think about their behavior. Like agoraphobia, social phobia can be characterized by avoidance of any situation that would stimulate the anxiety, and in this case situations such as parties, visits to the pub or having to talk to shop assistants might be avoided. Social phobia tends to develop at an earlier age than agoraphobia, and often has its roots in early adolescence.

Social phobia is often accompanied by depression. Ideally, the patient is offered cognitive behavioral therapy. The patient may benefit from analytical psychotherapy if the roots of the condition appear to have arisen in early childhood.

Simple (specific) phobia

In simple phobia the patient demonstrates an intense, but very specific, fear of a single trigger. Anxiety may otherwise not be a prominent part of that person's life. Typical triggers for simple phobias include subjects that tend to be generally seen in a negative or dangerous light by modern society, such as spiders, wasps, large dogs, snakes, heights, air travel and lightning. Fear of needles is a very common phobia, which has a particular impact on the practice of acupuncture. The rationale for some phobias is less obvious; for example, in phobias of cats, birds, feathers and wind the focus for the fear is one which would be commonly thought to be benign.

Simple phobias can have their origins in very early childhood, and do appear to run strongly in families. One theory is that there may be an inherited tendency in some people to have an excessive fear response, which, when experienced in an overwhelming way in early childhood, becomes internally linked to the original source of the fear response. As is the case for the other phobias, the core problem does not seem to be what the feared object can do in terms of harm, but rather that the resulting panic will become overwhelming. The phobia is again characterized by avoidance of trigger situations. Although described as simple, this sort of phobia can have an overwhelming impact on a person's day-to-day existence, particularly if the trigger, such as cats or dogs, is one that is a normal part of modern life.

Simple phobias can respond remarkably well to a cognitive behavioral approach, in which the patient is encouraged by the clinical psychologist to face up to increasingly close contact with the feared object. This approach, called graded exposure, is accompanied by education about the nature of the panic response, and encourages the patient to learn that they need not become overwhelmed by the fear.

Obsessive-compulsive disorder (OCD)

Obsessive-compulsive disorder (OCD) is a more complex anxiety disorder in which the avoidance of becoming overwhelmed by fear also plays a part. However, in OCD the trigger for the fear is often a thought or an idea about a situation, which seems to intrude into the patient's mind in such a way that the patient tends to find a behavior that will give them some relief from the anxiety induced by the thought. The intrusive, recurrent thoughts are termed obsessions in psychiatric language. They are often seen as senseless and futile by the patient, who nevertheless finds it impossible to resist them appearing. Compulsion is the term used to describe the behavior that is chosen to relieve the anxiety induced by the obsessions.

For example, a patient with OCD might be plagued by the thought that, having left their house, they might have left it unlocked. This very commonly experienced doubt can lead to anxiety. A normal response would be to return to the house to check the lock. However, in OCD, having checked once, the doubt recurs and recurs, so much so that the patient may find themself checking the locks over and over again. In this case, the obsessive thought is the house is unsafe and the compulsive behavior is the checking. In this sort of situation the person can be so disabled by the OCD that they may choose not to leave the house, rather than be trapped in the exhausting cycle of anxiety and checking.

Another common obsessive pattern of thought in OCD concerns fears of contamination. In this sort of case a patient might be plagued by concerns that germs or other dangerous influences are affecting their body or environment. The compulsive behavior in such a case is repetitive and excessive cleaning and disinfecting, and avoidance of potentially contaminated objects. This, too, can become exhausting and disabling, as the patient spends so much time washing and cleaning, and may avoid normal social situations.

Sometimes the obsessive thoughts have a slightly magical or superstitious quality, in that only by performing a behavior in a certain way will everything be alright. In this form of OCD, the affected patient might need the objects in their environment to be ordered "just so," or they may find themselves indulging in behaviors such as having to count as they go up the stairs, or always touching a certain gatepost as they walk to the shops. This sort of behavior is a very common and normal aspect of early childhood, but can become disabling and stigmatizing if it persists into adulthood.

OCD is a more complex problem to treat in conventional psychiatry, as the obsessive thoughts seem to pervade a person's values and ideals in a more profound way than is found in phobias. A person with OCD might have deep beliefs about personal security, or health and hygiene, or the interrelationship of events, all of which need exploring in much more depth than might be needed in the treatment of someone with a simple phobia. Often, the OCD will significantly affect all aspects of the person's life and cannot be easily avoided. Depression is very commonly found to be a complicating feature of OCD.

Ideally, OCD is treated with psychological approaches, including cognitive behavioral therapy. Analytical psychotherapy may be of benefit in certain individuals. It is believed that the SSRI antidepressants, such as paroxetine, can be of particular benefit, and so these may be prescribed, even if depression does not appear to be marked. Severe OCD is one of the rare examples of a mental health disorder in which psychosurgery may be of benefit. In OCD surgical approaches such as leucotomy, in which specific tracts of interconnecting nerve fibers in the brain are severed, may be performed, but this is done only as a last resort.

Post-traumatic stress disorder (PTSD)

Post-traumatic stress disorder (PTSD) is another anxiety disorder in which there is a deep fear of being overwhelmed by panic and avoidance of this, but in this case the trigger for the anxiety is a memory of a traumatic event. Typical events include physical or sexual abuse, involvement in a road traffic accident, witnessing a death or being involved in armed combat. It is known that PTSD develops in over 50 percent of rape victims, for example.

The patient with PTSD may avoid any behavior that might trigger the intrusion of the memory, and may develop panic symptoms if they begin to be reminded of the event. It is typical in PTSD for the patient to experience powerful flashbacks of the event, which can disturb sleep or interrupt normal life, as they can lead to overwhelming waves of fear, guilt, anger or grief. The affected patient can become watchful and nervous, and can startle easily. They may report a general sense of feeling numbed to life. Avoidant behavior can involve use of drugs and alcohol, which can greatly complicate the recovery from the initial trauma. Depression is also a very common aspect of PTSD.

Psychological treatment for PTSD ideally involves a cognitive behavioral approach to dealing with the panic. Cognitive behavioral approaches can greatly speed up recovery from PTSD, although not all cases will respond to treatment. The approach of encouraging the patient to face up to the memory in great detail, a technique known as flooding, is now largely outmoded, as in some cases it appeared to worsen the condition.

Generalized anxiety disorder (GAD)

In contrast to each of the previously described anxiety disorders, in generalized anxiety disorder (GAD) there may be no specific trigger for the anxiety. Instead, in GAD the anxiety is a pervasive aspect of the way in which the person experiences the world. A person with GAD will be known as a worrier. They might appear as nervous and jumpy, and may suffer from physical symptoms such as tremor, muscle tension, digestive disturbances, sweating and frequency of urination.

GAD is common. It has been estimated that GAD is present in 8 percent of people who visit their general practitioner (GP), although it probably affects just less than 3 percent of the general population. It is twice as common in women as in men. In general practice, GAD is likely to present as recurrent concerns about bodily symptoms, and so may not initially be diagnosed.

As GAD is a pervasive problem, the treatment is not straightforward. The patient might benefit to some degree from some simple cognitive behavioral approaches, but analytical psychotherapy might be more appropriate for dealing with the deep roots of this condition.

Information box 6.2d-I

Anxiety disorders: comments from a Chinese medicine perspective

From a Chinese medicine perspective, all the anxiety disorders are manifestations of the diverse Chinese syndromes that demonstrate Shen Disturbance. These include Blood Deficiency (Heart and Liver), Yin Deficiency (Heart, Liver, Lung, Kidney, Stomach and Spleen), Empty Heat, Liver Qi Stagnation, Blood Stagnation (Liver and Heart), Full Heat, Phlegm Fire and Wind.

Each of the anxiety disorders has its own flavor of Organ Imbalance depending on the nature of the individual symptoms. For example, the prominence of intrusive thoughts in OCD suggests that Spleen Pathology will be prominent. As worrying is a component in GAD, a Spleen Disorder might again be predicted. It could be expected that the trauma preceding PTSD might have had an impact on Heart and Kidney Qi, and thus these Organs may be more prominent in the differential diagnosis of cases of PTSD.

More specifically, Flaws and Lake (2001)[48] describe the Chinese disease categories of Anxiety and Thinking (Shan You Si), and also Susceptibility to Fear and Fright (Shan Kong and Shan Jing). Shan You Si includes diseases characterized by Spleen Pathology, including Spleen Qi Deficiency with Liver Qi Stagnation, Heart and Spleen Qi Deficiency, and Lung and Spleen Qi Deficiency.

Shan Kong and Shan Jing are characterized by Kidney, Gallbladder and Heart Pathology, including the Empty/Mixed patterns of Kidney Jing Deficiency, Qi and Blood Deficiency, Heart and Gallbladder Qi Deficiency, Liver Blood Deficiency with Qi Stagnation, and Kidney Deficiency. Phlegm Fire and Heart Fire can also lead to a susceptibility to fear, startling and palpitations.

The Chinese medical syndrome of "running piglet"[49] may also account for some manifestations of panic. In this syndrome the patient experiences an upsurging of energy or palpitations in the abdomen, and in Chinese medicine this is due to a relative insufficiency in Middle or Upper Burners from either Spleen or Heart Yang Deficiency or Liver Qi Stagnation and a fullness of Cold Qi in the Lower Burner. Shock or fright may typically cause the experience of running piglet as the Qi of the Heart, Liver or Kidney is Depleted.

Part II: Depression, somatoform disorders and eating disorders

Depression

THE SYNDROME OF DEPRESSION

Although in common usage the term depression describes a range of emotional states, from a medical perspective it is a syndrome with a number of defined characteristics. According to the range and intensity of these characteristics, depression can be graded as mild, moderate or severe (according to ICD-10), or as minor or major (according to DSM-5). The grading of depression has important consequences in how treatment is chosen.

The features of a depressive episode include characteristic emotions and thought patterns, which include:

- low mood
- inability to feel enjoyment
- poor attention and concentration
- ideas of guilt and worthlessness
- lowered energy and tiredness
- a belief that life is not worth living.

In severe depression, biological changes in body and brain function can occur. These include:

- loss of appetite, or abnormal appetite
- significant change in weight (usually loss, but can be gain)
- marked daily variation in mood, with it often being worse in the morning
- poor sleep, with early morning wakening
- physical agitation or, conversely, slowing down of movements.

According to DSM-5, if at least five of the above features (including low mood or inability to feel enjoyment) have been present every day for a two-week period, a diagnosis of a major depressive episode can be made. The ICD-10 diagnosis of severe depression is similar to this. This carries clinical weight because it is recognized that the risk of suicide is much higher in severe depression (occurring in up to 15 percent of patients with a major depressive episode) than in the less severe forms of depression. It is also important to note that the syndrome of major depression is common, affecting up to 26 percent of women and 12 percent of men in their lifetime.

Minor depression is characterized according to DSM-5 by low mood but with less than five of the above listed features present. According to ICD-10, in mild depression normal daily functioning is only slightly impaired, and in moderate depression daily functioning is more significantly impaired.

Depression is recognized as an episodic condition from which people can recover. After recovery, there is a 40–60 percent chance of relapse, but this need not necessarily occur. However, in some people a state of depression, even if mild, seems to be an ongoing condition. The diagnosis of dysthymia (ICD-10) is made if a person experiences low mood for most of the time over a two-year period or longer. If the only abnormal mood change that the patient experiences is towards depression, this is known as a unipolar mood disorder.

If the episodes of depression alternate with episodes of elevated mood (a state known as hypomania), this may be diagnosed as a form of bipolar mood disorder. This less common condition is explored in Section 6.2e.

In certain groups of patients, depression may be present but may not appear with the usual syndrome as described above. In children, depression might appear in the form of behavioral disturbance, poor academic performance or sexual promiscuity. In elderly people, depression can manifest in the form of memory loss, and difficulty in concentration and thinking. In this way it may appear to be like an early form of dementia (known as pseudo-dementia). It is of utmost importance to the patient that this reversible condition is differentiated from a dementia, because depression is treatable with appropriate support and antidepressant medication. Alternatively, depressed elderly people might not admit to a low mood, but might instead develop symptoms such as constipation, weight loss and excessive concern about their bodily symptoms.

THE CAUSATION OF DEPRESSION

It is clear that the tendency to develop depression can be inherited, and this suggests that there is a biological basis to depressive symptoms. It is currently believed that depression can result directly from reduced levels of certain neurotransmitters in the brain, including serotonin (5HT), and chemicals known as the amines. This theory is supported by the fact that drugs that are known to reduce levels of these neurotransmitters are also recognized to cause an experience of depression.

There are also well-founded psychological theories for the causation of depression. For example, it is recognized that negative life events in childhood, such as loss of a parent or the experience of sexual abuse, are associated with an increased risk of depression in adult life.

Research into the immediate triggers of depression has revealed that, in many cases, recent stressful life events led up to the onset of an episode (as is true for the onset of a wide range of psychological conditions). Bereavement (see later) is one example of a stressor that is well recognized to carry a high risk of depression. Childbirth is another major life event that can be followed by depression in one or both parents. While it is very likely that biological factors, such as changes in hormone levels, physical debility and loss of sleep, must play a part in postnatal depression, it is likely that the psychological impact of the arrival of a new baby will also play a part in the causation of this syndrome.

It is also well recognized that a number of physical illnesses are associated with depression. For example, it is known that the incidence of depression is much higher in hospitalized patients than in the general population. As is the case in postnatal depression, there may be a number of biological reasons why physical illness could manifest in depression. However, it also has to be appreciated that illness has social and psychological consequences, which could contribute to the causation of depression. The stress of constant pain or discomfort, and the fear of loss of health and livelihood, are psychological factors that may contribute to depression in the context of chronic illness.

It is also clear that personality factors play a part in the development of depression. What might be a depression-causing stressful event in one person might leave another relatively untouched. It is recognized that those people who can be described as having obsessional, dependent or histrionic personality types are more likely to develop depressive symptoms (see Section 6.2e).

TREATMENT OF DEPRESSION

Before treatment is begun, the degree of depression needs to be evaluated fully. Questionnaire scoring systems such as the Beck Depression Inventory or the Hamilton Rating Scale for depression may be useful in providing an objective measure of severity. Ideally, the medical practitioner should grade the symptoms into minor or major (DSM-5 grading) or mild, moderate or severe (ICD-10 grading) depression, and in particular, should explore the possibility of suicidal ideas and plans.

Suicidal ideas are common, particularly in major depression, but certain features indicate a greater risk that the patient might actually go on to attempt suicide.[50] In general, people who are solitary, male and elderly are more likely to attempt suicide and not survive the attempt. People who suffer from chronic illness or a substance misuse disorder are also at increased risk. Any evidence that the patient has made concrete plans for the attempt (e.g. purchased tablets, acquired a hosepipe for the car exhaust, made provision for family members who will be left behind) should be taken as extremely serious features.

According to the biopsychosocial model, ideally all the three domains (biological, psychological and social causes) will be attended to in the treatment of depression.

Medical treatment with antidepressant medication need not be the first line of action in minor or mild depression. In these less severe cases, ideally more conservative physical approaches, such as attention to healthy diet, sufficient sleep and regular exercise, should be recommended in the first instance. Any biological triggers, such as ongoing medication or recreational drug use, should be explored. Psychological and social causes may be attended to by means of appropriate counseling or psychotherapy.

In many cases cognitive behavioral therapy might be considered the most appropriate form of psychotherapy. In cognitive behavioral therapy the therapist will encourage the patient to assess their own negative thought patterns, and then challenge the patient about the validity of these thought patterns. The patient might be encouraged to keep diaries of negative thought patterns, and be recommended exercises in which they experiment with different ways of responding to stressful situations.

In moderate to severe depression, the patient may be considered unlikely to be able to respond to psychotherapy alone. One reason for this is that lifestyle change and engagement in psychotherapy are both dependent on the patient being able to focus and have the drive to generate change. Both these skills may be significantly impaired in more severe cases of depression.

If the severely depressed patient is not considered to be acutely at risk of a suicide attempt, they are likely to be offered a prescription of antidepressants. In this sort of case, the most commonly prescribed type of antidepressant is an SSRI (e.g. citalopram or fluoxetine).

If the depression is so severe that the patient is failing to take care of themselves adequately, or if there appears to be a very high risk of suicide, admission to a psychiatric unit may be considered to be the most appropriate option. In such cases it may be considered necessary to admit the patient using legal powers that allow for compulsory admission of patients with mental health illness. In situations in which urgent treatment is considered necessary, a brief course of electroconvulsive treatment (ECT) may be administered, because of the recognized delay in the action of antidepressants. In the UK the Mental Health Act (2007) provides safeguards that mean that sentient patients cannot be administered ECT without their express consent (unless they are deemed to lack the capacity to understand the rationale for the treatment).[51]

Most patients, however (60–70 percent), will respond to antidepressant medication, although some may need more time to find which type is best for them. Some patients might only respond to a prescription of two or more antidepressants, although this combined prescribing is usually only practiced by a psychiatrist with specialist experience.

Ideally, the improvement in symptoms will be such that the drug can be withdrawn, gradually, after a period of six to nine months. Some patients may find that they need to remain on a long-term prescription to keep negative symptoms at bay. In addition, some patients with profound mood changes might be prescribed lithium or one of the other mood-stabilizing drugs on a long-term basis to prevent further relapses.

BEREAVEMENT AND GRIEF

Prior to DSM-5, bereavement was not considered to be a psychiatric diagnosis. The low mood associated with bereavement is a recognized and normal reaction to loss. In the long term it may lead to acceptance of the loss in such a way that the bereaved person may be stronger and more mature as a result. The process of grief after bereavement has been clearly described by various psychologists in terms of certain key stages.

One of the most well-known descriptions of the stages of grief originates from the writings of the Swiss-born psychologist Elisabeth Kübler-Ross. In her book *On Death and Dying* (first published in 1969) she describes five responses that a patient might go through on being given the news of terminal illness.[52] These are:

- denial
- anger
- bargaining
- depression
- acceptance.

These stages are frequently seen in the process of developing acceptance of any type of loss, and can be a useful model for those involved in grief work. It is recognized that no one has to systematically progress through all these stages in order to arrive at acceptance of the loss. Zisook and Shear (2009) describe the stage of acceptance as "integrated grief," in that the sense of loss actually never leaves the bereaved person, but in acceptance they found a way of calmly relating to their loved one as deceased.[53]

However, these stages do not describe many of the commonly experienced responses to acute loss, including numbness, acute physical and mental pain, intrusive thoughts, guilt over what was not done, a sense of injustice and mood swings. It is also a normal response for someone who has been suddenly bereaved to experience hallucinations of the lost loved one, either in the form of seeing them or hearing their voice.

Normal bereavement leads to negative emotions, but these do not strictly equate to depression. Although it may be normal to have periods of sadness at the memory of the loss after bereavement, in normal bereavement the person is likely to have moved on from experiencing a continuous state of painful emotions within a year or so. However, DSM-5 makes it clear that if the features of depression are present in the context of bereavement, they should be considered as indicative of depression. This is in contrast to previous categorizations, in which a bereavement exclusion was appended to the definition of depression. There is much published criticism over this development, the concern being that normal emotional shifts in bereavement have now been medicalized in DSM-5.[54]

In abnormal or pathological grief, the bereavement leads to a decline in physical or mental health. The stage of acceptance or integrated grief is not reached. There might be little or no apparent emotional grieving, but instead, the development of bodily symptoms might occur. Alternatively, an excessively extreme grief response might develop into severe depression, with biological symptoms. In some cases grief might manifest in the form of a psychotic illness, with features of thought disorder (see Section 6.2e).

Normal grief is a gradual process, and a healthy progression to acceptance and reinvestment in life without the lost person can be enabled by supportive counseling. Grief counseling is a specialist discipline. In the UK access to grief counselors can be facilitated through contacting the charity Cruse Bereavement Care.[55]

Information box 6.2d-II

Depression: comments from a Chinese medicine perspective

In Chinese medicine, the symptoms of low mood and depression would sometimes fit into the category of diseases described as Frequent Sorrow or Shan Bei. These diseases have Lung Pathology in common, and the patterns include Lung and Heart Qi Deficiency, Liver Qi Stagnation with Fire Invading the Lungs, and Heart Qi Deficiency and Lung Fire. Flaws and Lake (2001)[56] suggest that the Lung Pathologies in Frequent Sorrow might result from excessive grief, overwork and chronic disease. Internally generated Heat resulting from Stagnant Liver Qi can flare upwards to damage the Lungs.

But depression is also referred to as Yu Zheng in Chinese. Greenwood (2004)[57] explains that the word Yu has the double meaning of depression or stagnation. This indicates the understanding that Liver Qi Stagnation is at the center of depression, and may then spread to cause pathology in other organs, and also lead to Blood Stasis, Heat, Phlegm and Phlegm Fire.

Depression also commonly overlaps with symptoms of Anxiety and Overthinking (Shan You Si in Chinese medicine), in which case Spleen Pathology would be recognized to coexist with the previously listed patterns. Agitation might suggest pathology of the Heart-Kidney axis.

It can be seen that depression might be a manifestation of either Empty or Mixed patterns.

Disorders manifesting in bodily functions (somatoform disorders)

The somatoform disorders are explained in ICD-10 as those conditions that are considered to have a root in a mental/emotional imbalance, but which manifest in physical symptoms as if they had originated in physical disease. In somatoform disorders the patient is not considered to have any willful control over the symptoms, which are believed to be generated unconsciously.

Information box 6.2d-III

Somatoform disorders: comments from a Chinese medicine perspective

In Chinese medicine, the physical basis, or otherwise, of a symptom does not have the relevance that it carries in conventional medicine. In all the somatoform disorders it would be the symptoms, the pulse and the tongue characteristics, rather than their physical roots, which would point to the underlying patterns.

MALINGERING AND FACTITIOUS DISORDER

Malingering and factitious disorder are two conditions in which physical symptoms are willfully created by the patient. Therefore, these are not somatoform disorders. In malingering, illness is feigned so that the patient can have some sort of material gain, such as leave from work duties or financial compensation. In factitious disorder there can also be feigning of symptoms, or even systematic and secretive self-harm (in which case the disorder is also known as Munchausen's syndrome), but in these disorders, the gain for the patient from feigning illness is less obvious. It may be that the gain for the patient is the medical attention these symptoms attract. Munchausen's syndrome by proxy is a sinister variant of factitious disorder in which the systematic harm is inflicted on a third party, usually a vulnerable person such as a child or an elderly person.

CONVERSION DISORDER

A conversion disorder is one in which there appears to be a loss or change of physical functioning that would ordinarily result from physical disease. However, on examination there are no signs of physical disease, and all tests reveal normal function. The symptoms in conversion disorder commonly mimic those of neurological disease (e.g. paralysis, loss of voice, blindness, fainting and epileptiform fits).

The term hysteria has been used to describe a condition in which an emotional disorder becomes manifest in the physical realm. This term, which originates from the Greek word for womb, is now largely outmoded because of its pejorative associations. Freud suggested that hysterical symptoms were the result of the conversion of emotional distress into a bodily symptom, which itself had symbolic significance for the patient. Psychological theory proposes that the development of the symptom somehow serves a purpose by diverting the anxiety of an emotional conflict for the patient.

In 1907 the French psychiatrist Charles Janet described patients with hysteria who appeared relatively unperturbed by the emergence of a symptom, such as paralysis, which in most people would have led to distress. Freud had already noted this phenomenon with a single patient with hysteria in 1895, and used the term *la belle indifférence* to describe an apparently happy state of indifference to the symptom.[58] This term is still used in psychiatry to describe this interesting feature that appears in some cases of conversion disorder, but is by no means characteristic.

True conversion disorder generally tends to resolve with time, often spontaneously. Psychoanalysis may be of value in exploring the roots of the origin of the symptoms, and a hypnosis-like treatment known as abreaction may also prove to be effective.

One subtype of conversion disorder is persistent somatoform pain disorder, in which the patient complains of persistent chronic pain for which no medical basis can be found. Common sites of the pain include the lower back, the head and, in women, the pelvic area. Persistent somatoform pain disorder is a very difficult condition to diagnose with confidence, and also to treat, without making the patient feel that the severity of their condition is being denied. Patients with chronic pain suffer considerable disability, and depression is very commonly part of the patient's experience. In some cases the pain can respond to a prescription of antidepressant medication such as amitriptyline or nerve-modulating medication such as gabapentin.

HYPOCHONDRIASIS

Hypochondriasis is a term now used in ICD-10 specifically for the tendency of the patient to worry that they may be suffering from one or more serious underlying diseases such as cancer or human immunodeficiency virus (HIV) infection. The patient might focus unduly on particular bodily symptoms, and may be unready to accept reassurance that these are benign. These patients might request medical tests and referrals to specialists, but even with normal results may still not be pacified.

The condition is characterized by anxiety, and can respond to cognitive behavioral therapy. Hypochondriasis differs from somatization (see below) in that the central cause of distress to the patient is the worry about the cause of the symptoms, rather than the discomfort of the symptoms themselves.

Body dysmorphic disorder (BDD) is a specific type of hypochondriasis in which there is excessive concern about a perceived defect in appearance, such as a wrinkle, a cleft in the chin, or the shape of the breasts. This can lead to social withdrawal, or the decision to undergo cosmetic surgery. Some authorities consider BDD to be a subtype of OCD, in that it is characterized by persistent negative thoughts and the compulsion to act to alter or cover the affected body part. BDD can also respond to cognitive behavioral therapy and also SSRI antidepressant medication.

SOMATIZATION DISORDER

Somatization is the medical term used to describe the pervasive tendency to experience mental or emotional distress as a physical symptom. Patients who somatize will often tend to seek help for their symptoms, which can for them be a source of long-term distress.

Somatization disorder is used to describe the long-term tendency for a patient to frequently attend their doctor complaining of a range of recurrent physical symptoms. This is possibly the most disabling of the somatoform disorders, in that its repercussions on the life of the patient may be lifelong, and it is also very resistant to psychological treatment. Typical symptoms in somatization include those listed in Table 6.2d-I. Although these symptoms are all common, at least eight have to be complained of before a diagnosis of somatization can be made.

Table 6.2d-I Somatization: typical symptoms experienced (eight or more need to be present for a diagnosis to be made)

Pain during urination	Diarrhea
Headaches	Pain in the arms or legs
Shortness of breath	Back pain
Palpitations	Joint pain
Chest pain	Vision changes
Dizziness	Paralysis or muscle weakness
Amnesia	Sexual apathy
Difficulty swallowing	Pain during intercourse
Vomiting	Impotence
Abdominal pain	Painful menstruation
Nausea	Irregular menses
Bloating	Excessive menstrual bleeding

Patients who tend to somatize may be referred inappropriately to a number of specialists for further investigations. All the symptoms tend to be functional in nature, and so medical tests often show no abnormalities. The symptoms generally tend to be resistant to medical treatments. Somatization is currently understood to be a manifestation of underlying unhappiness or depression, and is believed to have its roots in early childhood when patterns in illness behavior are formed. Patients may experience their doctors losing patience with their frequent consultations. Doctors often find somatization frustrating, as the cause of the problems is often elusive and medical treatments fail to benefit the patient. This frustration is expressed in the term "heartsink patient,"[59] which has been used by doctors to describe patients with somatization disorder.

Benefit might be achieved by means of cognitive behavioral therapy, which enables the patient to make links between their emotional feelings and their bodily symptoms. However, it is commonly found that patients with somatization disorder tend to resist exploration of the possible psychological roots of their symptoms.

Neurasthenia

Neurasthenia is a term that was first used by doctors over a century ago. The term embraces the syndrome of excessive fatigue, especially after mental effort or physical exertion, difficulty in concentration, and diverse symptoms including dizziness, headache, muscle pains and digestive disturbances. Although originally considered to be a somatoform disorder, and so one with a psychological basis, neurasthenia does carry a remarkable similarity to the chronic fatigue syndromes.

Dissociative disorders

Dissociative disorders are, like conversion disorders, conditions in which emotional distress is not directly experienced by the patient. However, instead of the distress manifesting in the physical realm, in dissociative disorders the condition manifests in terms of a problem of identity, memory or consciousness.

Total psychogenic amnesia is a rare dissociative disorder in which the patient suddenly loses the ability to remember essential personal information. The most usual trigger is extreme trauma. The amnesia may be total, or limited to a period of time surrounding the traumatic event. It may be selective so that only portions of the traumatic event can be remembered.

A psychogenic fugue is a very rare state. In such a state, a patient might travel and continue normal activities although they have lost some touch with the reality of who they are.

Multiple personality disorder is considered to be a rare form of severe dissociation.

The underlying reasons for both psychogenic amnesia and fugue can be explored by means of hypnosis and abreaction (a form of chemically induced hypnosis using the drug sodium thiopental).

Psychosomatic disorders

The term psychosomatic is commonly used with pejorative overtones, with the implication that a person's illness is all in their head. However, the precise medical use of the term is quite different. Psychosomatic illnesses are those very physically rooted conditions that also appear to have a strong interrelationship with intercurrent stress. Examples might include migraine, peptic ulcer, asthma and eczema, inflammatory bowel disease and rheumatoid arthritis.

Although the precise mechanisms of how the effects of stress are mediated in these very physical forms are unknown, the fact that stress can manifest in measurable physical illness is fully accepted by the conventional medical community.

Eating disorders

The eating disorders of anorexia nervosa and bulimia nervosa have some similarities with BDD, in that the primary issue for the patient appears to be an excessive focus on and dissatisfaction with bodily form. However, these two discrete disorders have so many features in common that they are considered to be in a category of their own. For this reason they are not classified as somatoform disorders. In ICD-10, eating disorders are classified as behavioral syndromes associated with a physiological disturbance, and in DSM-5 they are classified within a unique chapter entitled "Feeding and Eating Disorders."

Eating disorders carry one of the highest risks of ill health and death of all psychiatric diagnoses. There is undoubtedly a very strong social component in their causation. These disorders are likely to continue to cause a heavy burden of ill health until such a time as the popular adulation of excessive thinness in models, dancers and some athletes can be successfully challenged.

Anorexia nervosa

Anorexia nervosa is a condition that generally appears in teenage girls, although it also affects a smaller proportion of boys. It may have a later onset in adulthood in some cases. The primary concern for the patient is a fear of fatness and an excessive dissatisfaction with the amount of fat on their body. The concern is out of keeping with what would be considered an acceptable body shape by the general population, although it may be supported by similar concerns expressed in the patient's peer group or influence group.

The term anorexia is used in general medicine to describe loss of appetite which might occur for diverse medical reasons. However, its use in anorexia nervosa is somewhat inaccurate as loss of appetite is not the primary pathology in this condition, when, in fact, a preoccupation with food may co-exist with dietary restriction.

The fear of fatness and concern for a certain body form drives the patient with anorexia nervosa to restrict food intake, and in particular to avoid fattening foods. There may also be a drive to over-exercise and to misuse laxative medication. Low levels of nutrition and over-exercise will readily manifest in amenorrhea (cessation of periods) in young women.

Anorexia nervosa is diagnosed if there has been a weight loss of over 15 percent of the normal body weight, if the patient demonstrates a fear of becoming fat and has a distorted body image, and also, in women, if there is amenorrhea for more than three consecutive periods. Although the patient tends to avoid eating, it is often clear that there is excessive focus on and interest in food, an interest that can appear almost obsessional.

If anorexia persists, some characteristic physical changes appear, including dry skin and hair, downy body hair (lanugo), low body temperature, slow pulse rate and poor sleep. In the long term there is a risk of death from starvation or heart failure. There is also a high risk of suicide in patients with anorexia nervosa.

Psychological theories for the causation of anorexia suggest that the problem is more likely to develop with a background of low self-esteem. By achieving an ideal body weight, the anorexic patient can bolster a poor sense of self-worth. In addition, it is postulated that the person with anorexia finds some degree of control in their eating patterns, and this can provide a sense of comfort, particularly in the setting of a family in which expectations of performance are high. As anorexia progresses, there are marked similarities with OCD, in that the controlled eating behavior can pacify a welling anxiety regarding loss of control of weight.

The problem in treating anorexia nervosa is that it is often a hidden condition, and one that the patient may be reluctant to address. Some success may be achieved by forms of counseling that focus on self-esteem. If family dynamics are considered to be important in the causation, family therapy may be of value. Behavioral therapy, in which rewards are negotiated in response to adopting normalized eating patterns, can also be effective. Dietary advice is usually necessary. In some cases antidepressant medication can be of profound benefit. Full recovery occurs in 50 percent of patients, but in 20 percent the condition becomes chronic.

In extreme cases of near starvation or suicide risk, hospitalization may be deemed necessary, ideally in a dedicated unit. Compulsory admission is often necessary in these cases.[60]

BULIMIA NERVOSA

Bulimia nervosa is also a condition in which there is an excessive concern with fatness, but in this condition the eating patterns are more chaotic. The patient experiences urges to binge on food, particularly on carbohydrates, and then finds relief by inducing vomiting, or purging with diuretics, laxatives or enemas. At the time of the binge the patient experiences an overwhelming desire to keep eating, and has a sense of being out of control. In between binges a person with bulimia might achieve stringent control over

their diet, in a form akin to anorexia nervosa. Some cases of anorexia nervosa can progress to bulimia.

Although patients with bulimia tend to be of average weight, they can still suffer profound health consequences. The female patient with bulimia might also develop amenorrhea. Gastric acid can erode the teeth, and hands can develop sores from manual induction of vomiting. The salts in the blood can become imbalanced by the vomiting of fluids, and there is risk of death by heart attack.

Bulimia also primarily affects women, but is also fairly common in men, who account for up to a quarter of cases.

Patients with bulimia are more likely to seek help for their condition, as the sense of failure and guilt that accompanies the pattern can be overwhelming. However, this often comes after years of an ingrained pattern of eating, and so the condition may be very resistant to treatment.

It is considered that advice on proper nutrition and the medical consequences of vomiting and purging is an essential part of treatment. Psychotherapy for this condition focuses on issues of low self-esteem. Behavioral approaches can also be effective in the management of bulimia. Antidepressant medication can be effective for some people.

 Information box 6.2d-IV

Eating disorders: comments from a Chinese medicine perspective

From a Chinese medicine perspective, the underlying psychological factors in eating disorders clearly point to different elements in the Five Element system of diagnosis. Low self-esteem and a sense of needing to aspire to an ideal hint at Imbalance in the Metal Element. Over-concern with food relates to an imbalance of the Earth Element. Excessive need for control suggests an overactive Wood Element.

Hence, in anorexia nervosa there might be a primarily Deficient pattern of Lung and Spleen Qi or Yang Deficiency, together with Blood Deficiency. Liver Qi Stagnation could also be present. Prolonged starvation is likely to lead to Deficiency of Qi, Blood and Yin, and emotional disturbance is likely to be pronounced, resulting in Deficiency of the Organs, Qi Stagnation from Deficiency, and Rising Up of Empty Heat to Harass the Heart.

In bulimia nervosa, however, there may be a more mixed pattern. In addition to Deficiency of Blood and Yin, there may also be a buildup of Heat, Phlegm and Stagnation from overeating and induction of vomiting.

6.2e Psychoses, personality disorders and learning disability

The first half of this last section on mental health disorders considers psychoses and organic conditions. These are disorders in which a profound disorder of mental function and insight are apparent. Both these categories of disorder affect a patient in such a way that normal communication with another person may be severely disrupted. This disruption results from either thought disorder or clouded consciousness. Very often a patient suffering from one of these conditions in its acute form would be seen as either insane or very confused.

As stated in the previous section, the term neurosis is used to describe a mental health disorder in which a degree of insight into the condition is retained by the patient. In contrast, a psychosis is a condition characterized by a loss of insight by the patient.

There are two broad categories of mental disorder that involve a psychosis and in which the underlying process of disease is not yet clearly understood. These are schizophrenia and bipolar disorder (manic-depressive disorder). Because the underlying process of disease is poorly understood, these conditions are sometimes known as functional or idiopathic psychoses.

In contrast to functional mental health disorders, organic disorders are those in which the underlying cause is clearly rooted in a measurable physiological change in the function of the brain. Brain function can be affected by specific degenerative changes (the cause of the dementias), by drugs and toxins, and also by a wide range of bodily responses to disease. For example, the states of fever, uremia in kidney failure and hypoglycemia all have an impact on brain function. Organic disorders can result in a profound change in mental function, as they very often lead to confusion or altered consciousness. In this way they are more akin to psychoses than neuroses.

The second half of this section focuses on those conditions that seem to be clearly rooted in a person's constitution. These conditions are either congenital or develop very early in childhood. They include personality disorders, and the various causes of intellectual (learning) disability. The important developmental and behavioral disorders of childhood have already been summarized in Section 5.4e.

The conditions discussed in this section are:

Part I: Major mental disorders

- Schizophrenia and bipolar disorder:
  - schizophrenia
  - bipolar disorder (manic-depressive psychosis)
  - other psychotic disorders

- Organic psychiatric disorders:
  - dementia
  - confusional states and delirium.

Part II: Personality disorders and intellectual disability

- Personality disorders:
  - paranoid personality disorder
  - schizoid personality disorder
  - schizotypal personality disorder
  - antisocial personality disorder
  - borderline personality disorder (BPD)
  - histrionic personality disorder
  - narcissistic personality disorder
  - avoidant personality disorder
  - dependent personality disorder
  - obsessive-compulsive personality disorder (OCPD)
  - passive-aggressive behavior
- Intellectual disability.

Part I: Major mental disorders

Schizophrenia and bipolar disorder

Schizophrenia and bipolar disorder are two categories of functional psychoses. In both DSM-5 and ICD-10 they are classified as separate conditions. In ICD-10 bipolar disorder is classified, together with depression, as a mood disorder, and in DSM-5 it is given its own category. However, there are some strong similarities between the clinical features of schizophrenia and bipolar disorder, and also similarities in how they are treated medically.

SCHIZOPHRENIA

The term schizophrenia is derived from the Greek meaning split and mind. The name points at the lack of integration between thoughts, emotions and will that can be so apparent in schizophrenia. However, the term is commonly a source of confusion and stigma, as it is easily misinterpreted as meaning split personality, and, for some, conjures up images of an unpredictable Jekyll and Hyde character. This is totally erroneous in the case of schizophrenia. It is misunderstandings such as these that have led to inappropriate fear and avoidance of those given this diagnosis. Schizophrenia is a relatively common condition. One in 100 people in the UK will experience a schizophrenic breakdown in their lifetime.

As schizophrenia is a condition that tends to first develop in the late teens or early twenties, and may then persist in a disabling form for years, its impact on the health of a population is significant, and rivals the impact of the more physically based diseases of coronary heart disease or cancer. Although it is true that in 25 percent of cases a person will make a full recovery after an episode of schizophrenia, in two-thirds of cases symptoms will relapse and remit over the course of many years. In about 10–15 percent of cases there will be long-term disability as a direct result of the condition.

The symptoms of schizophrenia can be grouped into the more striking positive symptoms and the less remarkable, but arguably more disabling, negative symptoms.

The positive symptoms of schizophrenia include:

- delusions

- hallucinations

- incoherence and loosened associations.

Delusions

A delusion is, simply speaking, a false belief. In contrast to religious beliefs (which some might argue are erroneous), a delusion is not a belief that is understandable in the context of the person's culture, and nor is it one that can be shaken in the light of evidence that strongly suggests it is misguided. Delusions in schizophrenia are often paranoid in nature, and can involve beliefs that the person is somehow being watched or systematically harmed. Beliefs that the television is the source of a mechanism of surveillance of one's thoughts, or that poison has been secretly inserted into one's food, are examples of typical delusions in schizophrenia. Paranoid delusions can make life unbearable, and can lead the sufferer of such beliefs to withdraw socially. In severe cases they can drive the person to suicide.

For others, the delusions relate to their perception of the nature of their personality, and these can include the well-described delusions of grandeur (e.g. believing that they are the prime minister). Delusions that thoughts are being interfered with, transmitted, inserted, blocked or removed are particularly characteristic of schizophrenia. The delusional perception, a sudden appreciation of a delusional idea that seems to appear out of the blue after a sensory experience, is also very characteristic. A delusional perception is, for example, when, just after a thunderclap has been heard, it suddenly becomes clear to the patient that aliens are in control of the armed forces.

Hallucinations

A hallucination is a sensory perception that has not been triggered by a physical stimulus. Any sound, sight, smell, taste or bodily feeling is a hallucination if it is experienced with no obvious physical explanation. Auditory hallucinations (sounds) of voices are the most common hallucinations in schizophrenia. To the patient, the voices seem as if they are coming from an external source. Brain scans have proved that these voices are not figments of the imagination, as they are associated with increased brain activity in the region of the brain that deals with speech.

Incoherence and loosened associations

Another feature of schizophrenia is that thoughts may seem to ramble and not be related to thoughts that have gone before (loosening of associations). Speech can be difficult to follow (incoherence). Totally new words (neologisms) can appear, and strange patterns of speech or word play might be observed.

The negative symptoms of schizophrenia include:

- Catatonic behavior, where catatonic describes behavior that tends to total inaction. This can appear insidiously in the onset of schizophrenia. The affected person tends to withdraw from social contact, may neglect personal hygiene and basic bodily functions, and loses all volition.

- Flat or inappropriate affect (emotional responses). In schizophrenia the emotions may appear blunted, with a narrowing of the normal range of emotions, a state described as flattening of affect (affect is a technical term meaning mood). There can also be the unprompted inappropriate expression of emotions in the form of outbursts of laughter, tears or anger.

The diagnosis of schizophrenia is not one to be made lightly. According to DSM-5, it should be made if there have been persistent symptoms for at least six months of markedly reduced function in areas such as work, social relationships and self-care, together with at least one month's experience of two of the positive or negative symptoms listed above. If there are either particularly bizarre unshakeable delusions, or auditory hallucinations of voices talking to each other or commenting on the person's activity (e.g. "now he is going into the shop"), these alone are almost diagnostic of schizophrenia.

The onset of schizophrenia most commonly occurs in the late teens or early adulthood. There may be a period of gradual deterioration of function that precedes the appearance of more positively diagnostic features. In this period the person might tend to withdraw socially and their behavior might seem increasingly more bizarre. Speech can become vague and difficult to understand. Odd beliefs might become apparent. However, in other cases the onset may be quite abrupt.

It is clear that there can be an inherited vulnerability to schizophrenia. The identical twin of someone with schizophrenia has a 50 percent chance of developing the condition, even if raised in a totally different environment.

Siblings have a 15 percent chance. It is suggested that the inherited vulnerability might lie in the function of the serotonin-dopamine pathways in the brain, or in the structure of certain nerve membranes, as these are aspects of brain function that are known to be different in people with schizophrenia.

However, it is recognized that other triggers are required in addition to an inherited susceptibility. There are also theories that an early source of brain damage, such as birth trauma, head injury in childhood or a viral infection, might also lead to a vulnerability to a schizophrenic breakdown. For all these potential triggers there is epidemiological evidence to support the theory that they are relevant in the causation of schizophrenia.

There is no doubt that drugs can promote the development of schizophrenia. Cannabis use in early teens is increasingly implicated in the development of psychosis in young people. Amphetamines, hallucinogens and ecstasy may also be associated with the causation of psychosis. For this reason it is of the utmost importance that these triggers are avoided after a psychotic breakdown.

It is also known that extreme stress can lead to a schizophrenic breakdown, and can also be implicated in a relapse in someone who has recovered from schizophrenia. Studies of Afro-Caribbean people in the UK have shown that the incidence of schizophrenia is much higher in those who have moved to the UK than in those who remained in Trinidad and Barbados. The risk is even higher in second-generation immigrants. The implication of such studies is that the loss of cultural identity, social isolation and systematic racial abuse, which are most likely to affect second-generation immigrants, can be a very significant factor in the causation of schizophrenia in this group of people.[61]

The UK National Institute for Health and Care Excellence (NICE) has published guidelines for the management of psychosis and schizophrenia.[62] These emphasize that the management of the condition requires a detailed assessment of social, cultural, emotional and physical needs, thus involving a coordinated multidisciplinary approach. Treatments should be chosen with the consultation of the patient and any carers involved, and wherever possible, informed consent for treatment should be obtained.

The recommended treatment for an acute episode of schizophrenia is an initially low dose of an atypical antipsychotic drug such as amisulpride, olanzapine, quetiapine or risperidone. These drugs all have a markedly lower incidence of the more disabling side effects recognized to occur with the older antipsychotic drugs such as chlorpromazine and haloperidol.

The dose is gradually increased, and the drug is only changed if there is no significant response in six to eight weeks. In this case a second atypical antipsychotic drug

is prescribed. Only if two of the recommended atypical drugs fail to have sufficient effect is the drug clozapine prescribed. Although it is one of the most effective drugs available, clozapine carries the risk of inducing a dangerous drop in the white blood cells, and so the patient needs to be monitored with regular blood tests.

Most people will experience a reduction in both positive and negative symptoms with the first prescription of one of the newer antipsychotic medications. The current recommendation is that the drug is continued for one to two years and then withdrawn very gradually only if symptoms have resolved. The patient is then monitored for at least two more years. Approximately one in five people will suffer no further relapse with this treatment approach. Current practice is to treat an acute episode, or an acute relapse, of schizophrenia as a matter of urgency.

If the patient is failing to care for themselves adequately and if they are refusing to take medication, a decision may be made to admit the patient to a psychiatric inpatient unit. This admission may be made compulsory according to Sections 2 or 3 of the Mental Health Act 1983. It is not unusual for a first hospital admission for an acute psychosis to last for weeks to months. Ideally, while in hospital and also after discharge, the patient is offered a range of psychological and social therapies. In particular, cognitive behavioral therapy may be of benefit.

A patient who has suffered an acute psychotic breakdown may remain in a very vulnerable state for weeks to months. They will need a safe and stable environment in which to live, and may require a lot of support to cope with the routine activities of daily living.

Following the breakdown, a patient may need to be encouraged to avoid potentially stressful situations and recreational drugs, both of which are known to inhibit recovery. Because their condition often places them outside normal cultural norms of behavior, a patient who has suffered a schizophrenic breakdown may become victim to prejudice and physical abuse.

For all these reasons, whether the patient is in hospital or in the community, ideal care should involve the coordinated support of a team of mental health professionals, including a psychiatrist, community psychiatric nurses, occupational therapists and social workers. For some, placement in sheltered housing overseen by residential carers may be the most appropriate living environment in the medium to long term.

BIPOLAR DISORDER (MANIC-DEPRESSIVE PSYCHOSIS)

Bipolar disorder is a long-term condition characterized by episodes of elevated and depressed mood. A period of markedly elevated mood (by definition lasting for more than one week) is termed mania. Hypomania is the term reserved for a period of elevated mood lasting for more than four days that does not quite meet the criteria for mania (see below). If there is no history of an episode of either mania or hypomania, the diagnosis of bipolar disorder cannot be made.

Like schizophrenia, bipolar disorder is common, affecting 1 percent of the adult Western population in any one year. It, too, has a peak age of onset in the late teens and early adulthood. Unlike schizophrenia, bipolar disorder is more likely to be a lifelong condition, and as time progresses, the episodes of abnormal mood, which may initially be separated by long periods of normal mood, tend to become more prolonged and closer together. As time progresses, periods of depression also tend to predominate over the periods of elevated mood.

Bipolar disorder is subdivided into three categories in the DSM-5: bipolar I disorder, bipolar II disorder and cyclothymic disorder. These categories are distinguished by the severity of the mood swings. In bipolar I there may be marked episodes of mania interspersed by severe depression. In bipolar II elevated mood episodes are of the hypomanic variety, but the downswings can be very severe. In cyclothymic disorder the mood is very unstable and moves between hypomania and depression over the course of at least two years, but the depression is not of a severe form.

Mania is characterized by a prolonged period of high mood, and this is associated with three or more of the following features:

- increased energy, drive and restlessness

- racing thoughts

- rapid speech

- distractibility (the train of conversation may move rapidly from one topic to another, but the speech is never as disorganized as can be seen in schizophrenia)

- reduced need for sleep (less than three hours a night may seem sufficient)

- irritability

- an unrealistic perception of one's own abilities and powers, which may be so extreme as to be delusional (e.g. believing oneself to be the messiah or the US president)

- indulgence in extreme behavior that may be ultimately harmful (e.g. spending sprees, unwise sexual encounters, making foolish business investments)

- denial that anything is wrong with one's beliefs or behaviors

- hallucinations may also be experienced in some cases.

Although, by definition, these features have to be present for seven consecutive days, an episode of mania will often last for weeks to months, with four months being the average duration.

Hypomania is also characterized by high mood and driven behavior, but does not qualify for the diagnosis of mania as the indulgence in unwise behavior, and the experience of delusions and hallucinations, are not present.

The depressive episodes in bipolar disorder meet the same criteria as for unipolar depression, and by definition have to be present for 14 consecutive days. Psychotic features may become apparent in these episodes in the form of delusions of extreme low worth, poverty or illness, and the development of catatonia (extreme inactivity).

The episodes of mood disorder in bipolar disorder can be very disabling. In a state of mania personal and work relationships can break down, and there can be extreme financial and other material loss as a result or unwise behavior. The person can become both sexually and physically vulnerable. Once the episode has passed, the patient can experience deep embarrassment and remorse about what has happened during the episode. They may become unemployed and isolated as a result of the manic episode.

The periods of depression, which can become increasingly common, can be severe, and the risk of suicide is significant.

In 50 percent of cases of bipolar disorder there is a family history of psychosis (either bipolar disorder or schizophrenia), thus suggesting a biological basis to the condition and also some overlap in causation with schizophrenia. As in schizophrenia, stress and illicit drug and alcohol abuse may precipitate a relapse.

The aim of medical treatment for bipolar disorder is to stabilize mood. The atypical antipsychotics olanzapine and quetiapine, anticonvulsant drugs, such as carbamazepine and sodium valproate, and also lithium are all currently recommended as first treatments for bipolar disorder. All these drugs seem to inhibit the cycling of mood that is characteristic of the disorder, but each has its own unique but significant side effect profile. Antidepressants are not recommended as a first treatment in bipolar disorder, even for a depressive episode, as it is well recognized that they can precipitate mania. However, they may be used with caution if a depressive episode is not responding fully to the mood-stabilizing drugs, and if there is no known sensitivity to the drugs.

Ideally, mood is settled within six to eight weeks of commencing the mood-stabilizing drug. As is the case in acute schizophrenia, in both acute mania and profound depression a hospital admission may be considered necessary to ensure the patient is in a safe environment in which the basic needs of daily living can be attended to. It may be necessary to make this admission compulsory, as denial that there is anything wrong is characteristic of mania. If there is an incomplete response to medical treatment, a second mood-stabilizing drug may be added. If either the depression or mania is extremely severe or disabling, a course of electroconvulsive therapy (ECT) may be considered as a treatment option.

In the long term, continuous treatment with mood-stabilizing drugs may be the treatment of choice, and this is particularly the case if there have been two or more manic episodes, or if suicidal behavior is prominent. In both these cases the risks of a relapse are considered to outweigh the problems caused by the treatment. It is not currently considered appropriate to prescribe antidepressants in the long term for a person with bipolar disorder.

As is the case for schizophrenia, a person who has experienced an acute episode of bipolar disorder may well need support from a range of professionals, including a psychiatrist, community psychiatric nurse, social worker and occupational therapist. Structured psychological counseling, such as cognitive behavioral therapy, may be of benefit.

OTHER PSYCHOTIC DISORDERS

In some cases of functional psychosis the symptoms do not clearly fall into the categories of schizophrenia or bipolar disorder. Schizoaffective disorder is a condition in which the diagnostic features of schizophrenia are present together with a significant and episodic appearance of a mood disorder. As in bipolar disorder, the psychosis can be episodic. It is treated with either antipsychotic drugs or mood stabilizers, and may have a relatively good prognosis.

A brief psychotic episode or brief reactive psychosis describes a period of psychosis that often comes on suddenly but which, by definition, does not last for more than one month. It most often occurs in people aged 20–30 as a response to an acute shock or ongoing stress. This is the usual diagnosis in postnatal psychosis, which only rarely lasts for more than 30 days. The usual treatment is with antipsychotic medication.

Schizophreniform disorder is akin to schizophrenia, but does not meet the diagnostic criterion of lasting for more than six months.

Delusional disorder is a condition that tends to appear in slightly later life, and in which non-bizarre delusions, including a belief of being followed, harmed and conspired against, are persistently held despite evidence to the contrary. Delusions of jealousy, in which the person suspects that they are being betrayed by a loved one, can be particularly damaging, and have been known to be the cause of a violent vengeful response, including murder. If the delusions have bizarre characteristics, such as a belief in alien involvement, this is more typical of a schizophrenia-like illness than of delusional disorder. Delusional disorder does not appear to have any overlap with schizophrenia or

bipolar disorder in terms of causation or inheritance, but can respond to antipsychotic medication.

> ### Information box 6.2e-I
>
> ### Psychosis: comments from a Chinese medicine perspective
>
> In Chinese medicine, the features of psychosis are embraced by the syndromes of Dian Kuang (withdrawal and mania), Kuang Zhang (manic condition) and Chi Dai (feeble mindedness). The patterns that can be associated with these syndromes include Obstruction of the Orifices of the Heart by Phlegm, Damp Phlegm, Fire, Blood Stagnation and Qi Stagnation. In chronic psychosis there can be Depletion of Yin from Excessive Heat leading to a mixed picture of Yin Deficiency with Internal Heat.
>
> Although in most cases the patterns are mixed conditions, empty conditions can account for the negative symptoms and depression seen in the psychoses. These include Blood, Qi and Kidney Yang Deficiency, Heart Blood and Spleen Qi Deficiency, and Spleen and Kidney Yang Deficiency.
>
> Flaws and Lake (2001)[63] suggest that the origin of these patterns is a combination of constitutional Deficiency or Imbalance (of Yin or Yang) and expression of excessive emotions (leading to Qi Stagnation, Congealing of Phlegm, Fire and Blood Stagnation).

Organic psychiatric disorders

Organic psychiatric disorders are those syndromes that can be explained in terms of a clearly understandable problem in brain function or damage to the structure of the brain. There will be a clear link between the onset of the change in the function of the brain and the appearance of symptoms, which means that the symptoms can be attributed directly to the physical problem in the brain. Although the current psychiatric classification separates the organic from the functional psychiatric disorders, as more becomes known about disordered brain function in the functional conditions, the demarcation between the two is becoming more arbitrary.

DEMENTIA

Dementia is a term derived from the Latin meaning out of mind. It is used medically to refer to a number of conditions in which there is reduced mental functioning in a wide range of domains as a direct result of long-term change in brain structure. In the dementias, the physical problem can be located predominantly in the cortex of the brain. The cortex is the outer layer of the brain, which is responsible for the higher mental functions such as thinking, memory, insight, speech, inhibition of socially inappropriate behavior, processing of sensory information and purposeful movement. There is a range of causes of dementia, each of which has a specific physical causation and correspondingly characteristic range of symptoms.

A diagnosis of dementia is made when it can be demonstrated that, in a fully conscious person, new learning is impaired and there has been progressive decline in intellect, movement, speech, recognition of sensory information and performing complex activities. Dementia is usually a clinical diagnosis made without the need for confirmatory tests, although further tests can help to clarify the underlying cause. However, it is essential that reversible causes of confusion are excluded from the diagnosis (e.g. alcoholism, thyroid disease, normal pressure hydrocephalus). If there is any impairment of consciousness, the diagnosis should not be made, as this is more characteristic of a drug-induced state or a metabolic disorder. Severe depression in elderly people can also mimic dementia.

In most forms of dementia the onset is gradual, with the exception of the second most common cause, which is cerebrovascular disease. In this case the cause of the cortical damage is multiple areas of infarction of the brain, and these generally tend to develop very rapidly.

The most striking and universal aspect of dementia is memory impairment. In general, short-term memory is most profoundly affected initially, although long-term memory will also be eroded as the condition progresses.

Sometimes it appears as if memories are being erased in the opposite order in which they were laid down, and the patient becomes fixated on people and events from their early life. There is also increasing difficulty in complex tasks such as writing, addition, getting dressed and conversation. Physical movements can become clumsier, and gait unsteady. Urinary and fecal incontinence can develop. There is also gradual disinhibition of normal social control, and the patient becomes impulsive and emotionally unstable. There may be marked emotional or aggressive outbursts.

The different forms of dementia and the Chinese medicine correspondences are described in Section 4.1f.

CONFUSIONAL STATES AND DELIRIUM

Delirium is a term used to describe a particular organic syndrome in which clouded consciousness is the central feature. The term acute confusional state is synonymous with delirium. Consciousness can be impaired by degrees, and in the most extreme form would manifest as coma. In its more subtle forms there may be difficulty in sustaining attention, disorientation and some memory impairment.

Apart from confusion, other features of delirium include an abrupt onset and fluctuating intensity of symptoms

hour by hour. Hallucinations (especially visual in nature) can occur, as can persecutory delusions and misread visual images (illusions) (e.g. the curtains appearing to be like a threatening man in black). Agitation and anxiety can be common emotional components of delirium.

Impairment of consciousness has a wide range of causes, including head injury, stroke, brain infections, inadequate oxygen and glucose, the effect of drugs (and drug withdrawal) and the toxins that build up in chronic diseases. In contrast to dementia, if the cause is treated the delirium will subside. Children and elderly people are much more prone to delirium than the rest of the population. It has been estimated that this state affects up to 20 percent of elderly people admitted to a general hospital.

Some of the features of delirium are comparable to the symptoms of schizophrenia, but key differences are the fluctuating consciousness and the predominantly visual illusions and hallucinations in delirium.

The most important aspect of the treatment of delirium is elucidation of the cause. If the cause is not obvious, a range of tests (including full blood count, kidney and liver function, thyroid function, blood glucose, chest X-ray and infection screens) may be performed. A reversal of the cause (e.g. treatment of a urinary infection) can result in a remarkable resolution of the delirium with a rapidity that may appear close to miraculous to the patient's carers. Only in very extreme cases is medical sedation used, as sedative drugs can exacerbate the depression in consciousness. However, benzodiazepines are routinely used in the treatment of acute alcohol withdrawal to prevent the appearance of the confusional state known as delirium tremens.

 Information box 6.2e-II

Dementia and confusion: comments from a Chinese medicine perspective

From a Chinese medicine perspective, the dulled thinking and clouding of consciousness that appear in dementia and confusional states correspond to Shen Deficiency and Obstructed Shen, respectively, although it is possible that both of these pathologies of the Shen will coexist in both types of organic disorder.

Shen Deficiency can result from Deficiency of Kidney Essence, Kidney and Spleen Yang, Kidney Yin, and Qi and Blood.

The Shen can be obstructed by the Pathogenic Factors of Phlegm, Phlegm, Damp, Fire and Blood Stagnation.

Part II: Personality disorders and intellectual disability

Personality disorders

The mental health disorders so far described generally develop either in adolescence or in adult life. For each of the diagnoses studied so far, it would be possible to find cases in which the patient had a history of what would be called normal mental health before the disorder developed. In such cases one might expect that external biological factors, psychological factors or social factors might have played some part in the development of the condition. Two examples of disorders developing in a person with previously normal mental health would be the case of post-traumatic stress disorder (PTSD) following a car accident, and a case of depression following childbirth.

However, in many other cases, it might be clear that a vulnerability to conditions such as obsessive-compulsive disorder (OCD), panic disorder, depression or schizophrenia might have been apparent in the form of certain personality traits dating as far back as infancy. For example, a person with OCD might have a long-standing history of obsessive behavior and "magical" thinking from early childhood, and a person with panic disorder might have always tended to be fearful and anxious in social situations.

When certain personality traits are as extreme as to lead to a vulnerability to mental health disorder, or to cause problems for the patient in the context of their relationships, work or recreation, the term personality disorder is used. It must be remembered that the personality disorders listed below are common, affecting an estimated 10 percent of the population, and so it might be argued that to define 10 percent of the population as disordered is logically flawed. However, the classification of extreme personality traits can prove a useful tool, in that it can help with the understanding of the causation of certain mental illnesses.

By definition, a personality disorder, like personality itself, is deeply engrained and enduring, and dates back to early childhood. It is believed that personality disorder is either inherited, or is the result of pervasive psychological influences that deeply affected development early in life. Personality disorder is believed to be very resistant to treatment (and in the recent past was considered by some psychiatrists to be untreatable), but in many cases long-term psychotherapy of some form may be of significant benefit.

The German psychiatrist Kurt Schneider first categorized personality disorders in the 1930s, and this classification is recreated in ICD-10. DSM-5 classifies personality disorders slightly differently and lists ten types of personality disorders.

The DSM-5 personality disorders were grouped in DSM-IV into three clusters that are summarized below, as they help to show there are shared features between disorders in each cluster.

- DSM-IV Cluster A (characterized by odd or eccentric behavior):

    – paranoid personality disorder

    – schizoid personality disorder

    – schizotypal personality disorder

- DSM-IV Cluster B (characterized by dramatic, explosive, erratic or emotional behavior):

    – antisocial personality disorder

    – borderline personality disorder (BPD)

    – histrionic personality disorder

    – narcissistic personality disorder

- DSM-IV Cluster C (characterized by anxious, fearful, dependent or introverted behavior):

    – avoidant personality disorder

    – dependent personality disorder

    – obsessive-compulsive personality disorder (OCPD)

    – passive-aggressive personality behavior (no longer considered a personality disorder in DSM-5).

These disorders are considered in turn below.

PARANOID PERSONALITY DISORDER

Paranoid personality disorder is characterized by a belief that other people are threatening, devious and untrustworthy. Jealousy and contempt for others are prominent. A person with a paranoid personality disorder tends to read hidden, demeaning or threatening meanings into benign remarks or events, to hold grudges for a long time, and to avoid intimate relationships. They may perceive benign comments or reactions from other people as attacks on their character or reputation. They may be in the habit of making formal complaints. Particularly when in positions of power, they can consider others as beneath them.

A paranoid personality disorder is associated with a vulnerability to paranoid psychosis, anxiety and depression.

People with this personality disorder do not tend to ask for help. The development of a trusting therapeutic relationship will be difficult. Ideally, intensive psychotherapy is the treatment of choice.

SCHIZOID PERSONALITY DISORDER

A schizoid type is a person who has little desire to form relationships, has a restricted range of emotional expression (flattened affect), and chooses to spend their time in solitary activities and introspective thinking. They also may demonstrate little or no drive to seek out sexual experiences.

In this personality disorder, there also seems to be an indifference to the praise or criticism of others, so giving the impression of a striking self-sufficiency together with oddness, suspiciousness or emotional coldness.

A schizoid personality disorder is associated with a vulnerability to schizophrenia or delusional disorder.

The ideal treatment would be sensitively supervised group therapy, but someone with this sort of personality disorder is unlikely to seek treatment.

SCHIZOTYPAL PERSONALITY DISORDER

As is true for the schizoid type, the schizotypal personality disorder is characterized by a solitary lifestyle and difficulties with close personal relationships. However, in addition to the schizoid aspects, strange speech, odd beliefs and eccentric behavior are manifest. There may be suspicion and magical thinking, but the person does not meet the diagnostic criteria for schizophrenia. Often there is extreme discomfort in social company, possibly driven by paranoid fears.

A schizotypal personality disorder is associated with a vulnerability to anxiety, depression and episodes of psychosis.

Treatment is very difficult because of the problems the patient has in communicating with others and in forming relationships, but in some cases a cognitive behavioral approach can help the person modify some of their more stigmatizing behaviors. Antipsychotic medication may be considered to be of benefit in other cases.

ANTISOCIAL PERSONALITY DISORDER

In this disorder, the person has a lifelong tendency to behavior that appears to show total disregard for the needs and rights of others. Aggressive outbursts, lying, stealing and vandalism will have become apparent from early childhood, and from teenage years the child with this disorder will be in conflict with authority and the law. Remorse for this antisocial behavior is lacking. Impulsivity is characteristic, and features of attention deficit hyperactivity disorder (ADHD) are commonly present. It has been estimated that 65–75 percent of convicted criminals in US prisons could be given this diagnosis.

By definition, the diagnosis should not be made in children. The term conduct disorder is used to describe antisocial behavior in children.

A psychopath is a person who would qualify for the diagnosis of antisocial personality disorder, but has additional particularly chilling characteristics. A psychopath will indulge in violent and sadistic behavior that is planned, purposeful and emotionless. The person

will have an arrogant sense of elevated self-worth, and may even initially appear to be charming and charismatic. This is the diagnosis that would be applied to serial rapists or killers. However, psychopaths may find more acceptable outlets for their disregard for the well-being of others by attaining positions of political power or by joining the armed forces.[64]

An antisocial personality disorder is associated with a vulnerability to substance abuse and depression.

Group therapy may be the most appropriate treatment choice for a person with this disorder, and may be more effective if the group consists solely of people with this diagnosis. Often the person has never had the opportunity to form a close emotional relationship, and thus the therapeutic relationship can be very challenging, but if it can be established, it may have a powerful impact on the patient.

It is unlikely that psychopaths will be able to respond significantly to therapy, and imprisonment in a secure unit may often be the most positive possible treatment option.

BORDERLINE PERSONALITY DISORDER (BPD)

Borderline personality disorder (BPD) is the most prevalent of the personality disorders, affecting an estimated 1–2 percent of the general population. It occurs in women twice as often as it does in men. It is characterized by a triad of long-standing emotional instability, impulsive and unpredictable behavior, and poor self-image. The person with BPD may feel unclear about their identity, or their life direction. Mood swings are common, and relate to the feelings of low self-esteem. The mood is profoundly affected by relationships, and fears of rejection or abandonment. Relationships can be stormy, with acting out being a common feature. Close attachments may be made far too quickly, followed rapidly by deep disappointment and relationship breakdown.

Lack of joy or depression is the background mood, and although there can be sudden changes in mood (to anger, anxiety or euphoria), the patient with BPD may often return to suicidal ideation. The risk of suicide is significant, with up to 10 percent eventually dying as a result of suicide. Self-harm, binge eating and substance abuse are also very common in BPD.

Although it is a common disorder, and one that accounts for 20 percent of psychiatric hospital admissions in the US and one that is a significant cause of suicide deaths, BPD is not readily diagnosed. Often, on the surface, a person with BPD may seem to be functioning relatively normally, and it is only those who are closest to them who experience the consequences of their mood swings and impulsive behavior.

It is believed that the tendency to BPD is inherited, but in some cases a dysfunctional family background may be causative.

BPD is associated with a vulnerability to substance abuse, eating disorders (especially bulimia and obesity), anxiety and depression, suicide and psychosis.

The treatment of choice is intensive psychotherapy, in which the person with BPS is encouraged to explore the emotional roots to their impulsive and often damaging behavior.

HISTRIONIC PERSONALITY DISORDER

Histrionic is a term used to describe an overdramatic, almost theatrical, personality type. In this personality disorder, the affected person demonstrates exaggerated emotional responses and attention-seeking behavior. This personality type is uncomfortable whenever they are not the center of attention. They may use overdramatic speech and affected appearance to draw attention to themselves. There may be sexually seductive behavior, and a tendency to consider emotional relationships to be closer than they actually are.

The emotions and behavior of this personality type may be extremely affected by other people's actions and by external circumstances. Stormy interactions may be a consequence of an intense need for life to be less mundane than it is perceived to be. Illnesses and aches and pains are overdramatized, and their lives may be presented as if they are always in crisis. A person of the histrionic type is likely to blame other people and circumstances as the cause of their life's problems.

A histrionic personality disorder is associated with a vulnerability to conversion disorder, somatization disorder and depression.

In contrast to the other personality disorders, a histrionic type may readily present to a medical practitioner for support and affirmation. However, they may be resistant to change because of the tendency not to take responsibility for the way in which they react to the world around them. Ideally, intensive psychotherapy would be the most appropriate therapy for this disorder. Antidepressant medication can also be a helpful adjunct to therapy.

NARCISSISTIC PERSONALITY DISORDER

Narcissism is the term used to describe an overemphasized belief in one's own importance. In the narcissistic personality disorder this belief is accompanied by an extreme sensitivity to criticism. The narcissistic person will be preoccupied with fantasies of success, power or attractiveness, and may fabricate stories of past achievement and ongoing projects. There is a desire to relate to special and successful people, and a belief that more ordinary people are without value. The appearance is of someone who lacks empathy and who is arrogant and self-important. It follows that there is a tendency to exploit other people to meet calculated ends. In some cases this exploitation can be severe, and may involve extortion of money or planned harm to another person's well-being. If a narcissistic type experiences challenge or criticism, there can be extreme emotional outbursts or cold withdrawal.

A narcissistic personality disorder is associated with a vulnerability to depression and psychosis.

As is true for all the personality disorders, psychotherapy would be the treatment of choice, although it may be difficult to encourage the person to accept the need for therapy. Group therapy, in which the affected person is confronted with the reactions of others in a safe environment, might prove to be an appropriate treatment option.

AVOIDANT PERSONALITY DISORDER

A person with an avoidant personality type will tend to be anxious and fearful of social situations, with the consequence that they appear very shy and may tend to avoid activities that involve contact with others. They are particularly anxious in the context of new relationships, and prefer to make contact with people who are very familiar to them. In stark contrast to the isolated stance of a person of a schizoid type, the avoidant personality will be acutely sensitive to criticism, and fears social rejection. The isolation that can result from this fear is, in fact, the opposite of the safe closeness that a person with the avoidant personality desires.

Often, it can be recognized that many of these avoidant traits have been apparent from very early infancy, thus strongly suggesting an inherited tendency to this form of extreme shyness. Undoubtedly, negative experiences such as abuse in childhood can also result in social fearfulness in later life. It is likely that in most cases both biological and psychological factors have contributed to this personality type.

Avoidant personality disorder is associated with a vulnerability to social phobia, depression and anxiety.

Medical treatment, such as SSRI antidepressants and minor tranquillizers, may be prescribed to help the person cope with feelings of low self-esteem and anxiety. However, long-term psychotherapy is the ideal treatment choice, particularly as people with the avoidant tendency are likely to be very keen to uncover the roots of their anxiety and to try to deal with their fears.

DEPENDENT PERSONALITY DISORDER

In dependent personality disorder there is an excessive need for the support of others in meeting emotional and physical needs. A dependent type will tend to cling to known relationships and rely on those around them to help them to make decisions and to sort out problems. They may feel extreme anxiety if these relationships are threatened, and may choose to suffer abuse within relationships rather than challenge the emotional status quo. They may avoid the possibility of being alone and may become preoccupied with fears of being abandoned.

Dependent personality disorder is associated with a vulnerability to low mood and depression.

Psychotherapy may be of benefit in encouraging a person of this type to make their own choices in life. Cognitive behavioral therapy might be an appropriate mode of treatment.

Obsessive-compulsive personality disorder (OCPD)

It is important to make the distinction between obsessive-compulsive personality disorder (OCPD) and the previously discussed condition obsessive-compulsive disorder (OCD). The ritualistic (obsessive) behavior seen in OCD, and so often the cause for mental distress, is not the hallmark of OCPD. OCPD is characterized by a perfectionistic attitude to life and an extreme need to control and order events. It is more common in men than in women.

A person with OCPD will have very high personal standards and a preoccupation with attending to rules. They are often high achievers. They may become disturbed if their standards cannot be attained by themselves or others, or if the rules are broken. They may find it difficult to delegate, and may have difficulty in forming close relationships. They may also find it difficult to be generous or to throw things away.

In contrast to the other personality disorders, a person with OCPD may be able to function well in life without recourse to less healthy coping strategies such as recreational drugs or self-harm. The condition to which they are most vulnerable is depression.

There may be a good response to psychotherapeutic techniques that challenge the seemingly fixed value systems in OCPD.

Information box 6.2e-III

Personality disorders: comments from a Chinese medicine perspective

The personality diagnostic categories describe enduring tendencies in the ways in which a person might respond to the world. In this way they do share some parallels with the understanding in Five Element Constitutional Acupuncture that each person has a characteristic pattern of emotional responses, which may be described in terms of their Constitutional or Causative factor. For each of the personality types there are features that seem to reflect Imbalance in one or more of the Five Elements (Wood, Fire, Earth, Metal and Water). For example, the need of the dependent personality for support and encouragement might speak of an Imbalance in the Earth element, and the desire for attention and physical affection of the histrionic personality type might reflect an Imbalance in the Fire element.

A further parallel is that the personality types can be seen in terms of the way in which they embody a vulnerability to certain mental health disorders. Likewise, according to Five Element Constitutional Acupuncture, the constitutional types also correspond to the vulnerability to particular patterns of disease.

Passive-aggressive behavior

The tendency to passive-aggressive behavior was defined as a personality disorder in DSM-IV, but has been omitted from DSM-5 as a formal disorder because of its pervasive overlap with a wide range of other disorders. In passive aggression there is a long-term tendency to resist having to take responsibility or to be compliant to the demands of others. However, instead of outright confrontation, the passive-aggressive response is to appear to comply, and even to show willing, but then to sabotage the action by inefficiency or forgetfulness. The person may appear sullen and resentful, and particularly so if their behavior is challenged. There can be stormy outbursts. Others are usually blamed for life's problems.

A tendency to choose passive-aggressive responses is associated with a vulnerability to low mood, depression and substance abuse.

Psychotherapy may be of benefit in encouraging a person of this type to make their own choices in life. Cognitive behavioral therapy might be an appropriate mode of treatment.

Intellectual disability

Intellectual disability (formerly termed learning disability and mental retardation) is defined as an enduring state of low intellectual functioning that has persisted since childhood. Intelligence can be assessed in terms of the intelligence quotient (IQ), in which, by definition, an average person would score 100. In intellectual disability the IQ is more than two standard deviations below this mean value (i.e. less than 70). As well as reduced intellectual functioning, there may be impairments in other developmental areas, such as impairment of motor skills or speech. Intellectual disability affects 1–3 percent of the UK population.

Intellectual disability may first become apparent when a child fails to attain the normal developmental milestones in language, motor function and social skills. A lack of the expected levels of curiosity of childhood may be noticed, and also the fact that infantile behavior persists for longer than would be expected.

In only 25 percent of cases of intellectual disability can a specific cause be identified. In all other cases, the cause is unclear, and may be the result of a combination of inherited and environmental factors. There is a clear link between intellectual disability of unspecified cause and poverty and low socio-economic class. Some of the known causes of intellectual disability are summarized in Table 6.2e-I.

Table 6.2e-I The known causes of intellectual disability

Cause type	Specific causes
Trauma	Birth trauma (intracranial hemorrhage or lack of oxygen before, during or after birth)
	Head injury
Chromosomal abnormalities	Down syndrome
	Fragile X syndrome
	Prader Willi syndrome
Genetic abnormalities	Phenylketonuria
	Galactosemia
	Hunter syndrome
	Rett syndrome
Infections in childhood	Congenital rubella
	Meningitis and encephalitis
	Cytomegalovirus (CMV) and toxoplasmosis (congenital)
Listeria	Human immunodeficiency virus (HIV)
Metabolic disorders in infancy	Congenital hypothyroidism
	Raised levels of bilirubin
	Hypoglycemia
	Malnutrition
Effects of toxins in the fetus or in infancy	Alcohol and other recreational drugs
	Mercury
	Lead

TREATMENT OF INTELLECTUAL DISABILITY

Early recognition of possible intellectual disability can enable the initiation of early intervention. Maximizing educational and social intervention at an early stage in development can dramatically improve the outlook for children who have features of intellectual disability. As is the case for all children, a stimulating, safe and loving environment can have positive effects on development in all domains.

Young children with early features of intellectual disability need a particular emphasis on stimulation, because they tend to have less of the natural curiosity that provides most children with the stimulation they need to develop intellectually.

The emphasis is on treatment to enable individuals to reach their full potential and, ideally, to attain the social skills required for independent living. Throughout childhood the individual will need repeated assessment so that the most appropriate educational environment can be chosen, and also so that any coexisting mental health disorders, such as anxiety and depression, can be diagnosed and treated. It is clear that the outcome in terms of personal fulfillment and independence in adulthood is strongly related to the level of intervention and support the individual receives during childhood.

People with intellectual disability are also much more vulnerable to a wide range of physical illnesses, partly due to inherited constitutional weakness and disease, but also because of difficulties in maintaining self-care and taking part in disease prevention programs. Ideally an individual with intellectual disability is recognized as being at risk of deteriorating health, and is protected by means of a formal healthcare plan and the provision of key workers to ensure they take part in healthcare programs.

Other long-term problems for people with intellectual disability include social isolation and an inability to appropriately meet basic needs, such as shelter, nutrition, hygiene and friendship. In such cases the ideal solution would be some sort of sheltered lifestyle, such as a group residential home or community. As well as state-funded residential communities, in the UK there are independent communities, such as the Rudolf Steiner-inspired Camp Hill Communities and L'Arche Foundation, in which there is special emphasis on the personal value of each resident and the unique gifts they have to offer the rest of the community.

Information box 6.2e-IV

Learning disability: comments from a Chinese medicine perspective

From a Chinese medicine perspective, intellectual disability might result from a combination of constitutional Deficiency, in particular, of Kidney Essence, and Obstruction of the Shen, for example, by Phlegm, Phlegm Damp or Heat. Just as it is recognized that early intervention in terms of social and educational input can increase the chances of an individual reaching their full potential, so it makes sense that early intervention in terms of Chinese medicine treatment might well have a positive impact on the outcome of a child with early features of intellectual disability. An emphasis on nourishing Deficiency and clearing of Pathogenic Factors in theory could protect a child with an inherited constitutional defect from a downward spiral in both health and mental functioning. Scott and Barlow (1999) report very positive outcomes in this respect with early treatment of infants with Down syndrome.[65]

The red flags of mental health disorders

Some patients with mental health disorders will benefit from referral to a conventional doctor for assessment or treatment. Red flags are those symptoms and signs that indicate that referral should be considered. The red flags of mental health disorders are described in Table 6.2e-II. A summary of the red flags in a format designed for quick reference in clinical practice can be found in Appendix III. This gives advice on the degree of urgency of referral for each of the red flag conditions listed.

Table 6.2e-II A44: Red flags of mental health disorders

Red flag	Description	Reasoning
A44.1	Suicidal thoughts: with features that suggest serious risk (old age, male sex, social isolation, concrete plans in place)	This symptom may not be volunteered by a person suffering from depression. A question like "Have you ever thought life is not worth living?" may reveal suicidal ideation
		Thoughts that life is not worth living does not necessarily signify serious risk, but if present should lead you to question further about features that suggest seriousness of intent and a high-risk social situation
		High-risk factors include old age, male sex, isolation or marital separation, and concrete plans in place about how to end it all (e.g. clearly thought-out method, stockpiling medications, the writing of notes to those who will be left as a result of the suicide)
		If you have any concerns that your patient is at serious risk of suicide, you should urge them to discuss their situation with their doctor and seek treatment for their low mood. You may wish to discuss the situation with the doctor yourself, and should seek the patient's permission before you do this
		The patient may be resistant to the idea of referral. Only if you have grave concerns that the patient is a risk because of mental illness, or because others around them are at risk, does this becomes a situation when it may be appropriate to breach your normal practice of confidentiality. In such circumstances it would be advisable to first seek advice from the professional conduct officer of your professional body

A44.2	Hallucinations, delusions or other evidence of thought disorder, together with evidence of deteriorating self-care and personality change	These are all features of a psychosis such as schizophrenia. Suicide risk is high
		As it may be very difficult to fully assess this risk, it is advised that, unless absolutely sure of the patient's safety, you should refer them to professionals who are experienced in the treatment of mental health disorders. Ideally seek the patient's consent before speaking to a health professional
		Referral in such a situation may result in the serious outcome of the patient being compulsorily detained in hospital against their will
		The patient may be resistant to the idea of referral. Only if you have grave concerns that the patient is a risk because of mental illness, or because others around them are at risk, does this become a situation when it may be appropriate to breach your normal practice of confidentiality. In such circumstances it would be advisable to first seek advice from the professional conduct officer of your professional body
A44.3	Features of mania: increasing agitation, grandiosity, pressure of speech and sleeplessness with delusional thinking	Mania is a feature of bipolar disorder, and is a form of psychosis that carries a high risk of behavior that can be both socially and physically damaging to the patient and to those around them. Suicide risk is high
		As it may be very difficult to fully assess this risk, it is advised that, unless absolutely sure of the patient's safety, you should refer them to professionals who are experienced in the treatment of mental health disorders. Ideally seek the patient's consent before speaking to a health professional
		Referral in such a situation may result in the serious outcome of the patient being compulsorily detained in hospital against their will
		The patient may be resistant to the idea of referral. Only if you have grave concerns that the patient is a risk because of mental illness, or because others around them are at risk, does this become a situation when it may be appropriate to breach your normal practice of confidentiality. In such circumstances it would be advisable to first seek advice from the professional conduct officer of your professional body
A44.4	Evidence of an organic mental health disorder, e.g. confusion, deterioration in intellectual skills, loss of ability to self-care	Organic mental health disorders are, by definition, those that have a medically recognized physical cause, such as drug intoxication, brain damage or dementia. They are characterized by confusion or clouding of consciousness, and loss of insight. Visual hallucinations may be apparent, as in the case of delirium tremens (alcohol withdrawal)
		It is advised that, unless absolutely sure of the patient's safety, you should refer them to professionals who are experienced in the treatment of mental health disorders. Ideally seek the patient's consent before speaking to a health professional
		Referral in such a situation may result in the serious outcome of the patient being compulsorily detained in hospital against their will
		The patient may be resistant to the idea of referral. Only if you have grave concerns that the patient is a risk because of mental illness, or because others around them are at risk, does this become a situation when it may be appropriate to breach your normal practice of confidentiality. In such circumstances it would be advisable to first seek advice from the professional conduct officer of your professional body
A44.5	Severe depression/ obsessive-compulsive disorder (OCD) or anxiety: if not responding to treatment and seriously affecting quality of life	In certain cases of minor mental health disorder the symptoms of depression, obsessive thoughts or anxiety can be so overwhelming as to be disabling. Referral needs to be considered for psychiatric or psychological support if these symptoms appear to be seriously affecting quality of life (e.g. the patient is unable to leave their home)

A44.6	Severe disturbance of body image: if not responding to treatment, and resulting in features of progressive anorexia nervosa or bulimia nervosa (e.g. progressive weight loss, secondary amenorrhea, repeated compulsion to bring about vomiting)	Severe forms of eating disorder can result in progressive ill health, which can be so severe as to be life-threatening. If symptoms are not responding to treatment consider referral for professional psychiatric support The patient may be resistant to the idea of referral. Only if you have grave concerns that the patient is a risk because of mental illness, or because others around them are at risk, does this become a situation when it may be appropriate to breach your normal practice of confidentiality. In such circumstances it would be advisable to first seek advice from the professional conduct officer of your professional body
A44.7	Features of autism in a child: slow development of speech, impaired social interactions, little imaginative play, obsessional repetitive behavior	Mild degrees of autism may not be diagnosed until the child reaches secondary school age. Refer if you are concerned that the child is demonstrating impaired social interactions (aloofness), impaired social communication (very poor eye contact, awkward and inappropriate body language) and impairment of imaginative play (play may instead be dominated by obsessional behavior such as lining up toys or checking), as early diagnosis can result in the child being offered extra educational and psychological support
A44.8	Postnatal depression	Refer any case of depression developing in the postnatal period which is lasting for >3 weeks, and which is not responding to treatment. Refer straight away if the woman is experiencing suicidal ideas, or if you believe the health of the baby to be at risk The patient may be resistant to the idea of referral. Only if you have grave concerns that the patient is a risk because of mental illness, or because others around them are at risk, does this become a situation when it may be appropriate to breach your normal practice of confidentiality. In such circumstances it would be advisable to first seek advice from the professional conduct officer of your professional body
A44.9	Postnatal psychosis	Refer straight away if you suspect the development of postnatal psychosis (delusional or paranoid ideas and hallucinations are key features), as this condition is associated with a high risk of suicide or harm to the baby The patient may be resistant to the idea of referral. Only if you have grave concerns that the patient is a risk because of mental illness, or because others around them are at risk, does this become a situation when it may be appropriate to breach your normal practice of confidentiality. In such circumstances it would be advisable to first seek advice from the professional conduct officer of your professional body

Conclusions

6.3

6.3a The red flags of disease: a review

Throughout the study of the various diseases considered so far, the red flags of disease have been systematically introduced. In this section the rationale for describing certain clusters of symptoms and signs as red flags is clarified. The section continues with some guidance on how to prioritize patients who present with any combination of these warning symptoms and signs, and on how to refer patients to conventional medical practitioners. A summary of the red flags in a format designed for quick reference in clinical practice can be found in Appendix III.

The red flags of disease

Red flags are those symptoms and signs which, if elicited by an acupuncturist, merit referral to a conventional doctor. Referral is indicated because the presence of red flags indicates the possibility of a condition that either may not respond fully to non-medical treatment or may benefit further from conventional diagnosis, advice or treatment.

Referral may be considered for the following four broad reasons:

- to enable the patient to have access to treatment that will benefit their medical condition

- for investigations to exclude the possibility of serious disease

- for investigations to confirm a diagnosis and help guide treatment

- for access to advice on the management of a complex condition.

It is important to clarify at this stage that the red flags indicate those potentially serious conditions in which the patient would be in need of further tests, advice or treatment. Not all of the red flag conditions listed in this text indicate that the patient will need medical treatment. In some cases referral is advised so that the patient can have tests to exclude an unlikely but important treatable condition (e.g. a mole that might have features of skin cancer), or to obtain a medical diagnosis to guide in the future management of the condition (e.g. ascertaining the severity and cause of suspected anemia). In other situations it may be important to refer so that the patient can have access to detailed medical advice (e.g. on the complexity of assessing coronary risk and how this impacts on subsequent choice of medical treatment).

Use of acupuncture and red flags

There are very few examples of when acupuncture would not be beneficial to someone who is also receiving conventional investigation or treatment for a condition. Therefore, referral in response to a patient with red flag symptoms or signs does not mean that acupuncture need be discontinued, as long as the therapist is sure that the patient has given informed consent to this treatment.

The red flags as guides to referral

Red flags are guides to referral and not absolute indicators. Often the red flags described in this text specify a fixed, measurable point at which referral should be considered, for example, high fever (especially if over 40°C) not responding to treatment within two hours in a child. In reality, of course, disease falls somewhere along a spectrum that bridges the state of being of little concern and one of being of serious concern (see Figure 6.3a-I). A disease does not suddenly become serious once a fixed point has passed. Moreover, what might constitute a red flag in one individual may be of less concern in someone of a stronger constitution.

These red flags are guides for referral and not absolute indicators of serious disease

Figure 6.3a-I This illustrates the fact that red flags have to fall at a fixed point along the spectrum of symptoms of mild to serious disease

Bearing in mind the potential flexibility of interpretation of red flag syndromes, there may well be situations in which the clinical opinion of the acupuncturist is that referral is unnecessary even though a red flag is present. Conversely, if a nagging uncertainty persists in a clinical situation, even if the patient does not fit the criteria for any of the red flags, it is safest to trust clinical instincts and refer. The important thing is that there is an awareness of these indicators of possible serious disease, and that in every case time has been taken to consider their relevance for patients in the clinical situation.

Prioritization of the red flags

The various red flags merit different responses from the practitioner according to the nature of the underlying condition of which they may be an indication. To aid with decision-making in the clinical situation, the red flags listed in this text are assigned to one or more of three categories of urgency. These categories are:

* Non-urgent: A non-urgent referral means that the patient can be encouraged to make a routine appointment with a medical practitioner, and this ideally will take place within seven days at the most.

** High priority: A high priority referral means that a medical practitioner assesses the patient within the same day.

*** Urgent: The urgent category is for those situations when the patient requires immediate medical attention, and this may mean summoning an on-call doctor or calling paramedics to the scene.

The summaries of red flags that can be found in Appendix III indicate by means of the symbols * or ** or *** which category of urgency best fits each red flag. Again, this categorization is simply a guide to the degree of urgency rather than a fixed directive on the appropriate response in a particular clinical situation.

For many of the listed red flags, the labeling indicates a range of degrees of priority (e.g. */**). For these red flags, the precise level of priority depends on other characteristics of the individual case, which should become clear according to the particular clinical situation.

How to respond to the red flags

The response to a red flag in a clinical situation depends very much on what degree of urgency the response merits. The practicalities of this are described in Section 6.3c.

Non-urgent red flags

Some red flags are indicators of possible serious disease, and yet the patient does not require urgent treatment, even if the disease is actually present. An example of this is the patient who has features of anemia, including pallor, breathlessness and palpitations on exertion. Anemia can have serious underlying causes, for example, chronic gastrointestinal bleeding or pernicious anemia, some of which cannot be expected to respond fully to non-medical therapies. In a case of anemia, the patient obviously requires further investigation and may possibly require medical treatment according to the outcome of the investigations. However, if the symptoms have been developing over the course of weeks to months, the patient does not need to be seen by the doctor on the same day.

Another example of a non-urgent red flag is the well child who has symptoms that indicate occasional bouts of mild asthma. In this case referral is recommended more for confirmation of diagnosis, and so that the patient can have access to medical advice about how to manage a potentially serious condition, rather than simply for treatment. It will be obvious that in such a situation the child does not need to be seen urgently.

Most of the red flags of cancer have been prioritized as of non-urgent priority. This is because such features have usually taken weeks to develop, and one or two days' delay is not critical in the course of most cancers. For example, in the UK, the National Health Service (NHS) referral system is structured so that the patient demonstrating red flag signs of cancer is seen by a hospital specialist within two weeks of referral by their GP. Therefore the acupuncturist ideally needs to ensure that their patient with a red flag of cancer is seen by a GP within a maximum of a few days of referral in order to minimize the total wait, but there would usually be no need for an urgent response to finding the red flags. Of course, there will be some situations in which it would be appropriate to make a high priority referral for patients showing features of cancer, either because of rapidity of progression of symptoms, or in order to allay anxiety for the patient.

Those red flags that have been categorized as non-urgent will require non-urgent referral. In these situations it can be suggested to the patient to make a non-urgent appointment with their GP. This means that the patient will be seen within the next few days. In this situation a letter of referral can be prepared, although this may not be necessary if the patient is capable of passing on the essential information verbally. If a letter is needed, it can either be taken to the doctor by the patient (the most reliable approach) or can be sent by post to the practice (more likely to be delayed or to go astray). A guide to writing letters of referral to general practitioners (GPs) can be found in Section 6.3c.

High priority red flags

Some of the listed red flags are indicators of serious disease, and these merit seeking a medical opinion on the same day, because there is a possibility that the patient's condition might deteriorate rapidly without treatment. An example of a high priority case is hemoptysis (coughing up blood) in a patient who has lost two stone in weight over the past few months (strong indicators of lung cancer or tuberculosis). In this case, the potential of serious blood loss or the possibility of contagiousness makes the referral high priority.

In high priority situations, it may help with the referral for the acupuncturist to speak to the patient's medical doctor by telephone to explain the clinical situation. After discussion, if the GP agrees with the assessment of urgency, an appropriate appointment for the patient can be made.

Alternatively, it may be more appropriate that patients make these referrals themselves, and they should request a same-day appointment with their GP.

In such situations it is good practice to give the patient a letter describing the clinical findings and concerns to take to their GP before they leave the clinic (see also Section 6.3c).

Urgent red flags

In some cases the red flags indicate that the patient requires urgent medical assessment. In these cases it may be appropriate to request an emergency ambulance to take the patient to hospital. A less dramatic option is to telephone the patient's practice to ask to speak to a GP urgently in order to get their advice about referral to hospital. If there is some uncertainty, the GP may choose to visit the patient first, or ask for them to come to the practice to be seen before the paramedics are called.

In those urgent cases in which it is unlikely that the acupuncturist will meet the examining doctor, it will be helpful to produce a brief clinical summary letter to be taken with the patient to the hospital or to be given to the GP when they arrive (see also Section 6.3c).

Summaries of the red flags of disease

The red flags of disease are summarized in a format designed for easy access in Appendix III. Throughout the text, red flags have been systematically presented according to the physiological system of the body in which the disease they indicate might have become manifest. If the red flags are to be incorporated into a structured teaching clinical medicine program, this structure enables the red flags to be taught in a systematic way.

However, in the clinic situation, symptoms do not arise in a systematic way. Rather, in the clinic the question "Is this symptom/sign serious?" is more likely to be asked than "I wonder if there are any serious symptoms arising from this patient's digestive system?" For this reason, Appendix III presents the red flags according to symptom keywords to enable easy reference in a clinical situation.

6.3b Withdrawing from conventional medication

A review of the action of drugs on the body

This first section reviews the physical and energetic effects that drugs are understood to have on the body. These effects were first described in Sections 1.2c and 1.3b.

The physical effects of drugs on the body

The range of physical effects that drugs can have on the body was introduced in Section 1.2c, and are summarized in Table 6.3b-I below.

Table 6.3b-I The categorization of drugs according to mode of action in the body

Mode of action of drug	Examples of drugs
Replaces a deficient substance that is normally obtained from the diet	Iron (ferrous sulfate) in iron-deficiency anemia
Kills or suppresses the growth of infectious agents (microbes and other life forms that cause infection)	Benzylpenicillin sodium in meningitis
Toxic to rapidly dividing human cells, in particular, cancer cells	Vincristine in cancer chemotherapy
Replaces a substance that is normally produced by the body	Insulin in diabetes mellitus
Specifically stimulates the immune response by the introduction of an antigen	Polio vaccine
Other drugs that artificially stimulate natural bodily functions	Clomifene to stimulate ovulation
Suppresses natural bodily functions	Corticosteroids used to suppress the immune response in autoimmune disease
Counteracts the damage caused by toxins	Acetylcysteine in paracetamol overdose

The energetic effects of drugs on the body

It was explained in Section 1.3b that drugs can affect the energetics of the body in one or more of the following ways: cure, suppression, drug-induced disease and placebo. Table 6.3b-II illustrates the predominant energetic effect that may be associated with therapeutic results for each of the eight categories of drugs grouped by physical action in Table 6.3b-I. Table 6.3b-II does not mention the placebo effect, as this is likely to have some positive impact to some degree in all therapeutic prescriptions.

The three energetic effects that are most relevant to the withdrawal of prescribed medication are those of cure, suppression and drug-induced disease. When a complementary medical practitioner is faced with a patient who wants to withdraw from conventional medication, it is valuable first to take some time to consider which of these three effects may be most relevant for the patient.

Table 6.3b-II Energetic interpretations of the therapeutic effects of drugs according to the modes of drug action

Mode of action of drug	Energetic interpretation
Replaces a deficient substance that is normally obtained from the diet	Usually returns the body to a state of more balance: energetic cure
	However, if given without attention to a deeper underlying cause of deficiency: suppression
Kills or suppresses the growth of infectious agents (microbes and other life forms that cause infection)	In infections that are a manifestation of strong Evil (Xie Qi) Pathogenic Factor (in Chinese medicine terms) in a healthy individual, the drug may enable full clearance of the bacteria that are causing the manifestation of the infection, and so will enable the restoration of balance as the healthy body can then easily recover naturally: energetic cure
	In infections that have occurred as a result of an underlying imbalance in the individual, the treatment does not target the root cause, and so tends to be suppressive, even with full clearance of the bacterial overgrowth: suppression
	In some cases the end result is one of Residual Pathogenic Factor, and this means that symptoms will continue to present at a deeper energetic level: suppression
Toxic to rapidly dividing human cells	These treatments always target the manifestation (a tumor) of a deep underlying imbalance: suppression
	They also are very toxic to a wide range of healthy bodily tissues and are characterized by: marked drug-induced disease

Replaces a substance that is normally produced by the body	In cases in which the body will never be able to produce the essential substance ever again: energetic cure
	In cases when the body is under-producing an essential substance as a result of an ongoing deeper disease process: suppression
Specifically stimulates the immune response by introduction of an antigen	Drug-induced disease
Other drugs that stimulate natural bodily functions	If stimulants mask the symptoms of an imbalance then this is: suppression
	When used when there is no medical disease: drug-induced disease
Suppresses natural bodily functions	The suppression of a natural bodily function is not targeting the root cause of the problem: suppression
Counteracts the damage caused by toxins	These treatments reverse the damage that would have been caused by an external toxic substance: energetic cure

Withdrawal from suppressive medication

In Section 1.3b it is proposed that suppressive drugs are those that treat the manifest symptoms of a condition without dealing with the root cause. One drug that is suppressive according to this definition is salbutamol, which, when inhaled, can be remarkably effective in relieving an asthma attack. Salbutamol is known to act by means of stimulating the cellular receptors (beta receptors) in the bronchi and bronchioles, which normally respond to the action of the hormones adrenaline and noradrenaline. By acting at a chemical level, this drug induces a bodily change, in this case, relaxation of the smooth muscle that encircles the lining of the small airways in the lungs. This is how salbutamol causes relief of symptoms. However, by suppressing asthma, the stressor that has caused the asthma attack, which may actually be a combination of diverse factors such as environmental triggers and emotional disturbance, has not been treated. With symptomatic treatment such as salbutamol, the stressor is likely to remain, and so may possibly cause more subtle or intransigent symptoms at a later date.

It makes sense, then, that when suppressive medication is withdrawn, suppressed symptoms may well return. This can occur almost immediately, as would be the experience of the asthmatic patient who becomes wheezy once they have come to the end of their supply of salbutamol. However, this return of symptoms can be delayed. For example, following the withdrawal of some treatments, such as at the conclusion of cancer treatment, the suppressed symptoms (in this case, the cancer) do not return immediately, and may even not return at all. According to the theory of suppression, this is explained by the supposition that the original imbalance is either still likely to be present, but

is now expressed in a different way in the body (such as in the form of depression), or that the imbalance has been rectified by a different means, such as modification of harmful lifestyle factors. A move towards greater balance may therefore be accompanied by a recurrence of the original symptoms at a later date. However, a subsequent move towards balance need not always result in recurrence of the original symptoms.

It is important to take note that the conventional medical view is that when a drug causes suppression of symptoms, this has no lasting deleterious effect. The idea that an imbalance can be pushed away from the surface only to emerge in a different part of the body is not consistent with the conventional medical understanding of physiology.

From an energetic perspective, replacement therapy is an unusual example of a long-term prescription drug. In the case of some forms of replacement therapy (e.g. insulin in type 1 diabetes), the patient cannot survive without the drug. Although the replacement therapy certainly suppresses symptoms, it has been argued in this text that it cannot be described as energetically suppressive. Because there is no doubt that replacement therapy always returns a patient to a more balanced state, it has to be described as curative in nature.

To summarize, withdrawal from a suppressive drug might be expected from a holistic perspective to have the following consequences: recurrence of the original symptoms either immediately or at a later date, or persistence of the original imbalance expressed in some way at a deeper level. In some cases there might be no symptoms because of total resolution of the original imbalance, but this would only be expected if the patient had been making some positive emotional and lifestyle changes while taking the drug.

Withdrawal from medication that causes drug-induced disease

Most drugs also have side effects that are unrelated to the condition that they are prescribed to treat. For example, inhaled salbutamol has a range of short-term side effects, including tremor, palpitations and tachycardia. These can be explained in terms of the action of the drug in stimulating the beta receptors in other parts of the body, including the skeletal muscles and the heart muscle. These effects would occur in asthmatics and non-asthmatics alike. They are an example of drug-induced disease, and are not manifestations of suppression. If the drug is withdrawn, it would be expected that these less beneficial manifestations of drug-induced disease would, in most cases, subside.

However, there is one particular aspect of drug-induced disease that may lead to persistent problems for the patient, and this is the development of drug dependence.

Drug dependence

It is recognized that there are some drugs that cause the body to change in such a way that the patient comes to be reliant on the presence of that drug for a balanced existence. What this means is that, if the drug is withdrawn, the patient will experience a range of symptoms that, at least temporarily, will disturb their normal ability to cope with the stresses of everyday living. This effect is known as drug dependence.

Drug dependence may manifest primarily in the physical body. For example, withdrawal from certain types of antihypertensive medication can lead to a dangerous rise in blood pressure. It is as if the body has forgotten how to control blood pressure within a relatively safe range. This type of dependence is termed physical dependence.

Other drugs seem to have effects that are more pronounced in the emotional and mental realms. For example, withdrawal from nicotine can lead to a syndrome of psychological symptoms, including cravings for nicotine, irritability, insomnia and anxiety. This aspect of dependence is termed psychological dependence.

In reality, the distinction is not that clear-cut. Withdrawal from drugs of dependence will usually lead to a constellation of physical and psychological symptoms.

Addiction

Addiction is a term that is often used interchangeably with dependence. Medically speaking, the term addiction is used more precisely to mean a state of dependence that leads to drug-seeking behavior on withdrawal of the drug. A person who is addicted to a drug may spend a significant proportion of their time and effort in ensuring that the drug is in steady supply. Drugs of addiction are those that induce a powerful state of psychological dependence.

The mechanism of drug dependence

To understand what is happening to the body in drug dependence, it is helpful to consider the chemical changes that might occur in response to a drug. Conventional pharmacology describes the response of the body to a drug in terms of adaptation. Many drugs act by mimicking the action of one or more of the natural chemicals of the body. These natural chemicals include the hormones and neurotransmitters that connect with receptor proteins on the surface of certain cells to effect a physiological change. The drug salbutamol acts in this way, as does cortisone (an artificial corticosteroid hormone).

If a drug is present in the body for some time, in many cases the body adapts to its presence by reducing the production of the natural chemical that the drug is mimicking. For example, in the case of a long-term prescription of cortisone, the adrenal cortex ceases to produce the normal amounts of natural corticosteroids. In fact, the tissue of the adrenal cortex actually becomes wasted in someone who is taking a long-term prescription of cortisone. This adaptation is potentially fatal if the artificial cortisone is withdrawn suddenly. The shrunken adrenal cortex is no longer able to respond rapidly to produce the level of corticosteroids necessary for a healthy response to stress. From an energetic perspective, this bodily change is a clear example of drug-induced disease.

Other drugs stimulate the body to counteract their effects by increasing the number of protein receptors on the cell membranes of the tissues at which the drug is acting. This means that more of the drug is required to have the same effect as time goes on. This situation, known as tolerance, is very important to understand from the perspective of drug withdrawal. If tolerance to the drug has developed, on withdrawal the normal levels of the body chemicals that act at those tissues will be insufficient to effect a healthy response. Opiates (including morphine and heroin) are drugs that are known to induce a state of tolerance. Whether used medicinally for pain relief, or illicitly for their psychological effects, increasing doses of opiates are required over time to generate the same effect. It is well recognized that opiates mimic natural body chemicals, including the endorphins. As tolerance develops, it is believed that the numbers of cellular endorphin (opiate) receptors in the body increase. On withdrawal, the body is simply unable to produce sufficient quantities of natural endorphins to stimulate the increased numbers of receptors in the body, and the complex syndrome of opiate withdrawal is experienced.

Tolerance is a particular aspect of drug dependence. Once a person has become tolerant to a drug, withdrawal is very likely to lead to unpleasant symptoms. The development of tolerance is another example of drug-induced disease.

Recovery from drug dependence

The time for recovery from the physiological imbalances induced in drug dependence depends very much on the drug concerned. For example, it is generally accepted that physical recovery in acute withdrawal from alcohol and opiates occurs in a relatively short timescale of about two weeks, whereas recovery from a long-term prescription of a minor tranquillizer such as diazepam may take many more weeks. The timescale of the prescription is another important factor to take into consideration. The longer the body has been exposed to a drug, the more it will have adapted to accommodate that drug. This is why it is safe for a patient to withdraw suddenly from a short course of corticosteroids (less than one week), but if the course has lasted for weeks to months, the withdrawal must be extremely gradual.

Social reasons for drug dependence

So far drug dependence has been described in terms of the physiological adaptation to the chemical of the drug. However, in many cases of drug dependence there are some far more complex factors in the equation. In particular, cultural and social factors play a profound role in dependence on recreational drugs. This role is, by its very nature, difficult to explore or quantify. Although a heroin addict can withdraw physically from the habit over a period of a few days, an extreme vulnerability to returning to the habit remains for much longer, and sometimes for life. This suggests that the addict is left with a lasting belief that the drug has something to offer, and particularly so in certain settings. Animal experiments have suggested that a brief exposure to certain recreational drugs can lead to a lasting state of depletion of certain neurotransmitters in the brain. This physical phenomenon might explain, at least in part, the persistent state of vulnerability experienced by some drug users following withdrawal from a drug of addiction.

Drug rehabilitation programs aim to work at reducing this vulnerability. Such programs take place in a setting that separates the former addict from the factors that might increase their tendency to return to using the drug. A rehabilitation program often begins with a short period of medical support during the time of physical withdrawal from the drug, followed by weeks to months in which the former addict is encouraged to find a way of living that avoids those triggers that might lead to a return to the habit.

Although social factors might play a less significant role in the withdrawal from most prescribed medication, it is worth considering that they may be important in some cases. The use of a prescribed drug may, in some cases, bring rewards that are additional to the relief from symptoms. The possibility of an additional, less obvious benefit resulting from a treatment in this way is conventionally referred to as secondary gain. Reinforcement in the sick role and feelings of protection are two examples of the additional rewards, or secondary gain, that a prescription might bring.

When to consider withdrawal from medications

The possible negative consequences of drug withdrawal just discussed can be seen to result from two distinct processes. The first is the recurrence of symptoms. In the case of curative treatment, the recurrence of symptoms reflects the fact that cure has not taken place and the drug has been withdrawn too early. In the case of suppressive treatment, it is suppressed symptoms that reappear. In some situations these symptoms may be tolerable and responsive to positive lifestyle change, but in others they may be so severe as to overwhelm the patient.

The second process is the appearance of new symptoms as a consequence of a particular form of drug-induced disease known as drug dependence. In this case the symptoms of drug withdrawal can be profound, and in some cases, life-threatening.

It will be clear from this summary that withdrawal from medication is a process that needs to be managed with care. There are indeed many situations in which withdrawal is a perfectly safe prospect. However, an acupuncturist needs to be familiar with those situations in which it may not be reasonable to consider withdrawal from medication at all, and with those situations in which close medical supervision would be advisable. The remainder of this section is concerned with the practicalities of recognizing those situations when it is safe to withdraw from medication and, if it is recognized to be safe, supporting a patient through the process of withdrawal.

Withdrawing from prescribed medication: a practical approach

The basic principles

When considering withdrawal from long-term medication it is important to consider some basic principles:

- If the treatment is curative in nature, do not consider withdrawal.

- Withdrawal from suppressive medication is very likely to result in recurrence of the symptoms of the original condition, unless the patient has been able to make positive changes in lifestyle or emotions.

- Long-term adaptation of the body to the drug may give rise to an unpleasant withdrawal syndrome.

- In some cases, either the recurrence of the original symptoms or the withdrawal syndrome carries serious health consequences.

- There may be other social or cultural factors in the equation that have to be considered.

Categorization of drugs for withdrawal

Bearing the above-listed principles in mind, the various types of drugs can be categorized according to the main effects that can be expected on their long-term withdrawal. The categories are:

i. The underlying condition is not serious. Recurrence of symptoms is likely; there is no withdrawal syndrome.

ii. The underlying condition is not serious. Recurrence of symptoms is likely; the withdrawal syndrome is unpleasant, but does not seriously threaten health.

iii. Withdrawal may have serious physical or mental health consequences, either because the underlying condition is serious, or because the withdrawal syndrome is dangerous.

iv. Replacement therapy. Withdrawal will result in serious ill health or even death.

This categorization of the individual classes of drugs (ordered by the chapter in which they appear in the *British National Formulary* (BNF)[66]) is given in Appendix IV. This is designed to be a reference aid for use in clinical practice.

Practical aspects of withdrawing from medication

Now that the principles that underlie an approach to drug withdrawal have been clarified, the practical aspects of helping patients to withdraw from medication can be explored.

KNOWING WHEN NOT TO WITHDRAW FROM MEDICATION

When considering withdrawal from conventional medication, a fundamental question to ask is: "How much will the patient benefit from withdrawal from medication at the current time?" It may be that the answer to this question leads the practitioner to the conclusion that this is not the time to consider such a change.

Even for category (i) medications, withdrawal will necessarily result in some physical change in the body. Symptoms of the original condition are likely to recur, and will need to be dealt with. The patient needs to be prepared for this change, and willing to make the necessary changes to their lifestyle that will prevent recurrence of the original condition. If the drug is suppressive in nature, any residual symptoms that remain before withdrawal is initiated can only be expected to worsen on withdrawal, even if only temporarily. Therefore, ideally, it needs to be clear that the patient has been making good progress on the treatment before a reduction in medication is contemplated. If not, it

may be wise to defer withdrawal until residual symptoms have subsided.

This consideration is even more important for category (ii) and (iii) drugs. Withdrawal from these medications will result in additional distressing symptoms, as well as recurrence of the original symptoms. The patient needs to be in a good state to prepare for the inevitable period of physical and emotional imbalance that will occur on withdrawal.

Withdrawal from category (iv) medication should not, in general, be contemplated. This is absolutely the case if the replacement therapy is a substance that is normally produced by an organ whose function has failed totally. An example of this is insulin replacement therapy in type 1 diabetes mellitus. In the case of patients who are taking replacement therapy to support a failing organ, there is a possibility that complementary medical treatment can enable them to reduce the dose of medication. An example of this is the prescription of thyroxine in autoimmune hypothyroidism. However, in general, in such cases it is not usually necessary to be proactive in the reduction of medication. The dose of medication is balanced against the bodily requirements as measured by medical tests. If the body no longer requires such a high dose, the tests will indicate this, and the doctor will reduce the dose accordingly.

WITHDRAWAL FROM MEDICATION: PREPARATORY STAGES

In all cases of withdrawal from medication it is important to check that the patient is clear about the reasons for withdrawal, and is keen for the process to occur. To make a good decision the patient needs to be equipped with information about the advantages and disadvantages of medication, from both an alternative and a conventional medicine point of view.

If the patient is clear about the pros and cons relating to taking medication and definitely wants to come off the medication, the next stage is to ensure that the patient has the support of their doctor in this process. Most doctors are also keen to reduce medication, and are only reluctant not to if they believe there will be a worsening in the patient's condition as a result. In many cases, it is appropriate simply for the patient to meet with their doctor to explain that they wish to cut down on their medication. Acupuncturists may also wish to give the patient a supporting letter to take to the doctor, although in most cases of withdrawal from category (i) and (ii) medication this should not be necessary.

Most doctors, if they can see that the patient's symptoms have improved and that the patient is positive about making the change, will give the patient advice about how to set about the withdrawal process. For the acupuncturist this is the ideal situation; the patient can be supported through the process by means of acupuncture treatment, but the professional responsibility for withdrawal rests with the doctor who initiated the prescription.

It is unwise to set about withdrawal from category (iii) medication without the patient having the support of their doctor. Table IV-3 in Appendix IV indicates that medical supervision is deemed to be essential for the withdrawal of all classes of drug in this category. In such cases it will be appropriate for the acupuncturist to write to the patient's doctor to demonstrate awareness of the health consequences of withdrawal, and to indicate a commitment to monitor and support the patient through the withdrawal process. Guidance on how to write a letter on this topic is given in Section 6.3c.

SPEED OF WITHDRAWAL

Some drugs can be withdrawn abruptly, as long as the patient is in robust health and is prepared for the consequences of withdrawal. Drugs that can be withdrawn abruptly are those that are given for non-serious conditions and that do not induce a state of physical or emotional dependence. A return of the original symptoms is the main problem for the patient withdrawing from drugs that fit this description. These drugs fall exclusively into categories (i) and (ii), and are indicated by a single asterisk (*) in Tables IV-1 and IV-2 in Appendix IV.

Other drugs need to be withdrawn more slowly. Slow withdrawal will allow the return of the original symptoms to be more gradual, and the symptoms of any withdrawal syndrome to appear less abruptly. Slow withdrawal is very important in situations in which the previous condition has serious emotional or physical features. In general, it is also prudent that drugs that induce a state of dependence are withdrawn gradually.

However, not all drugs that induce dependence should be withdrawn slowly. For example, current medical advice is that people who are addicted to alcohol should withdraw abruptly, and then weather the storm of the inevitable withdrawal period with the aid of alternative physical and emotional support. For some drugs that are highly addictive, gradual withdrawal is less effective than abrupt withdrawal, probably because the drug's continued presence during the withdrawal process can stimulate an easy return to the original dose.

Slow withdrawal of most of the category (i) and (ii) drugs (indicated in Tables IV-1 and IV-2 in Appendix IV by a double asterisk (**)) can take place over the course of two to four weeks. In slow withdrawal it is advisable not to cut down the dose initially by more than one-third at a time, and to reduce by less if this is possible. The next step down should be made only when the patient has adjusted to the reduced dose, and when withdrawal symptoms have abated. For those drugs indicated by a treble asterisk (***) in the tables in Appendix IV, for example, long-term hypnotics or opiates, the reduction should be even more gradual, with a longer time interval between dose reductions. Full withdrawal may require a few months in some cases.

In many cases medication is given in tablets of fixed dose at prescribed times of the day. When the dose is reduced, the frequency must not be reduced. Instead, the amount given at each time interval needs to be gradually cut down. For example, if the dose is 400mg three times daily, a possible first reduction might be to 300mg three times daily.

Sometimes gradual dose reduction is limited by a tablet of a fixed size. If lower-dose tablets are available, the doctor might be willing to prescribe these. If not, most tablets can be cut in half and then into quarters to aid the gradual reduction process. Even better is for the patient to switch to a liquid preparation of the medication so that doses can be measured using a dosing syringe. Reducing the dose can become confusing for a patient who is used to a certain routine of taking tablets, so it is good practice to prepare a written schedule for the patient, which contains clear instructions about how the dose should be reduced.

ORDER OF WITHDRAWAL OF MEDICATION

Many people are concurrently taking a number of prescribed drugs. It is always safest to focus on withdrawing only one medication at a time so that if any withdrawal symptoms appear, it is clear exactly what has caused them.

WITHDRAWAL FROM CATEGORY (I) MEDICATION

Category (i) medication is prescribed to suppress unpleasant symptoms. It does not induce a significant state of drug dependence. Table IV-1 in Appendix IV indicates that all category (i) medications can either be withdrawn abruptly (*) or gradually over a relatively short period of time (**).

When discussing the withdrawal of a category (i) medication with a patient, it is important to ascertain the previous symptoms of the underlying condition. The patient needs to be advised that the symptoms may well recur after withdrawal, and may even be more severe for some time during the withdrawal process. The return of symptoms is less likely to be as severe if the patient has been making good progress on the treatment and has attended to those lifestyle factors that have been identified as contributing to the root cause of the condition.

Drugs marked with a single asterisk (*) can be withdrawn abruptly. Drugs marked with a double asterisk (**) should be withdrawn gradually (see above, "Speed of withdrawal"). Ideally, the patient is encouraged to inform the prescribing doctor of their decision to stop taking their medication.

WITHDRAWAL FROM CATEGORY (II) MEDICATION

Withdrawal from category (ii) medication is characterized not only by a return of the symptoms of the original condition, but also by the features of a withdrawal syndrome. With drugs that induce a state of physical dependence (see Table IV-2 in Appendix IV), the withdrawal syndrome may manifest in the form of a reappearance of the original symptoms. For example, withdrawal from a stimulant laxative may result in a period of constipation, which temporarily may be even more severe than the original condition. Withdrawal from a drug that induces psychological dependence will result in the appearance of symptoms of emotional imbalance, including anxiety, irritability and sleeplessness. Cravings for the drug may be very strong.

The withdrawal of a category (ii) medication should follow the same stages as described above for category (i) medication. However, acupuncture in the withdrawal period may be needed to address the symptoms of a withdrawal syndrome. It may be helpful for the patient to have prepared in advance some strategies for coping with these additional symptoms. For example, withdrawal from a stimulant laxative may require an intermediate period of taking another form of laxative. Emotional symptoms might be countered by approaches similar to those advised for people who give up smoking. Strategies such as taking up a program of gentle exercise, planning a range of activities to distract from cravings, and use of herbal substitutes might all be considered.

WITHDRAWAL FROM CATEGORY (III) MEDICATION

Withdrawal from category (iii) medication (see Table IV-3 in Appendix IV) again follows the same principles as described for category (i) medication. However, category (iii) medication has either been prescribed for a serious medical condition or may result in a dangerous withdrawal syndrome. For these reasons withdrawal from such medications should always be undertaken with the oversight of the patient's doctor.

In some cases the doctor may be reluctant to help the patient to withdraw from the drug. If this is the case, it may help if the acupuncturist writes a letter to the doctor, giving their professional viewpoint (see Section 6.3c). If the doctor can be assured in this way that treatment has brought about a positive change in the patient's condition, and that the patient has the ongoing support of their practitioner, they may agree to start reducing the medication.

There are some drugs in this category that are unlikely to be ever withdrawn by a doctor without very marked improvement in symptoms. This is because the threat to physical and mental health from withdrawal would be considered too severe to take the risk of withdrawal. These drugs are indicated with a quadruple asterisk (****).

6.3c Communicating with conventional medical practitioners

It is good for both patient care and interprofessional relationships that acupuncturists maintain contact with the conventional medical practitioners who are involved in the ongoing healthcare of their patients. The reasons for communicating include referral of red flags of serious disease, discussions about changes in treatment and acknowledgement of referrals from conventional medical practitioners. Moreover, if the communication is made in a way that is both valid in terms of patient care and respectful of the professional to whom it is directed, it can only serve to improve the ongoing relationship between complementary and conventional medical practitioners. In this way it can promote the ideal of integrated healthcare.

Choice of method of communication

There are three methods by which an acupuncturist might choose to communicate with a conventional medical doctor about a patient. In most cases the most appropriate and convenient method is to allow the patient to do the communicating by meeting with their doctor. Alternatively, the practitioner can telephone the practice or hospital to speak to the patient's healthcare professional in person. The most formal approach is to write a letter. These three approaches are considered below in turn.

Using the patient as the communicator

The identification of a non-urgent red flag of disease is a common situation in which it might help for the acupuncture patient to communicate with their doctor. For example, an elderly patient has mentioned that they have been more thirsty than usual for the past three months, and have been passing large amounts of urine (a red flag of type 2 diabetes).

In this situation the patient can be advised to make an appointment with their doctor so that the possibility of serious disease can be excluded or confirmed. At the appointment the patient can then explain to the doctor that their acupuncturist is concerned about their symptoms and that there is, for example, a possibility of diabetes. In many such situations a letter is not necessary.

Patients may also be the communicators when they have decided they want to withdraw from category (i) or (ii) medication. A confident patient can simply go to their doctor and say, for example, "I would like to see how I cope without my beclometasone inhaler as I have no symptoms now. How do you advise that I set about stopping it?"

As long as it is clear that the patient can effectively communicate the necessary information, this is the most empowering option for them.

Speaking to the doctor in person

Speaking to the patient's doctor in person is the preferred mode of communication either if the patient needs to be referred urgently or if there is a matter of some complexity that needs to be discussed. Most doctors would be prepared to discuss a problem concerning a patient over the telephone (e.g. "Mrs Jones, who lives alone, seems to have been getting progressively more confused. Are you aware of this?"). Whenever possible, it is important to ensure that the patient is told in advance what is going to be said, to ensure that there is no breach of confidentiality.

It is normal in most medical practices that there is a system whereby doctors will take telephone consultations on request, often at a particular time of the day. Moreover, in a situation of high urgency the duty doctor may be contacted straight away. If the call is made after office hours, in the UK it will be transferred to an on-call doctor when the general practice telephone number is called. It is important to bear in mind that the doctor who is contacted may not know the patient, although in office hours they should have access to the patient's records.

Communicating by letter or email

A written communication, ideally by letter, is often an appropriate method of referring patients with complex circumstances and also of explaining clinical information about a patient in a non-urgent situation. In the UK emails are not currently favored for the purposes of relaying detailed patient information as patient confidentiality cannot be guaranteed by this route; a written letter is still preferred, and will be attached to the patient's records. A letter is not appropriate if a reply is required from the doctor, as the process of writing a reply is inconvenient for a busy doctor and delays may be incurred if the letter is typed. If a problem needs to be discussed, such as Mrs Jones' confusion in the example above, the telephone is the best medium. If a brief message needs to be relayed, or a question asked, an email might be more suitable. If this is the case, best practice is to use anonymized patient information.

A letter is most useful when it either precedes or accompanies a patient who has made an appointment with the doctor. The letter can then communicate the additional information that it may be important to impart. Letters are also an accepted means of communication for indicating that a referral from a doctor has been accepted by the acupuncturist, and also to inform the doctor about the progress of a patient who has been treated following a referral.

The structure and content of the communication

Whenever a referral is made, after first ensuring that a letter will be handled in confidence, clear and succinct information needs to be imparted to the medical practitioner. Whether by spoken word or by letter, this is best done in a structured way, and with the information offered in an order that is familiar to the doctor. If it is necessary to communicate by telephone, it is worthwhile for the acupuncturist to prepare the order of the information to be imparted before making contact. The list of the categories of information summarized below can be a useful *aide-mémoire* to ensure that no important details are omitted from a telephone call or letter. Reference to this list will also help ensure that all the necessary information is given in a logical order. General practitioners (GPs) and hospital doctors tend to be overburdened with work and constrained for time, so it is important that telephone calls and referral letters offer information in a brief and accessible format. It helps to organize the information into short statements, and to keep a letter to less than one page in length.

In the UK there is legislation designed to protect the rights of patients to confidentiality so that sensitive information about them is stored in a safe way. The Data Protection Act (DPA) 1998[67] requires a practitioner to register if they intend to keep electronic records of sensitive information about patients. This is not necessary if electronic copies of letters are deleted once the letters have been printed out, in which case paper copies can be kept securely for the patient's records. Whether or not the practitioner is required to register, according to the Act all patients have a right to have their information kept confidential and secure, and also that only the absolute minimum of detail about them is recorded, which might be considered necessary for the delivery of clinical care.

Bearing this in mind, information to include when communicating about a patient to a medical practitioner is as follows:

- **Patient identifiers:** full name, date of birth and address. All three are required for medical records.

- **Brief summary of reason for referral:** in one sentence. For example: "I'd be grateful if you could assess this 28-year-old man who tells me he has had three episodes of nocturnal bedwetting."

- **More detailed history of the main complaint:** a brief synopsis of the key events in the history of the main complaint, including:

- **Symptoms:** describe the symptoms as described by the patient.

- **Signs:** describe any findings (including relevant negative findings such as "blood pressure was normal") from clinical examination.

- **Drug history:** summarize the medication the patient is currently taking (including contraceptives and non-prescribed medication such as indigestion remedies).

- **Social history:** list any relevant lifestyle factors (e.g. smoking, alcohol use) and occupational factors that might have impacted on the current condition.

- **Summarize what is wanted of the medical practitioner:** for example: "I am concerned that this man might be experiencing nocturnal seizures, and would value your opinion on whether he needs further investigations."

- **If appropriate, take the opportunity to describe how you have been treating the patient:** a referral is a good opportunity to explain more about what acupuncture involves. It is best not to use too much Chinese medical jargon in a referral, but a couple of sentences on why the patient is having acupuncture and how they are benefiting can do no harm.

IMPORTANT ADDITIONAL POINTS THAT APPLY TO LETTERS

The important points to follow when structuring letters are:

- **Headed notepaper:** this should include the practitioner's name, professional title and qualifications, address, telephone and/or mobile phone number, email address and website address.

- **Date:** the date of the letter is essential.

Box 6.3c-I is a simple guide to the basic information required in a professionally headed letter.

Box 6.3c-I A guide to the basic information required on a professionally headed letter

Dr George Jackson
The Springs Surgery
Reading RG2 3DD

Jane Goodson RGN LicAc MBAcC
Traditional Chinese Medicine
The Willows Clinic
Reading RG1 1OU
Tel: 01189 222222, Fax: 01189 222223
jgoodson@acupuncture.com

12 April 2017

Dear Dr Jackson

Re: [Include all patient identifiers here (i.e. name, address and date of birth)]

Contents of letter ....

....

Yours sincerely,
Jane Goodson

Choice of language

It will help with all communications if the practitioner aims to match the medical use of professional language as much as possible, and avoid using Chinese medical terminology, which may be misinterpreted or dismissed as meaningless.

Confidentiality

Although letters between conventional health professionals are often written and sent without the express permission of the patient, it is advisable whenever possible to ensure that the patient is happy for their acupuncturist to be writing to another professional about them, even if they have been referred to the acupuncturist by that professional. A helpful hint is to always write a letter that health professionals would be prepared for the patient to read. There should be very few situations in which health professionals wish to give information to the doctor without the patient knowing about it.

Sample letter formats

Boxes 6.3c-II to 6.3c-V give sample letter formats as a guide for letter design.

Box 6.3c-II Acceptance of a referral: sample letter

Dear Dr Jackson

Thank you for referring John Smith for treatment of recurrent migraine. I saw him in my clinic today.

History
Recurrent unilateral headaches felt over the left eye and temple that are associated with blurred vision and nausea.

Headaches worse at weekends.

Frequency of headaches increasing over the last six weeks associated with stress at work. He currently suffers a headache most weekends.

Alcohol: at least 40 units/week (wine).

Smoking: non-smoker.

Examination
Overweight (BMI 35).

Full red complexion.

BP 140/100.

Medication
Propranolol 80mg daily.

Sumatriptan and paracetamol during acute attacks.

Diagnosis
My diagnosis, based on his history, physical examination and pulse and tongue examination, is that he has features of a syndrome recognized in Traditional Chinese Medicine that is likely to respond to acupuncture treatments and also modifications to his diet and stressful lifestyle. The raised blood pressure is consistent with this diagnosis.

Treatment plan
Eight acupuncture treatments at weekly intervals.

I have advised him to reduce alcohol, and also the fatty and spicy food in his diet. He is also likely to benefit from gentle exercise and a less stressful approach to his working day.

I would hope that with treatment he may be able to reduce his need for propranolol, which makes him feel drowsy in the day, and he may discuss this with you in due course, assuming he makes good progress.

Yours sincerely,
Jane Goodson

Acceptance of referrals from medical practitioners

It is good practice to acknowledge a formally referred patient by sending a letter to the referring doctor after the first consultation (see Box 6.3c-II). In this letter it is good practice to thank the referring practitioner for the referral, and then to summarize the diagnosis and treatment plan.

After the last consultation, a letter can be sent in which the patient's response to treatment is summarized in terms of reduced symptoms and improvement in daily activities (see Box 6.3c-III).

Box 6.3c-III Discharge summary: sample letter

Dear Dr Jackson

Thank you for referring John Smith for treatment of irritable bowel syndrome. This was causing debilitating attacks of pain and diarrhea on a daily basis.

I have now seen him for the last of six fortnightly appointments.

Diagnosis
Constitutional weakness of his digestion, which is further weakened by certain dietary components such as raw foods, fatty foods and dairy products.

Ongoing stress from problems in current relationship also a contributory factor.

Treatment plan
Acupuncture to strengthen the constitutional weakness, with points to reduce the tension that he is experiencing.

Reduction of dairy products and raw foods in his diet.

Outcome
By the third treatment, the frequency and severity of attacks was reducing.

Currently he only gets mild attacks at less than weekly intervals.

Feels more able to confront the issues in his relationship, and feels less frustrated.

Future treatment
In view of his excellent response, regular but infrequent treatments could be sufficient to keep his symptoms under control. John knows to contact me should he require further treatment.

Yours sincerely,
Jane Goodson

Referring patients to medical practitioners

A standard format is advised for the referral of patients who merit the opinion of or treatment from a conventional practitioner (see Box 6.3c-IV). In such a letter it is important to clearly describe the red flags that are of concern. A medical diagnosis is not required in such a letter, as the red flags will usually speak for themselves.

In urgent situations a handwritten letter is perfectly acceptable. Handwritten letters should be structured in exactly the same way as typed letters.

Box 6.3c-IV Referral letter: sample letter

Dear Dr Jackson

I would be grateful if you could see John Smith with regard to unexplained back pain and weight loss.

I am treating him with acupuncture, but in view of his symptoms, I believe he needs further investigations.

History
Two years of increasing low back pain, which first came on while digging.

In recent months pain has been constant, and not responsive to simple painkillers.

Five weeks ago he booked an appointment with me for pain relief.

Loss of 3kg over the past year.

Poor appetite.

Night sweats and exhaustion over the past three months.

Examination
Pale, thin, general muscle wasting.

Abdominal exam: no obvious organ enlargement.

Very tender over the body of L3 vertebra with associated muscle spasm.

Medication
Co-codamol 1–2 tablets up to four times a day.

Treatment plan
I intend to see Mr Smith on a weekly basis. My treatments will involve gentle stimulation of general acupuncture points, and the use of points local to L3 to minimize pain.

This treatment would be entirely complementary to any treatment you may decide that he requires.

Many thanks for your help.

Yours sincerely,
Jane Goodson

Communicating about shared management of patients

An acupuncturist is not obliged to inform a patient's doctor of their treatment. However, to do so appropriately is likely to promote good relationships between the professions in general. It is reasonable that the more that acupuncture treatment impinges on a disease that is also being managed by a doctor, the more appropriate it would be to communicate about the treatment and its progress. There is less need for a structured letter in this situation (see Box 6.3c-V).

Box 6.3c-V Letter communicating about shared management of patients

Dear Dr Jackson

I have been treating John Smith with acupuncture for the past year. Over this time the treatment has been focused on managing his problems of long-standing anxiety and depression. He has made considerable progress, and is now expressing a desire to reduce, and eventually stop, his regular dose of sertraline 100mg daily that he has been taking for five years.

It is my opinion that, since commencing treatment, his mood has progressively become more stable and his anxiety is far less restrictive to his daily activities. He can now go shopping alone in town without a feeling of panic, for example. He now has no unbroken nights of sleep.

Continued acupuncture treatment is therefore likely to support him through a period of gradual withdrawal from sertraline. John is aware that the withdrawal process may have to be over the course of a few months. Throughout this time I will be seeing him regularly to monitor whether there is recurrence of his old symptoms.

I have asked him to make an appointment to discuss this with you, and if possible to plan with you how he can start gradually to reduce his dosage.

Yours sincerely,
Jane Goodson

6.3d Ethical issues

This final section is concerned with some of the broader issues that specifically relate to the situation of an acupuncturist who is offering therapy to a patient who is concurrently undergoing treatment from a conventional medical practitioner.

The section begins by considering two general principles to which it would be prudent for all practitioners to adhere. These are being attentive to keeping clear, contemporaneous records, and being prepared to seek professional advice in any situation in which there is ethical uncertainty.

To conclude the section, three broad areas in which ethical dilemmas are common are explored. These are maintaining good interprofessional relationships, advising patients on their medical treatments, and maintaining confidentiality.

General points

The importance of clear records

It is a cardinal rule that should an ethical dilemma arise in practice, clear documentation of all relevant issues is made at the time in the case notes. In particular, details should be recorded concerning the treatment and its rationale, any advice given, what has been discussed with the patient and the date. A practitioner's records are always used in an investigation of possible professional misconduct. If the records can demonstrate that the practitioner was following good practice as defined by their professional body in their dealings with a patient, the practitioner is unlikely to be disciplined.

For example, it would be advisable to keep clear records of any discussion that relates to withdrawal from conventional medication, such as tranquillizers. A practitioner should ensure that a clear record was made of the fact they had clearly discussed the pros and cons of withdrawing from tranquillizers with a patient. In particular, they could clarify that they described the possible consequences of a severe withdrawal syndrome and suggested that the patient discuss withdrawal from the medication with the prescribing doctor. If the patient later makes an official complaint that they did suffer from severe symptoms "as a result of advice given by their therapist," the fact that a discussion about possible complications was clearly recorded at the time will stand in the practitioner's favor (should the complaint come before an investigating committee).

For records to be seen to be reliable and contemporaneous, it is essential that practitioners never make alterations to clinical records at a later date, even if what is written down is accurate. If it is necessary to add extra information to earlier records, the additional notes need to be dated and signed. Altered records that are not dated as such will be seen as potentially falsified by an investigating committee. It is important to note that even tidying records, by reproducing in better writing an exact copy of original records, is enough to cast doubt on their authenticity.

If in doubt, seek advice

If a practitioner has any uncertainties about a particular case in practice, or if a complaint has been made about an aspect of treatment, it is wise for them to consult either the professional conduct officer of their professional body or their insurer before taking further action.

Areas in which ethical dilemmas are common

Maintaining good relationships with professional colleagues

It is an ethical responsibility for all health practitioners to ensure that they act in the best interests of their patient at all times, and this requires an acupuncturist to ensure that, whenever possible, their care is truly complementary to any medical treatment that is being offered concurrently. However, situations may arise in which the conventional medical advice patients may have been given conflicts in some way with Chinese medical wisdom.

In this situation, any therapeutic advice offered to the patient must be given to the patient with great care so that it is not understood to denigrate the professional standing of the doctor who might have given conflicting medical advice. This means that every effort should be made to ensure that the advice and treatment that is offered is based on unbiased research of the topic in question. If any advice or comment is offered about conventional medical treatment, it is the ethical duty of the practitioner to ensure that they are very knowledgeable about that treatment.

Moreover, advice given about acupuncture treatment should ideally be consistent with the views of the professional body to which the practitioner belongs, and if it is not, the practitioner should make this fact clear to the patient.

It is also important to bear in mind that whatever a patient says about their doctor is a personal view, and is not necessarily representative of what actually happened in a consultation. Therefore, it is wise for an acupuncturist not to collude with the patient and criticize a medical practitioner solely on the basis of what the patient alone has told them.

If an acupuncturist has serious concerns about what has been learned from the patient about the professional conduct of a medical practitioner, it is wise first to discuss this situation in confidence with the professional conduct officer of their professional body. If, following this discussion, it is agreed that a complaint is merited, this should be directed to the complaints manager of the employer of the practitioner, such as the practice manager at a general practice, the local primary healthcare trust complaints officer, or the registering body of the practitioner (e.g. the General Medical Council is the registering body for doctors in the UK[68]).

Helping a patient to reduce or change medical treatment

It is important for an acupuncturist to bear in mind when discussing with a patient the topic of withdrawal from conventional medication that this could be construed as undermining the considered opinion of another professional. It is wise to make efforts to ensure that this is not what either the patient or the prescribing doctor perceives. In most cases it is likely that the patient will be supported by their doctor in their desire to reduce medication.

If a patient requests support in making a change in medication that is against the advice of their medical doctor, it is prudent to ensure that the patient fully understands the risks and benefits of this choice, and that what has been explained to them about such risks and benefits is clearly documented.

To give balanced advice in this situation, it is essential that the practitioner has access to clear and up-to-date information on the risks and benefits of withdrawal from the treatment from a conventional perspective. If possible, the advice of another conventionally trained professional should be sought, and ideally this should be the prescribing doctor.

Maintaining confidentiality

All healthcare practitioners have a duty to keep all information concerning their patients, medical or otherwise, entirely confidential.[69] Such information should be released only with the explicit consent of the patient. This also applies to any views formed about the patient during consultations. To this end, when communicating with a doctor about a shared patient, it is advisable for practitioners to inform the patient in advance about the content of the letter or conversation, to ensure that they have given full consent to the information to be disclosed.

However, there are times when patient confidentiality needs to be breached. This should only be done when the practitioner is convinced it is in the best interests of the patient or of society at large. For example, there might be genuine concern that an elderly person is becoming too confused to look after themselves, whereas the patient insists they are managing perfectly well. In this instance it could be appropriate to make a telephone call to the patient's doctor to check that the practice is aware of the home situation of the elderly person, but ideally the prior consent of the patient is sought for this communication to take place.

If it is decided that it is in the best interests of the patient or the wider community to disclose information about a patient against their will, clear records should be made of how that decision was made. If a practitioner has any uncertainties about whether or not to disclose confidential information, it is advisable to discuss the situation first, in confidence, with their professional body. It must be emphasized that disclosure without consent is a very serious matter, and unless there is a serious risk of injury or harm to the public it can be very difficult to justify. For example, even suicide threats are not usually thought to be a serious enough reason to disclose unless the means suggested may impinge on other people (e.g. driving a car recklessly or jumping off a shopping center roof). Therefore, if there is any uncertainty about whether disclosure would be appropriate, it is advisable for the practitioner to consult in confidence with the professional conduct officer of their professional body.

Notes

1 Waugh, A. and Grant, A. (2014) *Ross and Wilson: Anatomy and Physiology in Health and Illness.* Twelfth Edition. Edinburgh: Elsevier, Chapter 14.

2 Waugh, A. and Grant, A. (2014) *Ross and Wilson: Anatomy and Physiology in Health and Illness.* Twelfth Edition. Edinburgh: Elsevier, Chapter 8.

3 Maciocia, G. (1989) *The Foundations of Chinese Medicine.* Edinburgh: Churchill Livingstone, p.80.

4 Waugh, A. and Grant, A. (2014) *Ross and Wilson: Anatomy and Physiology in Health and Illness.* Twelfth Edition. Edinburgh: Elsevier, Chapter 8.

5 Maciocia, G. (1989) *The Foundations of Chinese Medicine.* Edinburgh: Churchill Livingstone, p.97.

6 Acupuncture Safety Resource (2016) 'Basic safety principles.' Available at www.acupuncturesafety.org.uk/basic-safety-principles.html, accessed on 18 August 2016.

7 British Acupuncture Council (2016) *The Code of Safe Practice for Acupuncture.* Available at www.acupuncture.org.uk/index.php?option=com_k2&Itemid=40&id =1598_102ebd3b5289c5ec2ffb970d1def471f&lang=en&task=download&view=item, accessed on 10 February 2017.

8 Soll, D., Galask, R., Schmid, J., Hanna, C., Mac, K. and Morrow, B. (1991) 'Genetic dissimilarity of commensal strains of *Candida* spp. carried in different anatomical locations of the same healthy women.' *Journal of Clinical Microbiology 29*(8), 1702–1710. Available at www.ncbi.nlm.nih.gov/pubmed/1761692, accessed on 18 August 2016.

9 Fitz-Gibbon, S. *et al.* (2013) '*Propionibacterium acnes* strain populations in the human skin microbiome associated with acne.' *The Journal of Investigative Dermatology 133*(9), 2152–2160. Available at http://genome.wustl.edu/publications/detail/propionibacterium-acnes-strain-populations-in-the-human-skin-microbiome-associated-with-acne, accessed on 18 August 2016.

10 Flaws, B. and Sionneau, P. (2010) *The Treatment of Modern Western Diseases with Chinese Medicine.* Boulder, CO: Blue Poppy Press, Chapter 1.

11 Maciocia, G. (2004) *Diagnosis in Chinese Medicine: A Comprehensive Guide.* Edinburgh: Churchill Livingstone, Chapter 77.

12 Maciocia, G. (2004) *Diagnosis in Chinese Medicine: A Comprehensive Guide.* Edinburgh: Churchill Livingstone, Chapter 77.

13 Flaws, B. and Sionneau, P. (2010) *The Treatment of Modern Western Diseases with Chinese Medicine.* Boulder, CO: Blue Poppy Press, Chapter 68.

14 Flaws, B. and Sionneau, P. (2010) *The Treatment of Modern Western Diseases with Chinese Medicine.* Boulder, CO: Blue Poppy Press, Chapter 58.

15 Flaws, B. and Sionneau, P. (2010) *The Treatment of Modern Western Diseases with Chinese Medicine.* Boulder, CO: Blue Poppy Press, Chapter 64.

16 Dharmananda, S. (1999) 'Treatment of alopecia with Chinese herbs.' Available at www.itmonline.org/arts/alopecia.htm, accessed on 20 August 2016.

17 Wiseman, N. and Ye, F. (1999) *A Practical Dictionary of Chinese Medicine.* Brookline, MA: Paradigm, p.463.

18 Hammond, C. (2014) 'Do glasses weaken your eyesight?' Available at www.bbc.com/future/story/20140513-do-glasses-weaken-your-eyesight, accessed on 21 August 2016.

19 Bates Eye Exercises (2010) 'The Bates method.' Available at www.bateseyeexercises.com/bates_method.php, accessed on 21 August 2016.

20 Abelson, M. (2012) 'Of biomes, biofilm and the ocular surface.' *Review of Ophthalmology,* September. Available at www.reviewofophthalmology.com/article/of-biomes-biofilm-and-the-ocular-surface, accessed on 20 August 2016.

21 Dharmananda, S. (2004) 'Cataracts: Prevention and treatment with reference to Chinese medicine.' Available at www.itmonline.org/arts/cataracts.htm, accessed on 20 August 2016.

22 Maciocia, G. (1989) *The Practice of Chinese Medicine.* Edinburgh: Churchill Livingstone, Chapter 29.

23 James, N. (1994) 'A Historical Context.' In S. Bloch and B. Singh, *Foundations of Clinical Psychiatry.* Melbourne, VIC: Melbourne University Press, Chapter 1.

24 APA (American Psychiatric Association) (2013) *Diagnostic and Statistical Manual of Mental Disorders.* Fifth Edition. Washington, DC: APA.

25 Weir, K. (2012) *The Roots of Mental Illness: How Much of Mental Illness Can the Biology of the Brain Explain?* Washington, DC: American Psychological Association. Available at www.apa.org/monitor/2012/06/roots.aspx, accessed on 21 August 2016.

26 McLeod, S. (2007) 'Bowlby's attachment theory.' Available at www.simplypsychology.org/bowlby.html, accessed on 21 August 2016.

27 McLeod, S. (2013) 'Sigmund Freud.' Available at www.simplypsychology.org/Sigmund-Freud.html, accessed on 21 August 2016.

28 Royal College of Psychiatrists' Public Education Editorial Board (2013) 'Depression and men.' Available at www.rcpsych.ac.uk/healthadvice/problemsdisorders/depressionmen.aspx, accessed on 20 August 2016.

29 Flaws, B. and Lake, J. (2001) *Chinese Medical Psychiatry: A Textbook and Clinical Manual.* Boulder, CO: Blue Poppy Press, Book 1, Chapter 2.

30 Maciocia, G. (1989) *The Foundations of Chinese Medicine.* Edinburgh: Churchill Livingstone, Chapters 6–10.

31 Quoted in Bloch, S. and Singh, B. (1994) *Foundations of Clinical Psychiatry.* Melbourne, Australia: Melbourne University Press, Chapter 4.

32 WHO (World Health Organization) (1993) *ICD-10 Classification of Mental Health Disorders. Diagnostic Criteria for Research.* Available at www.who.int/classifications/icd/en/GRNBOOK.pdf, accessed on 24 August 2016.

33 APA (American Psychiatric Association) (2013) *Diagnostic and Statistical Manual of Mental Disorders.* Fifth Edition. Washington, DC: American Psychiatric Association.

34 APA (American Psychiatric Association) (2013) 'Frequently asked questions.' Available at www.dsm5.org/about/Pages/faq.aspx, accessed on 24 August 2016.

35 APA (American Psychiatric Association) (2016) *DSM-5 Resources: DSM-5 Contents.* Available at https://www.psychiatry.org/File%20Library/.../DSM/APA_DSM-5-Contents.pdf, accessed on 10 February 2017.

36 Pickersgill, M. (2014) 'Debating DSM 5: Diagnosis and the sociology of critique.' *Journal of Medical Ethics 40*, 521–525.

37 Hafal (2008) *Changes to Mental Health Legislation: A Brief Guide for Mental Health Service Users and Their Families.* Available at www.hafal.org/pdf/publications/Changes_to_Mental_Health_Legislation.pdf, accessed on 24 August 2016.

38 CSM (Committee on Safety of Medicines) (1988) 'Benzodiazepines, dependence and withdrawal symptoms.' *Current Problems*, No. 21, January.

39 Flaws, B. and Lake, J. (2001) *Chinese Medical Psychiatry: A Textbook and Clinical Manual.* Boulder, CO: Blue Poppy Press, Book 1, Chapter 2.

40 Rosenberg, Z. (2000) 'A Chinese look at Western pharmaceuticals.' Available at www.acupuncture.com/herbs/pharma.htm, accessed on 24 August 2016.

41 Greenwood, M.T. (2007) 'Drugs and acupuncture: The energetic impact of antihypertensives.' Available at www.paradoxpublishing.com/assets/files/publications/articles/aama/vol-19-antihypertensives.pdf, accessed on 27 February 2016.

42 NICE (National Institute for Health and Care Excellence) (2014) *Psychosis and Schizophrenia in Adults: Prevention and Management.* Clinical Guideline CG178. Available at www.nice.org.uk/guidance/cg178, accessed on 24 August 2016.

43 University of Maryland Medical Center (2016) *Complementary and Alternative Medicine Guide.* Available at http://umm.edu/health/medical/altmed, accessed on 24 August 2016.

44 Rosenberg, Z. (2000) 'A Chinese look at Western pharmaceuticals.' Available at www.acupuncture.com/herbs/pharma.htm, accessed on 24 August 2016; Flaws, B. and Lake, J. (2001) *Chinese Medical Psychiatry: A Textbook and Clinical Manual.* Boulder, CO: Blue Poppy Press, Book 1, Chapter 2; Greenwood, M.T. (2004) 'Drugs and acupuncture: The energetic impact of antidepressant medication.' Available at www.paradoxpublishing.com/assets/files/publications/articles/aama/vol-21-1-drugs-and-acupuncture.pdf, accessed on 24 August 2016.

45 Royal College of Psychiatrists (2015) 'Information about ECT.' Available at www.rcpsych.ac.uk/healthadvice/treatmentswellbeing/ect.aspx, accessed on 24 August 2016.

46 Greenwood, M.T. (2004) 'Drugs and acupuncture: The energetic impact of antidepressant medication.' Available at www.paradoxpublishing.com/assets/files/publications/articles/aama/vol-21-1-drugs-and-acupuncture.pdf, accessed on 24 August 2016.

47 Hafal (2008) *Changes to Mental Health Legislation: A Brief Guide for Mental Health Service Users and Their Families.* Available at www.hafal.org/pdf/publications/Changes_to_Mental_Health_Legislation.pdf, accessed on 24 August 2016.

48 Flaws, B. and Lake, J. (2001) *Chinese Medical Psychiatry: A Textbook and Clinical Manual.* Boulder, CO: Blue Poppy Press, Book 2, Chapters 4 and 6.

49 Flaws, B. and Lake, J. (2001) *Chinese Medical Psychiatry: A Textbook and Clinical Manual.* Boulder, CO: Blue Poppy Press, Book 2, Chapter 20.

50 Harding, M. (2014) 'Suicide risk assessment and threats of suicide.' Available at http://patient.info/doctor/suicide-risk-assessment-and-threats-of-suicide, accessed on 25 August 2016.

51 Mental Health Law Online (2015) 'Additional safeguards for ECT introduced in new S58A.' Available at www.mentalhealthlaw.co.uk/Additional_safeguards_for_ECT_introduced_in_new_s58A, accessed on 24 August 2016.

52 Kübler-Ross, E. (2014) *On Death and Dying: What the Dying Have to Teach Doctors, Clergy and Their Own Families.* New York: Scribner.

53 Zisook, S. and Shear, K. (2009) 'Grief and bereavement: What psychiatrists need to know.' *World Psychiatry 8*(2), 67–74. Available at www.ncbi.nlm.nih.gov/pmc/articles/PMC2691160, accessed on 24 August 2016.

54 Pies, R. (2014) 'The bereavement exclusion and DSM 5: An update and commentary.' *Innovations in Clinical Neuroscience 11*(7–8), 19–22. Available at www.ncbi.nlm.nih.gov/pmc/articles/PMC4204469, accessed on 24 August 2016.

55 Cruse Bereavement Care (2016) 'Home page.' Available at www.cruse.org.uk, accessed on 24 August 2016.

56 Flaws, B. and Lake, J. (2001) *Chinese Medical Psychiatry: A Textbook and Clinical Manual.* Boulder, CO: Blue Poppy Press, Book 3, Chapter 4.

57 Greenwood, M.T. (2004) 'Drugs and acupuncture: The energetic impact of antidepressant medication.' Available at www.paradoxpublishing.com/assets/files/publications/articles/aama/vol-21-1-drugs-and-acupuncture.pdf, accessed on 24 August 2016.

58 Stone, J., Smyth, R., Carson, A., Winlow, C. and Sharpe, M. (2006) '*La belle indifférence* in conversion symptoms and hysteria.' *The British Journal of Psychiatry 188*(3), 204–209. Available at http://bjp.rcpsych.org/content/188/3/204, accessed on 24 August 2016.

59 Moscrop, A. (2011) '"Heartsink" patients in general practice. A defining paper: Its impact and psychodynamic potential.' *The British Journal of General Practice 61*(586), 346–348. Available at www.ncbi.nlm.nih.gov/pmc/articles/PMC3080217, accessed on 24 August 2016.

60 Harding, M. (2015) 'Anorexia nervosa.' Available at http://patient.info/doctor/anorexia-nervosa-pro, accessed on 25 August 2016.

61 Cooper, B. (2005) 'Immigration and schizophrenia: The social causation hypothesis revisited.' *The British Journal of Psychiatry 186*(5), 361–363. Available at http://bjp.rcpsych.org/content/186/5/361, accessed on 24 August 2016.

62 NICE (National Institute for Health and Care Excellence) (2014) *Psychosis and Schizophrenia in Adults: Prevention and Management.* Clinical Guideline CG178. Available at www.nice.org.uk/guidance/cg178, accessed on 24 August 2016.

63 Flaws, B. and Lake, J. (2001) *Chinese Medical Psychiatry: A Textbook and Clinical Manual.* Boulder, CO: Blue Poppy Press, Book 3, Chapters 3 and 6.

64 Lipman, V. (2013) 'The disturbing link between psychopathy and leadership.' Available at www.forbes.com/sites/victorlipman/2013/04/25/the-disturbing-link-between-psychopathy-and-leadership/#57f0feed2740, accessed on 4 January 2017.

65 Scott, J. and Barlow, T. (1999) *Acupuncture in the Treatment of Children.* Seattle, WA: Eastland Press, Chapter 32.

66 British Medical Association and Royal Pharmaceutical Society (2016) *British National Formulary 71.* London: BMJ Group and Pharmaceutical Press.

67 ICO (Information Commissioner's Office) (2016) 'Register (notify) under the Data Protection Act.' Available at https://ico.org.uk/for-organisations/register, accessed on 25 August 2016.

68 General Medical Council (2016) 'Making a complaint about a doctor.' Available at www.gmc-uk.org/concerns/23339.asp, accessed on 25 August 2016.

69 CNHC (Complementary and Natural Healthcare Council) (2014) *Code of Conduct, Ethics and Performance.* Available at www.cnhc.org.uk/assets/pdf/1-033.pdf, accessed on 24 August 2016.

The Functions of the Organs: Correspondence Tables

The process of mapping the function of the conventionally recognized organs with their Chinese medical namesakes was introduced in Chapter 1.1. The tables in this appendix systematically summarize and compare the functions of some of the important organs as understood from both a conventional and a Chinese medicine perspective.

For clarity, the names of the physiological organs are written with a lower case initial letter. The names of the Organs of Chinese medicine, which are really constellations of functions rather than physical entities, are written with an upper case initial letter.

The tables have been drawn up by means of a very simple process. First, for each of a number of the important organs (as listed below), the functions as recognized by each of the two medical disciplines, conventional and Chinese, have been listed in a table of two columns for ease of comparison. The descriptions of functions of the Chinese organs are taken from the summaries made by Maciocia (1989),[1] who drew his descriptions from ancient Chinese texts including *The Yellow Emperor's Classic of Chinese Medicine* (Huang Ti Nei Jing Su Wen) and the *Spiritual Axis* (Ling Shu Jing).

Tabulating these functions alongside each other demonstrates the simple fact that they do not map to each other directly. For example, the conventionally recognized function of the spleen as being the site for the maturation of the white blood cells does not seem to correspond to any of the functions of the Organ named in Chinese medicine as the Spleen.

Then, for each of the functions listed in the tables, the following question has been asked: "To which organ in the contrasting medical viewpoint does this function most closely correspond?" For example, to what Organs in Chinese medicine does the known function of the spleen, the maturation of white blood cells, most closely correspond? As maturation of the white blood cells is important for a healthy immune system, and thus for the ability of the body to heal and also for the fighting of infection, this function would first seem to correspond more closely to the Kidney and Lung, in that these Organs are related in Chinese medicine to the ability of the body to withstand what would be conventionally described as infectious disease.

However, when considering the role of the immune system in the ability of the flesh to heal, this aspect would seem more closely associated with the role of the Spleen Organ. Therefore, the single function of the spleen of being the site for the maturation of white blood cells could reasonably be mapped to the Kidney, Lung and Spleen Organs in Chinese medicine. It is by asking this question of each of the functions in the tables that corresponding organs have been suggested. These are written in bold type after the description of each of the functions in the tables.

How can the tables be used in practice?

The tables can be used when considering the possible Chinese energetic consequences of a Western diagnosis. For instance, if a disease involves impaired kidney function, a quick glance at the Kidney table will give the information that disease of the kidney organ might manifest in a range of imbalances that could be attributed to a number of Chinese Organs (namely, the Kidney, Bladder, Heart, Triple Burner, Spleen and Small Intestine Organs). This process cannot, of course, replace a full diagnosis of patients in the clinic situation, but can help to make sense of the possible diagnoses that may be arrived at when treating patients with complex diseases.

The organs that are considered in the tables are presented in alphabetical order.

The functions of the organs: **The Bladder**

Functions of the bladder	Functions of the Bladder Organ
Receives urine from the kidneys via the ureters (**Bladder; receives dirty fluids from the Small Intestine Organ**)	"The bladder is like a district official: it stores the fluids so that they can be excreted by the action of Qi transformation"
Does not discharge urine until the volume of urine exceeds a certain amount (under voluntary control) (**Bladder, Triple Burner Organ**)	It removes water by means of Qi transformation (**kidney, ureters, bladder urethra**)
Discharges urine via the urethra by means of a coordinated contraction of its muscular wall (**Bladder, Triple Burner Organ, Liver**)	

The functions of the organs: **The Gallbladder**

Functions of the gallbladder	Functions of the Gallbladder Organ
Stores bile until it is appropriate for it to be released into the duodenum (upper small intestine) and thus aids in the digestion of fats (**Gallbladder, Small Intestine, Spleen and Liver Organs**)	"The Gallbladder is the upright official which takes decisions"
Bile contains waste products for excretion via the digestive system (**Small and Large Intestine Organs**)	It stores and excretes bile (**liver and gallbladder**)
	It controls judgment (**the brain**)
	It controls the sinews (and ensures proper movement and agility) (**muscles, tendons, ligaments and the nervous system**)

The functions of the organs: **The Heart**

Functions of the heart	Functions of the Heart Organ
Acts as a pulsatile pump to enable circulation of the blood (**Heart and Liver Organs**)	"The Heart is like the monarch and it governs the mind"
The origin of the heart muscle impulse (the pacemaker) (**Heart Organ**)	It governs blood (**bone marrow, heart, blood vessels**)
Contributes to the maintenance of blood pressure (**Heart Organ and Kidney Yang**)	It controls the blood vessels (**blood vessels, adrenal glands, autonomic nervous system**)
Will respond to bodily requirements by an alteration in strength and rate of pumping (**Heart Organ and Kidney Yang**)	It manifests in the complexion (**heart, blood vessels, blood, skin**)
Can lead to urination if the heart muscle becomes under strain by means of a release of a hormone from the atria which affects the kidneys (**Kidney Yang**)	It houses the mind (**brain**)
	It opens into the tongue (**digestive system**)
	It controls sweat (**skin, autonomic nervous system**)

The functions of the organs: **The Kidney**

Functions of the kidney	Functions of the Kidney Organ
Excretes waste products from the blood and forms urine (**Small Intestine, Kidney, Bladder and Triple Burner Organs**)	"The Kidneys are responsible for the creation of power. Skill and ability stem from them"
Maintains the balance of salts, water and acidity in the blood (**Kidney, Spleen and Triple Burner Organs**)	They store Essence and govern growth, reproduction and development (**constitutional strength, endocrine system and reproductive system**)
Aids in the maintenance of blood pressure by the secretion of renin (**Kidney and Spleen Organs**)	They produce Marrow, fill up the brain and control bones (**brain, spinal cord, bone marrow, skeleton, teeth and kidneys**)
Stimulates the increased production of red blood cells by the release of erythropoietin (**Heart and Kidney Organs**)	They govern water (**lungs, small and large intestines, kidneys, ureters, bladder and urethra**)
Converts vitamin D in the skin to its active form (**Kidney Organ**)	They control the reception of Qi (**inspiratory action of the lungs, adrenal gland, autonomic nervous system**)
	They open into the ears (**ears, acoustic nerve, brain**)
	They manifest in the hair (**the skin and hair follicles**)
	They control the two lower orifices (**urethra, genitalia, large intestine and anus**)
	They house willpower (**brain**)

The functions of the organs: **The Large Intestine**

Functions of the large intestine	Functions of the Large Intestine Organ
Receives the waste products of digestion from the small intestine and absorbs the bulk of the water from this residue (**Small Intestine and Large Intestine Organs**)	"The Large Intestine is the official responsible for transit. The residue of transformation stems from it"
Continues with the function of the small intestine by the absorption of a few nutrients (**Spleen and Small Intestine Organs**)	It receives transformed food and drink from the small intestine (**large intestine**)
Stores the final residue in the form of feces until the appropriate time for expulsion (**Large Intestine Organ**)	It absorbs the remaining food (**large intestine**)
Houses a large population of yeasts and microorganisms that are the source of vitamins and help to protect against disease (**Spleen, Small Intestine, Lung and Kidney Organs**)	It excretes dirty waste (**large intestine**)
Is the site of a local immune system for the protection against unwanted microorganisms and toxins (includes the lymphoid tissue of the appendix) (**Lung, Kidney Organs**)	

773

The functions of the organs: **The Liver**

Functions of the liver

Has an important role in the regulation of blood glucose (**Spleen, Small Intestine, Liver and Triple Burner Organs**)

Has an important role in the metabolism of fats and protein (**Spleen and Small Intestine Organs**)

Aids in the breakdown of aging blood cells (complementary function to the spleen) (**Heart, Liver and Spleen Organs**)

Cleanses the blood of toxins and foreign organisms originating from the digestive blood flow (**Small Intestine, Large Intestine, Kidney and Bladder Organs**)

Is the main heat-producing organ (**Gate of Vitality (Ming Men) and the Triple Burner Organ**)

It synthesizes vitamin A that benefits skin and eyes (**Lung and Liver Organs**)

It secretes bile and so aids in the digestion of fats (**Gallbladder, Spleen, Small Intestine and Liver Organs**)

It stores some vitamins (vitamins A, D, E and K, riboflavin, pyridoxine, folic acid and B12), iron and copper (**Stomach Spleen and Liver Organs**)

It carries a large volume of blood at any one time, particularly when the body is at rest (**Heart, Liver, Spleen and Kidney Organs**)

Functions of the Liver Organ

"The Liver is like an army general from whom the strategy is derived"

It stores Blood (and regulates blood volume and menstruation) (**blood vessels, liver, reproductive system and kidneys**)

It ensures the smooth flow of Qi (**lungs, digestive system, circulatory system, urinary system, reproductive system and nervous system**)

It controls the sinews (**muscles, tendons and ligaments**)

It manifests in the nails (**nails and skin**)

It opens into the eyes (**the eyes and brain**)

It houses the corporeal soul (**no correspondence to physiological body**)

The functions of the organs: **The Lung**

Functions of the lung

Involved in the process of external respiration that enables the exchange of oxygen and carbon dioxide between the circulation and the outside environment (**Lung and Kidney Organs**)

Helps to maintain a healthy balance of oxygen, carbon dioxide and acidity of the blood (**Lung and Liver Organs**)

Helps protect the body from noxious substances in the inhaled air (**Lung and Kidney Organs**)

Enables the production of a hormone (angiotensin) which is important in the maintenance of blood pressure (**Kidney, Spleen and Heart Organs**)

Very closely linked in structure and function to the heart on which they depend for an adequate supply of blood to oxygenate (**Heart, Kidney and Liver Organs**)

Provide a steady flow of air to power the production of speech from the larynx (**Lung, Liver and Heart Organs**)

Functions of the Lung Organ

"The Lungs are like a minister from whom policies are issued"

They govern Qi and respiration (**respiratory system, the process of "cellular respiration" which goes on in the mitochondria of all cells, the circulatory system**)

Control the channels and the blood vessels (**circulatory system**)

Control dispersing and descending (**immune system, the skin, large intestine, the bladder**)

They regulate the water passages (**circulatory system, kidneys and bladder**)

Control skin and (body) hair (**the skin, the immune system**)

The open into the nose (**nose and upper respiratory system**)

They house the corporeal soul (**no correspondence to a physiological organ**)

The functions of the organs: **The Ming Men**

Functions of the Ming Men (an Organ unique to Chinese medicine)

It is the root of the Original Qi (motive force for all the Organs and also aids in the formation of Qi and Blood) and the source of Fire for all the Yang Organs (**these functions could possibly correspond to all the metabolic processes within all cells through which energy is generated from nutrients and oxygen; also the thyroid gland, the adrenal gland, the hypothalamus and the pituitary gland**)

It warms the Lower Burner and the Bladder (and so prevents the accumulation of Damp and demae (**the kidneys, the bladder and the circulatory system**)

It warms the Stomach and Spleen to aid digestion (**the digestive system**)

It harmonizes the sexual function and warms the Essence and the Uterus (**the reproductive system, the hypothalamus and the pituitary**)

Assists the kidney function of the reception of Qi (**respiratory system, the adrenal gland, the autonomic nervous system**)

Assists the heart function of housing the mind (**the brain**)

The functions of the organs: **The Pericardium**

Functions of the pericardium	Functions of the Pericardium
It is a fibrous membrane that surrounds the heart and allows it free movement. It also protects from mechanical injury. The serous fluid it encloses contains protective antibodies and immune cells (**Heart, Liver and Kidney Organs**)	"The Pericardium is an ambassador and from it joy and happiness derive" Like the heart it governs blood (**bone marrow, heart, blood vessels**) Like the heart it houses the mind (**brain**) Together with the Kidney and Triple Burner Organs it has been associated with the Gate of Vitality (Ming Men) (**possibly the healthy function of the metabolic processes that go on in all the cells and particularly the sympathetic nervous system**)

The functions of the organs: **The Small Intestine**

Functions of the small intestine	Functions of the Small Intestine Organ
Receives partly digested food from the stomach (**Small Intestine Organ**)	"The Small Intestine is the official in charge of receiving, being filled and transforming"
It is the site of further breakdown of food (**Spleen and Small Intestine Organs**)	It controls receiving and transforming (**stomach, small intestine, gallbladder and liver**)
Absorption of sugars, simple fats, amino acids, vitamins, minerals and water (**Stomach, Spleen and Small Intestine Organs**)	It separates fluids (**stomach, small intestine, large intestine and kidneys**)
Site of local immune system to protect against microorganisms in food and drink (**Spleen, Wei Qi and Kidney**)	

The functions of the organs: **The Spleen**

Functions of the spleen

Aids in the breakdown of aging red blood cells (complementary function to the liver) (**Heart, Liver and Spleen Organs**)

It is the site for the maturation of the white blood cells and thus the generation of an appropriate immune response (akin to a large lymph node) (**Lung, Kidney, Spleen, Upright Qi of all the organs**)

It can function, together with the liver, as an additional site to the bone marrow for the formation of the blood cells (**Heart, Liver, Spleen and Kidney Organs**)

Functions of the Spleen Organ

"The Spleen is the granary official from whom the five tastes are derived"

It governs transformation and transportation (**all of the digestive system and also the urinary system**)

It controls the blood (**the blood vessels, the bone marrow, the clotting function of the blood and the health of the soft tissues**)

It controls the muscles and the four limbs (**muscles, tendons and ligaments and the nervous system**)

It opens into the mouth and manifests in the lips (**the digestive system**)

It controls the "raising Qi" (**integrity of the smooth muscle within the hollow organs and their supporting soft tissue**)

It houses thought (**the brain**)

The functions of the organs: **The Stomach**

Functions of the stomach

Receives chewed food from the mouth via the esophagus and begins the digestion of protein through the release of acid and pepsin (**Stomach, Spleen and Small Intestine Organs**)

Stores partly digested food until it is appropriate for it to be released into the duodenum (upper small intestine) (**Stomach and Spleen Organs**)

Functions of the Stomach Organ

"The Stomach is the official in charge of food storage and from whom the five flavors are derived"

It controls the rotting and ripening of food (**the mouth, stomach, pancreas, liver, gallbladder and small intestine**)

It controls the transportation of food essences (**the small intestine, the circulatory system and the liver**)

It controls the descending of Qi (**the integrity of the smooth muscle of the digestive tract and the autonomic nervous system**)

It is the origin of fluids (**the mouth and the stomach**)

The functions of the organs: **The Thyroid**

Functions of the thyroid (not a named non-physical organ in Traditional Chinese Medicine)

The thyroid gland is an endocrine organ that secretes into the bloodstream thyroid hormones together with a lesser known hormone, calcitonin. These hormones serve to help regulate the diverse aspects of metabolism of the body and also the calcium balance in the bones and blood. The functions of these hormones include:

Regulation of the rate at which the metabolic processes of all the bodily cells take place, leading to an increase in cellular activity and generation of heat (**Kidney Yang and the Ming Men**)

Enabling the basic nutrients to be utilized for growth (**Spleen, Small Intestine and Kidney Organs**)

The normal functioning of the cardiovascular and nervous systems (**Heart and Kidney Organs**)

Stimulation of the muscular movement of the digestive system (**Spleen, Small Intestine, Large Intestine and Liver Organs**)

The regulation of the female reproductive system and the production of milk (**Kidney, Liver, Heart and Spleen Organs, Ren Mai and Chong Mai Channels**)

Control of the uptake of calcium into the bone (**Kidney Organ**)

The functions of the organs: **The Triple Burner**

Functions of the Triple Burner Organ (an Organ unique to Traditional Chinese Medicine)

"The Triple Burner is the official in charge of irrigation and it controls the water passages"

It ensures a smooth "letting out" of Qi at the various stages of energy production (i.e. Wei Qi in the Upper Burner, Nutritive Qi in the Middle Burner, and Body Fluids in the Lower Burner)

It is an avenue for the Original Qi, the motive force between the kidneys. It thus influences digestion and excretion of food wastes

It is a summarization of the function of all the Yang organs (Stomach, Gallbladder, Small Intestine, Large Intestine, Bladder) and also the Lungs and Spleen in the three divisions of the body. It enables the mutual assistance and inter-transformation of Gathering Qi (Upper Burner), Central Qi (Middle Burner) and Original Qi (Lower Burner) (**respiratory system, digestive system, bladder and urethra, cellular respiration, immune system**)

Worked Examples of the Six-Step Method for Interpreting the Energetic Action of Drugs

The six-step method for interpreting the energetic action of drugs

This method involves gathering information in six steps (see Chapter 1.3b):

1. *How does the drug give relief of symptoms?*

   First describe how the drug gives relief of symptoms.

2. *What is the Chinese medicine interpretation of the disease?*

   Give a simple Chinese medicine interpretation of the disease being treated.

3. *How does the drug alleviate disease in Chinese medicine terms?*

   Explain the alleviation of this disease in Chinese medicine terms.

4. *What are the common side effects of this drug?*

   List the common side effects of the medication (use a formulary such as the *British National Formulary*[2])

5. *What is a simple Chinese medicine interpretation of the side effects?*

   Explain side effects in Chinese medicine terms.

6. *Into what category of mode of action does the drug fit?*

   Decide if the drug might have caused suppressed symptoms in addition to drug-induced disease.

The same method can be applied to any form of treatment (i.e. not necessarily a drug treatment). For example, it could be applied to surgery or any form of physical therapy or counseling. The prerequisite is simply knowledge about both the way in which the treatment improves the symptoms of a condition and also its side effects.

Worked examples

This appendix gives three worked examples of the method for three commonly prescribed drugs:

- atorvastatin (a statin) for lowering lipids
- atenolol (a beta blocker) for hypertension
- penicillin (an antibiotic) for tonsillitis.

The energetic action of atorvastatin when prescribed for hyperlipidemia

1. *How does atorvastatin give relief of symptoms?* Very simply speaking, atorvastatin does not treat overt symptoms, but the BNF tells us it acts at the liver to interfere with cholesterol synthesis. In this way it reduces the levels of lipids in the blood. It is used to treat hyperlipidemia.

2. *What is the Chinese medicine interpretation of hyperlipidemia?* This condition starts with no symptoms but if severe may lead to cholesterol plaques on the skin. It is associated with increased cholesterol plaques and atheroma in the blood vessels and eventually thrombosis.

   In Chinese medicine this might be described in terms of Phlegm Damp and eventually Blood Stagnation.

3. *How does atorvastatin alleviate hyperlipidemia in Chinese medicine terms?* Atorvastatin might be described as Clearing Damp Phlegm and Moving of Blood.

4. *What are the common side effects of atorvastatin?* The BNF lists the common side effects as back pain, nosebleeds, high blood sugar and sore throat. Joint ache, muscle inflammation, depression, hair

loss and fatigue are not described as common but instead as "frequency not known."

5. *What is a simple Chinese medicine interpretation of the side effects?* Atorvastatin is associated with musculoskeletal side effects that could readily be described in terms of Stagnation of Liver Qi and Blood Stagnation if severe. High blood sugar suggests that there has been a negative impact on Spleen Qi with accumulation of Damp. Nosebleeds and sore throat suggest Heat affecting the Lungs.

6. *Into what category of mode of action does the drug fit?* Atorvastatin is suppressive in nature; it does not deal with the root cause of hyperlipidemia that is known to result from a combination of inborn tendency and lifestyle factors.

   Atorvastatin also causes drug-induced disease.

Summary: Atorvastatin is a powerful drug that appears to have Moving qualities in that it can clear the manifestation of Phlegm Damp in the blood vessels. However, its side effects suggest it is Heating, Damp Forming, and can Damage Spleen and Stagnate Liver Qi and Blood.

The energetic action of atenolol in treating hypertension (high blood pressure)

1. *How does atenolol give relief of symptoms?* Atenolol is a member of the class of drugs known as beta blockers. These act by blocking the action of the hormone adrenaline (which stimulates tissue cells that carry the protein receptor known as the beta adrenoceptor). Atenolol counteracts the cardiovascular effects of adrenaline, which are to increase arterial resistance and raise the heart rate. In this way atenolol causes a drop in blood pressure and also pulse rate. However, atenolol does not deal with the root cause of hypertension; instead, it counteracts the action of a hormone that contributes to the hypertensive state.

2. *What is the Chinese medicine interpretation of hypertension?* Raised blood pressure can mainly be differentiated in terms of Excess (Phlegm/Damp or Hyperactivity of Liver Fire) and Deficiency (Kidney and Liver Yin or Kidney Yin and Yang).

3. *How does atenolol alleviate hypertension in Chinese medicine terms?* It would make sense from our knowledge of the physiological action of atenolol that it acts energetically by reducing excess rather than by boosting deficiency. It is suggested in Section 3.2d that the action of excessive adrenaline might be seen as a manifestation of Liver Fire, and so we could conclude that atenolol is Cooling in action and subdues Liver Fire. It slows the heart rate, and this may be expressed as a subduing of Heart and Kidney Yang, which is also in keeping with the Cooling nature.

4. *What are the common side effects of atenolol?* The BNF lists the common side effects of atenolol as heart failure, asthma, poor circulation and chilly extremities, fatigue and depression.

5. *What is a simple Chinese medical interpretation of these side effects?* Heart failure could well be a manifestation of subdued Heart and Kidney Yang (see Section 3.2f), and if extreme could develop into Water Overflowing to the Heart and Lungs. Poor circulation and depression and fatigue can both be expressions of Heart and Kidney Yang Deficiency. The Heart Yang Deficiency would embrace Deficiency of Chest (Zong) Qi, which is particularly associated with poor circulation to the extremities. Zong Qi Deficiency could also manifest as asthma failure as could failure of the Kidneys to receive Lung Qi, and this would fit with the interpretation of Subduing of Kidney Yang.

6. *Into what category of mode of action does the drug fit?* As atenolol treats hypertension by dealing with the manifestation and not the root cause, by definition it acts in a suppressive manner. Therefore, there is a possibility that atenolol may lead to the imbalances that originally gave rise to the hypertension found expressed elsewhere in the body. In this case, subdued Kidney Yang deficiency might well contribute to some of the side effects described in steps 4 and 5.

   Atenolol also causes drug-induced disease.

Summary: In hypertension atenolol appears to be Cooling in action in that it subdues Liver Fire and it also appears to subdue Heart and Kidney Yang. The side effects of cold extremities, heart failure and depression are in keeping with Heart and Kidney Yang Deficiency becoming apparent in other bodily systems. Atenolol causes asthma as well as heart failure, which may be attributed to Depletion of Chest (Zong) Qi and Depletion of Kidney Yang.

The energetic action of penicillin in treating tonsillitis

1. *How does penicillin give relief of symptoms?* Simply speaking, penicillin inhibits the growth of certain bacteria by interfering with the formation of the bacterial cell wall. In bacterial tonsillitis the inflamed tonsil is a result of bacterial infection, and so elimination of the bacteria will promote resolution of the inflammation.

2. *What is the Chinese medicine interpretation of tonsillitis?* In Chinese medicine, tonsillitis is clearly a condition of Heat, and traditionally can be attributed to Lung Heat or Stomach Heat. If severe it may be described as Fire Poison.

3. *How does penicillin alleviate tonsillitis in Chinese medicine terms?* By promoting resolution of tonsillitis, penicillin would appear to Clear Heat and therefore have a Cooling action.

4. *What are the common side effects of penicillin?* The BNF lists the common side effects as allergic sensitivity (rashes, anaphylaxis) fever, damage to blood cells and diarrhea. It is known that penicillin can cause imbalance of the healthy bacteria found in the body (the microbiome) and this may result in long-term side effects of digestive problems and vaginal candidiasis.

5. *What is a simple Chinese medicine interpretation of the side effects?* Allergic reactions suggest that Wei Qi has been depleted and therefore permitted Invasion of Wind Heat/Wind Water. Fever and damage to blood cells suggests Heat at a deep level. Diarrhea could be a result of the Cooling action, and subsequent damage to Spleen Qi. Vaginal candidiasis may either result from Damp Heat or Damp Cold.

6. *Into what category of mode of action does the drug fit?* Tonsillitis is the result of an invasion of bacteria or viruses into the tonsils. In many cases tonsillitis develops when a person's immunity is low, and may be recurrent. It does not seem to have the epidemic qualities of a truly infectious disease such as malaria.

For this reason, penicillin in this situation is suppressive in nature as it doesn't target the true root cause of disease. It also causes drug-induced disease.

Summary: In bacterial tonsillitis penicillin acts by clearing Pathogenic Heat, but its Cooling action may have the side effect of Depleting Spleen Qi and Accumulation of Damp. It also appears to Deplete Wei Qi, in that it is commonly associated with allergic reactions and rashes. Heat can become apparent at a deep level in the form of fever and damage to Blood Cells. One possible explanation for this is suppression of Pathogenic Heat. Another explanation is that Depletion of Spleen Qi has led to Accumulation of Damp. Stagnation of Damp predisposes to Heat.

Either way penicillin is a Cooling medicinal that leads to Damp Accumulation and also appears to promote generation of Heat at a deep level.

Red Flag Conditions:
A Guide for Acupuncturists

The tables of red flag symptoms and signs given in this appendix are intended as a guide for use in clinical practice. The listed syndromes (i.e. clusters of symptoms and signs) point to possible conditions which, if present, might merit referral to a medical practitioner. All these symptoms and signs have been included in the guide simply because the author considers that, in seeing a medical practitioner, the patient with these red flags of serious illness is likely to benefit over and above the benefit they will be receiving from acupuncture alone.

Very few of these syndromes are absolute indicators of the need to refer a patient to a doctor. They are listed here because they reflect current medical opinion about when evidence suggests that further tests may be needed, or treatment should be instigated. Each syndrome is referenced to its location in the red flag tables in the main body of the text. The rationale for the inclusion of each syndrome in the tables can be found in these corresponding tables so that it may be understood why these symptoms and signs have been included. The information in this guide is simply intended to help in making as informed a decision about referral as possible.

Please note that not all of the conditions listed in this guide might require medical treatment. In some cases referral is advised so that the patient can have tests to exclude an unlikely but important treatable condition (for example, a mole that might have features of skin cancer), or to obtain a medical diagnosis to guide in the future management of the condition (for example, ascertaining the severity and cause of suspected anemia). In other situations it may be important to refer so that the patient can have access to detailed medical advice (for example, on the complexity of assessing coronary risk and how this impacts on subsequent choice of medical treatment).

In summary, referral may be considered for the following four broad reasons:

- to enable the patient to have access to medical treatment that might benefit their condition

- to access investigations to exclude the possibility of serious disease

- to access investigations to confirm a diagnosis and help guide treatment

- to receive expert advice on the management of a complex condition.

Not all of the listed conditions by any means merit emergency referral, and so the guide also offers a broad indication of with what sort of level of priority a referral might need to be made.

Priority of referral of patients with red flag symptoms and signs

In this guide the urgency of referral of patients with red flag symptoms and signs is described as falling into one or more of three categories: non-urgent, high priority and urgent.

These three categories reflect the three different ways in which a patient can access a medical consultation in a conventional medical setting.

See Chapter 6.3 for guidance on communicating with conventional medical practitioners by letter or telephone when referring patients with red flag conditions.

- **Non-urgent referral (*):** This means the patient can be encouraged to make a routine appointment with a medical practitioner (general practitioner, GP), and this ideally will take place within seven days at the most.

  In most situations with a non-urgent red flag condition a patient can self-refer. If a formal referral may be preferred, this is when a structured typed referral letter would be appropriate. The patient might be advised to take this letter to the appointment with their doctor to eliminate any delays that might result from relying on the postal service or email communication.

- **High priority referral (**):** This means the patient needs to be assessed by a medical practitioner on the same day, either as a home visit or at the medical practice.

  The patient can request this sort of appointment, but if the acupuncturist wishes to explain their concerns, they can either ask to speak to the attending doctor by telephone or give the patient a handwritten letter to take with them.

- **Urgent referral (***):** This category is for those situations when the patient requires immediate medical attention, and this may mean summoning an on-call doctor or calling the paramedics to the scene. In these cases information has usually to be imparted by telephone, but a handwritten note of information to go with the patient can be a useful additional means of communication.

For many of the red flag conditions listed in the tables it is not possible to be absolute about the priority of referral, and often two categories of priority are suggested. The decision about which is the most appropriate category will depend on the unique characteristics of the case in question. For example, in most cases of referral to exclude a possible diagnosis of cancer it might be appropriate to refer non-urgently (i.e. the patient is seen within the week, but not necessarily on the same day). However, if the patient is very anxious, or if the symptoms seem to be progressing rapidly, a same-day referral might be more beneficial.

Use of acupuncture when referring

In most situations, even if an urgent referral has been made, it is still entirely acceptable for a practitioner to continue to administer acupuncture to their patient, as long as it is clear that informed consent has been given. Those rare situations in which continued acupuncture treatment might be hazardous are when the patient is either at a risk of increased bleeding (due to thrombocytopenia or clotting failure) or increased risk of infection (due to bone marrow failure or immunosuppression).

Red flags ordered by symptom keyword: Index		Page number
B1	Red flags of abdominal pain and swelling	783
B2	Red flags of anemia	785
B3	Red flags of anxiety or agitation	785
B4	Red flags of bleeding or blood loss	786
B5	Red flags of disorders of the breast	787
B6	Red flags of breathlessness or difficulty in breathing	787
B7	Red flags of bruising and purpura	788
B8	Red flags of chest pain	789
B9	Red flags particular to childhood diseases	790
B10	Red flags of collapse and loss of consciousness	791
B11	Red flags of confusion and clouding of consciousness	792
B12	Red flags of cough	794
B13	Red flags of dehydration	795
B14	Red flags of depression and exhaustion	795
B15	Red flags of dizziness	796
B16	Red flags of diseases of the ear	796
B17	Red flags of edema	797
B18	Red flags of diseases of the eye	797
B19	Red flags of fever	798
B20	Red flags of headache	799
B21	Red flags of hypertension	800

B22	Red flags of infections	801
B23	Red flags of jaundice	802
B24	Red flags of lumps, masses and glands	802
B25	Red flags of disorders of menstruation	804
B26	Red flags of disorders of the mouth	804
B27	Red flags of muscle tremor and spasms	805
B28	Red flags of numbness	805
B29	Red flags of pain in the bones, joints or muscles	806
B30	Red flags of palpitations or abnormal pulse rate	807
B31	Red flags of pregnancy and the puerperium	808
B32	Red flags of diseases of the skin	809
B33	Red flags of disorders of speech	811
B34	Red flags of disorders of swallowing	811
B35	Red flags of thirst	812
B36	Red flags of urinary disorders	812
B37	Red flags of visual disturbance	813
B38	Red flags of vomiting and/or passage of feces	814
B39	Red flags of weakness/paralysis	815
B40	Red flags of weight loss or weight gain	816

B1: Red flags of abdominal pain and swelling

Symptoms and signs	Priority	Chapter reference
Severe abdominal pain with collapse (the acute abdomen): the pain can be constant or colicky (coming in waves); rigidity, guarding and rebound tenderness are serious signs. Includes: • Acute pancreatitis: presents as acute abdomen with severe central abdominal and back pain, vomiting and dehydration • Ruptured aortic aneurysm: acute abdominal or back pain with collapse; features of shock (low blood pressure and rapid pulse) may be coexistent • Right hypochondriac pain (pain under the right ribs) that is very intense and comes in waves. May be associated with fever, vomiting and jaundice. This is one of the manifestations of acute abdomen	***/**	A6: Red flags of diseases of the stomach (3.1c) A7: Red flags of diseases of the pancreas (3.1d) A9: Red flags of diseases of the gallbladder (3.1d) A10: Red flags of diseases of the small intestine and large intestine (3.1e) A11: Red flags of diseases of the blood vessels (3.2c)
Pelvic inflammatory disease (acute form): low abdominal pain with collapse and fever. Offensive vaginal discharge may be an additional feature	***/**	A35: Red flags of sexually transmitted diseases (5.2d)
Acute testicular pain: radiates to groin, scrotum or lower abdomen. May be vomiting and collapse	***/**	A36: Red flags of structural disorders of the reproductive system (5.2g)
Acute loin pain (pain in flanks radiating round to pubic region): comes in waves. May be vomiting, agitation and collapse. Suggests obstructed kidney stone	***/**	A30: Red flags of diseases of the ureters, bladder and the urethra (4.3d)

Severe abdominal pain in pregnancy: refer as emergency if any signs of shock are apparent (low blood pressure, fainting, rapid pulse). If periodic mild cramping sensations in later pregnancy (lasting no more than a few seconds) are becoming regular and intensifying, these might signify early labor (by definition, before week 36 of pregnancy)	***/**	A37: Red flags of pregnancy (5.3d)
Pre-eclampsia/HELLP syndromes in pregnancy: headache, abdominal pain, visual disturbance, nausea and vomiting and edema (in middle to late pregnancy)	***	A37: Red flags of pregnancy (5.3d)
Right hypochondriac pain (pain under the right ribs) with malaise for >3 days suggests chronic biliary or hepatic disease	**/*	A8: Red flags of diseases of the liver (3.1d) A9: Red flags of diseases of the gallbladder (3.1d)
Recurrent or persistent urinary tract infection: episodes of symptoms including some or all of cloudy urine, burning on urination, abdominal discomfort, blood in urine and fever, especially if occurring in men. If occurring in women, no need to refer if settling down within 5 days	**/*	A30: Red flags of diseases of the ureters, bladder and the urethra (4.3d)
Signs of an inguinal hernia: swelling in groin that is more pronounced on standing, especially if uncomfortable	**/*	A10: Red flags of diseases of the small intestine and large intestine (3.1e)
Pelvic inflammatory disease (chronic form): vaginal discharge, gripy abdominal pain, pain on intercourse, dysmenorrhea, infertility	**/*	A35: Red flags of sexually transmitted diseases (5.2d)
Pelvic pain or deep pain during intercourse. Suggests ovarian or uterine inflammation	**/*	A36: Red flags of structural disorders of the reproductive system (5.2g)
Early shingles: intense, one-sided abdominal pain, with overlying rash of crops of fluid-filled reddened and crusting blisters. The pain may precede the rash by 1–2 days. Refer for early consideration of antiviral treatment	**	A25: Red flags of diseases of the spinal cord and peripheral nerves (4.1g)
Stable aortic aneurysm: pulsatile tubular mass in abdomen >5cm in diameter. Usually affects people >50 years, and is associated with the degenerative changes of atherosclerosis	*	A11: Red flags of diseases of the blood vessels (3.2c)
Chronic pancreatitis: central abdominal and back pain, weight loss and loose stools over weeks to months	*	A7: Red flags of diseases of the pancreas (3.1d)
Epigastric pain or dyspepsia: only if for the first time in someone >40 years or if resistant to treatment after 6 weeks	*	A6: Red flags of diseases of the stomach (3.1c)
Abdominal swelling: discrete suprapubic or inguinal mass. Possible fibroids, ovarian cyst, tumor, pregnancy	*	A36: Red flags of structural disorders of the reproductive system (5.2g)
Abdominal swelling: generalized and painless. Possible fluid accumulation from a tumor (ascites)	*	A1: Red flags of cancer (2.3) A36: Red flags of structural disorders of the reproductive system (5.2g)
Chronic dull testicular pain: may radiate to groin, scrotum or lower abdomen. Possible epididymitis or varicocele	*	A36: Red flags of structural disorders of the reproductive system (5.2g)

B2: Red flags of anemia

Anemia is the term describing any state in which the oxygen-carrying ability of the red blood cells is reduced and the concentration of hemoglobin in the blood is lower than normal

Symptoms and signs	Priority	Chapter reference
Bone marrow failure: severe progressive anemia, recurrent progressive infections or bruising, purpura and bleeding	***/**	A1: Red flags of cancer (2.3) A20: Red flags of leukemia and lymphoma (3.4e)
Severe anemia: pallor, extreme tiredness, breathlessness on exertion, feeling of faintness, depression, sore mouth and tongue. Excessive bruising and severe visual disturbances There may also be features of strain on the cardiovascular system: chest pain on exertion, features of tachycardia and increasing edema	**	A18: Red flags of anemia (3.4c)
Pernicious anemia (vitamin B12 deficiency): tiredness, lemon-yellow pallor and gradual onset of neurological symptoms (numbness, weakness)	**/*	A18: Red flags of anemia (3.4c)
Long-standing anemia: pallor, tiredness, breathlessness on exertion, feeling of faintness, depression, sore mouth and tongue	*	A18: Red flags of anemia (3.4c)
Anemia in pregnancy: pallor, tiredness, breathlessness on exertion. The risks of bleeding during labor are higher in women with anemia, so refer for treatment	*	A37: Red flags of pregnancy (5.3d)

B3: Red flags of anxiety or agitation

Symptoms and signs	Priority	Chapter reference
Hypoglycemia (due to effects of insulin or antidiabetic medication in excess of bodily requirements): agitation, sweating, dilated pupils, confusion and coma	***	A32: Red flags of diabetes mellitus (5.1d)
Hallucinations, delusions or other evidence of thought disorder, together with evidence of deteriorating self-care and personality change. All features of a psychosis such as schizophrenia. Suicide risk is high. Refer urgently if behavior is posing a risk to the patient or others	***/**	A44: Red flags of mental health disorders (6.2e)
Mania: increasing agitation, grandiosity, pressure of speech and sleeplessness with delusional thinking. All features of bipolar disorder, a form of psychosis, which carries a high risk of behavior that can be both socially and physically damaging to the patient. Suicide risk is high. Refer urgently if behavior is posing a risk to the patient or others	***/**	A44: Red flags of mental health disorders (6.2e)
Postnatal psychosis: delusional or paranoid ideas and hallucinations are key features. This condition is associated with a high risk of suicide or harm to the baby. Refer urgently	***/**	A38: Red flags of the puerperium (5.3e)
Organic mental health disorder (i.e. due to underlying gross physical abnormality): confusion, agitation, deterioration in intellectual skills, loss of ability to care for self (possible organic brain disorder such as drug intoxication, brain damage or dementia)	***/**	A44: Red flags of mental health disorders (6.2e)
Hyperthyroidism: irritability, anxiety, sleeplessness, increased appetite, loose stools, weight loss, scanty periods and heat intolerance. Signs: sweaty skin, tremor of the hands, staring eyes and rapid pulse	**/*	A31: Red flags of diseases of the thyroid gland (5.1c)
Severe depression/obsessive-compulsive disorder or anxiety: if not responding to treatment and seriously affecting quality of life	*	A44: Red flags of mental health disorders (6.2e)
Severe disturbance of body image: resulting in features of progressive anorexia nervosa or bulimia nervosa (e.g. progressive weight loss, secondary amenorrhea, repeated compulsion to bring about vomiting)	*	A44: Red flags of mental health disorders (6.2e)

B4: Red flags of bleeding or blood loss

Symptoms and signs	Priority	Chapter reference
Severe blood loss leading to shock: if the following symptoms and signs have been present for more than a few minutes (i.e. not just simple faint) or are worsening: dizziness, fainting and confusion. Rapid pulse of >100 beats/minute. Blood pressure <90/60mmHg. Cold and clammy extremities	***	A19: Red flags of hemorrhage and shock (3.4d)
Bone marrow failure: symptoms of progressive anemia, recurrent progressive infections, progressive bruising, purpura and bleeding	***/**	A20: Red flags of leukemia and lymphoma (3.4e)
Vomiting of fresh blood or altered blood (hematemesis): if blood is altered it looks like dark gravel or coffee grounds in the vomit	***/**	A6: Red flags of diseases of the stomach (3.1c) A8: Red flags of diseases of the liver (3.1d)
Altered blood in stools (melena): stools look like black tar. Suggests large amount of bleeding from stomach	***/**	A6: Red flags of diseases of the stomach (3.1c)
Any episode of vaginal bleeding in pregnancy: refer as an emergency if any signs of shock are apparent (low blood pressure, fainting, rapid pulse), as internal bleeding may not become immediately apparent. Otherwise refer as a high priority for investigation of cause	***/**	A37: Red flags of pregnancy (5.3d)
Postpartum hemorrhage: if bleeding after childbirth is any more than a blood-stained discharge. A profuse bleed of >500ml or the symptoms of shock (low blood pressure, fainting, rapid pulse rate) constitutes an emergency	***/**	A38: Red flags of the puerperium (5.3e)
Continuing blood loss: any situation in which significant bleeding is continuing for more than a few minutes without any signs of abating (e.g. nosebleed), except within the context of menstruation	***/**	A19: Red flags of hemorrhage and shock (3.4d)
Unexplained bleeding: either from the surface of the skin or emerging from an internal organ, such as the bowel, bladder or uterus	**	A1: Red flags of cancer (2.3)
Dysentery or food poisoning: any episode of diarrhea and vomiting in which food is suspected as the origin, or in which blood appears in the stools. This is a notifiable disease	**	A10: Red flags of diseases of the small intestine and large intestine (3.1e)
Blood mixed in with stools: fresh blood mixed in with the stools suggests colonic or rectal origin. Note: Blood that drips after passage of stools is anal in origin and is usually benign (no need to refer)	**	A10: Red flags of diseases of the small intestine and large intestine (3.1e)
Coughing up of blood (hemoptysis): only amounts more than a teaspoon in volume are significant	**	A17: Red flags of lower respiratory disease (3.3e)
Tuberculosis infection: chronic productive cough, weight loss, night sweats, blood in sputum for >2 weeks	**	A17: Red flags of lower respiratory disease (3.3e)
Blood in the urine or sperm: refer all cases in men. Refer in women except in the case of acute urinary infection, in which case it is usually benign	**/*	A29: Red flags of diseases of the kidneys (4.3c) A30: Red flags of diseases of the ureters, bladder and the urethra (4.3d)

B5: Red flags of disorders of the breast

Symptoms and signs	Priority	Chapter reference
Mastitis in pregnancy or puerperium: if not responding to treatment in 2 days or if features of an abscess (inflamed mass with severe malaise) present	**/*	A38: Red flags of the puerperium (5.3e) A39: Red flags of diseases of the breast (5.3f)
Inflamed breast tissue but not breastfeeding: rare to develop inflammation if not breastfeeding; may suggest underlying tumor	**/*	A39: Red flags of diseases of the breast (5.3f)
Insufficient breast milk: if the mother is considering stopping breastfeeding because of insufficient milk, refer to midwife for breastfeeding advice, as once a baby becomes reliant on formula milk it is often an irreversible decision	**/*	A38: Red flags of the puerperium (5.3e)
Lump in the breast: always refer for investigation. One in ten breast lumps is cancerous	*	A39: Red flags of diseases of the breast (5.3f)
Eczema of nipple region: may be due to Bowen's disease (form of breast cancer)	*	A39: Red flags of diseases of the breast (5.3f)
Lactation but not breastfeeding: might suggest pituitary disorder	*	A39: Red flags of diseases of the breast (5.3f)
Hypopituitarism: inappropriate lactation, loss of libido, infertility, menstrual disturbances, tiredness, low blood pressure	*	A33: Red flags of the less common endocrine diseases (5.1e)

B6: Red flags of breathlessness or difficulty in breathing (see also B12: Red flags of cough)

Symptoms and signs	Priority	Chapter reference
Severe asthma: at least two of the following – rapidly worsening breathlessness, >30 respirations/minute (or more if a child[1]), heart rate >110 beats/minute, reluctance to talk because of breathlessness; need to sit upright and still to assist breathing. Cyanosis is a very serious sign	***	A17: Red flags of lower respiratory disease (3.3e)
Infection of the alveoli (pneumonia): cough, fever, malaise, >30 respirations/minute (or more if a child[1]), heart rate >110 beats/minute, reluctance to talk because of breathlessness; need to sit upright and still to assist breathing. Cyanosis is a very serious sign	***/**	A17: Red flags of lower respiratory disease (3.3e)
Progression of respiratory infection to the lower respiratory tract. Breathlessness with malaise suggests the involvement of the bronchi or lower air passages. Usually accompanied by cough and fever, but may be the only symptom of an infection in elderly people or those who are immunocompromised	***/**	A16: Red flags of upper respiratory disease (3.3c)
Pulmonary embolism: sudden onset of pleurisy (chest pain exacerbated by breathing in), with breathlessness, cyanosis, collapse and blood in sputum	***	A17: Red flags of lower respiratory disease (3.3e)
Sudden lung collapse (pneumothorax): onset of severe breathlessness, may be some pleurisy (chest pain exacerbated by breathing in), and collapse if very severe	***	A17: Red flags of lower respiratory disease (3.3e)
Stridor (harsh noisy breathing heard on both the in-breath and out-breath): suggests obstruction to upper airway. Patient will want to sit upright and still. Don't ask to examine the tongue	***/**	A16: Red flags of upper respiratory disease (3.3c)
Any new onset of difficulty breathing in a young child (<8 years). Possible asthma (suggested by the presence of cough), chest infection, foreign body in airway, allergic reaction. All need assessing, but some may require urgent treatment	***/**/*	A16: Red flags of upper respiratory disease (3.3c)

Unstable angina or heart attack: sustained intense chest pain associated with fear or dread. Palpitations and breathlessness may be present. The patient may vomit or develop a cold sweat. Beware: In elderly people can present as sudden onset of breathlessness, palpitations or confusion, but without pain	***	A13: Red flags of angina and heart attack (3.2e)
Acute heart failure: sudden onset of disabling breathlessness and watery cough	***	A14: Red flags of heart failure and arrhythmias (3.2f)
Any sudden or gradual onset of muscle weakness that might be affecting muscles of respiration. Needs to be referred urgently, as condition may progress to respiratory failure	***	A25: Red flags of diseases of the spinal cord and peripheral nerves (4.1g)
Severe chronic heart failure: marked swelling of ankles and lower legs, disabling breathlessness, cough and exhaustion. There may also be palpitations and chest pain on exertion	**	A14: Red flags of heart failure and arrhythmias (3.2f)
Mild chronic heart failure: slight swelling of ankles, slight breathlessness on exertion and when lying flat, cough, but no palpitations or chest pain	*	A14: Red flags of heart failure and arrhythmias (3.2f)
Stable angina: central chest pain related to exertion, eating or the cold that improves with rest. Pain is heavy and gripping (rather than sharp or stabbing), and can radiate down neck and arms. Beware: In elderly people can present as episodes of breathlessness/chest tightness, but without pain	**/*	A13: Red flags of angina and heart attack (3.2e)
Complicated pericarditis: sharp central chest pain that is worse on leaning forward and lying down. Fever. Associated palpitations and breathlessness are more serious features	**	A15: Red flags of pericarditis (3.2g)
Pleurisy: localized chest pain that is associated with inspiration and expiration. Refer if associated with fever and breathlessness, as this is an indication of underlying pneumonia	**	A17: Red flags of lower respiratory disease (3.3e)
Long-standing anemia: pallor, tiredness, breathlessness on exertion, feeling of faintness, depression, sore mouth and tongue	**/*	A18: Red flags of anemia (3.4c)
Unexplained persistent blockage of nostril on one side. In an adult this suggests possible nasopharyngeal carcinoma; refer for investigations if persisting for >3 weeks. In a child this suggests obstruction by a foreign body; refer as a high priority	*/**	A16: Red flags of upper respiratory disease (3.3c) A40: Red flags of the diseases of childhood (5.4e)

1 *Categorization of respiratory rate in children*
The normal range for respiratory rate in children varies according to age.
The following rates indicate moderate to severe breathlessness:
> Newborn (0–3 months) >60 breaths/minute
> Infant (3 months to 2 years) >50 breaths/minute
> Young child (2–8 years) >40 breaths/minute
> Older child to adult >30 breaths/minute.

B7: Red flags of bruising and purpura[1]

Symptoms and signs	Priority	Chapter reference
Bone marrow failure: severe progressive anemia, recurrent progressive infections or bruising, purpura and bleeding	***/**	A1: Red flags of cancer (2.3) A20: Red flags of leukemia and lymphoma (3.4e)
Severe headache with fever and with a bruising and non-blanching rash: suggests meningococcal meningitis	***	A23: Red flags of headache (4.1e)

Bruising and non-blanching rash with severe malaise: suggests meningococcal septicemia	***	A11: Red flags of diseases of the blood vessels (3.2c)
Purpura or bruising rash (non-blanching): suggests a bleeding disorder or vasculitis	***/**	A41: Red flags of diseases of the skin (6.1c)
Edema, bruising and confusion in someone with known liver disease: suggests liver disease has progressed to a serious stage, and the patient is at risk of coma	**	A8: Red flags of diseases of the liver (3.1d)
Severe anemia: extreme tiredness and breathlessness on exertion, excessive bruising and severe visual disturbances. There may also be features of **strain on the cardiovascular system**: chest pain on exertion, tachycardia and increasing edema	**	A18: Red flags of anemia (3.4c)

1 Purpura is pinpoint bruising that appears as a rash of small, red, non-blanching macules. It may result from low platelets or from inflammation of the blood vessels (vasculitis).

B8: Red flags of chest pain

Symptoms and signs	Priority	Chapter reference
Unstable angina or heart attack: sustained intense chest pain associated with fear or dread. Palpitations and breathlessness may be present. The patient may vomit or develop a cold sweat. Beware: In elderly people can present as sudden onset of breathlessness, palpitations or confusion, but without pain	***	A13: Red flags of angina and heart attack (3.2e)
Pulmonary embolism: sudden onset of pleurisy (chest pain related to breathing in) with breathlessness, cyanosis, collapse and blood in sputum	***	A17: Red flags of lower respiratory disease (3.3e)
Sudden lung collapse (pneumothorax): breathlessness; may be some pleurisy and collapse if very severe	***	A17: Red flags of lower respiratory disease (3.3e)
Complicated pericarditis: sharp central chest pain that is worse on leaning forward and lying down. Fever. Associated palpitations and breathlessness are more serious features	***/**	A15: Red flags of pericarditis (3.2g)
Dissecting aortic aneurysm: sudden onset, tearing chest pain with radiation to back. Features of shock may be present (faintness, low blood pressure, rapid pulse)	***	A13: Red flags of angina and heart attack (3.2e)
Stable angina: central chest pain related to exertion, eating or the cold and that improves with rest. Pain is heavy and gripping (rather than sharp or stabbing), and can radiate down neck and arms. Beware: In elderly people can present as episodes of breathlessness/chest tightness, but without pain	**/*	A13: Red flags of angina and heart attack (3.2e)
Uncomplicated pericarditis: sharp central chest pain that is worse on leaning forward and lying down. Fever should be slight and pulse rate no more than 100 beats/minute	**	A15: Red flags of pericarditis (3.2g)
Pleurisy: localized chest pain that is associated with inspiration and expiration. Refer if associated with breathlessness, as this is an indication of associated pneumonia or pulmonary embolism	**	A17: Red flags of lower respiratory disease (3.3e)
New onset of chronic cough or deep persistent chest pain in a smoker: this could be the first sign of bronchial carcinoma	**/*	A17: Red flags of lower respiratory disease (3.3e)
Early shingles: intense, one-sided pain, with overlying rash of crops of fluid-filled reddened and crusting blisters. The pain may precede the rash by 1–2 days. Refer for early consideration of antiviral treatment	**	A25: Red flags of diseases of the spinal cord and peripheral nerves (4.1g)

B9: Red flags particular to childhood diseases

This table lists only those red flags that are particular to children. Many of the red flags listed in the other tables could also apply to children, and these are not repeated here.

Symptoms and signs	Priority	Chapter reference
Dehydration in an infant: dry mouth and skin, loss of skin turgor (firmness), drowsiness, sunken fontanel (soft spot in region of DU-24) and dry diapers	***/**	A40: Red flags of the diseases of childhood (5.4e)
Febrile convulsion in child: ongoing	***	A40: Red flags of the diseases of childhood (5.4e)
Severe diarrhea and vomiting if lasting >24 hours in infants	***/**	A6: Red flags of diseases of the stomach (3.1c)
High fever in a child (<8 years) not responding to treatment within 2 hours	**	A40: Red flags of the diseases of childhood (5.4e)
Any fever if present in an infant (especially if <3 months old): treat with caution; may be the only sign of serious disease	**	A2: Red flags of infectious diseases: vulnerable groups (2.4c)
Febrile convulsion in child: recovered	**	A40: Red flags of the diseases of childhood (5.4e)
Complications of acute otitis media: persistent fever/pain/confusion for >3–4 days after the onset of the earache (may indicate spread of the infection, e.g. mastoiditis or brain abscess)	**	A40: Red flags of the diseases of childhood (5.4e)
Mastoiditis: fever, with a painful and swollen mastoid bone	**	A43: Red flags of diseases of the ear (6.1e)
Discharge from the eye: if severe, prolonged for >5 days and painful, or if seen in the newborn or a malnourished child	**	A42: Red flags of diseases of the eye (6.1d)
Malabsorption syndrome: loose, pale stools and malnutrition; weight loss, thin hair, dry skin, cracked lips and peeled tongue. Will present as failure to thrive in children	**/*	A7: Red flags of diseases of the pancreas (3.1d) A10: Red flags of diseases of the small intestine and large intestine (3.1e)
Unexplained injury; child not thriving; child miserable: refer any situation in which you suspect the possibility of physical or sexual abuse as a high priority. If in the UK call the NSPCC helpline for confidential advice in the first instance	**	A40: Red flags of the diseases of childhood (5.4e)
Vaginal discharge or itch before puberty: refer any situation in which you suspect the possibility of sexual abuse as a high priority. Call the NSPCC helpline for confidential advice in the first instance	**	A40: Red flags of the diseases of childhood (5.4e)
Epilepsy: refer any child who has suffered a suspected blank episode (absence) or seizure	*	A40: Red flags of the diseases of childhood (5.4e)
New onset of difficulty hearing in a child: if lasting for >3 weeks (especially if interfering with school and social interactions)	*	A40: Red flags of the diseases of childhood (5.4e)
Squint: in any child if previously undiagnosed	*	A40: Red flags of the diseases of childhood (5.4e)

Soiling of stool (in underwear or bed): if affecting a previously continent child	*	A40: Red flags of the diseases of childhood (5.4e)
Bedwetting: if persisting over age 5 years	*	A40: Red flags of the diseases of childhood (5.4e)
Primary amenorrhea: after age 16 years	*	A34: Red flags of the diseases of menstruation (5.2c)
Delayed puberty: secondary sexual characteristics not apparent by age 15 in girls and 16 in boys	*	A36: Red flags of structural disorders of the reproductive system (5.2g)
Precocious puberty: secondary sexual characteristics before age 8 in girls and 9 in boys	*	A36: Red flags of structural disorders of the reproductive system (5.2g)
Autism in a child: slow development of speech, impaired social interactions, little imaginative play, obsessional repetitive behavior	*	A40: Red flags of the diseases of childhood (5.4e)

B10: Red flags of collapse and loss of consciousness (see also B11: Red flags of confusion and clouding of consciousness)

Symptoms and signs	Priority	Chapter reference
Cardiac arrest: collapse with no palpable pulse	***	A14: Red flags of heart failure and arrhythmias (3.2f)
Loss of consciousness (continuing loss of brain function): diverse causes include stroke, metabolic disease, brain infection, intoxication	***	A22: Red flags of brain hemorrhage, stroke and brain tumor (4.1d)
Rapid increase in intracranial pressure: a rapid deterioration of consciousness leading to coma. Irregular breathing patterns and pinpoint pupils are a very serious sign	***	A21: Red flags of raised intracranial pressure (4.1c) A22: Red flags of brain hemorrhage, stroke and brain tumor (4.1d)
First ever epileptic seizure. Generalized tonic-clonic seizure: convulsions, loss of consciousness, bitten tongue, emptying of bladder and/or bowels. This is an emergency if the fit does not settle down within 2 minutes. Refer as high priority if fit has settled down	***	A24: Red flags of dementia, epilepsy and other disorders of the central nervous system (4.1f)
Febrile convulsion in child: ongoing	***	A3: Red flags of infectious diseases: fever, dehydration and confusion (2.4c)
Hypoglycemia (due to effects of insulin or antidiabetic medication in excess of bodily requirements): agitation, sweating, dilated pupils, confusion and coma	***	A32: Red flags of diabetes mellitus (5.1d)
Pulmonary embolism: sudden onset of pleurisy (chest pain on breathing in), with breathlessness, cyanosis, collapse	***	A17: Red flags of lower respiratory disease (3.3e)
Sudden lung collapse (pneumothorax): onset of severe breathlessness, may be some pleurisy (chest pain on breathing in) and collapse if very severe	***	A17: Red flags of lower respiratory disease (3.3e)

General symptoms of shock: dizziness, fainting and confusion. Rapid pulse of >100 beats/minute. Blood pressure <90/60mmHg. Cold and clammy extremities. Refer if these symptoms are worsening or sustained (more than a few seconds)	***	A19: Red flags of hemorrhage and shock (3.4d)
Addison's disease: increased pigmentation of skin, weight loss, muscle wasting, tiredness, loss of libido, low blood pressure, diarrhea and vomiting, confusion, collapse with dehydration	***/**	A33: Red flags of the less common endocrine diseases (5.1e)
Febrile convulsion in child: recovered	**	A40: Red flags of the diseases of childhood (5.4e)
Unexplained falls or faints in elderly person: may be the result of an arrhythmia (cardiac syncope)	**/*	A14: Red flags of heart failure and arrhythmias (3.2f)
A temporary loss of brain function (usually <2 hours long): recovery from loss of consciousness, loss of vision, unsteadiness, confusion, loss of memory, loss of sensation or limb weakness	**	A22: Red flags of brain hemorrhage, stroke and brain tumor (4.1d)
Simple fainting: dizziness, temporary collapse (no more than a few seconds) and temporary confusion. Normal or slowed pulse rate. Blood pressure <90/60mmHg. Cold and clammy extremities. Patient starts to recover in seconds to a minute. No need to refer	–	A19: Red flags of hemorrhage and shock (3.4d)

B11: Red flags of confusion and clouding of consciousness (see also B10: Red flags of collapse and loss of consciousness)

Symptoms and signs	Priority	Chapter reference
General symptoms of shock: dizziness, fainting and confusion. Rapid pulse of >100 beats/minute. Blood pressure <90/60mmHg. Cold and clammy extremities. Refer if these symptoms are worsening or sustained (more than a few seconds)	***	A19: Red flags of hemorrhage and shock (3.4d)
Hypoglycemia (due to effects of insulin or antidiabetic medication in excess of bodily requirements): agitation, sweating, dilated pupils, confusion and coma	***	A32: Red flags of diabetes mellitus (5.1d)
Confusion/coma with dehydration (hyperglycemia)	***	A32: Red flags of diabetes mellitus (5.1d)
Unusual drowsiness in infants (especially if <3 months old): may signify underlying serious illness	***/**	A2: Red flags of infectious diseases: vulnerable groups (2.4c)
Organic mental health disorder (a mental health condition due to an underlying gross physical cause): acute confusion, agitation, visual hallucinations, deterioration in intellectual skills, loss of ability to care for self (these suggest organic brain disorder such as metabolic disease, drug intoxication, brain damage or dementia)	***/**	A44: Red flags of mental health disorders (6.2e)
A persisting loss of brain function: including loss of vision, unsteadiness, confusion, loss of memory, loss of sensation or muscle weakness (possible stroke or multiple sclerosis)	***	A22: Red flags of brain hemorrhage, stroke and brain tumor (4.1d) A24: Red flags of dementia, epilepsy and other disorders of the central nervous system (4.1f)

Hallucinations, delusions or other evidence of thought disorder, together with evidence of deteriorating self-care and personality change: all are features of a psychosis such as schizophrenia. Suicide risk is high	***/**	A44: Red flags of mental health disorders (6.2e)
Mania: increasing agitation, grandiosity, pressure of speech and sleeplessness with delusional thinking: all are features of bipolar disorder, a form of psychosis that carries a high risk of behavior that can be both socially and physically damaging to the patient. Suicide risk is high	***/**	A44: Red flags of mental health disorders (6.2e)
Postnatal psychosis: delusional or paranoid ideas and hallucinations are key features. This condition is associated with a high risk of suicide or harm to the baby.	***/**	A38: Red flags of the puerperium (5.3e)
Acute confusion in an elderly person: can result from an underlying medical condition, such as stroke, heart attack, infection or pain	***/**	A2: Red flags of infectious diseases: vulnerable groups (2.4c)
Confusion in older children and adults with fever	**	A3: Red flags of infectious diseases: fever, dehydration and confusion (2.4c)
Slow increase in intracranial pressure: progressive headaches and vomiting over the timescale of a few weeks to months. The headaches are worse in the morning and the vomiting may be effortless. Blurring of vision and confusion may be additional symptoms	**	A21: Red flags of raised intracranial pressure (4.1c)
Loss of brain function that is progressive over the course of days to weeks: may include confusion. This is more suggestive of a brain tumor than a stroke	**	A22: Red flags of brain hemorrhage, stroke and brain tumor (4.1d)
Pernicious anemia: tiredness, lemon-yellow pallor and gradual onset of neurological symptoms (numbness, weakness, confusion)	**/*	A18: Red flags of anemia (3.4e)
A temporary loss of brain function (usually <2 hours long): recovery from loss of consciousness, loss of vision, unsteadiness, confusion, loss of memory, loss of sensation or limb weakness (possible transient ischemic attack)	**/*	A22: Red flags of brain hemorrhage, stroke and brain tumor (4.1d) A24: Red flags of dementia, epilepsy and other disorders of the central nervous system (4.1f)
Progressive decline in mental and social functioning: increasing difficulty in intellectual function, memory, concentration and use of language	*	A22: Red flags of brain hemorrhage, stroke and brain tumor (4.1d) A24: Red flags of dementia, epilepsy and other disorders of the central nervous system (4.1f)
First-ever epileptic seizure (complex partial). Generalized absence or complex partial seizures: defined periods of vagueness or loss of awareness, or mood or personality changes. Refer any child who has suffered a suspected blank episode (absence) or seizure	*	A24: Red flags of dementia, epilepsy and other disorders of the central nervous system (4.1f)
Simple fainting: dizziness, temporary collapse (no more than a few seconds) and temporary confusion. Normal or slowed pulse rate. Blood pressure <90/60mmHg. Cold and clammy extremities. Patient starts to recover in seconds to a minute. No need to refer	–	A19: Red flags of hemorrhage and shock (3.4d)

B12: Red flags of cough (see also B6: Red flags of breathlessness and difficulty in breathing)

Symptoms and signs	Priority	Chapter reference
Acute heart failure: sudden onset of disabling breathlessness and watery cough	***	A14: Red flags of heart failure and arrhythmias (3.2f)
Infection of the alveoli (pneumonia): cough, fever, malaise, >30 respirations/minute (or more if a child[1]), heart rate >110 beats/minute, reluctance to talk because of breathlessness; need to sit upright and still to assist breathing. Cyanosis is a very serious sign	***/**	A17: Red flags of lower respiratory disease (3.3e)
Progression of infection to the lower respiratory tract: breathlessness[1] with malaise suggests the involvement of the bronchi or lower air passages. Usually accompanied by cough and fever, but may be the only symptom of an infection in elderly people or those who are immunocompromised	***/**	A16: Red flags of upper respiratory disease (3.3c)
Any new onset of difficulty breathing in a young child (<8 years): possible asthma (suggested by coughing as well as difficulty breathing), chest infection; foreign body in airway, allergic reaction. All need assessing, but some may require urgent treatment	***/**/*	A16: Red flags of upper respiratory disease (3.3c)
Progressive upper respiratory infection in susceptible people (e.g. frail elderly people, those who are immunocompromised and people with pre-existing disease of the bronchi and bronchioles): cough and fever, or new production of yellow-green phlegm, each persisting for >3 days	**	A16: Red flags of upper respiratory disease (3.3c) A17: Red flags of lower respiratory disease (3.3e)
Tuberculosis infection: chronic productive cough, weight loss, night sweats, blood in sputum for >2 weeks	**	A17: Red flags of lower respiratory disease (3.3e)
New onset of chronic cough or deep persistent chest pain in a smoker	**/*	A17: Red flags of lower respiratory disease (3.3e)
Severe chronic heart failure: marked swelling of ankles and lower legs, disabling breathlessness, cough and exhaustion. There may also be palpitations and chest pain on exertion	**	A14: Red flags of heart failure and arrhythmias (3.2f)
Mild chronic heart failure: slight swelling of ankles, slight breathlessness on exertion and when lying flat, cough, but no palpitations or chest pain. Dry cough may be the only symptom in sedentary elderly people	*	A14: Red flags of heart failure and arrhythmias (3.2f)

1 Categorization of respiratory rate in adults
Normal respiratory rate in an adult: 10–20 breaths/minute (one breath is one inhalation and exhalation).
Moderate breathlessness in an adult: >30 breaths/minute.
Severe breathlessness in an adult: >60 breaths/minute.
Categorization of respiratory rate in children
The normal range for respiratory rate in children varies according to age.
The following rates indicate moderate to severe breathlessness:
    Newborn (0–3 months) >60 breaths/minute
    Infant (3 months to 2 years) >50 breaths/minute
    Young child (2–8 years) >40 breaths/minute
    Older child to adult >30 breaths/minute.

B13: Red flags of dehydration

Symptoms and signs	Priority	Chapter reference
Dehydration in an infant: signs include dry mouth and skin, loss of skin turgor (firmness), drowsiness, sunken fontanel (soft spot in the region of DU-24) and dry diapers	***/**	A3: Red flags of infectious diseases: fever, dehydration and confusion (2.4c)
Type 1 diabetes or poorly controlled type 2 diabetes: short history of thirst, weight loss and excessive urination, which is rapidly progressive in severity. Can progress to confusion/coma, with dehydration (due to hyperglycemia)	***/**	A32: Red flags of diabetes mellitus (5.1d)
Addison's disease: increased pigmentation of skin, weight loss, muscle wasting, tiredness, loss of libido, low blood pressure, diarrhea and vomiting, confusion, collapse with dehydration	***/**	A33: Red flags of the less common endocrine diseases (5.1e)
Dehydration in older children and adults if severe or lasting >48 hours: signs include dry mouth and skin, loss of skin turgor, low blood pressure, dizziness on standing and poor urine output	**	A3: Red flags of infectious diseases: fever, dehydration and confusion (2.4c)

B14: Red flags of depression and exhaustion

Symptoms and signs	Priority	Chapter reference
Severe anemia: extreme tiredness and breathlessness on exertion, excessive bruising, and severe visual disturbances. There may also be features of strain on the cardiovascular system: chest pain on exertion, features of tachycardia and increasing edema	**	A18: Red flags of anemia (3.4c)
Long-standing anemia: pallor, tiredness, breathlessness on exertion, feeling of faintness, depression, sore mouth and tongue	**/*	A18: Red flags of anemia (3.4c)
Type 2 diabetes: general feeling of unwellness, with thirst and increased need to urinate large amounts of urine, which develop over the course of weeks to months	**/*	A32: Red flags of diabetes mellitus (5.1d)
Hypothyroidism (symptoms and signs tend to be progressive over the course of a few months). Symptoms: tiredness, depression, weight gain, heavy periods, constipation and cold intolerance. Signs: dry puffy skin, dry and thin hair, slow pulse	*	A31: Red flags of diseases of the thyroid gland (5.1c)
Pernicious anemia: tiredness, lemon-yellow pallor and gradual onset of neurological symptoms (numbness, weakness, confusion)	**/*	A18: Red flags of anemia (3.4c)
Hypopituitarism: loss of libido, infertility, menstrual disturbances, tiredness, low blood pressure, inappropriate lactation	**/*	A33: Red flags of the less common endocrine diseases (5.1e)
Suicidal thoughts with features that suggest serious risk: old age, male sex, social isolation, concrete plans in place	**	A44: Red flags of mental health disorders (6.2e)
Postnatal depression lasting >3 weeks that is not responding to treatment: refer straight away if the woman is experiencing suicidal ideas, or if you believe the health of the baby to be at risk	**	A38: Red flags of the puerperium (5.3e)
Severe disturbance of body image: if not responding to treatment, and resulting in features of progressive anorexia nervosa or bulimia nervosa (progressive weight loss, secondary amenorrhea, or repeated compulsion to bring about vomiting)	*	A44: Red flags of mental health disorders (6.2e)

B15: Red flags of dizziness

Symptoms and signs	Priority	Chapter reference
Shock: dizziness, fainting and confusion. Rapid pulse of >100 beats/minute. Blood pressure <90/60mmHg. Cold and clammy extremities. Refer if these symptoms are worsening or sustained (more than a few seconds)	***	A19: Red flags of hemorrhage and shock (3.4d)
Vertigo[1] in young person: usually due to benign labyrinthitis and will settle down. Refer if lasting >6 weeks or if so severe as to be causing recurrent vomiting. Refer if patient is at increased risk of thromboembolic disease (e.g. in pregnancy) so that the possibility of stroke can be excluded	**/*	A43: Red flags of diseases of the ear (6.1e)
Vertigo for the first time in older person (>45 years): refer for high priority medical opinion. Stroke is a more likely cause in this age group. If the vertigo is persisting and profound refer urgently	**/***	A43: Red flags of diseases of the ear (6.1e)
Simple fainting: dizziness, temporary collapse (no more than a few seconds) and temporary confusion. Normal or slowed pulse rate. Blood pressure <90/60mmHg. Cold and clammy extremities. Patient starts to recover in seconds to a minute. No need to refer	–	A19: Red flags of hemorrhage and shock (3.4d)

1 Vertigo is the medical term used to describe a sensation of dizziness in which the world appears to be spinning. The patient may lose balance or feel acutely nauseous. The term vertigo is also sometimes used to mean fear of heights; but strictly speaking should only be used to describe a state in which there is a sensation of movement. The term dizziness is commonly used simply to mean light-headedness; it is important diagnostically to distinguish dizziness from true vertigo.

B16: Red flags of diseases of the ear

Symptoms and signs	Priority	Chapter reference
Sudden onset of absolute deafness (one-sided or bilateral): needs same-day, specialist assessment	**	A43: Red flags of diseases of the ear (6.1e)
Complications of acute otitis media: persistent fever/pain/confusion for >3–4 days after the onset of the earache (may indicate spread of the infection, e.g. mastoiditis or brain abscess)	**	A43: Red flags of diseases of the ear (6.1e)
Mastoiditis: fever, with a painful and swollen mastoid bone. Serious infection; needs same-day assessment and treatment	**	A43: Red flags of diseases of the ear (6.1e)
Earache in an adult for >3 weeks: may suggest nasopharyngeal pathology; refer to exclude cancer	*	A43: Red flags of diseases of the ear (6.1e)
Persistent discharge (lasting >2 weeks) from the ear (chronic otitis media/otitis externa): risk of permanent damage to the ear from chronic inflammation; refer for assessment and treatment	*	A43: Red flags of diseases of the ear (6.1e)
Gradual onset of relative deafness in adult for >7 days (exclude earwax as a cause if possible): deafness from respiratory infection should have cleared by this time; refer to exclude progressive cause, including acoustic neuroma	*	A43: Red flags of diseases of the ear (6.1e)
Tinnitus, if progressive (constant or variable tinnitus is common and usually benign): refer to exclude progressive cause, including acoustic neuroma	*	A43: Red flags of diseases of the ear (6.1e)
New onset of difficulty hearing in a child lasting for >3 weeks (especially if interfering with school and social interactions): prolonged deafness can affect the development of a child; refer for assessment and treatment if not responding	*	A43: Red flags of diseases of the ear (6.1e)

B17: Red flags of edema

Symptoms and signs	Priority	Chapter reference
Progressive swelling of the soft tissues of the face and neck (angio-edema) and/or urticaria (nettle rash): refer urgently if there are any features of respiratory distress (itchy throat/wheeze)	***	A41: Red flags of diseases of the skin (6.1c)
Severe chronic heart failure: marked swelling of the ankles and lower legs, disabling breathlessness, cough and exhaustion	**	A14: Red flags of heart failure and arrhythmias (3.2f)
Unexplained edema (excess tissue fluid, manifesting primarily as ankle swelling extending to >2cm above the malleoli): possible acute or chronic kidney disease	**	A29: Red flags of diseases of the kidneys (4.3c)
Severe anemia: extreme tiredness and breathlessness on exertion, excessive bruising, and severe visual disturbances. There may also be features of strain on the cardiovascular system: chest pain on exertion, features of tachycardia and increasing edema	**	A18: Red flags of anemia (3.4c)
Edema, bruising and confusion in someone with known liver disease: suggests liver disease has progressed to a serious stage	**	A8: Red flags of diseases of the liver (3.1d)
Edema in pregnancy: swelling of ankles is common, but refer if extending >2cm above the malleoli or if facial edema is apparent	**	A37: Red flags of pregnancy (5.3d)
Mild chronic heart failure: slight swelling of the ankles, slight breathlessness on exertion and when lying flat, cough, but no palpitations or chest pain	*	A14: Red flags of heart failure and arrhythmias (3.2f)

B18: Red flags of diseases of the eye

Symptoms and signs	Priority	Chapter reference
Painful, red and swollen eyes and eyelids: patient (often a child) very unwell (orbital cellulitis)	***	A42: Red flags of diseases of the eye (6.1d)
Sudden onset of painless blurring or loss of sight in one or both eyes, accompanied by one-sided headache in patient >50 years: suggestive of temporal arteritis; high risk of further loss of sight or stroke. Refer for urgent treatment with corticosteroids	***	A42: Red flags of diseases of the eye (6.1d)
An intensely painful and red eye: iritis, choroiditis, acute glaucoma, corneal ulcer or keratitis	***/**	A42: Red flags of diseases of the eye (6.1d)
Sudden onset of painless blurring or loss of sight in one or both eyes: refer as soon as possible, as may result from treatable retinal tear	***/**	A42: Red flags of diseases of the eye (6.1d)
A painful eye with no obvious inflammation: deep, intense pain exacerbated by eye movement is characteristic of optic neuritis or choroiditis	**	A42: Red flags of diseases of the eye (6.1d)
Foreign body in the eye	**	A42: Red flags of diseases of the eye (6.1d)
Inability to close the eye: occurs in severe Bell's palsy or thyroid eye disease. The conjunctiva is at risk of ulceration	**	A42: Red flags of diseases of the eye (6.1d)
Recent onset of double vision in an adult	**	A42: Red flags of diseases of the eye (6.1d)
Discharge from the eye. If severe, prolonged for >5 days and painful, or if seen in the following vulnerable groups: • newborns • immunocompromised people • malnourished people	**	A42: Red flags of diseases of the eye (6.1d)

Gradual onset of painless blurring or loss of sight in one or both eyes: possible refractive error, cataract, glaucoma or macular degeneration	*	A42: Red flags of diseases of the eye (6.1d)
Thyroid eye disease: staring eyes (whites visible above and below pupils), inflamed conjunctiva; symptoms of hyperthyroidism (tremor, agitation, weight loss, palpitations)	*	A42: Red flags of diseases of the eye (6.1d)
Squint: in any child if previously undiagnosed	*	A42: Red flags of diseases of the eye (6.1d)
Recent onset of drooping eyelid (ptosis)	*	A42: Red flags of diseases of the eye (6.1d)

B19: Red flags of fever

Symptoms and signs	Priority	Chapter reference
Meningococcal septicemia: acute onset of a purpuric rash, possibly accompanied by headache, vomiting and fever	***	A11: Red flags of diseases of the blood vessels (3.2c)
A severe headache that develops over the course of a few hours to days, with fever, and together with either vomiting or neck stiffness: suggests acute meningitis or encephalitis	***	A23: Red flags of headache (4.1e)
Febrile convulsion in child: ongoing	***	A3: Red flags of infectious diseases: fever, dehydration and confusion (2.4c)
High fever in a child (<8 years) if high (>38.5°C) and not responding to treatment within 2 hours	**	A3: Red flags of infectious diseases: fever, dehydration and confusion (2.4c)
High fever in an older child or adult if high (>38.5°C) that does not respond to treatment within 48 hours	**	A3: Red flags of infectious diseases: fever, dehydration and confusion (2.4c)
Fever in pregnancy if high (>38.5°C) and no response to treatment in 24 hours: refer early, as risk to fetus	**	A37: Red flags of pregnancy (5.3d)
Fever in the puerperium: any case of fever developing in the first 2 weeks of the puerperium (temperature >38°C for >24 hours). Refer early, as possible uterine infection	**	A38: Red flags of the puerperium (5.3e)
Fever of any level in an infant (especially if <3 months old): treat with caution, as could be the only sign of serious underlying disease. Refer if you have any uncertainty about the case	**	A2: Red flags of infectious diseases: vulnerable groups (2.4c)
Fever of any level in an elderly person: treat with caution, as could be the only sign of serious underlying disease. Refer if you have any uncertainty about the case	**	A2: Red flags of infectious diseases: vulnerable groups (2.4c)
Fever of any level in an immunocompromised person: treat with caution, as could be the only sign of serious infection. Refer if you have any uncertainty about the case	**	A2: Red flags of infectious diseases: vulnerable groups (2.4c)
Fever of any level in anyone with a recent history of travel to a tropical country (within the past month): treat with caution, as could be a sign of tropical disease. Refer if you have any uncertainty about the case	**	A2: Red flags of infectious diseases: vulnerable groups (2.4c)

Any fever that persists or recurs for >2 weeks: possible chronic infection, inflammatory process or cancer	**	A1: Red flags of cancer (2.3) A3: Red flags of infectious diseases: fever, dehydration and confusion (2.4c)
Febrile convulsion in child: recovered	**	A3: Red flags of infectious diseases: fever, dehydration and confusion (2.4c)

B20: Red flags of headache

Symptoms and signs	Priority	Chapter reference
A sudden very severe headache that comes on out of the blue: the patient needs to lie down, and may vomit. There may be neck stiffness (reluctance to move the head) and dislike of bright light. This suggests subarachnoid (intracranial) hemorrhage	***	A23: Red flags of headache (4.1e)
Severe headache that develops over the course of a few hours to days, with fever, together with either vomiting or neck stiffness: there may be a bruising and non-blanching rash. Suggests acute meningitis or encephalitis	***	A23: Red flags of headache (4.1e)
Malignant hypertension: diastolic hypertension >120mmHg, with symptoms including recently worsening headaches, blurred vision, chest pain	***/**	A12: Red flags of hypertension (3.2d)
Pre-eclampsia/HELLP syndromes: headache, abdominal pain, visual disturbance, nausea and vomiting and edema (in middle to late pregnancy)	***	A37: Red flags of pregnancy (5.3d)
Severe, one-sided headache over the temple occurring for the first time in an elderly person or in someone with polymyalgia rheumatica: possible temporal arteritis. Blurring or loss of sight are very serious signs	***/**	A23: Red flags of headache (4.1e)
Long history of worsening (progressive) headaches: especially with generalized symptoms such as fever, loss of appetite, exhaustion or neurological symptoms. Suggests malignancy or brain abscess	**/*	A23: Red flags of headache (4.1e)
Slow increase in intracranial pressure: progressive headaches and vomiting over the timescale of a few weeks to months. The headaches are worse in the morning and the vomiting may be effortless. Blurring of vision and confusion may be additional symptoms	**	A21: Red flags of raised intracranial pressure (4.1c) A22: Red flags of brain hemorrhage, stroke and brain tumor (4.1d)
Growth of a pituitary tumor: progressive headaches, visual disturbance and double vision	**/*	A33: Red flags of the less common endocrine diseases (5.1e)
Acromegaly (growth hormone excess): thickening of facial features and soft tissues, enlarged hands and feet, headaches, high blood pressure	**/*	A33: Red flags of the less common endocrine diseases (5.1e)
Trigeminal neuralgia (and other forms of one-sided facial pain): lancinating pain, on one side of the face, which radiates out from a focal point in response to defined triggers. May be associated with twitching (tic douloureux)	*	A25: Red flags of diseases of the spinal cord and peripheral nerves (4.1g)

B21: Red flags of hypertension

Symptoms and signs	Priority	Chapter reference
Malignant hypertension: diastolic hypertension >120mmHg, with symptoms including recently worsening headaches, blurred vision, chest pain	***/**	A12: Red flags of hypertension (3.2d)
Pre-eclampsia/HELLP syndromes: headache, abdominal pain, visual disturbance, nausea and vomiting, and edema (in middle to late pregnancy). Often follows a rise in blood pressure	***	A37: Red flags of pregnancy (5.3d)
Seriously high hypertension: systolic pressure ≥220mmHg, diastolic pressure ≥120mmHg, but no symptoms	**	A12: Red flags of hypertension (3.2d)
Severe hypertension: systolic pressure ≥180mmHg, diastolic pressure ≥110mmHg. Refer as high priority if major risk factors[1] are present. Otherwise, refer for treatment if there is no improvement in 2 weeks	*	A12: Red flags of hypertension (3.2d)
Moderate hypertension: systolic pressure ≥160mmHg and <180mmHg, diastolic pressure ≥100mmHg and <110mmHg. Refer for assessment if risk factors are present, otherwise only refer if there is no improvement within 4 weeks	*	A12: Red flags of hypertension (3.2d)
Mild hypertension: systolic pressure ≥140mmHg and <160mmHg, diastolic pressure ≥90mmHg and <100mmHg. Refer for assessment if risk factors are present, otherwise refer only if there is no improvement within 3 months	*	A12: Red flags of hypertension (3.2d)
Moderate to severe pregnancy-induced hypertension: diastolic pressure >100mmHg or systolic pressure >140mmHg. Arrange same-day assessment with midwife	**	A37: Red flags of pregnancy (5.3d)
Mild pregnancy-induced hypertension: diastolic pressure 90–99mmHg, systolic pressure <140 mmHg	*	A37: Red flags of pregnancy (5.3d)
Potential pregnancy-induced hypertension: systolic pressure is 30mmHg or diastolic pressure is 15mmHg above any measurement taken previously in pregnancy	*	A37: Red flags of pregnancy (5.3d)
Hypertension of any level with established kidney disease	**/*	A12: Red flags of hypertension (3.2d)
Hypertension of any level with diabetes	**/*	A12: Red flags of hypertension (3.2d)
Cushing's syndrome: weight gain, weakness and wasting of limb muscles, stretch marks and bruises. Mood changes, hypertension, red cheeks, acne	*	A33: Red flags of the less common endocrine diseases (5.1e)
Acromegaly (growth hormone excess): thickening of facial features and soft tissues, enlarged hands and feet, headaches, high blood pressure	*	A33: Red flags of the less common endocrine diseases (5.1e)

1 In this case major risk factors are features that are known to be associated with increased risk of a cardiovascular event in the presence of hypertension. These include diabetes, past history of heart disease, chronic leg ischemia and kidney disease.

B22: Red flags of infections

Symptoms and signs	Priority	Chapter reference
Bone marrow failure and current infection: severe progressive anemia, recurrent progressive infections or bruising, purpura and bleeding	***/**	A1: Red flags of cancer (2.3) A20: Red flags of leukemia and lymphoma (3.4e)
Severe headache that develops over the course of a few hours to days, with fever, together with either vomiting or neck stiffness: there may be a bruising and non-blanching rash. Suggests acute meningitis or encephalitis	***	A23: Red flags of headache (4.1e)
Pelvic inflammatory disease (acute form): low abdominal pain with collapse, fever	***	A35: Red flags of sexually transmitted diseases (5.2d)
Unexplained infection or spreading areas of inflammation in an infant (especially if <3 months old): treat with caution as the immune system is immature and infections can take hold easily	**	A2: Red flags of infectious diseases: vulnerable groups (2.4c)
Unexplained infection or spreading areas of inflammation in elderly people: treat with caution as the immune system is deficient and infections can take hold easily	**	A2: Red flags of infectious diseases: vulnerable groups (2.4c)
Unexplained infection or spreading areas of inflammation in an immunocompromised person: treat with caution as the immune system is deficient and infections can take hold easily	**	A2: Red flags of infectious diseases: vulnerable groups (2.4c)
Unexplained infections in pregnancy: treat with caution as certain infections can damage the embryo/fetus	**	A2: Red flags of infectious diseases: vulnerable groups (2.4c)
A rapidly advancing region or line of redness tracking up the skin of a limb (following the pathway of a lymphatic vessel): cellulitis and/or lymphangitis. Deep tissue infection; may need antibiotic treatment to prevent spread	**	A41: Red flags of diseases of the skin (6.1c)
A rapidly enlarging patch(es) of painful, crusting or swollen red skin: most likely to be a bacterial infection (impetigo or erysipelas). Very contagious, and may require antibiotic treatment if not settling down. Refer with some urgency if this occurs in someone with eczema; possible viral infection causing the serious condition of eczema herpeticum	**	A41: Red flags of diseases of the skin (6.1c)
Generalized macular rash (flat red spots): refer if you suspect rubella, measles or scarlet fever (notifiable diseases)	**	A41: Red flags of diseases of the skin (6.1c)
Early shingles: intense, one-sided pain, with overlying rash of crops of fluid-filled reddened and crusting blisters. The pain may precede the rash by 1–2 days. Early antiviral therapy can reduce the severity of post-herpetic neuralgia; important to consider for elderly people	**	A41: Red flags of diseases of the skin (6.1c)
Complications of acute otitis media: persistent fever/pain/confusion for >3–4 days after the onset of the earache (may indicate spread of the infection, e.g. mastoiditis or brain abscess)	**	A43: Red flags of diseases of the ear (6.1e)
Mastoiditis: fever, with a painful and swollen mastoid bone. This deep bone infection is unlikely to settle without antibiotic therapy	**	A43: Red flags of diseases of the ear (6.1e)
Discharge from the eye. If severe, prolonged for >5 days and painful, or if seen in the following vulnerable groups: • newborns • immunocompromised people • malnourished people	**	A42: Red flags of diseases of the eye (6.1d)

Pronounced features of candidal infection (thrush) of the skin or mucous membranes of the mouth: suggests underlying diabetes or immune deficiency	*	A4: Red flags of diseases of the mouth (3.1c) A41: Red flags of diseases of the skin (6.1c)
Pelvic inflammatory disease (chronic form): vaginal discharge, gripy abdominal pain, pain on intercourse, dysmenorrhea, infertility	**/*	A35: Red flags of sexually transmitted diseases (5.2d)
Discharge from penis: may indicate sexually transmitted disease	**	A35: Red flags of sexually transmitted diseases (5.2d)
Fever with rash in the first trimester of pregnancy: refer suspected rubella or chickenpox so that the health of the embryo/fetus can be monitored	**	A37: Red flags of pregnancy (5.3d)
Offensive, fishy, watery discharge in pregnancy (possible bacterial vaginosis): can increase risk of early labor	**	A35: Red flags of sexually transmitted diseases (5.2d)
Fever with rash in the last trimester of pregnancy: refer if chickenpox or shingles suspected, as there is a risk of fatal fetal varicella infection	**	A37: Red flags of pregnancy (5.3d)
Outbreak of genital herpes in the last trimester of pregnancy: refer because if apparent during labor herpes virus can be transmitted to the baby. Planned cesarean section may be indicated	*	A35: Red flags of sexually transmitted diseases (5.2d)
Poor wound healing, especially in the feet and legs: might suggest diabetes mellitus or immune deficiency	**/*	A32: Red flags of diabetes mellitus (5.1d)
Increased tendency to infections such as cystitis, boils and oral thrush (candidiasis): might suggest diabetes mellitus or immune deficiency	*	A32: Red flags of diabetes mellitus (5.1d)

B23: Red flags of jaundice

Symptoms and signs	Priority	Chapter reference
Right hypochondriac pain that is very intense and comes in waves; associated with jaundice. Acute cholecystitis: may be associated with fever and vomiting. This is one of the manifestations of the acute abdomen	***/**	A9: Red flags of diseases of the gallbladder (3.1d)
Jaundice (yellowish skin, yellow whites of the eyes, and possibly dark urine and pale stools): itch may be a prominent symptom. Always refer any case of jaundice, as it more often than not results from serious disease of the liver, gallbladder, pancreas or blood	**	A7: Red flags of diseases of the pancreas (3.1d) A8: Red flags of diseases of the liver (3.1d) A9: Red flags of diseases of the gallbladder (3.1d)

B24: Red flags of lumps, masses and glands

Symptoms and signs	Priority	Chapter reference
A single, grossly enlarged tonsil: patient unwell, feverish and has foul-smelling breath. This suggests quinsy, which is a surgical emergency as breathing may be compromised	***/**	A16: Red flags of upper respiratory disease (3.3c)
Tender or inflamed gums or salivary glands that do not respond within days to treatment	**	A4: Red flags of diseases of the mouth (3.1c)
Any unexplained lump >1cm in diameter: especially if hard, irregular, fixed and painless	*	A1: Red flags of cancer (2.3)

A single markedly enlarged lymph node (>2cm in diameter) with no obvious cause	*	A1: Red flags of cancer (2.3) A20: Red flags of leukemia and lymphoma (3.4e)
Multiple enlarged painless lymph nodes (>1cm in diameter) with no other obvious cause (e.g. known glandular fever infection)	*	A1: Red flags of cancer (2.3) A20: Red flags of leukemia and lymphoma (3.4e)
A single, grossly enlarged tonsil: patient generally well. If patient appears well, lymphoma is a possible diagnosis. Systemic symptoms may include fever, night sweats and weight loss	*	A16: Red flags of upper respiratory disease (3.3c)
Painless enlargement of a salivary gland over weeks to months: possible salivary tumor	*	A4: Red flags of diseases of the mouth (3.1c)
Painful or painless enlargement of a salivary gland immediately after eating: suggests salivary gland stone; refer if does not settle down in a week, or sooner if painful	*	A4: Red flags of diseases of the mouth (3.1c)
Goiter: refer only if symptoms of hyperthyroidism or hypothyroidism are present, or if the goiter is tender, irregular or noticeably enlarging. Small, smooth, rubbery goiters are common and benign	*	A31: Red flags of diseases of the thyroid gland (5.1c)
Any lump in the breast: refer, as one in ten of all breast lumps show malignant change	*	A39: Red flags of diseases of the breast (5.3f)
Any lump in the testis: refer as, although usually benign, early diagnosis of testicular cancer has a very good prognosis	*	A36: Red flags of structural disorders of the reproductive system (5.2g)
Breast tissue development in adult men (gynecomastia): although common, benign and transitory in teenage boys, breast lumps in men should be referred to exclude cancer	*	A39: Red flags of diseases of the breast (5.3f)
Abdominal swelling: discrete mass in suprapubic or iliac fossa regions: possible fibroids, ovarian cyst, tumor, pregnancy	*	A36: Red flags of structural disorders of the reproductive system (5.2g)
Signs of an inguinal hernia: swelling in groin that is more pronounced on standing, especially if uncomfortable	*	A10: Red flags of disorders of the small intestine and large intestine (3.1e)
Painless lump felt in anus: refer to exclude serious conditions of anal warts and anal carcinoma	*	A10: Red flags of disorders of the small intestine and large intestine (3.1e)
Painful lump felt in anus: refer to exclude strangulated hemorrhoid, which will require a surgical opinion	**/*	A10: Red flags of disorders of the small intestine and large intestine (3.1e)
Any lumps/moles with features suggestive of malignancy: irregularity, a tendency to bleed, crusting, >5mm in diameter, intense black color	*	A41: Red flags of diseases of the skin (6.1c)

B25: Red flags of disorders of menstruation

Symptoms and signs	Priority	Chapter reference
Postpartum hemorrhage: refer if bleeding is any more than a blood-stained discharge after childbirth. A profuse bleed of >500ml or the symptoms of shock (low blood pressure, fainting, rapid pulse rate) constitutes an emergency	***/**	A38: Red flags of the puerperium (5.3e)
Menorrhagia with features of severe anemia (tiredness, breathlessness, palpitations on exertion)	**	A34: Red flags of menstruation (5.2c)
Vaginal discharge: if irregular, blood stained or unusual smell	**/*	A35: Red flags of sexually transmitted diseases (5.2d)
Hyperthyroidism. Symptoms: irritability, anxiety, sleeplessness, increased appetite, loose stools, weight loss, scanty periods and heat intolerance. Signs: sweaty skin, tremor of the hands, staring eyes and rapid pulse	**/*	A31: Red flags of diseases of the thyroid gland (5.1c)
Postmenopausal bleeding: any unexplained bleeding after the menopause	*	A34: Red flags of menstruation (5.2c)
Vulval itch or vaginal discharge in postmenopausal women	*	A36: Red flags of structural disorders of the reproductive system (5.2g)
Pelvic inflammatory disease (chronic form): vaginal discharge, gripy abdominal pain, pain on intercourse, dysmenorrhea, infertility	*	A35: Red flags of sexually transmitted diseases (5.2d)
Primary amenorrhea: after age 16	*	A34: Red flags of menstruation (5.2c)
Secondary amenorrhea: for >12 months	*	A34: Red flags of menstruation (5.2c)
Metrorrhagia: bleeding between periods that has no regular pattern. This includes postcoital bleeding (bleeding after intercourse)	*	A34: Red flags of menstruation (5.2c)
Severe disturbance of body image: with features of progressive anorexia nervosa or bulimia nervosa (e.g. progressive weight loss, secondary amenorrhea, or repeated compulsion to bring about vomiting) and not responding to your treatment in 3 weeks	*	A44: Red flags of mental health disorders (6.2e)
Hypopituitarism: loss of libido, infertility, menstrual disturbances, tiredness, low blood pressure, inappropriate lactation	*	A33: Red flags of the less common endocrine diseases (5.1e)

B26: Red flags of disorders of the mouth

Symptoms and signs	Priority	Chapter reference
Painful ulceration of mouth: if persistent or if preventing proper hydration	**/*	A4: Red flags of diseases of the mouth (3.1c)
Enlarged or inflamed gums or salivary glands that do not respond within days to treatment	**/*	A4: Red flags of diseases of the mouth (3.1c)
Long-standing anemia: pallor, tiredness, breathlessness on exertion, feeling of faintness, depression, sore mouth and tongue	**/*	A18: Red flags of anemia (3.4c)
Persistent oral thrush (candidiasis) (appearing as a thick white coating on tongue or palate): suggests underlying diabetes mellitus or immune deficiency	*	A4: Red flags of diseases of the mouth (3.1c)
Persistent, painless, white plaque (leukoplakia) on the tongue (appearing as a coat that appears to sit on the surface of the sides of the tongue): this is a premalignant change	*	A4: Red flags of diseases of the mouth (3.1c)

B27: Red flags of muscle tremor and spasms

Symptoms and signs	Priority	Chapter reference
Tremor with features of hyperthyroidism (symptoms and signs tend to be progressive over the course of a few months). Symptoms: irritability, anxiety, sleeplessness, increased appetite, loose stools, weight loss, scanty periods and heat intolerance. Signs: sweaty skin, staring eyes and rapid pulse	**/*	A31: Red flags of diseases of the thyroid gland (5.1c)
First-ever epileptic seizure – focal simple seizures: episodes of coarse twitching of one part of the body	**	A22: Red flags of brain hemorrhage, stroke and brain tumor (4.1d)
Progressive coarse tremor appearing in middle to late life: possible Parkinson's or Huntingdon's disease (coarse tremor); distinguish from benign essential tremor (a fine tremor that worsens with anxiety), which does not require referral	*	A24: Red flags of dementia, epilepsy and other disorders of the central nervous system (4.1f)

B28: Red flags of numbness

Symptoms and signs	Priority	Chapter reference
An unexplained temporary loss of brain function (usually <2 hours long): including loss of consciousness, loss of vision, unsteadiness, confusion, loss of memory, loss of sensation or limb weakness. This is a transient ischemic attack until proved otherwise. Could also be the first presentation of migrainous aura	**	A22: Red flags of brain hemorrhage, stroke and brain tumor (4.1d) A24: Red flags of dementia, epilepsy and other disorders of the central nervous system (4.1f)
A persisting loss of brain function: including loss of vision, unsteadiness, confusion, loss of memory, and loss of sensation or muscle weakness. This could be the result of a stroke, or a relapse of multiple sclerosis	**	A22: Red flags of brain hemorrhage, stroke and brain tumor (4.1d) A24: Red flags of dementia, epilepsy and other disorders of the central nervous system (4.1f)
A loss of brain function that is progressive over the course of days to weeks: this is more suggestive of a brain tumor than a stroke	**	A22: Red flags of brain hemorrhage, stroke and brain tumor (4.1d)
Any other sudden or gradual onset of unexplained severe numbness or pins and needles: all possible causes of polyneuropathy or mononeuropathy merit investigation	**	A25: Red flags of diseases of the spinal cord and peripheral nerves (4.1g)
Intervertebral disc prolapse and severe nerve root irritation: sudden onset of low back pain that is so severe that walking is impossible (severe sciatica). Sciatica alone is not absolute indication for referral. Refer if there is difficulty in urinating or defecating, or if the condition is progressive or not responding to treatment	**	A27: Red flags of localized diseases of the joints, ligaments and muscles (4.2e)
Pernicious anemia: tiredness, lemon-yellow pallor and gradual onset of neurological symptoms (numbness, weakness, confusion)	**/*	A18: Red flags of anemia (3.4c)

B29: Red flags of pain in the bones, joints or muscles

Symptoms and signs	Priority	Chapter reference
Limb infarction (suddenly extremely pale, painful, mottled and cold limb): results from a clot in major artery. The life of the limb is threatened	***	A11: Red flags of diseases of the blood vessels (3.2c)
Polymyalgia rheumatica with new onset of one-sided headache: prolonged pain and stiffness of the muscles of the hips and shoulders, associated with malaise and depression. Refer urgently if there is a sudden onset of a severe, one-sided temporal headache or visual disturbances (possible temporal arteritis)	***/**	A28: Red flags of generalized diseases of the joints, ligaments and muscles (4.2f)
Severely compromised circulation to the extremities: pain in the calf that is related to exercise and relieved by rest. Pain in the calf in bed at night relieved by hanging the leg out of bed (i.e. not cramp). Cold, purplish, shiny skin. Areas of blackened skin (gangrene)	**/*	A11: Red flags of diseases of the blood vessels (3.2c)
Deep vein thrombosis: hot, swollen, tender calf; can be accompanied by fever and malaise. Increased risk after air travel and surgery, in pregnancy and cancer, and if on the oral contraceptive pill	**	A11: Red flags of diseases of the blood vessels (3.2c)
Bone pain: characteristically fixed and deep. It may have either an aching or a boring quality. Tenderness on palpation and on percussion. Refer to exclude underlying inflammation or fracture of the bone, both of which result from serious conditions	**/*	A26: Red flags of diseases of the bones (4.2d)
Inflammatory arthritis: symmetrical pain, stiffness and swelling of the joints, or symmetrical stiffness and pain in the sacroiliac joint. May be associated with fever or a sense of malaise	**/*	A28: Red flags of generalized diseases of the joints, ligaments and muscles (4.2f)
Septic or crystal arthritis: a single, hot, swollen and very tender joint. The patient is unwell. Risk of inflammatory damage to the joint	**	A27: Red flags of localized diseases of the joints, ligaments and muscles (4.2e)
Degenerative arthritis that may benefit from joint replacement: severe disability from long-standing pain and stiffness in the hips, knees or shoulders	*	A28: Red flags of generalized diseases of the joints, ligaments and muscles (4.2f)
Traumatic injury to a muscle or joint (which may require surgical treatment or immobilization): sudden onset of pain or swelling in a joint (possible hemarthrosis); sudden severe pain and swelling around a joint, with reluctance to move (sprain or strain or possible fracture); locking of the knee joint (meniscal cartilage tear); sudden onset of tender swelling in a muscle (possible hematoma)	**	A27: Red flags of localized diseases of the joints, ligaments and muscles (4.2e)
Intervertebral disc prolapse and severe nerve root irritation: sudden onset of low back pain that is so severe that walking is impossible (severe sciatica). Difficulty urinating or defecating	**	A27: Red flags of localized diseases of the joints, ligaments and muscles (4.2e)
Pubic symphysis pain in pregnancy: refer if the patient is significantly hindered in activities of daily living	**	A37: Red flags of pregnancy (5.3d)
Persistent loin pain (i.e. pain in the flanks either side of the spine between the levels of T11 and L3): pain might be radiating from the kidneys	**	A29: Red flags of diseases of the kidneys (4.3c)

B30: Red flags of palpitations or abnormal pulse rate

Symptoms and signs	Priority	Chapter reference
Unstable angina or heart attack: sustained, intense chest pain associated with fear or dread. Palpitations and breathlessness may be present. The patient may vomit or develop a cold sweat. Beware: In elderly people can present as sudden onset of breathlessness, palpitations or confusion, but without pain	***	A13: Red flags of angina and heart attack (3.2e)
General symptoms of shock: dizziness, fainting and confusion. Rapid pulse of >100 beats/minute. Blood pressure <90/60mmHg. Cold and clammy extremities. Refer if these symptoms are worsening or sustained (more than a few seconds)	***	A19: Red flags of hemorrhage and shock (3.4d)
A very rapid pulse (140–250 beats/minute): most likely to be supraventricular tachycardia or atrial fibrillation. Refer urgently if ongoing, and as a high priority if it has settled down but was the first-ever episode	***/**	A14: Red flags of heart failure and arrhythmias (3.2f)
A very slow pulse (40–50 beats/minute) (complete heart block): refer if either of recent onset or if associated with features of shock, such as dizziness, light-headedness or fainting	***/**	A14: Red flags of heart failure and arrhythmias (3.2f)
Severe chronic heart failure: marked swelling of the ankles and lower legs, palpitations, disabling breathlessness, exhaustion	**	A14: Red flags of heart failure and arrhythmias (3.2f)
Complicated pericarditis: palpitations, fever and sharp central chest pain that is worse on leaning forward and lying down. There may be breathlessness due to acute cardiac failure. This is a serious sign	**	A15: Red flags of pericarditis (3.2g)
An irregularly irregular pulse (atrial fibrillation): refer, as there is a risk of embolic stroke as small blood clots can develop in chaotically contracting atria of the heart	**/*	A14: Red flags of heart failure and arrhythmias (3.2f)
Palpitations in pregnancy: refer if it seems that there is any form of arrhythmia in pregnancy. The increased cardiac output in pregnancy can expose previously undiagnosed congenital heart disease	**	A37: Red flags of pregnancy (5.3d)
Hyperthyroidism (symptoms and signs tend to be progressive over the course of a few months). Symptoms: irritability, palpitations, anxiety, sleeplessness, increased appetite, loose stools, weight loss, scanty periods and heat intolerance. Signs: sweaty skin, tremor of the hands, staring eyes and rapid pulse	**/*	A31: Red flags of diseases of the thyroid gland (5.1c)
A pulse that is regular but skips beats at regular intervals (i.e. one out of every 3–5 beats is missing): suggests incomplete heart block. This is an arrhythmia that may precede more serious arrhythmias. Refer for investigation of cause	*	A14: Red flags of heart failure and arrhythmias (3.2f)
Hypothyroidism (symptoms and signs tend to be progressive over the course of a few months). Symptoms: tiredness, depression, weight gain, heavy periods, constipation and cold intolerance. Signs: dry puffy skin, dry and thin hair, slow pulse	*	A31: Red flags of diseases of the thyroid gland (5.1c)

B31: Red flags of pregnancy and the puerperium

Symptoms and signs	Priority	Chapter reference
Pre-eclampsia/HELLP syndromes: headache, abdominal pain, visual disturbance, nausea and vomiting, and edema (in middle to late pregnancy). These symptoms and signs are serious indicators of the dangerous syndromes of eclampsia and hemolysis/liver abnormalities and low platelets, both of which can threaten the life of the mother and the fetus	***	A37: Red flags of pregnancy (5.3d)
Thromboembolism: pain in the calf, swollen or discolored leg, or breathlessness with chest pain, or blood in sputum in pregnancy or the puerperium. These symptoms and signs are serious at all times, but are listed here as they are more likely to develop in pregnancy and the puerperium, as there is an increased tendency for the blood to form clots at these stages	***	A37: Red flags of pregnancy (5.3d)
Abdominal pain: refer any episode of sustained abdominal pain in pregnancy as an emergency, particularly if any signs of shock are apparent (low blood pressure, fainting, rapid pulse), as internal bleeding may not be immediately apparent. Abdominal pain may be the first sign of pre-eclampsia. Periodic mild cramping sensations in later pregnancy (lasting no more than a few seconds) are likely to be Braxton Hicks contractions, but if becoming regular and intensifying, beware that these might signify premature labor (by definition, before week 36 of pregnancy)	***	A37: Red flags of pregnancy (5.3d)
Bleeding: refer any episode of vaginal bleeding in pregnancy. Refer as an emergency if any signs of shock are apparent (low blood pressure, fainting, rapid pulse), as internal bleeding may not be immediately apparent	***/**	A37: Red flags of pregnancy (5.3d)
Postnatal psychosis: delusional or paranoid ideas and hallucinations are key features. This condition is associated with a high risk of suicide or harm to the baby	***/**	A38: Red flags of the puerperium (5.3e)
Nausea and vomiting with dehydration for >1 day in pregnancy	**	A37: Red flags of pregnancy (5.3d)
Moderate to severe pregnancy-induced hypertension: refer as a high priority if the diastolic pressure is >100mmHg or if the systolic pressure is >140mmHg	**	A37: Red flags of pregnancy (5.3d)
Mild pregnancy-induced hypertension: refer for assessment if diastolic pressure is 90–99mmHg and systolic pressure is <140mmHg	**	A37: Red flags of pregnancy (5.3d)
Fever with rash in the first trimester of pregnancy: refer suspected rubella or chickenpox so that health of the embryo/fetus can be monitored	**	A37: Red flags of pregnancy (5.3d)
Fever with rash in the last trimester of pregnancy: refer if chickenpox or shingles is suspected, as there is a risk of fatal fetal varicella infection	**	A37: Red flags of pregnancy (5.3d)
Offensive, fishy, watery discharge: possible bacterial vaginosis; there is an increased risk of stillbirth and premature labor	**	A35: Red flags of sexually transmitted diseases (5.2d)
Any watery vaginal leakage in middle to late pregnancy: this is amniotic fluid until proved otherwise	**	A37: Red flags of pregnancy (5.3d)
Fever in the puerperium: refer any case of fever developing in the first 2 weeks of the puerperium (temperature >38°C for >24 hours) as there is a risk this could result from uterine infection	**	A38: Red flags of the puerperium (5.3e)
Mastitis when breastfeeding, if not responding to treatment in 2 days, or if there are features of an abscess: mastitis is very debilitating, and if not settling may need antibiotic treatment	**/*	A38: Red flags of the puerperium (5.3e)

Insufficient breast milk or sore nipples: if the mother is considering stopping breastfeeding because of insufficient milk or soreness, refer to the midwife, health visitor or breastfeeding counselor for breastfeeding advice; the problem may be in the technique, and not a true reflection of low milk production	**/*	A38: Red flags of the puerperium (5.3e)
Postnatal depression lasting for >3 weeks and not responding to treatment: refer straight away if the woman is experiencing suicidal ideas, or if you believe the health of the baby to be at risk	**/*	A38: Red flags of the puerperium (5.3e)
Itching (severe), especially of the palms and soles in pregnancy: may result from cholestasis (buildup of bile salts); refer, as there is a theoretical risk to the health of the fetus if levels rise too high	**	A41: Red flags of diseases of the skin (6.1c)
Edema in pregnancy: refer all but mild ankle swelling; may result from a kidney or heart problem	*	A37: Red flags of pregnancy (5.3d)
Pubic symphysis pain in pregnancy: refer if the patient is significantly hindered in activities of daily living, as the prescription of a pelvic brace can be a great help	*	A37: Red flags of pregnancy (5.3d)
Anemia in pregnancy: the risks of bleeding during labor are higher in women with anemia, so refer for assessment and advice about treatment	*	A37: Red flags of pregnancy (5.3d)
Outbreak of genital herpes in the last trimester of pregnancy: may be an indication for a cesarean section to prevent the baby contracting the herpes virus (can be fatal) as it passes through the birth canal	*	A35: Red flags of sexually transmitted diseases (5.2d)
Potential pregnancy-induced hypertension: refer for assessment if systolic pressure has risen by 30mmHg or diastolic pressure by 15mmHg above any measurement taken previously	*	A37: Red flags of pregnancy (5.3d)

B32: Red flags of diseases of the skin		
Symptoms and signs	**Priority**	**Chapter reference**
Progressive swelling of the soft tissues of the face and neck (angio-edema) and/or urticaria (nettle rash): refer urgently if there are any features of respiratory distress (itchy throat, wheeze)	***	A41: Red flags of diseases of the skin (6.1c)
Meningococcal septicemia: acute onset of a purpuric rash, possibly accompanied by headache, vomiting and fever	***	A11: Red flags of diseases of the blood vessels (3.2c)
Bruising and non-blanching rash, together with a severe headache that develops over the course of a few hours to days with fever: suggests meningococcal meningitis	***	A23: Red flags of headache (4.1e)
Purpura or bruising rash (non-blanching): suggests a bleeding disorder or vasculitis. Refer if unexplained, and as a high priority if extensive or rapidly extending	***/**	A41: Red flags of diseases of the skin (6.1c)
Large areas of redness affecting most (>90%) of the body surface (erythroderma): refer because of the risk of dehydration and loss of essential salts	***/**	A41: Red flags of diseases of the skin (6.1c)
A rapidly enlarging patch(es) of painful, crusting or swollen red skin (impetigo or erysipelas): if spreading, refer as a high priority for antibiotic treatment. Refer with some urgency if this occurs in someone with eczema (possible viral eczema herpeticum)	**	A41: Red flags of diseases of the skin (6.1c)
Early shingles: intense, one-sided pain, with an overlying rash of crops of fluid-filled reddened and crusting blisters. The pain may precede the rash by 1–2 days. The pain and rash correspond in location to a neurological dermatome. Refer for early consideration of antiviral treatment	**	A41: Red flags of diseases of the skin (6.1c)

A rapidly advancing region or line of redness tracking up the skin of a limb (following the pathway of a lymphatic vessel): cellulitis and/or lymphangitis	**	A41: Red flags of diseases of the skin (6.1c)
Any new skin ulcer: refer any break in the skin that is not starting to heal within 3 days, or earlier if the margins of the break are widening, or if there are any signs of infection (pus and offensive smell). Be particularly cautious in elderly people and those with diabetes	**	A41: Red flags of diseases of the skin (6.1c)
Cold, purplish, shiny skin suggesting severely compromised circulation to the extremities: may be associated with pain in the calf that relates to exercise and is relieved by rest. Pain in the calf in bed at night relieved by hanging the leg out of bed (i.e. not cramp). These are serious signs of narrowing of the arteries in the pelvis and legs. Refer as high priority if there are areas of blackened skin (gangrene)	**/*	A11: Red flags of diseases of the blood vessels (3.2c)
Generalized macular rash (flat red spots): refer for notification if you suspect rubella, measles or scarlet fever (rash accompanied by significant fever)	**/*	A41: Red flags of diseases of the skin (6.1c)
Lumps/moles with features suggestive of malignancy: • irregularity • recently changing • tendency to bleed • crusting • >5mm in diameter • intense black color	*	A41: Red flags of diseases of the skin (6.1c)
Hirsutism (unexplained hairiness): refer to exclude endocrine disease or polycystic ovary syndrome	*	A41: Red flags of diseases of the skin (6.1c)
Itching (severe), especially of the palms and soles in pregnancy: possible cholestasis; refer, as high levels of bile salts may damage the fetus if prolonged	*	A41: Red flags of diseases of the skin (6.1c)
Generalized itch: refer if cause unknown	*	A41: Red flags of diseases of the skin (6.1c)
Pronounced features of candidal infection (thrush) of the skin or mucous membranes of the mouth: suggests underlying diabetes or immunodeficiency	*	A41: Red flags of diseases of the skin (6.1c)
Vaginal itch, if persisting for >3 weeks: the most common cause is candidiasis (thrush), but this should be self-limiting. If persisting, refer to exclude an underlying cause, such as immunodeficiency, malignancy or lichen sclerosus	*	A35: Red flags of sexually transmitted disease (5.2d)
Anal itch, if persisting for >3 weeks: the most common cause is hemorrhoids with skin tags. If persisting, refer to exclude a serious underlying cause, such as anal carcinoma or lichen sclerosus	*	A41: Red flags of diseases of the skin (6.1c)
Eczema of the nipple region (possible Paget's disease)	*	A39: Red flags of diseases of the breast (5.3f)

B33: Red flags of disorders of speech

Symptoms and signs	Priority	Chapter reference
Persistent loss of ability to speak clearly: might result from a persistent loss of brain function (other features include loss of vision, unsteadiness, confusion, loss of memory, loss of sensation, or muscle weakness). Most likely cause is stroke (thrombotic or hemorrhagic). Needs referring urgently for rapid access to hospital treatment	***	A22: Red flags of brain hemorrhage, stroke and brain tumor (4.1d) A24: Red flags of dementia, epilepsy and other disorders of the central nervous system (4.1f)
Brief loss of ability to speak clearly: suggests a temporary loss of brain function (usually <2 hours), such as loss of consciousness, loss of vision, unsteadiness, confusion, loss of memory, loss of sensation or limb weakness. If migraine not previously diagnosed, most likely cause is transient ischemic attack	**	A22: Red flags of brain hemorrhage, stroke and brain tumor (4.1d) A24: Red flags of dementia, epilepsy and other disorders of the central nervous system (4.1f)
Progressive loss of ability to speak clearly: may result from a loss of brain function that is progressive over the course of days to weeks. This is more suggestive of a brain tumor than a stroke. Could also result from multiple sclerosis or motor neuron disease	**	A22: Red flags of brain hemorrhage, stroke and brain tumor (4.1d)
Unexplained hoarseness lasting for >3 weeks: may be the first symptom of laryngeal or lung cancer (particularly in smokers >50 years)	*	A17: Red flags of lower respiratory disease (3.3e)

B34: Red flags of disorders of swallowing

Symptoms and signs	Priority	Chapter reference
Difficulty swallowing (dysphagia) that is worse with solids (in particular, if progressive over days to weeks): suggests a physical obstruction and, if progressive, esophageal cancer is a possible diagnosis (weight loss is strongly suggestive of this). Other possible causes are esophageal stricture, esophageal web (can form in severe anemia) and candidiasis of the esophagus (a feature of AIDS). Neurological disease (e.g. stroke and motor neuron disease) can also cause dysfunctional swallowing, and in this case even swallowing of fluids may be difficult. Refer for diagnosis and treatment. Discomfort in swallowing that does not affect the eating of solids or drinking is very likely to be benign, and does not merit referral	**/*	A5: Red flags of diseases of the esophagus (3.1c)
Difficulty swallowing (dysphagia) associated with enlarged lymph nodes in the neck: lymph node enlargement suggests the possibility of cancer or an inflammatory mass in the neck (e.g. tuberculous abscess)	**/*	A5: Red flags of diseases of the esophagus (3.1c)
Swallowing associated with central chest pain (behind the sternum): may result from esophageal inflammation, an esophageal tear or a lodged foreign body (fish bone). Refer if persisting for more than a day, or if getting worse	**	A5: Red flags of diseases of the esophagus (3.1c)

B35: Red flags of thirst

Symptoms and signs	Priority	Chapter reference
Type 1 diabetes or poorly controlled type 2 diabetes: short history of thirst, weight loss and excessive urination, which is rapidly progressive in severity	***/**	A32: Red flags of diabetes mellitus (5.1d)
Type 2 diabetes: general feeling of unwellness, with thirst and increased need to urinate large amounts of urine. These symptoms develop over the course of weeks to months	**/*	A32: Red flags of diabetes mellitus (5.1d)

B36: Red flags of urinary disorders

Symptoms and signs	Priority	Chapter reference
Type 1 diabetes or poorly controlled type 2 diabetes: short history of thirst, weight loss and excessive urination, which is rapidly progressive in severity	***/**	A32: Red flags of diabetes mellitus (5.1d)
Type 2 diabetes: general feeling of malaise, with thirst and increased need to urinate large amounts of urine. These symptoms develop over the course of weeks to months	**/*	A32: Red flags of diabetes mellitus (5.1d)
Urinary tract infection (cloudy urine, painful urination, low abdominal pain, fever) in someone in one of the following vulnerable groups: • pre-existing disorder of the urinary system • diabetes • pregnancy	**	A30: Red flags of diseases of the ureters, bladder and the urethra (4.3d)
Vesico-ureteric reflux disease in a child: any history of recurrent episodes or a current episode of cloudy urine or burning on urination should be taken seriously in a prepubescent child	**/*	A29: Red flags of diseases of the kidneys (4.3c) A30: Red flags of diseases of the ureters, bladder and the urethra (4.3d)
Recurrent or persistent urinary tract infection: recurrent episodes of symptoms including some or all of cloudy urine, burning on urination, abdominal discomfort, blood in urine and fever, especially if occurring in men. Need to exclude an underlying cause	**/*	A30: Red flags of diseases of the ureters, bladder and the urethra (4.3d)
Acute pyelonephritis: fever, malaise, loin pain and cloudy urine suggest an infection of the kidneys	**	A29: Red flags of diseases of the kidneys (4.3c) A30: Red flags of diseases of the ureters, bladder and the urethra (4.3d)
Blood in the urine (hematuria) or sperm (hemospermia): refer all cases in men. Refer in women, except in the case of acute urinary infection	**/*	A30: Red flags of diseases of the ureters, bladder and the urethra (4.3d)
Intervertebral disc prolapse and severe nerve root irritation: sudden onset of low back pain that is so severe that walking is impossible (severe sciatica); difficulty urinating or defecating	**	A27: Red flags of localized diseases of the joints, ligaments and muscles (4.2e)
Cauda equina syndrome: numbness of the buttocks and perineum (saddle anesthesia), with bilateral numbness or sciatica in the legs. Difficulties in urination or defecation are serious symptoms	**	A25: Red flags of diseases of the spinal cord and peripheral nerves (4.1g)
Moderate prostatic obstruction: enlargement of the prostate gland leads to symptoms such as increasing difficulty urinating and the need to get up at night to urinate (nocturia). Refer to assess severity and to exclude prostate cancer	*	A30: Red flags of diseases of the ureters, bladder and the urethra (4.3d)

Bedwetting, if persisting over the age of 5: refer to exclude a physical or emotional cause	*	A30: Red flags of diseases of the ureters, bladder and the urethra (4.3d)
Incontinence, if unexplained or causing distress: refer for investigations and advice from an incontinence specialist nurse	*	A30: Red flags of diseases of the ureters, bladder and the urethra (4.3d)

B37: Red flags of visual disturbance

Symptoms and signs	Priority	Chapter reference
Blurred vision in malignant hypertension: diastolic pressure >120mmHg, with symptoms including recently worsening headaches, blurred vision and chest pain	***/**	A12: Red flags of hypertension (3.2d)
Blurred vision in pre-eclampsia/HELLP syndromes: headache, abdominal pain, visual disturbance, nausea and vomiting, and edema (in middle to late pregnancy)	***	A37: Red flags of pregnancy (5.3d)
Sudden blurring of vision with a one-sided headache in an older person: consider temporal arteritis if there is no history of migraine. Refer urgently for steroid treatment, as the risk of blindness and stroke is high	***	A42: Red flags of diseases of the eye (6.1d)
A temporary, persisting or progressive loss of clarity of sight due to brain dysfunction: may result from loss of brain function in migraine, transient ischemic attack or stroke. Other symptoms include loss of consciousness, loss of vision, unsteadiness, confusion, loss of memory, loss of sensation or limb weakness. Refer urgently if the loss of brain function is persisting and as a high priority if temporary	**/***	A22: Red flags of brain hemorrhage, stroke and brain tumor (4.1d) A24: Red flags of dementia, epilepsy and other disorders of the central nervous system (4.1f)
Painless sudden loss of sight: may result from retinal detachment, vitreous detachment or retinal artery thrombosis. Refer as a high priority to the emergency department, as retinal detachment is treatable if caught early	**	A42: Red flags of diseases of the eye (6.1d)
Visual disturbance from the growth of a pituitary tumor: features include progressive headaches, visual disturbance and double vision	**/*	A33: Red flags of the less common endocrine diseases (5.1e)
Severe anemia: extreme tiredness and breathlessness on exertion, excessive bruising and severe visual disturbances suggest that the anemia is very severe. There may also be features of strain on the cardiovascular system: chest pain on exertion, features of tachycardia and increasing edema	**	A18: Red flags of anemia (3.4c)
Thyroid eye disease (vision only affected if very advanced). Symptoms: irritability, anxiety, sleeplessness, increased appetite, loose stools, weight loss, scanty periods and heat intolerance. Signs: sweaty skin, tremor of the hands, staring eyes and rapid pulse	**/*	A31: Red flags of diseases of the thyroid gland (5.1c)
Optic neuritis: blurred vision with deep aching pain in the eye. Associated with multiple sclerosis. Refer for diagnosis	**	A42: Red flags of diseases of the eye (6.1d)

B38: Red flags of vomiting and/or passage of feces

Symptoms and signs	Priority	Chapter reference
Severe headache that develops over the course of a few hours to days, with fever, together with either vomiting or neck stiffness: possible acute meningitis or encephalitis	***	A23: Red flags of headache (4.1e)
Meningococcal septicemia: acute onset of purpuric rash, possibly accompanied by headache, vomiting and fever	***	A11: Red flags of diseases of the blood vessels (3.2c)
Diarrhea and vomiting associated with features of dehydration	***/**	A6: Red flags of diseases of the stomach (3.1c)
Severe diarrhea and vomiting if lasting >24 hours in infants or elderly people	***/**	A6: Red flags of diseases of the stomach (3.1c)
Projectile vomiting persisting for >2 days	***/**	A6: Red flags of diseases of the stomach (3.1c)
Vomiting of fresh blood or altered blood (looks like dark gravel or coffee grounds)	***/**	A6: Red flags of diseases of the stomach (3.1c) A8: Red flags of diseases of the liver (3.1d)
Right hypochondriac pain that is very intense and comes in waves: may be associated with fever and vomiting. May be associated with jaundice. This is one of the manifestations of the acute abdomen	***/**	A9: Red flags of diseases of the gallbladder (3.1d)
Addison's disease: increased pigmentation of skin, weight loss, muscle wasting, tiredness, loss of libido, low blood pressure, diarrhea and vomiting, confusion, collapse with dehydration	***/**	A33: Red flags of the less common endocrine diseases (5.1e)
Diarrhea and/or vomiting in an elderly person: treat with caution, as elderly people are prone to dehydration, and diarrhea and vomiting may be presenting features of more serious underlying disease	**	A2: Red flags of infectious diseases: vulnerable groups (2.4c)
Diarrhea and/or vomiting in infants (especially if <3 months old): treat with caution, as infants are prone to dehydration, and diarrhea and vomiting may be presenting features of more serious underlying disease	**	A2: Red flags of infectious diseases: vulnerable groups (2.4c)
Diarrhea and/or vomiting in an immunocompromised person: treat with caution; diarrhea and vomiting may be features of a serious infection in people who are immunocompromised	**	A2: Red flags of infectious diseases: vulnerable groups (2.4c)
Diarrhea and vomiting if continuing for >5 days in otherwise healthy adults: most mild infections should have settled down in 2–3 days; needs further investigation	**	A6: Red flags of diseases of the stomach (3.1c)
Diarrhea with mucus or gripy pain if not responding to treatment within a week: possible inflammatory bowel disease or parasitic infection	**	A10: Red flags of diseases of the small intestine and large intestine (3.1e)
Altered bowel habit lasting for >3 weeks in a patient >50 years	**/*	A10: Red flags of diseases of the small intestine and large intestine (3.1e)
Dysentery or food poisoning (any episode of diarrhea and vomiting in which food is suspected as the origin or in which blood appears in the stools): notifiable diseases	**	A10: Red flags of diseases of the small intestine and large intestine (3.1e)
Nausea and vomiting with dehydration (dry skin, dry mouth, low blood pressure, low skin turgor) for >1 day in pregnancy: patient may need fluid replacement	**	A37: Red flags of pregnancy (5.3d)
Cauda equina syndrome: numbness of the buttocks and perineum (saddle anesthesia), with bilateral numbness or sciatica in the legs; difficulty in urination or defecation are serious symptoms	**	A25: Red flags of diseases of the spinal cord and peripheral nerves (4.1g)

Soiling of stool or anal discharge (in underwear or bed) in a previously continent child or adult: may signify constipation in both children and elderly people, and also emotional distress in a child. In adults anal discharge may be a sign of anorectal carcinoma	*	A10: Red flags of diseases of the small intestine and large intestine (3.1e)
Slow increase in intracranial pressure: progressive headaches and vomiting over a timescale of a few weeks to months. The headaches are worse in the morning, and the vomiting may be effortless. Blurring of vision and confusion may be additional symptoms	**	A21: Red flags of raised intracranial pressure (4.1c)
Vertigo in young person: usually due to benign labyrinthitis and will settle down. Refer if lasting for >6 weeks, or if so severe as to be causing recurrent vomiting. Refer if patient is at increased risk of thromboembolic disease (e.g. in pregnancy) so that the possibility of stroke can be excluded	**/*	A43: Red flags of diseases of the ear (6.1e)
Vertigo in an older person (>45 years): refer for medical assessment straight away. Although still more likely to be a result of inner ear disease, stroke is also a possible cause in this age group	**	A43: Red flags of diseases of the ear (6.1e)
Hyperthyroidism. Symptoms: irritability, anxiety, sleeplessness, increased appetite, loose stools, weight loss, scanty periods and heat intolerance. Signs: sweaty skin, tremor of the hands, staring eyes and rapid pulse	**/*	A31: Red flags of diseases of the thyroid gland (5.1c)

B39: Red flags of weakness/paralysis

Symptoms and signs	Priority	Chapter reference
Any sudden or gradual onset of muscle weakness that might be affecting muscles of respiration: refer urgently	***	A25: Red flags of diseases of the spinal cord and peripheral nerves (4.1g)
Addison's disease: increased pigmentation of skin, weight loss, muscle wasting, tiredness, loss of libido, low blood pressure, diarrhea and vomiting, confusion, collapse with dehydration	***/**	A33: Red flags of the less common endocrine diseases (5.1e)
Weakness that results from a temporary, progressive or persisting loss of brain function: suggested by accompanying symptoms such as loss of consciousness, loss of vision, unsteadiness, confusion, loss of memory or loss of sensation. Possible stroke, transient ischemic attack or brain tumor. Refer urgently if persisting and high priority if temporary	**/***	A22: Red flags of brain hemorrhage, stroke and brain tumor (4.1d) A24: Red flags of dementia, epilepsy and other disorders of the central nervous system (4.1f)
Any sudden or gradual onset of muscle weakness that can be objectively assessed (i.e. not just the patient's perception of weakness): refer to exclude serious muscular or neurological condition (e.g. myasthenia gravis, polymyositis, peripheral neuropathy or mononeuropathy, motor neuron disease)	**/*	A25: Red flags of diseases of the spinal cord and peripheral nerves (4.1g)
Cauda equina syndrome: numbness of the buttocks and perineum (saddle anesthesia), with bilateral numbness, weakness or sciatica in the legs. Difficulty in urination or defecation are serious symptoms	**	A25: Red flags of diseases of the spinal cord and peripheral nerves (4.1g)
Bell's palsy: sudden onset of facial weakness; almost always unilateral. Refer for same-day treatment with antiviral and steroid medication	**	A25: Red flags of diseases of the spinal cord and peripheral nerves (4.1g)
Cushing's syndrome: weight gain, weakness and wasting of limb muscles, stretch marks and bruises. Mood changes, hypertension, red cheeks, acne	*	A33: Red flags of the less common endocrine diseases (5.1e)

B40: Red flags of weight loss or weight gain

Symptoms and signs	Priority	Chapter reference
Progressive unexplained symptoms over weeks to months (e.g. weight loss, recurrent sweats, fevers, poor appetite): may be cancer, HIV or tuberculosis	**/*	A1: Red flags of cancer (2.3)
Malabsorption syndrome (loose, pale stools and malnutrition): weight loss, thin hair, dry skin, cracked lips and peeled tongue. Will present as failure to thrive in children. Causes include celiac disease and chronic pancreatitis	**/*	A7: Red flags of diseases of the pancreas (3.1d) A10: Red flags of diseases of the small intestine and large intestine (3.1e)
Tuberculosis infection: chronic productive cough, weight loss, night sweats, blood in sputum for >2 weeks	**	A17: Red flags of lower respiratory disease (3.3e)
Hyperthyroidism (symptoms and signs tend to be progressive over the course of a few months). Symptoms: irritability, anxiety, sleeplessness, increased appetite, loose stools, weight loss, scanty periods and heat intolerance. Signs: sweaty skin, tremor of the hands, staring eyes and rapid pulse	**/*	A31: Red flags of diseases of the thyroid gland (5.1c)
Severe disturbance of body image: if not responding to your treatment, and resulting in features of progressive anorexia nervosa or bulimia nervosa (e.g. progressive weight loss, secondary amenorrhea, or repeated compulsion to bring about vomiting)	*	A44: Red flags of mental health disorders (6.2e)
Hypothyroidism (symptoms and signs tend to be progressive over the course of a few months). Symptoms: tiredness, depression, weight gain, heavy periods, constipation and cold intolerance. Signs: dry puffy skin, dry and thin hair, slow pulse	*	A31: Red flags of diseases of the thyroid gland (5.1c)
Cushing's syndrome: weight gain, weakness and wasting of limb muscles, stretch marks and bruises. Mood changes, hypertension, red cheeks, acne	*	A33: Red flags of the less common endocrine diseases (5.1e)

Tables Showing Categories of Drugs for Withdrawal from Medication

The following tables group drugs into four categories according to how safe and uncomplicated withdrawal is likely to be. The four categories, which are explained in detail in Chapter 6.3, are:

i. Underlying condition not serious. Recurrence of symptoms is likely; no withdrawal syndrome (see Table IV-1).

ii. Underlying condition not serious. Recurrence of symptoms is likely; withdrawal syndrome is unpleasant, but does not seriously threaten health (see Table IV-2).

iii. Withdrawal may have serious physical or mental health consequences, either because the underlying condition is serious or because the withdrawal syndrome is dangerous (see Table IV-3).

iv. Replacement therapy. Withdrawal will result in serious ill health or death (see Table IV-4).

In the tables in this appendix the drugs are ordered by physiological system and section headings according to the system used in the online version of the *British National Formulary* (BNF).[3] This means that it is possible to locate which table applies to a drug if its BNF section is known.

However, as the section headings are general descriptive terms, even without access to the BNF it should be straightforward to determine to which category a particular drug should be assigned. For example, ispaghula husk is a bulk-forming laxative. This is listed in Section 1.6.1 in the BNF, and as such can be found in Table IV-1 in this appendix. Furthermore, knowledge of the physiological system on which the drug acts (gastrointestinal) and its action (bulk-forming laxative) can also be used to locate the drug to Table IV-1.

Each class of drug listed in the four tables is labeled with one or more asterisks. These labels signal the ideal speed and safety implications of withdrawal from this class of medications. The key to this labeling is as follows:

*	Safe to withdraw abruptly.
**	Withdraw gradually over 2–4 weeks.
***	Withdraw very slowly over a few months.
****	Do not consider withdrawal unless there has been a very marked improvement in symptoms. Always to be initiated by doctor.
Asterisks in brackets (e.g. (**)) indicate that withdrawal should only be undertaken under the close supervision of the prescribing doctor.	

Table IV-1: Category (i) medications. Underlying condition not serious. Recurrence of symptoms likely, but no withdrawal syndrome

BNF chapter	BNF section	Class of drug	How to withdraw
1. Gastrointestinal system	1.1	All antacids	*
	1.2	All antispasmodics	**
	1.3	All ulcer-healing drugs, unless the patient is on the drug to protect them from the effect of another drug	*
	1.4	Most antidiarrheal drugs	**
		Not including codeine, which if used long term can induce a state of dependence: Category (ii)	
	1.6.1	Bulk-forming laxatives	**
	1.7	Preparations for hemorrhoids	*
	1.9.1	Drugs acting on the gallbladder	*
3. Respiratory system	3.1	Bronchodilators, when used in mild asthma only	**
	3.3	Cromoglicate, when used for mild asthma only	**
	3.4	Antihistamines for allergic rhinitis	**
	3.7	Mucolytics	*
	3.8	Aromatic inhalations	*
	3.9	Cough suppressants	*
		Not including codeine, which if used long term can induce a state of dependence: Category (ii)	
		Not including opiates, such as diamorphine, which if used long term can induce a serious state of dependence: Category (iii)	
4. Central nervous system	4.3	Antidepressant drugs. It is increasingly recognized that, although antidepressants are not addictive, abrupt withdrawal after a period of more than one month of taking them can lead to a syndrome of nausea, digestive disturbance, anxiety and headache. For this reason they should be classed in Category (ii)	**
	4.6	Drugs used in the treatment of nausea and vertigo	**
	4.7.1	Non-opioid analgesics	**
	4.7.3	Drugs for trigeminal neuralgia	**
5. Infections	All sections	The decision to withdraw from a medium- to long-term course of antibiotics has to be made on the basis of the underlying condition	
		It is not advisable to withdraw from a prescription which has the aim of total eradication of a serious infection (e.g. anti-tubercular antibiotics). Premature withdrawal from the treatment aimed to eradicate any infection may encourage the growth of drug-resistant strains of bacteria	
		Some prescriptions are given to keep a serious underlying condition at bay (e.g. antiretroviral therapy in the treatment of HIV infection, or erythromycin for recurrent urinary infections in children). In these sorts of situation it is inadvisable to withdraw without agreement from the patient's doctor	
		Antibiotics prescribed for the treatment of less serious conditions (e.g. tetracycline for acne) can be withdrawn safely	
		Antibiotics do not usually induce a state of dependence	

6. Endocrine system	6.4.1.2	Progestogens	*
	6.4.3	Anabolic steroids	*
	6.5.1	Anti-estrogens used in anovulatory infertility	*
	6.6	Drugs affecting bone metabolism	*
	6.7	Other endocrine drugs: bromocriptine, danazol, gestrinone and gonadorelin analogues	*
7. Drugs used in obstetrics, gynecology and urinary disorders	7.2	Treatment of vaginal and vulval conditions	*
	7.3	Combined oral contraceptives and progesterone-only contraceptives; counsel the patient about the need for alternative contraceptive measures on withdrawal of these preparations	*
	7.4	Drugs used in urinary frequency, enuresis and incontinence	**
9. Drugs affecting nutrition and blood	9.1	Preparations for deficiency anemias, including oral iron, vitamin B12 and folic acid Not including injected vitamin B12: Category (iv) All these should only be withdrawn if you are sure that the deficiency has been adequately treated (this requires confirmation from the doctor)	*
	9.5	Minerals for deficiency states All these should only be withdrawn if you are sure that the deficiency has been adequately treated	*
	9.6	Vitamins for deficiency states All these should only be withdrawn if you are sure that the deficiency has been adequately treated	*
10. Drugs used in musculoskeletal disorders	10.1.1	Non-steroidal anti-inflammatory drugs	**
	10.2.2	Quinine for nocturnal cramp	*
	10.3.2	Topical anti-rheumatic preparations	*
11. Drugs acting on the eye	11.3	Anti-infective eye preparations: see notes above for BNF Chapter 5	
	11.4.2	Other anti-inflammatory eye preparations	**
12. Drugs used in the treatment of diseases of the ear, nose and oropharynx	12.1	Drugs acting on the ear	*
	12.2.1	Drugs acting in nasal allergy Not including inhaled nasal corticosteroids: Category (ii)	**
	12.3	Drugs acting on the oropharynx	*
13. Drugs acting on the skin	13.2	Emollient and barrier preparations	**
	13.5.1	Preparations for eczema	**
	13.5.2	Preparations for psoriasis Not including immunosuppressants: Category (iv)	**
	13.6	Preparations for acne	*
	13.7	Preparations for warts and calluses	*
	13.9	Shampoos and some other scalp preparations	**
	13.10	Anti-infective skin preparations: see notes above for BNF Chapter 5	

Table IV-2: Category (ii) medications. Underlying condition not serious. Recurrence of symptoms is likely; withdrawal syndrome is unpleasant, but does not seriously threaten health

BNF chapter	BNF section	Class of drug	How to withdraw
1. Gastrointestinal system	1.4	Codeine phosphate: physical and psychological dependence	**
	1.6.2	Stimulant laxatives: physical dependence	**/***
3. Respiratory system	3.9	Codeine phosphate: physical and psychological dependence	**
	3.10	Nasal decongestants: physical dependence	**
4. Central nervous system	4.1	Hypnotics Not included if a long-term prescription, as this can result in a serious withdrawal syndrome: Category (iii)	**/***
	4.3	Antidepressants when prescribed for mild-moderate depression and when prescription is long term (i.e. >1 month) Not including monoamine oxidase inhibitors: Category (iii)	**
	4.5	Appetite suppressants: psychological dependence	**
	4.7.1	Opioid analgesics: physical and psychological dependence Not included if long-term prescription, as this can give rise to a serious withdrawal syndrome: Category (iii)	**/***
6. Endocrine system	6.4.1.1	Female sex hormones prescribed for menopausal symptoms	*
12. Drugs used in the treatment of diseases of the ear, nose and oropharynx	12.1.1	Topical corticosteroids for otitis externa: physical dependence	**
	12.2.1	Inhaled corticosteroids used in nasal allergy	**
	12.2.2	Topical nasal decongestants: physical dependence	**
13. Drugs acting on the skin	13.4	Topical corticosteroids: physical dependence	**/***

Table IV-3: Category (iii) medications. Withdrawal may have serious physical or mental health consequences, either because the underlying condition is serious or because the withdrawal syndrome is dangerous

BNF chapter	BNF section	Class of drug	How to withdraw
1. Gastrointestinal system	1.5	Drugs used in the treatment of chronic diarrhea: can result in a serious relapse of inflammatory bowel disease if withdrawn suddenly	(****)
2. Cardiovascular system	2.1	Positive inotropes	(**/***)
	2.2	Diuretics	(**)
	2.3	Anti-arrhythmics	(****)
	2.4	Beta blockers	(**/***)
	2.5	ACE inhibitors and other anti-hypertensives	(**/***)
	2.6	Nitrates, calcium channel blockers, potassium channel activators	(**/***)
	2.7	Sympathomimetics	(**)
	2.8	Anticoagulants	(****)
	2.9	Anti-platelets	(****)
	2.11	Lipid-lowering drugs	(*)

3. Respiratory system	3.1	Bronchodilators, when used in all but the most mild cases of asthma	(**)
	3.2	Corticosteroid inhalers	(**)
	3.3	Cromoglycate, when used in all but the most mild cases of asthma	(**)
	3.9	Opiates for cough suppression in terminal care	(**)
4. Central nervous system	4.1	Hypnotics, if after a long-term prescription	(***)
	4.2	Drugs used in psychoses and other related disorders	(****)
	4.3.1 4.3.3 4.3.4	Antidepressants, when the underlying depression has been severe (e.g. suicidal ideation, extreme social withdrawal)	(**/***)
	4.3.2	Monoamine oxidase inhibitor (MAOI) antidepressants	(**/***)
	4.4	Central nervous system stimulants	(**)
	4.7.2	Long-term prescription of opioid analgesics	(**/***)
	4.7.4.2	Drugs for prophylaxis of migraine	(**)
	4.8	Anti-epilepsy medication	(****)
	4.9	Anti-Parkinson's disease medication	(****)
	4.10	Drugs used in substance dependence	(**/***)
5. Infections	See BNF Chapter 5 notes in Table IV-1, Category (i) medication		**/***
6. Endocrine system	6.2.1	Anti-thyroid medication	(**)
	6.3.1	Oral corticosteroid medication (detailed advice given in the BNF concerning the dangers of withdrawal)	(**/***)
	6.4.2	Male sex hormones prescribed for testicular failure	(****)
7. Drugs used in obstetrics, gynecology and urinary disorders	7.4.1	Drugs used in urinary retention	(**/***)
8. Malignant disease and immuno-suppression	8.1	Cytotoxic drugs	(****)
	8.2	Drugs affecting the immune response, including cytotoxics, corticosteroids, immunostimulants and interferons	(****)
	8.3	Sex hormone and hormone antagonists in malignant disease	(****)
10. Drugs used in musculoskeletal disorders	10.1.2	Corticosteroids for inflammatory arthritis	(**/***)
	10.1.3	Drugs that suppress the rheumatic process	(**/***)
	10.1.4	Drugs used to suppress the recurrence of gout	(*/**)
	10.2	Drugs used in neuromuscular disorders Not including quinine: Category (i)	(**/***)
11. Drugs acting on the eye	11.4.1	Topical corticosteroids for uveitis and scleritis	(**)
	11.6	Drugs used in the treatment of glaucoma	(****)
13. Drugs acting on the skin	13.5.2	Immunosuppressants for psoriasis	(****)

Table IV-4: Category (iv) medications. Replacement therapy. Withdrawal will result in serious ill-health or death

BNF chapter	BNF section	Class of drug	How to withdraw
1. Gastrointestinal system	1.9.4	Pancreatic enzymes for chronic pancreatitis and cystic fibrosis	(****)
6. Endocrine system	6.1.1	Drugs used in diabetes: insulin and oral hypo-glycemics	(****)
	6.2.1	Thyroid hormones	(****)
	6.3.1	Corticosteroid replacement therapy in Addison's disease and hypopituitarism	(****)
	6.4.1.1	Female sex hormones for premature ovarian failure	(****)
	6.5.2	Posterior pituitary hormones for diabetes insipidus	(****)
9. Drugs affecting nutrition and blood	9.1.2	Injected vitamin B12 for pernicious anemia	(****)
	9.1.3	Erythropoietin in chronic renal failure	(****)
	9.2.1	Oral potassium and bicarbonate	(****)
	9.8	Drugs used in metabolic disorders	(****)

Notes

1 Maciocia, G. (1989) *The Foundations of Chinese Medicine*. Edinburgh: Churchill Livingstone.

2 National Institute for Health and Care Excellence (2016) *British National Formulary*. Available at www.evidence.nhs.uk/formulary/bnf/current, accessed on 16 May 2016.

3 For more details on the conventional medical correspondences of these functions of the Small Intestine Organ, see the concluding pages of Section 3.1a, "The physiology of the gastrointestinal system."

Index

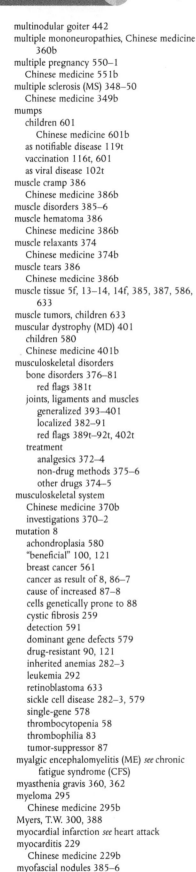